To Barbara
with my
highest regards

Nelson Ervin, M.D.
Aug 18, 83

Editor
EDWIN L. KENDIG, JR., M.D., Sc.D. (Hon.)

Professor of Pediatrics, Medical College of Virginia,
Health Sciences Division,
Virginia Commonwealth University, Richmond, Virginia;
Director, Child Chest Clinic,
Medical College of Virginia Hospitals;
Director, Department of Pediatrics, St. Mary's Hospital,
Richmond, Virginia

Associate Editor
VICTOR CHERNICK, M.D., F.R.C.P.(C)

Professor and Head, Department of Pediatrics,
The University of Manitoba.
Faculty of Medicine, Winnipeg, Manitoba, Canada;
Pediatrician-in-Chief,
Health Sciences Center,
Winnipeg, Manitoba, Canada

Disorders
of the
Respiratory
Tract
in Children

Third Edition

1977

W. B. SAUNDERS COMPANY
Philadelphia • London • Toronto

W. B. Saunders Company: West Washington Square
                          Philadelphia, Pa.   19105

                          1 St. Anne's Road
                          Eastbourne, East Sussex BN21 3UN, England

                          1 Goldthorne Avenue
                          Toronto, Ontario M8Z 5T9, Canada

Library of Congress Cataloging in Publication Data

Kendig, Edwin L ed.

Disorders of the respiratory tract in children.

Includes index.

1. Pediatric respiratory diseases.   I. Chernick, Victor,
   joint ed.   II. Title. [DNLM: 1. Respiratory tract
   diseases — In infancy and childhood. WS280 D612]

RJ431.K42 1978   618.9′22   76–41538

ISBN 0–7216–5378–2

Disorders of the Respiratory Tract in Children   ISBN   0-7216-5378-2

Last digit is the print number: 9   8   7   6   5   4   3   2   1

CONTRIBUTORS

WILLIAM CURTIS ADAMS, M.D.

Medical Director, Emergency Department, Southeast Alabama Medical Center, Dothan, Alabama.

Hypostatic Pneumonia

MARY ELLEN AVERY, M.D.

Thomas Morgan Rotch Professor of Pediatrics, Harvard Medical School. Physician-in-Chief, Children's Hospital Medical Center, Boston, Massachusetts.

The Functional Basis of Respiratory Pathology

FELICIA B. AXELROD, M.D.

Associate Professor of Pediatrics, New York University School of Medicine. Director, Dysautonomia Treatment and Evaluation Center, New York University Medical Center, New York, New York.

Familial Dysautonomia

C. WARREN BIERMAN, M.D.

Clinical Professor of Pediatrics and Chief, Division of Allergy, Department of Pediatrics, Children's Orthopedic Hospital and Medical Center and The University of Washington School of Medicine, Seattle, Washington.

Nonasthmatic Allergic Pulmonary Disease

JAMES W. BROOKS, M.D.

Professor of Surgery, The Medical College of Virginia, Health Sciences Division, Virginia Commonwealth University. Attending Surgeon, Division of Cardiac and Thoracic Surgery, Medical College of Virginia, Richmond, Virginia.

Foreign Bodies in the Air Passages; Tumors of the Chest; Disorders of the Respiratory Tract due to Trauma

VICTOR CHERNICK, M.D., F.R.C.P.(C.)

Professor and Head, Department of Pediatrics, University of Manitoba Faculty of Medicine. Pediatrician-in-Chief, Health Sciences Center, Winnipeg, Manitoba, Canada.

The Functional Basis of Respiratory Pathology: Intensive Care of Respiratory Disorders; Pleurisy and Empyema; Liquid and Air in the Pleural Space

AMOS CHRISTIE, M.D.

Professor Emeritus of Pediatrics, Vanderbilt University School of Medicine, Nashville, Tennessee.

Histoplasmosis

HENRY G. CRAMBLETT, M.D.

Professor of Pediatrics and Medical Microbiology, and Dean, College of Medicine, The Ohio State University College of Medicine. Attending Staff, Children's Hospital and The Ohio State University Hospitals, Columbus, Ohio.

Croup (Epiglottitis; Laryngitis; Laryngotracheobronchitis); Viral Etiology of Respiratory Illness

JOSEPH DANCIS, M.D.

Professor and Chairman, Department of Pediatrics, New York University School of Medicine, New York, New York.

Familial Dysautonomia

SUSAN COONS DEES, M.D.

Professor of Pediatrics (Allergy), Duke University Medical Center, Durham, North Carolina.

Asthma

FLOYD W. DENNY, M.D.

Professor and Chairman, Department of Pediatrics, The University of North Carolina School of Medicine. Attending Pediatrician, North Carolina Memorial Hospital, Chapel Hill, North Carolina.

Viral Pneumonia; Infections of the Respiratory Tract due to Mycoplasma pneumoniae

FRANK E. EHRLICH, M.D., F.A.C.S.

Richmond, Virginia.

Congenital Malformations of the Lower Respiratory Tract

BARRY D. FLETCHER, M.D., C.M.

Professor of Radiology, Case Western Reserve University. Director, Division of Pediatric Radiology, University Hospitals of Cleveland, Cleveland, Ohio.

Diagnostic Pulmonary Radiology

ROBERT A. GOOD, M.D., Ph.D.

Director and Professor of Pathology, Sloan-Kettering Division, Graduate School of Medical Science, Cornell University; Professor of Medicine and Pediatrics, Cornell University Medical College; Professor of Pediatrics, University of South Alabama College of Medicine, Mobile; and Adjunct Professor, Rockefeller University. Attending Physician, Departments of Medicine and Pediatrics, Memorial Hospital for Cancer and Allied Diseases; Attending Pediatrician, New York Hospital; Visiting Physician, Rockefeller University; Director of Research, Memorial Hospital for Cancer and Allied Diseases and Memorial Sloan-Kettering Cancer Center; President and Director, Sloan-Kettering Institute for Cancer Research, New York, New York.

Chronic Granulomatous Disease of Childhood

BEULAH HOLMES GRAY, Ph.D.

Associate Professor of Microbiology, University of Minnesota School of Medicine, Minneapolis, Minnesota.

Chronic Granulomatous Disease of Childhood

VINCENT V. HAMPARIAN, Ph.D.

Professor of Pediatrics and Medical Microbiology, The Ohio State University College of Medicine. Executive Director, The Children's Hospital Research Foundation, Columbus, Ohio.

Viral Etiology of Respiratory Illness

DOUGLAS C. HEINER, M.D., Ph.D.

Professor of Pediatrics, UCLA School of Medicine, Harbor General Hospital Campus. Director, Division of Immunology and Allergy, Harbor General Hospital, Torrance, California.

Pulmonary Hemosiderosis

ROBERT H. HIGH, M.D.

Clinical Professor of Pediatrics, The University of Michigan Medical School, Ann Arbor. Senior Pediatrician, Henry Ford Hospital, Detroit, Michigan.

Pulmonary Abscess; Idiopathic Pulmonary Alveolar Microlithiasis; Psittacosis (Ornithosis); Q Fever; Idiopathic Histiocytosis (Histiocytosis X)

JAMES C. HOGG, M.D., Ph.D., F.R.C.P.(C.)

Professor of Pathology, McGill University Faculty of Medicine. Assistant Pathologist, Royal Victoria Hospital, Montreal, Quebec, Canada.

Age as a Factor in Respiratory Disease

WILLIAM A. HOWARD, M.D.

Clinical Professor of Pediatrics, The George Washington University School of Medicine. Chairman, Department of Allergy, and Senior Attending Pediatrician, Children's Hospital National Medical Center, Washington, D.C.

Tonsillitis and Adenoiditis (The Tonsil and Adenoid Problem); Cytomegalic Inclusion Disease; Tularemia; Visceral Larva Migrans; Loeffler's Syndrome

WALTER T. HUGHES, M.D.

Eudowood Professor of Pediatrics and Director, Division of Infectious Diseases, Johns Hopkins Hospital, Baltimore, Maryland.

Pneumocystis Carinii Pneumonitis

EDWIN LAWRENCE KENDIG, Jr., M.D., Sc.D.(Hon.)

Professor of Pediatrics, The Medical College of Virginia, Health Sciences Division, Virginia Commonwealth University. Director, Child Chest Clinic, Medical College of Virginia Hospitals; Director, Department of Pediatrics, St. Mary's Hospital, Richmond, Virginia.

Tuberculosis; Infections with the Atypical Mycobacteria; Sarcoidosis

BARRY V. KIRKPATRICK, M.D.

Assistant Professor of Pediatrics and Director, Newborn Intensive Care Unit, The Medical College of Virginia, Health Sciences Division, Virginia Commonwealth University, Richmond, Virginia.

Bronchopulmonary Dysplasia

JEROME O. KLEIN, M.D.

Professor of Pediatrics, Boston University School of Medicine. Associate Director, Department of Pediatrics, Boston City Hospital, Massachusetts.

Antimicrobial Therapy

WILLIAM E. LAUPUS, M.D.

Professor and Chairman, Department of Pediatrics, and Dean, School of Medicine, East Carolina University, Greenville, North Carolina.

Bronchopulmonary Dysplasia

RICHARD JOHN LEMEN, M.D.

Assistant Professor of Pediatrics and Physiology, Tulane University School of Medicine. Director of Pulmonary Laboratories, Section of Pulmonary Diseases (Pediatrics), Tulane Medical Center, New Orleans, Louisiana.

Pulmonary Function Testing in the Office and Clinic

F. STANFORD MASSIE, M.D.

Associate Professor of Pediatrics and Director, Pediatric Allergy Training Program, Medical College of Virginia, Health Sciences Division, Virginia Commonwealth University, Richmond, Virginia.

Nonasthmatic Allergic Pulmonary Disease

ROBERT B. MELLINS, M.D.

Professor of Pediatrics, Columbia University College of Physicians and Surgeons. Attending Pediatrician, Presbyterian Hospital, New York, New York.

Lung Injury from Hydrocarbon Aspiration and Smoke Inhalation; Pulmonary Edema

VICTOR G. MIKITY, M.D., F.A.C.R.

Professor of Pediatric Radiology, University of Southern California School of Medicine. Chief, Diagnostic Radiology, Pediatric Pavilion, Los Angeles County–USC Medical Center, Los Angeles, California.

Chronic Respiratory Distress in the Premature Infant (Wilson-Mikity Syndrome)

JEROME H. MODELL, M.D.

Professor and Chairperson, Department of Anesthesiology, J. Hillis Miller Health Center, University of Florida College of Medicine. Shands Teaching Hospital and Veterans Administration Hospital, Gainesville, Florida.

Drowning and Near-Drowning

ROSA LEE NEMIR, M.D.

Professor of Pediatrics, New York University School of Medicine. Attending Pediatrician, University Hospital and Bellevue Hospital Center; Director, Children's Chest Clinic, Bellevue Hospital Center, New York, New York.

Bronchiectasis; Atelectasis; Varicella Pneumonia; Measles Pneumonia; Pertussis Pneumonia; Pertussoid Eosinophilic Pneumonia; Salmonella Pneumonia; Rheumatic Pneumonia

JACQUELINE A. NOONAN, M.D.

Professor and Chairman, Department of Pediatrics, University of Kentucky College of Medicine. Chief, Pediatric Service, Albert B. Chandler Medical Center, Lexington, Kentucky.

Cor Pulmonale

REYNALDO D. PAGTAKHAN, M.D., M.Sc., F.C.C.P.

Assistant Professor of Pediatrics, University of Manitoba Faculty of Medicine. Associate Director, Pediatric Respirology, and Director, Cystic Fibrosis Program, Children's Centre, Health Sciences Centre, Winnipeg, Manitoba, Canada.

Intensive Care of Respiratory Disorders; Pleurisy and Empyema; Liquid and Air in the Pleural Space

BYUNG HAK PARK, M.D.

Professor of Pediatrics, State University of New York at Buffalo. Director, Immunobiology Laboratory, Children's Hospital, Buffalo, New York.

Chronic Granulomatous Disease of Childhood

ROBERT H. PARROTT, M.D.

Professor and Chairman, Department of Child Health and Development, The George Washington University. Director, Children's Hospital National Medical Center and Research Foundation of Children's Hospital, Washington, D.C.

Influenza

WILLIAM E. PIERSON, M.D.

Clinical Professor of Pediatrics, The University of Washington School of Medicine. Co-Director, Allergy Clinic, Children's Orthopedic Hospital and Medical Center, Seattle, Washington.

Nonasthmatic Allergic Pulmonary Disease

ARNOLD C. G. PLATZKER, M.D.

Associate Clinical Professor of Pediatrics, University of Southern California School of Medicine. Attending Physician and Head, Neonatal-Respiratory Diseases Division, Children's Hospital of Los Angeles, California. Head, Neonatology, USC–Children's Hospital of Los Angeles–Hollywood Presbyterian Hospital Regional Perinatal Center, California.

Pulmonary Involvement in the Rheumatic Disorders (So-called Collagen Diseases) of Childhood

HARRIS D. RILEY, Jr., M.D.

Distinguished Professor of Pediatrics, The University of Oklahoma College of Medicine. Chief, Infectious Disease Service, Children's Memorial Hospital, University of Oklahoma Health Sciences Center, Oklahoma City, Oklahoma.

Pulmonary Alveolar Proteinosis

SAMI I. SAID, M.D.

Professor of Internal Medicine and Pharmacology, University of Texas Health Science Center at Dallas Southwestern Medical School. Chief, Pulmonary Disease Section, Veterans Administration Hospital, Dallas, Texas.

Metabolic and Endocrine Functions of the Lung

ARNOLD M. SALZBERG, M.D.

Professor of Surgery and Chairman, Division of Pediatric Surgery, The Medical College of Virginia, Health Sciences Division, Virginia Commonwealth University. Attending Pediatric Surgeon, The Medical College of Virginia Hospitals, St. Mary's Hospital, and Richmond Memorial Hospital, Richmond, Virginia.

Congenital Malformations of the Lower Respiratory Tract; Foreign Bodies in the Air Passages; Disorders of the Respiratory Tract due to Trauma

JOHN HOLLISTER SEABURY, M.S., M.D.

Professor Emeritus of Medicine, Louisiana State University Medical Center. Consultant in Medicine, Southern Louisiana Community Health Care Corporation, New Orleans, Louisiana.

The Mycoses (Excluding Histoplasmosis)

HARRY SHWACHMAN, M.D.

Professor Emeritus of Pediatrics, Harvard Medical School. Senior Associate in Medicine and Chief, Clinical Nutrition Division, Emeritus, Harvard Medical School, and The Children's Hospital Medical Center, Boston, Massachusetts.

Cystic Fibrosis

BERNHARD H. SINGSEN, M.D.

Assistant Clinical Professor of Pediatrics, University of Southern California School of Medicine. Division of Rheumatology, Children's Hospital of Los Angeles, California. Consulting Attending Physician, Pediatric Rheumatology, Rancho Los Amigos Hospital, Downey, California and Los Angeles County Medical Center, California.

Pulmonary Involvement in the Rheumatic Disorders (So-called Collagen Diseases) of Childhood

MARGARET H. D. SMITH, M.D.

Professor of Pediatrics and Preventive Medicine, New Jersey Medical School. Director, Children's Hospital of Newark, New Jersey.

Bacterial Pneumonias: Gram-Positive; Bacterial Pneumonias: Gram-Negative

MILDRED T. STAHLMAN, M.D.

Professor of Pediatrics, Vanderbilt University School of Medicine. Professor of Pediatrics and Director, Division of Neonatology/Director of Nurseries, Vanderbilt University Medical Center, Nashville, Tennessee.

Respiratory Disorders in the Newborn

S. ALEX STALCUP, M.D.

Visiting Fellow, Pediatric Pulmonary Division, Department of Pediatrics, Columbia University College of Physicians and Surgeons, New York, New York.

Pulmonary Edema

SAMUEL STONE, M.D.

Professor of Clinical Pediatrics, New York University School of Medicine. Attending Pediatrician, Bellevue and University Hospitals, New York, New York.

Giant Cell Pneumonia

RICHARD C. TALAMO, M.D.

Professor of Pediatrics, The Johns Hopkins University School of Medicine. Pediatrician, The Johns Hopkins Hospital, Baltimore, Maryland.

Emphysema and Alpha₁-Antitrypsin Deficiency

WILLIAM M. THURLBECK, M.D., Ch.B., F.R.C.P.(C.), F.R.C. Path.

Professor and Head, Department of Pathology, University of Manitoba Faculty of Medicine. Head, Department of Pathology, Health Science Centre, Winnipeg, Manitoba, Canada.

Cryptogenic or Idiopathic Fibrosing Alveolitis (Usual Interstitial Pneumonia); Desquamative Interstitial Pneumonia and Other Variants of Interstitial Pneumonia

J. A. PETER TURNER, M.D., F.R.C.P.(C.)

Professor of Pediatrics, The University of Toronto Faculty of Medicine. Chief, Division of Pulmonary Diseases, Hospital for Sick Children, Toronto, Ontario, Canada.

Bronchitis

WILLIAM W. WARING, M.D.

Professor of Pediatrics and Chief, Section of Pulmonary Diseases, Department of Pediatrics, Tulane University School of Medicine. Senior Visiting Physician, Charity Hospital of Louisiana; Staff Pediatrician, Tulane Medical Center Hospital and New Orleans Children's Hospital, New Orleans, Louisiana.

The History and Physical Examination; Diagnostic and Therapeutic Procedures

MARY ELLEN B. WOHL, M.D.

Assistant Professor of Pediatrics, Harvard Medical School. Associate, Pulmonary Division, The Children's Hospital Medical Center, Boston, Massachusetts.

Bronchiolitis

PREFACE

This is the third edition of *Disorders of the Respiratory Tract in Children.* The objective of the third edition is the same as that of the two preceding editions: to provide an answer to almost any question about respiratory diseases in children raised by the practitioner, resident or intern in pediatrics, the chest physician, the roentgenologist, the medical student, or the family practitioner. However, there has been some modification in the approach. Consideration will be given to disorders involving the tonsils and adenoids, but this edition will be otherwise limited to disorders of the lower respiratory tract. There will be no volume on pediatric otolaryngology.

With this edition, Dr. Victor Chernick has become associate editor of *Disorders of the Respiratory Tract in Children.* There are twenty-one new contributors, and all chapters have been rewritten by new authors or revised and brought up to date. Particular note should be made of the expansion of chapters dealing with the fundamental basis of pulmonary pathology. There are seven new chapters: Diagnostic Pulmonary Radiology; Pulmonary Function Testing in the Office and Clinic; Antimicrobial Therapy; Drowning and Near-Drowning; Cor Pulmonale; Emphysema and Alpha$_1$-Antitrypsin Deficiency; and Nonasthmatic Allergic Pulmonary Disease.

The editors would like to express their appreciation to the contributors who have made this book possible. We are most grateful for their willingness, dedication, and expert attention to their assignment.

We should like to express our gratitude, too, to Dr. John Chapman, Dr. Louis Siltzbach, Dr. Donald Brummer, and Dr. Rosa Lee Nemir, who have generously read and criticized specific chapters of the book. Dr. Marc O. Beem has also contributed valuable advice.

Judith Howell, R.N., has assisted in the collection of case material for several of the chapters, and Mrs. Judith Gauldin has assisted in the proofreading and typing of manuscripts.

The editors are most grateful to Mr. Brian Decker and the staff of the W. B. Saunders Company for their helpful advice and willing cooperation.

EDWIN L. KENDIG, JR., M.D.
VICTOR CHERNICK, M.D.

CONTENTS

Section I

GENERAL CONSIDERATIONS

Chapter One

THE FUNCTIONAL BASIS OF RESPIRATORY PATHOLOGY 3
Victor Chernick, M.D., and Mary Ellen Avery, M.D.

Definitions and Symbols 3
Properties of Gases 4
Lung Morphology and Growth 5
Lung Volumes 11
Mechanics of Respiration 14
Alveolar Ventilation 25
Diffusion 30
Transport of Oxygen 32
Oxygen Therapy 35
Carbon Dioxide Transport and Acid-Base Balance 37
Tissue Respiration 41
Ventilation-Perfusion Relations 44
Pulmonary Circulation 48
Regulation of Respiration 52
Clinical Application of Pulmonary Function Studies 60

Chapter Two

METABOLIC AND ENDOCRINE FUNCTIONS OF THE LUNG 62
Sami I. Said, M.D.

Some Pulmonary Cells of Importance in Metabolic Function
    and Dysfunction 62
Some Metabolic and Endocrine Functions of the Lung 69
Illustrations of the Metabolic Basis of Pulmonary Disease 72

Chapter Three

THE HISTORY AND PHYSICAL EXAMINATION 77
William W. Waring, M.D.

The History 77
The Physical Examination 83

Chapter Four

DIAGNOSTIC AND THERAPEUTIC PROCEDURES 105
William W. Waring, M.D.

Diagnostic Procedures 105
Therapeutic Procedures 109

Chapter Five

DIAGNOSTIC PULMONARY RADIOLOGY 133
Barry D. Fletcher, M.D., C.M.

Radiation Hazards 134
Imaging Methods 134
Technical Factors Affecting Radiologic Interpretation 137
Radiology of the Neck and Thoracic Inlet 139
The Chest Wall and Diaphragm 142
The Pleura and Fissures 144
The Mediastinum 147
The Bronchi 150
The Hila and Pulmonary Vessels 152
Pulmonary Consolidation 154
Interstitial Disease 157
Decreased Lung Volume 160
Increased Lung Volume 162

Chapter Six

PULMONARY FUNCTION TESTING IN THE OFFICE AND CLINIC 166
Richard J. Lemen, M.D.

Chapter Seven

AGE AS A FACTOR IN RESPIRATORY DISEASE 177
J. C. Hogg, M.D.

Normal Lungs... 177
Diseased Lungs 183

Section II

INTENSIVE CARE OF RESPIRATORY DISORDERS

Chapter Eight

INTENSIVE CARE OF RESPIRATORY DISORDERS.................................... 191
Reynaldo D. Pagtakhan, M.D., and Victor Chernick, M.D.

Functional Classification of Respiratory Disorders.................................. 191
Recognition of Respiratory Failure.. 192
Resuscitation... 194
Resuscitation of the Newborn Infant 199
Immediate Postresuscitation Phase 199
Continuing Respiratory Care.. 200
Monitoring 208
Summary 210

Section III
RESPIRATORY DISORDERS IN THE NEWBORN

Chapter Nine

CONGENITAL MALFORMATIONS OF THE LOWER
RESPIRATORY TRACT 213
    Arnold M. Salzberg, M.D., and Frank E. Ehrlich, M.D.

    Pectus Carinatum (Pigeon Breast) 213
    Sternal Clefts (Fissura Sterni Congenita) 213
    Pectus Excavatum (Funnel Chest) 214
    Congenital Absence of Ribs 217
    Congenital Anterior Diaphragmatic Hernia (Morgagni) 218
    Congenital Diaphragmatic Hernia of Bochdalek 219
    Congenital Eventration of the Diaphragm 222
    Congenital Hiatal Diaphragmatic Hernia 224
    Chylothorax 225
    Tracheal Agenesis and Stenosis 226
    Tracheomalacia 227
    Vascular Ring 228
    Tracheoesophageal Fistula without Esophageal Atresia 231
    Esophageal Atresia 232
    Congenital Bronchial Stenosis 237
    Bronchogenic Cyst 237
    Pulmonary Agenesis, Aplasia and Hypoplasia 240
    Congenital Pneumatocele (Pulmonary Hernia) 242
    Congenital Pulmonary Cysts 242
    Lobar Emphysema 245
    Pulmonary Sequestration 247
    Congenital Cystic Adenomatoid Malformation of the Lung 250
    Congenital Pulmonary Lymphangiectasis 251
    Pulmonary Arteriovenous Fistula 252

Chapter Ten

RESPIRATORY DISORDERS IN THE NEWBORN 271
    Mildred T. Stahlman, M.D.

    Evaluation of the Infant with Respiratory Difficulty 271
    Effects of a Transitional Circulation on Neonatal Respiratory Distress 274
    Respiratory Depression, Asphyxia and Resuscitation 276
    Intrauterine Aspiration Pneumonia (Massive Aspiration Syndrome,
        Meconium Aspiration Pneumonia) 278
    Emphysema, Pneumothorax and Pneumomediastinum (Air Block) 280
    Hyaline Membrane Disease 283
    Type II Respiratory Distress Syndrome 290
    Infections of the Lung 292
    Pulmonary Hemorrhage 296
    Congenital Lobar Emphysema 297
    Lung Cysts and Pneumatoceles 299
    Agenesis and Hypoplasia of the Lungs 299
    Congenital Diaphragmatic Hernia 300
    Vascular Rings 301
    Esophageal Atresia and Tracheoesophageal Fistula 301
    Micrognathia with Glossoptosis 303
    Choanal Atresia 303
    Nonpulmonary Causes of Respiratory Symptoms in the Newborn 304
    Congenital Cardiac Disease 305
    Assisted Ventilation in Neonatal Lung Disorders 309

Chapter Eleven

BRONCHOPULMONARY DYSPLASIA 314
Barry V. Kirkpatrick, M.D., and William E. Laupus, M.D.

Mechanical Ventilation 314
Clinical-Radiographic-Histologic Correlation 317

Chapter Twelve

CHRONIC RESPIRATORY DISTRESS IN THE PREMATURE INFANT
(WILSON-MIKITY SYNDROME) 324
Victor G. Mikity, M.D.

Section IV

INFECTIONS OF THE RESPIRATORY TRACT

Chapter Thirteen

ANTIMICROBIAL THERAPY 331
Jerome O. Klein, M.D.

The Penicillins 331
Antimicrobial Agents Used as Alternatives to Penicillins 335
Drugs Effective Against Infections Due to Gram-Negative Bacilli 338
Important Aspects of Administration of Antibiotics 339
What to Look for When Antimicrobial Therapy Fails.......................... 344

Chapter Fourteen

TONSILLITIS AND ADENOIDITIS (THE TONSIL AND
ADENOID PROBLEM) 347
William A. Howard, M.D.

Chapter Fifteen

CROUP (EPIGLOTTITIS; LARYNGITIS;
LARYNGOTRACHEOBRONCHITIS).. 353
Henry G. Cramblett, M.D.

Chapter Sixteen

BRONCHITIS... 361
J. A. Peter Turner, M.D.

Chapter Seventeen

BRONCHIOLITIS... 367
Mary Ellen B. Wohl, M.D.

Bronchiolitis Obliterans 375

Chapter Eighteen

BACTERIAL PNEUMONIAS: GRAM-POSITIVE.. 378
Margaret H. D. Smith, M.D.

General Considerations 378
Pneumococcal Pneumonia.. 380
Meningococcal Pneumonia.. 386
Streptococcal Pneumonia 386
Staphylococcal Pneumonia 388

Chapter Nineteen

BACTERIAL PNEUMONIAS: GRAM-NEGATIVE 398
Margaret H. D. Smith, M.D.

Pneumonia Due to *Hemophilus influenzae* 398
Aerobic Gram-Negative Bacillary Pneumonia... 400

Chapter Twenty

PNEUMOCYSTIS CARINII PNEUMONITIS.. 403
Walter T. Hughes, M.D.

Chapter Twenty-One

VIRAL ETIOLOGY OF RESPIRATORY ILLNESS 412
Vincent V. Hamparian, Ph.D., and Henry G. Cramblett, M.D.

Picornaviruses.. 414
Adenoviruses.. 416
Orthomyxoviruses 418
Paramyxoviruses... 419
Coronaviruses 420
Comment 421

Chapter Twenty-Two

VIRAL PNEUMONIA... 423
Floyd W. Denny, M.D.

Chapter Twenty-Three

INFECTIONS OF THE RESPIRATORY TRACT DUE TO
MYCOPLASMA PNEUMONIAE 433
Floyd W. Denny, M.D.

Chapter Twenty-Four

INFLUENZA... 442
Robert H. Parrott, M.D.

Chapter Twenty-Five

BRONCHIECTASIS.. 446
Rosa Lee Nemir, M.D.

Chapter Twenty-Six

PULMONARY ABSCESS.. 470
Robert H. High, M.D.

Chapter Twenty-Seven

PLEURISY AND EMPYEMA.. 475
Reynaldo D. Pagtakhan, M.D., and Victor Chernick, M.D.

Section V

NONINFECTIOUS DISORDERS OF THE RESPIRATORY TRACT

Chapter Twenty-Eight

LUNG INJURY FROM HYDROCARBON ASPIRATION AND
SMOKE INHALATION.. 491
Robert B. Mellins, M.D.

Lung Injury From Hydrocarbon Aspiration 491
Respiratory Complications of Smoke Inhalation 493

Chapter Twenty-Nine

DROWNING AND NEAR-DROWNING.. 498
Jerome H. Modell, M.D.

Pathophysiology 499
Therapy.. 504

Chapter Thirty

HYPOSTATIC PNEUMONIA 511
William Curtis Adams, M.D.

Chapter Thirty-One

FOREIGN BODIES IN THE AIR PASSAGES................................. 513
James W. Brooks, M.D., and Arnold M. Salzberg, M.D.

Chapter Thirty-Two

CRYPTOGENIC OR IDIOPATHIC FIBROSING ALVEOLITIS
(Usual Interstitial Pneumonia) 518
William M. Thurlbeck, M.B., Ch.B.

CONTENTS

Chapter Thirty-Three

DESQUAMATIVE INTERSTITIAL PNEUMONIA AND OTHER
VARIANTS OF INTERSTITIAL PNEUMONIA.. 523
William M. Thurlbeck, M.B., Ch.B.

Desquamative Interstitial Pneumonia (DIP) 523
Lymphoid Interstitial Pneumonia (LIP)... 527
Giant Cell Interstitial Pneumonia (GIP).. 528
Bronchiolitis Obliterans (Bronchiolitis Obliterans with
    Interstitial Pneumonia — BIP).. 528

Chapter Thirty-Four

PULMONARY ALVEOLAR PROTEINOSIS 530
Harris D. Riley, Jr., M.D.

Chapter Thirty-Five

IDIOPATHIC PULMONARY ALVEOLAR MICROLITHIASIS......................... 535
Robert H. High, M.D.

Chapter Thirty-Six

PULMONARY HEMOSIDEROSIS.. 538
Douglas C. Heiner, M.D.

Isolated Primary Pulmonary Hemosiderosis.. 538
Primary Pulmonary Hemosiderosis with Cardiac or Pancreatic
    Involvement 546
Primary Pulmonary Hemosiderosis with Glomerulonephritis
    (Goodpasture's Syndrome) 546
Primary Pulmonary Hemosiderosis with Sensitivity to Cow Milk 547
Pulmonary Hemosiderosis Secondary to Heart Disease..................................... 549
Pulmonary Hemosiderosis as a Manifestation of Diffuse Collagen-
    Vascular or Purpuric Disease... 549

Chapter Thirty-Seven

ATELECTASIS.. 553
Rosa Lee Nemir, M.D.

Nonobstructive Atelectasis.. 565
Massive Pulmonary Collapse... 566

Chapter Thirty-Eight

PULMONARY EDEMA... 573
Robert B. Mellins, M.D., and S. Alex Stalcup, M.D.

Chapter Thirty-Nine

EMPHYSEMA AND ALPHA$_1$-ANTITRYPSIN DEFICIENCY............................. 593
Richard C. Talamo, M.D.

Chapter Forty

LIQUID AND AIR IN THE PLEURAL SPACE.. 602
Reynaldo D. Pagtakhan, M.D., and Victor Chernick, M.D.

Liquid in the Pleural Space 602
Air in the Pleural Space.. 610

Chapter Forty-One

ASTHMA 620
Susan C. Dees, M.D.

Chapter Forty-Two

NONASTHMATIC ALLERGIC PULMONARY DISEASE 670
C. Warren Bierman, M.D., William E. Pierson, M.D., and
F. Stanford Massie, M.D.

Hypersensitivity Pneumonitis or Extrinsic Allergic Alveolitis 670
Allergic Bronchopulmonary Disease 684
Pulmonary Hypersensitivity States Due to Chemical Agents and Drugs.............. 688

Chapter Forty-Three

TUMORS OF THE CHEST.. 697
James W. Brooks, M.D.

Pulmonary Tumors... 697
Mediastinal Tumors.. 710
Primary Cardiac and Pericardial Tumors 734
Tumors of the Diaphragm... 734
Primary Tumors of the Chest Wall.. 734

Section VI

**OTHER DISEASES WITH A PROMINENT RESPIRATORY
COMPONENT**

Chapter Forty-Four

COR PULMONALE.. 747
Jacqueline A. Noonan, M.D.

Parenchymal Lung Disease.. 747
Extrinsic Factors Resulting in Hypoventilation 750
Deformities of the Thoracic Chest.. 751
Pulmonary Vascular Disease.. 753
Summary 757

Chapter Forty-Five

CYSTIC FIBROSIS... 760
Harry Shwachman, M.D.

Chapter Forty-Six

TUBERCULOSIS... 787

Edwin L. Kendig, Jr., M.D.

Classification of Tuberculosis.. 811
Positive Tuberculin Reaction 812
Primary Pulmonary Tuberculosis 813
Progressive Primary Pulmonary Tuberculosis..................................... 816
Tuberculous Pneumonia (Hematogenous) 818
Obstructive Lesions of the Bronchi (Tuberculous Bronchitis or
    Lymph Node–Bronchial Tuberculosis).. 818
Tuberculosis in the Newborn 823
Acute Miliary Tuberculosis 825
Pleurisy with Effusion.. 826
Chronic Pulmonary Tuberculosis 829
Other Tuberculous Involvement of the Respiratory Tract 830
Extrapulmonary Tuberculosis.. 831
The Prevention of Tuberculosis... 838

Chapter Forty-Seven

INFECTIONS WITH THE ATYPICAL MYCOBACTERIA 844

Edwin L. Kendig, Jr., M.D.

Chapter Forty-Eight

SARCOIDOSIS... 852

Edwin L. Kendig, Jr., M.D.

Chapter Forty-Nine

HISTOPLASMOSIS 865

Amos Christie, M.D.

Chapter Fifty

THE MYCOSES (EXCLUDING HISTOPLASMOSIS) 879

John H. Seabury, M.D.

General Methods of Microbiologic Diagnosis...................................... 880
Actinomycosis 883
Nocardiosis.. 889
North American Blastomycosis 893
South American Blastomycosis (Paracoccidioidomycosis).................. 899
Coccidioidomycosis 902
Pulmonary Cryptococcosis... 910
Opportunistic Fungus Infections... 917
Treatment of Systemic Mycoses 925

Chapter Fifty-One

CYTOMEGALIC INCLUSION DISEASE.. 936

William A. Howard, M.D.

Chapter Fifty-Two
PSITTACOSIS (ORNITHOSIS) 942
Robert H. High, M.D.

Chapter Fifty-Three
Q FEVER 948
Robert H. High, M.D.

Chapter Fifty-Four
TULAREMIA... 950
William A. Howard, M.D.

Chapter Fifty-Five
VARICELLA PNEUMONIA... 955
Rosa Lee Nemir, M.D.

Chapter Fifty-Six
MEASLES PNEUMONIA 966
Rosa Lee Nemir, M.D.
Atypical Measles Pneumonia 977

Chapter Fifty-Seven
GIANT CELL PNEUMONIA 983
Samuel Stone, M.D.

Chapter Fifty-Eight
PERTUSSIS PNEUMONIA.. 986
Rosa Lee Nemir, M.D.

Chapter Fifty-Nine
PERTUSSOID EOSINOPHILIC PNEUMONIA 994
Rosa Lee Nemir, M.D.
Pertussis Syndrome.. 995

Chapter Sixty
SALMONELLA PNEUMONIA.. 998
Rosa Lee Nemir, M.D.

Chapter Sixty-One
RHEUMATIC PNEUMONIA 1006
Rosa Lee Nemir, M.D.

Chapter Sixty-Two
VISCERAL LARVA MIGRANS 1019
William A. Howard, M.D.

Chapter Sixty-Three

LOEFFLER'S SYNDROME 1023
William A. Howard, M.D.

Chapter Sixty-Four

IDIOPATHIC HISTIOCYTOSIS (HISTIOCYTOSIS X) 1027
Robert H. High, M.D.

Chapter Sixty-Five

PULMONARY INVOLVEMENT IN THE RHEUMATIC DISORDERS
(SO-CALLED COLLAGEN DISEASES) OF CHILDHOOD 1031
Bernhard H. Singsen, M.D., and Arnold C. G. Platzker, M.D.

Systemic Lupus Erythematosus 1034
Scleroderma 1043
Dermatomyositis.. 1046
Juvenile Rheumatoid Arthritis.. 1048
Mixed Connective Tissue Disease 1050
Wegener's Granulomatosis 1052
Vasculitis Syndromes... 1055
Summary 1057

Chapter Sixty-Six

FAMILIAL DYSAUTONOMIA... 1061
Felicia B. Axelrod, M.D., and Joseph Dancis, M.D.

Chapter Sixty-Seven

CHRONIC GRANULOMATOUS DISEASE OF CHILDHOOD 1067
Byung Hak Park, M.D., Beulah Holmes Gray, Ph.D., and
Robert A. Good, M.D., Ph.D.

Chapter Sixty-Eight

DISORDERS OF THE RESPIRATORY TRACT DUE TO TRAUMA 1077
Arnold M. Salzberg, M.D., and James W. Brooks, M.D.

Sternal Fractures... 1077
Fractured Ribs 1078
Traumatic Pneumothorax.. 1082
Hemothorax 1084
Tracheobronchial Trauma 1085
Pulmonary Compression Injury (Traumatic Asphyxia) 1086
Post-Traumatic Atelectasis (Wet Lung)... 1087
Cardiac Trauma... 1087
Injuries to the Esophagus 1091
Thoracoabdominal Injuries.. 1091

INDEX 1095

SECTION I

GENERAL CONSIDERATIONS

CHAPTER ONE

THE FUNCTIONAL BASIS OF RESPIRATORY PATHOLOGY

Victor Chernick, M.D., and Mary Ellen Avery, M.D.

A knowledge of normal function is fundamental in considering the effect of pathologic processes on the patient. Over the past three decades, pulmonary physiology has been undergoing a revolution in concepts and terminology. As in most revolutions, there have been stages of confusion that precede stages of clarification. Agreement on terminology, which ended one aspect of confusion, was achieved by a committee of American pulmonary physiologists in 1950. The increasing use of classic physical and engineering concepts has added another order of clarity. And finally, technological advances have increased the precision and availability of measurements of blood gases, pressures and flows, for example, so that functional evaluations are widely available to clinicians.

When tools are available, and physiologic principles elucidated, the translation of the new findings and their ultimate application in illness become the task and obligation of the clinician. The purpose of this opening section of a volume on disorders of the respiratory tract in children is to attempt the translation of relevant physiologic concepts. The principles involved are straightforward. The terminology, once defined, is logical. It is our belief that the physician will find the differential diagnosis of pulmonary problems and the rationale of therapy immensely simplified once a problem is approached with the question, What is the nature of the functional derangement? Quantification of the functional derangement is most helpful in the evaluation of therapy and in documenting the course of chronic pulmonary diseases.

DEFINITIONS AND SYMBOLS

The principal variables for gases are as follows:

V = gas volume
P = pressure
F = fractional concentration in dry gas
R = respiratory exchange ratio, V carbon dioxide/V oxygen
f = frequency
D_L = diffusing capacity of lung

The designation of which volume or pressure is cited requires a small capital letter after the principal variable. Thus V_{O_2} = volume of oxygen; P_B = barometric pressure.

I = inspired gas   T = tidal gas
E = expired gas   D = dead space gas
A = alveolar gas   B = barometric pressure

When both location of the gas and its species are to be indicated, the order is $V_{I_{O_2}}$, which means the volume of inspired oxygen. A dot above any symbol represents an amount per unit of time; thus, $\dot{V}_E$ = amount of air expired per minute.

STPD = standard temperature, pressure, dry (0°C., 760 mm. Hg)

BTPS = body temperature, pressure, saturated with water vapor

ATPS = ambient temperature, pressure, saturated with water vapor

The principal designations for blood are as follows:

S = Percentage saturation of gas in blood

C = content of gas per 100 ml. of blood

Q = volume of blood

Q̇ = blood flow per minute

a = arterial

v̄ = mixed venous

c = capillary

All sites of blood determinations are indicated by lower case initials. Thus Pa_{CO_2} = partial pressure of carbon dioxide in arterial blood. $P\bar{v}_{O_2}$ = partial pressure of oxygen in mixed venous blood. Pc_{O_2} = partial pressure of oxygen in a capillary. (Standardization of definitions and symbols in respiratory physiology is from *Federation Proceedings*, 9:602–605, 1950.)

PROPERTIES OF GASES

Gases behave as an enormous number of tiny particles in constant motion. Their behavior is governed by the gas laws, which are essential to the understanding of pulmonary physiology.

① DALTON'S LAW. This law states that the total pressure exerted by a gas mixture is equal to the sum of the pressures of the individual gases. The pressure exerted by each component is independent of the other gases in the mixture. For instance, at sea level, air saturated with water vapor at a temperature of 37°C. has a total pressure equal to the atmospheric pressure (P_B = 101.3 kilopascals or 30 inches of mercury or 760 mm. Hg), with the partial pressures of the components as follows:

P_B = 760 mm. Hg = P_{H_2O} (47 mm. Hg + P_{O_2} (149.2 mm. Hg) + P_{N_2} (563.5 mm. Hg) + P_{CO_2} (0.3 mm. Hg).

The gas in alveoli contains 5.6 per cent carbon dioxide, BTPS. If P_B = 760 mm. Hg, then:

Pa_{CO_2} = 0.056 (760 − 47) = 40 mm. Hg.

The terms "partial pressure" and "tension" are interchangeable for gases. ② BOYLE'S LAW states that at constant temperature the volume of any gas varies inversely as the pressure to which the gas is subjected: PV = k. Since respiratory volume measurements may be made at different barometric pressures, it is important to know the barometric pressure, and convert to standard pressure, which is considered to be 760 mm. Hg. ③ CHARLES'S LAW states that if the pressure is constant, the volume of a gas increases in direct proportion to the absolute temperature. At absolute zero (−273°C), molecular motion ceases. With increasing temperature, molecular collisions increase, so that at constant pressure, volume must increase.

In all respiratory calculations, water vapor pressure must be taken into account. The partial pressure of water vapor increases with temperature, but is independent of atmospheric pressure. At body temperature (37°C.), fully saturated gas has P_{H_2O} = 47 mm. Hg.

Gases may exist in physical solution in a liquid, escape from the liquid, or return to it. At equilibrium, the partial pressure of a gas in a liquid medium exposed to a gas phase is equal in the two phases (Henry's Law). Note that in blood the sum of the partial pressures of all the gases does not necessarily equal atmospheric pressure. For example, in venous blood: P_{O_2} has fallen from the 100 mm. Hg of the arterial blood to 40 mm., while P_{CO_2} changes from 40 to 46 mm. Hg. Thus, the sum of the partial pressures of O_2, CO_2 and N_2 in venous blood equals 655 mm. Hg. sis, and space-occupying materials as in effusion, edema and tumors. Thus the

④ HENRY'S LAW OF DIFFUSION. The diffusion rate for gases in a liquid phase is directly proportional to their solubility coefficients. For example, in water:

$$\frac{\text{Solubility of } CO_2}{\text{Solubility of } O_2} = \frac{0.592}{0.0244} = \frac{24.3}{1}$$

Therefore, carbon dioxide diffuses more than 24 times as fast as oxygen.

The diffusion rate of a gas in the gas phase is inversely proportional to $\sqrt{\text{molecular weight}}$ (Graham's Law). Therefore, in the gas phase:

$$\frac{\text{rate for } CO_2}{\text{rate for } O_2} = 0.85.$$

That is, carbon dioxide diffuses slower in the gas phase than oxygen.

Combining Henry's and Graham's Laws for a system with both a gas phase and a liquid phase, e. g., alveolus and blood: carbon dioxide diffuses (24.3 × 0.85 or) 20.7 times as fast as oxygen.

LUNG MORPHOLOGY AND GROWTH

Some aspects of lung growth and morphology are relevant and indeed necessary to the understanding of lung function. For example, the prematurely born infant's survival may be limited by ① the inability of the lung to distend adequately ② retain air at the end of expiration, or ③ be perfused with sufficient blood to permit gas exchange.

Embryology and Histology

The lung arises as an outpouching of gut at 24 days, and undergoes progressive bronchial proliferation in the first weeks of fetal life. Inductive interaction between epithelium and mesenchyme occurs. Epithelium, isolated in vitro, does not undergo morphogenesis; when it is recombined with pulmonary mesenchyme, development resumes. Branching proceeds chiefly by a heightened mitotic activity in the epithelium

compared with that of the mesenchyme. The mesenchyme differentiates into cartilage, smooth muscle and connective tissue around the epithelial tubes. By the sixteenth week the lung has its full complement of bronchial generations. Bronchial generations are fewer in the upper lobes and more numerous in the lower lobes, where there are 25 segmental branches. Before the sixteenth week, the glandular appearance of passages lined with cuboidal epithelium predominates. From the sixteenth to the twenty-fourth week, a canalicular phase predominates, and thereafter clusters of terminal air spaces with attenuated epithelium appear (Fig. 1). After birth, respiratory passages elongate. It is not until the sixth to eighth week of postnatal life that typical sharply curved alveoli can be identified.

The internal surface of the airways is lined by cells in all phases of lung development. The trachea and bronchi are lined by pseudostratified epithelium of four types ① ciliated cells (present from the tenth week) ② goblet cells (found first at thirteen to fourteen weeks) ③ brush cells, and ④ short (basal) cell. The bronchioles contain ciliated cells, but here the goblet cells are replaced by another columnar cell with small apical secretory droplets. The last cells to appear in lung development are those most specific to the lung, and farthest removed from the pharyngeal area. They are the lining cells of the most terminal air spaces, which are first evident in the sixth month of gestation. At least two types of alveolar lining cells can be distinguished: ① an attenuated epithelial cell which may have cytoplasmic continuity with cuboidal cells of the bronchiole (type I cell), the other a more granular cell with many mitochondria, osmiophilic inclusions, Golgi apparatus and other organelles (type II cell). Both alveolar cells rest on a continuous basement membrane (Fig. 2). Macrophages may also be seen fixed to the cell wall or free in the lumen, and these are presumably the cells that can be seen with the light microscope and found by the

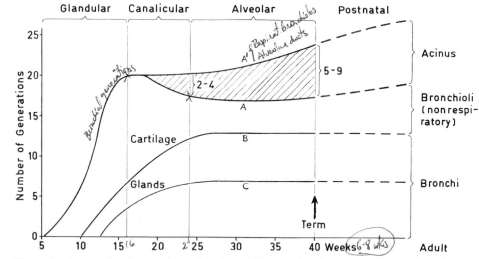

Figure 1. Intrauterine development of the bronchial tree. Line *A* represents the number of bronchial generations, and *A'* the respiratory bronchioles and alveolar ducts. *B* is the extension of cartilage along the bronchial tree, and *C* the extension of mucous glands. (From Bucher, U., and Reid, L.: *Thorax*, 16:267, 1961.)

millions in sputum. Their relation to the granular alveolar lining cell or type II cell remains uncertain.

The larger airways are rich in mucous glands from early development. Acid mucopolysaccharides are abundant in the trachea of an 18-week fetus, and persist through the first year of life in relatively greater amount than found in adults.

The pulmonary artery arises from aortic arches and nourishes the lung bud. Capillary proliferation becomes most abundant at 26 to 28 weeks of gestation, and it is during this phase of development that the lung becomes the most vascular of all organs of the body. Before that time the pulmonary vascular bed is not able to accommodate the whole of the cardiac output, and it is reasonable to consider the maintenance of life, dependent on the lung for gas exchange, not possible before the stage of capillary proliferation.

Fetal Lung at Term

The fetal lung contains a liquid that differs in composition from blood and amniotic liquid, and therefore is thought to be a secretory product of the lung itself. The pH is about 6.4, the bicarbonate concentration is lower than that of plasma, and hydrogen ion concentration is greater. Its protein content is about 300 mg. per 100 ml. The amount of liquid in the fetal lung increases during gestation until at term it is estimated to approximate a functional residual capacity, about 10 to 25 ml. per kilogram of body weight.

The assessment of lung function in early stages of development is based chiefly on measurements in lambs, which provides insight into the direction of changes with time, although exact analogies to the human subject are hazardous. The distensibility of the lung early in gestation is much less than at term. When peak volumes are expressed as milliliters per gram of lung tissue, it is evident that the potential air space is small with respect to lung mass. The ability to retain air at end-expiration, which depends on the presence of the pulmonary surfactant, is not evident until later in the canalicular stage of development. In the lamb it is at 120 to 130 days of a 147-day gestation. In the human being it is probably about the twentieth to twenty-fourth week of gestation, with a wide scatter. The dis-

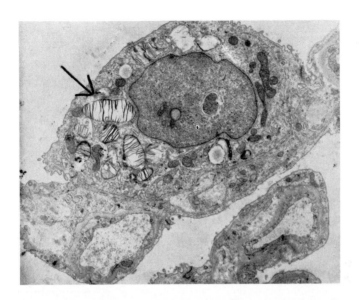

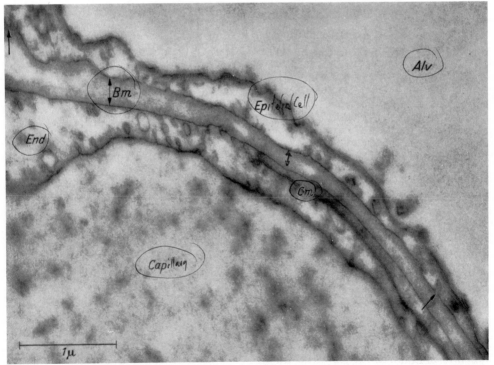

Figure 2. *Upper,* Electron micrograph of one type of cell that lines the alveolus. This particular cell is from a dog's lung, but is similar to those found in all mammalian lungs. The air space is in the upper portion of the figure. The arrow points to the osmiophilic inclusions that are thought to be associated with the alveolar lining substance. The cell rests on a basement membrane that separates it from the capillary endothelium in the lower part of the picture. (Photograph courtesy of E. S. Boatman and H. B. Martin, University of Washington Medical School, Seattle, Washington.)

Lower, Normal human lung showing the attenuated alveolar cytoplasm. Abbreviations: *Alv,* alveolus; *Ep,* cytoplasmic layer of an epithelial cell; *Bm,* basement membrane; *End,* capillary endothelium; *Cm,* erythrocyte cell membrane; *Cap,* capillary. (Published with permission from Schultz, H.: *The Submicroscopic Anatomy and Pathology of the Lung.* Berlin, Springer-Verlag, 1959.)

distensibility of the vascular bed likewise increases with fetal age. Little blood flow is possible even at high perfusion pressures in the early fetal lung. As term approaches, the capacity and distensibility of the vascular bed increase. The morphologic counterpart of these changes is seen in the greater wall-lumen ratios in the fetal lung compared with those in postnatal life. After about ten days of extrauterine life the lumens are wider, regardless of the time of birth. The events of birth have little effect on other aspects of lung development, including histochemical changes.

It is useful to remember that the lung has the most abundant lymphatics of any organ of the body. They are located beneath the pulmonary pleura, in perivascular and peribronchial connective tissue sheaths, and within the bronchial walls. They do not form a network around the alveoli, although their endings are within a few microns of the terminal air sacs. They form a plexiform network with simple valves that direct flow centripetally. The vessels gain in connective tissue and smooth muscle near the pulmonary hilus and resemble the thoracic duct. They form a closed system and are the main pathway for removal of fine particulate matter and protein from air spaces. Aggregates of lymphoid tissue are located along the bronchi, particularly at sites of branching, but lymph nodes are found chiefly at lobar bronchial branches.

Postnatal Lung

The postnatal growth of the lung continues until approximately eight years of age, with an increase in numbers of alveoli and the dimensions of all the air spaces. Some further increase in dimensions of terminal air spaces may proceed to 40 years of age. The lung of the newborn infant is not the miniature of the adult; tracheal diameter approximately triples, alveolar dimensions increase about fourfold, and alveolar numbers increase about tenfold, while body mass increases some 20-fold. The obvious advantage of relatively large airways is to facilitate the movement of air. The relatively smaller alveoli permit a larger surface area per volume of lung, which is essential for gas transfer. Indeed, the internal surface area of the lung bears a close relation to body mass, approximately 1 square meter per kilogram of body weight, which would appear to be a useful design to permit the area for gas exchange to follow changes in amounts of metabolizing tissue.

Other gross anatomic relations of the infant's and child's lung are similar to those of the adult (Figs. 3 and 4). The proportion of total lung weight represented by each lobe is remarkably constant from infancy to adulthood. Average values of lung lobe weight expressed as a percentage of total and based on a study of normal human lungs are as follows: right upper lobe, 19.52; right middle lobe, 8.34; right lower lobe, 25.26; left upper lobe, 22.48; left lower lobe, 24.61. Lobular septa are better developed in the apical regions of the lung and beneath sharp margins than they are near the costal or lateral surfaces and lower lobes. It has been suggested that those areas with many septa would have less collateral ventilation, and hence be more susceptible to atelectasis. Collateral ventilatory pathways, the alveolar pores of Kohn, are also fewer in number in the infant's lung, and increase with advancing age.

The influence of lung growth on respiratory disease is discussed in detail in Chapter 7 of this section.

Muscles of Respiration

The movement of air in and out of the lungs in normal breathing requires an increase and decrease in size of the thorax, which is achieved by the coordinated movements of the muscles that surround it. Their geometric arrangements and the details of their action are so complex as to defy thorough analysis at this time.

The diaphragm is the principal mus-

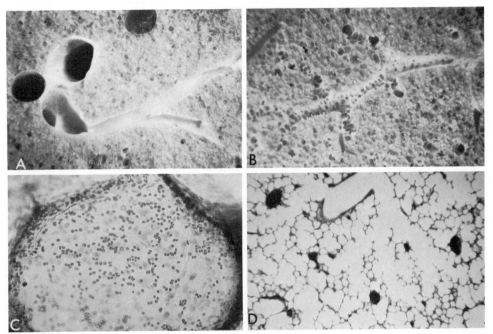

Figure 3. The architecture of the lung. *A,* Fresh frozen cat lung (4×). Segmental cartilaginous bronchus and branches. The pulmonary artery is close to the airway; the pulmonary vein is in a more peripheral location. *B,* Fresh frozen cat lung (4×). Terminal bronchiole with many alveolar ducts arising from it. *C,* Thick section of cat lung (100×). A single alveolar wall is in the plane of focus. Individual red cells in alveolar capillaries are clearly seen. *D,* Guinea pig (15×), fixed thin section. The terminal respiratory unit, with alveoli shown as outpouchings of the alveolar duct, arises from the terminal bronchiole at the top of the picture. Note that three vessels, probably pulmonary veins, mark the distal boundaries of the unit. (Reproduced by permission of Dr. Norman Staub, University of California Medical Center, San Francisco. All but *A* appeared in color in *Anesthesiology, 24*:831, 1963.)

cle of respiration; however, it is not essential for breathing in the awake state. During deep anesthesia it is essential because the other muscles of respiration become inactive. Its contraction causes descent of its dome, and aids in elevation of the lower ribs in adults. In infants with a very compliant rib cage, descent of the diaphragm may oppose elevation of the lower ribs and result in paradoxical subcostal retractions. In the preterm infant it has been proposed that such paradoxical movement of the chest wall may trigger an intercostal-phrenic inhibitory reflex responsible for recurrent apnea, particularly during the REM stage of sleep when the normal stabilizing influence of the intercostal muscles on the chest wall is lost.

The force exerted by the diaphragm during maximal inspiration in adults is about 100 cm. of water when its fibers shorten by about 50 per cent of their initial length. Its motor innervation is from the third to fifth cervical roots through the phrenic nerve.

The main portion of the intercostal muscles is arranged to facilitate inspiration by elevating the lower ribs. Contraction of the external intercostals occurs in inspiration; the internal intercostals are active chiefly in expiration. However, if the intercostals alone are paralyzed, there is little decrease in exercise tolerance, since expiration is normally passive.

The abdominal muscles are the most powerful muscles of expiration. The external and internal oblique muscles compress the abdomen, flex the trunk, and help to depress the lower ribs. The recti draw the lower rib cage toward the pubis and further decrease abdom-

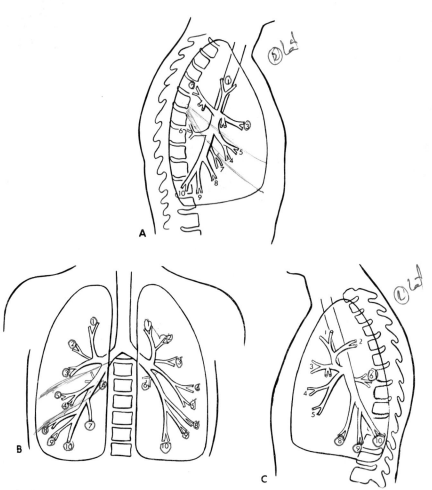

Figure 4. The nomenclature of bronchopulmonary anatomy, adapted from report by the Thoracic Society in 1950. (Adapted from Negus.)

Right lung	**Left lung**
Upper lobe	*Upper lobe*
1. Apical	1.⎫
2. Posterior	2.⎭ Apicoposterior
3. Anterior	
Middle lobe	3. Anterior
4. Lateral	4.⎫ Lingula
5. Medial	5.⎭
Lower lobe	*Lower lobe*
6. Apical	6. Apical
7. Cardiac (medial basal)	7. − − absent
8. Anterior ⎫	8. Anterior ⎫
9. Lateral ⎬ basal	9. Lateral ⎬ basal
10. Posterior ⎭	10. Posterior ⎭

inal volume. In most normal subjects there is no participation of the abdominal muscles in quiet breathing. In some persons the abdominal muscles contract at end-inspiration and set a limit to further expansion of the lung.

The scalenes act to elevate the first two ribs even in quiet breathing. Elevation of the sternum is achieved by contraction of the sternocleidomastoid muscles; they are not usually active in quiet breathing in adults. When inspiratory efforts are marked, their activity is significant; in fact, they are considered the most important accessory muscles of inspiration. Elevation and prominence of the upper portion of the sternum is a common observation in infants with respiratory distress, presumably from contraction of the sternocleidomastoid muscles.

Other muscles of respiration include the costal levators and the suprahyoid group. The latter probably stabilize the trachea and larynx when during deep inspiration the descent of the diaphragm acts to draw the lung caudad. It can readily be shown that although the hili do descend slightly during deep inspiration, the larynx barely moves. The action of the sacrospinalis, trapezius, pectorals, and serratus anterior and posterior superior is to enlarge the thorax; the posterior inferior serratus decreases thoracic volume.

Some additional accessory muscles aid inspiration by reducing the resistance to air flow in the upper airway. These include the alae nasi, cheek muscles, platysma, and tongue muscles.

LUNG VOLUMES

Nomenclature

The partition of lung volumes and the nomenclature can be appreciated

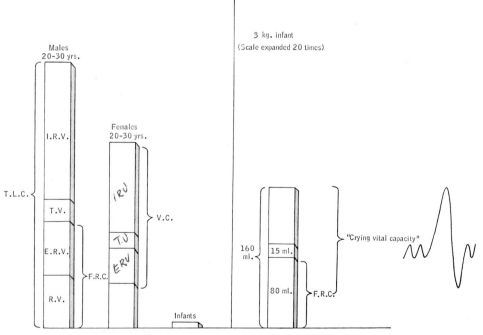

Figure 5. The lung volumes. A volume is a single subdivision; a capacity is more than one subdivision. Abbreviations: *T.L.C.*, total lung capacity (6 liters in an average male, 4.2 liters in an average female); *I.R.V.*, inspiratory reserve volume; *T.V.*, tidal volume; *E.R.V.*, expiratory reserve volume; *R.V.*, residual volume; *F.R.C.*, functional residual capacity. The spirogram shown on the right is a tracing from a revolving drum attached to a water-filled spirometer. T.V., I.R.V., E.R.V. and vital capacity can be measured from such a tracing.

from Figure 5. The spirogram on the right is a tracing from a rotating drum marked by an ink writer attached to a spirometer.

The concept of lung volumes and capacities, rather than a single volume, derives from the fact that sometimes more or less air is moved, some air is always present in normal lungs, and it is useful to apply labels to the portions of the total gas volume that are under discussion. For example, if it is desired to study lung growth with age, a measure of total lung capacity is appropriate. (A capacity is more than one lung volume.) If an index of the degree of overexpansion of the lungs in chronic lower airway obstructive disease is desired, either the functional residual capacity or residual volume would be helpful. If a patient has a restriction to lung expansion from thoracic disease or a pulmonary fibrotic process, the pertinent measurement would be the largest breath he is capable of taking or his vital capacity.

Methods of Measurement

The tidal volume, inspiratory and expiratory volumes and vital capacity can be measured by asking a patient to breathe quietly, and take in the biggest possible breath and blow it all out.

The measurement of functional residual capacity and residual volume requires another approach. Since both include the air in the lungs that the patient does not normally exhale, they must be measured indirectly. One method uses the principle of dilution of the unknown volume with a known concentration of a gas that is foreign to the lung and only sparingly absorbed, such as helium. The patient breathes from a container with a known volume and concentration of helium in oxygen-enriched air. After sufficient time has elapsed for the gas in his lung to mix and equilibrate with the gas in the container, the concentration of helium in the container is remeasured. Since initial volume times concentration of helium equals final volume times concen-

tration of helium, the final volume, which includes gas in the lungs, can be calculated. Correction factors can be applied for the volumes of oxygen absorbed or carbon dioxide released during the period of equilibration. Another commonly used method involves measurement of the nitrogen in the lung after it has come into equilibrium with inspired pure oxygen.

If some gas is "trapped" within the lungs, its volume will not be reflected in the helium dilution measurement. There is, however, a method of measurement of total gas volume within the thorax which depends on the change in volume that occurs with compression of the gas with the glottis closed. Practically, this measurement requires the patient to be in a body plethysmograph, and to make a forced inspiration (Mueller maneuver) or forced expiration (Valsalva maneuver) against an obstruction. The change in pressure can be measured in the mouthpiece; the change in volume can be recorded on a spirometer attached to the body plethysmograph: $V = P\Delta V/\Delta P$. This method has the advantage of being repeatable several times a minute. It has the disadvantage of including some abdominal gas in the measurement.

Interpretation

The vital capacity is one of the most valuable measurements that can be made in a functional assessment, although it cannot be interpreted without some additional knowledge of the patient. For example① it is a function of body size and②correlates most closely with body height; therefore, it should be expressed as a percentage of the predicted value for height (Table 1). It may be decreased by poor patient cooperation, which must be determined by the examiner. It can be decreased by a wide variety of disease processes, such as ①weakness of the muscles of respiration, ②loss of lung tissue as after lobectomy, ③obstruction of portions of the airways, ④changes in lung distensibility as in fibro-

TABLE 1. NORMAL VALUES FOR LUNG VOLUMES (LITERS)

Height (cm.)	Males			Females		
	VC	FRC	TLC	VC	FRC	TLC
92	0.68	0.38	0.88	0.66	0.41	0.88
94	0.72	0.40	0.94	0.70	0.44	0.93
96	0.77	0.43	1.00	0.74	0.47	0.99
98	0.82	0.46	1.07	0.79	0.50	1.05
100	0.87	0.49	1.14	0.84	0.54	1.12
102	0.93	0.53	1.21	0.89	0.57	1.18
104	0.98	0.56	1.28	0.94	0.61	1.25
106	1.04	0.60	1.36	0.99	0.64	1.32
108	1.10	0.64	1.44	1.05	0.68	1.40
110	1.16	0.68	1.52	1.11	0.72	1.47
112	1.23	0.72	1.60	1.17	0.76	1.55
114	1.30	0.76	1.69	1.23	0.81	1.63
116	1.37	0.81	1.78	1.29	0.85	1.72
118	1.44	0.85	1.88	1.36	0.90	1.81
120	1.52	0.90	1.98	1.43	0.95	1.90
122	1.59	0.95	2.08	1.50	1.00	1.99
124	1.67	1.01	2.19	1.57	1.05	2.09
126	1.76	1.06	2.29	1.65	1.10	2.19
128	1.84	1.12	2.41	1.73	1.16	2.29
130	1.93	1.18	2.52	1.81	1.22	2.40
132	2.02	1.24	2.64	1.89	1.28	2.50
134	2.12	1.30	2.77	1.97	1.34	2.62
136	2.21	1.36	2.89	2.06	1.40	2.73
138	2.31	1.43	3.03	2.15	1.47	2.85
140	2.42	1.50	3.16	2.24	1.54	2.97
142	2.52	1.57	3.30	2.34	1.61	3.10
144	2.63	1.65	3.44	2.43	1.68	3.23
146	2.74	1.72	3.59	2.53	1.75	3.36
148	2.86	1.80	3.74	2.64	1.83	3.49
150	2.98	1.88	3.90	2.74	1.91	3.63
152	3.10	1.97	4.06	2.85	1.99	3.78
154	3.23	2.05	4.22	2.96	2.07	3.92
156	3.35	2.14	4.39	3.07	2.16	4.07
158	3.49	2.24	4.57	3.19	2.25	4.23
160	3.62	2.33	4.74	3.31	2.34	4.38
162	3.76	2.43	4.93	3.43	2.43	4.54
164	3.90	2.53	5.11	3.56	2.53	4.71
166	4.05	2.63	5.30	3.69	2.62	4.88
168	4.20	2.74	5.50	3.82	2.72	5.05
170	4.35	2.85	5.70	3.95	2.83	5.23
172	4.51	2.96	5.91	4.09	2.93	5.41
174	4.67	3.07	6.12	4.23	3.04	5.59
176	4.83	3.19	6.34	4.37	3.15	5.78
178	5.00	3.31	6.56	4.52	3.26	5.98
180	5.17	3.44	6.78	4.67	3.38	6.17

From Cook and Hamann: *J. Pediatr.*, 59:710, 1961.

vital capacity is not a useful tool to discriminate between types of lesions. Its chief role is to assign a value to the degree of impairment and to document changes with therapy or in time.

The functional residual capacity or the residual volume reflects the degree of distention of lung. Overdistention is usually compensatory for partial lower airway obstruction. When the lung volume is increased, intrathoracic airways enlarge, and widespread partial obstruction may be relieved by the assumption of a large resting lung volume. The increase in the antero-posterior diameter of the chest noted in asthma or cystic fibrosis is accompanied by a large functional residual capacity. A decrease in functional residual capacity is associated with conditions in which alveolar collapse is prominent, such as hyaline membrane disease. Since clinical and roentgenographic signs permit a rough estimate of the functional residual capacity, it is rarely helpful to measure it in infants and children.

MECHANICS OF RESPIRATION

Alterations in the mechanics of breathing account for most of the respiratory complaints and many of the abnormal findings on physical examination. Shortness of breath, tachypnea, stridor, wheezing, retractions and rales are all associated with abnormal ventilatory mechanics. A cough, sometimes deliberate, sometimes involuntary, is associated with a sequence of mechanical events that accelerate the air column and exert a milking action on the tracheobronchial tree.

It is traditional, and useful, to consider mechanical events under two main categories① the static-elastic properties of the lungs and chest wall, and ② the flow-resistive or dynamic aspects of moving air. Changes in one category may be associated with compensatory changes in the other. Thus, many diseases affect both static and dynamic behavior of the lungs. Often the principal derangement is in the elastic properties of the tissues or in the dimensions of the airways, and the treatment or alleviation of symptoms depends on distinguishing them.

Static-Elastic Forces

The lung is an elastic structure that tends to reduce its size at all volumes. It is the elastic recoil of the lung that makes it tend to pull away from the chest wall with a resultant subatmospheric pressure in the pleural "space." The word "space" refers to a potential space; in health the pleural surface of the lung is apposed to the pleura lining the chest wall, held firm by the molecular forces of the thin layers of liquid that cover the two surfaces. The subatmospheric pressure that surrounds the lung (often called negative pressure) is not the same over all surfaces of the lung. Forces are applied to the lung by supporting structures, and gravity. In general, pleural pressures are lower in the apices than in the bases. The effect is exaggerated by the height of the person, and further increased during head-forward acceleration.

The elasticity of the lung depends on ① the structural components (although elastic fibers are not essential for normal performance② the geometry of the terminal air spaces, and③ the presence of an air-liquid interface. When a lung is made airless, then inflated with liquid, the elastic recoil at large volumes is less than half that of a lung inflated to the same volume with air. Thus, the most significant determinant of the elastic properties of the lung is the presence of an air-liquid interface. A further demonstration of the role of the interface is the absence of subatmospheric pleural pressure in the fetus, whose lungs contain liquid, but no air. After the few first breaths, pleural pressure is subatmospheric.

The increase of elastic recoil in the presence of an air-liquid interface is from the forces of surface tension. What is surface tension? When molecules are aligned at an air-liquid interface, they lack opposing molecules on one side. The intermolecular attractive forces are then unbalanced, and the resultant force tends to move molecules away from the interface. The effect is to reduce the area of the surface to a minimum. In the lungs, whose surface area in square meters approximates body weight in kilograms, the forces at the air-liquid interface operate to reduce the internal surface area of the lung, and thus augment elastic recoil. A remarkable property of the material at the alveolar interface, the alveolar lining layer or pulmonary surfactant, is the ability to achieve a high surface tension at large lung volumes, and a low tension at low volumes. It is a phospholipid-protein complex which can form insoluble folded surface films of low surface tension on compression, as can be shown on a surface film balance. The ability to achieve a low surface tension at low lung volumes tends to stabilize the air spaces and prevent their closure (Fig. 6). Lacking such a stabilizing substance or emulsifying agent, the smaller alveoli would tend to empty into the larger in accord with the Laplace relationship, which relates the pressure across a surface (P) to surface tension (T) and radius (R) of curvature. For a spherical surface, $P = \dfrac{2T}{r}$. The smaller the radius, the greater is the tendency to collapse.

The elasticity of the lung is described by measuring static volume-pressure relations. These can be done in vivo with a needle in the pleural space to record the transpulmonary pressure at known volumes; alternately, and more safely for the patient, the pressure within the esophagus can be used as an index of pleural pressure. If the changes in pressure at points of no flow are related to the resultant changes in volume, $\Delta V/\Delta P$, it is referred to as the dynamic lung compliance, a measure of the elastic recoil of the lung.

The compliance will depend on the initial lung volume from which the change in volume is measured, the ventilatory events immediately preceding the measurement, as well as the properties of the lung itself. At large lung volumes the compliance is lower, since the lung is near its elastic limit. If the subject has breathed with a fixed tidal volume for some minutes, portions of the lung are not participating in ventilation, and the compliance may be reduced. A few deep breaths, with return to the initial volume, will increase the compliance. Thus, a careful description of associated events is required for interpretation of the measurement.

Changes in lung compliance occur with age (Table 2). Of course, the smaller the subject, the smaller is the change in volume, so that $\Delta V/\Delta P$ is 4 to 6 ml. per centimeter of water in infants, and 125 to 190 ml. per centimeter of water in adults. It is more rele-

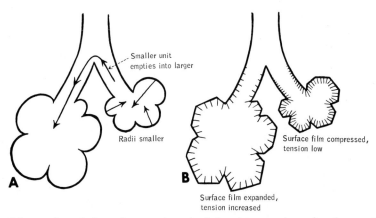

Figure 6. Schema of terminal ventilatory units and relations between size and surface tension. *A.* Effect of deficient surface film is for smaller unit to empty into larger, since radii are smaller, if surface tension of both units were the same.

$$P = \frac{2T}{r}$$

B. Effect of film is to lessen the role of different radii, since surface tension (T) decreases as r decreases. The shape of alveoli tends to be polygonal rather than spherical when the surfactant is present.

TABLE 2. LUNG COMPLIANCE
(C$_L$) WITH AGE

	ml./cm. H$_2$O	C$_L$/FRC
Newborns		
3 hours	4.75 ± 1.67	0.041 ± 0.01
24 hours	6.24 ± 1.45	0.055 ± 0.01
Infants		
1 month–2 years	7.9	0.038
Children		
Average age 9 years	77	0.063
Young adult males	184	0.050
Young adult females	125	0.053
Adults over 60 years	191	0.041

vant to a description of the elastic properties of the lung to express the compliance per unit of lung volume, such as the FRC. In Table 2, note that the compliance of the lung/FRC, or specific compliance, changes very little with age.

The elastic properties of the thorax can be measured by considering the pressure difference between pleural space or esophagus and the atmosphere, per change in volume. At resting lung volume (FRC), the elastic recoil of the thorax is equal and opposite to that of the lungs. The lungs tend to reduce their size, and the thorax tends to expand.

Significant changes in thoracic compliance occur with age. In the range of normal breathing, the thorax of the infant is nearly infinitely compliant. The pressures measured at different lung volumes are about the same across the lung as those measured across lung and thorax together. The functional significance of the very compliant thorax of the fetus is evident if consideration is given to the effect of an outward recoil of the thorax when the lung lacks an air-liquid interface. The fetal lung would then contain an even greater volume of liquid, which would compound the problem of the removal of lung liquid at birth. Alternately, liquid would fill the pleural space, where it would be even more difficult to resorb at birth.

With advancing age the thorax becomes relatively stiffer. Changes in volume-pressure relations are profitably

considered only if referred to a reliable unit, either a unit of lung volume or a percentage of total lung capacity. When the compliance of the thorax is considered on a percentage basis, it is evident that it has a decreasing compliance with age. How much is contributed by changes in tissue properties such as increasing calcification of ribs and connective tissue changes, and how much is a disproportionate growth of the chest wall relative to the lung remain unclear (Fig. 7).

Description of the passive elastic characteristics of the thorax does not allow one to predict adequately how the thorax will respond to an added elastic load. The elastance (elastance = compliance^{-1}) of the respiratory system in preterm and term newborn infants has been measured during added elastic loads. The elastance measured with this method is called the effective elastance and has been found to be surprisingly high. Presumably, this response is related to a vagal reflex resulting in recruitment of intercostal muscle activity and is brisk and forceful in the newborn infant, perhaps in association with the active Hering-Breuer reflex found at birth.

Dynamic Forces

Most of the work of quiet breathing is used to overcome the static-elastic forces that depend on the tissue properties of lungs and thorax. About one third of the total work is expended to overcome the frictional resistance of the movement of air and tissue. In any disease that compromises the airway dimensions, or results in an increased respiratory rate, resistive forces assume much greater importance.

The laws governing the resistance of flow of gases in tubes apply to pulmonary resistance just as they do in engineering. The equation for calculating the pressure gradient required to maintain streamlined flow of air through a tube is given by Poiseuille's Law:

$$P = \frac{\dot{V}\,(8l)\eta}{\pi r^4}$$

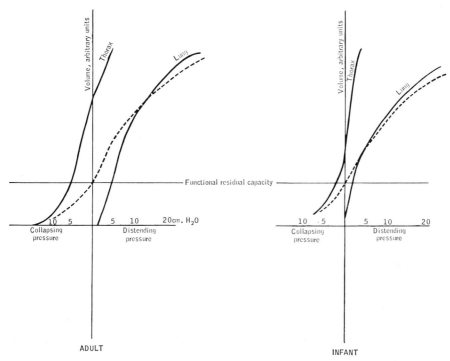

Figure 7. Pressure-volume relations of lungs and thorax in an adult on the left, in an infant on the right. The dashed line represents the characteristic of lungs and thorax together. Transpulmonary pressure at the resting portion (functional residual capacity) is less in the infant, and thoracic compliance is greater in the infant.

where P equals pressure; $\dot{V}$, flow; l, length; r, radius of the tube; and η the viscosity of the gas. The viscosity of air is 0.000181 poise at 20°C., 0.0001708 poise at 0°C. The viscosity of water, for comparison, is 0.0100 poise at 20°C., or nearly 100 times that of air. Resistance is pressure/flow. It is clear that the most important determinant of resistance will be the radius of the tube, which is raised to the fourth power in the denominator of the equation. Since flow is not always laminar, but often turbulent, the Poiseuille Law is not strictly applicable to all circumstances. It will underestimate resistance to turbulent flow.

MEASUREMENT OF RESISTANCE. Resistance is calculated from the relation $R = \dfrac{\text{driving pressure}}{\text{airflow}}$. The pressure must be measured at the two ends of the system—in the case of the lung, at the mouth and at alveoli—and the corresponding flow recorded. Alveolar pressure presents the greatest problem. If pleural pressure is substituted, the result is a measure of both airway and lung tissue viscous resistance (total nonelastic resistance). In health, tissue viscous resistance is about 20 per cent of the total.

Several methods have been used to measure alveolar pressure. The most commonly used method employs a body plethysmograph. The patient in this airtight chamber breathes air from the outside environment through a tube containing a shutter while pressures inside the chamber and at the mouth are recorded. The shutter is then closed so that the airway is completely obstructed and mouth pressure is identical to alveolar pressure. The subject makes an expiratory effort against the closed shutter, which compresses the air in the lungs and decompresses the air in the chamber. This results in simultaneous changes in mouth pressure, alveolar pressure, and chamber pressure, and the ratio of alveolar pressure to chamber pressure is determined. The shutter is then opened and the patient breathes through an unobstructed airway while airflow and changes in chamber pressure are recorded. Since the ratio of alveolar pressure to chamber pressure is known, alveolar pressure may be related to a given airflow and a value for airway resistance may be calculated.

Airway resistance changes with lung volumes. At large volumes the airways are distended, and resistance is low. Near the residual volume after forced expiration, resistance becomes infinite as airways are closed by high pleural pressures (Fig. 8).

Estimates of total nonelastic resistance (tissue viscous resistance plus airway) have been obtained on infants by use of dynamic pressure-volume curves. Airflow can be calculated from the slope of the volume tracing versus time, since flow is volume per unit of time. The pressure change is measured on the corresponding esophageal pressure tracing at points of equal volume on inspiration and expiration. That portion of pressure change required to overcome elastic forces is subtracted from the total. Measurements of total lung resistance by this method on in-

fants through the first year of life show a wide scatter, with an average value of 29 cm. of water per liter per second. The average value for airway resistance in infants, measured by the plethysmographic method, is 18 cm. of water per liter per second, suggesting that tissue resistances in the infant are nearly half of the total resistance. By contrast, the adult with larger airways has a much lower airway resistance, 1 to 3 cm. of water per liter per second at resting lung volume.

Recently, a simple method of measuring total pulmonary resistance has been used in infants and children and it is called the forced oscillation technique. This measurement includes airway resistance plus the tissue viscous resistance of the lung and chest wall. Nasal resistance is also included in the measurement if the infant is breathing through his nose. Advantages of this method are that it does not require a body plethysmograph or estimates of pleural pressure. It can be done quickly enough to be used on ill patients, is easily repeatable and does not require any patient cooperation. A sinusoidal pressure applied at the upper airway changes airflow, and the ratio of pressure change to flow change is used to calculate resistance. When the forced oscillations are applied at the so-called resonant frequency of the lung (3 to 5

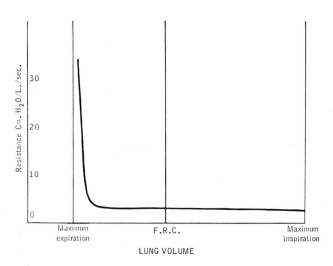

Figure 8. The relation of airway resistance to lung volume in the normal adult. Resistance remains low through the range of normal breathing, and increases greatly at residual volume, where airways are smallest.

cycles per second), it is assumed that the force required to overcome elastic resistance of the lung and the force required to overcome inertia are equal and opposite so that all of the force is dissipated in overcoming flow resistance. This technique has demonstrated that infants with bronchiolitis have about a twofold increase in inspiratory pulmonary resistance and a threefold increase in expiratory resistance.

SITES OF RESISTANCE. The contribution of the upper airway to total resistance is substantial. The average nasal resistance of infants by indirect measurement is 13 cm. of water per liter per second, or nearly half of total respiratory resistance, as is the case in adults. It is hardly surprising that any compromise of the dimensions of the nasal airway in an infant who is a preferential nose-breather will result in retractions and labored breathing. Likewise, even mild edema of the trachea or larynx will impose a significant increase in airway resistance, since the total resistance will increase by at least the fourth power of any reduction in radius of the upper airway.

In the adult lung, about 80 per cent of the resistance to airflow resides in airways greater than 2 mm. in diameter. The vast number of small peripheral airways provides a large cross-sectional area for flow and therefore contributes less than 20 per cent to the airway resistance. Thus, these airways may be the site of disease that may severely impair ventilation of distal air spaces without appreciably altering the total airway resistance. In the infant lung, however, small peripheral airways may contribute as much as 50 per cent to the total airway resistance, and this proportion does not decrease until about five years of age. Thus, the infant is particularly severely affected by diseases that affect the small airways, e.g., bronchiolitis. The methods of assessment of peripheral airway resistance will be discussed below.

FACTORS THAT MAY AFFECT AIRWAY RESISTANCE. Airway resistance is determined by the diameter of the airways, the velocity of airflow and the physical properties of the gas breathed. The diameter is determined by the balance of forces tending to narrow the airways and those tending to widen them. One of the forces tending to narrow airways is exerted by the contraction of bronchial smooth muscle. The neural regulation of bronchial smooth muscle tone is mediated by efferent impulses through autonomic nerves. Sympathetic impulses relax the airways, and parasympathetic impulses constrict them. Bronchi constrict reflexly from irritating inhalants such as sulfur dioxide and some dusts; by arterial hypoxemia and hypercapnia; by embolization of the vessels; by cold; and by some drugs such as acetylcholine and histamine. They dilate in response to an increase in systemic blood pressure through baroreceptors in the carotid sinus, and to sympathomimetic agents such as isoproterenol and epinephrine. The airways are probably in tonic contraction in health, since in unanesthetized adults atropine or isoproterenol will decrease airway resistance by nearly 50 per cent.

Another force tending to narrow airways is the peribronchial pressure; forces tending to keep airways open are the intraluminal pressure and the tethering action of the surrounding lung. The relationship between these forces is particularly important during forced expiration when pleural pressure is elevated above atmospheric pressure. The intraluminal pressure must decrease along the pathway of airflow from the alveoli to the mouth where it becomes equal to atmospheric pressure. However, at some point in the airway, intraluminal pressure must equal pleural pressure (equal pressure point or EPP). Downstream from the EPP, pleural pressure exceeds intraluminal pressure and thus is a force that tends to narrow airways. Indeed, during periods of maximum expiratory flow, pleural pressure exceeds the critical closing pressure of airways and they become narrowed to a slit. Despite cartilaginous support of the larger airways, the membranous portion of the wall of the trachea and large bronchi invaginates under pressure to occlude the airways. Maximum flow under this circumstance is therefore determined by the resistance of the airways that are located upstream from the equal pressure point, and the driving pressure is the difference between the alveolar pressure and the pressure at the EPP. In disease states in which there is an increased airway resistance, the equal pressure point moves toward the alveoli because of the greater intraluminal pressure drop. Thus, small airways are now compressed during forced expiration with severe flow limitations. With the measurement of pressure-flow and flow-volume curves during forced expiration, it is now possible to calculate resistance upstream and downstream from the point of critical closure or EPP. Increasing the lung volume increases the tethering action of the surrounding lung on airways, and therefore close attention must be paid to the lung volume at which resistance measurements are made during these studies.

Airway closure apparently occurs at low lung volumes and may be measured by measuring nitrogen washout from the lung following an inspiration of 100 per cent oxygen from residual volume. Those airways that are open receive less oxygen than those that are closed, and therefore contain a high P_{N_2}. At the point of airway closure, the expired concentration of nitrogen therefore rises sharply. The volume above residual volume at which this occurs is called the closing volume; the closing volume plus residual volume is called the closing capacity. Closing volume is high in young children and older individuals and may exceed the FRC in children under six years of age. It is evident that any property of a gas which will tend to increase friction will increase airway resistance. Thus, breathing gases with a low density, such as helium, will tend to decrease resistance; gases such as sulfur hexafluoride will increase resistance. In addition, barometric pressure influences the den-

sity of gas so that at high altitudes airway resistance is decreased, and at underwater depths it is increased.

The effect of gas density on airway resistance is caused by an effect on the resistance to turbulent gas flow, since the resistance to streamlined, or laminar, gas flow is not affected by gas density. Thus, comparison of airway resistance of flow-volume curves during air and helium/oxygen breathing has been used to assess the contribution of small peripheral airways, where flow is laminar, to the total airway resistance.

RELATIONSHIP BETWEEN AIRWAY RESISTANCE AND COMPLIANCE.   The rate at which an area of the lung will fill and empty is related to both airway resistance and compliance. A decrease in airway dimension will increase the time required for air to reach the alveoli; a region of low compliance will receive less ventilation per unit time than an area with high compliance. The product of resistance times compliance (time constant) is approximately the same in health for all ventilatory pathways. The unit of resistance times compliance is time. Note:

$$\text{Resistance} = \text{pressure/flow} = \frac{\text{cm. } H_2O}{\text{liters/sec.}}$$

$$\text{Compliance} = \frac{\Delta \text{ volume (liters)}}{\Delta \text{ pressure (cm. } H_2O)}$$

The product, then, is a unit of time, analogous to the time constant in an electrical system, and represents the time taken to accomplish 67 per cent of the volume change.

As mentioned previously, peripheral airways contribute little to overall airway resistance after about five years of age. However, in the presence of small airway disease, some areas of the lung will have high time constants while others are normal. This is particularly evident as the frequency of respiration increases. With increasing frequency air will go to those areas of the lung with low time constants, that is, with the least airway resistance. These areas then become relatively overdistended, and a greater transpulmonary pressure is required to inspire the same volume of air because alveoli in these relatively normal areas are reaching their elastic limit. Thus, a decreased dynamic compliance with increasing frequency of respiration is used as a test of small airway disease and indeed may be the only mechanical abnormality detectable in the early stages of diseases such as emphysema or cystic fibrosis.

CLINICAL EVALUATION OF AIRWAY RESISTANCE. Careful physical examination can usually provide information on both the degree and site of airway obstruction. Exaggerated inspiratory efforts, with little airflow, are the hallmark of upper airway obstruction. In the absence of venoatrial shunts, cyanosis in such a situation is reason for urgent intervention with either an oral airway if the obstruction is nasal, or a tracheostomy if it is laryngeal. Indeed, if carbon dioxide retention is evident by an elevation in Pa_{CO_2}, intervention should take place before the appearance of cyanosis, which signals serious respiratory failure.

A prolonged expiratory phase, with forced expirations, denotes lower airway obstruction. Usually there is some increase in inspiratory effort as well, associated with retractions of the soft tissues. The principal physiologic derangement is in expiration, when airways are normally of smaller caliber. When pleural pressures are raised in an effort to assist expiration, transmural pressure across the airways may result in their closure. Air trapping ensues, evidenced by an increase in chest volume. The assumption of a larger lung volume promotes distention of the airways, and is a regular compensatory device in patients with lower airway obstruction such as bronchiolitis, asthma and emphysema. Although a larger lung volume is appropriate to distend airways, when extreme it requires much larger pressures to achieve effective ventilation, since the lungs and thorax are nearer their elastic limit. It is usual to observe an increase in anteroposterior diameter of the chest in patients with lower airway obstruction,

associated with an obvious increase in the work of breathing.

Simple tests of the degree of airway obstruction have extensive use in cooperative subjects. The one-second forced expiratory volume (FEV_1) is a measure of the percentage of the expiratory vital capacity that can be moved by maximal effort in one second. Children can usually expire more than 90 per cent of the total in one second, adults more than 80 per cent of the total. Reduction in the amounts that can be expired per unit of time reflects either poor cooperation, muscle weakness or lower airway obstruction. A normal inspiratory flow rate and slow expiratory rate are indicative of weak-walled airways or check valves. Some decrease in both flow rates is more common in organic narrowing of the lumens. Flow meters are available for measurement of the peak expiratory flow rate, and have the advantage over the one-second volume in young children of not requiring a sustained effort (Fig. 9).

Since expiratory flow rates are greatly influenced by lung volume, there has been an increased use of expiratory flow-volume curves to evaluate airway resistance. The technique is simple and involves plotting the expired volume during a vital capacity maneuver against flow. Although peak flow and total volume may be nearly normal, in the presence of small airway disease flow is markedly diminished at lower lung volumes. Analysis of these curves yields more information than estimates of FFV, FEV_1, or peak flow rates.

Artificial Respiration

A logical outgrowth of recent advances in understanding the mechanics of respiration is the application of the knowledge to assisted respiration. Perhaps the first practical application of the measurement of volume-pressure relations of lungs and thorax was the change in teaching of artificial respiration. No longer is it admissible to try to maintain ventilation by use of the ex-

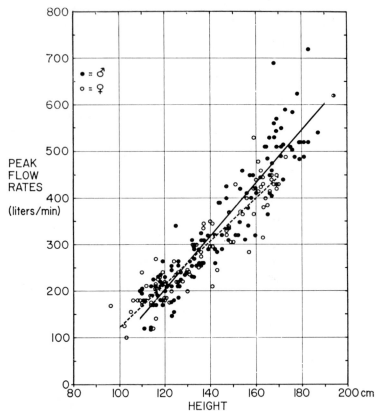

Figure 9. Peak flow rates as a function of body height. The regression lines for boys (————————) and girls (-------------------) are shown. (From Murray, A. B., and Cook, C. D.: *J. Pediatr.*, *62*:186, 1963.)

piratory reserve volume as in the prone back-pressure method of artificial respiration. The pressures applied must be dangerously large to move adequate volumes of air. The inspiratory reserve volume is a more compliant portion of the respiratory system, and is of course the one used in health. Effective assisted breathing requires movement of air into this volume. In the case of the adult with normal lungs, adequate volumes can be moved by tilting as in the rocking bed. The infant, with a shorter abdominal length, cannot be adequately ventilated in this manner.

Active inflation of the lungs can be achieved by a variety of methods, most of which are in everyday use in hospitals. The anesthetist may do it by intubation and the exertion of pressure on a bag of gas which displaces the gas into the chest. The elastic recoil of the distended lungs and thorax raises alveolar pressure, and air is expired through a valve to prevent rebreathing. In the delivery room it is customary to assist the initiation of breathing either with devices that apply positive pressure to a mask over the nose and mouth, or more effectively in the severely distressed infant by intubation, suction of the trachea, and mouth-to-tube or bag-to-tube application of positive pressure. For patients who require long-term assisted respiration, a variety of respirators are available, some delivering positive pressure to the trachea, others achieving lung expansion by lowering the pressure around the body with respect to that at the nose and mouth. An important consideration in long-term assisted breathing is the ability to give an occasional deep breath to overcome the tendency toward atelectasis with fixed tidal volumes.

PRINCIPLES OF ARTIFICIAL RESPIRATION. Movement of air into the lungs requires that the pressure at the mouth be greater than that in the alveoli. Movement of air from the lungs is passive, since at the beginning of expiration alveolar pressure will exceed mouth pressure. Normally, the pressure differences between mouth and alveoli are 4 to 8 cm. of water in adults, probably about 2 to 6 cm. in infants, after the initiation of respiration. Since the movement of air depends only on a pressure difference between two regions, it will be the same regardless of whether the pressure is raised at one point or lowered at another. From the aspect of lung distention, the effect of positive pressure at the mouth is identical with that of negative pressure around the body. The only circumstance in which the effects on the lung could be different is in the event of an air-containing space, such as a cyst or pneumothorax, temporarily not in communication with the airway. With negative pressure around the chest, its volume would temporarily increase; with positive pressure at the mouth, its volume would tend to decrease. This single exception is so unusual, however, that the principle can be emphasized that the effects on airways and alveoli are identical with either positive pressure at the mouth or negative pressure around the body.

The effects of the two kinds of assisted respiration on the circulation are the same, but they differ significantly from the circulatory effects of normal breathing. In normal breathing the decrease in pressure in the thorax, and thus around the heart and great vessels, facilitates return of blood from systemic veins. In positive-pressure breathing, venous return tends to be impeded. Likewise, in body respirators the usual inspiratory augmentation of venous return via the inferior vena cava is not present, since the systemic vessels are also exposed to negative

pressure. However, venous return from the head will continue to be enhanced during inspiration. When the lungs are normal, the applied pressures required to produce a normal tidal volume by either method are not sufficiently great to cause circulatory embarrassment. When the lungs are diseased, and high pressures are required to move air, venous return is reduced, cardiac output falls, and pulmonary blood flow is decreased. Patients in circulatory collapse, as after barbiturate poisoning, patients in shock, and sometimes infants with severe respiratory distress may not tolerate artificial respiration without appropriate circulatory support.

The adverse circulatory effects can be reduced if the time of applied pressure is short, less than 50 per cent of the respiratory cycle, and mask pressures during expiration are atmospheric so that the average increase in intrathoracic pressure is minimal.

On the other hand, recent experience with artificial ventilation in conditions associated with reduced lung compliance and a tendency to develop atelectasis, such as hyaline membrane disease and the "shock lung" syndrome in adults, indicates that the intermittent sigh is inadequate to keep air spaces open. The use of a positive end-expiratory pressure of 5 to 8 cm. H_2O prevents airway closure and enhances gas exchange, particularly oxygenation of blood, without any deleterious effects on the circulation. This suggests that in conditions with a decreased lung compliance, pleural pressure is not influenced by airway pressure to the same extent it is in the normal lung. Indeed, in hyaline membrane disease it has been possible to avoid artificial respirators by maintaining a continuous positive transpulmonary pressure of 5 to 15 cm. H_2O either by a positive pressure at the mouth or a negative pressure around the chest wall. The infant is able to breathe spontaneously, but airway closure at end-expiration is prevented and oxygenation is markedly improved.

APPARATUS. Several types of respirators have been designed that overcome most of the problems of artificial ventilation of infants and children. It is imperative that the dead space of the equipment not be excessive. Since the anatomic dead space of a patient is approximately equal in milliliters to body weight in pounds, a mask or tubing of 6 to 8 ml. in an infant will be equivalent to one of 150 ml. in an adult, and significant rebreathing may occur. Either a circle arrangement for the flow of air past an orifice or suitably miniaturized valves can overcome the equipment dead space problem.

Control of the amount of air delivered can be on the basis of a predetermined volume, pre-set pressure limit, or time and flow control. Any one of the three can be effective if the sensitivity of the adjustments is adequate to make the small changes that may be necessary in an infant whose tidal volume is 10 to 20 ml. Usually the volume adjustments depend on a degree of trial and error. Observation of the degree of excursion of the chest wall, the presence of breath sounds bilaterally, and the general response of the infant permit the first estimate of efficacy. Thereafter the only adequate way to evaluate the respirator is to measure the partial pressure of carbon dioxide in arterial or arterialized capillary blood. Hyperventilation is indicated by a low carbon dioxide tension, which can be dangerous at levels under 25 mm. of mercury because of both the associated alkalosis and the decrease in cerebral blood flow. Hypoventilation is indicated by an elevated carbon dioxide tension. Over 50 mm. of mercury, the concomitant acidosis and (at higher levels) cerebral depression are dangerous.

A potentially useful feature available in both positive and negative pressure respirators is a sensing device to permit an infant or child to cycle the respirator. With each inspiratory effort he gets an assist. In the event of apnea, automatic timers trigger the respirator.

Another requirement of a respirator, especially in the young infant, is that it not be so cumbersome that it precludes other supportive and monitoring procedures, and that it can be attached to an infant in an incubator, or be itself an integral part of an incubator. The maintenance of environmental temperature sufficient to keep the infant at a normal body temperature without the expenditure of calories for added metabolism is essential in distressed infants. A thermal stress further increases oxygen consumption, and hence ventilatory requirements.

The actual setting of the controls of a respirator cannot be prescribed for all circumstances. The first consideration is whether the need for assisted breathing is due to central respiratory failure or muscle weakness with reasonably normal lungs, or whether pulmonary disease underlies the need. With normal lungs, low pressures are adequate. The actual pressure setting depends on where the pressure is measured. If the manometer is far upstream from the mouth, there will be some flow resistance in the tubing, and 10 to 20 cm. of water may be appropriate. If the pressure sensing device is near the mouth, about 10 cm. of water may be suitable. If a patient has diseased lungs, much higher pressures are appropriate, up to 40 cm. at the mouth. If the respirator is adjusted by a volume control, the setting depends on the size of possible leaks. A loose-fitting endotracheal tube allows some advantage in that it effectively lessens the dead space, but the volume setting will have to allow for a variable leak, and may need repeated adjustments. When the inspiratory flow rate and time are pre-set, the pressures and volumes are dependent variables.

With pressure-limited respirators, any change in dynamic compliance, such as that which occurs with accumulation of secretions in airways, will cause a decrease in tidal volume. Thus, positive pressure respirators have the advantage that lung rupture is less likely to occur but the disadvantage that alveolar ventilation may decrease without any change in respirator settings.

In contrast, volume-limited respirators continue to deliver a pre-set tidal volume even though compliance decreases. Pressure increases and may be enough to rupture the lung. However, careful mointoring of inspiratory pressures will indicate to the nurse that compliance has changed, and the simple maneuver of suctioning the endotracheal tube may be all that is necessary to correct the problem. It is beyond the scope of this chapter to review the particular advantages and disadvantages of various types of commercially available respirators used for infants and children. It is quite clear that an awareness of the limitations of a particular respirator and a familiarity with its use are the most important considerations.

ALVEOLAR VENTILATION

The preceding sections have been devoted to the problems of lung growth, volumes, and the mechanical aspects of moving air. Clearly, the purpose of the lung is for gas exchange, i.e., the introduction of oxygen and removal of carbon dioxide from the blood that perfuses it. This section and the following ones focus on the fate of air once introduced into the lung, and aspects of gas transport and tissue respiration.

In Figure 10 the partial pressures of oxygen, carbon dioxide and nitrogen are depicted at various stages of the pathway from ambient air to the tissues. Since nitrogen is inert, changes in its partial pressure in the gas phase depend on changes in the partial pressures of oxygen and carbon dioxide, gases that are utilized and excreted, respectively. In contrast, P_{N_2} in blood and tissue is identical because nitrogen is inert. The rather complex influences of dead space, alveolar ventilation, ventilation-perfusion relationships and tissue metabolism on the partial pressures of oxygen and carbon dioxide will be discussed in some detail, and frequent reference to Figure 10 will be useful in clarifying some of the concepts.

Dead Space

A portion of each inspired breath remains in the conducting airways (consisting of the nose, mouth, pharynx, larynx, trachea, bronchi and bronchioles) where no significant exchange of oxygen and carbon dioxide with blood takes place. The volume of the conducting airways is called the anatomic dead space (V_D anat), and is filled by about 25 per cent of each tidal volume. The remainder of each tidal volume goes to the alveoli, where rapid exchange of oxygen and carbon dioxide occurs, and the proportion of ventilation that undergoes gas exchange is known as the alveolar ventilation (V_A). When some alveoli are relatively underperfused with blood, as in some disease states, a proportion of alveolar air does not undergo gas exchange, but acts as if it were in a dead space. It is called the alveolar dead space (V_D alv). Thus:

$$V_T \text{ (tidal volume)} = V_D \text{ anat} + V_D \text{ alv} + V_A$$

V_D anat + V_D alv is called the physiologic dead space.

In health, anatomic dead space and physiologic dead space are nearly identical, since the distribution of air and blood in alveoli is nearly uniform. Anatomic dead space in milliliters is roughly equal to the weight of the subject in pounds (for a 7-pound baby, 7 or 8 ml.; for an adult, 150 ml.) and is normally less than 30 per cent of V_T. In the normal premature infant, anatomic dead space is slightly higher than 30 per cent, and physiologic dead space may be over 40 per cent. In the infant with respiratory distress, physiologic dead space may be more than 70 per cent of the tidal volume.

Anatomic dead space may be measured by making use of the following argument originally developed by Bohr:

Volume CO_2 expired per breath = volume CO_2 in the dead space + volume CO_2 in the alveoli

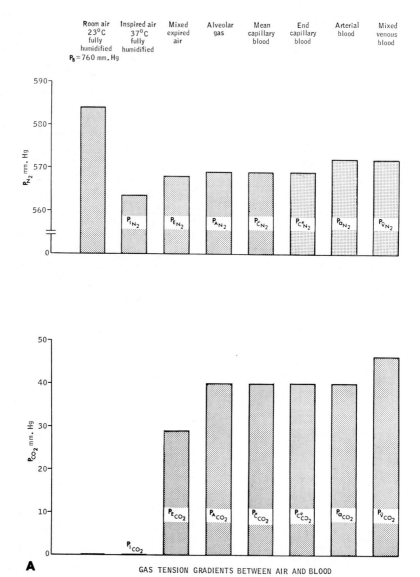

Figure 10. Partial pressures of nitrogen and carbon dioxide at different portions of the airway and blood.

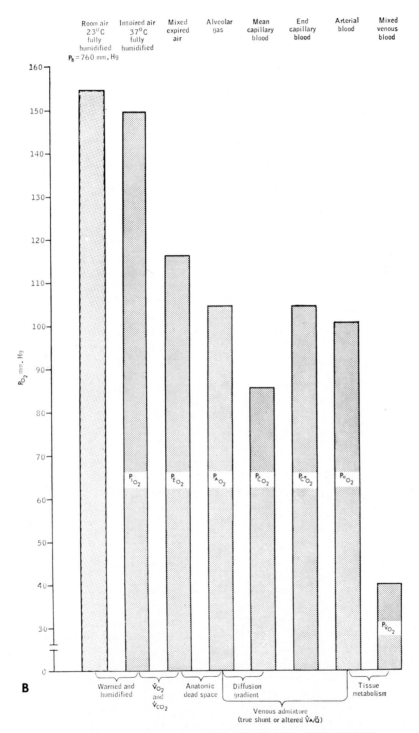

PARTIAL PRESSURE OF OXYGEN AT DIFFERENT PORTIONS OF THE AIRWAY AND BLOOD

Figure 10. *Continued.*

The volume of carbon dioxide is equal to the volume of a compartment times the fractional concentration of carbon dioxide. Thus:

$$F_{E_{CO_2}} V_E = F_{D_{CO_2}} V_D + F_{A_{CO_2}} V_A$$

Since the dead space at end-inspiration is filled with air containing no significant amount of carbon dioxide,

$$F_{D_{CO_2}} V_D = 0;$$

and since $V_A = V_E - V_D$,

$$F_{E_{CO_2}} V_E = F_{A_{CO_2}} (V_E - V_D),$$

$$F_{A_{CO_2}} V_D = (F_{A_{CO_2}} - F_{E_{CO_2}}) V_E, \text{ and}$$

$$V_{D_{anat}} = \frac{(F_{A_{CO_2}} - F_{E_{CO_2}}) V_E}{F_{A_{CO_2}}} \quad \begin{array}{l}\text{(anatomic}\\\text{dead space).}\end{array}$$

Since

$$P_{A_{CO_2}} = F_{A_{CO_2}} \times (P_b - 47)$$

and

$$P_{A_{CO_2}} = Pa_{CO_2}$$

$$V_{D_{phys}} = \left(\frac{Pa_{CO_2} - P_{E_{CO_2}}}{Pa_{CO_2}}\right) V_E \quad \begin{array}{l}\text{(physiologic}\\\text{dead space).}\end{array}$$

The concentration of carbon dioxide in the alveolus ($F_{A_{CO_2}}$) can be measured from an end-tidal sample, which represents the average alveolar carbon dioxide concentration. V_E is measured by collecting expired gases, and $F_{E_{CO_2}}$ can be measured on an aliquot of mixed expired air. The amount of dilution of $F_{A_{CO_2}}$ is proportional to the size of the dead space; the larger it is, the lower is $F_{E_{CO_2}}$. For physiologic dead space, the partial pressure of carbon dioxide in arterial blood is used instead of the end-expired sample. A discrepancy in the two determinations, using end-tidal versus arterial blood, implies the presence of portions of the lung that are ventilated and not perfused. That is, $P_{A_{CO_2}}$ is diluted by alveolar dead space and is therefore lower than Pa_{CO_2}.

Another method of measuring the anatomic dead space, Fowler's method, requires that a single breath of oxygen be inspired. On expiration, both the volume of expired gas and percentage of nitrogen are measured. The first portion of the expired gas comes from the dead space and contains little or no nitrogen. As the breath is expired, the percentage of nitrogen increases until it "plateaus" at the alveolar concentration. By assuming that all the initial part of the breath comes from the anatomic dead space and all the latter portion from the alveoli, the anatomic dead space can be calculated. The same measurements can be made by monitoring the expired carbon dioxide concentration.

In practice anatomic dead space is difficult to define accurately, since it depends on lung volume (greater at large lung volumes when the airways are more distended) and on body position (being smaller when supine). It is now quite clear that $V_{D_{phys}}$ must be defined according to the gas being measured. Since oxygen is more diffusible in the gas phase than is carbon dioxide, physiologic dead space using oxygen or various inert gases is different from the CO_2 dead space. However, $V_{D_{phys}}$ measurements using CO_2 are in common use in pulmonary function laboratories and are helpful in assessing patients because they do reflect the portion of each breath that participates in gas exchange, particularly with respect to CO_2.

From the foregoing discussion it is apparent that a tidal volume must be chosen that will allow adequate alveolar ventilation. For example, an adult might breathe 60 times a minute with a tidal volume of 100 ml. for a minute ventilation of 6 liters. Nevertheless alveolar ventilation under these circumstances is zero, since only the dead space is ventilated. When selecting suitable volumes and rates for patients on respirators, it is useful to approximate normal values, and consider adequate alveolar ventilation rather than total ventilation.

Alveolar Gases

The amount of alveolar ventilation per minute must be adequate to keep the alveolar P_{O_2} and P_{CO_2} at values that will promote the escape of carbon dioxide from the venous blood and the uptake of oxygen by venous blood. In health this means that $P_{A_{O_2}}$ is approximately 105 to 110 mm. and $P_{A_{CO_2}}$ 40 mm. Hg (Fig. 11).

Since inspired air is "diluted" in the alveoli by the functional residual capacity of air containing carbon dioxide and water vapor, the partial pressure of ox-

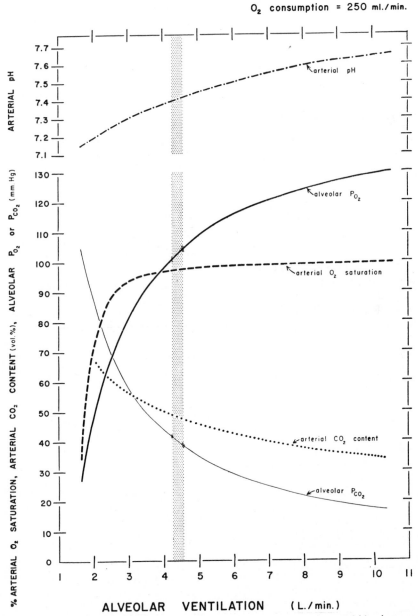

Figure 11. The effect of changing alveolar ventilation on alveolar gas and arterial blood oxygen, carbon dioxide and pH. (From Comroe, J. H., and others: *The Lung*. 2nd Ed. Chicago, Year Book Medical Publishers, Inc., 1962.)

ygen in alveolar gas must be less than that of the inspired air (see Dalton's Law, p. 4). $P_{A_{O_2}}$ may be calculated from the alveolar air equation. When oxygen consumption equals carbon dioxide production, then:

$$P_{A_{O_2}} = P_{I_{O_2}} - P_{A_{CO_2}}$$

$$P_{I_{O_2}} = 0.2093 \times (P_b - 47 \text{ mm. Hg}) = 150 \text{ mm. Hg}$$

If $P_{A_{CO_2}}$ is 40 mm. of mercury, then $P_{A_{O_2}}$ is 110 mm. Usually R is 0.8, or more oxygen is consumed than carbon dioxide eliminated, thereby decreasing $P_{A_{O_2}}$ slightly more than would be expected from the dilution of $P_{A_{CO_2}}$. To account for changes in R, a useful form of the alveolar air equation for clinical purposes is:

$$P_{A_{O_2}} = P_{I_{O_2}} - \frac{P_{A_{CO_2}}}{R}$$

When $P_{A_{CO_2}}$ is 40 and R is 0.8, $P_{A_{O_2}}$ is 99 mm. of mercury. Note that 40 per cent oxygen raises $P_{A_{O_2}}$ to 235 mm.

Since the partial pressures of alveolar gases must always equal the same total pressure, any increase in one must be associated with a decrease in the other. For example, if Pa_{CO_2} is 80 mm. Hg and the patient is breathing room air, assuming an R of 0.8, the highest $P_{A_{O_2}}$ can be is 50 mm. Hg.

Arterial P_{O_2} is markedly affected by the presence of right-to-left vascular shunts and therefore it is not a good measurement of the adequacy of pulmonary ventilation. Pa_{CO_2} is minimally affected in the presence of shunts because $P\bar{v}_{CO_2}$ is 46 mm. and Pa_{CO_2} is 40 mm. of mercury. If one third of the cardiac output is shunted, this raises Pa_{CO_2} to only 42 mm. of mercury. Thus the arterial P_{CO_2} is the optimum measurement of the adequacy of alveolar ventilation. When alveolar ventilation halves, Pa_{CO_2} doubles; when alveolar ventilation doubles, then Pa_{CO_2} halves. Hyperventilation is defined as a Pa_{CO_2} less than 35 mm. Hg, hypoventilation as a Pa_{CO_2}

TABLE 3. ILLUSTRATIVE CAUSES OF HYPOVENTILATION

Respiratory Center Depression
General anesthesia; excessive doses of drugs such as morphine, barbiturates or codeine; severe or prolonged hypoxia, cerebral ischemia, high concentrations of CO_2; electrocution; cerebral trauma; increased intracranial pressure

Conditions Affecting the Airways and Lung
UPPER OR LOWER AIRWAY OBSTRUCTION
Foreign body, large tonsils and adenoids, vocal cord paralysis, croup, endobronchial tuberculosis, chronic bronchitis, emphysema, asthma, bronchiectasis, cystic fibrosis, bronchiolitis
DECREASED LUNG COMPLIANCE
Vascular diseases such as emboli, polyarteritis, mitral stenosis; parasitic infiltrations; interstitial disease such as sarcoid, Hamman-Rich syndrome, pneumoconioses, lupus, rheumatoid arthritis, berylliosis, histicytosis X, radiation fibrosis, idiopathic pulmonary hemosiderosis
EXTENSIVE LOSS OF FUNCTIONING LUNG TISSUE
Atelectasis, tumor, pneumonia, cystic fibrosis, surgical resection
LIMITATION OF MOVEMENT OF LUNGS
Pleural effusion, pneumothorax, fibrothorax

Conditions Affecting the Thorax
DECREASED CHEST WALL COMPLIANCE
Arthritis, scleroderma, kyphoscoliosis, fractured ribs, thoracoplasty, thoracotomy, pickwickian syndrome, phrenic nerve paralysis
DISEASES OF RESPIRATORY MUSCLES
E.g., muscular dystrophy
PARALYSIS OF RESPIRATORY MUSCLES
Poliomyelitis, peripheral neuritis, spinal cord injury, myasthenia gravis; curare, succinylcholine botulinus and nicotine poisonings

greater than 45 mm. Hg. Some of the causes of hypoventilation are listed in Table 3.

DIFFUSION

Principles

The barriers through which a gas must travel when diffusing from the alveolus to the blood include the alveolar epithelial lining, basement membrane, capillary endothelial lining, plasma and the red blood cell. As observed on electron micrographs of lung tissue, the thinnest part of the barrier is 0.2 micron, but may be as much as three times this distance.

Fick's Law of diffusion modified for gases states:

$$Q/min. = \frac{K \ S \ (P_1 - P_2)}{d}$$

The amount of gas (Q) diffusing through a membrane is directly proportional to the surface area available for diffusion (S), the pressure difference of the two gases on either side of the membrane, and a constant (K) that depends on the solubility coefficient of the gas and the characteristics of the particular membrane and liquid used; and inversely proportional to the distance (d) through which the gas has to diffuse. In the lung of a given subject, exact values for K, S and d are unknown. Therefore, for the lung, Bohr and Krogh suggested the term "diffusion capacity" (D_L). For oxygen:

$$D_{L_{O_2}} \text{ (ml./min./mm. Hg)} = \frac{V_{O_2}}{P_{A_{O_2}} - P\bar{c}_{O_2}}$$

where $P_{A_{O_2}}$ is the alveolar oxygen tension and $P\bar{c}_{O_2}$ is the average capillary oxygen tension. Therefore, the denominator represents the average "driving" pressure for oxygen across the alveolar-capillary pathway.

Carbon dioxide diffuses nearly 21 times faster than oxygen in a gas-liquid system. Therefore, for all practical purposes, there is never any impairment of diffusion for carbon dioxide from the blood to the alveolus.

Measurement

For the measurement of the diffusing capacity of oxygen in the lung, oxygen uptake and the alveolar oxygen tension are easily determined. The average capillary oxygen tension $(P\bar{c}_{O_2})$ is difficult to assess, however, since we cannot measure it directly. $P\bar{c}_{O_2}$ will vary according to $P\bar{v}_{O_2}$, the diffusing capacity and the time available for diffusion to take place (mean transit time of a red blood cell through a lung capil-

lary has been estimated at rest to be 0.75 second). With a measurement of $P_{A_{O_2}}$ and a knowledge of the transit time through the pulmonary capillary, a special technique called the Bohr integration procedure can be used to determine $P\bar{c}_{O_2}$. We can easily measure the arterial P_{O_2}, but it is influenced by both the diffusing capacity and the amount of right-to-left shunt present. When low concentrations of oxygen are inspired (12 to 14 per cent), the effect of a right-to-left shunt on arterial P_{O_2} is minimal because of the shape of the oxyhemoglobin dissociation curve, and any difference between $P_{A_{O_2}}$ and $P_{a_{O_2}}$ is assumed to be related to a diffusion defect (see Transport of Oxygen). When breathing low concentrations of oxygen, therefore, $P_{a_{O_2}}$ is considered to be identical with the P_{O_2} at the end of the pulmonary capillary after gas exchange has taken place. It is now possible to calculate $P\bar{c}_{O_2}$ using the Bohr integration technique and $P_{A_{O_2}} - P\bar{c}_{O_2}$. This driving pressure is considered to be identical with that while breathing room air, and $D_{L_{O_2}}$ is calculated by dividing the oxygen consumption measured during room air breathing by this driving pressure. Although this method has been extensively used in adults, it has not been used widely in children.

Carbon monoxide (CO), however, has been used extensively in children to test diffusing capacity. The advantage of using carbon monoxide is due to its remarkable affinity for hemoglobin, some 210 times that of oxygen, and therefore the capillary P_{CO} is negligible and offers no back pressure for diffusion. Many different techniques have been used, but the differences between them will not be discussed here.

In order to calculate $D_{L_{CO}}$, one need only know the amount of carbon monoxide taken up per minute and $P_{A_{CO}}$. $D_{L_{CO}}$ is linearly related to lung growth and has been found to be closely correlated with height or total lung capacity.

The reaction rate between hemoglobin and carbon monoxide is affected by the level of alveolar P_{O_2}; if high, this

slows down the formation of carbon
monoxide hemoblogin; if low, then carbon monoxide and hemoglobin combine more rapidly. If one performs the
test at two levels of $P_{A_{O_2}}$, it is possible
to separate the $D_{L_{CO}}$ into two components, the membrane diffusing capacity
and the red blood cell component. For
both children and adults, approximately half of the resistance to diffusion of carbon monoxide resides in the
alveolar membrane and half in the red
blood cell.

Clinically, a reduction in diffusing capacity may be due to an increased
thickness of the alveolar-capillary membrane, as seen with interstitial pulmonary fibrosis, sarcoid, pneumoconioses,
scleroderma, pulmonary edema or pulmonary hemosiderosis. A reduction in
the surface area available for diffusion
will reduce the diffusion capacity, as
found in patients after lobectomy, or
with emphysema when alveolar walls
are destroyed. Patients with cystic fibrosis may have much of the lung unavailable for gas exchange and, therefore, a reduced diffusing capacity.

It is important to point out that an
impaired diffusion of oxygen from the
alveolar air to the pulmonary capillary
is rarely the cause of a low Pa_{O_2}. Hypoxemia in pulmonary disease usually
results from alveolar hypoventilation or
impaired relationship between ventilation and perfusion in the lung; this
relationship is discussed later in this
chapter. With the possible exception of
the two-level oxygen and carbon monoxide tests described previously, most
techniques for the measurement of diffusing capacity merely reflect these abnormalities in gas exhange rather than
a true diffusion defect.

TRANSPORT OF OXYGEN

Dissolved Oxygen and Oxyhemoglobin

Once oxygen molecules have passed
from the alveolus into the pulmonary

capillary, they are transported in the
blood in two ways. A small proportion
of the oxygen exists as dissolved oxygen in the plasma and water of the
red blood cell. For 100 ml. of whole
blood equilibrated with a P_{O_2} of 100
mm. of mercury, 0.3 ml. of oxygen is
present as dissolved oxygen. If this
represented the total oxygen-carrying
capacity of blood, then cardiac output
would have to be greater than 80 liters
per minute in order to allow 250 ml. of
oxygen to be consumed per minute.
During 100 per cent oxygen breathing,
Pa_{O_2} is approximately 650 mm. of mercury and 100 ml. of blood contains 2.0
ml. of oxygen, and would require a cardiac output of about 12 liters per minute if no hemoglobin were present.

Since 1 gm. of hemoglobin can combine with 1.34 ml. of oxygen, between
40 and 70 times more oxygen is carried
by hemoglobin than by the plasma and
enables the body to achieve a cardiac
output at rest of 5.5 liters per minute
with an oxygen uptake of 250 ml. per
minute.

The potential usefulness of hyperbaric oxygen (i.e., oxygen under very
high pressures) for a variety of clinical
conditions is due to the fact that at a
pressure of 3 atmospheres (absolute)
($P_{A_{O_2}}$ about 1950 mm. of mercury),
approximately 6.0 ml. of oxygen is dissolved in 100 ml. of whole blood, and
this amount can meet the metabolic demands of the tissues under resting
conditions even when no hemoglobin is
present.

The remarkable oxygen-carrying
properties of blood depend not on the
solubility of oxygen in plasma, but on
the unusual properties of hemoglobin.
Figure 12 illustrates the oxyhemoglobin
dissociation curve, showing that hemoglobin is nearly 95 per cent saturated at
a P_{O_2} of 80 mm. of mercury. The steep
portion of the curve, up to about 50
mm., permits large amounts of oxygen
to be released from hemoglobin with
small changes in P_{O_2}. Under normal
circumstances, 100 per cent oxygen
breathing will raise the amount of oxygen carried by the blood by only a

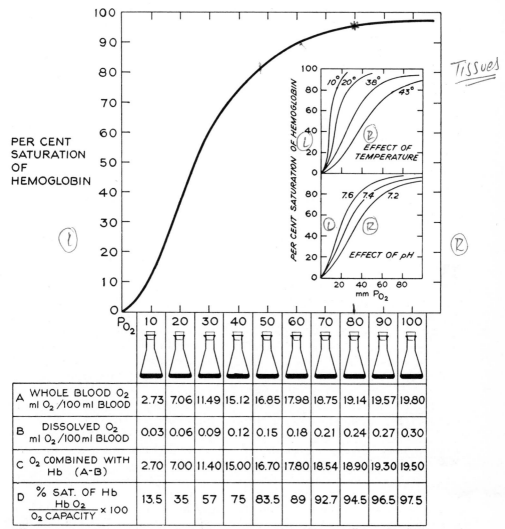

	Pₒ₂	10	20	30	40	50	60	70	80	90	100
A	WHOLE BLOOD O₂ ml O₂/100 ml BLOOD	2.73	7.06	11.49	15.12	16.85	17.98	18.75	19.14	19.57	19.80
B	DISSOLVED O₂ ml O₂/100 ml BLOOD	0.03	0.06	0.09	0.12	0.15	0.18	0.21	0.24	0.27	0.30
C	O₂ COMBINED WITH Hb (A-B)	2.70	7.00	11.40	15.00	16.70	17.80	18.54	18.90	19.30	19.50
D	% SAT. OF Hb $\frac{Hb\,O_2}{O_2\,CAPACITY} \times 100$	13.5	35	57	75	83.5	89	92.7	94.5	96.5	97.5

Figure 12. Oxyhemoglobin dissociation curves. The large graph shows a single dissociation curve, applicable when the pH of the blood is 7.40 and temperature is 38°C. The blood oxygen tension and saturation of patients with carbon dioxide retention, acidosis, alkalosis, fever or hypothermia will not fit this curve because it shifts to the right or left when temperature, pH or P_{CO_2} is changed. Effects on the oxyhemoglobin dissociation curve of change in temperature *(upper right)* and in pH *(lower right)* are shown in the smaller graphs. A small change in blood pH occurs regularly in the body; e.g., when mixed venous blood passes through the pulmonary capillaries, P_{CO_2} decreases from 46 to 40 mm. of mercury, and pH rises from 7.37 to 7.40. During this time, blood changes from a pH of 7.37 dissociation curve to a pH of 7.40 curve. (From Comroe, J. H.: *Physiology of Respiration.* Chicago, Year Book Medical Publishers, Inc., 1965.)

small amount, since at a P_{O_2} of 100 mm. of mercury, hemoglobin is already 97.5 percent saturated. Even with air breathing one is on the flat portion of the curve. The presence of a right-to-left shunt markedly affects P_{O_2}, but may reduce the percentage saturation only minimally. For example, a 50

per cent shunt with venous blood containing 15 ml. of oxygen per 100 ml. will only reduce the oxygen content of 100 ml. of blood from 20 ml. to 17.5 ml. The blood is still 88 per cent saturated, but Pa_{O_2} is now 60 mm. instead of 100 mm. of mercury. Thus, the change in oxygen content is linearly related to the amount of right-to-left shunt, but the change in P_{O_2} is not because of the S-shaped hemoglobin-oxygen curve. It is also apparent that at levels greater than 60 mm. Hg, Pa_{O_2} is a more sensitive measure of blood oxygenation because neither percentage saturation nor oxygen content changes as much as P_{O_2} in this range. However, below about 60 mm. Hg P_{O_2}, relatively small changes in P_{O_2} produce large changes in saturation and content, and in this range the measurement of content may be more reliable than the measurement of P_{O_2}.

The oxyhemoglobin dissociation curve is affected by changes in pH, P_{CO_2} and temperature. A decrease in pH, increase in P_{CO_2} (Bohr effect) or an increase in temperature shifts the curve to the right, particularly in the 20- to 50-mm. of mercury range. Thus, for a given P_{O_2} the saturation percentage is less under acidotic or hyperpyrexic conditions. In the tissues, carbon dioxide is added to the blood, and this facilitates the removal of oxygen from the red blood cell. In the pulmonary capillaries, carbon dioxide diffuses out of the blood, facilitating oxygen uptake by hemoglobin. An increased temperature has a similar effect to an increase in P_{CO_2} and thus facilitates oxygen removal from the blood by the tissues. Note that a patient who is pyrexic with carbon dioxide retention could not have a normal oxygen saturation during air breathing because of the Bohr and temperature effects on the oxyhemoglobin dissociation curve.

The fetal hemoglobin dissociation curve is shifted to the left of the adult curve at a similar pH. Thus, at a given P_{O_2}, fetal blood contains more oxygen than adult hemoglobin. This property ensures that an adequate amount of oxygen will get to fetal tissues, since the fetus in utero has a Pa_{O_2} about 30 mm. of mercury. The affinity of fetal hemoglobin for oxygen is not a result of the structure of hemoglobin, but depends on an intact fetal red blood cell membrane, for free fetal hemoglobin in solution has the same oxygen-carrying capacity as adult hemoglobin. Fetal hemoglobin disappears from the circulation shortly after birth, and by a few months of age less than 2 per cent is present. Normal fetal development is not dependent on differences in maternal and fetal hemoglobins, since in some species they are identical.

Recent evidence has indicated a role of the erythrocyte concentration of D-2,3-diphosphoglycerate (DPG) in accounting for shifts in oxyhemoglobin dissociation curves. DPG and hemoglobin are present in about equimolar concentrations in adult human red cells. There is strong binding between DPG and deoxyhemoglobin, and this complex is highly resistant to oxygenation. Shifts of the dissociation curve to the right associated with an increased DPG concentration—for example, in anemia—facilitates the release of oxygen to the tissues. Since erythrocyte DPG concentration can change within a matter of hours, a regulatory role for DPG in maintaining optimal tissue oxygenation has been suggested. Studies in fetal and adult human red cells do not indicate a difference in DPG concentration, but DPG binds less well to hemoglobin F and likely has much less influence on oxygen binding.

Abnormal hemoglobins differ in their oxygen-carrying capacity. Hemoglobin S has a curve shifted to the right, so that at 100 mm. of mercury P_{O_2} it is only 80 per cent saturated. It is insoluble when deoxygenated, and at low P_{O_2} crystallizes within the erythrocyte. This produces the well known "sickle" cell shape of the cell in this disorder. Hemoglobin H, with 12 times the affinity for oxygen as hemoglobin A, does not release oxygen readily to the tissues. Hemoglobin M is oxidized by oxygen to methemoglobin, which does not release oxygen to the tissues; a large amount is incompatible with life. The formation of methemoglobin by agents such as nitrates, aniline, sulfonamides, acetanilid, phenylhydrazine or primaquine may also be life-threatening. Congenital deficiency of an enzyme, hemoglobin reductase, is also associated with large amounts of methemoglobin, and these patients are cyanotic in room air. Sulfhemoglobin is, likewise, unable to transport oxygen.

Since carbon monoxide has 210 times more affinity for hemoglobin than oxygen, it is important to note that P_{O_2} may be normal in carbon monoxide poisoning, while oxygen content is markedly reduced.

Thus, a variety of factors may affect the position of the oxyhemoglobin dissociation curve. The position of the curve may be described by measuring the P_{O_2} at which there is 50 per cent saturation, the so-called P_{50}. In situations where the curve is shifted to the left, the P_{50} will be low; if shifted to the right, P_{50} will be elevated.

Cyanosis

The degree of visible cyanosis depends on the amount of unsaturated hemoglobin present in the blood perfusing superficial vessels. In polycythemia adequate amounts of oxygen may be present, but the patient appears cyanotic because not all his hemoglobin is saturated. Conversely, in anemia, a patient may be hypoxic, but not appear cyanotic. The clinical assessment of oxygenation is hazardous in part because a poor peripheral circulation may result in peripheral cyanosis when the arterial blood is well oxygenated. Thus, the most reliable estimate of the oxygen content of arterial blood involves direct measurement, since both hypoxemia and hyperoxemia cannot be reliably assessed by clinical observation.

OXYGEN THERAPY

Increased Inspired Mixtures

Increased inspired mixtures of oxygen are required when tissue oxygenation is inadequate. The response to increased inspired oxygen depends on which cause of hypoxia is present (Table 4). Most of the conditions characterized by hypoxemia respond well to added oxygen. Patients with venoatrial

TABLE 4. FOUR TYPES OF HYPOXIA AND SOME CAUSES

(1) **Hypoxemia (low P_{O_2} and low oxygen content)**
Deficiency of oxygen in the atmosphere
Hypoventilation (see Table 3)
Uneven distribution of alveolar gas and/or pulmonary blood flow
Diffusion impairment
Venous to arterial shunt

(2) **Deficient Hemoglobin (normal P_{O_2} and low oxygen content)**
Anemia
Carbon monoxide poisoning

(3) **Ischemic Hypoxia (normal P_{O_2} and oxygen content)**
General or localized circulatory insufficiency
Tissue edema
Abnormal tissue demands

(4) **Histotoxic Anoxia (normal P_{O_2} and oxygen content)**
Poisoning of cellular enzymes so that they cannot use the available oxygen (e.g., cyanide poisoning)

shunts will respond less well, since the shunted blood does not perfuse alveoli. Even so, tissue oxygenation may be improved by the addition of oxygen to the blood, which does undergo gas exchange in the lung. A direct attack on the underlying disorder in anemia, ischemia and poisonings is clearly indicated; oxygen therapy may be lifesaving during the time required to treat the disease.

Oxygen therapy can be utilized to facilitate the removal of other gases loculated in body spaces, such as air in pneumothorax, pneumomediastinum and ileus. High inspired oxygen mixtures effectively wash out body stores of nitrogen. With air breathing, the blood that perfuses the tissue spaces has an arterial oxygen tension of 100 mm. of mercury and a venous tension of 40 mm. With oxygen breathing, although arterial tensions rise to 600 mm. of mercury, venous oxygen tensions do not rise above 50 to 60 mm. because of oxygen consumption and the shape of the dissociation curve. With air breathing, arterial and venous nitrogen tensions are the same, about 570 mm. of mercury. If the loculated gas were air at atmospheric pressure, the gradient for the movement of nitrogen to the blood would be very small. After nitrogen washout, with oxygen breathing, the lack of high elevation in venous oxygen tension permits movement of both nitrogen and oxygen into the blood. The increased pressure differences increase the rate of absorption of loculated air some fivefold to tenfold.

Hazards of High Oxygen Mixtures

Hypoxemia in conditions associated with hypoventilation, such as chronic pulmonary disease and status asthmaticus, may be overcome by enriched oxygen mixtures without concomitant lessening of the hypercapnia. The patient may appear pink, but become narcotized under the influence of carbon dioxide retention. In chronic respiratory acidosis, respiration may be maintained chiefly by the hypoxic drive, and correction of the hypoxemia may result in a cessation of respiration. Frequent measurements of arterial gas tensions are invaluable in such patients. Only as much oxygen should be given as is needed to keep the arterial oxygen tension in the range of 40 to 60 mm. of mercury (75 to 90 per cent saturated).

Excessive oxygenation of the blood can be dangerous. Human volunteers in pure oxygen at one atmosphere experience symptoms in about 24 hours, chiefly substernal pain and paresthesias. Some animals, exposed for longer periods, die of pulmonary congestion and edema in four to seven days. The toxicity of oxygen is directly proportional to its partial pressure. Symptoms occur within minutes under hyperbaric conditions, and may not be present after one month in pure oxygen at one third of an atmosphere. Some of the effects of oxygen are to decrease minute ventilation and cardiac output slightly, and constrict retinal and cerebral vessels and the ductus arteriosus. Cerebral vasoconstriction may lead to irrevers-

ible brain damage. Retinal vasoconstriction does not seem to be a significant problem in mature retinas that are richly vascularized. In premature infants, however, the vasoconstriction may lead to ischemia. After the cessation of oxygen therapy, or with maturation of the infant, neovascularization of the retina occurs. The disorderly growth and scarring may cause retinal detachments and fibroplasia, which appears behind the lens; hence, the name "retrolental fibroplasia." This manifestation of oxygen toxicity, restricted to prematurely born infants and some animals, depends on the level of oxygen in the arterial blood that perfuses the retina. High oxygen mixtures in infants with large right-to-left shunts do not put the infant at risk of retrolental fibroplasia unless the arterial oxygen tensions are elevated above normal.

During the past decade there has been considerable experience with the use of high concentrations of oxygen in both adults and newborn infants who require prolonged respirator therapy. The use of concentrations of oxygen above 60 to 70 per cent for more than four or five days is associated with the appearance of a diffuse interstitial fibrosis of the lung and alterations of bronchiolar epithelium known as bronchopulmonary dysplasia. (See Chapter 11.) In both animal studies and in patients there appears to be a wide difference in susceptibility between subjects. Improved methods of oxygenation of the blood enabling a decrease of inspired oxygen concentration to less than 60 per cent are now being introduced in an effort to avoid this complication (see Artificial Respiration).

Pure oxygen breathing predisposes to atelectasis in the presence of any airway obstruction. Just as it facilitates removal of air from loculated spaces as in pneumothorax, so can it facilitate removal of air from alveoli that are not in communication with the airway. The hazard is greater with breathing pure oxygen mixtures at a reduced total pressure, such as the one third of an atmosphere, which is the environment of our space capsules. Absorption of air from the nasal sinuses and middle ear in the event of obstruction may result in painful pressure differences and even hemorrhage.

The mechanism of oxygen's toxic effect on cells is incompletely understood. The oxygen molecule may also exist in a high energy state called superoxide. An enzyme, superoxide dismutase, which catalyzes the formation of hydrogen peroxide, may be extremely important in preventing tissue damage from the superoxide anion. It further has a paramagnetic effect which may affect electron motion of neighboring molecules. Some enzyme systems, such as dehydrogenases in the central nervous system, do not function in hyperoxic environments, a fact which may underlie the occurrence of convulsions.

Hyperbaric Oxygen

All the toxic effects that may be seen in pure oxygen breathing at one atmosphere are exaggerated and occur sooner under hyperbaric conditions. Nevertheless, hyperbaric oxygenation has a role in oxygen therapy of a few disease states such as coronary occlusion and shock, to enhance the effects of radiation in tumor therapy, in the treatment of some infections with anaerobic organisms such as gas gangrene, and in carbon monoxide poisoning. Some advantage has been found in cardiac surgery when the period of cardiac arrest can be prolonged. Effective oxygenation by hyperbaric pressure can be achieved even in the face of severe pulmonary insufficiency as in hyaline membrane disease, although it has not been associated with recovery of the patient in that disease.

The procedure requires a rigid chamber capable of withstanding several atmospheres of pressure, and suitable ports for monitoring equipment. For cardiac surgery it also requires space for a complete operating team. Oxygen toxicity and fire are ever-present hazards.

CARBON DIOXIDE TRANSPORT AND ACID-BASE BALANCE

Buffering and Transport

Acids are normally produced in the body at the rates of 15 to 20 moles of carbonic acid and 80 millimoles of fixed acids per day. For the cells to maintain their normal metabolic activity, the pH of the environment of the cells must be close to 7.40. The understanding of the regulation of hydrogen ion concentration requires knowledge of the buffering action of the chemical constituents of the blood and the role of the lungs and kidney in the excretion of acids from the body.

The constituents that are of most importance for acid-base regulation are the sodium bicarbonate and carbonic acid of the plasma, the potassium bicarbonate and carbonic acid of the cells, and hemoglobin.

The concentration of carbonic acid is determined by the partial pressure of carbon dioxide, and the solubility coefficients of carbon dioxide in plasma and in red cell water. Carbonic acid in aqueous solution dissociates as follows:

$$CO_2 + H_2O \rightleftarrows H_2CO_3$$
$$H_2CO_3 \rightleftarrows H^+ + HCO_3^-$$

The law of mass action describes this reaction:

$$\frac{(H^+)(HCO_3^-)}{(H_2CO_3)} = K$$

In plasma, K has the value of $10^{-6.1}$. Equivalent forms of this equation are

$$pH = pK + \log \frac{(HCO_3^-)}{H_2CO_3}$$

By definition $pH = -\log(H^+)$; $pK = -\log K = 6.1$ for plasma. Applied to plasma, where dissolved carbon dioxide exists at a concentration 1000 times that of carbonic acid, the equation becomes

$$pH = 6.1 + \log \frac{(HCO_3^-)}{0.03 P_{CO_2}}$$

This form of the equation is known as the Henderson-Hasselbalch equation. A clinically useful form of this equation is:

$$\frac{H^+}{\text{(nanomoles/liter)}} = 24 \times \frac{P_{CO_2}}{HCO_3^-}$$

Thus, at a normal bicarbonate concentration of 24 mEq./liter, when Pa_{CO_2} is 40 mm. Hg, hydrogen ion concentration is 40 nanomoles/liter.

Just as oxygen has a highly specialized transport mechanism in the blood in order to ensure an adequate delivery to tissues under physiologic conditions,

carbon dioxide produced by the tissues has a special transport system to carry it in the blood to the lung, where it is expired. The amount of carbon dioxide in blood is related to the P_{CO_2} in a manner shown in Figure 13. Unlike oxygen, the relation between P_{CO_2} and carbon dioxide content is nearly linear, and therefore doubling alveolar ventilation halves Pa_{CO_2}; conversely, halving alveolar ventilation doubles Pa_{CO_2}. Oxygenated hemoglobin shifts the carbon dioxide dissociation curve to the right (Haldane effect), so that at a given

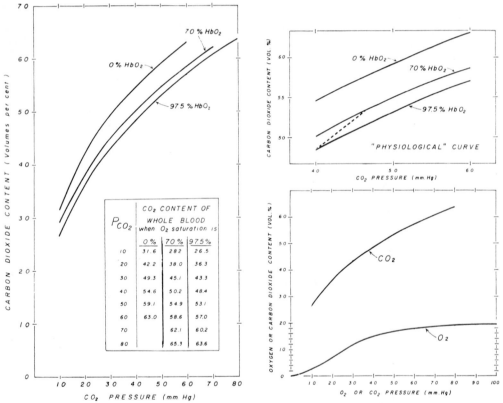

CARBON DIOXIDE DISSOCIATION CURVES FOR WHOLE BLOOD

Figure 13. The carbon dioxide dissociation curve. The large graph shows the relation between P_{CO_2} and carbon dioxide content of whole blood; this varies with changes in saturation of hemoglobin with oxygen. Thus, P_{CO_2} of the blood influences oxygen saturation (Bohr effect), and oxygen saturation of the blood influences carbon dioxide content (Haldane effect). The oxygen–carbon dioxide diagram gives the correct figure for both carbon dioxide and oxygen at every P_{O_2} and P_{CO_2}. *Above, right,* Greatly magnified portion of the large graph to show the change that occurs as mixed venous blood (70 per cent oxyhemoglobin, P_{CO_2} 46 mm. of mercury) passes through the pulmonary capillaries and becomes arterial blood (97.5 per cent oxyhemoglobin, P_{CO_2} 40 mm. of mercury). Dashed line is a hypothetical transition between the two curves. *Below right,* Oxygen and carbon dioxide dissociation curves plotted on same scale to show the important point that the oxygen curve has a steep and a flat portion and that the carbon dioxide curve does not. (From Comroe, J. H., Jr., and others: *The Lung.* Chicago, Year Book Medical Publishers, Inc., 1963.)

P_{CO_2} there is less carbon dioxide content. This effect aids in the removal of carbon dioxide from the blood in the lung when venous blood becomes oxygenated. The average arterial carbon dioxide tension (Pa_{CO_2}) in adults is 40 mm. of mercury, in infants closer to 35 mm., and venous levels are normally 6 mm. of mercury higher. Thus, the effect of venous admixture on arterial P_{CO_2} is very small.

The processes involved in the uptake of carbon dioxide in the blood and tissues are as follows:

① Carbon dioxide diffuses into the blood from the tissue. Some carbon dioxide is dissolved in the plasma water in physical solution.

② Carbon dioxide hydrates slowly in the plasma to form a small amount of carbonic acid.

③ Most of the carbon dioxide enters the red cells. A small amount is dissolved in the water of the red cell. A fraction combines with hemoglobin to form a carbamino compound.

④ A larger fraction in the red cell hydrates rapidly, because of the presence of carbonic anhydrase, to form carbonic acid, which dissociates into H^+ plus HCO_3^-.

⑤ Bicarbonate diffuses into plasma because of the concentration gradient, and Cl^- ions enter the cell to restore electrical neutrality.

Hemoglobin is important in the transport of carbon dioxide because of two properties of the molecule. First, it is a good buffer. This property permits blood to take up carbon dioxide with only a small change in pH. Second, it is a stronger acid when oxygenated than when it is reduced. Thus, when oxyhemoglobin is reduced, more cations are available to neutralize HCO_3^-. Carbon dioxide exists in two forms in the red cell because of this property of hemoglobin, as bicarbonate ion and as hemoglobin carbamate ($HbNHCOO^-$).

$$KHbO_2 + H_2CO_3 \rightleftarrows$$
$$HHb + O_2\uparrow + KHCO_3$$
$$KHbO_2 NH_2 + CO_2 \rightleftarrows$$
$$HHb \cdot NHCOOK + O_2\uparrow$$

An enzyme in the red cell, carbonic anhydrase, accelerates the reaction

$$CO_2 + H_2O \rightleftarrows H^+ + HCO_3^-$$

some 13,000 times. A concentration gradient between red cell and plasma causes the bicarbonate ion to leave the red cell. Because the red blood cell membrane is relatively impermeable to Na^+ and K^+, the chloride ion and water move into the red cell to restore electrical neutrality (chloride or Hamburger shift). Thus, although the larger portion of the buffering occurs within the red cell, the largest amount of carbon dioxide is in the plasma as HCO_3^- (Table 5).

In the lung the reverse process to that just described takes place because carbon dioxide diffuses out of the blood and into the alveoli. Since diffusion of CO_2 is rapid, the equilibrium between the P_{CO_2} of the pulmonary capillary and alveolar air is promptly achieved. About 30 per cent of the CO_2 that is exchanged is given up from hemoglobin carbamate. When hemoglobin is oxygenated in the pulmonary capillary, chloride and water shift out of the red cell and bicarbonate diffuses in and combines with hydrogen ion to form H_2CO_3, which is in turn dehy-

TABLE 5. CARBON DIOXIDE IN THE BLOOD

	Arterial Blood		Venous Blood	
	MM./L. BL.	%	MM./L. BL.	%
Total	21.9		24.1	
Plasma				
Dissolved CO_2	0.66	3	0.76	3
HCO_3^-	14.00	64	15.00	63
Cells				
Dissolved CO_2	0.44	2	0.54	2
HCO_3^-	5.7	26	6.1	25
$HbNHCOO^-$	1.2	5	1.8	7

The table gives normal values of the various chemical forms of CO_2 in blood with an assumed hematocrit level of 46. Approximately twice as much CO_2 exists in the plasma as in the red cells, chiefly as HCO_3^-.

drated to form carbon dioxide. CO_2 then diffuses out of the cell into the plasma and alveolar gas.

Although red blood cells from newborn infants have less carbonic anhydrase activity than adult cells, no defect in carbon dioxide transport is apparent. In patients receiving a carbonic anhydrase inhibitor such as acetazolamide (Diamox), the loss of carbon dioxide from the pulmonary capillaries and the uptake of carbon dioxide from the tissues may be incomplete, leading to an increased arterial and tissue P_{CO_2}. Also, on breathing 100 per cent oxygen, less reduced hemoglobin is present in venous blood, and therefore less buffering capacity for H^+ is present, leading to an increased P_{CO_2}. This is an important consideration during hyperbaric oxygenation when the venous blood may remain almost completely saturated with oxygen, H^+ is less well buffered, and tissue P_{CO_2} rises.

Acid-Base Balance

A reduction in pH, acidosis, may be caused by a reduction in HCO_3^- (metabolic acidosis) or an increase in P_{CO_2} (respiratory acidosis). An elevation of pH, alkalosis, may be caused by an elevation of bicarbonate (metabolic alkalosis) or a reduction of P_{CO_2} (respiratory alkalosis) (Table 6).

Metabolic acidosis is found in such conditions as diabetes, in which there is an accumulation of keto acids, in renal failure when the kidney is unable to excrete hydrogen ion, in diarrhea from loss of base, or in tissue hypoxia asso-

ciated with lactic acid accumulation. When pH falls, respiration is stimulated so that P_{CO_2} will fall and tend to compensate for the reduction in pH. This compensation is usually incomplete, and pH remains below 7.35. The pH, carbon dioxide content (HCO_3^- + P_{CO_2}), HCO_3^- and P_{CO_2} are all reduced.

Metabolic alkalosis occurs most commonly after excessive loss of Cl^- in vomiting (as in pyloric stenosis) or after an excessive citrate or bicarbonate load. The carbon dioxide content is elevated, and the P_{CO_2} will be normal or elevated, depending on the chronicity of the alkalosis.

Acute respiratory acidosis is secondary to respiratory insufficiency and accumulation of carbon dioxide within the body. The associated acidosis may be compensated by renal adjustments that promote retention of HCO_3^-. Compensation may require several days. Patients with chronic respiratory acidosis, in whom therapy may improve alveolar ventilation, often have a rapid fall of Pa_{CO_2}. The adjustment in bicarbonate may be much slower, with a resultant metabolic alkalosis of several days' duration. Such a sequence of events has been noted in emphysema and cystic fibrosis.

Similarly, acute respiratory alkalosis, for example, secondary to fever, psychogenic hyperventilation, or a pontine lesion with meningoencephalitis, will be associated with a high pH, low P_{CO_2} and normal bicarbonate. Renal compensation in time leads to an excretion of bicarbonate and a return of pH toward normal.

TABLE 6. BLOOD MEASUREMENTS IN VARIOUS ACID-BASE DISTURBANCES

	pH	Pa_{CO_2} (mm. Hg)	HCO_3^- (mEq./L.)	CO_2 Content (mEq./L.)
Metabolic acidosis	↓	↓	↓	↓
Acute respiratory acidosis	↓	↑	↔	Slight ↑
Compensated respiratory acidosis	(↔ or slight ↓)	↑	↑	↑
Metabolic alkalosis	↑	Slight ↑	↑	↑
Acute respiratory alkalosis	↑	↓	↔	Slight ↓
Compensated respiratory alkalosis	(↔ or slight ↑)	↓	↓	↓
Normal values	7.35–7.45	35–45	24–26	25–28

It is important to point out that the lung excretes some 300 mEq./kg. of acid per day in the form of carbon dioxide, the kidney 1 to 2 mEq./kg. per day. Thus the lung plays a large role in the acid-base balance of the body, and in fact provides rapid adjustment when necessary. The Henderson-Hasselbalch equation may be thought of as:

$$pH\alpha\ \frac{Kidney}{Lung}$$

Difference Between Addition of CO_2 to Blood in Vitro and in Vivo

An appreciation of the difference between the so-called in vitro and in vivo CO_2 dissociation curves is necessary in order to clarify the confusion that has arisen regarding the interpretation of measurements of acid-base balance, particularly during acute respiratory acidosis (acute hypoventilation). When blood in vitro is equilibrated with increasing concentration of CO_2, bicarbonate concentration also increases because of the hydration of carbon dioxide. If, for example, blood with a P_{CO_2} of 40 and a bicarbonate concentration of 24 mEq./liter were equilibrated with a P_{CO_2} of 100 mm. Hg, the actual bicarbonate concentration would be measured as 34 mEq./liter. In the commonly used Astrup nomogram, a correction for this increased bicarbonate due to CO_2 alone is made and the standard bicarbonate (bicarbonate concentration at a P_{CO_2} of 40 mm. Hg) is considered as 24 mEq./liter or a base excess of zero. With this correction, one can readily see that the metabolic (renal) component of acid-base balance is normal. However, confusion has arisen because the in vitro correction figures have been incorrectly applied to the situation in vivo. Unlike equilibration in the test tube, when there is acute hypercapnia in vivo the additional bicarbonate generated not only is distributed to water in red cells and plasma but also equilibrates with the interstitial fluid space; that is, bicarbonate ion equilibrates with extracellular water.

If the interstitial fluid represents 70 per cent of extracellular water, then 70 per cent of the additional bicarbonate generated will be distributed to the interstitial fluid. Thus, an arterial sample taken from a patient with an acute elevation of P_{CO_2} to 100 mm. Hg would have an actual bicarbonate concentration of 27 mEq./liter. If 10 mEq./liter were subtracted according to the in vitro correction, the standard bicarbonate would be reported as 17 mEq./liter or a base excess of −7, indicating the presence of a metabolic acidosis as well as a respiratory acidosis. This is in fact incorrect, and bicarbonate concentration in vivo is appropriate for the P_{CO_2}. The situation is worse in newborn infants because of the high hematocrit and large interstitial fluid space. Base excess values of as much as −10 mEq./liter (standard bicarbonate 14 mEq./liter) may be calculated despite the fact that the in vivo bicarbonate concentration is appropriate for the particular P_{CO_2} and there is no metabolic component to the acidosis. Thus, the appropriate therapy is to increase alveolar ventilation and not the administration of bicarbonate.

TISSUE RESPIRATION

Aerobic Metabolism

The ultimate function of the lung is to provide oxygen to meet the demands of the tissues and to excrete carbon dioxide, a by-product of metabolic activity. Thus, respiratory physiologists have been concerned with the assessment of respiration at the tissue level and the ability of the cardiopulmonary system to meet the metabolic demands of the body.

One method is to measure the amount of oxygen consumed by the body per minute ($\dot{V}_{O_2}$). This is equal to the amount necessary to maintain the life of the cells at rest, plus the amount necessary for oxidative combustion required to maintain a normal body temperature, as well as that used for the metabolic demands of work above the resting level. The basal metabolic rate is a summation of many component energy rates of individual organs and tissues and is defined as the amount of energy necessary to maintain the life of the cells at rest, under conditions in which there is no additional energy expenditure for temperature regulation or additional work.

In practice, $\dot{V}_{O_2}$ is measured after an overnight fast, the subject lying supine in a room at a comfortable temperature. This "basal" metabolic rate has a wide variability ($\pm$ 15 per cent of predicted $\dot{V}_{O_2}$). Since absolutely basal conditions are difficult to ensure, the measurement of basal metabolic rate is not widely used at present.

The performance of the cardiopulmonary system can be more adequately assessed and compared with normal measurements under conditions of added work, such as exercise. The healthy lung does not limit the ability to increase oxygen consumption to meet the demands of the body, since even during severe exercise the maximal breathing capacity is not reached. Rather, the inability of cardiac output to exceed a certain level limits exercise tolerance. Performance can be increased by physical fitness, and athletes are able to increase their cardiac output by sixfold or sevenfold. Athletic conditioning also increases the diffusing capacity of the lung and in some manner, not well understood, increases the efficiency of oxygen extraction from the blood in the tissues at a given cardiac output. Few studies have been done in children, but in general the relation between work capacity, ventilation and oxygen consumption is the same as that of the adult. The maximal $\dot{V}_{O_2}$ that can be achieved increases throughout childhood, reaches its peak of 50 to 60 ml. per minute per kilogram between 10 and 15 years of age, and thereafter declines slowly with age.

At the tissue level, the ability for a given cell to receive an adequate oxygen supply depends on the amount of local blood flow, the distance of that cell from the perfusing capillary and the difference between the partial pressure of oxygen in the capillary and in the cell. The critical mean capillary P_{O_2} appears to be in the region of 30 mm. of mercury for children and adults. Exercising muscle has 10 to 20 times the number of open capillaries as resting muscle does.

Anaerobic Metabolism

The adequacy of oxygen supply to the tissues has more recently been assessed by measuring blood lactate, a product of anaerobic metabolism (Embden-Meyerhof pathway). When there is insufficient oxygen supply to the tissues from insufficient blood flow, or a decreased oxygen content of blood, lactic acid concentration within the tissues and blood rises. In the blood this accumulation leads to a metabolic acidosis.

During moderate to heavy muscular exercise, the cardiac output cannot meet the demands of the muscles, and an oxygen debt is incurred, which is repaid upon cessation of exercise. During this period lactic acid accumulates and therefore severe exercise is often associated with a metabolic acidosis. There is an excellent correlation between the serum lactate level and the oxygen debt. Since oxygen debt is not measurable at rest and is difficult to measure during exercise, the adequacy of tissue oxygenation appears to be accurately reflected in the serum lactate level. In adult man, blood lactate is less than 1 mEq. per liter, but may rise to 10 or 12 mEq. per liter during very heavy exercise.

Relation Between $\dot{V}_{O_2}$ and $\dot{V}_{CO_2}$

In the normal subject in a steady state, the amount of carbon dioxide excreted by the lung per minute is dependent upon the basal metabolism activity of the cells and the type of substrate being oxidized. The volume of carbon dioxide exhaled divided by the amount of oxygen consumed is known as the ventilatory respiratory quotient (R). For the body as a whole the ratio is 1 if primarily carbohydrate is being metabolized, 0.7 for fat, and 0.8 for protein. Normally the ratio is 0.8 at rest and approximately 1.0 during exercise. The ventilatory respiratory quotient may vary considerably with changes in alveolar ventilation and metabolism and therefore must be measured in the steady state, i.e., with a steady alveolar ventilation and a steady metabolic rate. For an individual organ, the metabolic respiratory quotient (R.Q.) is nearly constant, but may vary from 0.4 to 1.5, depending on the balance of anabolism and catabolism in a particular organ. Thus, the measurement of R represents the resultant of many component metabolizing organs and tissues. In the first few days after birth, R falls from nearly 1 to 0.7, indicating a loss of carbohydrate stores; as feeding is started, R approaches 0.8.

With the introduction of modern equipment which can monitor breath-by-breath CO_2 and N_2 concentrations, it is now possible to calculate R on a breath-by-breath basis. Using this technique it is possible more precisely to define the workload at which anaerobic metabolism begins (threshold for anaerobic metabolism). As lactic acid begins to accumulate in the blood, the carbon dioxide dissociation curve shifts to the right and there is a sudden increase in expired CO_2. R therefore suddenly increases from about 1.0 to above 1.0. It has been shown that the threshold for anaerobic metabolism in both normal adults and children can be increased by training. This technique is particularly useful in children, since it does not require blood sampling and can be readily applied to cooperative subjects with a variety of pulmonary and cardiac problems.

Temperature Effects

Increasing emphasis has recently been placed on the relation between metabolism and body temperature, particularly in the newborn infant. Van't Hoff's Law for simple chemical reactions states that the reaction rate is directly proportional to the temperature at which the reaction is taking place. In a biologic system, for each $10°$ C. rise in temperature, reaction rate increases by twofold to threefold (Q_{10} effect). Homeothermic mammals, however, do not obey van't Hoff's Law because as temperature decreases, oxygen consumption increases to maintain a normal body temperature, until hypothermic levels are reached (below a body temperature of $30°$ C, V_{O_2} decreases with decreasing temperature). Under a cold stress the adult becomes exhausted after a few hours. Since it is likely that the newborn with a relatively large surface area and poor insulation would fail to maintain a normal body temperature even sooner, the optimum thermal environment for premature and term infants has undergone considerable recent investigation. Since fat is a good insulator, the premature infant with deficient subcutaneous fat is in a more precarious position with respect to temperature control than is the full-term infant. Evidence that premature infants with a low body temperature have a higher mortality rate has necessitated careful regulation of the environmental temperature.

Normal newborn infants do not exhibit a Q_{10} effect; i.e., they increase V_{O_2} with decrease in environmental temperature (Fig. 14). The optimum or neutral environmental temperature, i.e., the temperature at which oxygen consumption is minimal, has been found to vary with the weight and age of the infant. Within the first few days of life, neutral environmental temperature for infants less than 1.5 kg. birth weight is between 33.5 and $34.5°$ C.; between 1.5 and 2.5 kg. it ranges from 32 to $34°$ C., and in full-term infants it ranges between 31 and $34°$ C. Thus the range of neutral temperature is narrow in newborn infants, decreasing with decreasing size of the infant compared with the unclothed adult who does not start to increase oxygen consumption

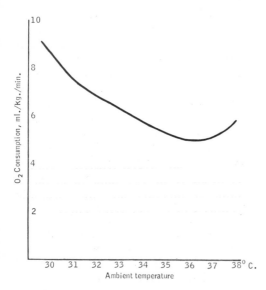

Figure 14. The relation of oxygen consumption and environmental temperature in a typical infant of 1.5 to 2 kg. of body weight. (Adapted from the data of Mestayn and others.)

until ambient temperature falls below 27 or 28° C. At the neutral environmental temperature, the skin temperature of the anterior abdominal wall is 36 to 36.5° C. or about 1° C. below deep body (core) temperature.

In contrast to the adult, the newborn infant does not increase oxygen consumption during a thermal stress by shivering. Nonshivering thermogenesis is stimulated by noradrenaline, which increases the activity of brown fat located at the nape of the neck, around the heart, and around the interscapular and retrosternal areas. Noradrenaline activates a lipase in brown fat, which causes the breakdown of triglyceride to fatty acids and glycerol. This reaction is highly exothermic and adds heat to the blood. Although glycerol is released to the circulation, fatty acids are recycled to form triglyceride. This increased activity of brown fat requires oxygen and results in the increased oxygen consumption seen during thermal stress in the newborn infant.

A consideration of thermal stress and associated increased oxygen requirements is important in the management of older children with impaired respiratory function. A common sight on any pediatric ward is the child with respiratory distress lying in the cold, albeit oxygenated and humidified, environment of the oxygen tent. The addi-

tional thermal stress may be life-threatening.

VENTILATION–PERFUSION RELATIONS

The efficiency of pulmonary gas exchange is remarkable when one considers that air must be properly distributed to several hundred million alveoli in correct proportion to the amount of blood perfusing these alveoli. It is this nearly perfect matching of blood flow ($\dot{Q}$) and alveolar ventilation ($\dot{V}_A$) within millions of respiratory units that enables the healthy lung to maintain blood gas tensions that are nearly constant. For the adult lung, $\dot{V}_A$ is 4 liters per minute and $\dot{Q}$ is 5 liters per minute. The relation between ventilation and perfusion is expressed as the ratio:

$$\frac{\dot{V}_A}{\dot{Q}} = 0.8$$

This ratio reflects the relation of ventilation to perfusion for the lung as a whole. Even in health not all alveoli have a perfect match of $\dot{V}_A$ and $\dot{Q}$. Within an individual alveolus, ventilation may be in excess of the blood flow ($\dot{V}_A/\dot{Q}$ greater than 0.8) or blood flow may be in excess of the ventilation ($\dot{V}_A/\dot{Q}$ less than 0.8). What is the effect on alveolar and blood gas tension of grossly altered $\dot{V}_A/\dot{Q}$? Consider two extreme examples: (1) one lung has normal ventilation, but no blood flow ($\dot{V}_A/\dot{Q} = \infty$); (2) one lung has no ventilation, but normal blood flow ($\dot{V}_A/\dot{Q} = 0$).

In the first situation, if one lung receives 2.0 liters per minute of ventilation, but does not receive any blood supply ($\dot{V}_A/\dot{Q} = \infty$), no gas exchange can occur, and the ventilation enters an alveolus that acts as if it were dead space. If the other lung received 2.0 liters per minute alveolar ventilation, half of the total, but now had 5 liters per minute blood flow (instead of 2.5), the blood leaving the lung would have an elevated P_{CO_2} of about 80 mm. of mercury and a P_{O_2} decreased to approximately 60 mm. of mercury (about 80 per cent saturated). If alveolar ventilation is doubled to compensate for the shift in blood flow, the arterial P_{CO_2} and P_{O_2} will return to normal, yet a sample of mixed alveolar gas will not have normal gas tensions. Normally, the alveolar gas from each lung, each with the same P_{CO_2} and P_{O_2}, would mix in the trachea and emerge with a P_{O_2} of 100 mm. and a P_{CO_2} of 40 mm. of mercury. In the above-mentioned example, when 50 per cent of the alveolar ventilation goes to alveolar dead space, the mixing of alveolar gas from the two lungs produces a P_{CO_2} of $\frac{40 + 0}{2}$ or 20 mm. of mercury, much lower than the arterial P_{CO_2}. Mixed alveolar P_{O_2} will be higher $\left(\frac{100 + 150}{2} = 125 \text{ mm. Hg}\right)$. Note that Pa_{CO_2} is greater than $P_{A_{CO_2}}$ and $P_{A_{O_2}}$ greater than Pa_{O_2}. These gradients form the basis for the measurement of alveolar dead space ($V_D$alv) (see p. 25).

In the second situation, when one lung has no ventilation and normal blood flow ($\dot{V}_A/\dot{Q} = 0$), while the other lung has a normal $\dot{V}_A/\dot{Q}$, the blood flowing through the nonventilated lung acts as shunted blood, mixes with the arterial blood, and lowers the P_{O_2} and

oxygen content (hypoxemia). For example, if mixed venous blood contained 12 ml. of oxygen per 100 ml. of blood and arterial blood coming from the ventilated lung contained 20 ml. of oxygen per 100 ml. of blood, the mixture of equal parts (50 per cent shunt) would have an arterial oxygen content of $\frac{20 + 12}{2} = 16$ ml. per 100 ml. of blood. The arterial oxygen tensions would be reduced from 100 mm. to about 45 mm. of mercury and the saturation reduced to 80 per cent. There is little effect on P_{CO_2}, since arteriovenous P_{CO_2} differences are only 6 mm. of mercury. An increased alveolar ventilation to the one ventilated and perfused lung, or an increased inspired oxygen concentration would have practically no effect on the oxygen content of the blood coming from that lung, since it was previously nearly fully saturated with oxygen.

The same principles apply to less extreme examples of ventilation-perfusion derangements, such as alveoli that receive slightly more ventilation than perfusion. Here a portion of $\dot{V}_A$ is wasted and acts as if dead space were ventilated. If there is less ventilation than blood flow to an alveolus ($\dot{V}_A/\dot{Q}$ less than 0.8), the blood does not undergo complete gas exchange. The effect is similar to that of an anatomic shunt which permits venous to arterial circulation. The blood from such an alveolus can be considered a mixture of normally arterialized blood and pure venous blood. Indeed, in patients with pulmonary disease, the commonest cause of hypoxemia is improper matching of blood and gas in the lung.

Measurement of Distribution of Ventilation

Nitrogen has been used to determine the distribution of inspired gas within the lung because it is poorly soluble and does not pass quickly in large amounts from the pulmonary capillaires to the alveoli. One test requires the inhalation of a single breath of 100 per cent oxygen and measurement of the concentration of nitrogen in the expired air. The concentration of nitrogen at the beginning of expiration is low; as expiration continues, it increases to alveolar tensions and "plateaus" at this value. When there is altered distribution of ventilation, some alveoli get only a small amount of oxygen, while others receive more than their share. Thus there is no representative alveolar nitrogen concentration, and it continues to rise during expiration, since the hypoventilated areas empty last.

Another standard test is to inspire 100 per cent oxygen and watch the fall in alveolar nitrogen concentration that occurs as it is washed out of the lung. For the normal adult, nitrogen concentration should be less than 2.5 per cent after seven minutes of oxygen breathing. With poor distribution of ventilation, this value is much higher. In normal children, nitrogen concentration falls much more rapidly and is below 2.5 per cent after only two minutes of oxygen breathing. In the normal newborn infant, this level is reached in one minute. These two methods measure only the distribution of inspired air to alveoli, without reflecting the relation between $\dot{V}_A$ and $\dot{Q}$.

Several methods are used to examine the distribution of ventilation in relation to perfusion. One of the commonest is the measurement of physiologic dead space. When alveolar ventilation is in excess of blood flow in many areas of the lung, physiologic dead space (anatomic dead space plus alveolar dead space) is elevated.

Another method of assessing $\dot{V}_A/\dot{Q}$, the measurement of a-A nitrogen tension gradients, has recently been developed. Since nitrogen is inert, fluctuations in alveolar nitrogen tension ($P_{A_{N_2}}$) are passive and depend on changes in oxygen and carbon dioxide tension. Alveolar gas in areas with a low $\dot{V}_A/\dot{Q}$ has a high nitrogen tension because more oxygen is absorbed and less carbon dioxide excreted. On expiration the small amount of ventilation from these

areas mixes with a large amount of ventilation from normal areas, and only slightly raises the average $P_{A_{N_2}}$. A relatively large amount of blood from the area of low $\dot{V}_A/\dot{Q}$ in equilibrium with the high $P_{A_{N_2}}$ present mixes with a smaller amount of blood from normal areas, resulting in an elevation of the Pa_{N_2}. Thus, the effect of many areas containing a low $\dot{V}_A/\dot{Q}$ is to produce an a-A P_{N_2} gradient. Since nitrogen is inert, P_{N_2} is the same in all biologic fluids. It may be measured, using gas chromatography, in both blood and urine. In normal children the a-A P_{N_2} gradient averages 3 mm. of mercury (less than 10 mm.). In conditions, however, with severe abnormality in $\dot{V}_A/\dot{Q}$, such as cystic fibrosis, the gradient increases some fivefold to tenfold. Moderate a-A P_{N_2} gradients are found in normal newborn infants during the first day of life, returning to normal by the second day.

Mechanism of Nonuniform Ventilation

The use of radioactive gases such as oxygen, carbon dioxide and xenon has recently enabled investigators to describe $\dot{V}_A/\dot{Q}$ relations of different areas of the lung. Geographic mapping of $\dot{V}_A/\dot{Q}$ from the apex to the base of the lung has supported the previous indirect methods which suggested that $\dot{V}_A/\dot{Q}$ was altered by gravitational forces. Indeed, in normal upright man, $\dot{V}_A/\dot{Q}$ may vary from 0.6 at the base to more than 2.0 at the apex. The influence of gravity on pulmonary blood flow will be described later. Gravity also plays an important role in the distribution of ventilation, particularly in the upright posture, because the weight of the lung produces regional differences in pleural pressure. In upright man, at FRC pleural pressure at the apex is about −10 cm. H_2O and rises at about the rate of 0.25 cm. H_2O per cm. vertical distance down the lung. Thus, at the base of the lung pleural pressure is only −2.5 cm. H_2O. Because of these differences in transpulmonary pressure, the alveoli at the apex are more expanded than the alveoli at the bottom of the lung. The apical alveoli are nearer their elastic limit and therefore less compliant than basal alveoli. Thus, during inspiration a greater proportion of the tidal volume goes to the base of the lung.

Within a given region of lung, the distribution of ventilation largely depends on the relationship between the resistance of the airways and the compliance of the alveoli. The importance of the notion of time constants has already been discussed earlier in this chapter (see page 20). Inhomogeneity of time constants within the lung is the primary cause of altered distribution of ventilation. Almost any disease process in the lung will alter time constants in the affected areas and therefore will result in uneven distribution of ventilation. Despite the variance of $\dot{V}_A/\dot{Q}$ in normal man, little effect on blood gases is seen until greater inhomogeneity is present.

Measurement of the Distribution of Blood Flow

The amount of venous admixture that is present can be estimated from the shunt equation:*

$$\frac{\dot{Q}_S}{\dot{Q}_T} = \frac{Ca_{O_2} - Cc_{O_2}}{C\bar{v}_{O_2} - Cc_{O_2}}$$

---

*Since the amount of oxygen in arterial blood equals the amount of oxygen in blood that has passed through pulmonary capillaries (Q_C) plus the amount of oxygen in shunted blood (Q_S), and

Amount of oxygen = content of oxygen/1. (C_{O_2}) × blood flow ($\dot{Q}$)

Therefore, $Ca_{O_2}\dot{Q}_t = Cc_{O_2}\dot{Q}_C + C\bar{v}_{O_2}\dot{Q}_s$

(where Q_t = total blood flow)

Since $\dot{Q}_C = \dot{Q}_t - \dot{Q}_s$

$Ca_{O_2}\dot{Q}_t = Cc_{O_2}\dot{Q}_t - Cc_{O_2}\dot{Q}_s + C\bar{v}_{O_2}\dot{Q}_s$

and $\dfrac{\dot{Q}_s}{\dot{Q}_t} = \dfrac{Cc_{O_2} - Ca_{O_2}}{C\bar{v}_{O_2} - Cc_{O_2}}$

where $\dot{Q}_S/\dot{Q}_T$ is the fraction of total cardiac output that is shunted.

In normal subjects, up to 6 per cent of the cardiac output may be shunted from right to left primarily through bronchial veins, which empty into the left side of the circulation. A small portion comes from the thebesian veins, which drain the coronary circulation directly into the left ventricle. During exercise there is less than 3 per cent venous admixture. An increased venous admixture can be due to low $\dot{V}_A/\dot{Q}$, anatomic right-to-left shunt within the lung, or a cardiac abnormality. Breathing 100 per cent oxygen will obliterate the shunt effect of low $\dot{V}_A/\dot{Q}$, leaving only anatomic shunt, and is used as a test to differentiate between the two effects. Pa_{O_2} should be greater than 500 mm. of mercury during oxygen breathing in the absence of anatomic shunt.

Causes of Nonuniform Pulmonary Blood Flow

1. Gravity. Adult man in the upright position does not perfuse the apices of the lung. Since gravity does not affect the distribution of ventilation to the same degree, the apices have a high $\dot{V}_A/\dot{Q}$. Children have a relatively higher pulmonary artery pressure and therefore a more uniform distribution of pulmonary blood flow in the upright position.

2. Partial or complete occlusion of the pulmonary artery or arterioles by arteriosclerosis, endarteritis, collagen disease, congenital abnormalities, thrombosis or embolism of blood clots, fats, gas bubbles (caisson disease), tumor cells.

3. Compression of pulmonary vessels by masses, pulmonary exudate, pneumothorax.

4. Reduction in the size of the pulmonary vascular bed,

5. Closure of some pulmonary vessels due to a low pulmonary artery pressure, which may occur in shock.

6. Overexpansion of some alveoli and collapse of others.

7. Regional congestion of vessels as in left-sided heart failure.

(8) Anatomic pulmonary artery to pulmonary venous shunts, as with pulmonary hemangiomas. The distribution of blood that flows to the capillaries may be uniform, but some mixed venous blood completely bypasses the capillaries and reduces the oxygen content of arterial blood.

Intrinsic Regulation of Regional $\dot{V}_A/\dot{Q}$

Abnormalities of $\dot{V}_A/\dot{Q}$ may be caused by either too much or too little ventilation to an area, although the blood flow may be normal; too much or too little blood flow, although ventilation may be normal; or a combination of both effects. Whatever the absolute amount of regional ventilation and perfusion, the lung has intrinsic regulatory mechanisms that are directed toward the preservation of the "ideal" $\dot{V}_A/\dot{Q}$ of 0.8. In areas where $\dot{V}_A/\dot{Q}$ is high, the low carbon dioxide concentration results in local constriction of airways, and tends to reduce the amount of ventilation to that area. When $\dot{V}_A/\dot{Q}$ is low, the high alveolar carbon dioxide concentration results in local airway dilatation and a tendency to increase ventilation to the area. Furthermore, a low $\dot{V}_A/\dot{Q}$ with an associated low alveolar oxygen concentration causes regional pulmonary vasoconstriction. Effects on airways and vessels from changing gas tensions tend to preserve a normal $\dot{V}_A/\dot{Q}$, but they are limited mechanisms, and derangements are common.

PULMONARY CIRCULATION

The contributions of anatomists, pathologists, cardiologists and respiratory physiologists to our understanding of the pulmonary circulation have been numerous in recent years. The following section cannot be an exhaustive review of the subject, but rather is biased toward those aspects of the pulmonary circulation that are significant in the evaluation of lung function and pathologic changes in the infant and the child.

Anatomy

The main pulmonary arteries and their branches that accompany the cartilaginous bronchi into the lobes of the lung are elastic arteries, characterized by laminations of elastic tissue in the medial layers, similar to the aorta. They branch to form the smaller muscular arteries, with a circular layer of smooth muscle bounded by external and internal elastic laminae. The muscular arteries of the lung have thinner media than their counterparts in the systemic circulation, and range from 100 to 1000 microns in diameter. Arterioles branch from the muscular arteries and are discernible by the lack of a muscular layer. Their walls are composed of some supporting collagen, an elastic layer and a thin adventitia.

Fetal muscular arteries have a thick medial layer that increases during the latter half of gestation; at birth the muscular wall represents about 50 per cent of the total vessel diameter and then gradually becomes thinner, or the wall-lumen ratio decreases. The adult ratio of 0.20 is reached at different ages in different persons, from two to six months after birth.

The lungs have a double circulation. The pulmonary arteries carry nearly all the cardiac output to the lungs. The nutrient vessels of the lung, the bronchial arteries, are small arteries that arise from the aorta or intercostals and follow the dorsal portion of each primary bronchus. They lose their identity along the respiratory bronchioles; the capillaries they supply drain with the alveolar capillary network into the rich peribronchial venous network, which empties into the pulmonary veins. Unlike systemic veins, which usually follow the course of the artery, pulmonary veins follow the interlobular connective-tissue planes. The direct connections of veins to adjacent limiting membranes of lung tissue are the anatomic device that makes their diameters reflect changes in lung volume. Less than 6 per cent of the cardiac output bypasses the alveoli through bronchial vessels and the thebesian veins in the left side of the heart.

Hemodynamics

PRESSURES, FLOWS, RESISTANCES. In the fetal circulation, only about 12 per cent of the output of the right ventricle goes to the lungs: the remainder goes through the ductus arteriosus to the aorta. With the initiation of air breathing at birth, pulmonary blood flow increases. The action of increasing oxygen tensions and falling carbon dioxide tensions decreases the tone of the pulmonary vessels, but facilitates closure of the ductus. The changing geometry of the alveoli and vessels which accompanies the creation of an air-liquid interface is a major factor in decreasing pulmonary vascular resistance and therefore also promotes increased blood flow.

Left and right ventricular pressures in the fetal heart are nearly the same. Mean pulmonary artery and aortic pressures in fetal lambs are 50 to 70 mm. of mercury. After birth there is a persistent pulmonary hypertension relative to values at an older age. Mean pulmonary artery pressures in normal term infants are between 20 and 50 mm. of mercury, mean aortic pressures usually 40 to 50 mm. in the first hours of life. Mean pulmonary artery pressure begins to fall within hours after birth, and the upper limit of normal adult values is reached in four to ten days. During infancy and childhood, the tendency is for a gradual increase in systemic pressures and decrease in pulmonary artery pressures.

The pulmonary vessels are capable of dilatation and compression. The degree of distention will depend on the tone of the vessel wall, and the difference in pressure across it, the transmural pressure. In the lung, the pressure outside a vessel may vary greatly during the respiratory cycle. The pressure outside the large arteries and veins is pleural pressure, whereas the pressure outside the alveolar capillaries is approximately alveolar pressure. The blood vessels within the lung parenchyma are also subjected to direct forces from the attachments of the pulmonary tissue. Thus, the elasticity of the lung tissue exerts a "radial traction" on vessel walls, which increases with lung volume. The pulmonary vascular bed may be thought of as existing in two compartments: one which expands with increasing lung volume and presumably includes all vessels outside the alveolar walls, and the other which is compressed at large lung volumes and presumably contains alveolar vessels.

It is apparent that evaluations of pulmonary vascular resistance (pressure/flow) will be complicated by the different pressure relations existing across parts of the pulmonary vascular bed. Much of the confusion in the literature about pressure-flow relations in the lung has been overcome by an appreciation of the so-called vascular waterfall phenomenon. The simile implies that upstream pressure and flow are independent of changes downstream in a system of collapsible vessels as long as the downstream pressure is less than that which surrounds the collapsible member. Since the pressure outside the collapsible pulmonary alveolar capillaries is approximately alveolar pressure, when the pressure in the pulmonary veins is less than alveolar pressure, pulmonary blood flow will depend on the difference between pulmonary artery and alveolar pressure. When pulmonary venous pressure is greater than alveolar pressure, pulmonary blood flow will be determined by the difference in pressure between artery and vein.

EFFECT OF GRAVITY. The pressure is not the same in similar vessels in an upright person at the apex of the lung as at the base, and the magnitude of the difference is related to the height of the person. Since the pulmonary artery enters about the midportion of the lung, the systolic arterial pressure of 15 to 20 mm. of mercury is adequate to perfuse the apices during systole, but not during diastole if the distance is greater than the diastolic pressure. The vessels in the lung bases are exposed to pulmonary artery pressure, plus the pressure generated by the weight of the column of blood, which may be another 15 cm. of water. Thus, in any situation in which transudation is favored, more fluid will be found in the bases than in the apices in the upright posture. The relative underperfusion of the apices in upright man results in a slightly higher mean alveolar P_{O_2}, and a lower P_{CO_2} in apical alveolar air. One important clinical application of this effect of gravity is that the higher P_{O_2} in apical segments favors the growth of the tubercle bacillus and is thought to be the basis for the apical localization of tuberculosis in adults. The smaller size of the child makes the hydrostatic effects of gravity less and may underlie the random localization of the primary tuberculosis complex in the child. From the foregoing discussion, it is apparent that the lung may be divided into three zones with regard to the pulmonary circulation: Zone I at the apex, where there is little or no blood flow; Zone II or the vascular waterfall zone, where pulmonary venous pressure is less than alveolar pressure; and Zone III, where venous pressure exceeds alveolar pressure. (The physiologic consequences of the forces of gravity on the distribution of the circulation and ventilation are discussed on page 46).

Movement of Liquid in the Lung

The forces that tend to move liquid from capillary to air space are the positive pressure within the capillary, the negative pericapillary tissue pressures and, in the case of the lung, the pressure exerted by the forces of surface tension at the air-liquid interface. The force that opposes these pressures, and normally keeps liquid in the capillary along its entire length, is the colloid osmotic pressure of the blood (Fig. 15).

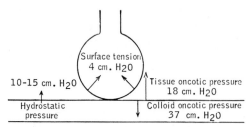

Figure 15. Forces that maintain water balance between alveolus and capillary.

The amount of edema formation will depend also on the permeability of the capillaries and their filtration area. The area will in turn depend on any nervous, chemical or physical change in blood vessel tone. In general, increased distention of the capillaries will also increase the permeability.

Some of the causes of pulmonary edema are categorized in Table 7. It can be initiated by a variety of insults to several systems, and the mechanism of edema formation may differ accordingly. Most commonly, left ventricular failure and an elevation in capillary hydrostatic pressure underlie pulmonary

TABLE 7. SOME CAUSES OF PULMONARY EDEMA

Hemodynamic derangements
   Coronary occlusion
   Left ventricular outflow obstruction
   Left atrial occlusion
   Mitral valve disease
   Hypervolemia
   Hemorrhage and shock
   Embolism
   Pulmonary venous obstruction, high altitude
Central nervous system disorders
Vagotomy
Respiratory system disorders
   Airway obstruction
   Hypoxia
   Burns
   Drowning
   Injury
Pharmacologic agents
   Epinephrine
   Histamine
   Acetylcholine
   Irritant gases
   Other agents such as alloxan

edema. Humoral agents, vagotomy, alterations in capillary wall integrity and many pharmacologic agents can also induce pulmonary edema.

The pulmonary functional derangements in edema affect both gas exchange and pulmonary mechanics. Usually a diffusion impairment can be demonstrated before there are significant mechanical changes. One of the earliest changes is a thickening of the alveolar-capillary membranes. Arterial hypoxemia is present, and may be ameliorated by forcible inflation of the lungs, suggesting that some of the venous admixture is from blood flow through poorly ventilated portions of the lungs. Edematous lungs lack the pulmonary surfactant, which is either denatured by movement of fluid across alveolar membranes or washed out by the foaming that accompanies acute pulmonary edema. Lung compliance is greatly reduced, airway resistance is increased, and respiratory work increases manyfold.

Some water exchange occurs in normal lungs. In the resting state, net water loss from the lung is about 0.63 to 0.65 mg. per milliliter of oxygen absorbed. Flux of water in the lung is much greater.

Drowning

The inhalation of liquid into the lung is associated with immediate reflex laryngospasm. If this is sustained to the point of severe hypoxia, the larynx opens, and more liquid may enter the lung. The physiologic consequences depend on the nature of the liquid aspirated. If it is fresh water, which is hypotonic (about 20 milliosmoles) with respect to the blood (310 milliosmoles), about 1 ml. per kilogram is absorbed in two to three minutes. Significant amounts absorbed lead to hypervolemia, hemolysis, hyperkalemia and ventricular fibrillation. If salt water, which is hypertonic (about 1100 milliosmoles) with respect to the blood, enters the alveoli, further movement of liquid from blood to lung occurs with pulmonary

edema and hemorrhage. Hypovolemia and systemic hypotension ensue.

The physiologic sequelae may be profound, even with small amounts aspirated, from reflex irritation of the airways and the obstructive effects of foam. The major problem is that of pulmonary edema and asphyxia, and intermittent positive-pressure breathing may be lifesaving.

Regulation

Some of the passive regulatory events with changes in lung volume have been cited above. Active changes in pulmonary vascular resistance can occur with changes in blood gases, with neural stimulation and with drugs. Low oxygen tensions tend to constrict pulmonary vessels, both reflexly and locally. Increased hydrogen ion concentrations potentiate the vasoconstrictive effects of hypoxia, but have little effect in the absence of hypoxia. Reflex vasoconstriction accompanies elevated left atrial pressures, and thus operates to prevent pulmonary edema.

Many drugs affect the pulmonary vasculature, including the arteriolar constrictors norepinephrine, epinephrine, histamine, angiotensin and serotonin. Isoproterenol and acetylcholine are examples of agents that tend to dilate constricted arterioles. Both the fetal and neonatal pulmonary circulations are exquisitely sensitive to vasoconstrictors and respond with a prompt and marked increase in pulmonary vascular resistance. Similarly, at this stage the pulmonary circulation is very responsive to vasodilator agents. In older children and adults, the effects of neural and chemical stimuli are qualitatively similar but quantitatively much less than in the neonatal infant.

Methods of Evaluation

The chest radiograph remains the most widely used tool to determine the possible presence of pulmonary vascular disease. Prominence of the pulmonary outflow tract and increased or decreased vascular markings may be noted. Regional pulmonary angiography further delineates localized disturbance in blood flow, although the procedure requires cardiac catheterization. Direct measurements of pulmonary artery and "wedge" or capillary pressures add further information. Occasionally drugs can be infused into the pulmonary artery to evaluate the potential reversibility of pulmonary vasoconstriction.

Recently, embolization of a minute but uniformly distributed portion of the pulmonary vascular bed with macroaggregated albumin tagged with ^{131}I has permitted direct visualization of regional blood flow. The tagged molecules are metabolized within a few hours, and excreted by six to eight hours. The radioactivity can be recorded with suitable scanners. It has been shown that the density of the radioscan correlates with oxygen uptake. Thus differential lung perfusion can be evaluated, even in infants, with this technique.

Measurements of pulmonary blood flow with an inert gas method are becoming more widely used and are applicable to infants. The method depends on the solubility of nitrous oxide in blood. The patient inspires a mixture of 80 per cent nitrous oxide and 20 per cent oxygen. From the measured volumes and concentrations of the inspired and expired mixtures, the amount absorbed can be calculated. The alveolar nitrous oxide concentration is measured from the end-tidal level read on a continuous analyzer. The formula used is as follows:

$$Q_C = \frac{V_{N_2O} \times f}{[\alpha]^{37°N_2O}} \times F_{A_{N_2O}}$$

where Q_c represents pulmonary capillary blood flow per minute, V_{N_2O} volume of nitrous oxide absorbed per heart beat, f heart rate per minute, and $F_{A_{N_2O}}$ nitrous oxide in the alveolar or end-tidal gas. $[\alpha]^{37°}$ is the solubility coefficient of nitrous oxide in blood at 37° C. and 760 mm. of mercury pressure, and is 0.47 ml. of nitrous oxide per milliliter of blood. The uptake of nitrous oxide will be restricted to those portions of lung which are both ventilated and perfused; thus, the measurement is of "effective pulmonary blood flow" and may underestimate total blood flow. In adults the normal value is 5.9 liters per minute, with some increase toward the end of inspiration, and a decrease toward the end of expiration, and is pulsatile during the cardiac cycle.

Estimates from dye studies indicate that about 20 per cent of the total blood volume is in the lungs at any one time, but the distribution of blood between the pulmonary and systemic vascular beds varies with posture and the relative resistances of the two beds, and also depends on the relationship between intra-abdominal and intrathoracic pressure. About 30 per cent of the total pulmonary blood volume is in arteries, 10 per cent is in capillaries and 60 per cent is in veins. Capillary blood volume increases with increasing venous pressure and may go up three- to fourfold during exercise.

REGULATION OF RESPIRATION

Over the past 15 years, the classic concepts concerned with the respiratory control system have been challenged and broadened in many areas. It is appropriate for pediatricians to have an understanding of the normal respiratory control mechanisms, since alterations in respiratory frequency or alveolar ventilation are a frequent concomitant of many diseases in childhood.

Two main systems are involved in the regulatory process: (1) a neural system which is responsible for the maintenance of a coordinated, rhythmic respiratory cycle and the regulation of the depth of respiration, and (2) a chemical (neurohumoral) system which regulates alveolar ventilation and maintains normal blood gas tensions.

Neural System

The respiratory center is now recognized to consist of four areas in the brain stem, two pontine and two medullary areas (Fig. 16). The pneumotaxic center is located in the rostral few millimeters of the pons. Section of the pons below this level results in a slowing and an increase in amplitude of respiration. If, in addition, the vagi are cut, respiration stops at a maximal inspiratory position called apneusis. The pneumotaxic center has no intrinsic rhythmicity, but functions to modulate respiratory frequency and depth, since ablation produces respiratory slowing and stimulation accelerates respiration. It is also responsible for periodic inhibition of the apneustic center in the pons.

The apneustic center is located in the middle and caudal pons. This area produces a tonic inspiratory spasm and is modulated through feedback mechanisms by the pneumotaxic center, medullary respiratory centers and vagal afferent impuslses. Total removal of the pons abolishes apneusis and produces rhythmic respirations that are generally gasping and not well coordinated.

The medullary respiratory centers consist of an inspiratory center situated caudally in the ventral portion of the medullary reticular formation, and an expiratory center situated dorsal and cephalad to the inspiratory center. It is now accepted that the medullary centers are intrinsically rhythmic, but are modulated by pontine and vagal discharges.

Proprioceptive vagal impulses from receptors in the lung parenchyma (Hering-Breuer reflex) result in inhibition of inspiration as the lung distends. Cutting the vagi results in slow, deep rhythmic respiration. Therefore, vagal reflexes serve to accelerate the central neural mechanism. At slow respiratory rates the stretch receptors increase in-

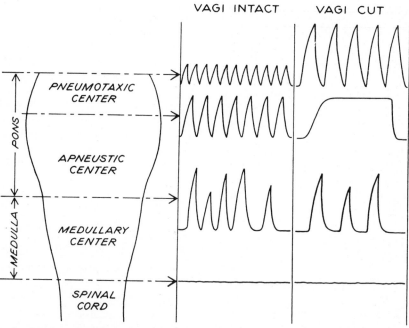

Figure 16.   Patterns of respiration after brain stem sections. The four patterns are representative of those that follow complete sections at each level. Section below the medulla results in complete apnea. (From Comroe, J. H.: *Physiology of Respiration*. Chicago, Year Book Medical Publishers, Inc., 1965.)

spiration slightly, while at rapid frequencies they inhibit inspiration. Thus, the peripheral component of the neural system complements the activity of the central neural centers. Stimulation of these receptors in conditions such as pulmonary edema and interstitial pulmonary fibrosis results in tachypnea. Although this reflex is active in normal animals and newborn infants, it seems to play no role in limiting inspiration in the adult human unless tidal volume is greater than one liter.

It is worthwhile noting that brain stem hemorrhage, although usually resulting in apnea, may initially be associated with tachypnea.

The respiratory control areas are also influenced by higher centers. Tachypnea, associated with fever, is presumably mediated by the influence of the hypothalamus on the brain stem centers. Furthermore, voluntary control of ventilation is possible within limits.

It is now apparent that the background of different stimuli through the medullary reticular system is important in maintaining the ability of respiratory neurons to discharge spontaneously. This concept of "neuronal traffic" has been implicated as an important mechanism in the newborn infant who begins to breathe spontaneously in association with the sensory stimuli associated with the birth process, and perhaps explains the lack of sustained respiration in utero.

A variety of peripheral reflexes are known to affect respiration. Hyperpnea may be produced by stimulation of pain, temperature or mechanoreceptors in the limbs. Visceral reflexes are usually associated with apnea, e.g., distention of the gallbladder or traction on the gut. Afferent impulses from muscle spindles of the intercostal muscles and diaphragm may play a role in determining the optimum response of the muscles of ventilation to various respiratory stimuli. In both neonatal animals and humans, an inspiratory gasp may be elicited by distention of upper airways. Although this reflex is mediated by the vagus, it is the opposite to that of the Hering-Breuer reflex inhibition of inflation and is known as Head's paradoxical reflex. It has been suggested that this inspiratory gasp reflex is important in the initial inflation of the lung at birth.

Chemical System

The neurohumoral system is primarily concerned with the regulation of alveolar ventilation and blood gases. This chemical control is mediated by two sets of specialized neural structures which are susceptible to changes in pH, P_{CO_2} and P_{O_2}, one, the central receptors, and the other, chromaffin tissue along the great vessels.

The exact location of the central chemoreceptors is uncertain. The most recent evidence suggests that chemoreceptive tissue is located along the ventral lateral medulla near the area postrema. Direct stimulation of this area by increased P_{CO_2} or H^+ produces an increase in ventilation, and conversely, a decreased P_{CO_2} or H^+ concentration causes a depression of ventilation. It has been suggested that this area is influenced primarily by the acid-base composition of cerebrospinal fluid and that the delay in ventilatory response to changes in arterial P_{CO_2} and bicarbonate is due to the time required to change the cerebrospinal fluid H^+ concentration. Carbon dioxide, which diffuses into the cerebrospinal fluid in a few minutes, has a rapid effect on the central chemoreceptors. Changes in blood bicarbonate are much less rapidly reflected in the cerebrospinal fluid (24 to 48 hours). Thus, with acute metabolic acidosis, arterial P_{CO_2} falls along with cerebrospinal fluid P_{CO_2}. Hyperventilation is produced by the H^+ stimulation of peripheral chemoreceptors, but this stimulus is inadequate to compensate fully for the metabolic acidosis because of inhibition from the decreased H^+ concentration in the cerebral spinal fluid. After 24 hours, cerebrospinal fluid bicarbonate falls and restores cerebrospinal fluid pH to normal. There is a further fall in arterial P_{CO_2}, and arterial pH returns toward normal. From these observations it has been suggested that the control of alveolar ventilation is a function of the central chemoreceptors which are under the influence of cerebrospinal fluid or brain interstitial fluid H^+, acting in association with the peripheral chemoreceptors, which are directly under the influence of the arterial blood (Table 8).

The peripheral chemoreceptors are embryologic remnants of the primitive gill system of respiration and are found in man along the structures associated with the branchial arches. Two sets of chemoreceptors appear to be of greatest physiologic importance: (1) the carotid bodies, located at the division of the common carotid artery into its internal and external branches, and (2) the aortic bodies, which lie between the ascending aorta and the pulmonary artery. Afferent nerves from the carotid body join the glossopharyngeal (IX) nerve; those from the aortic bodies join the vagosympathetic trunk along with the recurrent laryngeal nerves.

The carotid and aortic bodies are responsive primarily to changes in oxygen tension. At rest they are tonically active, signifying that some ventilatory drive exists even at a Pa_{O_2} of 100 mm. of mercury. Inhalation of 33 per cent oxygen reduces ventilation; inhalation of low oxygen mixtures is associated with a significant increase in ventilation when the Pa_{O_2} is less than 60 mm. of mercury. Potentiation of the hypoxic stimulus is achieved by an increase in Pa_{CO_2}. For example, at a Pa_{CO_2} of 50 mm. of mercury, ventilation is significantly increased when Pa_{CO_2} is lowered to 80 mm. Hypoxia and hypotension presumably act together to decrease the oxygen supply of the chemoreceptor tissue, resulting in a greater ventilatory response to hypoxia.

The response of the peripheral chemoreceptors to P_{CO_2} is rapid (within seconds), but ventilation increases only slightly until Pa_{CO_2} is increased by 10 mm. of mercury or more. More important than the amplitude of change may be the rate of change of Pa_{CO_2}. Recent evidence supports the hypothesis that the carotid bodies respond more to an oscillating Pa_{CO_2} than to a steady Pa_{CO_2} at the same mean level, because these chemoreceptors adapt to a constant stimulus in the same manner as do thermal or touch sensory receptors of the skin. Part of the hyperventilation of exercise may be accounted for on this basis, since oscillations of arterial P_{CO_2} of about 7 mm. of mercury accompany moderate exercise. The peripheral chemoreceptors play a minor role in the stimulation of respiration when there is central depression because they adapt to the constant Pa_{CO_2}, and respiration is maintained for the most part by the hypoxic drive alone.

The peripheral chemoreceptors, also

TABLE 8. ACID-BASE RELATIONSHIPS IN CEREBROSPINAL FLUID AND ARTERIAL BLOOD

		pH	P_{CO_2}	HCO_3^-	$\dot{V}_E$
Normal	Arterial blood	7.40	40	25	↔
	Cerebrospinal fluid	7.32	43	21	
Acute metabolic acidosis	Arterial blood	↓↓	↓	↓↓	↑
	Cerebrospinal fluid	↑	↓	↔	
Chronic metabolic acidosis	Arterial blood	↓	↓↓	↓↓	↑↑
	Cerebrospinal fluid	↔	↓↓	↓	
Acute hypoxia	Arterial blood	↑	↓	↔	↑
	Cerebrospinal fluid	↑	↓	↔	
Chronic hypoxia, as at high altitude	Arterial blood	↑↑	↓↓	↓	↑↑
	Cerebrospinal fluid	↔	↓↓	↓	

responsive to changes in arterial pH, increase ventilation in association with a fall of 0.1 pH unit, and produce a twofold to threefold increase with a fall of 0.4 pH unit. Some investigators believe that the peripheral chemoreceptor response is mediated through changes in intracellular hydrogen ion concentration. Direct proof of this hypothesis is lacking.

Response to Hypercapnia and Hypoxia in the Newborn Infant

There is special interest in the control of breathing in the newborn infant, since this is the period of transition from the intrauterine apneic state to extrauterine existence, which depends on the lung as the organ of gas exchange.

Infants are known to increase ventilation in response to inspired carbon dioxide. When infants (both premature and full-term) and adults are compared by ventilation per kilogram of body weight, all infants breathe more at a given P_{CO_2} than adults do, presumably because of a higher P_{CO_2} production per kilogram and less buffering capacity of the blood. Yet the change in ventilation per millimeter of mercury change in P_{CO_2} is the same in infants and adults, suggesting that their neurochemical apparatus has the same sensitivity, but that the ventilatory response is a function of body mass. Recently, this concept has been challenged, since it has been pointed out that the ventilatory response to CO_2 may be impaired because of mechanical factors such as a stiff lung or chest wall. Measurements using a new approach to the estimate of respiratory center output, by measuring the mouth pressure generated during brief airway occlusion, suggest that pre-term infants may not respond as well as the term infant or adult to inspired CO_2. Maturation of this response is a function of gestational age as well as of postnatal age.

Peripheral chemoreceptors are functional in newborn infants as demonstrated by a slight decrease in $\dot{V}_E$ with 100 per cent oxygen breathing. The effect of hypoxia as a stimulant may differ in the first 12 hours of life; 12 per cent of oxygen in the first 12 hours of life fails to stimulate ventilation. Presumably the atypical response reflects persistent fetal shunts which affect the oxygen tensions of blood perfusing the carotid body. In addition, the pre-term infant has been found to increase his ventilation only transiently to a hypoxic stimulus, whereas the term infant and the adult will have a sustained increase in ventilation.

Derangements

PERIODIC BREATHING. Periodic breathing is commonly seen in otherwise normal premature infants. It is characterized by a period of apnea lasting three to 10 seconds followed by a period of ventilation for 10 to 15 seconds. The average respiratory rate is 30 to 40 per minute; the rate during the ventilatory interval is 50 to 60 per minute. It is rarely seen during the first 24 hours of life and disappears by 38 to 40 weeks postconceptual age. Periodic breathing may appear intermittently interspersed by long periods of regular breathing. During periodic breathing infants appear more wakeful, with tremors of the tongue and extremities, and movements of the eyes. This resembles the rapid eye movement (REM) stage of sleep in the adult, which can also be associated with periodic or Cheyne-Stokes respiration. Also, as in the adult with Cheyne-Stokes respiration, periodic breathing is associated with mild hyperventilation, resulting in slightly alkalotic arterial blood (mean pH 7.44) compared with regular breathers (mean pH 7.39). Average arterial P_{CO_2} is approximately 3 to 4 mm. of mercury lower during periodic breathing. During the apneic period, P_{CO_2} increases by 6 to 7 mm. of mercury, and this increased cyclic change in Pa_{CO_2} may be responsible for the slight hyperventilation (see peripheral chemoreceptors, p. 55). Immaturity of the central integrating mechanism responsible for the integration of chemical and nonchemical ventilatory stimuli may be responsible for periodic breathing. Another possibility is that inhibition of normal intercostal reflexes during the REM stage of sleep may lead to periodicity.

APNEIC SPELLS. Apneic spells, characterized by more than 20 seconds of apnea with bradycardia, occur frequently in distressed premature infants and may be repetitive. They denote serious underlying disease. In one series, 70 per cent of premature infants died after a prolonged apneic spell, in contrast to 15 per cent of full-term infants. A decrease in arterial oxygen saturation from 95 to 81 per cent follows 25 seconds of apnea, with concomitant carbon dioxide retention and acidosis.

The cause is obscure. Some attacks follow feeding and appear to be associated with aspiration; some may be secondary to central nervous system depression. Of those who die, 33 per cent have associated intracranial hemorrhage, but whether the bleeding is primary or secondary to the prolonged apnea remains obscure. Paradoxical movement of the chest wall has recently been described in some pre-term infants, particularly during REM sleep. That is, the lower rib cage retracts instead of expanding during inspiration. It has been suggested that such a distortion, if rapid, may stimulate an intercostal-phrenic inhibitory reflex, leading to prolonged apnea.

DYSAUTONOMIA (RILEY-DAY SYNDROME). This rare disease, first recognized in 1949, is characterized by some degree of mental and physical retardation, deficient lacrimation, excessive sweating, transient hypertension, postural hypotension, attacks of cyclic vomiting, absent knee jerks, absence of the papillae of the tongue, and blotchy skin. It occurs predominantly in Jewish children and may or may not be associated with mental deficiency. Recurrent pulmonary infiltrations are thought to be the result of a defective swallowing mechanism with associated aspiration. Studies of the control of

breathing in these patients show that they are less responsive to changes in Pa_{CO_2} and oxygen tensions than normal subjects are, perhaps from peripheral chemoreceptor dysfunction. Since they do not have a normal ventilatory drive from changes in arterial P_{CO_2} and P_{O_2}, protection from high altitude and a warning against breath-holding during swimming may be important considerations.

PICKWICKIAN SYNDROME (PRIMARY ALVEOLAR HYPOVENTILATION). This condition, although common in obese adults, is rarely seen in children. It is characterized by extreme obesity and an elevated arterial P_{CO_2}, which may result in somnolence. In these patients, gastric distention following a meal may acutely elevate the Pa_{CO_2}. The hypoventilation is probably due to the increased work of breathing produced by chest wall obesity or gastric distention; presumably in order to do less respiratory work, the body adjusts to an elevated arterial P_{CO_2} with retention of bicarbonate.

Respiratory Stimulants and Depressants

Some of the factors known to influence alveolar ventilation are presented in Table 9.

Non–Gas Exchange Function of the Respiratory Tract

A chapter devoted to the functional basis of respiratory disease would be incomplete without a brief consideration of some of the non–gas exchange functions of the respiratory tract that are important in the understanding of the pathogenesis of pulmonary disease. The respiratory apparatus designed for gas exchange with the environment in the adult man requires that over 9000 liters of air be ventilated daily. The respiratory tract therefore provides a major source of contact between man and his environment and must contain an elaborate defensive mechanism to

TABLE 9. SOME FACTORS KNOWN TO INFLUENCE RESPIRATION

Stimuli	Depressants
CORTICAL	
Anxiety	Increased intracranial pressure
Pontine lesions	Electrocution
Cerebral hemorrhage	Cerebral hemorrhage
Voluntary control is possible within limits	
THERMAL	
Gram-negative septicemia	Hibernation
Fever	Sudden chilling
Sudden chilling	
CHEMICAL	
Arterial P_{CO_2} up to about 80 mm. Hg	Arterial P_{CO_2} over 80 mm. Hg
Rapid rate of change of arterial P_{CO_2}	Arterial pH less than 6.9 or over 7.5
Arterial pH 7.0–7.4	Profound hypoxia
Arterial P_{O_2} less than about 60–80 mm. Hg (in adults)	
(Newborn infants with only mild hypoxemia are stimulated by inspired oxygen)	
PHARMACOLOGIC	
Epinephrine	Morphine
Lobeline	Barbiturates
Nicotine	Chloramphenicol
Salicylates	Neomycin
Picrotoxin	Anesthetic gases, etc.
Nikethamide	
Progesterone	
PULMONARY REFLEXES	
Deflation receptors (Hering-Breuer)	Stretch receptors
Stretch receptors (Head's reflex)	Aortic arch and carotid sinus stretch receptors
PRESSORECEPTORS	
Decrease in blood pressure	Increase in blood pressure
BONES AND JOINTS	
Stretch receptors in muscles	Tactile responses
Tactile responses	

protect itself against such damaging agents as bacteria and other particles or noxious gases that may pollute the atmosphere.

The lung defenses against noxious gases are poor and include a reflex apnea on exposure to an irritant gas, absorption of a gas such as sulfur dioxide on the moist epithelial surface of the nasal cavity or tracheobronchial tree, or local detoxification.

The respiratory tract is better equipped to deal with inhaled particles. Because of turbulence and inertial impaction, particles larger than 10 μ in diameter are largely filtered out in the nose; those between 2 and 10 μ settle out onto the mucous blanket of the tracheobronchial epithelium. Ninety per cent of the particles greater than 2 to 3 μ settle out on the mucociliary blanket. Smaller particles in the range of 0.5 to 3 μ penetrate to the alveolar ducts and alveoli where 90 per cent are deposited by gravitational forces and, to a lesser extent, by Brownian movement. Smaller particles show no appreciable deposition and are exhaled. Humidification of incoming air causes hygroscopic particles to increase in size and thus impact at a higher point in the tracheobronchial tree.

Once deposited, particles are subject to several excretory transport mechanisms. The mucous lining layer is propelled by ciliary activity at the rate of 10 to 20 mm. per minute so that 90 per cent of the material deposited on the mucosa is physically cleared within an hour. Particles deposited distal to the ciliated columnar epithelium are cleared much more slowly and depend on the rate of phagocytosis by alveolar or interstitial macrophages and the rate of fluid transport from alveoli to the mucociliary blanket. Fluid transport is probably the mechanism for the clearance of about 50 per cent of the deposited material in 24 hours. The second phase of alveolar clearance has a half-life of 100 hours and may reflect interstitial fluid flow mechanisms. The third phase has a half-life of 60 to 100 days and is likely due to movement of particles to perivascular channels where removal is very slow.

Ciliary activity carries particles and macrophages on the mucous lining layer of the respiratory epithelium to larger bronchi where the cough reflex is important in clearance. Ciliary activity is influenced by numerous agents. Ciliary motion is stimulated by acetylcholine, inorganic ions, weak acids and low concentrations of local anesthetics. It is inhibited by low humidity, alcohol, cigarette smoke, oxygen and other noxious gases.

In addition to these transport mechanisms, the lung is capable of detoxifying potentially injurious particles such as bacteria. Phagocytosis by alveolar macrophages and tissue histiocytes is the major defensive response to particles less than 3μ and has been shown to be impaired by smoking, air pollutants such as ozone, and high concentrations of oxygen. Immunoglobulins such as IgA in normal lung and IgM and IgG in inflamed lung appear to have opsonic activity and thus enhance phagocytosis. In addition, recent studies have indicated that IgA on epithelial surfaces, such as the respiratory tract, contains specific neutralizing antibodies and is the major determinant of immunity against viral infection. IgA is actively secreted onto respiratory epithelium and requires the addition of a secretory "piece" (S) to two molecules of circulating IgA. Thus, although serum IgA levels may be normal, there may be an impaired ability to secrete IgA onto epithelial surfaces. Deficient secretory IgA has been described in normal newborn infants, in patients with recurrent sinopulmonary infection, and in ataxic telangiectasia.

In addition to an elaborate defense mechanism, the lung has other non–gas exchange functions. The lung is a site of active metabolism. It has been estimated that this organ normally utilizes as much as 10 per cent of the total oxygen consumed, and this level appears to increase with pulmonary disorders such as cancer and tuberculosis. This high level of oxygen consumption is not surprising because of the presence of cellular elements possessing high metabolic activity. One of these is the type II cell responsible for surfactant biosynthesis. Alveolar macrophages have a high respiratory rate, some ten times that of the polymorphonuclear leukocyte and three times that of the monocyte. It has been estimated that the lung contains some 600,000,000 alveolar macrophages.

Another aspect of the metabolic activity of the lung is its ability to influence the circulating level of certain vasoactive substances. The lung is capable of inactivating circulating bradykinin, prostaglandins, serotonin and histamine, but it has little effect on epinephrine. The lung also contains an enzyme that is responsible for converting the relatively inactive polypeptide angiotensin I to the potent vasoconstrictor angiotensin II and is capable of this conversion even in early fetal life. The lung is capable of synthesizing certain vasoactive substances such as histamine and prostaglandins.

Consideration of some of the non–gas exchange functions of the lung has only recently received increasing attention but is of obvious importance in our understanding of pulmonary disease. These functions are considered in greater detail in Chapter 2.

CLINICAL APPLICATION OF PULMONARY FUNCTION STUDIES

Changing dimensions of lung structure with age, the mechanical properties of the lungs, properties of gases and gas exchange, consideration of blood flow to the lungs, aspects of the regulation of respiration, and a brief consideration of non–gas exchange functions of the lung compose the substance of this chapter. The preceding sections are a distillate of an extensive literature, largely accumulated since World War II.

It remains to evaluate the role of measurements of lung function, only briefly discussed, in the practice of pediatrics. The pediatrician who approaches a child with respiratory symptoms relies first on an etiologic classification of disorders in differential diagnosis. Are the symptoms the result of an infection, foreign body aspiration, trauma, congenital malformation, allergic manifestation or tumor? Another question concerns the anatomic localization of the disease. Is the upper or lower respiratory tract primarily affected? The majority of respiratory illnesses can be successfully diagnosed and managed without recourse to measurements of lung function.

The role of the pulmonary function laboratory is chiefly to quantify the severity of the derangement and the response to therapy. In practice, the most useful measurement is the partial pressure of carbon dioxide in arterial or "arterialized" capillary blood, since the most important question concerns the adequacy of ventilation. An unconscious patient, or one with respiratory muscle weakness or severe pulmonary disease, will need assisted ventilation when the P_{CO_2} rises to narcotic levels. The only way to monitor the efficacy of a respirator is to follow the arterial carbon dioxide tensions. The carbon dioxide–combining power alone is not an adequate determination. Metabolic acidosis is frequently present in conditions that cause respiratory failure, and the carbon dioxide–combining power may be normal or low in combined respiratory and metabolic acidosis.

Measurements of arterial oxygen saturation or tension are of value in assessing the magnitude of venous admixture that may exist with severe ventilation-perfusion imbalance, or anatomic shunts. Oxygen measurements are important in guiding appropriate oxygen administration. Since too little oxygen is lethal and too much is associated with toxic effects, serial measurements are necessary.

The only other widely used measurement is the vital capacity. Since patient cooperation is required, the measurement has limited usefulness in very sick patients, and is not usually feasible in those under five years of age. Its value is in following the course of chronic pulmonary disease.

The timed vital capacity, or one-second forced expiratory volume, has the same limitations as the vital capacity. It is useful as an index of lower airway obstructive disease. The timed vital capacity and peak flow rate are the most simple measurements to evaluate the role of bronchodilators, e.g., in asthma.

Angiography and cardiac catheterization contribute essential information in delineating malformations of the pulmonary vessels and the presence of pulmonary hypertension.

Bronchoscopy and bronchography are indispensable tools in localizing abnormalities in the major airways.

The other functional evaluations, such as measurement of diffusion capacity, distribution of ventilation, radioscans, functional residual capacity, compliance and resistance, require more elaborate instrumentation and experience. Such measurements can be done in selected children, and are clinically useful in a few rare situations. For practical purposes, they should be considered research and teaching tools.

It behooves the student of pulmonary diseases to understand the physiologic derangements that contribute to the symptoms; to appreciate the necessity of measuring blood gases; and to know when further functional evaluations are pertinent.

REFERENCES

Avery, M. E., and Fletcher, B. D.: *The Lung and Its Disorders in the Newborn Infant.* 3rd Ed. Philadelphia, W. B. Saunders Company, 1974.

Aviado, D.: *Lung Circulation.* Vols. I and II. New York. Pergamon Press, 1965.

Bates, D. V., MacKlem, P. T., and Christie, R. V.: *Respiratory Function in Disease.* 2nd Ed. Philadelphia, W. B. Saunders Company, 1971.

Cherniack, R. M., Cherniack, L., and Naimark, A.: *Respiration in Health and Disease.* 2nd Ed. Philadelphia, W. B. Saunders Company, 1972.

Comroe, J. H., Jr.: *Physiology of Respiration.* Chicago, Year Book Medical Publishers, Inc., 1962.

Comroe, J. H., Jr., and others: *The Lung: Clinical Physiology and Pulmonary Function Tests.* 2nd Ed. Chicago, Year Book Medical Publishers, Inc., 1962.

Cunningham, D. J. C., and Lloyd, B. B.: *The Regulation of Human Respiration* (J. S. Haldane Centenary Symposium). Oxford, Blackwell Scientific Publications, 1963.

Davenport, H.: *The ABC of Acid Base Chemistry.* 4th Ed. Chicago, University of Chicago Press, 1958.

De Reuck, A. V. S., and O'Conner, M. (Eds.): *Ciba Foundation Symposium on Pulmonary Structure and Function.* London, J. & A. Churchill, Ltd., 1961.

De Reuck, A. V. S., and Porter, R. (Eds.): *Ciba Foundation Symposium on Development of the Lung.* London, J. & A. Churchill, Ltd., 1967.

Fenn, W. O., and Rahn, H. (Eds.): *Handbook of Physiology:* Section 3, Respiration. Vols. I and II. Washington, D. C., American Physiological Society, 1964, 1965.

Green, G. M.: In defense of the lung. *Am. Rev. Resp. Dis., 102*:691, 1970.

Negus, V.: *The Biology of Respiration.* Baltimore, Williams & Wilkins Company, 1965.

Rossier, P. H., Buhlman, A. A., and Wiesinger, K.: *Respiration. Physiological Principles and Their Clinical Applications.* Translated by P. C. Luchsinger and K. M. Moser. St. Louis, C. V. Mosby Company, 1960.

Safar, P. (Ed.): *Respiratory Therapy.* Philadelphia, F. A. Davis Company, 1965.

Said, S. I.: The lung as a metabolic organ. *N. Engl. J. Med., 279*:1330, 1968.

CHAPTER TWO

METABOLIC AND ENDOCRINE FUNCTIONS OF THE LUNG

SAMI I. SAID, M.D.

In examining the mechanisms and effects of pulmonary diseases (in children or in adults), it is helpful to view the lung not merely in terms of its ability to perform the vital processes of ventilation and gas exchange, but also as an organ with multiple metabolic and endocrine activities. These activities play an important role in the maintenance of normal structure and function, and in the pathogenesis or mediation of many pulmonary disorders.

SOME PULMONARY CELLS OF IMPORTANCE IN METABOLIC FUNCTION AND DYSFUNCTION

The lung is made up of numerous cell types; some of these that are especially related to metabolic events in the lung are listed here, with comments on their probable function or role in disease.

Large Alveolar Cell (great alveolar cell, type II alveolar cell, granular pneumonocyte)

Having an abundant cytoplasm that is rich in mitochondria, endoplasmic reticulum and lamellated, electron-dense inclusion bodies (Fig. 1), this cell is credited with the biosynthesis and secretion of alveolar surfactant. Massive injury to this cell, or its immaturity, is associated with large-scale atelectasis, as in the respiratory distress syndrome (hyaline membrane disease). This is also the one alveolar epithelial cell that can proliferate in response to alveolar injury.

Flat Alveolar Cell (small, type I pneumonocyte)

By contrast, this cell has a thin shell of cytoplasm with few cytoplasmic organelles (Fig. 1), and has no known specific metabolic activity. Flat epithelial cells constitute the major portion of alveolar surface area, and are vulnerable to the toxic effects of high P_{O_2} and inhaled chemical irritants, but are incapable of mitotic division. Regeneration of these cells takes place by division of type II cells, and their subsequent transformation into type I cells.

Alveolar Macrophage

The lung's chief defense against invading bacteria and other foreign particles, this cell functions like other phagocytic cells (e.g., the monocyte), but has distinguishing morphologic and metabolic features (Fig. 2). The proteo-

62

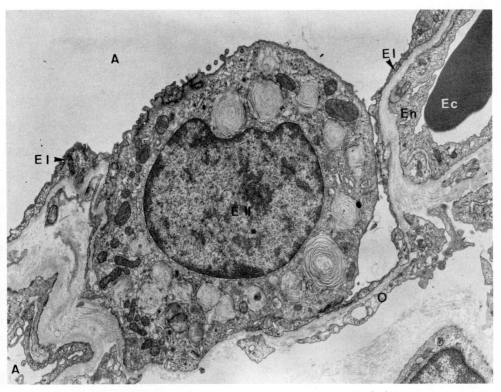

Figure 1.   Alveolar epithelial type II cell *(E II)* showing numerous lamellar bodies. Shown also are epithelial type I cells *(E I)* and a capillary. (*A*, Alveolar space; *Ec,* erythrocyte in capillary; *En,* endothelium.) (Human lung, × 13,340; courtesy of Drs. Ewald R. Weibel, M. Bachofen, and Joan Gil, Bern, Switzerland.)

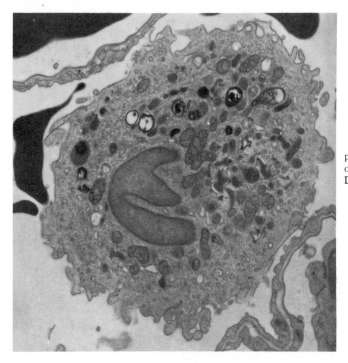

Figure 2. Alveolar macrophage (rat lung, × 3400; courtesy of Dr. Rolland C. Reynolds, Dallas, Texas.)

lytic and other hydrolytic enzymes normally contained within the lysosomal granules of these cells may, if released, cause profound lung damage and destruction.

Endothelial Cell

This cell (Fig. 3) appears to play a key role in the pulmonary metabolism of vasoactive hormones, e.g., the activation of angiotensin I to angiotensin II, and the inactivation of bradykinin.

Mast Cell

Located in bronchial mucosa (Fig. 4) and alveolar wall, around small blood vessels and in the pleura, this cell is packed with metachromatic, electron-dense granules that contain biogenic amines, heparin, and various enzymes. The mast cell is the chief target cell for immediate hypersensitivity reactions, typical of hay fever and extrinsic asthma.

Smooth Muscle and Other Contractile Elements

Throughout the tracheobronchial tree there are smooth muscle cells that contract or relax in response to neurohumoral influences, causing narrowing or dilatation of the airways. Smooth muscle also occurs in alveolar ducts, and its contraction leads to expulsion of air. Although there is no smooth muscle in alveoli, alveolar walls contain special "contractile interstitial cells."

Mucus-secreting and Other Glandular Cells

Normal bronchial secretion results from contribution from cells secreting mucus and others secreting serous fluid. Abnormalities in bronchial secretion could result from altered proportions or properties of these two constituents. Examples are increased mucus production, as in chronic bronchitis (where goblet cells are increased in number and size and may extend to

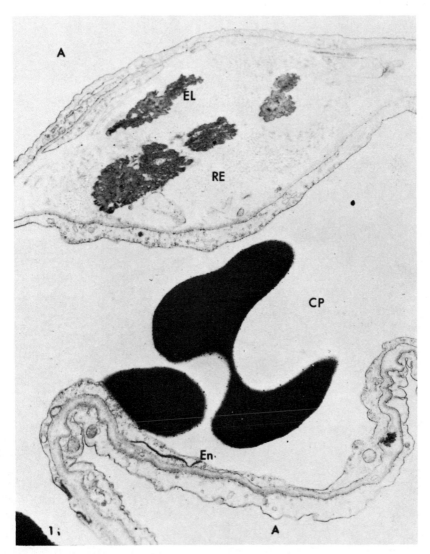

Figure 3. Portion of alveolar-capillary septum, showing capillary *(CP)*, endothelium *(En)*, and connective tissue. *(EL,* Elastin; *RE,* reticulin; *A*, alveolar space.) (Human lung, × 8400; courtesy of Dr. Rolland C. Reynolds, Dallas, Texas.)

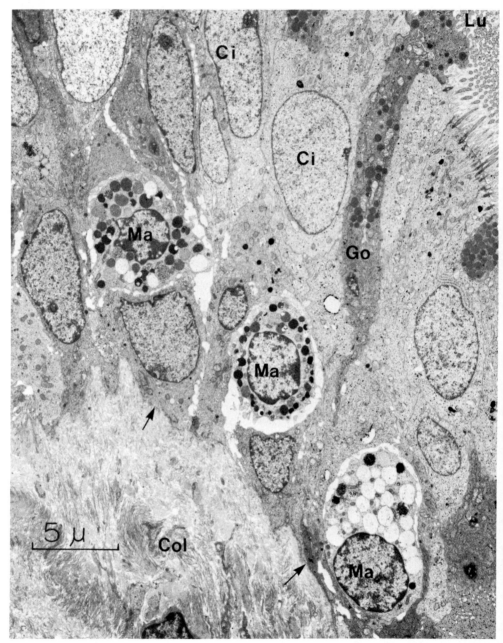

Figure 4. Section of lung biopsy from an asthmatic subject, showing mast cells *(Ma)* within the bronchial mucosa. The mast cells are wedged between ciliated *(Ci)* and goblet *(Go)* cells, and are distributed along the basement membrane *(arrows)*. *(Col,* Collagen deposit beneath the basement membrane; *Lu* lumen.) (× 6000; courtesy of Dr. Ernest Cutz, Toronto. Reproduced with permission from Lichtenstein, L. M., and Austen, K. F. (Eds.): *Asthma: Physiology, Immunopharmacology and Treatment.* Vol. 2. New York, Academic Press [in press].)

terminal bronchioles); decreased water content, as from excessive evaporation through a tracheostomy; and qualitative changes, as in cystic fibrosis.

Ciliary Epithelium

Ciliated epithelial cells (Fig. 5), extending distally just short of the alveolar ducts, provide the coordinated, rhythmic force that propels the overlying "mucus blanket" toward the upper respiratory passages and the oropharynx.

Connective Tissue

Comprising ground substance (proteoglycans), elastin, elastic fibers, collagen and reticulin, connective tissue is present in the airways, lung parenchyma and blood vessels (Fig. 3). Normal connective tissue provides structural support for the lung and airways, and abnormalities of connective tissue are of central importance in certain lung diseases, especially emphysema and interstitial fibrosis (fibrosing alveolitis).

Neuroendocrine Cells

In addition to the mast cells, which have neuroendocrine properties and characteristics, the lung contains cellular elements that synthesize, store or secrete neurohumoral products. Among these cells is the *Kulchitsky cell*. Morphologically similar to its counter-

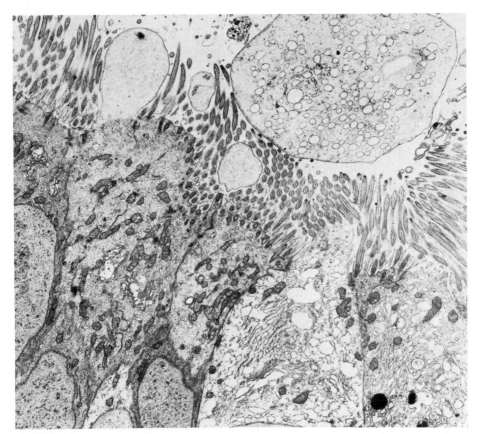

Figure 5. Ciliated bronchial epithelium. A goblet cell is seen in section. (Human lung, × 8000; courtesy of Dr. Rolland C. Reynolds, Dallas Texas.)

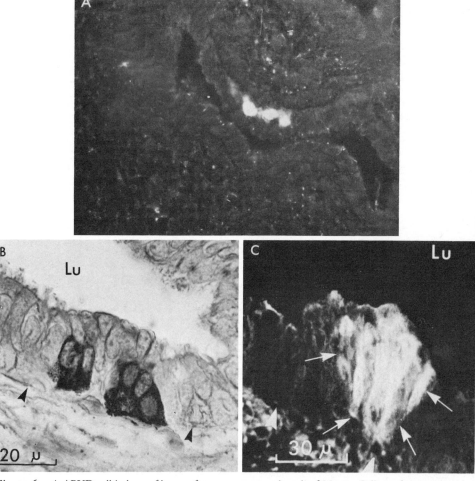

Figure 6.   *A,* APUD-cell in lung of human fetus, crown-rump length of 95 mm. Cell was demonstrated by formaldehyde-induced fluorescence, which depends on the presence of catecholamines. (× 40; courtesy of Dr. Esther Hage, Odense, Denmark.) *B,* Group of argyrophilic cells forming a "neuroepithelial body" within the bronchial mucosa of human lung. The cells are resting on the basement membrane *(arrows)* and do not extend to the lumen *(Lu).* (Grimelius' silver-nitrate stain, × 1000.) *C,* Intensely fluorescent, amine-containing cells *(arrows)* within the bronchial mucosa of rabbit lung. The apical surfaces of these cells are in contact with the lumen *(Lu).* (L-DOPA incubation, formaldehyde-induced fluorescence, × 640. B and C courtesy of Dr. Ernest Cutz, Toronto. Reproduced with permission from Lichtenstein, L. M., and Austen, K. F. (Eds.): *Asthma: Physiology, Immunopharmacology and Treatment.* Vol. 2. New York, Academic Press [in press].)

part by the same name in the gastrointestinal tract, this cell is believed to give rise to bronchial carcinoid tumors, as well as to oat cell carcinoma.

Other neuroendocrine cells have been referred to as *APUD cells,* an acronym derived from certain cytochemical features they have in common: amine-content, amine-precursor uptake, and decarboxylation. The APUD cells occur in many organs that are apparently unrelated, e.g., pituitary, thyroid (C cells), pancreatic islets, adrenal medulla, stomach and small intestine. In addition to the histochemical features that earned them their name, these cells also share in the presence of characteristic electron-dense granules, in their ability to secrete polypeptide hormones, and in their probable common embryologic ancestry from neural ectoderm.

APUD cells are demonstrable in fetal, newborn and mature lungs (Fig. 6). More recently, clusters of cells with probable neuroendocrine function have been described in bronchial and bronchiolar epithelium. These groups of cells, called "neuroepithelial bodies," are ultrastructurally similar to the APUD cells, and contain argyrophilic, serotonin-rich granules that are depleted on exposure to hypoxia. The likely neuroendocrine role of neuroepithelial bodies is accented by their rich afferent and efferent innervation.

SOME METABOLIC AND ENDOCRINE FUNCTIONS OF THE LUNG

Biosynthesis and Secretion of the Surface-active Lipoprotein that Forms Alveolar Surfactant

The alveoli of human and other mammalian lungs are lined with a thin layer of surface-active material, which regulates surface tension at the air-liquid interface. Investigation into the composition, biosynthesis, cellular origin,

secretion, and metabolism of surfactant has been a major stimulus to the study of pulmonary metabolism as a whole.

The main component of alveolar surfactant is dipalmitoyl lecithin (phosphatidylcholine), probably present as a complex with a protein. The main mechanism for de novo synthesis of this phospholipid is the phosphorylation of choline, followed by its conversion to cytidine diphosphate, and the incorporation of the latter compound with a diglyceride molecule to form phosphatidylcholine (lecithin). Another biosynthetic pathway, the formation of phosphatidylethanolamine and its subsequent methylation, appears to be of minor importance in human lung.

Surfactant is probably synthesized and secreted by the great alveolar cell. The primary function of surfactant is to stabilize the alveoli by preventing excessive increases or unevenness in alveolar surface forces. Reduction of surface tension by surfactant reduces the pressure required to fill the alveoli during inspiration and helps to maintain alveolar patency at a given pressure during expiration. Surfactant is also a factor in guarding against transudation of fluid into the alveoli. Thus, its absence or deficiency predictably leads to large-scale atelectasis and pulmonary edema.

The formation and maintenance of normal surfactant depends upon several factors, including the maturity of the great alveolar cells and their biosynthetic enzyme systems, the adequacy of blood flow to the alveolar walls (normally from the pulmonary arterial circulation) a normal rate of turnover, and the absence of inhibitors. There are other influences of possible physiologic importance. For example, glucocorticoids and thyroid hormone, in pharmacologic doses, can accelerate the maturation of the great alveolar cells and the secretion of surfactant in fetal lungs (see section on Metabolic Basis of Pulmonary Disease). The possible effect of innervation on function of alveolar cells is unknown.

Numerous clinical and experimental

situations are associated with inadequacy of surfactant. This inadequacy could be due mainly to insufficient formation (e.g., in prematurity); to inactivation as by certain constituents of serum and by some lipids (e.g., in pulmonary edema and alveolar proteinosis); or to both factors (e.g., after pulmonary arterial occlusion and in the "respiratory distress syndrome" of infants or adults). Excessively rapid depletion and incomplete regeneration of surfactant may complicate breathing at extremes of lung volumes. The relative importance of surfactant deficiency in these and similar states is difficult to ascertain. Even if it is not the sole or the primary lesion, however, this deficiency is certain to contribute to compromised lung function.

Defense Against Infectious Agents and Other Foreign Particles

This important function depends on the combined effects of several mechanisms:

1 CAPACITY OF ALVEOLAR MACROPHAGES TO PHAGOCYTOSE BACTERIA AND OTHER PARTICULATE MATTER. The phagocytic and bactericidal effectiveness of alveolar macrophages depends in part on the presence of stimulated lymphocytes. Such lymphocytes induce activation of macrophages, enhancing their phagocytic and bactericidal abilities.

2 MUCOCILIARY TRANSPORT. Responsible for clearance of the airways, this mechanism, in turn, depends on the presence of mucus with normal viscoelastic properties, ciliary contractile proteins and an adequate source of energy for their contraction. Ciliotoxic agents include high CO_2 concentrations, sulfur dioxide, cigarette smoke, alcohol, hypoxia, some viruses and *Mycoplasma pneumoniae*. Despite the apparent importance of ciliary function, its absence, reported in patients with Kartagener's syndrome, is not incompatible with life.

3 IMMUNE MECHANISMS. These include blood-borne immunoglobulins; local (secretory) immunoglobulins, principally IgA; and the T cell–mediated reactions that constitute cell-mediated (delayed) immunity.

Metabolism, Synthesis and Release of Vasoactive Hormones

The lung has the only capillary bed through which the entire blood flow passes, making the pulmonary capillary circulation uniquely suited for exercising a controlling influence on circulating vasoactive hormones. These hormones have many and diverse actions on all smooth muscle organs, such as the blood vessels, the bronchi and alveolar ducts, the gastrointestinal system and the uterus. Certain vasoactive substances (e.g., the prostaglandins and catecholamines) also affect various metabolic functions throughout the body, including metabolism of lipids, carbohydrates and the cyclic nucleotides.

Some vasoactive compounds are normal constituents of blood; others are formed or activated only in abnormal circumstances, e.g., as a consequence of tissue injury or inflammation. In either case, pulmonary handling of a given active agent can modulate its physiologic or pharmacologic effects. A summary of the metabolic alterations of some vasoactive agents by lung is given in Table 1. The conversion of angiotensin I to angiotensin II is the only known example of biologic activation by passage through the pulmonary circulation. Angiotensin II, up to 50 times more active than its precursor, is unaf-

TABLE 1. PULMONARY METABOLISM OF VASOACTIVE HORMONES

Activation
  Angiotensin I to angiotensin II
Inactivation
  Highly effective: Bradykinin, serotonin
    (5-hydroxytryptamine), PGE and $PGF_{2\alpha}$
  Partial: Norepinephrine, (?)histamine
Little or No Change
  Epinephrine, angiotensin II, vasopressin
    (ADH), PGA, VIP

fected by passage through the lung. The angiotensin-converting activity of lung is many times greater than that of plasma. Many vasoactive materials are partially or completely inactivated by the lung. Among those that are almost completely (more than 80 per cent) removed or inactivated are serotonin (5-hydroxytryptamine), bradykinin, adenosine 5′-triphosphate (ATP), and prostaglandins E_1, E_2 and $F_{2\alpha}$. Norepinephrine and histamine are taken up to lesser degrees.

Vasoactive hormones that pass through the lung without significant loss or gain in activity include epinephrine, prostaglandins A_1 and A_2, some bradykinin-like peptides such as eledoisin and polisteskinin, angiotensin II, vasopressin (ADH), and the recently isolated vasoactive intestinal peptide (VIP).

An interesting feature of the pulmonary metabolism of vasoactive hormones is its high selectivity. One member of a given group of substances (e.g., catecholamines, prostaglandins, kinins) may be removed in one passage, while another member of the same group is permitted to go through without change. In the case of compounds such as serotonin and norepinephrine, loss of activity in passage across the lung is mainly due to uptake and storage. In other instances the inactivation is by enzymic action (e.g., by a specific dehydrogenase acting on prostaglandins E and F) and by a peptidase breaking down bradykinin. Economy is another feature of the metabolism of vasoactive substances by the lung. Thus, the same enzyme that inactivates the vasodepressor bradykinin can also activate angiotensin I.

Although the cellular sites of these metabolic alterations are still undetermined, the endothelial cell, in intimate contact with blood, is a likely candidate. There is evidence that the pinocytotic vesicles of this cell, many of which communicate directly with the capillary lumen, take up ATP and other adenine nucleotides. Other cells, including the macrophage, the Kulchitsky and other neuroendocrine cells, and the mast cells, may participate in the metabolism of vasoactive hormones.

Vasoactive substances that are normally stored or synthesized within the lung may be discharged into the circulation in large quantities under certain pathologic influences. In anaphylaxis, for example, the lung releases histamine, "slow-reacting substances," bradykinin, prostaglandins and other pharmacologically active substances. Certain other pathologic conditions, including pulmonary embolism, mechanical distortion of the lung, respiratory alkalosis, alveolar hypoxia and pulmonary edema, stimulate the synthesis and release of potent chemicals, which may then contribute to the pathogenesis of such complications as systemic hypotension, pulmonary hypertension, and bronchial and alveolar duct constriction (see section on Metabolic Basis of Pulmonary Disease). For some actions of vasoactive agents, see Table 2.

TABLE 2. NATURE AND ACTIONS OF VASOACTIVE AGENTS

Agent	Action
Biogenic Amines	
Histamine Serotonin (5-HT)	Bronchoconstriction, alveolar duct constriction; increased capillary permeability
Polypeptides	
Bradykinin	Inflammation, increased capillary permeability
Angiotensin	Vasoconstriction, raised blood pressure, aldosterone release
Vasoactive lung peptides	Bronchoconstriction, systemic vasodilation
Proteins	
Kallikrein	Release of bradykinin
Complement	Immunologic injury
Lipids	
Prostaglandins (PGs) PG endoperoxides	Constriction of bronchi, alveolar ducts, pulmonary vessels; systemic vasodilation (PGE)
Thromboxanes	As above (more potent), plus platelet aggregation

Other vasoactive agents that are known to occur in lung tissue (and could therefore be released or activated following tissue damage) include kallikrein, newly identified vasoactive lung peptides, and probably other incompletely identified substances.

ILLUSTRATIONS OF THE METABOLIC BASIS OF PULMONARY DISEASE

Altered metabolic function may be a factor in the causation, or at least in the perpetuation or aggravation, of certain pulmonary disorders. Following are some examples.

Hyaline Membrane Disease (HMD)

This condition is estimated to affect at least 40,000 newborn babies in the United States annually. The incidence is directly related to the degree of prematurity, judged by gestational age or by birth weights below 2500 grams, and is as high as 81 per cent when birth weight is between 1001 and 1250 grams. Aside from prematurity, other factors predisposing to increased incidence of HMD include cesarean section and perinatal asphyxia.

Major advances have been made in recent years in the prenatal diagnosis, prevention and treatment of HMD. These advances have resulted directly from (1) discovery of the association and causal relationship between HMD and deficiency of pulmonary surfactant; (2) identification of dipalmitoyl lecithin (phosphatidylcholine) as the main surface-active component; (3) elucidation of the biosynthetic pathways of this compound by the mature and developing lung; and (4) the demonstration that amniotic fluid lipids could reveal evidence of pulmonary maturity.

Thus, it is now possible to predict fetal lung maturity from a determination of the ratio of lecithin to sphingomyelin (L/S) in amniotic fluid, obtained by amniocentesis. If the ratio is 2 or higher, HMD is extremely unlikely (less than 1 per cent). L/S ratios of less than 2 imply an increased likelihood of HMD, with an average incidence of approximately 45 to 55 per cent. Such a finding should call for a therapeutic response in the form of delaying delivery, if possible, or use of pharmacologic agents to enhance lung maturation. The latter approach is based on the observations that cortisol-receptors are present in fetal lung cells, and that cortisol can induce certain key enzymes of lecithin biosynthesis. Experimental and clinical trials show that intramuscular administration of the glucocorticoid betamethasone to expectant mothers with less than 32 completed weeks of gestation, more than 24 hours before delivery, reduces the incidence and mortality of HMD.

Another therapeutic advance has been the use of continuous positive pressure respiration, which prevents the lungs from reaching critically low volumes during expiration (thus guarding against atelectasis) and conserves alveolar surfactant (by avoiding its overcompression and disruption at minimal lung volumes).

Bronchial Asthma

In allergic bronchial asthma, the basic disease process is an interaction of inhaled, extrinsic antigens with tissue mast cells and basophil leukocytes in the presence of specific antibodies of the IgE class. This union sets off a cascade of metabolic reactions inside the mast cells, culminating in the release of biologically active mediators that bring about the episodic bronchoconstriction, increased mucus secretion and eosinophilic infiltration.

The identities of these mediators, their possible interactions, and the factors governing their formation and release are still under investigation. Much has been learned recently, some of it directly applicable to the treatment and prevention of this disease, but our knowledge remains incomplete. The best-known and, in many ways, the prototype of these mediators is *histamine*. It is concentrated within the granules of the mast cells and basophils, may be released from these cells or from lung tissue with appropriate immunologic challenge, and can induce some of the changes characteristic of an asthmatic attack—bronchoconstriction and increased capillary permeability. It seems unlikely, however, that histamine is the most important mediator, for it is well known that antihistaminics (antagonists of H_1-receptors) are practically useless in the treatment of asthma.

A variety of other chemical agents are now known to be released in the immediate hypersensitivity state, some of which have been fully identified but others only partially purified and characterized. The group includes, in addition to histamine and *serotonin, bradykinin*, the *"eosinophil-chemotactic factor* of anaphylaxis" (ECF–A), prostaglandins of the E and F series, and the much discussed, but still unidentified, *"slow-reacting substance of anaphylaxis."*

Very recently, three new groups of compounds have been discovered as potential mediators of bronchoconstriction and the associated changes in the asthmatic reaction. These are the *endoperoxides*, intermediate compounds formed during the biosynthesis of the prostaglandins, and approximately 10 times more potent than the PGs as bronchoconstrictors; the *thromboxanes*, which are about 100 times as potent as the PGs; and a newly isolated lung peptide that contracts most smooth muscle structures, known as the *spasmogenic lung peptide*. No pharmacologic antagonists are yet available to counter the effects of these newly identified, powerful substances, and so their relative importance as mediators remains to be determined.

Other Immunologic Disorders

In many other pulmonary diseases, the basic underlying disorder is an immunologic reaction. Such pulmonary diseases include:

GOODPASTURE'S SYNDROME. In this syndrome, an example of type II (cytotoxic) allergic reactions, injury to the alveolar and glomerular basement membranes results from the interaction of a tissue antigen and an antibody against both basement membranes.

EXTRINSIC ALLERGIC ALVEOLITIS. An example of type III (immune-complex) allergic disease, extrinsic allergic alveolitis results from inhaled antigens, most commonly thermophilic actinomycetes. Some of the entities belonging to this group are farmer's lung, bagassosis, and hypersensitivity pneumonitis due to contamination of ventilation and air conditioning systems.

EOSINOPHILIC PNEUMONIA. "Pulmonary infiltrates, eosinophilia and asthma," or *"eosinophilic pneumonia,"* most commonly results from a hypersensitivity to *Aspergillus fumigatus*, hence the name "allergic bronchopulmonary aspergillosis."

DISEASES RELATED TO CELL-MEDIATED (DELAYED) Hypersensitivity. T cell-mediated immunity and hypersensitivity are important mechanisms in the pulmonary defenses against intracellular organisms, e.g., *Mycobacterium tuberculosis, M. intracellulare* (Battey disease), *Histoplasma capsulatum, Coccidioides immitis, Cryptococcus neoformans, Listeria monocytogenes*, and the viruses of varicella, influenza and mumps. These reactions depend on activated lymphocytes secreting a number of soluble factors (lymphokines), which bring about the spectrum of responses constituting cell-mediated immunity and hypersensitivity.

Decreased or absent cell-mediated immunity (as manifested by absent skin reactivity to tuberculin and other allergens) is commonly seen in certain disorders, such as Hodgkin's disease and sarcoidosis.

Emphysema

Experimental evidence in animals and observations in human subjects suggest that a relative excess of proteolytic enzymes with a potential for attacking lung connective tissue, in relation to protease-inhibitors available for counteracting these enzymes, may be an underlying mechanism of emphysema. This protease-pathogenesis hypothesis offers great promise for understanding this disease, but it does not readily explain more than a fraction of the emphysema population.

Vascular Disorders

In a number of disorders of the pulmonary circulation, various vasoactive (and otherwise biologically active) substances may be released from the lung. This release, along with possible impairment of normal pulmonary inactivation of these substances, could have important effects on the lung and on the systemic circulation (Table 3), and could thus play an important contributory role in the pathogenesis of such vascular disorders as pulmonary thromboembolism, pulmonary microembolism (intravascular platelet aggregation), pulmonary edema, and the respiratory distress syndrome.

TABLE 3. SOME POSSIBLE EFFECTS
OF ALTERED PULMONARY
METABOLISM OF VASOACTIVE
HORMONES

Pulmonary
  Bronchoconstriction, alveolar duct constriction; pulmonary vasoconstriction; inflammation; increased capillary permeability; platelet aggregation.
Systemic
  Peripheral vasodilation, hypotension and shock; (?)hypertension; (?)other.

Endotoxin Shock and Other Conditions Associated with the Respiratory Distress Syndrome

Septic (endotoxin) shock is accompanied by the release of prostaglandins (especially PGE compounds) that contribute to the systemic hypotension and pulmonary hypertension.

Some of the features of endotoxin shock may be explained by the effects of two intravenous injections of endotoxin (spaced a day apart) in experimental animals. This procedure results in widespread fibrin thrombi in pulmonary and glomerular vessels, with bilateral renal cortical necrosis (generalized Shwartzman reaction). This reaction depends on the presence of granular leukocytes, which, together with the endotoxin, trigger the intravascular clotting.

The syndrome of disseminated intravascular coagulation may also complicate lung injury, presumably because lung tissue is rich in thromboplastin.

Other forms of shock and trauma may predispose to the respiratory distress syndrome (dyspnea, diffuse infiltrates, increasing arterial hypoxemia, with progressive stiffening of the lungs). Altered metabolic function of lung is probably an important pathogenetic factor in these conditions, but the precise alterations (e.g., release of active mediators) have not been defined.

Paraneoplastic Syndromes

Hypersecretion of hormones by pulmonary tumors may result in a variety of endocrine syndromes. These hormones are usually polypeptides or biogenic amines, and the tumors are most often of the oat cell variety. Table 4 gives a listing of the more common endocrine syndromes, together with the associated hormonal secretions and anatomic lesions.

Cystic Fibrosis

One of the more common and more serious diseases of children, this is an

TABLE 4.   HORMONAL SECRETION BY PULMONARY TUMORS:
PARANEOPLASTIC SYNDROMES

Hormone	Syndrome	Lesion
ACTH	Hypokalemic alkalosis, edema, Cushing's syndrome	Oat cell carcinoma, adenoma
ADH (arginine vasopressin)	Hyponatremia (SIADH)	Oat cell carcinoma, adenoma; also, tuberculosis, pneumonia, aspergillosis
PTH or related peptide	Hypercalcemia	Squamous cell carcinoma, adenocarcinoma and large-cell undifferentiated carcinoma
Gonadotropins	Gynecomastia (adults), precocious puberty (children)	Large-cell anaplastic carcinoma
Calcitonin	No clinical findings	Adenocarcinoma, squamous and oat cell carcinoma
VIP or related peptide	Watery diarrhea or no symptoms	Squamous, oat or large-cell carcinoma
Growth hormone(?)	Hypertrophic osteoarthropathy	Squamous cell carcinoma
Serotonin, kinins (and PGs)	"Carcinoid"	Bronchial adenoma, oat cell carcinoma
Insulin-like peptide	Hypoglycemia	Mesenchymal cell tumors
Glucagon or related peptide	Diabetes	Fibrosarcoma
Prolactin	Galactorrhea (or no symptoms)	Anaplastic cell carcinoma
Combination of above	Multiple syndromes	Anaplastic cell carcinoma

Abbreviations: ACTH, adrenocorticotropic hormone; SIADH, syndrome of inappropriate secretion of antidiuretic hormone; PTH, parathyroid hormone; PGs, prostaglandins; VIP, vasoactive intestinal polypeptide.

inherited disorder of all exocrine glands, but the cause of death is usually respiratory insufficiency. The basic underlying defect remains unknown, but there are some indications that metabolic alterations may be at play. Such alterations may account, in part, for the increased viscosity of bronchial and other secretions, and for the abnormal humoral factors reported in serum and other body fluids (inhibiting ciliary activity and sodium reabsorption, and enhancing degranulation of leukocytes).

Patent Ductus Arteriosus

It has recently been demonstrated that indomethacin, an inhibitor of prostaglandin biosynthesis, can induce the closure of patent ductus arteriosus in premature infants. The pharmacologic basis of this action is that prostaglandins, especially PGE compounds, increase ductal flow, apparently by dilating the ductus. This simple means of closing the ductus could be an important advance in the management of the respiratory distress syndrome of the newborn, where ductal shunt can aggravate cardiopulmonary dysfunction.

REFERENCES

Austen, K. F.: Reaction mechanisms in the release of mediators of immediate hypersensitivity from human lung tissue. *Fed. Proc., 33*:2256, 1974.

Austen, K. F., and Becker, E. L.: *Biochemistry of the Acute Allergic Reactions.* Oxford, Blackwell Scientific Publications, 1971.

Avery, M. E.: Pharmacological approaches to acceleration of fetal lung maturation. *Br. Med. Bull., 31*:13, 1975.

Cutz, E., Chan, W., Wong, V., and Conen, P. E.: Ultrastructure and fluorescence histochemistry of endocrine (APUD-type) cells in tracheal mucosa of human and various animal species. *Cell Tissue Res., 158*:425, 1975.

Di Sant'Agnese, P. A., and Davis, P. B.: Research in cystic fibrosis. *N. Engl. J. Med., 295*:481; 534; 597, 1976.

Farrell, P. M., and Avery, M. E.: Hyaline membrane disease. *Am. Rev. Resp. Dis., 111*:657, 1975.

Green, G. M.: The J. Burns Amberson Lecture—In defense of the lung. *Am. Rev. Resp. Dis.*, *102*:691, 1970.

Hage, E.: Endocrine cells in the bronchial mucosa of human foetuses. *Acta. Pathol. Microbiol. Scand.* [*A*], *80*:225, 1972.

Hall, T. C. (Ed.): Paraneoplastic syndrome. *Ann. N.Y. Acad. Sci.*, *230*:1, 1974.

James, L. S.: Perinatal events and respiratory distress syndrome. Editorial. *N. Engl. J. Med.*, *292*:1291, 1975.

Kaltreider, H. B.: Expression of immune mechanisms in the lung. *Am. Rev. Resp. Dis.*, *113*:347, 1976.

Kueppers, F., and Black, L. F.: Alpha₁-antitrypsin and its deficiency. *Am. Rev. Resp. Dis.*, *110*:176, 1974.

Lenfant, C. (Ed.): Monographs on *Lung Biology in Health and Disease.* New York, M. Dekker, Inc. 1976.

McCombs, P. P.: Diseases due to immunologic reactions in the lungs. *N. Engl. J. Med.*, *286*:1186, 1972.

Mittman, C. (Ed.): *Pulmonary Emphysema and Proteolysis.* New York, Academic Press, 1972.

Newhouse, M., Sanchis, J., and Bienenstock, J.: Lung defense mechanisms. *N. Engl. J. Med.*, *295*:990; 1045, 1976.

Said, S. I.: The lung as a metabolic organ. *N. Engl. J. Med.*, *279*:1330, 1968.

Said, S. I.: The lung in relation to vasoactive hormones. *Fed. Proc.*, *32*:1972, 1973.

Said, S. I.: The endocrine role of the lung in disease. *Am. J. Med.*, *57*:453, 1974.

Said, S. I.: The prostaglandins in relation to the lung: regulators of function, mediators of disease or therapeutic agents? *Bull. Physiopathol. Resp. (Nancy)*, *10*:411, 1974.

Said, S. I.: Metabolic event in the lung. In *Pathophysiology: Altered Regulatory Mechanisms in Disease.* 2nd Ed. Philadelphia, J. B. Lippincott Company, 1976, pp. 189–207.

Van Golde, L. M. G.: Metabolism of phospholipids in the lung. *Am. Rev. Resp. Dis.*, *114*:977, 1976.

Wood, R. E., Boat, T. F., and Doershuk, C. F.: Cystic fibrosis. *Am. Rev. Resp. Dis.*, *113*:833, 1976.

CHAPTER THREE

THE HISTORY AND PHYSICAL EXAMINATION

WILLIAM W. WARING, M.D.

THE HISTORY

GENERAL AIMS

All physicians know that history-taking for disease in a specific organ cannot be divorced from a general history. When the complaints are primarily pulmonary, however, parts of the general history should be emphasized in order to answer several broad questions:

1) Is the Present Episode Acute or Chronic and Is It Recurrent?

Certain diseases are self-limited, whereas others naturally tend to run protracted courses. A knowledge of the duration of symptoms or signs, therefore, can be of considerable diagnostic help. One may arbitrarily divide diseases of the respiratory tract of children into acute, subacute and chronic on the basis of presumed or known duration. A process of less than three weeks' duration may be termed "acute." A "subacute" process may persist from three weeks to three months, and any disease lasting more than three months should be considered "chronic." Frequently, such timing is based on the history of cough duration, but it may also be dated from a chest roentgenographic abnormality, abnormal pulmonary function test, any other test or sign, or any combination of these.

In setting duration, the physician should have good reason to believe that the disease has been continuous, such as a cough heard every day for a certain period. On the other hand, if there is a significant discontinuity of signs or symptoms, the disease is presumed to be "recurrent." In such cases, a factor predisposing to recurrence should be searched for, such as allergy or immunologic incompetence. Recurrent pulmonary disease may itself be classified as acute, subacute or chronic according to the above criteria.

The closer the symptom or sign is to birth, the greater the possibility that it is a manifestation of inherited disease or secondary to a congenital malformation.

2. Is the Process a Life-Threatening One, Either Immediately or Ultimately?

The threat to life has both diagnostic and therapeutic implications. The presence of cyanosis or severe stridor, for example, may indicate a presently dangerous situation. On the other hand, a progressive pulmonary opacification on a chest roentgenogram with increasing tachypnea implies diminishing pulmonary reserve and a serious long-term outlook. When the physician has decided that there is a substantial life-threatening potential involved, no diagnostic or therapeutic stone can be left unturned. Although the cause may not be known, there is diagnostic weight in the manner in which life is threatened, and this manner in turn frequently suggests appropriate therapy—intubation or tracheostomy for stridor or oxygen for cyanosis, for example.

3. What Is the "Inertia" of the Process?

The concept of inertia of a disease is implicit in medicine, but calls for some amplification. Disorders with low inertia begin and end rapidly, either naturally or artificially. Those with high inertia are more ponderous, being slower in onset and harder to stop. The term "inertia" has nothing to do with severity. Diseases of low inertia can be either mild or serious, as, for example, the common cold and acute lobar pneumococcal pneumonia. On the other hand, severe staphylococcal pneumonia and asymptomatic pulmonary histoplasmosis differ in severity, but both have greater inertia than the first two examples. A judgment on disease inertia is helpful in setting both the type and expected duration of treatment in each case. Advanced diseases of high inertia may require weeks or months of vigorous therapy.

4. Can the Process Be Categorized as Mainly Airway Obstructive or Space-Occupying (Restrictive) in the Chest?

The pulmonary function laboratory has been helpful in classifying pulmonary disease into either restrictive or obstructive components. Diseases that stiffen the lungs are termed "restrictive," whereas those that produce encroachment on the airways, either upper or lower, are "obstructive." Both types of abnormalities may exist in the same patient simultaneously. Patients with restrictive diseases are usually clinically recognizable by their fast, shallow respirations, whereas obstructive disease patients breathe noisily (wheeze or stridor) and, if the process diffusely involves lower airways, demonstrate a barrel-chest deformity and a relatively prolonged expiratory phase.

5. Does Infection Appear to Be Present?

The most helpful historical criteria of infection are fever, cervical lymphadenitis, and purulent discharges from the nares, ears or lungs (sputum).

6. What Has Been the Effect of Any Prior Treatment?

Careful attention should be given to the types of therapy that the patient has previously received. A history of paroxysmal wheezing relieved promptly by subcutaneous epinephrine establishes a past history of asthma and may shed light on the present wheezing or middle lobe atelectasis. Similarly, an illness suggesting pneumonia that has not responded to penicillin is probably not due to a pneumococcus.

7. Is the Patient's Disease a Familial One?

The health of the family should be investigated in all cases because there may be direct or indirect associations between it and the patient's disease. So-called ping-pong infections are frequently seen within the family. Familial disease may be explained by a common genetic background or by exposure to common infectious or physical agents. The same organism commonly has different and nonpulmonary manifestations. For example, a history of breast abscess in the mother or furuncles in siblings may suggest the staphylococcal origin of an infant's pneumonia.

Heredity undoubtedly plays a prominent role in many diseases of the lungs, extending in a spectrum from rare mendelizing diseases at one end to more common diseases of mixed environmental and genetic causation. Table 1 lists hereditary diseases of the lungs in accordance with the above spectral concept. They are the (1) mendelizing group, (2) intermediate group and (3) polygenic group.

If the parents are intelligent and observant, much information can be obtained under these several categories, and the physical examination can then be made with more definite ideas of the nature of the process and its prognosis.

TABLE 1.   HEREDITARY DISEASES OF THE LUNGS

Mendelizing Diseases and Modes of Inheritance

Agammaglobulinemia (Bruton's disease)	Sex-linked recessive
	Autosomal recessive
Ataxia-telangiectasia syndrome	Autosomal recessive
Chronic granulomatous disease	Sex-linked recessive
	Autosomal recessive
Cystic fibrosis	Autosomal recessive
Familial dysautonomia	Autosomal recessive
Familial emphysema (homozygous deficiency of	
alpha$_1$-antitrypsin)	Autosomal recessive
Familial interstitial fibrosis	Autosomal dominant
Familial pulmonary alveolar microlithiasis	Autosomal recessive
Familial spontaneous pneumothorax	Autosomal dominant
Hunter syndrome	Sex-linked recessive
Hurler's syndrome	Autosomal recessive
Kartagener's syndrome	Autosomal recessive
Lung in Marfan syndrome	Autosomal dominant
Primary pulmonary hypertension	Autosomal recessive
Pulmonary arteriovenous fistulas	Autosomal dominant
Tuberous sclerosis	Autosomal dominant

Intermediate Diseases (Familial Aggregation with Genetic Contribution to Etiology)

Chronic bronchitis and bronchiectasis	Susceptibility to repeated infection and to action of irritants
Familial emphysema	Heterozygous alpha$_1$-antitrypsin deficiency and possibly others producing "susceptibility of lung to action of an irritant"
Miscellaneous rare diseases	Data on inheritance meager; some may be simple Mendelian disorders
Obesity-hypoventilation syndrome	
Potter's syndrome	
Pulmonary cystic lymphangiectasis	
Scimitar syndrome	
Tracheobronchomegaly	
Wolman's disease	
Williams-Campbell syndrome	
(bronchial cartilage	
deficiency)	
Letterer-Siwe disease	

Polygenic Diseases (with Mixed Genetic and Environmental Factors)

Allergic respiratory disease (asthma, rhinitis)	Inherited allergic diathesis
Sarcoidosis	Unknown, but familial aggregation reported
Tuberculosis	Increased susceptibility to bacterial invasion
Other communicable diseases	Increased susceptibility or genetically determined "low resistance"

Adapted from McKusick, V. A., and Mutalik, G. S.: Genetics and pulmonary disease. In Liebow, A. A., and Smith, D. E. (Eds.): *The Lung*. Baltimore, Williams and Wilkins Company, 1968.

Since much of the examination of the chest and lungs consists of inspection of the undisturbed child, it is helpful to take the history in a warm examining room as the child, stripped to the waist, sits on his parent's lap. In this way one can make important observations as he proceeds with the history.

The *chief complaint* serves the prime purpose of initiating the dialogue and also of determining what most disturbs the parents. Chronology is most important, since it yields information on the chronicity and inertia of the disorder. In any detailed chronology, the specific symptoms and signs volunteered by the informant should be noted, while additional information is obtained through careful, nonleading questions. At each important episode, answers should be obtained as to (1) what the patient did, (2) what the family did and (3) what any "other doctor" did. When the chronologic account has been completed, the informant is psychologically ready for certain "finishing" questions, such as those asked in a review of the cardiorespiratory and other systems. The remainder of the past history follows and, finally, the more intimate family and environmental history.

SPECIFIC POINTS OF IMPORTANCE IN PRESENT AND PAST ILLNESSES

Informants often have information under the following headings, but may not volunteer it.

The Nature of the Cough

Is the cough productive or tight? It is necessary to make clear that expectoration is not the only criterion of a productive cough. Rather, its discontinuous sound informs even the nonmedical observer that fluid (mucus, pus, blood or aspirated liquid) is present in the tracheobronchial tree. Under what circumstances is the cough heard? A nonproductive nocturnal cough suggests an allergic or viral causation. A productive cough, especially on getting up in the morning, indicates the bronchorrhea of chronic bronchitis or bronchiectasis. A paroxysmal cough suggests pertussis or a foreign body. Recurrent cough with wheeze implies tracheobronchial obstruction, as seen in asthma, foreign body, mediastinal tumors or occasionally cystic fibrosis. A cough associated with swallowing points toward aspiration of contents into the tracheobronchial tree, due to incoordination of the swallowing and breathing mechanisms, anomaly or mass in the hypopharyngeal area, achalasia of the esophagus or tracheoesophageal fistula. Cough with aphonia or dysphonia should suggest hypopharyngeal or laryngeal foreign body, papilloma of

the larynx, croup (infectious or allergic) or psychoneurosis. Cough with a ringing or "brassy" quality suggests tracheal irritation, as exemplified by the tracheitis of rubeola. The "croupy" cough, which sounds like the bark of a seal or dog, is an indication of involvement of the glottic and subglottic areas. Is the cough heard every day, or may the child be totally free of cough for days or weeks?

Labored Breathing

A history of difficult breathing should first suggest airway obstruction. Has the dyspnea been getting steadily worse, as in bronchiolitis, or does it seem to come and go, as in asthma? Was its onset sudden, as, for example, when a previously well toddler is found suddenly coughing and retracting with peanuts in his mouth? Can the dyspnea be consistently related to signs of infection? Perhaps the child has always had labored breathing, as in anomalies of the lungs or heart. Can the child play vigorously without distress, or does he avoid a situation in which increased ventilation would be demanded?

Difficult breathing may also occur in nonobstructive pulmonary disease, such as large pleural effusion, pneumothorax or diaphragmatic paralysis. It may also be produced by pain on chest expansion, regardless of its cause, as in rib fracture or lobar pneumonia. In such cases it may be more accurately described as "shortness of breath." The child at rest may not be greatly distressed, whereas exercise tolerance is sharply reduced.

Noisy Breathing

The informant may have noted various respiratory noises. If so, what sort of noise has been heard and with what phase of respiration has it been associated? Typical *snoring* during sleep may be present in normal children only with acute coryza or may be more or less constant in those with adenoidal hypertrophy, posterior choanal obstruction, nasal polyposis, nasal foreign body or the Pierre Robin syndrome. Most intelligent informants can differentiate the snore of nasal obstruction and the harsh stridor of laryngeal or tracheal obstruction.

Wheezing

Wheezing is a prolonged, high-pitched, rather musical sound of varying intensity; it is frequently audible without a stethoscope. It is most common on expiration and indicates partial obstruction in one or more of the larger bronchi. Its paroxysmal occurrence is typical of asthma. Persistent wheezing of sudden onset should suggest an aspirated foreign body. It is most important that this possibility be thoroughly investigated. Slowly progressive wheezing should suggest increasing bronchial obstruction caused, for example, by lymphoma or tuberculous lymphadenitis. If bronchodilators, such as epinephrine, have been administered, information on the response of the patient should be obtained, since prompt disappearance of wheezing after use of a bronchodilator is indicative of a relaxation of the bronchospasm of asthma.

The association of labored breathing and wheezing suggests either a single high obstruction (trachea or main bronchus) or multiple lower obstructions (lobar, segmental or subsegmental bronchi).

Grunting

Grunting is frequently a sign of chest pain and suggests an acute pneumonic process with pleural involvement. It is also seen in pulmonary edema, regardless of its cause, and is a regular accompaniment of the neonatal respiratory distress syndrome.

Cyanosis

The distribution, degree and duration of blueness should be ascertained.

In peripheral circulatory stasis, as in a chilled newborn infant, it may have little cardiorespiratory significance. But cyanosis of the lips, mouth, face and trunk almost always indicates cardiorespiratory disease and may demand emergency treatment. It is produced by (1) acute or chronic alveolar hypoventilation (airway obstruction, depressed respiratory center or respiratory muscle weakness), (2) uneven distribution of gas and blood throughout the lungs (bronchopneumonia), (3) anatomic right-to-left shunts of blood (congenital cyanotic heart disease, congenital arteriovenous aneurysms of the lung) or rarely (4) disturbances of alveolocapillary diffusion (interstitial pneumonia or pulmonary fibrosis).

If oxygen was administered to the cyanotic patient, did the informant note that his color improved markedly? If it did not, it is likely that one or more right-to-left shunts are responsible for the cyanosis, since the above-noted other causes of cyanosis respond to increases in the partial pressure of oxygen in inspired air.

Chest Pain

Older children may have complained of chest pain. The physician should consider disease of the esophagus, pericardium, diaphragmatic and parietal pleuras, or chest wall. In the esophagus, foreign body, achalasia, lye stricture and ulceration may be responsible, and the pain is dull, deep and usually referred anteriorly. Parietal pleural pain is usually localized and lies more or less over the involved area. The pain of diaphragmatic pleural irritation may be referred to the base of the neck posteriorly and laterally, or even to the abdomen, where it may cause great diagnostic confusion. Pleural pain is frequently related to respiration, in which case the respirations are rapid and shallow, and there may be an expiratory grunt. Severe chest pain may be produced by the myositis of pleurodynia, by chest wall trauma, or by intercostal neuralgia, as in herpes zoster.

Sputum

The age at which a child can spit out coughed-up sputum varies considerably. Expectoration, literally taken as removal of sputum from the lungs by ciliary activity and cough, certainly occurs at all ages. During infancy, such "expectorated" material is universally swallowed and undoubtedly composes at least some of the "cold" or mucus noted in vomitus and stools. Occasionally, older infants with chronic lung disease, e.g., patients with cystic fibrosis, may use their own index fingers to "hook out" viscous mucopurulent material from the oropharynx. Only in the supervised older child, however, can the volume of spit-out sputum be expected to approach the volume leaving the lungs. Nevertheless, the physician should ask for information on the volume, color, viscosity and odor of sputum. Changes in these characteristics are guides to the presence of fresh bacterial infection. The "rusty" sputum of acute pneumococcal pneumonia is unusual in childhood, as is massive pulmonary hemorrhage, but streaks of pink or brownish pink blood are not uncommon in bronchiectasis.

Clubbing

Observant parents may have noted the signs of clubbing and should be directly questioned on progressive changes in the nail curvature and in the shape of the terminal phalanges. The presence of clubbing has etiologic significance, and its duration may throw light on the chronicity of the process.

Bad Breath

A chronically malodorous breath may be noted in children with bronchiectasis, lung abscess, paranasal sinusitis, nasal foreign body, adenoidal infection and allergic rhinitis.

Previous Chest Roentgenograms and Laboratory Data

If the child has had chest roentgenograms in the past, it is helpful to elicit the date and interpretation of each and, if possible, to inspect the films themselves. Differentiation may sometimes be clearly made between congenital and acquired diseases by review of former x-ray films. In chest disease of chronic, recurrent or obscure nature, every effort must be made to locate such roentgenograms for comparison with current films.

All other available data on the patient's past pulmonary illnesses should be sought; such data include past pulmonary function tests, blood counts, sweat tests, skin tests and clinical chemistries.

NONSPECIFIC SIGNS OF RESPIRATORY DISEASE

Failure to thrive may be a manifestation of severe, chronic respiratory disease. It may appear as failure to gain or even as loss of weight. Weights at birth and subsequent ages can be requested for plotting on appropriate weight-age graphs. A sudden deviation from the established growth channel of a child may indicate the approximate time of onset of his disease. Stature can be similarly handled if heights at earlier ages are known. Other nonspecific signs include sallowness, pallor, lethargy, subnormal school performance and emotional disturbances.

THE PATIENT'S ENVIRONMENT

The social, psychologic and physical characteristics of the sick child's environment may illuminate the nature of the disease or for other reasons may be important for the physician to know. Information of possible importance includes the status of the parents' marriage, the income of the family and its debts, its recreations and its religion. Where does the family live, and does its location near industry, dump or stable help explain the patient's disease? Has the family lived in areas of endemic fungous infection? Does the patient have his own bed and his own room, and what means exist of heating, cooling, humidifying and dust-freeing the sleeping area, in which he spends a third or more of his life? Is there gross air pollution in the neighborhood? Are there conditions of crowding, low income, poor nutrition, ignorance, and lack of routine immunizations and skin testing such that infectious disease can quickly spread throughout the family, remain unrecognized for long periods, and be almost ineradicable?

Are there abnormal exposures to the environment, such as that produced by dirt-eating? Is there a possibility that the patient's illness has been caused by "battering," such as thoracic trauma or purposeful exposure to the elements?

THE PHYSICAL EXAMINATION

The physical examination is traditionally divided into categories of inspection, palpation, percussion-auscultation, and olfaction, for each of which the examiner uses a different organ of sense. Such a division serves basic pedagogic purposes, but in practice, one sense is seldom used exclusively. *The senses, as well as the tools actually used, always subserve the goals of examination of the lungs, which are to determine (1) the pattern of respiration, (2) the adequacy of gas exchange and (3) the localization of disease, if it exists.*

The following discussion is in accordance with these goals. Physical findings will be correlated with the causative disturbances of function.

PATTERN OF RESPIRATION

Knowledge of the pattern of respiration is best acquired by careful observation of the sleeping or quietly awake child. This general term "pattern" includes an evaluation of rate, depth, ease and rhythm of breathing.

Rate of Respiration

The physician should reach a conclusion as to whether the respiratory rate is normal for this patient, abnormally or disproportionately rapid (tachypnea, polypnea) or abnormally slow (bradyp-

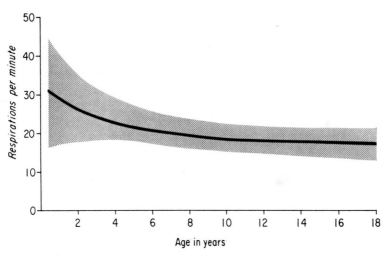

Figure 1. Normal resting respiratory rates from Table 2 are plotted against age to show more clearly the rapid decrease that occurs during the first two years of life. Since there is no significant difference in rates between boys and girls, a single regression is applicable to both sexes. The shaded area represents the approximate area of normal variation (two standard deviations above and below the mean at each age). (Iliff and Lee.)

nea, oligopnea). Data on the expected rates for age are shown in Figure 1 and Table 2 and indicate a rapid decline from early infancy to about two years of age, and then a slower, steady fall for the rest of childhood and adolescence. Data on normal respiratory rates in both sleeping and awake white subjects from a high socioeconomic group in New Orleans are shown in Table 3. These observations indicate the variability of the respiratory rate, as well as the importance of counting such rates in the sleeping or resting unaware child.

The respiratory rate, when properly observed under controlled conditions, however, is a simple and useful, although nonspecific, pulmonary function test of thoracic and pulmonary compliance. Diseases of the thorax and lungs that act to stiffen them are associated with significantly higher rates. The course of low-compliance (high stiffness) processes, such as interstitial or other pneumonias, pleural effusion and pulmonary edema, can be simply and accurately evaluated by careful serial observations of rate (Fig. 2). Decreases toward normal indicate improvement, whether occurring spontaneously or induced by treatment. Rapid rates are also observed with anxiety, exercise, fever, severe anemia, metabolic acidosis (severe diarrhea, diabetes) and respiratory alkalosis (psychoneurosis, salicylates, central nervous system disturbances).

Bradypnea is less commonly observed, but may be seen, for example, with metabolic alkalosis (pyloric stenosis) and respiratory acidosis due to central nervous system depression (morphine overdosage, increased intracranial pressure).

For ordinary clinical purposes, the rate may be counted for a minute, but when the rate is being used to follow the progress of a patient, several resting steady-state counts should be made and the mean rate per minute computed. It is always preferable for the child to be ignorant of the counting

TABLE 2. NORMAL RESTING RESPIRATORY RATE PER MINUTE

Age (Years)	Boys Mean ± SD	Girls Mean ± SD
0- 1	31 ± 8	30 ± 6
1- 2	26 ± 4	27 ± 4
2- 3	25 ± 4	25 ± 3
3- 4	24 ± 3	24 ± 3
4- 5	23 ± 2	22 ± 2
5- 6	22 ± 2	21 ± 2
6- 7	21 ± 3	21 ± 3
7- 8	20 ± 3	20 ± 2
8- 9	20 ± 2	20 ± 2
9-10	19 ± 2	19 ± 2
10-11	19 ± 2	19 ± 2
11-12	19 ± 3	19 ± 3
12-13	19 ± 3	19 ± 2
13-14	19 ± 2	18 ± 2
14-15	18 ± 2	18 ± 3
15-16	17 ± 3	18 ± 3
16-17	17 ± 2	17 ± 3
17-18	16 ± 3	17 ± 3

Data of Iliff and Lee from both fed, sleeping and fasting, awake children. SD = one standard deviation of the mean.

TABLE 3. RESPIRATORY RATES PER MINUTE OF NORMAL CHILDREN, BOTH SEXES, SLEEPING AND AWAKE

Age	Sleeping No.	Mean	Range	Awake No.	Mean	Range	Mean Difference Between Sleeping and Awake
6–12 months	6	27	22–31	3	64	58–75	37
1– 2 years	6	19	17–23	4	35	30–40	16
2– 4 years	16	19	16–25	15	31	23–42	12
4– 6 years	23	18	14–23	22	26	19–36	8
6– 8 years	27	17	13–23	28	23	15–30	6
8-10 years	19	18	14–23	19	21	15–31	3
10–12 years	11	16	13–19	17	21	15–28	5
12–14 years	6	16	15–18	7	22	18–26	6

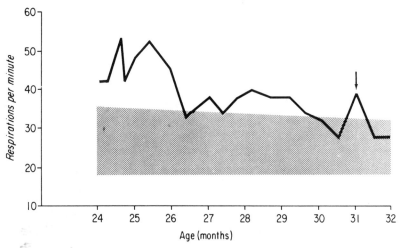

Figure 2. Respiratory rate per minute in a child with chronic diffuse interstitial fibrosis of the lung (Hamman-Rich syndrome). The diagnosis was confirmed by open biopsy, and treatment consisted of progressively decreasing oral doses of prednisone. Rates were carefully counted during serial visits to the Chest Clinic. Each point is the mean of two or more one-minute counts. Auscultation of the lungs never revealed abnormal breath sounds or rales during the depicted period. The return toward normal of the child's rate of breathing strongly suggests that the process is in part reversible. The arrow indicates tachypnea produced by an intercurrent, acute respiratory infection with fever.

process and for the physician to be at a low-anxiety distance. Usually, thoracic excursions are sufficiently discrete for counting by inspection, but occasionally a stethoscope must be used. In a sleeping child breathing shallowly, respirations may be counted without touching him by auscultating with a stethoscope a short distance below the patient's nose.

Most parents can be shown how to count respirations and how to maintain a sleeping respiratory rate log on their children. Such logs are extremely useful in monitoring the course of chronic restrictive pulmonary disease.

Depth of Respiration

The physician now attempts to decide whether, for the rate observed, the child is breathing at a normal depth, too deeply (hyperpnea) or too shallowly (hypopnea). Such a clinical estimate of minute volume (the volume of air expired each minute) can be recognized as abnormal only at the extremes. For example, the hyperpnea with metabolic acidosis in the course of diarrhea or diabetes mellitus is easily detected. Sim-

ilarly, the hypoventilation with metabolic alkalosis can sometimes be sensed, although it is more easily missed because most physicians have not trained themselves to evaluate effortless, shallow breathing. Between these extremes, much variation may pass undetected.

Hyperpnea occurs with fever, severe anemia, salicylism, metabolic acidosis and respiratory alkalosis, and in those diseases of the lungs in which there is increased physiologic dead space. Hypopnea occurs with metabolic alkalosis (pyloric stenosis) and with respiratory acidosis (e.g., bilateral diaphragmatic paralysis or central nervous system depression).

The depth of respiration is generally estimated from the amplitude of thoracic and abdominal excursions. Initial impressions, gained from inspection, may be reinforced by palpation and auscultation. The palm of the hand held a short distance in front of the mouth and nose may reveal increased or decreased tidal volumes. Auscultation of a generalized increase or decrease in amplitude of breath sounds of normal quality similarly helps to confirm initial impressions. In hyperpnea, the faint inspiratory and expiratory sounds of large tidal volumes can be easily heard without a stethoscope.

Ease of Respiration

The physician should also evaluate with what ease respiration is being effected. Effortless breathing (eupnea) indicates that no significant airway obstruction is present. Difficult or labored respiratory efforts (dyspnea) mean that increased work is being performed by the muscles of respiration toward ensuring normal alveolar ventilation. The greatest increases in work of breathing are caused by airway obstruction.

Dyspnea is both a sign and a symptom. If a patient is aware of even the slightest distress in breathing, he is dyspneic. Such subtlety is obviously not generally applicable to infants and children, and the pediatrician accordingly seeks signs of distressed breathing or extraordinary respiratory effort before deciding that dyspnea is present. These advanced signs include orthopnea, intercostal retractions and bulging, flaring of the alae nasi, head-bobbing, wheezing and grunting. Each of these will be briefly discussed.

Orthopnea

Children with pulmonary edema or asthma, for example, appear unable to tolerate recumbent positions and will spontaneously prop themselves upright with their arms behind in the so-called tripod position. For both comfort and improved gas exchange, such children should be propped in a semi-sitting position.

Intercostal Retractions and Bulging

The term "retraction" indicates an inspiratory sinking-in of soft tissues in relation to the cartilaginous and bony thorax. Slight intercostal depressions are normal and can easily be seen between the lower ribs, becoming slightly more marked as the child inspires. In disease, especially when airway obstruc-

tion is severe, retractions may become extreme and extend to the jugular notch and supraclavicular and infraclavicular areas. In infants, whose thoraces are more pliable, the lower sternum may be depressed with each inspiratory effort.

Whether physiologic or pathologic, retractions are produced by differences in pressure existing at any moment between the intrapleural space (intrathoracic) and that outside the thorax (atmospheric) (Fig. 3, *inspiration*). Greater than normal decreases of intrathoracic pressure occur during inspiration with airway obstruction and with increased lung stiffness. The greater the pressure decrease below atmospheric, the more the flexible intercostal soft tissues will yield, and the more conspicuous will be the resulting intercostal retractions. In accord with this concept of retractions, it is not the location of any obstruction within the respiratory tract that controls the particular soft tissue retracted, but rather the degree of that obstruction, which in turn affects the magnitude of the decrease in intrathoracic pressure necessary for ventilation.

It is thus clear that retractions, when abnormal, indicate increased *inspiratory* effort. It is not generally appreciated, however, that inspection of the interspaces can also yield evidence of greater than normal *expiratory* effort, which is common in asthma, bronchiolitis and cystic fibrosis. Normally, intrathoracic pressure is subatmospheric throughout expiration. With widespread bronchial obstruction, however, increased expiratory muscular effort is required to force air *out* of the lungs. Under such circumstances, intrathoracic pressure may exceed atmospheric pressure, and in obedience to the outward pressure gradient, the intercostal space will be noted to flatten and sometimes to bulge out (Fig. 3, *expiration*). Intercostal bulging is thus always to be taken as a sign of greater than normal expiratory effort.

Movements of intercostal soft tissues are best observed when light is al-

Inspiration   Expiration

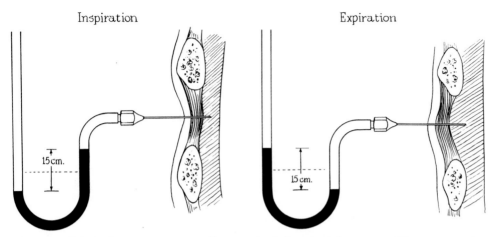

Figure 3.   Relation between movement of intercostal soft tissues and the pressure difference across them. Differences in pressure between the intrapleural space and the atmosphere during obstructed inspiration and expiration are depicted diagrammatically. A simple water manometer is attached to a needle whose tip lies between the parietal and visceral pleuras. Simultaneous pressure differences and movements of the intercostal soft tissues are noted.

Inspiration.   During partially obstructed inspiration, the intrapleural pressure is shown decreasing to 15 cm. of water below that of the atmosphere. (A normal tidal inspiration does not usually produce a difference of more than 8 cm. of water.) This larger than normal pressure difference, greater on the outside, forces in the pliable intercostal soft tissues, resulting in retractions, which the physician sees on physical examination.

Expiration.   During partially obstructed expiration, as in asthma, intrapleural pressure, which is normally always less than atmospheric, may equal or exceed it. In this diagram, intrapleural pressure is 15 cm. of water greater than that of the atmosphere. This results in a pressure gradient from inside out, and as pressure rises, the pliable tissues at first flatten and finally bulge outward.

together from a direction roughly perpendicular to the plane of the middle ribs, as, for example, from a ceiling light a few feet above and in front of the sitting or standing patient. In general, the intercostal spaces that can be observed most satisfactorily are the eighth and ninth in the posterior axillary line.

If the patient is both retracting and bulging his intercostal spaces, a curious flickering bar of light and shadow may occur in the same interspace as the space alternately becomes dark with the retraction during inspiration and bright with the bulge during expiration. The uninitiated observer may erroneously ascribe this "intercostal flicker" to sudden downward rib movement with expiration. Palpation of the "flickering" interspace will indicate at once that rib movements are too slight and gradual to explain the effect.

Subcostal retractions seen at the lower costal margins anteriorly should be differentiated from all other retractions, since their significance and interpretation are not the same. Subcostal retractions indicate a flattened diaphragm, a considerable portion of whose action is being directed not toward lowering the "floor" of the thorax but, rather, toward pulling in its "walls." Such diaphragmatic flattening most commonly is seen in diseases producing diffuse lower airway obstruction, but also is seen in very extensive restrictive pulmonary diseases.

Flaring of the Alae Nasi

Flaring of the alae nasi exists when an enlargement of both nares occurs during inspiration. It is due to contraction of the anterior and posterior dilatores naris muscles, which are supplied by the facial nerves. The appearance of flaring indicates that accessory muscles are being recruited for inspiration. Since flaring implies that greater than normal work is required for breathing, it is an excellent sign of dyspnea. In many cases, its presence suggests that inspiratory efforts are being abnormally shortened by pain, as in pleuritis or thoracic trauma. Unilateral flaring is a sign of facial paralysis on the opposite side, in addition to its usual significance.

Head-Bobbing

This is a sign of dyspnea best observed in an exhausted or sleeping infant lying in its mother's arms. The head must be unsupported except for the suboccipital area, which rests on the mother's forearm. In synchrony with each inspiration, the head is noted to bob forward owing to neck flexion. The phenomenon is probably explained by contraction of the scalene and sternocleidomastoid muscles, which are accessory muscles of inspiration. Counteraction from the extensor muscles of the neck is insufficient to fix the cervical spine and head. The result is that nonrespiratory work is done in flexing the neck instead of raising the sternum and the first two ribs.

Wheezing and Grunting

Wheezing indicates partial obstruction, usually expiratory, and may be caused by single or multiple points of narrowing within the airways. Usually, such obstruction exists in larger (segmental or lobar) bronchi because the necessary critical velocities of air flow for wheeze production probably occur only in larger airways. It is likely that such velocities cannot be reached in the smaller bronchi, even with deep rapid breathing. For this reason, an audible wheeze is not a characteristic sign of bronchiolitis, in which airway obstruction is diffuse and primarily involves the smallest airways. It is commonly heard, however, in patients with asthma or tracheobronchial foreign bodies.

Auscultation at the open mouth may reveal faint wheezes and crepitations, since sounds from even small bronchi travel easily up the airway.

Grunting, as mentioned previously, is associated with pneumonia and chest pain, but in the neonatal period it is commonly observed in the respiratory distress syndrome.

Rhythm of Respiration

Respiration is not absolutely regular in either health or disease. The depth of separate breaths may vary significantly, and the intervals between them are not fixed. Occasional deep breaths, *sighs*, occur in all normal persons and probably serve an important antiatelectatic function.

Periodic breathing occurs so frequently in premature infants as to be considered a normal finding. It usually appears after 24 hours and is characterized by acyanotic apneic periods lasting five to ten seconds, followed by periods of ventilation lasting up to 15 seconds. The phenomenon lacks the crescendo-decrescendo pattern characteristic of Cheyne-Stokes breathing, and is probably explained by the immaturity of integrating pathways in the central nervous system.

Premature infants may also show a more serious type of respiratory irregularity, *apneic spells*, that may last more than 20 seconds. Bradycardia is usually present, and cyanosis may occur. Infants with apneic spells have a high mortality.

Classic *Cheyne-Stokes breathing* is characterized by a waxing and waning of the depth of tidal volumes with periods of apnea between each such sequence. The cause is not certain, although it is an abnormal type of respiratory arrhythmia. It is seen in children with congestive heart failure, cerebral trauma and increased intracranial pressure.

Biot's breathing is more ominous and consists of one or several breaths of irregular depth with interspersed apneic periods of varying lengths. It generally signifies severe brain damage.

ADEQUACY OF GAS EXCHANGE

The primary function of the lungs is gas exchange, i.e., getting sufficient oxygen into the body to satisfy metabolic needs and removing carbon dioxide thereby produced. Insufficiency of the lungs' oxygen-supplying role causes hypoxia, and insufficiency of their carbon dioxide–eliminating role causes hypercapnia. In disease, both gases may be insufficiently exchanged. Hypoxia may occur without hypercapnia, however, and vice versa. For example, disturbances of distribution of blood and gas throughout the lungs may produce hypoxia without hypercapnia, and oxygen therapy in a patient with overall alveolar hypoventilation may relieve hypoxia, but it will not lessen hypercapnia and may indeed make it worse.

It would be of inestimable clinical value to be able to detect the presence of hypoxia or hypercapnia, or both, on physical examination. Unfortunately, the recognition of both types of disturbance is difficult owing to nonspecificity of their manifestations, variations among patients, and differences in the severity and duration of inadequate gas exchange.

The signs and symptoms of hypoxia, listed in Table 4, are cyanosis, tachycardia, exertional dyspnea, and those due to depression of the central nervous system. Dyspnea at rest probably does not occur in hypoxia without hypercapnia. The ability of an observer to perceive cyanosis varies greatly. Some persons may detect cyanosis when arterial oxygen saturation has dropped to 85 per cent from its sea-level normal of 96 per cent. The majority of observers, however, will not perceive cyanosis unless arterial oxygen saturation is 80 per cent or less.

The signs of hypercapnia should be especially sought in those clinical situations in which reduced depth of respiration is expected or has been observed. Careful studies in adults indicate that signs of hypercapnia appear in relation to an increase in tension of mixed venous carbon dioxide above that which is usual for each person. In other words, *chronic* mild or moderate elevations of carbon dioxide tension may not be detectable on physical examination, but *acute progressive* elevations of carbon dioxide tension

TABLE 5. SIGNS OF PROGRESSIVE HYPERCAPNIA*

Hot hands (+5)

Rapid bounding pulse (+10)
Small pupils (+10)

Engorged fundal veins (+15)
Confusion or drowsiness (+15)
Muscular twitching (+15)

Depressed tendon reflexes (+30)
Extensor plantar responses (+30)
Coma (+30)

Papilledema (+40)

*Figures in parentheses are the approximate elevations above *usual* levels of mixed venous carbon dioxide tension (mm. Hg) at which each sign may first appear. Thus, hot hands may be observed in a patient whose mixed venous P_{CO_2} is only 5 mm. Hg above the value usual for him, whereas the presence of papilledema probably indicates that his P_{CO_2} has risen 40 mm. Hg, or more, above the usual level.

Since mixed venous P_{CO_2} is usually about 6 mm. higher than simultaneously observed arterial P_{CO_2} in the same subject, these signs may also be applied to relative changes in arterial P_{CO_2}.

TABLE 4. SIGNS AND SYMPTOMS OF HYPOXIA

Mild
None or decreased efficiency only

Moderate
Mood changes: euphoria or depression
Decreased efficiency and impaired judgment
Headache
Hypertension
Exertional dyspnea
Hyperpnea, variable
Cyanosis
Tachycardia
Polycythemia (chronic exposure)

Severe
Hypertension or hypotension
Dimness of vision
Somnolence, stupor, coma

above usual levels may be associated with increasingly serious signs; these are listed in Table 5. Although similar correlations have not been reported in infants and children, and although differences undoubtedly exist among various age groups, it is probable that the general pattern of signs is sufficiently similar to make Table 5 of value for children.

LOCALIZATION OF DISEASE

The third main goal of examination of the lungs is to determine the location of disease, if it is present. Considerable information has already been developed on the nature of the process from the history and from judgments made of the nature and adequacy of respiration earlier in the physical examination. Clubbing of the fingers is often a good clue to the presence of significant and commonly destructive disease, whereas several other signs are useful in an attempt at its localization.

Clubbing

There is an old physical diagnostic adage that says, "Examination of the lungs begins at the fingertips." There are perhaps two characteristic hallmarks of every examination by a chest physician: careful examination of the ends of the fingers and palpation of the position of the trachea.

In the case of advanced clubbing, casual inspection by an inexperienced observer is sufficient, but the early changes of clubbing can be most subtle. The basic characteristic of a clubbed digit is a lifting of the nail base by tissue proliferation on the dorsal surface of the terminal phalanx. Figure 4 indicates the progressive stages of the clubbing process and one method for its quantitation. A more precise method is shown in Figure 5, in which the depth of a plaster cast of the index finger at the nail base is compared with its depth at a standard and unaffected point, the terminal interphalangeal fold. Careful

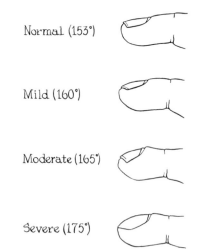

Figure 4. Stages of clubbing. These profiles are drawn from casts made of the terminal phalanges of children seen in a chest clinic. The number in parentheses for each stage of clubbing represents the angle formed above the finger at the skin-nail junction by straight lines drawn to it from equidistant points in front of and behind the junction. An angle greater than 160 degrees and decided curvature of the nail are good criteria of the presence of clubbing. The "moderate" and "severe" examples are from patients with cystic fibrosis.

serial measurements of such casts can be used to quantitate the clubbing phenomenon. Rapidly worsening clubbing in a patient with cystic fibrosis, for example, frequently indicates a poor prognosis. In this disease also, significant unclubbing can be produced by vigorous pulmonary therapy. Clubbing will disappear altogether with complete resection of bronchiectatic segments or lobes.

At the bedside, the presence of clubbing is best observed by holding the child's index finger in such a way as to estimate the relative finger depths indicated in Figure 5. The various conditions associated with clubbing are listed in Table 6.

The observation of nonfamilial clubbing should have a certain significance for the pediatrician. If congenital cyanotic heart disease and the various nonpulmonary causes can be eliminated, it is reasonable to conclude that there exists significant chronic, organic lung disease that may be either localized or

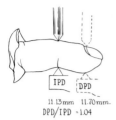

IPD   DPD
11.13mm 11.70mm.
DPD/IPD = 1.04

Figure 5. Method of measuring casts of the index finger with a metric micrometer. A depth at the nail base (distal phalangeal depth = DPD) is compared with another at the interphalangeal fold (interphalangeal depth = IPD). Values of DPD/IPD greater than 1.0 at all ages are considered indicative of clubbing.

generalized. In such cases, bronchiectasis is the most common cause. The appearance of clubbing in "asthma" probably indicates that either the diagnosis is incorrect or that complicating disease is coexistent, such as atelectasis with bronchiectasis. Observation for clubbing is an absolute essential in the examination of a child with chronic cough, and its discovery is a mandate for extensive additional investigation.

The pathogenesis of the clubbing phenomenon is unknown, and in the light of the variety of its disease associa-

TABLE 6. DISEASES COMMONLY ASSOCIATED WITH ACQUIRED CLUBBING IN CHILDREN

Pulmonary
Bronchiectasis
Pulmonary abscess
Empyema
Chronic pneumonias, various
Neoplasms, primary and metastatic

Cardiac
Congenital cyanotic heart disease
Subacute bacterial endocarditis

Hepatic
Biliary cirrhosis

Gastrointestinal
Chronic ulcerative colitis
Regional enteritis
Chronic dysentery, amebic and bacillary
Polyposis, multiple

Other
Thyrotoxicosis

tions (Table 6), more than one mechanism may be acting. It is possible that a potent vasoactive substance is either elaborated in the diseased lung or not inactivated there. Its subsequent presence in the systemic circulation causes clubbing by opening small arteriovenous connections in the tips of the fingers and toes.

Trepopnea

A child is described as trepopneic if he is more comfortable in one lateral recumbent position than in the other. Trepopnea indicates severe, predominantly unilateral disease, and the patient prefers to keep uppermost the better functioning lung.

Tracheal Palpation

The trachea can be viewed as the needle of a gauge whose function is the detection of differences in pressure or volume between the two sides of the thorax. The tracheal needle pivots on its fixation in the neck (where differences in thoracic pressure or volume produce little lateral movement) and swings its arrow in an arc at the carina (where lateral movement is maximal). The sign loses sensitivity because the examiner is not able to palpate the position of the trachea at the level of the carina but must content himself with palpation at the suprasternal notch. Nevertheless, with a little experience in tracheal palpation, it is possible to detect relatively small degrees of mediastinal shift.

Discovery of a shift does not alone indicate in which hemithorax the volume or pressure change has occurred, but it does indicate an abnormal inequality between the two sides of the chest. For example, a foreign body in the left main bronchus might completely occlude the bronchus and produce atelectasis of the entire left lung. As air is absorbed from the alveoli of the lung, its volume decreases and intrapleural pressure becomes more negative. The mediastinum with the trachea shifts

obediently to the left from an area of
higher pressure and greater volume to
one of lower pressure and smaller volume. On the other hand, a pneumothorax on the right adds volume to the
right hemithorax and makes less negative (increases) intrapleural pressure on
that side; the mediastinum and trachea
therefore still shift to the left. Other
portions of the examination should indicate the side responsible for the observed shift.

There are two different methods of
tracheal palpation. The first is most
useful in infants and small children and
is performed with one finger (Fig. 6).
The other, applicable to older children
and adults, involves inspection and two-
finger palpation (Fig. 7). In both
methods, the patient should slightly extend the neck without the slightest lateral tilt or rotation from a midline position. The head of the patient can be

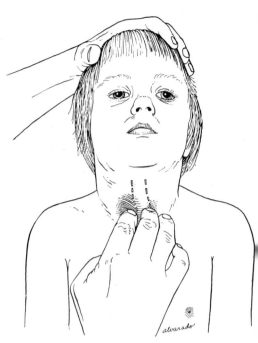

Figure 7. Technique of determining tracheal
position in an older child. Inspection of the suprasternal area may show asymmetry of the fossae
bounded laterally by the sternocleidomastoid muscles and medially by the trachea. In this case, the
fossa on the right is larger than that on the left, as
indicated by its larger shadow. It is concluded that
the trachea has been shifted to the left. The impression gained from inspection is then tested by
two-finger palpation of the relative size of the two
fossae. As shown, the index finger fits easily between
the right sternomastoid and trachea, but the middle
finger is too large for the corresponding space on
the left.

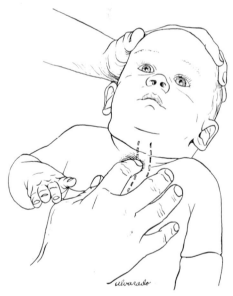

Figure 6. Technique of determining tracheal
position in an infant. The index finger of the pal-
pating hand is placed in the suprasternal notch and
gently slid inward in the midsagittal plane. It is
essential that the head be fixed in a neutral position,
and the neck slightly extended. If the finger consistently slides off one side of the trachea, it can be
concluded that the trachea is deviated in the opposite direction. In this illustration, the trachea is
shifted to the left. This method can also be applied
to older children.

fixed in the left hand of the examiner
as he palpates with his free right hand.

An additional observation can be
made during tracheal palpation. The
examiner can sense the distance between the jugular notch of the manubrium and the anterior wall of the
trachea. Diseases associated with
chronic expiratory obstruction, producing barrel-chest deformity, displace the
sternum away from the trachea. ("The
sternum leaves the trachea behind.")

Thoracic Configuration

As the various characteristics of respiration are being noted, the examiner

should also evaluate the form and symmetry of the chest. Although palpation and actual measurement may be required to complete such evaluation, especially of the lower costal angle, careful inspection can detect all but the most subtle changes. Readily seen are absence of the pectoral muscles, pigeon breast (pectus carinatum), funnel chest (pectus excavatum), barrel chest (pectus profundum), kyphoscoliosis and left-sided chest bulge due to enlargement of the right ventricle.

The symmetry of inspiration should be noted because those diseases producing unequal ventilation of the two lungs will be manifested by lagging or shallower expansion of the involved hemithorax.

The clinician should ask himself whether the chest shape of a patient deviates significantly from normal for that age. Traditionally, such judgments have been based on the two generally appreciated facts that the chests of infants are rounder than those of older children and that chronic diffuse air-way obstruction produces an abnormally rounded or "barrel-shaped" chest. It is possible, however, to refine clinical judgment considerably by serial chest measurements that can be made a part of every office visit. Chest circumference, although easily measured, is not a determinant of chest shape. In order to follow changes in shape, it is necessary to measure one or more thoracic diameters. An obstetrical caliper (pelvimeter) and a metal tape measure are the only necessary tools (Fig. 8). Of most importance is a measure of the anteroposterior diameter of the thorax, because overinflation of the lungs affects this dimension more than any other. With a little practice, sufficiently accurate and reproducible results can be obtained. The anteroposterior diameter can be correlated with age, height or another thoracic measure, such as transverse diameter. The thoracic index (depth-width ratio) is obtained by dividing the anteroposterior diameter by the transverse diameter (Tables 7 and 8). In severe obstructive lung dis-

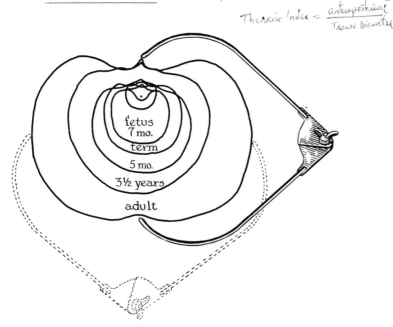

Figure 8.   Changes in chest shape at different ages, and their measurement with obstetrical calipers. The relatively round chest of the fetus and term infant gradually flattens dorsoventrally with age. Measurements should be made in either the recumbent (infants) or standing (children) position, never in the sitting position. Maximum dimensions are measured in both cases without regard to the level or phase of respiration, but care must be taken to place the calipers in a true transverse plane. The distance between the caliper tips is then measured with a steel centimeter rule.

TABLE 7.   NORMAL THORACIC DIMENSIONS, BOYS

Age Group	Anteroposterior* Mean ± SD (cm.)	Transverse* Mean ± SD (cm.)	Thoracic Index† Mean
0 – 3 months	10.2 ± 0.7	12.1 ± 0.9	0.84
3 – 6 months	11.2 ± 0.8	13.8 ± 0.9	0.81
6 – 9 months	11.6 ± 0.8	14.7 ± 0.9	0.79
9 –12 months	12.0 ± 0.7	15.4 ± 0.7	0.78
1 –1¼ years	12.2 ± 0.8	15.7 ± 0.8	0.77
1¼–1½	12.5 ± 0.9	16.1 ± 0.8	0.78
1½–1¾	12.6 ± 0.8	16.2 ± 0.7	0.78
1¾– 2	12.7 ± 0.7	16.6 ± 0.9	0.77
2 – 2¼	12.7 ± 0.8	16.7 ± 0.9	0.76
2¼– 2½	12.6 ± 0.7	16.7 ± 0.5	0.75
2½– 2¾	12.5 ± 0.8	16.8 ± 1.0	0.74
2¾–3	12.6 ± 0.7	16.9 ± 0.8	0.75
3 – 3½	12.7 ± 0.6	17.1 ± 0.8	0.74
3½– 4	12.9 ± 0.7	17.4 ± 0.8	0.74
4 – 4½	13.2 ± 0.6	17.6 ± 0.8	0.75
4½– 5	13.3 ± 0.7	17.8 ± 0.8	0.75
5 – 5½	13.6 ± 0.8	18.2 ± 0.9	0.75
5½– 6	13.8 ± 0.9	18.5 ± 1.0	0.75
6 – 6½	14.1 ± 1.0	18.7 ± 1.0	0.75
6½– 7½	14.5 ± 1.0	19.3 ± 1.1	0.75
7½– 8½	15.0 ± 1.1	20.0 ± 1.2	0.75
8½– 9½	15.4 ± 1.1	20.8 ± 1.4	0.74
9½–10½	15.9 ± 1.2	21.6 ± 1.6	0.74
10½–11½	16.3 ± 1.3	22.1 ± 1.7	0.74
11½–12½	17.0 ± 1.5	22.9 ± 1.9	0.74
12½–13½	17.8 ± 1.7	24.0 ± 1.8	0.74
13½–14½	18.6 ± 1.7	25.1 ± 2.1	0.74
14½–15½	19.3 ± 1.7	26.0 ± 2.1	0.74
15½–16½	20.0 ± 1.7	27.0 ± 1.9	0.74
16½–17½	20.7 ± 1.7	27.7 ± 2.0	0.75
17½–18½	21.5 ± 1.7	28.3 ± 1.7	0.76

Data of Meredith for white Iowa City boys.
*Measured at the level of the nipples.
†Thoracic index was obtained by dividing mean anteroposterior diameter by mean transverse diameter.

ease, this index or ratio may approach, reach or rarely exceed 1.0.

In children with chronic obstructive disease, serial determinations of thoracic index or thoracic anteroposterior diameter may furnish valuable clues to the course of the disease or possibly the efficacy of a treatment regimen (Fig. 9). Graphs for serial thoracic measurements are available.*

Thoracic and Abdominal Respirations

At the time that movements of intercostal soft tissue are being observed,

the physician should also look for *Litten's phenomenon.* This is not a sign of dyspnea, but an occasionally very helpful sign of diaphragmatic contraction and mobility. If the light source is properly adjusted, it can be seen in most normal nonobese children. The phenomenon consists of a slight shadow that moves down the lower intercostal spaces during inspiration, rising upward during expiration. It is related to movements of the diaphragm and is best seen in the posterior axillary line. The sign is probably best explained by the progressive downward extension during inspiration of negative intrapleural pressure as the diaphragm leaves the inner surface of the

*Medical Research Department, Mead Johnson Research Center, Evansville, Indiana 47721.

TABLE 8. NORMAL THORACIC DIMENSIONS, GIRLS

Age Group	Anteroposterior* Mean ± SD (cm.)	Transverse* Mean ± SD (cm.)	Thoracic Index† Mean
3 months	10.5 ± 1.0	12.5 ± 0.9	0.84
6 months	11.2 ± 0.8	13.7 ± 1.0	0.82
9 months	11.5 ± 0.8	14.2 ± 0.8	0.81
1 year	11.9 ± 0.8	14.9 ± 0.8	0.80
1¼	12.3 ± 0.7	15.3 ± 0.7	0.80
1½	12.4 ± 0.7	15.5 ± 0.8	0.80
1¾	12.4 ± 0.8	16.0 ± 0.7	0.78
2	12.4 ± 0.7	16.1 ± 0.8	0.77
2¼	12.4 ± 0.7	16.1 ± 0.8	0.77
2½	12.5 ± 0.7	16.3 ± 0.8	0.77
2¾	12.4 ± 0.8	16.3 ± 0.8	0.76
3	12.5 ± 0.8	16.7 ± 0.8	0.75
3½	12.7 ± 0.7	17.1 ± 0.9	0.74
4	12.8 ± 0.7	17.4 ± 1.0	0.74
4½	12.9 ± 0.7	17.6 ± 1.1	0.73
5	12.9 ± 0.8	17.8 ± 1.1	0.72
5½	12.9 ± 0.9	18.1 ± 1.1	0.71
6	13.2 ± 1.0	18.2 ± 1.1	0.73
7	13.4 ± 1.0	18.6 ± 1.2	0.72
8	13.8 ± 1.3	19.2 ± 1.3	0.72
9	14.1 ± 1.2	19.6 ± 1.5	0.72
10	14.5 ± 1.2	20.3 ± 1.4	0.71
11	15.3 ± 1.6	21.1 ± 1.5	0.73
12	16.1 ± 1.6	22.1 ± 1.8	0.73
13	16.8 ± 1.7	23.1 ± 1.7	0.73
14	17.4 ± 2.0	24.1 ± 2.0	0.72
15	17.8 ± 2.3	24.6 ± 2.2	0.72
16	18.0 ± 2.1	24.8 ± 2.0	0.73
17	17.8 ± 1.9	24.9 ± 1.8	0.71
18	17.7 ± 1.6	24.7 ± 1.7	0.72

Data of Boynton for white Iowa City girls.
*Measured at the level of the xiphoid.
†Thoracic index was obtained by dividing mean anteroposterior diameter by mean transverse diameter.

chest wall. Its absence suggests absolute or relative immobility of the diaphragm (paralysis, eventration, pleural effusion), especially if it is clearly seen on the opposite side. It must be emphasized that this is a subtle sign that can be observed only by looking for it with care.

Inspection of the thorax and upper part of the abdomen of the breathing child indicates the relative importance of thoracic expansion and diaphragmatic contraction. In all normal persons, both processes are at work, but in younger ones, especially infants, the role of the diaphragm is of greater importance. Hence, the normal infant is seen to protrude the upper part of the abdomen with inspiration, and this movement is larger than that of thoracic expansion. In bilateral phrenic nerve paralysis or diaphragmatic eventration, the abdomen may actually sink during inspiration, and the thorax is simultaneously observed to enlarge significantly. In such cases, careful inspection for Litten's sign, percussion of the lower lung margins and palpation of the lower costal angle are indicated to confirm the activity and position of the diaphragms.

Lower Costal Angle

At the xiphoid there originates an angle whose sides are formed by the lower edges of the ribs. Normally, this angle increases with inspiration and

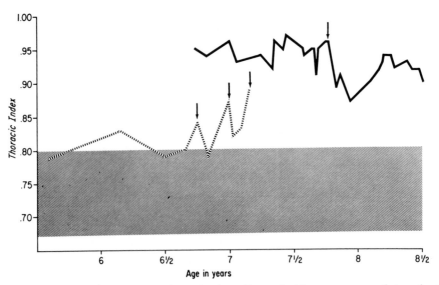

Figure 9. Thoracic index in chronic obstructive lung disease. Serial measurements of chest depth and width can be made easily in children. In this figure, thoracic index (depth-width ratio) is plotted against age for two children with severe obstructive lung disease due to cystic fibrosis.

The first patient (broken line) had considerable fluctuation of thoracic index, but the slope is generally upward, suggesting progressive overinflation of the lungs, which could be only temporarily relieved by intensive care during hospitalizations (arrows). Death occurred during the last hospitalization.

The second patient (solid line) has more severe overinflation than the first does, as shown by higher thoracic indices, but the slope of the serial measurements is generally downward. The rather abrupt decrease in thoracic index beginning at the arrow coincides with a period of intensive combined antibiotic, mucolytic aerosol and physical therapy.

Both patients illustrate the probable value of such measurements for purposes of prognostication and evaluation of therapy in obstructive lung disease.

decreases with expiration, owing to symmetrical expansion of the lower part of the thorax. Changes in this angle are best appreciated by laying the thumbs along both lower costal margins, their tips meeting at the xiphoid process. The angle changes with respiration, owing to combined action of the diaphragm and of the intercostal and scalene muscles. It increases normally during inspiration because the combined action of the intercostal-scalene group and the domed diaphragm elevates the lower ribs. If the diaphragm is flattened by obstructive lung disease, its mechanical advantage acts transversely rather than vertically, and there may be no increase in the angle with inspiration, or occasionally a paradoxical decrease with inspiration. Unilateral diaphragmatic flattening,

due to pleural effusion or pneumothorax, causes asymmetrical increase of the lower costal margin on inspiration with less movement on the involved side.

Boundaries and Divisions of the Lungs

By means of percussion, the boundaries of the lungs can be clearly delineated and marked with a wax pencil on the skin of the chest (Fig. 10). The divisions within each lung should be mastered if the physician desires to diagnose and treat chest disease in children with any finesse. Fortunately, there is a remarkably constant division of each lung into lobes (Fig. 11), and of each lobe into segments (Fig. 12). Although segmental anatomy is most easily learned from a three-dimensional model,* it can also be learned from diagrams. Efforts to remember exact rib and interspace boundaries of the lobes and segments, and their changes with age, are usually wasted because they are soon forgotten. It is much more to the point to be able to transfer the boundaries of the lobes and segments from a figure to a living chest wall in order to get them proportion-

*For example, the Huber Lung Model, manufactured by the Clay-Adams Company, 141 E. 25th St., New York, N.Y. 10010.

ately within the limits of the lungs, as determined by percussion. The technique is similar to learning how to carve a turkey from a diagram in a book. If the diagram is mastered, the dotted "cut here" lines, proportionately expanded, show up in the mind's eye on the steaming Thanksgiving turkey. Once the examiner has mastered the relative sizes of the segments, he "sees" the dotted lines that outline the segments on any chest, regardless of its size. He is then able to percuss and auscultate according to the anatomic divisions of the lungs.

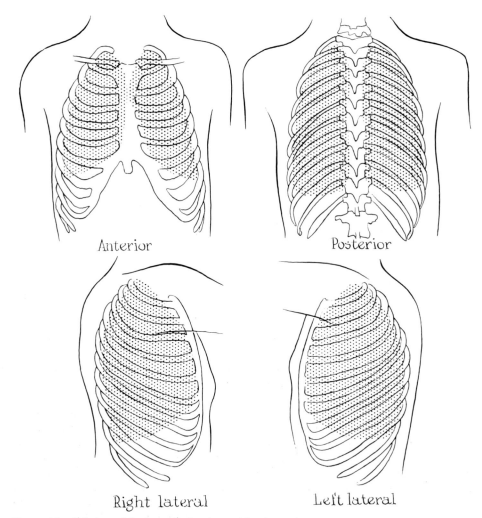

Anterior

Posterior

Right lateral

Left lateral

Figure 10. Relation of the lungs to the thorax. This figure depicts the approximate areas of resonance produced by air-containing lung tissue within the thorax of an older child. The lungs of infants are of different shapes and proportions, conforming with the previously discussed age changes of the thorax.

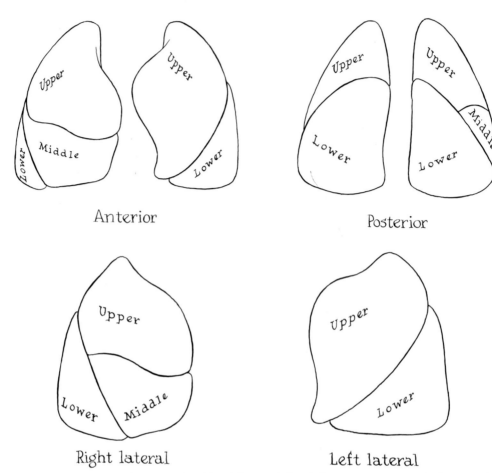

Anterior   Posterior

Right lateral   Left lateral

Figure 11. Division of the lungs into lobes. Minor variations in fissures may occur, producing somewhat different lobar proportions, incompletely separated lobes or supernumerary lobes. The patterns above are the most common, however.

Percussion of the chests of children is best done by the indirect method, in which a fingertip (plexor) of the examiner's dominant hand taps sharply on a terminal phalanx (pleximeter) of the other hand. The action of the percussing hand is altogether at the wrist; there should be little or no forearm motion. The tap should be just forceful enough to produce an audible note.* It is a mistaken notion to correlate increases in resonance with increases in amplitude (loudness) of the percussion note. The relation is between increas-ing resonance and decreasing pitch. In this sense, percussion can be compared with notes on a musical scale, with the resonant notes in the bass clef, dull notes in the treble clef, and flat notes even higher. There is a physiologic variation in percussion of the normal lung, slightly lower notes being heard toward the base and higher notes toward the apex. The transition is smooth, and sudden changes in pitch should suggest a pathologic state.

Although variably developed among physicians, a sense of touch is also involved in percussion, resonance being more easily felt than dullness.

In lobar or segmental consolidation, the transitions from dullness to reso-

*This is particularly important if the chest of the child is touching another resonating object, such as the mother's chest.

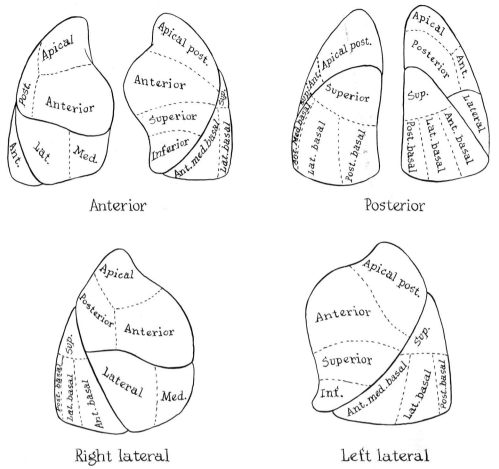

Anterior   Posterior

Right lateral   Left lateral

Figure 12. Division of the lobes into segments. The projections here correspond to those of Figures 10 and 11. The segments of each lung have been labeled. There are ten segments in the right lung, all of which touch the inner thoracic wall, with the exception of the medial basal segment of the lower lobe. On the left there are eight segments (or nine, depending on notation), all of which touch the thorax, except for the medial portion of the anteromedial basal segment of the lower lobe. The physical diagnostic significance of these facts is that almost all the segments can be percussed and auscultated.

nance should correspond to the "dotted lines" that indicate lobar and segmental boundaries. Thus, precise anatomic localization of the disease may be possible.

Palpation of the thorax as an aid to localizing disease is generally less helpful in infants than in older children. Areas of increased tactile fremitus may correspond to the topographic anatomy of consolidated lobes or segments. Decreased or absent fremitus may be noted over a hemithorax with pleural effusion or pneumothorax.

Segmental Auscultation

The pediatrician has often been afflicted with acoustically inferior stethoscopes on the grounds of an alleged need for miniaturization. This need has been exaggerated, since his patients extend from the premature through the adolescent, and he must have a stethoscope applicable to all or face the necessity of a stethoscope for each of several age groups. The situation is further complicated by the need for both a bell and a diaphragm in order to extend the range of sound perception to cover both very low and very high frequencies. The stethoscope diaphragm is generally used for most pulmonary auscultation because of its weighted frequency response toward higher frequencies, breath sounds being higher pitched than heart sounds. There are now available greatly improved instruments whose increased cost is easily justified by the very importance and frequency of use of the tool itself. Accordingly, the first and most important rule of auscultation is to procure a bell-diaphragm stethoscope with modern responsiveness.* By proper selection of earpieces, it should be made to fit both snugly and comfortably into the external ear canals. Comfortable, soft rubber earpieces are now available that effectively exclude most of the undesirable background noise.† Finally, it should be both sturdy and light.

A second rule, almost universally ignored, is to relate auscultation to bronchopulmonary anatomy, as was done for percussion. A busy physician could theoretically listen to every available segment in both lungs in 17 respiratory cycles. In practice, he should listen, preferably with the diaphragm, for one or two complete respirations over each of the bronchopulmonary segments, spending most time on those that the history and preceding portions of the examination have suggested as sites of disease. In infants it is convenient to begin auscultation on the back, since this produces less anxiety than a frontal approach. The infant may remain quietly, breast to breast, in his mother's arms. Every lobe is covered by listening to each of its various segments before proceeding to another one. Using a conventional stethoscope, the observer should sequentially compare the homologous segments of the two lungs—that is, first listen over the right posterior basal segment, then over the left posterior basal segment, moving in this fashion from side to side until all segments have been auscultated. The assumption in such segmental auscultation is that the relations of the segments within the lobe and the lobes within the lung are constant and have not been grossly disturbed by disease. This assumption is reasonable in most instances, since bronchopulmonary segmentation is remarkably constant. It would obviously be open to error in the presence of major lung-shifting processes, such as gross anomalies, large tension cysts, atelectasis, pneumothorax and pleural fluid collections, as well as in patients who have had substantial resections of lung tissue.

It follows that the physician's records should indicate by description or diagram the presumably involved lobe and segment. If a child has persistent crackles in the posterior basal segment of the right lower lobe, heard on repeated office visits, the implications are clearly not the same as those of crackles heard in *different* segments on repeated visits. *Careful, serial recording of anatomically related physical findings is the best means of diagnosing significant, structural lesions in the lungs.*

One of the problems of pediatric pulmonary auscultation is that posed by insufficiently deep breaths. Older children, like adults, can be shown how to breathe deeply through the mouth. Smaller children can be asked to "pant like a puppy dog" or to pretend to blow out candles on a birthday cake. In others, expiration may be reinforced by compression of the thorax between the hand holding the stethoscope on one side and the remaining hand on the other. After such an assisted expiration, especially if well timed, the next inspiration is usually deeper. This maneuver may also reveal undetected wheezes by increasing expiratory flow rate. If all else fails, the deep respira-

---

*One such stethoscope is the Littmann, manufactured by 3M Company, Medical Products Service Center, 3M Center Building 518, St. Paul, Minnesota 55101. The larger model for adults is preferred to the smaller one designed for children because of its superior diaphragm. It works perfectly well on infants and children.

†Flexible Ear Tips, #4216, Bard-Parker, Division of Becton, Dickinson and Company, Rutherford, New Jersey 07070.

tions just before and during crying may produce diagnostically sufficient inspiratory depths and provide an excellent chance for careful examination at the height of inspiration.

Breath Sounds

Since breath sounds are not transmitted alike through different stethoscopes, an examiner should always use the same stethoscope. It requires experience to become familiar with the nature of breath sounds heard at different ages. The spectrum of breath sounds that range from vesicular to tracheal is most easily appreciated by noting differences in the expiratory phase, although the pitch of inspiration is also quite different. The tubular quality of *tracheal* breathing is easily learned by placing the diaphragm over the examiner's own trachea and listening to the high-pitched "tubular" sound that is audible throughout both phases of respiration. This is easily contrasted with the *vesicular* breath sounds heard in the examiner's own axilla. The inspiratory note is softer and lower pitched, and expiration is essentially soundless. Between these two extremes range both the normal and abnormal breath sounds of infancy and childhood.

Bronchovesicular breath sounds are characterized by a soft, rather low-pitched expiratory note heard during the early part of expiration. Breath sounds may change from vesicular to bronchovesicular in a child if the depth of ventilation is increased. The inspiratory note of bronchovesicular breathing is slightly higher pitched than that of vesicular breathing. *Bronchial breath sounds* fall between bronchovesicular and tracheal and are characterized by a tubular note throughout all of expiration, but this tubular quality is less than that heard in tracheal breathing.

As a rule, the closer the stethoscope is to a large airway, the more audible and tubular will be the expiratory note. The bronchial breath sounds of lobar consolidation are based on the excellent transmission through fluid-filled alveoli of sounds made by air moving in the trachea and main bronchus of that lung.

If the examiner is in doubt about whether breath sounds in an area are normal, he should compare the area in question with a corresponding area of the opposite lung, as suggested previously. Clear differences may quickly reinforce his suspicions.

The term *suppressed breath sounds* implies diminished ventilation of that area of the lung being auscultated. Its use is usually based on the amplitude (audibility) of the inspiratory note. Breath sounds may be exaggerated or suppressed without being abnormal in quality. In atelectasis, for example, breath sounds may be vesicular and sharply suppressed over the involved lobe, owing to the relatively great distance from the stethoscope of normally ventilating lung.

Rales and Rhonchi

There exist several conflicting classifications of rales and rhonchi. This author prefers exclusive definitions of the two (Table 9). Rales are discontinuous, nonmusical, crackling or bubbling, soft or loud, inspiratory or expiratory, palpable or impalpable sounds produced by air bubbling through fluid in the lungs or more commonly by the snapping open of approximated airway walls. A rhonchus is a continuous, musical, soft or loud, usually expiratory, usually nonpalpable sound produced by air moving with velocity past a fixed obstruction in the airway. The nature of the obstruction may vary, including

TABLE 9. CLASSIFICATION OF RALES AND RHONCHI

Rales
Fine
Medium
Coarse
Rhonchi
Sibilant
Sonorous

foreign body, vascular anomaly, bronchospasm, inspissated mucopurulent secretions, or combinations of these. Regardless, it must present a relatively *solid* partial obstruction to airflow.

Terms such as "crepitant," "dry" and "moist" are apt to be confusing and are better replaced with *fine, medium and coarse*, although the usefulness of such descriptions is doubtful. Fine rales imply sounds originating in or below the terminal bronchioles, whereas medium and coarse rales originate in the proportionately larger divisions of the airway. Care should be taken to differentiate coarse, frequently palpable rales from friction rubs.

Rhonchi are either sibilant or sonorous, depending on pitch. Sibilant rhonchi are soft and high-pitched, whereas sonorous rhonchi are louder and lower pitched, such differences being due presumably to differences in flow rates past the point of obstruction. In addition to their significance as indicators of obstruction in the airways, the auscultation of rhonchi implies that larger bronchi are involved, because

TABLE 10. CLASSIFICATION OF CRACKLES AND WHEEZES

Crackles
Fine
Medium
Coarse
Wheezes
High-pitched
Low-pitched

only in the larger bronchi is there sufficient velocity of air movement to produce a musical sound.

Because of the frequent confusion of the terms "rales" and "rhonchi," it has been suggested by Forgacs (1969) that the simpler and therefore preferable words "crackles" and "wheezes" be substituted. Table 10 shows an alternate classification equivalent to that of Table 9.

Differential Auscultation

Serious chest pediatricians should add differential auscultation to their

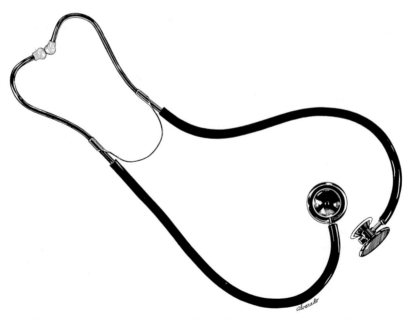

Figure 13. The double stethoscope of Scott Alison. This instrument can be easily made by purchasing two identical bell-diaphragm heads of good acoustic properties and attaching them to a standard earpiece yoke with equal lengths of plastic or rubber tubing.

diagnostic armamentarium. This technique was first described more than 100 years ago in London by Alison (1861) but has recently been justifiably exhumed. The double stethoscope differs from the conventional binaural instrument by division into a double, separate and matched system — each ear having its own bell-diaphragm chest piece (Fig. 13). The instrument is used to compare homologous parts of each lung simultaneously. With practice, a physician can on a single breath in such paired segments compare the amplitude, pitch and phasing of inspiratory breath sounds, as well as localize adventitious sounds. When these parameters are identical in simultaneously auscultated homologous segments, a state of *homophony* exists, which almost always indicates normality. If there are significant differences in amplitude, pitch or phasing of inspiratory breath sounds in simultaneously auscultated homologous segments (or if adventitious sounds exist), a state of *heterophony* is present, which almost always indicates pulmonary disease.

With double auscultation, far more information can be obtained in approximately half the time. The author uses the double stethoscope exclusively and adheres to a standard pairing of the segments of the two lungs for differential segmental auscultation (Table 11).

TABLE 11. PAIRING OF SEGMENTS FOR DIFFERENTIAL SEGMENTAL AUSCULTATION

Breath	Back of Chest	
	LEFT LOWER LOBE	RIGHT LOWER LOBE
1	Posterior basal	Posterior basal
2	Lateral basal	Lateral basal
3	Anterior basal	Anterior basal
4	Superior	Superior
	LEFT UPPER LOBE	RIGHT UPPER LOBE
5	Posterior	Posterior
6	Apical	Apical
	Front of Chest	
	RIGHT MIDDLE LOBE	LEFT UPPER LOBE
7	Medial	Inferior lingular
8	Lateral	Superior lingular
	RIGHT UPPER LOBE	
9	Anterior	Anterior

The placing of the two chest pieces in differential auscultation is in accordance with standard segmental auscultation (see Fig. 12).

REFERENCES

Alison, S. S.: *The Physical Examination of the Chest in Pulmonary Consumption and Its Intercurrent Diseases.* London, John Churchill, 1861.

Avery, M. E., and Fletcher, B. D.: *The Lung and Its Disorders in the Newborn Infant.* 3rd Ed. Philadelphia, W. B. Saunders Company, 1974.

Boynton, B.: *The Physical Growth of Girls.* University of Iowa Studies in Child Welfare. Volume XII, No. 4, 1936.

Cherniack, R. M., Cherniack, L., and Naimark, A.: *Respiration in Health and Disease.* 2nd Ed. Philadelphia, W. B. Saunders Company, 1972.

Commey, J. O. O., and Levison, H.: Physical signs in childhood asthma. *Pediatrics, 58*:537, 1976.

Comroe, J. H., Jr., and Botelho, S.: The unreliability of cyanosis in the recognition of arterial anoxemia. *Am. J. Med. Sci., 214*:1, 1947.

Dawson, J. B.: Auscultation and the stethoscope. *Practitioner, 193*:315, 1964.

Ertel, P. Y., Lawrence, M., Brown, R. K., and Stern, A. M.: Stethoscope acoustics. I. The doctor and his stethoscope. *Circulation, 34*:889, 1966.

Fischer, D. S., Singer, D. H., and Feldman, S. M.: Clubbing, a review, with emphasis on hereditary acropachy. *Medicine (Baltimore), 43*:459, 1964.

Forgacs, P.: Lung sounds. *Br. J. Dis. Chest, 63*:1, 1969.

Gross, N. J., and Hamilton, J. D.: Correlation between the physical signs of hypercapnia and the mixed venous P_{CO_2}. *Br. Med. J.,2*:1096, 1963.

Hall, G. H.: The cause of digital clubbing. Testing a new hypothesis. *Lancet, 1*:750, 1959.

Harrison, V. C., Heese, H. de V., and Klein, M.: The significance of grunting in hyaline membrane disease. *Pediatrics, 41*:549, 1968.

Horowitz, L.: Expiratory thrust, an aid in physical diagnosis. *Am. J. Dis. Child., 105*:116, 1963.

Howatt, W. F., and DeMuth, G. D.: The growth of lung function. II. Configuration of the chest. *Pediatrics, 35*:177, 1965.

Iliff, A., and Lee, V. A.: Pulse rate, respiratory rate, and body temperature of children between two months and eighteen years of age. *Child Dev., 23*:237, 1952.

Krahl, V. E.: Anatomy of the mammalian lung. In *Handbook of Physiology*, Section 3: Respiration. Vol. 1. Washington, D.C., American Physiological Society, 1964, pp. 213–284.

McKusick, V. A., and Mutalik, G. S.: Genetics and pulmonary disease. In Liebow, A. A., and Smith, D. E. (Eds.): *The Lung.* Baltimore, Williams and Wilkins Company, 1968, pp. 187–202.

Meredith, H. V.: *The Rhythm of Physical Growth.* A study of eighteen anthropometric measurements on Iowa City white males ranging in age between birth and eighteen years. University of Iowa Studies. No. 3, Vol. XI, 1935.

Waring, W. W., Wilkinson, R. W., Wiebe, R. A., Faul, B. C., and Hilman, B. C.: Quantitation of digital clubbing in children. Measurement of casts of the index finger. *Am. Rev. Resp. Dis.,* *104*:166, 1971.

CHAPTER FOUR

DIAGNOSTIC AND THERAPEUTIC PROCEDURES

WILLIAM W. WARING, M.D.

It is possible to divide all procedures pertaining to respiratory disease into the categories of prophylaxis, diagnosis and therapy. Only those that are felt to deserve special comment will be discussed in this chapter. Some procedures can be performed without assistance by any physician, while others require specialized skills or other physicians or laboratory workers. Radiologic procedures are discussed in Chapter 5, and pulmonary function testing is covered in Chapter 6.

DIAGNOSTIC PROCEDURES

BRONCHOSCOPY

Bronchoscopy is a procedure performed to visualize and manipulate the surface of the larger branches of the tracheobronchial tree. The trachea and main bronchi can thus be directly approached in a child of any age. With a conventional rigid bronchoscope, depending on the size of the patient and the type and size of instrument, the lower lobe bronchi, the orifices of the upper and middle lobe bronchi, and the orifices of the lower lobe segmental bronchi are accessible.

The availability within the past ten years of the flexible bronchofiberscope has revolutionized adult pulmonary medicine, but the role of this instrument in the pediatric age range is less well defined and for mechanical rea-

sons has serious limitations. The technologic achievement common to all fiberscopes is their ability to transmit light and images around corners. An excellent review has been written by Sackner (1975) on bronchofiberscopy. The standard fiberscope can be used in childhood at about 11 years, but generally not at younger ages because of its space occupation of the airway. Smaller instruments (3 mm.) exist, but lack a channel for instillation of solutions, aspiration of secretions and passage of brushes or biopsy forceps. Nevertheless, they are of value, frequently in conjunction with a rigid scope, for more distal exploration of the airways.

Bronchoscopy most frequently is electively performed under general anesthesia, but in emergency states, especially in a small or unconscious patient, it may be carried out without anesthesia. In such cases, a trained team is essential in order to carry out the procedure as quickly and as gently as possible.

Bronchoscopy seldom requires more than 15 minutes. The operator is usually a surgeon, most frequently an otolaryngologist or thoracic surgeon. The bronchofiberscope generally requires less training for safe and efficient use than does the rigid scope, and increasing numbers of pediatricians have begun to use the new instrument. Nevertheless, regardless of the tool, considerable skill and experience are required to obtain maximal benefit, since the anatomy of the tracheobronchial tree can be confusing, and landmarks can be altered by volume shifts within the thorax. Prolonged or clumsy bronchoscopy may traumatize the larynx and be followed by dangerous edema and upper airway obstruction. A "mist tent" during the immediate postoperative period may lessen laryngeal edema. During bronchoscopy, the patient's color, pulse and respirations should be carefully monitored, since dangerous hypoxemia may occur in children with severe unilateral or bilateral disease. This is especially true of the bronchofiberscope, whose construction does not permit ventilation or airway management through the instrument itself. Even with the rigid bronchoscope, which can be modified for effective ventilation, there can be considerable airway obstruction. Significant arrhythmias have been reported in adults undergoing bronchoscopic examination, and a monitoring cardioscope is thus recommended.

Bronchoscopy is performed when disease is known or presumed to involve the bronchi observable thereby, and when less heroic diagnostic and therapeutic procedures have failed. From a diagnostic standpoint, in addition to direct observation of the tracheobronchial tree, the operator may identify and localize foreign bodies and the origin of bleeding or purulent secretions. Fluid or tissue may be removed for culture, cytologic study or histologic examination. Anomalies or sites of compression may be definitively identified.

Therapeutically, bronchoscopy is the ideal means of removing aspirated foreign bodies from the major airways, and here the rigid bronchoscope is clearly the instrument of choice as employed by a skilled endoscopist. Such removal is facilitated by preoperative assessment of the nature, number and location of such foreign material. This type of information is generated by a probing history, careful physical examination, inspiration and expiration chest roentgenograms, and frequently by fluoroscopy. A skilled team composed of a pediatric pulmonologist and endoscopist, working together before, during and after bronchoscopic removal of a foreign body, can make the difference between a smooth, complete recovery and a nightmare.

Tenacious or mucopurulent secretions may be directly aspirated through a bronchoscope with relief of atelectasis or obstructive overinflation, especially when the lower lobes are involved. Simultaneous atelectasis of the right middle and right lower lobes almost always indicates obstruction of the bronchus intermedius, a particularly common site for the lodgement of foreign bodies. Collapse of the upper lobes or right middle lobe is generally less susceptible to direct bronchoscopic attack because of the awkward locations and orientations of these lobar bronchi, although the flexibility of the bronchofiberscope is beginning to render these bronchi accessible to examination and, in older children, to manipulation. Small particles of foreign material, such as partly chewed popcorn, can also be bronchoscopically aspirated from the tracheobronchial tree when cough, the mucociliary escalator and postural bronchial drainage have been ineffective.

Localized lobar or segmental lavage with dilute N-acetylcysteine (5 to 10 per cent in normal saline) may assist in removing mucoid bronchial plugs beyond the sight of the bronchoscopist. Multiple bronchial lavage has recently been employed, especially in patients with cystic fibrosis, with both the rigid and flexible bronchoscopes, although there is still disagreement as to its indication and efficacy.

Nice judgment may be required for the timing of either diagnostic or therapeutic bronchoscopy. For example, in known foreign body aspiration of longer than acute duration, judicious delay of two or three days for good medical preparation (antibiotics, expectorants, aerosols and others) may make a subsequent bronchoscopy both safer and more likely to retrieve the offending foreign body than would have been the case with immediate intervention.

In acute atelectasis of either lower

lobe, as in infants with otherwise un-complicated pneumonia, it is safe to try vigorous medical therapy for one week before resorting to bronchoscopy. A lesser delay seems reasonable when there is collapse of both the right mid-dle and lower lobes, and collapse of an entire lung usually calls for prompt in-tervention. Regardless of the duration of the collapse, one or more bronchos-copies should be performed prior to abandoning therapy or considering surgical intervention. Failure to recog-nize lobar collapse during pneumonia and to take the medical and broncho-scopic steps to rectify it is a common cause of bronchiectasis in childhood.

LUNG PUNCTURE

This diagnostic procedure probably deserves selective, wider application, since it can yield information not other-wise easily obtained. Lung puncture has been used to obtain a lung aspirate for either histologic study or culture. The technique is simple. A short-bevel 20-gauge needle is attached to a 10-ml. syringe which contains 1 ml. of sterile isotonic saline solution. *It is essential that the saline contain no bacteriostatic agent.* An intercostal space is locally anesthetized, and a quick stab is made through the space, across the pleurae, and into the lung to a depth of 3 to 4 cm. The saline is injected to assure pa-tency of the needle, and negative pres-sure is produced in the syringe-needle system by withdrawing the plunger of the syringe. Simultaneously, the needle is withdrawn so that tissue fluid is drawn into the needle and syringe. The needle remains in the lung only a few seconds, preferably for less than one respiratory cycle. The contents of the needle and syringe may then be smeared on slides for special staining, or may be transferred to a liquid cul-ture medium by drawing up the me-dium into the syringe through the aspirating needle and thence returning it to its original container. If the sample is sufficient, both may be accomplished.

It should be emphasized that the method has been successfully used to isolate viruses, mycoplasma and tuber-cle bacilli, in addition to conventional bacterial pathogens.

Lung puncture may be the only way of obtaining an organism for antibiotic sensitivity testing in a child with pneu-monia. In such patients, physical ex-amination and chest roentgenograms allow the physician to aspirate the most involved segment of the lung. The procedure should be especially considered in critically ill children, in those who have failed to respond to therapy based on upper respiratory bacterial flora, and in those whose pneumonias are secondary to other un-derlying diseases or drugs that limit host defense. The method has also been of value in diagnosing obscure, in-terstitial pneumonopathies, such as idiopathic pulmonary hemosiderosis.

The procedure has certain theoreti-cal dangers: pulmonary hemorrhage, empyema and pneumothorax. In prac-tice, the only complications have been transient, slight pneumothorax when the tap has been made into air-contain-ing lung and rare minimal hemoptysis. One death related to the procedure has been reported by Sapington and Favor-ite (1936) in a series of 2000 lung taps. Pneumothorax can usually be avoided by choosing a densely consolidated seg-ment for puncture.

LUNG BIOPSY

Biopsy of the lung is occasionally necessary when protracted pulmonary disease cannot be explained by other means, although careful and intelligent use of less extreme diagnostic proce-dures makes it uncommonly necessary. When indicated, lung biopsy is usually performed under general anesthesia with an endotracheal airway, by which normal pulmonary ventilation is main-tained and collapse of the lung pre-vented. Open thoracotomy is per-formed at a site corresponding to known involvement, and sufficient pulmonary tissue is removed for all required studies. Even critically ill (hypoxic, anemic, thrombocytopenic, leukopenic) patients have successfully withstood open lung biopsy. Percutaneous lung biopsy with a Vim-Silverman or Franklin-Silverman needle and by trephine has been reported in adults, but is not at present recommended for infants and children.

PNEUMOPERITONEUM

The injection of 200 to 300 ml. of air into the peritoneal cavity sharply demarcates the position of the diaphragm on subsequent chest roentgenography of the erect patient. It is occasionally useful in differentiating eventration of the diaphragm from supradiaphragmatic lesions, such as extralobar sequestration. In cases of this type, confirmation of an asymptomatic localized eventration might obviate a formal surgical exploration.

PULMONARY FUNCTION TESTS

This subject is fully discussed in Chapter 6.

ARTERIAL PUNCTURE

The physician in his office cannot quantitate the effects of respiratory failure: hypoxemia and hypercapnia. Such an assessment requires precise analysis of the partial pressure of oxygen (P_{O_2}) and carbon dioxide (P_{CO_2}) in arterial blood—that is, blood that has been acted on by the lungs but before its gaseous composition has been altered by passage through the tissues. "Arterialized" capillary or venous blood has been used, but serious underestimates of P_{O_2} may result, especially in critically ill patients. Since blood gas analyzers are universally available in hospitals, pediatricians should be able both to obtain an anaerobic sample of

arterial blood and to interpret blood gas data returning from the laboratory.

Vessels that can be sampled include the temporal (neonates), brachial, radial and femoral arteries. The brachial and radial vessels are to be preferred in older infants and children, and use of femoral artery should be avoided because of post-tap arterial spasm.

Radial arteripuncture is a relatively simple and safe procedure at all ages, although it is wise to test the efficacy of the ulnar collateral arterial supply by compressing the radial artery and noting that the palm does not blanch. A 2 ml. glass syringe (with a plunger that slides easily in the barrel) and attached small-gauge needle (23–24 gauge) are rinsed with a solution of sodium heparin (1000 units/ml.), leaving only the dead space of the syringe and needle filled.

The author prefers to use local anesthesia (2 per cent lidocaine *without* epinephrine) in small volume so as not to disturb the vessel position or size. The puncture is made at an angle of about 45 degrees between the tips of the operator's index and middle fingers. Occlusion of the vessel with the downstream finger helps to dilate the artery (Fig. 1). The needle is pointed upstream with the bevel pointed down. As the artery is entered, blood will appear in the syringe, which will fill slowly and spontaneously if the plunger is properly fitted and moistened with heparin. One should attempt to collect a full 2 ml. of blood, since significant errors in P_{CO_2} occur with small samples that are diluted by dead-space heparin. The needle is removed as soon as the sample is collected, and any small air bubbles are immediately expelled. The system is then sealed by embedding the needle tip in a rubber stopper. Heparin and blood sample are mixed by vigorous rotary movement of the syringe between the palms, and the syringe is dropped into a small pan containing ice and water. Analyses should be made within minutes after collection for greatest accuracy.

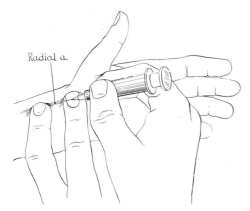

Figure 1. Radial arteripuncture. See text for details. (From Waring, W. W., and Jeansonne, L. O., III: *Practical Manual of Pediatrics.* St. Louis, C. V. Mosby Co., 1975.

The laboratory is usually prepared to report P_{O_2}, P_{CO_2} and pH, as well as to calculate certain secondary parameters, such as standard bicarbonate, base excess, and arterial oxygen saturation. These latter and other data can be obtained from the Severinghaus slide rule* or from the nomograms of Olszowka (1973).

Outside of the neonatal period, the author has found Table 1 of value in interpreting blood gas results. The monograph of Shapiro (1973) should be consulted for greater details on blood gas analysis and interpretation.

THERAPEUTIC PROCEDURES

BRONCHIAL (POSTURAL) DRAINAGE AND PHYSICAL THERAPY

These methods of treating disease of the bronchi will receive considerable emphasis here because they are neither practiced as effectively nor used as frequently as they should be. Bronchial drainage is indicated in any clinical situation in which excessive fluid in the

---

*Radiometer Blood Gas Calculator, London Co., Cleveland, Ohio 44145.

TABLE 1. BLOOD GAS AND ACID-BASE INTERPRETATION

pH
(Normal = 7.350–7.450)

ACIDOSIS		ALKALOSIS	
Mild:	7.300–7.350	Mild:	7.450–7.500
Mod.:	7.250–7.300	Mod.:	7.500–7.550
Severe:	<7.250	Severe:	>7.550

P_{CO_2}
(Normal = 35–45 mm. Hg)

HYPERCAPNIA		HYPOCAPNIA	
Mild:	45–50	Mild:	30–35
Mod.:	50–60	Mod.:	25–30
Severe:	>60	Severe:	<25

P_{O_2}
(Sea level, room air, normal = >85 mm. Hg)

HYPOXEMIA	
Mild:	55–85
Mod.:	40–55
Severe:	<40

Standard Bicarbonate
(Normal = 22–28 mEq./liter)

DEPRESSION		ELEVATION	
Mild:	19–22	Mild:	28–31
Mod.:	17–19	Mod.:	31–35
Severe:	<17	Severe:	>35

Base Excess
(Normal = −3 to +4)

DEPRESSION		ELEVATION	
Mild:	−3 to −7	Mild:	+4 to +8
Mod.:	−7 thru −10	Mod.:	+8 thru +12
Severe:	<−10	Severe:	>+12

bronchi is not being removed by normal ciliary activity and cough. Determination of the presence of excessive bronchial fluid and its localization are most easily accomplished by segmental auscultation of the lungs. Persistent crackles in a given segment or lobe constitute sufficient indication in themselves for drainage of the involved bronchi.

Examination of the anatomy of the tracheobronchial tree (Fig. 2) indicates that in the erect position the segments of the middle lobe, of the lingular division of the left upper lobe, and of both lower lobes normally must drain against gravity. Only the segments of the right upper lobe and the nonlingular portions of the left upper lobe receive gravitational assistance in erect man. Normally, such a situation does not interfere with the body's ability to maintain patency of the tracheobronchial tree. Special loads, however, may be placed on the clearing mechanisms of the relatively small bronchi of children by viscous or excessive mucus and pus. It is axiomatic that infection is ultimately superimposed on bronchial obstruction due to any cause and that infection increases obstruction. Although

bronchial drainage may not be the principal or sole therapy, it can be of invaluable assistance. After bronchoscopic removal of a foreign body, after administration of a bronchodilator to an asthmatic child, or during the resolution of a pneumonia, excessive fluid may remain in one or more lobar or segmental bronchi. The affected bronchi can be identified by the topographical distribution of crackles, as well as roentgenographically. The physician then can determine the position in which to place the patient that best promotes drainage of involved bronchi (Figs. 3 and 4).

Bronchial drainage is carried out three or four times daily, usually before meals and at bedtime, in periods not

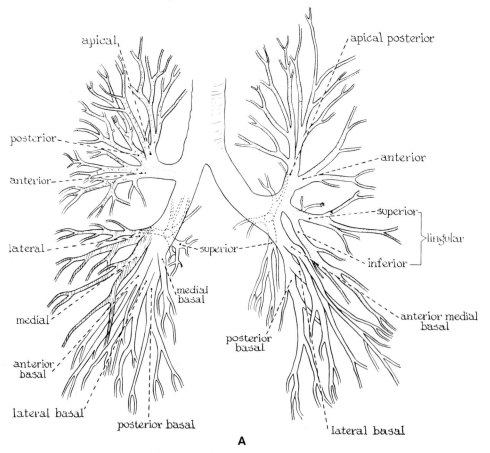

Figure 2. *A,* Posteroanterior projection. Distribution of lobar and segmental bronchi. Upper lobe bronchi are stippled, middle lobe bronchi are diagonally lined, and lower lobe bronchi are outlined only. Segmental bronchi are labeled.

Illustration continued on the following page

exceeding 30 minutes. Up to four positions may be used, since more than this number tends to exceed reasonable limits of cooperation. The exact arrangements for drainage vary with the situation: the physical therapy department or treatment room if the child is hospitalized, the bedroom if the child is at home. Infants may be positioned on the lap and legs of a parent, and small children may be effectively drained on a padded ironing board.

Children with chronic bronchial disease, such as cystic fibrosis or bronchiectasis, may require daily periods of drainage over many months. They will profit from specially constructed tables or platforms, the surfaces of which can be padded for comfort and adjusted to the different angles required to drain all involved segments (Fig. 5). Comfort is important because adequate drainage depends on relaxation and cooperation in each position over a period of five to 15 minutes. Therapy may be discontinued when auscultation reveals that no excessive bronchial fluid remains and when the chest roentgenogram indicates clearing of the disease.

In all cases, the exact positions, as well as their order, duration and frequency, should be explained to the person (parent, nurse or therapist) who will be working with the child. At least one treatment should be demonstrated on the patient to parents or others who are unfamiliar with the techniques. Positions for drainage are varied sub-

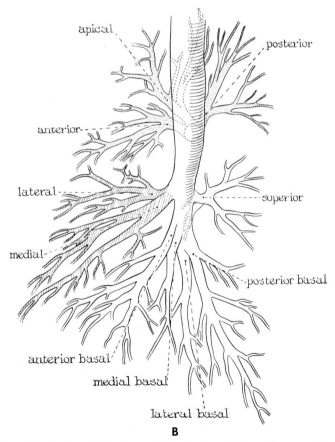

B

Figure 2. *B,* Lateral projection of right bronchi. Distribution of lobar and segmental bronchi. Upper lobe bronchi are stippled, middle lobe bronchi are diagonally lined, and lower lobe bronchi are outlined only. Segmental bronchi are labeled.

Illustration continued on the following page

sequently by the physician in conformity with shifting patterns of bronchial disease. The family should have diagrams (Fig. 3 or 4) to which reference may be made until they are thoroughly familiar with the prescribed positions.

If bronchorrhea is diffuse without any particularly specific localization, it is reasonable to recommend positions that will drain major dependent bronchi when the child is in the erect position, i.e., the posterior basal segments, the middle lobe, and the lingula, in that order. Drainage positions for the upper lobes may also be of importance for predominantly recumbent infants.

Certain physical therapeutic maneuvers are of great help when combined with bronchial drainage. Indeed, the modern concept of bronchial drainage implies the use of such maneuvers in addition to simple positioning of the patient. Viscid secretions may not drain from bronchi by gravity alone. The simile is frequently used of a freshly opened catsup bottle. Although the bottle is inverted, i.e., properly positioned for drainage, no catsup may flow until it is ejected by repeated blows on the bottom of the bottle; once started, however, flow may continue with little further agitation.

The maneuvers that may assist the removal of fluid by gravity include deep breathing, reinforced cough, thoracic "squeezing," "cupping" and vibration. Each will be briefly described.

After the child has been placed in position for drainage and has been encouraged to relax, he is asked to take

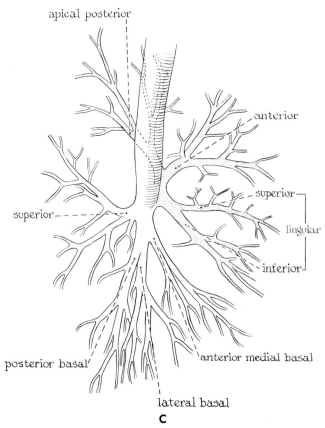

apical posterior

anterior

superior

superior

lingular

inferior

posterior basal

anterior medial basal

lateral basal

C

Figure 2.   *C,* Lateral projection of left bronchi. Distribution of lobar and segmental bronchi. Upper lobe bronchi are stippled, middle lobe bronchi are diagonally lined, and lower lobe bronchi are outlined only. Segmental bronchi are labeled.

Illustration continued on the following page

several deep breaths. Since deep inspiration enlarges the tracheobronchial tree, air may penetrate around and through secretions that would not be affected by usual tidal volumes. Expiration following such a deep breath may carry secretions in the desired direction and may even initiate a productive cough.

The child should be taught not to suppress his cough and not to waste his strength with repeated feeble, and therefore ineffective, coughs. Instead, he should take a deep breath and cough once or twice as *hard* as he can. Such anticipated coughs can be reinforced by the hands of the operator encircling and synchronously compressing the sides of the lower half of the chest. The cough may thus be less fatiguing and more effective. Many children are not able to cough well in a dependent position. These children should be allowed to sit up after several minutes of drainage for a further trial of repeated, reinforced coughs. Sputum produced should be spit out into a container so that the productivity of the treatment can be demonstrated to both the child and the physician.

With the child in a bronchial drainage position, another maneuver, the "squeeze," may be tried. The child is asked to take a deep breath and then exhale through the mouth as completely and rapidly as possible, as he

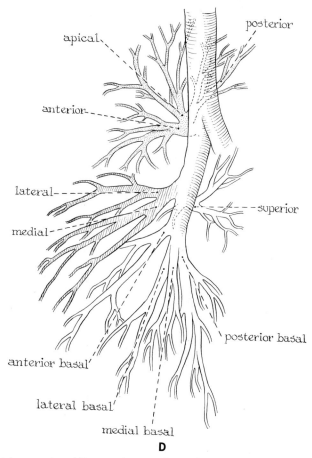

apical

posterior

anterior

lateral

superior

medial

posterior basal

anterior basal

lateral basal

medial basal

D

Figure 2. *D,* Right posterior oblique projection of right bronchi. Distribution of lobar and segmental bronchi. Upper lobe bronchi are stippled, middle lobe bronchi are diagonally lined, and lower lobe bronchi are outlined only. Segmental bronchi are labeled.

Illustration continued on the following page

would do for a forced expiratory volume determination. The depth of expiration is increased by brief, firm pressure from the operator's hands compressing the sides of the thorax. The goal is to decrease maximally the volume of the tracheobronchial tree. Secretions may thus be expressed from the "open ends" of the bronchi, similar to the squeezing of toothpaste from a tube. The subsequent inspiration may be followed by a most productive cough, which should again be "reinforced" by the operator.

The maneuver known as "cupping" or "clapping" is performed intermittently several times in each drainage position. One or both of the cupped hands of the operator vigorously and repeatedly strike that part of the chest

under which the segments being drained are located. Although "cupping" should be vigorous, it is painless if performed properly. The patient should wear a light cotton undershirt to avoid irritation of the skin of the chest. Care should be taken not to slap the chest with the fingers or palm, but to make the cupped hand conform exactly to the contour of the chest wall. No jewelry should be worn on the hands of the therapist. The entire circumference of the hand should touch the chest at the same instant. A proper "cupping" emits a definitely hollow sound. The effect of "cupping" is related partly to the compression of air between the operator's hand and the patient's chest wall. This compression wave is presumably transmitted to the underlying bronchi

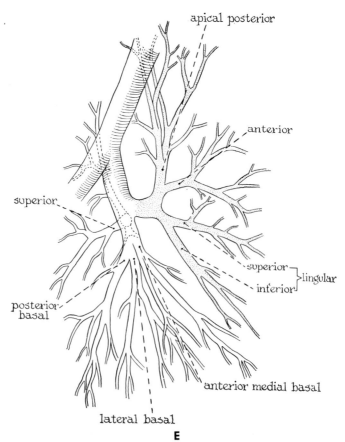

E

Figure 2. *E*, Left posterior oblique projection of left bronchi. Distribution of lobar and segmental bronchi. Upper lobe bronchi are stippled, middle lobe bronchi are diagonally lined, and lower lobe bronchi are outlined only. Segmental bronchi are labeled.

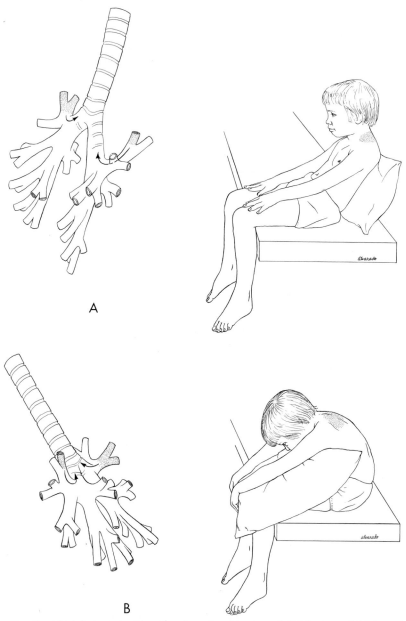

Figure 3. Bronchial drainage positions for the major segments of all lobes on a child. In each position, a model of the tracheobronchial tree is projected beside the child in order to show the segmental bronchus being drained (stippled) and the flow of secretions out of the segmental bronchus (*arrow*). The drainage platform is padded but firm, and pillows are liberally used to maintain each position with comfort. The platform is horizontal unless otherwise noted. A stippled area on the child's chest indicates the area to be "cupped" or vibrated by the therapist (see text). *A*, Apical segment of right upper lobe and apical subsegment of apical-posterior segment of left upper lobe. Drainage moves secretions into main bronchi from which they can be more easily expelled (*curved arrows*). *B*, Posterior segment of right upper lobe and posterior subsegment of apical-posterior segment of left upper lobe. Drainage moves secretions into main bronchi from which they can be more easily expelled (*curved arrows*).

Illustration continued on the following page

and aids the gravitational flow of secretions from them.

Vibration is a more difficult procedure and, therefore, is usually effectively executed only by a therapist. A rapid vibratory impulse is transmitted through the chest wall from the flattened hands of the operator by an almost isometric contraction of forearm flexor and extensor muscles. Vibration may be used directly over the involved area, or it may be applied to the sides of the chest in performing the chest "squeeze" maneuver.

If the operator is a parent, he can easily be taught the maneuvers of deep breathing, reinforced coughing, and "cupping." More advanced techniques

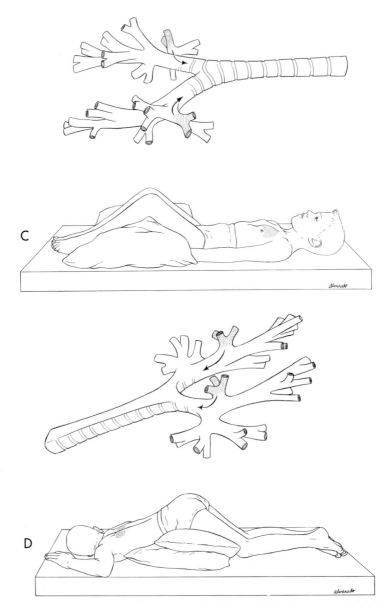

Figure 3. *C,* Anterior segments of both upper lobes. The child should be rotated slightly away from the side being drained. *D,* Superior segments of both lower lobes. Although the platform is flat, pillows are used to raise the buttocks moderately.

Illustration continued on following page

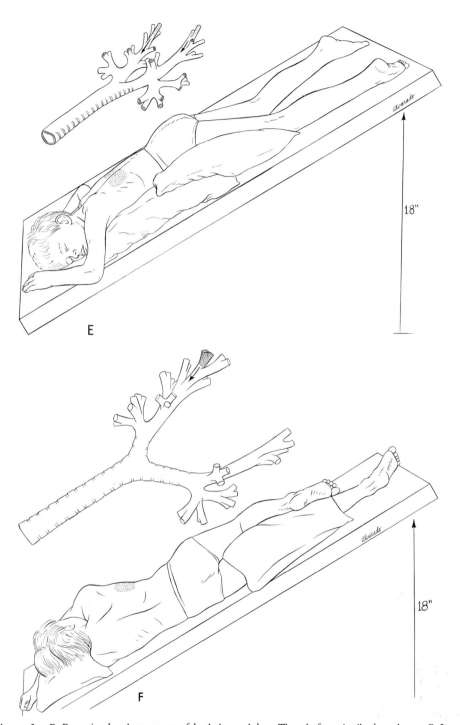

Figure 3. *E,* Posterior basal segments of both lower lobes. The platform is tilted as shown. *F,* Lateral basal segment of the right lower lobe. The platform is tilted as shown. Drainage of the lateral basal segment of the left lower lobe would be accomplished by a mirror image of this position (right side down).

Illustration continued on the following page

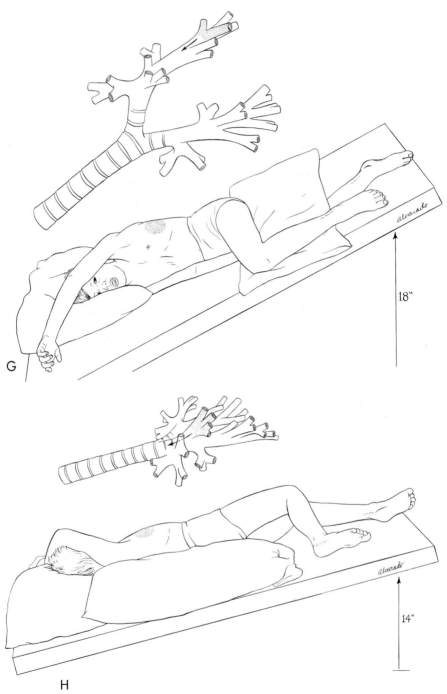

Figure 3. *G,* Anterior basal segment of the left lower lobe. The platform is tilted as shown. *H,* Right middle lobe. The platform is tilted as shown.

Illustration continued on the following page

should be reserved for the trained therapist or for the intelligent parent with a child who requires bronchial drainage over months or years.

Since bronchial drainage is both fatiguing and time-consuming, efforts have been made to introduce mechanical vibration of various types as a substitute for cupping and vibrating. These have ranged from simple "barber shop" massage-vibrators, through modified saber-saws with a piston and padded cushion replacing the blade, to percussion "vests" containing several percussing units. The evaluation of such equipment is extremely difficult. It probably ranges from ineffective to less effective than a trained therapist. However, the saber-saw type is probably the most effective and can be employed by adolescents away from home or in those cases in which parents are unable to carry out the procedure at home because of conflicting work hours, arthritis, or other situations that prevent parental assistance.

Bronchial drainage has also been advocated as a means of removing aspirated foreign bodies from the tracheobronchial tree. The method is not without hazard, however, and should never be employed outside of a hospital setting in which emergency endoscopy is immediately available.

Although many experts feel that drainage procedures of the types described above are effective in clinical situations associated with bronchorrhea, there is division of opinion as to their prophylactic value in patients who are expected, because of their disease (cystic fibrosis), to develop chronic bronchitis and bronchiectasis. Nevertheless, many physicians routinely prescribe prophylactic bronchial drainage as soon as a diagnosis of cystic fibrosis is made, even in the absence of any evidence of pulmonary disease.

BREATHING EXERCISES

Breathing exercises have not been widely applied to children, but may be of value in certain patients, including those with kyphoscoliosis, cystic fi-

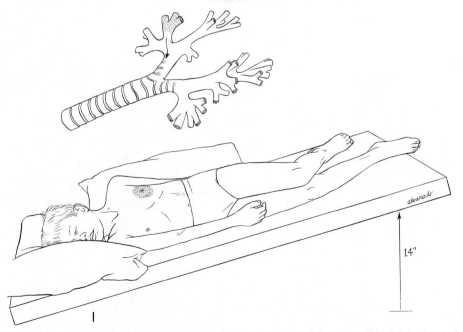

Figure 3. *1,* Lingular segments of the left upper lobe (homologue of the right middle lobe). The platform is tilted as shown.

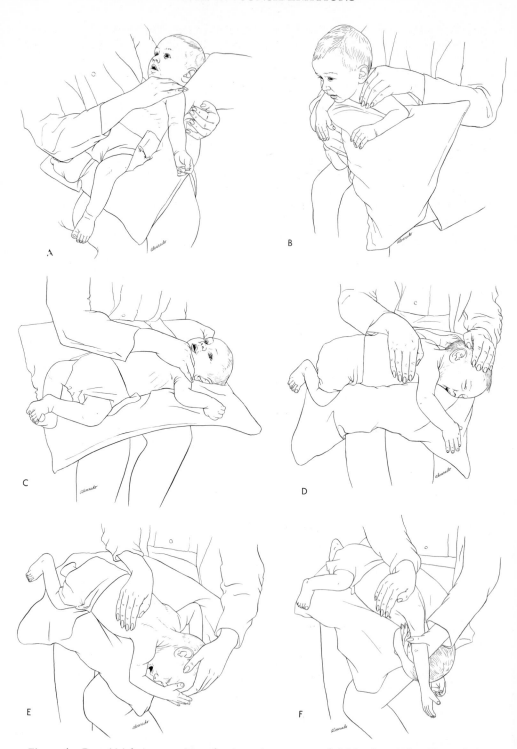

Figure 4. Bronchial drainage positions for the major segments of all lobes in an infant. The procedure is most easily carried out in the therapist's lap. The therapist's hand on the chest indicates the area to be "cupped" or vibrated (see text). *A,* Apical segment of the left upper lobe. *B,* Posterior segment of the left upper lobe. *C,* Anterior segment of the left upper lobe. *D,* Superior segment of the right lower lobe. *E,* Posterior segment of the right lower lobe. *F,* Lateral segment of the right lower lobe.

Illustration continued on the following page

brosis, asthma and bronchiectasis, as well as those who have had extensive resections of diseased lung. There are few data available with which to support efficacy of the various exercise programs. If applied, however, exercises should be a part of a total therapeutic program that frequently also includes correction of posture, bronchial drainage, and various types of inhalation therapy. Breathing exercises are conveniently done during and after bronchial drainage.

Goals of the exercises include (1) development of more effective diaphragmatic and lower costal breathing, (2) relaxation of all muscles, but especially those of the upper part of the chest, shoulder girdle and neck, and (3) attainment of a good, easy posture.

The precise manner of proceeding with retraining must depend on the age, motivation and strength of the child, as well as his disease, the extent of the physiologic disturbance, and his emotional reactions to the therapist. In addition to being experienced, the therapist should be cheerful, positive and firmly gentle. A parent should be present for the exercises so that they can be continued correctly at home.

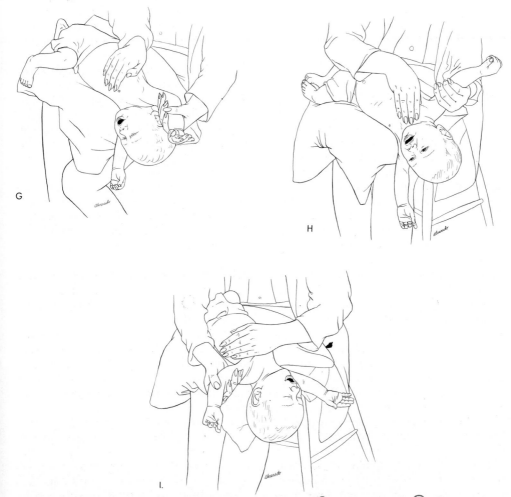

Figure 4. *G,* Anterior basal segment of the right lower lobe. *H,* Right middle lobe. *I,* Lingular segments of the left upper lobe.

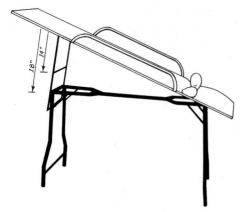

Figure 5. Adjustable table for bronchial (postural) drainage (Greater Cleveland Cystic Fibrosis Chapter, 3098 Mayfield Road, Cleveland, Ohio 44118). The surface measures 15½" × 71" and is padded but firm. The top adjusts from horizontal to two inclinations, a shallow one for lingula and right middle lobe and a deep one for the basal segments of the lower lobes.

INHALATION THERAPY

The term "inhalation therapy" is an inclusive one that covers the theory and practice of treating a patient by certain changes in the composition, volume or pressure of inspired gases. Such alterations include ① increases in the fractional concentration of oxygen (oxygen therapy) ② replacement of a part of the nitrogen with another inert gas with more desirable properties (oxygen-helium mixture) ③ increases in the water vapor content of inspired gas (humidification) ④ constant increases in the total pressure of administered gases (hyperbaric therapy) ⑤ removal of undesirable air-borne material, such as dust and bacteria (filtration) ⑥ the addition of air-borne particles with beneficial properties (aerosol therapy), and ⑦ various means of assisting or controlling respiration (intermittent positive pressure breathing, various respirators). A full discussion of the indications for these different types of inhalation therapy and of their application to children would require a text in itself. Only certain aspects of this field can be alluded to here, but the physician caring for children with respiratory disease is urged to become familiar with the goals and methods of inhalation therapy and with a few specific items of equipment.

Oxygen therapy is usually administered in the hospital; its use at home is not generally recommended, although the author has employed it on several occasions in the home management of near-terminal children with cystic fibrosis. Oxygen is indicated when significant reductions in its partial pressure in arterial blood are present and when such reductions can be significantly elevated by increasing alveolar oxygen concentrations. Children with anatomic right-to-left shunts, such as those with tetralogy of Fallot, may neither require nor benefit from oxygen. The presence of cyanosis remains the best single clinical criterion for supplemental oxygen. It is a late sign, however, since a considerable drop in the partial pressure of oxygen in arterial blood must occur before cyanosis is detectable. Oxygen alone will not relieve dyspnea, and, depending on the cause of dyspnea, more rational therapy might be a bronchodilator agent administered in the form of an aerosol.

When oxygen is indicated, it may be given by mask, face tent, nasal catheter or cannula, oxyhood, intermittent positive pressure apparatus or conventional oxygen tent. The method of choice depends on the ventilatory status of the child, the percentage of oxygen desired in the inspired air, and the anticipated duration of need. For most conditions, an inspired oxygen concentration of 40 to 50 per cent ($F_{I_{O_2}}$ of 0.4 to 0.5) is satisfactory. Simple open-top tents may give effective concentrations of oxygen for an infant, while a nasal cannula or face tent may be well tolerated by an older child.

The adequacy of oxygen therapy can be monitored by determinations of the concentration of oxygen within a tent by devices that employ principles of thermal conductivity, paramagnetic susceptibility, or membrane diffusion in an electrode. It is obviously also possible to monitor arterial oxygen saturation or partial pressure within the patient himself (blood gas analysis).

Oxygen should not be continued after the indication for its use has ceased. To the extent that it reduces the partial pressure of nitrogen in alveoli, oxygen increases the rate of lung collapse in the event of airway obstruction. Excessive and prolonged concentrations are related to the production of retrolental fibroplasia and play a significant role in so-called bronchopulmonary dysplasia in newborn infants. Moreover, the lungs can be injured at *any* age by excessive and prolonged inspired oxygen concentrations.

Since oxygen is dry, whether it is supplied from cylinders or from a central hospital system, some provision must be made to humidify it.

It is also good practice to measure at regular intervals the temperature of the gases within a tent to avoid an uncomfortably hot environment for a sick child.

Aerosol therapy is designed to prevent or treat respiratory disease by the inhalation and subsequent deposition of airborne water particles. In addition, these particles may contain specific bronchodilating, decongestant, mucolytic, antimicrobial or other agents. Particle sizes range from a fraction of a micron in diameter to droplets larger even than 50 microns. Aerosol therapy may be intermittent and brief (less than a minute) or continuous and prolonged (hours at a time). The former technique is usually employed for the purpose of delivering a specific pharmacologic agent to the respiratory tract. The latter is always used to deliver water to the airways, usually with the goal of thinning secretions.

It is implicit in all forms of aerosol therapy that the nebulized material is distributed in accordance with gas flow patterns within the lung. Unventilated areas of the lung thus receive none of the aerosol; this is important in the use of aerosols in obstructive lung disease, especially if atelectasis is present.

Aerosols for clinical use are produced by nebulizers, which act as repositories for the solution to be nebulized and also generate visible aerosol mists when connected to a source of gas under pressure (oxygen cylinder, hand bulb, or powered oil-free air compressor). By suitable internal construction, a nebulizer can be made to baffle out large particles and deliver a spectrum of particles over the desired range of diameters.

The kind of equipment chosen for aerosol therapy is largely dependent on whether the physician wants to treat the patient continuously (hours at a time) or intermittently (20 or 30 minutes). Equipment suitable for continuous treatment is shown in Figure 6. Such a "mist tent" can be used either in the hospital or at home when one desires to thin tracheobronchial secretions that are thickened by disease (cystic fibrosis, bronchiectasis).

Water may exist in inspired air either in the form of vapor or in the form of droplets. Regardless of its initial water content or initial temperature, inspired air is warmed to body temperature and essentially is fully saturated with water in the upper respiratory tract. The alveoli thus receive air containing about 44 mg. of water in invisible vapor form per liter of gas. Since air holds more water when fully saturated at 37° C. than at room temperature, full saturation of inspired air under ordinary conditions can occur only by an obligatory transfer of water from the mucosa of the respiratory tract. Only about 20 to 25 per cent of the heat and water transferred to inspired air is normally recovered during expiration. This obligatory transfer can be diminished, however, by warming and fully saturating inspired air. Additionally, if water is added to inspired gas in the form of particles, it is possible to achieve a positive net delivery of water to the respiratory tract.

Such a net positive water delivery is obtainable, however, with the inhalation of very dense aerosol mists whose total water content (vapor plus aerosol) at ambient conditions exceeds that of fully saturated air at 37° C. Such con-

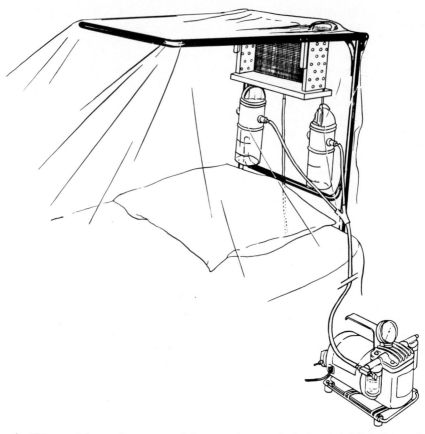

Figure 6. "Mist tent" for continuous aerosol therapy at home or in the hospital. A light frame of tubular aluminum at the head of the bed supports an ice cannister (with drain) for cooling and two nebulizers. Clear, light plastic sheeting covers the frame and tucks snugly under the mattress when the tent is in use. The nebulizers are powered with compressed, filtered air from a portable, continuously running diaphragm-type compressor. Two such nebulizers should deliver about 200 ml. of aerosol per eight hours with a mean particle size of less than 5 microns. The equipment, as illustrated, should maintain a water concentration in the tent in the range of 26 mg. per liter. A concentration of 33 mg. per liter could be achieved with a larger compressor, and an ultrasonic nebulizer could maintain a water concentration of up to 75 mg. per liter.

centrations are obtained by ultrasonic nebulizers, which can maintain water concentrations of 44 to 75 mg. per liter in a standard mist tent. Mechanical nebulizers operating on a jet principle with compressed gas, either oxygen or air, maintain water concentrations in a tent considerably below 44 mg. of water per liter of air (Fig. 6). The total water content is of more than academic interest, since it undoubtedly has some effect on the amount of the mist utilized for the obligatory saturation of air as its temperature is increased. In theory, the entire aerosol output of a mechanical nebulizer system supplying a mist tent could be converted into vapor in the upper respiratory tract and thus not penetrate in droplet form to the lower tracheobronchial tree. It is probable, however, that there is some small amount of peripheral distribution, and it is possible that this is sufficient to alter the viscoelastic properties of sputum or mucus in a way that encourages their removal by mucociliary activity, cough or postural bronchial drainage.

Aside from the total water output of the nebulizers, the distribution of the aerosol mass into various sizes of particles is certainly a critical factor in considering levels of deposition. Particles larger than 10 microns probably do not penetrate beyond the upper airway, whereas intermediate particles (measuring 1 to 10 microns) achieve deeper penetration, and submicronic (smaller than 1 micron) particles in theory reach the alveolar level. The largest particles are deposited by inertial impaction, the intermediate are deposited by sedimentation, and the smallest are subject to diffusion forces.

Of interest, therefore, is a knowledge for a *particular* nebulizer of its output in terms of particle size distribution. Particle size measurement is itself a difficult task with considerable variations in results, depending on the exact sampling parameters and methods employed. Comparisons between nebulizers of particle size spectra are thus frequently misleading because of nonuniform sampling and analysis techniques. Moreover, there may be differences between count mean, mode and median particle diameters. Probably the best index of particle size is the mass median diameter (MMD) — the particle size that divides the mass of water output into two equal parts. Since a 10-micron particle weighs 1000 times more than a 1-micron particle, a nebulizer producing only a relatively small number of large particles and a relatively large number of small particles could still have a large MMD. In such a case, the addition of more effective baffling to remove the large particles would reduce the MMD considerably. At the same time total water output would be reduced. Presumably, clinical efficacy would be unchanged, but the patient's bed would be less wet. MMD is the best indicator of how much of the aerosol will be deposited and in what part of the upper airway and lungs.

In continuous aerosol therapy, distilled water is probably most commonly used. Propylene glycol in a 10 per cent aqueous solution is also widely employed, especially in jet-type nebulizers. This mixture has been thought to stabilize the particles and thus favor their

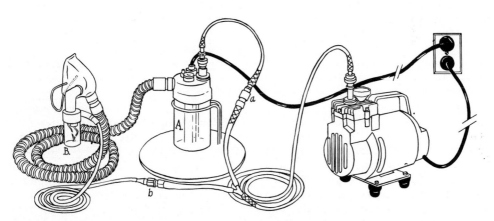

Figure 7. Equipment for semicontinuous tepid aerosol therapy with provision for addition of special aerosols into the main stream. A single, portable compressor powers both nebulizers (*A* and *B*) by dividing its output through a **Y** tube. Airflow regulators (*a* and *b*) control the volume of air going to the respective nebulizers. Nebulizer *A* is of large capacity, similar to those shown in Figure 6, and usually contains 10 per cent propylene glycol in water. An immersion heater (electric cord attached) within the nebulizer warms the contained fluid to approximately 140°F. Air passes through regulator *a* and aerosolizes the hot solution. Warm mist thus generated passes through the large-caliber corrugated hose to a light plastic mask over the patient's nose and mouth. The aerosol is cooled in its passage through the tubing, but is inhaled at a temperature above that of the body (100 to 110°F.). Condensation of water occurs in the tubing with cooling; by placement of the mask at a level above nebulizer *A,* fluid thus formed drains back into the nebulizer for reuse. Nebulizer *B* is of small capacity and is designed to inject unheated agents, such as an antibiotic, into the side of the mask where it mixes and is inhaled with the tepid aerosol.

deposition, but increased retention has not been noted when such was actually measured.

When it is desired to administer by aerosol small quantities of an agent for a specific pharmacologic action, the equipment is necessarily different from the "mist tent." A small nebulizer with a capacity of less than 10 ml. is required (nebulizer B, Fig. 7), which should nebulize about 2 ml. per ten minutes. Such a nebulizer for use at home can be powered by a small electric compressor or even a bicycle pump. Hand bulbs are not satisfactory except for bronchodilators. Some patients may require both continuous and intermittent aerosol therapy—i.e., during the night they sleep in a tent for general tracheobronchial wetting and during the day receive intermittent treatment with an antibiotic or mucolytic agent from a small nebulizer.

Solutions for aerosolization may also be heated so that they are inhaled at temperatures slightly warmer than that of the body (Fig. 7). Such tepid aerosols are fully saturated with water and thus diminish or eliminate the obligatory loss of water from the mucosa of the airway. Tepid aerosols cannot be used in a tent because of their heat, but the attachment of a face tent may allow more prolonged treatments than in the usual intermittent administration of aerosols. Although theoretically more effective than aerosols delivered at ambient temperature, heated aerosols in chronic obstructive lung disease in childhood may be enervating, especially if treatment is prolonged.

With regard to the clinical efficacy of aerosol therapy, there is a large body of clinical, primarily testimonial, evidence that it is beneficial in certain disease states (Table 2). It has been widely used in the treatment of both upper and lower respiratory tract disease, including croup, tracheobronchitis, bronchiolitis, pneumonia, bronchiectasis, atelectasis, cystic fibrosis, asthma and others.

Controversy centers around the treatment of the lungs of patients with

TABLE 2. VARIOUS CLINICAL SITUATIONS IN WHICH AEROSOL THERAPY MAY BE INDICATED

Asthma
Cystic fibrosis
Laryngotracheobronchitis
Bronchiectasis
Pneumonia, especially with atelectasis
Weakness of muscles of respiration (poliomyelitis, paraplegia, amyotonia)
Traumatic croup (postintubation)
Any state in which upper airway is bypassed (intubation, tracheostomy, and so on)

cystic fibrosis. At present, some physicians inaugurate a night mist tent program for such patients at the time of diagnosis. There exist clinical studies both to support and to refute this practice, but the bulk of evidence appears to indicate that prolonged mist tent therapy is not a critical factor in the management of children with cystic fibrosis.

Mist therapy in croup appears to be beneficial, but controlled data are lacking. In asthma, continuous water mist tent therapy seems to have a variable effect. Patients with hyperreactive tracheobronchial trees may respond with worsening of their bronchospasm. The same patient at a later stage in his attack, or other patients during acute attacks, appear to be benefited. Intermittent aerosol therapy for the purpose of delivering a specific bronchodilating agent, such as isoproterenol, has a definite beneficial effect, promptly improving airway mechanics but paradoxically, in some patients, causing increased unevenness in ventilation-perfusion relationships. Recently, aerosolized racemic epinephrine, delivered either by intermittent positive pressure apparatus or by nonpressure nebulizer, has been advocated for the treatment of infectious croup and postintubation laryngeal edema and tracheitis.

Aerosol therapy also appears to have an important role in maintaining normal airway patency in patients with tracheostomies and in patients with other types of artificial airways, such as orotracheal or nasotracheal tubes, especially if they are also being mechanically ventilated. However, aerosols are not required if inspired gas can be delivered fully saturated with water at body temperature.

The application of aerosol therapy to pulmonary disease prophylaxis has also been employed and strongly advocated in cystic fibrosis, in which the transition is from normal lungs to severe end stages of bronchiectasis, obstructive overinflation, mucoid impaction and chronic pneumonitis. The evidence for its prophylactic application has been theoretical and supported by epidemiologic studies indicating improved survival rates when patients are so handled after early diagnosis.

Aerosol therapy does not appear to have a beneficial role in the treatment of respiratory distress syndrome or bronchiolitis of viral causation in infancy.

Intermittent inhalation of aerosols of 20 per cent or less N-acetylcysteine has been advocated and widely used for a mucolytic action. Although considerable testimonial evidence supports its beneficial action, studies have failed to show improvement in pulmonary function after its aerosolization.

With regard to the harmful effects of aerosol therapy, there is strong circumstantial evidence relating excessive use of isoproterenol aerosols and asthma deaths. In addition, failure to control bacterial growth in aerosol equipment or in nebulized solutions has led to serious and even fatal gram-negative bacterial infections. Nebulizers should be cleaned and sterilized daily in the hospital, and parents should be given detailed instruction on their cleaning and sterilization at home. The availability of disposable equipment has undoubtedly been valuable in reducing nosocomial infections.

There is a definite relation between aerosol therapy and bronchial drainage. Drainage is much more effective if it *immediately follows* effective aerosol therapy.

BRONCHIAL AND PULMONARY LAVAGE

The instillation of varying quantities of liquids into the tracheobronchial tree has been advocated in adults for the treatment of pulmonary alveolar proteinosis and obstructive pulmonary diseases (chronic bronchitis and status asthmaticus). In children, the technique has been advocated as a radical form of therapy in cystic fibrosis. The techniques have varied widely and have ranged from limited lobar lavage, through multifocal bilateral lavages, to total unilateral bronchoalveolar lavage (with a Carlens catheter to ventilate the contralateral lung).

The purpose of lavage in cystic fibrosis is to wash out trapped accumulations of mucopus from extensively bronchiectatic airways. Patients have been selected in various ways but usually include children with ① failure to respond to conventional but vigorous medical therapy, ② diffuse pulmonary disease, presumably bronchiectasis, and ③ decreased pulmonary function without respiratory failure.

Lavage should not be attempted on critically ill or terminal patients or in the absence of expert pediatric anesthetic assistance and intensive care facilities.

In one study, isotonic sodium chloride solution has been reported to be somewhat safer than 10 per cent N-acetylcysteine as a lavage agent, although larger quantities of the former removed less material than smaller quantities of the latter.

Transient decreases in pulmonary function and post-lavage pneumonias are commonly observed, and considerable mortality has been encountered, especially in unreported series. The latter has led to abandonment of the procedure in some centers.

Although it is quite possible that selective lavage (both with respect to patient and technique) is an effective form of therapy in cystic fibrosis, it should not be attempted lightly and never in the absence of a necessary combination of experienced personnel and intensive care facilities.

PLEURAL SPACE DRAINAGE AND INTRACAVITARY (MONALDI) DRAINAGE

The insertion of a soft catheter between the ribs, for drainage of either the pleural space or of a cavity within the lung, is frequently indicated in certain complications of staphylococcal pneumonia. This procedure may be done in a treatment room, if necessary, but is best performed semielectively in an operating room. Such drainage serves to remove fluid or gas that may ① restrict pulmonary function, ② unduly prolong a septic process, or ③ cause fibrotic imprisonment of the lung in a partially collapsed state.

Soft rubber catheters are generally used, since they are available in a variety of sizes and have the desirable combination of flexibility and relative incompressibility. Several additional holes are cut near the tip so that drainage will not be stopped by occlusion of a single orifice. The catheter is secured to the chest wall and is usually connected to a drainage-suction system that is simultaneously capable of removing large volumes of gas, collecting effluvia, and applying a negative pressure of 15 to 18 cm. of water at the catheter holes.

The insertion of such tubes is always indicated in pyopneumothorax, tension pneumothorax and large tension pneumatoceles (intracavitary drainage). Their application to empyema without pneumothorax is less absolute, since some prefer to use intermittent thoracentesis to drain empyemas in childhood. It is true that almost all pleural effusions in the course of acute pneumonias in childhood can be easily drained by one or two needle aspirations, since they are thin and usually sterile. But if the fluid is frankly purulent and is present in more than trace quantities, needle drainage is usually inadequate, and the more effective tube should be inserted.

In empyema without bronchopleural fistula, the tube should remain until drainage has ceased and the patient's temperature is essentially normal. In late empyema, the tendency of the pus to loculate in various parts of the pleural space may require repositioning of a catheter or insertion of another. In most patients it is possible to discontinue pleural drainage after one week. In pyopneumothorax, the tube must remain until the bronchopleural fistula has closed; this may require in some cases three weeks or more of suction. Depending on the adequacy of antibiotic therapy, it is usually possible to remove the tube in less than ten days when closure of the fistula is indicated by cessation of bubbling of the underwater portion of the system. Prior to its removal in pyopneumothorax, it is wise to clamp the tube for 24 hours, at the end of which a chest roentgenogram will indicate whether the fistula is truly closed.

TRANSTRACHEAL CATHETERIZATION

The development of mucolytic drugs, such as N-acetylcysteine, has led to the exploration of ways in which they can be introduced directly into the tracheobronchial tree. It is presumed that N-acetylcysteine, for example, is more effective when thus given in large quantities than in the relatively small amounts achievable by aerosol techniques.

Transtracheal catheterization is relatively easily performed by threading a small-bore plastic catheter into the lower cervical trachea through a needle, after the pretracheal soft tissues have been anesthetized. The needle is then removed and the catheter fixed by tape or suture, or both. Injection of a minute amount of bronchographic contrast medium allows positioning of the catheter's tip, either above the carina or in either main bronchus. At any time thereafter, small quantities (1 to 3 ml.) of diluted mucolytic agent can be injected. Proper positioning of the child at the time of injection ensures delivery of the agent to the desired bronchus.

Such injection is usually followed by a brief, hard paroxysm of coughing, which is now more productive than it would be without the agent. Several such injections can be made three or four times daily and can be followed by bronchial drainage and chest "cupping." Since the removal of both the mucolytic agent and the resulting liquefied secretions is largely dependent on the effectiveness of the child's cough, this procedure is contraindicated in children with extreme exhaustion, central nervous system depression, or respiratory muscle weakness due to any cause. It is of definite value in children with atelectasis, especially of an upper lobe or middle lobe, in whom bronchoscopic aspiration may be impossible or unsuccessful.

BRONCHOTOMY

Occasionally a lobar or segmental bronchus may harbor obstructing material that can be removed only by a direct surgical attack on the involved bronchus at the point of obstruction. Successful bronchotomy demands exact anatomic localization of the pathologic process prior to operation. Such precision is usually possible by combining information from physical examination, chest roentgenography, bronchoscopy and bronchography. It is presumed that the lung distal to the point of obstruction is not permanently damaged, because if it were, the treatment of choice would be segmental or lobar resection.

TRACHEOSTOMY

Tracheostomy may be a lifesaving procedure, the indications for which may be divided into six categories: (1) mechanical obstruction of the upper airway (croup, foreign body, laryngeal paralysis); (2) disease of the central nervous system (head injury, craniotomy, drug depression); (3) neuromuscular disease (poliomyelitis, tetanus, myasthenia gravis, amyotonia congenita); (4) secretional obstruction (debility with weak cough, painful thoracic or abdominal incision); (5) intrinsic acute or chronic disease with disturbances of gas diffusion or distribution (blunt chest injuries, smoke inhalation, widespread pneumonia); and (6) prophylaxis (radical head and neck surgery).

Tracheostomy may be combined with mechanical ventilation in children with pulmonary insufficiency (hypercapnia and hypoxia), but in such cases care must be taken not to add excessive dead space by improper selection of equipment. The management of such patients, especially infants, calls for serial determinations of arterial P_{CO_2}, P_{O_2} and pH, as well as minute volumes.

The procedure itself is best done on an elective basis, and even in an emergency, an endotracheal airway (bronchoscope or endotracheal tube) can almost always be inserted prior to the operation. The importance of early tracheostomy has undoubtedly been overemphasized by the expression, "When you begin to wonder whether a tracheostomy is necessary, you should have done it already." Nevertheless, the basis of such a statement is the well recognized danger of excessive delay, as opposed to the few risks of an orderly operation. If in doubt, the physician should not hesitate to call for emergency consultation. In all cases, objective serial observations of the nature of respiration, color, pulse rate and blood pressure should be made and recorded by a trained observer in constant attendance. Increasing pulse and respiratory rates, as recorded every few minutes, are perhaps the best signs of increasing hypoxia. Stridor and retractions may diminish as the child weakens, and if oxygen is being given, cyanosis may not appear until too late.

The type of tube still most commonly used is the silver cannula with a removable inner liner. If a seal is required between the cannula and the trachea for purposes of positive pressure ventilation, the conventional silver cannula may be provided with an inflatable rubber cuff. Cuffed tubes of all types are generally considered more hazardous because of greater tracheal irritation.

Conventional, flexible endotracheal tubes of the anesthesia type, either cuffed or uncuffed, are not recommended for tracheostomy, because of plugging at the tip and difficulties in proper positioning.

The size of the cannula can be preselected, but for all patients the tube must be large enough for effortless gas exchange without excessive pressure inside the trachea. The operator should have cannulas both larger and smaller than the size anticipated. The smaller sizes are available in three lengths and in two angles. Prompt postoperative anteroposterior and lateral roentgenograms are essential; they allow the physician to determine the exact position of the cannula with respect to the trachea and carina, then to make any necessary adjustments or revisions. They also reveal the presence and extent of pneumothorax and pneumomediastinum.

The postoperative care of a child with a tracheostomy is crucial. He requires psychologic and physical support, best supplied by a nurse experienced in tracheostomy care in constant attendance. Vital signs must be regularly monitored. The trachea should be suctioned gently by special sterile catheters. The attendant must be aware of the need to suction the oropharynx occasionally, since vomitus and secretions accumulating there may be aspirated into the lungs between a loose-fitting cannula and the inner wall of the trachea. The inner tube is cleaned and replaced as often as needed, and the outer cannula should be replaced every two days.

A spare cannula and obturator of the proper size should be kept at the bedside in the event that the tube becomes dislodged and requires replacement. A dislodged cannula during the first two days may be extremely difficult to replace. A good light, soft tissue "spreaders" and skill are quickly required in such a circumstance. After two days, a tract is usually sufficiently established to allow easy reinsertion.

Provision should be made for humidifying inspired gas, since the wetting, warming and filtering functions of the upper airway are now inoperative. Although plastic "collars" that allow aerosols to be delivered directly to a tracheostomy are available, they may not be applicable to infants or young children. A "mist tent" (Fig. 6) is then probably the best compromise. Instillation of saline, sodium bicarbonate or other solutions into the trachea does not alone prevent drying and crusting within the airway.

The tracheostomy tube should be removed as soon as it is no longer needed. In general, the longer a tube remains in the trachea, the more difficult will be the process of decannulation. Processes of short duration (foreign body, croup) usually permit prompt removal of the tube, whereas others of chronic nature (poliomyelitis) may take much longer.

Although opinions differ on the best way to remove a tube, the more common practice is to reduce the size of the cannula daily. When a small tube (perhaps two or more sizes smaller than the original) is reached without difficulty, it is then plugged. If the child has no difficulty after 24 hours, the plugged tube may be removed. Subsequent air leaks through the wound nearly always cease within 72 hours. In small infants, the mother may partially occlude the tracheostomy tube with her finger while rocking and cuddling the baby. The infant may thus be slowly adapted to decannulation.

The complications of tracheostomy can be divided into immediate (operative) and late (postoperative) categories. Operative complications, usually in children less than five years old, include wound bleeding, pneumothorax, pneumomediastinum, tracheoesophageal fistula, subcutaneous emphysema, cardiac or respiratory arrest, and apnea immediately after provision of a good airway. Late complications include infection, atelectasis, cannula occlusion, tracheal bleeding, expulsion of the cannula, tracheal ulceration and granulation, tracheal stenosis, aerophagia, and delayed healing of the stoma.

RESECTION OF LUNG TISSUE

Advances in diagnostic and surgical methods have made it possible to remove diseased segments or lobes, as well as an entire lung. Such operations are indicated when it has been established ① that the process is creating significant present or potential morbidity, ② that it is not treatable by other means, ③ that it is sufficiently localized that its resection will leave adequate pulmonary reserve, and ④ that the resection is technically feasible and does not constitute a risk out of proportion to the disease itself.

Surgery should be preceded by adequate bronchograms and, if possible, pulmonary function testing in order to establish the anatomic and physiologic extent of the disease.

The most common indication for resection is bronchiectasis, with or without atelectasis, though asymptomatic bronchiectasis, especially of an upper lobe, and so-called cylindrical bronchiectasis almost never require resection. Other indications include anomalies, tuberculosis and neoplasms.

Postoperative complications are common in small children, especially atelectasis and pneumonia. Unless these complications can be avoided or promptly handled by enlightened management, the procedure may be responsible for more harm than good. Scrupulous attention should be given to maintaining good tracheobronchial toilet. This usually requires continuous or intermittent aerosol therapy and physical therapy (e.g., bronchial drainage, breathing exercises, controlled cough, thoracic "cupping") and may necessitate bronchoscopy, tracheostomy, assisted ventilation or transtracheal catheterization.

REFERENCES

Bronchoscopy

Atkins, J. P.: Bronchoscopic problems of infancy and childhood. *Arch. Otolaryngol.,* 79:152, 1964.

Burman, S. O., and Gibson, I. C.: Bronchoscopy and cardiorespiratory reflexes. *Ann. Surg.,* 157:134, 1963.

Sackner, M. A.: Bronchofiberscopy. *Am. Rev. Resp. Dis.,* 111:62, 1975.

Lung Puncture

Finland, M.: Diagnostic lung puncture. *Pediatrics,* 44:471, 1969.

Gellis, S. S., Reinhold, J. L. D., and Green, S.: Use of aspiration lung puncture in diagnosis of idiopathic pulmonary hemosiderosis. *Am. J. Dis. Child.,* 85:303, 1953.

Hughes, J. R., Sinha, D. P., Cooper, M. R., Shah, K. V., and Bose, S. K.: Lung tap in childhood. Bacteria, viruses, and mycoplasmas in acute lower respiratory tract infections. *Pediatrics,* 44:477, 1969.

Klein, J. O.: Diagnostic lung puncture in the pneumonias of infants and children. *Pediatrics,* 44:486, 1969.

Sapington, S. W., and Favorite, G. O.: Lung puncture in lobar pneumonia. *Am. J. Med. Sci.,* 191:225, 1936.

Lung Biopsy

Roback, S. A., Weintraub, W. H., Nesbit, M., Spanos, P., Burke, B., and Leonard, A. S.: Diagnostic open lung biopsy in the critically ill child. *Pediatrics,* 52:605, 1973.

Weng, T.-R., Levison, H., Wentworth, P., Simpson, J., and Moes, C. A. F.: Open lung biopsy in children. *Am. Rev. Resp. Dis.,* 97:673, 1968.

Arterial Puncture

Olszowka, A. J., Rahn, H., and Farhi, L. E.: *Blood Gases: Hemoglobin, Base Excess and Maldistribution.* Philadelphia, Lea and Febiger, 1973.

Shapiro, B. A.: *Clinical Application of Blood Gases.* Chicago, Year Book Medical Publishers, 1973.

Bronchial Drainage and Physical Therapy

Cotton, E. K., Abrams, G., Vanhoutte, J., and Burrington, J.: Removal of Aspirated Foreign Bodies by Inhalation and Postural Drainage. *Clin. Pediatr.,* 12:270, 1973.

Doyle, B.: Physical therapy in the treatment of cystic fibrosis. *Phys. Ther. Rev.,* 39:24, 1959.

Fountain, F. P., and Goddard, R. F.: Breathing exercises for children with chronic respiratory diseases. *Lovelace Clinic Review,* 1:159, 1963.

Gaskell, D. V., and Webber, B. A.: *The Brompton Hospital Guide to Chest Physiotherapy.* 2nd Ed. London, Blackwell Scientific Publications, 1973.

Mellins, R. B.: Pulmonary physiotherapy in the pediatric age group. *Am. Rev. Resp. Dis.,* 110 (Suppl.):137, 1974.

Rattenborg, C. C., and Holaday, D. A.: Lung physiotherapy as an adjunct to surgical care. *Surg. Clin. North Am.,* 44:219, 1964.

Tecklin, J. S., and Holsclaw, D. S.: Evaluation of bronchial drainage in patients with cystic fibrosis. *Phys. Ther.,* 55:1081, 1975.

Thacker, E. W.: *Postural Drainage and Respiratory Control.* London, Lloyd-Luke (Medical Books), Ltd., 1959.

Inhalation (Respiratory) Therapy

Adair, J. C., Ring, W. H., Jordan, W. S., and Elwyn, R. A.: Ten-year experience with IPPB in the treatment of acute laryngotracheobronchitis. *Anesth. Analg., 50*:649, 1971.

Batson, R., and Young, W. C.: The administration of oxygen to infants and small children. An evaluation of methods. *Pediatrics, 22*:436, 1958.

Campbell, E. J. M.: Oxygen administration. *Anesthesia, 18*:503, 1963.

Chang, N., Levison, H., Cunningham, K., Crozier, D. N., and Grossett, O.: An evaluation of nightly mist tent therapy for patients with cystic fibrosis. *Am. Rev. Resp. Dis., 107*:672, 1973.

Comroe, J. H., Jr., and Dripps, R. D.: *The Physiological Basis for Oxygen Therapy.* Springfield, Illinois, Charles C Thomas, 1950.

Denton, R.: The clinical use of continuous nebulization in bronchopulmonary disease. *Dis. Chest, 28*:123, 1955.

Doershuk, C. F., Matthews, L. W., Gillespie, C. T., Lough, M. D., and Spector, S.: Evaluation of jet-type and ultrasonic nebulizers in mist tent therapy for cystic fibrosis. *Pediatrics, 41*:723, 1968.

Heaf, P. J. D.: Deaths in asthma: a therapeutic misadventure? *Br. Med. Bull., 26*:245, 1970.

Jordan, W. S., Graves, C. L., and Elwyn, R. A.: New therapy for post-intubation laryngeal edema and tracheitis in children. *J.A.M.A., 212*:585, 1970.

Kory, R., Bergmann, J. C., Sweet, R. D., and Smith, J. R.: Comparative evaluation of oxygen therapy techniques. *J.A.M.A., 179*:767, 1962.

Lough, M. D., Doershuk, C. F., and Stern, R. C.: *Pediatric Respiratory Therapy.* Chicago, Year Book Medical Publishers, 1974.

Morrow, P. E.: Some physical and physiological factors controlling the fate of inhaled substances. I. Deposition. *Health Phys., 2*:366, 1960.

Pierce, A. K., Sanford, J. P., Thomas, G. D., and Leonard, J. S.: Long-term evaluation and decontamination of inhalation-therapy equipment and the occurrence of necrotizing pneumonia. *N. Engl. J. Med., 282*:528, 1970.

Tizard, J. P. M.: Indications for oxygen therapy in the newborn. *Pediatrics, 34*:771, 1964.

Wells, R. E., Perera, R. D., and Kinney, J. M.: Humidification of oxygen during inhalational therapy. *N. Engl. J. Med., 268*:644, 1963.

Wolfsdorf, J., Swift, D. L., and Avery, M. E.: Mist therapy reconsidered; an evaluation of the respiratory deposition of labelled water aerosols produced by jet and ultrasonic nebulizers. *Pediatrics, 43*:799, 1969.

Bronchial Lavage

Cezeaux, G., Jr., Telford, J., Harrison, G., and Keats, A. S.: Bronchial lavage in cystic fibrosis. A comparison of agents. *J.A.M.A., 199*:15, 1967.

Hacket, P. R., and Reas, H. W.: A radical approach to therapy for the pulmonary complications of cystic fibrosis. *Anesthesiology, 26*:248, 1965.

Kylstra, J. A., Rausch, D. C., Hall, K. D., and Spock, A.: Volume-controlled lung lavage in the treatment of asthma, bronchiectasis, and mucoviscidosis. *Am. Rev. Resp. Dis., 103*:651, 1971.

Ramirez-R., J., Kieffer, R. F., and Ball, W. C.: Bronchopulmonary lavage in man. *Ann. Intern. Med., 63*:819, 1965.

Thompson, H. T., and Pryor, W. J.: Bronchial lavage in the treatment of obstructive lung disease. *Lancet, 2*:8, 1964.

Pleural Space Drainage and Intracavitary (Monaldi) Drainage

Greenwood, M. E.: *An Illustrated Approach to Medical Physics.* Philadelphia, F. A. Davis Company, 1963, pp. 99–102.

Rakower, J., and Wayl, P.: Monaldi drainage in the management of postinfectious pulmonary cysts. *J. Pediatr., 52*:573, 1958.

von Hippel, A.: *Chest Tubes and Chest Bottles.* Springfield, Illinois, Charles C Thomas, 1970.

Webb, W. R.: Chairman: Management of nontuberculous empyema. A statement of the Subcommittee on Surgery, American Thoracic Society. *Am. Rev. Resp. Dis., 85*:935, 1962.

Tracheostomy

Crawford, O. B.: The anesthesiologist's responsibilities in tracheostomy. *Anesthesiology, 22*:86, 1961.

Dugan, D. J., and Samson, P. C.: Tracheostomy: present day indications and technics. *Am. J. Surg., 106*:290, 1963.

Eigen, H., and Waring, W. W.: Tracheostomy care. In Shirkey, H. C. (Ed.): *Pediatric Therapy.* 5th Ed. St. Louis, C. V. Mosby Company, 1975, pp. 681–685.

Fennell, G.: Management of tracheotomy in infants. *Lancet, 2*:808, 1962.

Glas, W. W., King, O. J., Jr., and Lui, A.: Complications of tracheostomy. *Arch. Surg., 85*:57, 1962.

Head, J. M.: Tracheostomy in the management of respiratory problems. *N. Engl. J. Med., 264*:587, 1961.

Oliver, P., Richardson, J. R., Clubb, R. W., and Flake, C. G.: Tracheotomy in children. *N. Engl. J. Med., 267*:631, 1962.

Resection

Filler, J.: Effects upon pulmonary function of lobectomy performed during childhood. *Am. Rev. Resp. Dis., 89*:801, 1964.

Massion, W. H., and Schilling, J. A.: Physiological effects of lung resection in adult and puppy dogs. *J. Thorac. Cardiovasc. Surg., 48*:239, 1964.

Nanson, E. M.: Pulmonary resection in infancy and childhood. *Can. Med. Assoc. J., 87*:275, 1962.

Quinlan, J. J., Schaffner, V. D., and Hiltz, J. E.: Lung resection for tuberculosis in children. *Can. Med. Assoc. J., 87*:1362, 1962.

CHAPTER FIVE

DIAGNOSTIC PULMONARY RADIOLOGY

Barry D. Fletcher, M.D., C.M.

The purpose of this chapter is to explain some of the basic concepts used in the interpretation of chest radiographs, particularly those which most frequently apply to pulmonary diseases of children. In this respect, minor modifications of the principles of radiologic interpretation found in standard textbooks, most of which are directed toward diagnosis of disease in the adult, are necessary. Obviously, a complete course in pulmonary radiology cannot be offered in the space allotted. I have, therefore, based my choice of the subjects to follow on their importance in the day-to-day practice of radiology as well as on the frequency with which the meaning and importance of certain radiologic findings are queried by my clinical colleagues. Specific disease entities will be discussed when they are illustrative of the more important anatomic or pathophysiologic principles necessary for successful radiologic diagnosis, but no attempt has been made to duplicate the detailed accounts of these disorders that are to be found in other sections of this book.

The experienced observer develops a systematic approach to interpretation of chest radiographs, which is designed to ensure that assessment is complete in the face of an apparently normal examination and that additional information is not overlooked when there is an obvious lesion. Individual systems of examination may differ considerably, but all are designed to promote accurate observation of all of the structures dis-

TABLE 1. BASIC APPROACH TO ASSESSMENT OF CHEST RADIOGRAPHS

1 **Technique**
  Are the views appropriate for the information sought?
  Are there technical variations or faults that might influence your interpretation?

2 **Chest Wall**
  Does the appearance of the soft tissues suggest any disturbance of growth, nutrition, and so on?
  Are there congenital or acquired defects of the ribs or spine?
  Are the spine and sternum intact on lateral view?

3 **Diaphragm**
  Are the diaphragmatic outlines intact or is there a positive silhouette sign?
  Are the diaphragmatic domes in normal position?

4 **Pleura**
  Are the costophrenic angles sharply outlined?
  Is there a pneumothorax?
  Are the fissures in normal position?

5 **Mediastinum**
  Is the mediastinum in normal position?
  Is the heart large?
  Is it really cardiomegaly or is it due to thymus or an expiration film?
  Is the aortic arch on the left?
  Are the heart borders clearly visible?
  Is the cervical airway visible?
  Is it, and are the major airways normal?

6 **Hila and Pulmonary Vessels**
  Are the hila normal in size and position?
  Are the pulmonary vessels normal in caliber and sharply defined?

7 **Lungs**
  Are there any abnormal densities?
  Is there an air bronchogram?
  Is there a positive silhouette sign?
  Is the area behind the heart normal?
  Are there Kerley lines?
  Is there a "spine sign"?
  Are there any areas of hyperaeration or atelectasis?

played on the films. One such personal approach is offered in Table 1 for the use and modification by the reader.

RADIATION HAZARDS

The evidence for somatic damage caused by x-radiation is derived from a number of sources, including animal experiments, data from radiation accidents and the Atomic Bomb Casualty Commission, as well as epidemiologic studies. Although there is no definitive information on the effects of low-range diagnostic doses (Margulis, 1973), careful protection of the more immature gonads of the infant and child is essential. The thyroid gland, ocular lens and bone marrow are also relatively radiosensitive structures, and therefore deserve protection as well. Unnecessary exposure of both patients and personnel to diagnostic radiation occurs frequently and is related to overexposure of radiographs, overutilization of radiologic services, improper columnation of the x-ray beam and absence of appropriate lead shielding.

The overall x-ray dose during childhood can be further reduced by eliminating the practice of routine chest screening and hospital admission radiographs and curtailing the custom of routine preoperative chest radiographs.

IMAGING METHODS

Fluoroscopy

Fluoroscopy is performed using an image intensifier which electronically increases the brightness level so that the image can be displayed on a television monitor. "Spot films" are radiographs made at desired times during fluoroscopy. Cinefluoroscopy can also be carried out, but necessitates an increased radiation dosage, particularly when high frame speeds are employed. A decline in the use of cinefluoroscopy has coincided with the increased resolution now attainable with modern image tubes, television systems and video tapes. Photofluorography with 70 to 105 mm. film exposed directly from the output phosphor of the image intensifier produces high-quality films with considerably lower radiation exposure than "spot films." Fluoroscopy is principally used in order to study diaphragmatic excursion and respiratory motion of the lungs or for examination of the barium-filled esophagus in order to delineate mediastinal abnormalities.

Radiography

The methods for obtaining chest films vary throughout infancy and childhood. Except for routine follow-up of chronic disease, when a frontal projection may be sufficient, lateral views should be obtained. In x-ray departments, three-phase generators that provide high milliamperage and, conversely, very short exposure times are now frequently available. Exposure times of less than 10 milliseconds can be achieved even with portable units. The radiographs of newborn infants are usually exposed with the baby in the incubator, using portable x-ray equipment. We have found that a vertical beam anteroposterior view taken through the Plexiglas cover and a lateral view made with a horizontally directed beam require the least handling of fragile newborn infants. Metallic devices such as electrocardiogram electrodes, which may obscure significant portions of the chest, should be removed.

In the older infant, anteroposterior supine and vertical beam lateral views can be obtained in the x-ray department. Since the patient is radiographed on the x-ray table, the tube film distance is considerably decreased from the usual six-foot distance used for older children. The distorting effect of magnification at the shorter distance is not significant in these patients (Davis, 1967), and shorter exposure times can be achieved. Upright views of the chest can be obtained in cooperative young children with the use of various supporting devices that usually fix the child in a sitting position. These, however, will not completely eliminate slumping of the body in the younger child, so that the recumbent position described above is preferable in those up to two to three years of age. After the patient is able to sit or stand unsupported, conventional posteroanterior and lateral radiographs can be made at a distance of 72 inches (Fig. 3 *B*).

Special Views

Forty-five degree oblique views aid in the spatial perception of thoracic lesions and are frequently used in assessing cardiac chambers. These projections are also sometimes helpful in evaluation of the lungs of patients with severe chest wall deformities or scoliosis. Evaluation of pneumothorax and pleural effusion is facilitated by lateral decubitus views, which are made with a horizontal x-ray beam and the patient lying on one side (see also p. 145). A frontal projection of the chest made at the end of expiration is used chiefly to demonstrate air-trapping in patients with suspected foreign body aspiration. Since exact timing of the exposure may be difficult in these patients, fluoroscopic evaluation is more precise. Apical-lordotic views are made in the supine position with an exaggerated extension of the spine. These are helpful for the visualization of upper lobe lesions and the demonstration of middle lobe disease.

"High KV" films refer to radiographs on which increased penetration of the x-rays results in a relative decrease in radiographic density of the bones, thus accentuating the air-containing structures, such as the trachea and major bronchi (see Fig. 5). The assessment of airway narrowing, bronchial anomalies and mediastinal masses is, therefore, facilitated.

Tomography

Tomograms or laminograms are produced by simultaneous motion of the tube and film at varying levels so that all structures not included in a predetermined plane are blurred. The structures that remain stationary are, therefore, viewed independently of superimposed tissues. Thickness of the "cuts" can be reduced to the range of 1 mm., although for studies of the lungs, thicker sections approximating 1 cm. are more commonly used (Bernard and coworkers, 1967). Even with short tube travel distances, which result in thick sections, exposure times considerably exceed those of conventional radiography, so that tomography is generally reserved for children who are old enough to be able to voluntarily suspend respirations. In younger patients, the required information can often be obtained by the high KV techniques described above.

Esophagram

This is a valuable adjunct to diagnosis of chest diseases and is used principally to define mediastinal masses that may cause esophageal displacement, as well as swallowing disorders and malformations such as tracheoesophageal fistula. Colloidal barium is preferred over water-soluble contrast media, since it is more palatable and less irritating should it enter the tracheobronchial tree. The barium esophagram is usually performed under fluoroscopic control.

Bronchography

This procedure is now less commonly used than previously, and its value has been seriously questioned (Avery, 1970). In the past, bronchography was commonly employed in the evaluation of chronic lung disease, and its decline has coincided with the diminishing need for surgical therapy and the availability of greater information from other radiologic and isotope methods. This procedure, however, is invaluable in the demonstration and mapping of bronchiectasis and is mandatory if surgical resection is being contemplated. Bronchography can be safely carried out under general anesthesia using small amounts of propyliodone (Dionosil) in either an oily or aqueous base. An opaque catheter is inserted via the orotracheal tube and positioned under fluoroscopic control. A small amount of contrast medium is then injected. Separate examination of each lung is recommended, particularly if pulmonary function is abnormal. Alternate contrast agents include tantalum dust (Nadel and coworkers, 1970), which is not yet in general use, and barium sulfate (Nice and associates, 1964). Both substances tend to be retained in the lungs for a longer period of time than Dionosil.

Angiography

Aside from the investigation of various anomalies of the pulmonary vasculature (Gooding, 1974), pulmonary angiography has not found many applications in childhood. Recently, Fellows and colleagues (1975) have used bronchial arteriography to localize sites of hemoptysis in patients with cystic fibrosis in whom bronchoscopy could not be done. Franken and co-

workers (1973) have pointed out the advantages of pulmonary angiography over bronchography in the investigation of causes of unequal aeration of the lungs.

Isotope Scanning

Lung scans delineate defects in pulmonary arterial perfusion as well as diseased areas of lung that are occasionally not appreciated on radiographs (Pendarvis and Swischuk, 1969). Perfusion defects are seen in patients during acute asthmatic attacks (Mishkin and Wagner, 1968). An example of multiple defects in an asthmatic child with a "normal" chest radiograph is shown in Figure 1. Isotope studies are particularly helpful in children with suspected foreign body aspiration in whom a definitive, radiographic and fluoroscopic assessment of obstructive emphysema cannot be made. After intravenous injection of macroaggregated albumin labeled with technetium or ^{131}I, a perfusion defect can be seen on the scan corresponding to the involved portion of lung. The experimental data of Rudavsky and coworkers (1973) suggest that the lung scan may not be positive within the first 24 hours of bronchial obstruction and that the perfusion defect will resolve within several days of

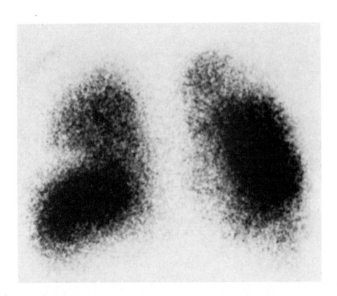

Figure 1. An isotope scan showing perfusion defects in the lungs of an asthmatic patient.

bronchoscopic removal of the offending foreign body. Inhalation scans using radioactive aerosols or xenon gas provide similar information.

Intervention

Wesenberg and Struble (1972) have recommended selective bronchial catheterization and lavage under fluoroscopic control for newborn infants with lobar atelectasis. Fluoroscopic visualization may also be helpful for localization of sites for needle aspiration and biopsy.

TECHNICAL FACTORS AFFECTING RADIOLOGIC INTERPRETATION

Exposure

The quantity and quality of the x-ray exposure is determined by two factors: kilovoltage (KV), which controls the penetration of the beam, and milliamperage (MA), upon which contrast is dependent. On a well exposed frontal view of the chest, the vertebrae should be fairly clearly seen; at the same time, water density structures, such as the pulmonary vascular markings, should also be easily visible. Excess contrast material results in a radiograph in which the bones and soft tissue structures are chalklike with considerable loss of detail.

Motion

The most common cause of loss of image sharpness is respiratory motion due to ineffective immobilization of the child and lengthy exposure times. This technical fault is recognized by blurring of the diaphragmatic domes.

Rotation

Since the spinous processes of children have varying degrees of ossifica-

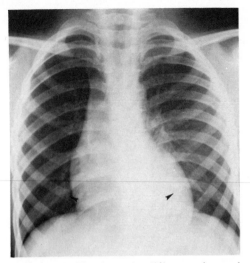

Figure 2. The thorax is mildly rotated toward the right posterior oblique position. The anterior ends of the fifth ribs are marked. Note the relative lucency of the right lung.

tion, and since some twisting of the upper thorax frequently occurs, it is not practical to compare the distance between the proximal ends of the clavicles and the spinous processes as is done in adults. Rotation can be more effectively judged by comparing the position of the anterior ends of the lower ribs (Fig. 2). Rotation produces considerable diagnostic confusion. If, for example, the thorax is rotated toward the right, the mediastinum is projected over the right hemithorax, and the right lung will appear more lucent. The hila, pulmonary vessels and anterior rib ends of the left side are also magnified in this position. On lateral views, variable lengths of the posterior rib ends can be seen if the patient is rotated.

Respiratory Cycle

The level to which the diaphragmatic domes descend on full inspiration depends to some extent on the age of the child. The degree of inspiratory effort is usually judged according to the position of the top of the right diaphragmatic dome with respect to the adjacent rib. In general, if the right diaphragmatic dome is projected at the level of the sixth rib anteriorly and the ninth to tenth ribs posteriorly, a satisfactory inspiratory film has been made. Expiration films result in crowding of the bronchovascular markings and are a frequent cause of overdiagnosis of pulmonary abnormalities.

Magnification

Magnification using a very small focal spot as a source of the x-ray beam is a useful technique to increase radiographic information. When this happens inadvertently with the more commonly used large focal spot tubes, lack of clarity as well as undesirable enlargement of structures occurs. Magnification may result from rotation of the thorax and may also occur when a short focal-film distance is used. The latter situation occurs mainly with portable or recumbent radiographs of larger children. However, minor degrees of magnification can be easily tolerated in small children, since recumbent views may be more desirable for other reasons (Fig. 3).

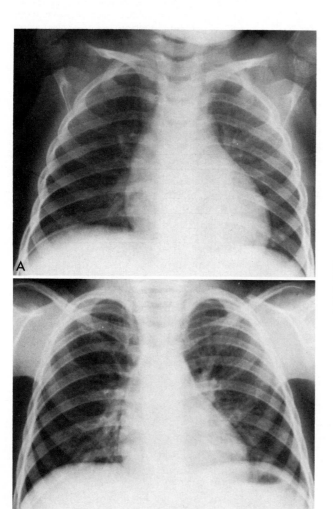

Figure 3. Normal chest radiographs of the same patient. Note the differences in heart size in *A*, anteroposterior supine position, and *B*, posteroanterior erect position made with a longer focal-film distance.

RADIOLOGY OF THE NECK AND THORACIC INLET

Technique

Frequently, the lower cervical area is exposed on routine anteroposterior and lateral radiographs. While excessive exposure of radiosensitive organs such as the thyroid should be avoided on a routine basis, a glimpse of the cervical airway can be very helpful in determining a cause of respiratory distress. When an obstructive airway lesion is suspected clinically, high KV radiographs provide excellent visualization. Dunbar (1970) utilizes anteroposterior and lateral views taken during inspiration and expiration. Joseph and coworkers (1976) have recently worked out a method for high KV magnification radiography of the neck.

For specific purposes (to be discussed later), a barium esophagram may be a useful additional examination.

Normal

The amount of air contained in the pharynx varies with the respiratory cycle and is expelled with swallowing. When air-filled, the vallecula and epiglottis are distinctly outlined and the pyriform sinuses are distended. Enlarged palatine tonsils can be seen, superimposed on the pyriform sinuses in lateral projection (Fig. 4).

When the laryngeal ventricles are air-filled, they are recognizable as a lucent diamond-shaped shadow on anteroposterior or lateral projections situated at approximately the same level as the inferior angle of the pyriform sinuses. The subglottic portion of the trachea is seen on anteroposterior views as an archlike structure. Below this, the trachea should be of uniform caliber to the level of the thoracic inlet, where its anteroposterior diameter may normally decrease up to 50 per cent in a struggling or crying infant. There is little change in caliber with quiet breathing (Wittenborg and coworkers, 1967).

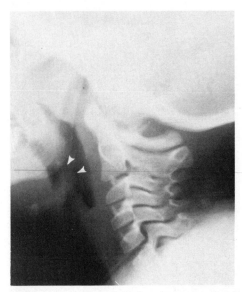

Figure 4. Lateral view of neck showing prominent adenoid tissue and palatine tonsils. The epiglottis (*arrows*) is normal in size (compare with Fig. 8).

It is important to note that in babies and young children, the cervical trachea is redundant and, therefore, may buckle anteriorly and to the right, particularly if the neck is flexed (Fig. 5). Occasionally, this normal finding may lead to the erroneous diagnosis of a cervical mass. The normal trachea will, however, straighten when the neck is extended.

Immediately below the thoracic inlet, the trachea deviates to the right owing to the normal left-sided aortic arch. Since the infant is held in a somewhat exaggerated lordotic position, the carina is projected high in the thorax, immediately below the aortic "knob."

Besides visualization of tracheal changes that are directly caused by an upper airway lesion, there are several general principles that are helpful in deciding whether respiratory distress is due to upper airway obstruction or pulmonary disease. Upper airway obstruction should be suspected when (1) tracheal collapse occurs with quiet breathing; (2) the pharynx is distended (Meine and coworkers, 1974); (3) there

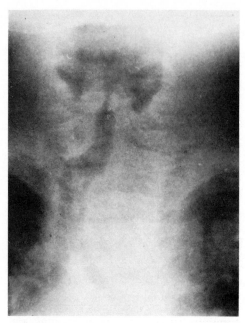

Figure 5. Film of normal infant's neck showing deviation of the trachea to the right. Note the arch-like appearance of the normal subglottic portion of the trachea.

is a paradoxical change in heart size during respiration (i.e., the transverse cardiac diameter is smaller on expiration than on inspiration) (Capitanio and Kirkpatrick, 1973); ④ the lung volume is decreased; ⑤ a large amount of swallowed air is present in the esophagus (Fig. 6); or ⑥ there is indrawing of the anterior chest wall.

It is worthwhile to note that the latter two findings also occur in neonates with respiratory distress syndrome who tend to swallow air (Keats and Smith, 1974).

Croup

On the rare occasion when the clinical diagnosis is in doubt, the diagnosis of laryngotracheobronchitis can be made because of its distinctive radiologic appearance. The normal subglottic arch becomes obliterated owing to submucosal edema so that a diffuse narrowing, in the shape of an inverted "V," is seen on anteroposterior projections (Fig. 7). Distention of the supraglottic airway and secondary tracheal collapse may be visible on lateral views. However, there is no direct correlation between the severity of the radiologic and clinical findings (DeLevie and coworkers, 1972). Edema due to tracheal intubation will produce a similar appearance, as will congenital subglottic stenosis (Grünebaum, 1975). Subglottic hemangiomas are usually asymmetric and cause a more discrete indentation of the trachea.

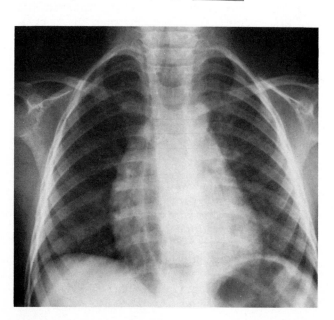

Figure 6. Esophageal distention due to swallowed air, and decreased lung volume in acute epiglottitis.

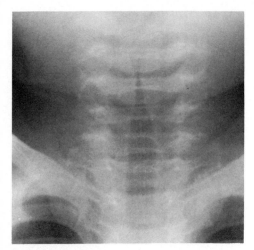

Figure 7. Subglottic narrowing due to croup.

Epiglottitis

Lateral radiographs of the neck are extremely helpful in confirming this diagnosis. While radiography is less traumatic than direct visualization, attempts to position the child in a recumbent position may trigger further airway obstruction. For this reason, a lateral radiograph is made, with the patient sitting. In epiglottitis, marked swelling of the epiglottis and aryepiglottic folds is evident (Fig. 8).

Masses

Tumors arising from the retropharyngeal and retrotracheal soft tissues will compress the trachea, as will large foreign bodies that have become lodged in the cervical esophagus (Smith and coworkers, 1974). The latter diagnosis can be established by means of a barium swallow.

Retropharyngeal cellulitis will cause posterior compression of the pyriform sinuses and anterior deviation of the trachea. Except in the case of traumatic perforation, an air-containing retropharyngeal abscess is rarely encountered.

Congenital Laryngeal Stridor

Anteroinferior displacement and buckling of the aryepiglottic folds and

posterior deflection of the epiglottis have been convincingly demonstrated in this disorder by Dunbar (1970). These changes occur on inspiration simultaneously with inspiratory stridor. If stridor is not audible at the time of examination, other causes of upper airway obstruction must be excluded.

Vascular Rings

Vascular rings encircling the trachea may be responsible for symptoms of airway obstruction. The two common types of vascular rings are double aortic arch, and right aortic arch with an aberrant left subclavian artery. In the latter disorder, traction by the ductus arteriosus presumably creates the tracheal compression (Felson and Palayew, 1963). In either of the above types of vascular ring, the right-sided aortic component causes deviation of the tra-

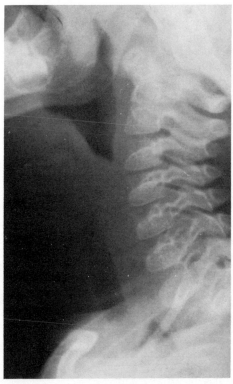

Figure 8. Marked swelling of the epiglottis and aryepiglottic folds in a patient with acute epiglottitis.

chea to the left at the level of the aortic "knob." The abnormal tracheal deviation should be carefully sought in a child with signs or symptoms of upper airway obstruction (Fig. 9). A more exact determination of the type of aortic anomaly can be made by means of a barium esophagram.

THE CHEST WALL AND DIAPHRAGM

Chest Wall

The changes in configuration of the chest wall that occur with growth are reflected on both anteroposterior and lateral chest radiographs. During infancy, the thorax is circular and has a relatively greater anteroposterior diameter than transverse diameter. The latter becomes relatively larger as the child grows. The ribs of the infant are aligned horizontally. On the supine radiograph, which is often obtained with the patient in an exaggerated lordotic position, the anterior rib ends may be projected over or even slightly above the posterior aspects of the ribs. In this position, the clavicles are projected well above the first ribs.

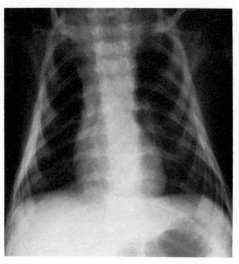

Figure 10. Bell-shaped thorax due to Werdnig-Hoffmann disease.

The shape of the chest wall may also reflect the volume of the lungs. Hyperaeration produces anterior bowing of the sternum and an increase in the anteroposterior diameter of the chest as well as flattening of the diaphragmatic domes. A decrease in lung volume is accompanied by a reduction in width of the intercostal spaces. A "bell-shaped" thorax may be the result of muscular weakness (Fig. 10).

There are several misleading images produced by structures of the chest wall. In babies, skin folds on the back produce slightly curved lines that may simulate a pneumothorax. Recognition of pulmonary vessels peripheral to these lines and careful examination of their course will usually clarify this artifact. On lateral radiographs, made with the patient's arms extended over the head, the axillary folds are prominent and produce a homogeneous density overlying the posterior aspect of the chest that may be mistaken for an intrathoracic abnormality. Also on lateral projection, the density cast by the scapulae may simulate a posterior mediastinal mass (Alazraki and Friedman, 1972). The scapulae also overlie the upper lung fields on anteroposterior projections and their shadows may be

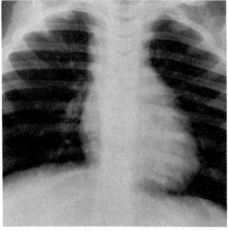

Figure 9. The "mass" to the right of the trachea is produced by a right aortic arch.

mistaken for pneumonia or pleural effusion.

Spine

The thoracic and upper lumbar spines are well visualized on adequately exposed chest radiographs, and examination of these vertebrae is one of the most important aspects of chest radiology. The vertebral bodies are particularly well demonstrated on lateral views, enabling assessment of congenital and acquired disorders such as fusion and compression. On frontal projection, recognition of a significant scoliosis may be equally as important as the observation of intrathoracic disease. Significant disturbance of segmentation of the vertebrae and defects in their bodies or neural elements occur with such anomalies as enteric duplications (Neuhauser and coworkers, 1958), intraspinal lesions and meningomyelocele. Inflammatory processes such as tuberculosis (Fig. 11) or neoplasms such as neuroblastoma may produce a paraspinal mass.

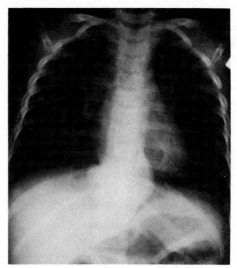

Figure 11. Lower thoracic paraspinal mass due to tuberculosis.

Diaphragm

The diaphragm descends on full inspiration so that the higher right diaphragmatic dome is projected at the level of the ninth to tenth ribs pos-

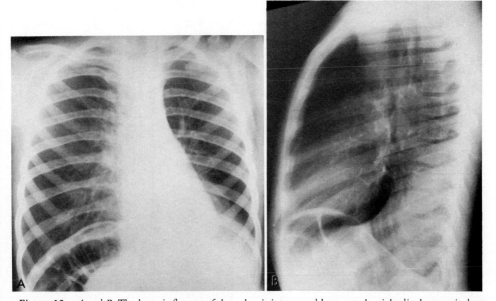

Figure 12. *A* and *B*, The hepatic flexure of the colon is interposed between the right diaphragmatic dome and liver. The haustral markings serve to distinguish colon from free intraperitoneal air. Left lower lobe atelectasis has caused leftward shift of the heart, loss of the left diaphragmatic outline and posterior displacement of the major fissure.

teriorly. Consistent elevation of both diaphragmatic domes occurs when there is abdominal distention or a large intra-abdominal mass. A large amount of gas in the stomach elevates the left hemidiaphragm. The colon is sometimes interposed between the liver and right diaphragmatic dome (Fig. 12). Elevation of a hemidiaphragm is seen in phrenic nerve paralysis and eventration. Paradoxical movement will occur in either condition, while a subphrenic abscess will usually cause decreased or absent excursion of the adjacent diaphragmatic dome.

It is very helpful to be able to differentiate between right and left diaphragmatic domes on lateral views of the chest. Their relative height may be misleading owing to variations in position of the central x-ray beam. Identification of the gastric air bubble is helpful, since it cannot be projected above the left hemidiaphragm. Also, because of the levoposition of the heart, the superior surface of the left diaphragmatic dome is obscured anteriorly (see Silhouette Sign, p. 156), whereas the outline of the right hemidiaphragm can be traced to the anterior chest wall.

THE PLEURA AND FISSURES

The lungs are surrounded by two layers of pleura—the visceral and parietal—between which there is a potential space. The fissures are formed by two apposed layers of visceral pleura that separate the lobes. When the x-ray beam is directed tangentially to them, the fissures can be visualized as thin curvilinear densities.

The oblique or major fissures run from the posterior surface of the lungs, at about the level of the fourth thoracic vertebra, downward and anteriorly, where their pleural surfaces become continuous with the visceral pleura of the diaphragmatic surfaces of the lungs. For purposes of anatomic locali-

zation, it is helpful to note that the right major fissure usually extends more anteriorly at its inferior end than does the left.

On occasion, the inferior portion of the major fissure may have a more vertical course than normal, allowing it to be visualized on frontal projections. This occurs particularly in association with cardiomegaly (Davis, 1960).

The minor or horizontal fissure extends from the right major fissure at approximately its midpoint to the anterior surface of the lung, thus dividing the upper and middle lobes. The juncture of the two fissures is an important landmark on lateral chest radiographs, since it serves to identify the right lung. The minor fissure may be absent, bilateral or left-sided, particularly with congenital heart disease and abnormal situs (Landing and coworkers, 1971).

The azygos fissure (Fig. 13) is the most frequently visualized accessory fissure. It is seen as a curvilinear density

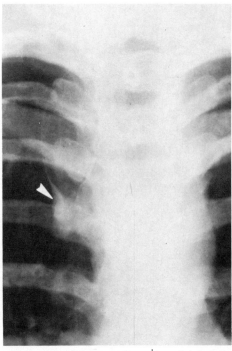

Figure 13. The azygos fissure extends inferiorly to envelope the aberrantly positioned azygos vein (*arrow*).

coursing downward and medially from the apex of the lung, blending inferiorly with the teardrop-shaped density that is formed by the azygos vein. The vein is surrounded by both visceral and parietal pleura. The azygos "lobe," which is the portion of the lung medial to the fissure, may occasionally appear opaque. The opacity is more likely caused by the pleural layers than by disease within the accessory "lobe."

Pleural Effusion

Intrapleural fluid accumulates primarily below the diaphragmatic surface of the lung, then causes blunting of the posterior costophrenic angle on lateral views. Small amounts of pleural fluid can also be detected between the convex surface of the lung and chest wall on lateral decubitus views. Larger accumulations are readily visible on frontal projections owing to blunting of the lateral costophrenic angles. Fluid also may be seen in the mediastinal pleural space as a triangular density to the left of the lower thoracic spine and also between the visceral pleural layers of the fissures. A variable amount of the superior surface of the diaphragmatic dome becomes obliterated, depending on the size of the effusion. Superiorly, the intrapleural fluid seems to terminate as a concave meniscus.

Since many small children are radiographed in the supine position, pleural fluid tends to collect posteriorly, and if large enough, will cause an increase in density of the hemithorax (Fig. 14 B). The fluid may also cap the lung apex because of the lordotic position of the supine infant.

Any type of pleural fluid, i.e., exudate, transudate, blood or even chyle, produces similar radiographic densities. However, empyema due to staphylococcus should be suspected in an infant with a large unilateral effusion. Lack of change in the configuration of pleural effusion with alteration of the position of the patient suggests loculation or organization. The presence of a horizontal air-fluid level rather than a meniscus superiorly indicates the presence of a hydropneumothorax.

Since the distribution of pleural effusion is also related to lung elasticity, atypical configurations will occur when there is underlying pulmonary disease (Fleischner, 1963). It is also important to recognize that a large volume of intrapleural fluid will obscure the ipsilateral lung and cause the mediastinum to shift to the opposite side. Absence of shift, then, indicates the presence of atelectasis of the underlying lung.

Subpulmonic Effusion

With the patient erect, fluid accumulates below the visceral pleura of the diaphragmatic surface of the lung. When this reaches a large enough proportion, the fluid upon which the lung is floating will visibly widen the space between the visceral and diaphragmatic pleura. The superior aspect of the fluid then resembles a hemidiaphragm, but its "dome" tends to be more lateral in position than the normal diaphragmatic dome. Moreover, there is a wider than normal distance between the inferior surface of the lung and the gastric air bubble on the left side. The presence of an infrapulmonary collection of fluid can be readily confirmed by means of lateral decubitus views (Dunbar and Favreau, 1959) (Fig. 14).

Pneumothorax

The presence of air outside the visceral pleura on the convex aspect of the lung indicates a pneumothorax. In older children, this pleural surface is usually readily visible. An increase in density of the lung due to compression by the surrounding air further contributes to the diagnosis of a pneumothorax. This difference in densities can be enhanced on films obtained in expiration.

Intrapleural air is often less obvious on supine radiographs of infants, since the air tends to rise over the anterior surface of the lung (Fig. 15). In these patients, lateral decubitus views may be

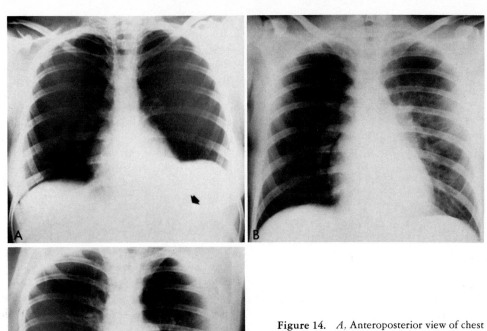

Figure 14. *A,* Anteroposterior view of chest shows apparently elevated left diaphragmatic dome, which is separated from the stomach bubble (*arrow*). *B,* In supine position, the left pleural effusion has caused a diffuse increase in density of the hemithorax. *C,* The left lateral decubitus view demonstrates the extent of subpulmonic effusion.

Figure 15. A pneumomediastinum elevates the sail-like thymic lobes away from the pericardium. The air surrounding the lung apices also indicates bilateral pneumothoraces.

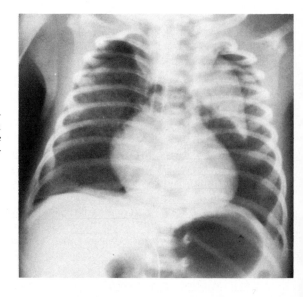

necessary to demonstrate the presence and extent of a pneumothorax (Mac-Ewan and coworkers, 1971). This method is helpful even in the presence of bilateral pneumothoraces. Also, a collection of air medial to the lung may simulate a pneumomediastinum (Moskowitz and Griscom, 1976). In this case, lateral decubitus views will again help to clarify the diagnosis.

THE MEDIASTINUM

The mediastinum includes those structures that are encased in the parietal pleura between the two lungs. The pleural reflections of a number of mediastinal structures can be visualized on plain chest radiographs. It is beyond the scope of this chapter to discuss mediastinal anatomy in detail. The heart and thymus, however, are frequently sources of confusion in the interpretation of chest radiographs, and some of their features will be described below. Other anatomic details are shown in Figure 16.

The mediastinum is arbitrarily divided, for descriptive purposes, into three compartments: the anterior, containing lymph nodes and the thymus gland; the middle, which contains the heart and great vessels, esophagus, trachea and major bronchi; and the posterior, which includes the descending aorta, azygos venous system and sympathetic chain.

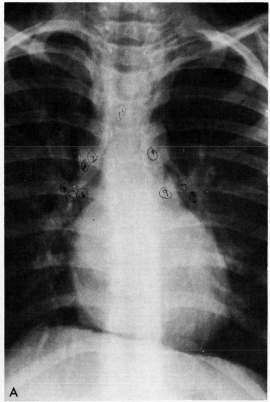

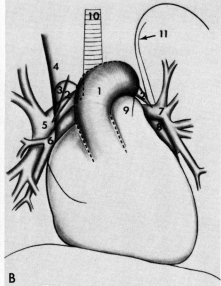

Figure 16. *A* and *B,* Normal mediastinal structures outlined by a small pneumomediastinum. (1, Aorta; 2, thymus; 3, azygos vein; 4, superior vena cava; 5, right pulmonary artery; 6, right bronchi; 7, left pulmonary artery; 8, left bronchus; 9, main pulmonary artery; 10, trachea; 11, mediastinal pleura.)

Anterior Mediastinum

The major structure of the anterior mediastinal compartment, the thymus, is a source of endless confusion because of its protean configuration. While the thymus gland continues to grow throughout childhood until prepubescence, it is relatively most prominent in the infant and small child in whom it can simulate a mediastinal tumor or cardiomegaly. A number of characteristics, however, help to elucidate this polymorphous structure:

1. *Sail sign* (Kemp and coworkers, 1948). The thymus projects laterally (usually to the right) of the upper mediastinum and its shape is reminiscent of a triangular sail. Its sharply defined lateral and lower borders as well as absence of an air bronchogram help to distinguish it from upper lobe consolidation (Fig. 17).

2. *Wave sign* (Mulvey, 1963). Since the edge of the thymus is indented by the costal cartilages, its lateral border has a wavelike contour.

3. *Retraction.* Under fluoroscopy, the edge of the thymus can be seen to retract momentarily during a deep inspiration. At this time, the wavelike configuration of its lateral border becomes apparent.

4. *Absence of mediastinal displacement.* Thymic tissue is relatively compliant and should not compress or displace adjacent structures.

5. *Anterior position.* On lateral projections, the gland tends to obliterate the space between the posterior border of the sternum and the anterior surface of the right ventricle. When a dense shadow is present in this area and there is a normal retrocardiac space, it is likely that cardiomegaly, if suspected on an anteroposterior film, is due instead to a large thymus (Fig. 18).

6. *Effect of steroids.* Exogenous steroids have been given in order to produce thymic involution and thus rule out a mediastinal tumor (Caffey and diLiberti, 1959; Caffey and Silbey, 1960), although continuing experience with the various appearances of the thymus has reduced the need for this test.

ABSENCE OF THYMUS. Along with anomalies of the aortic arch and absence of the parathyroids, the thymus may also be missing, as in the DiGeorge syndrome. The thymus is also dysplastic in a number of immune deficiency dis-

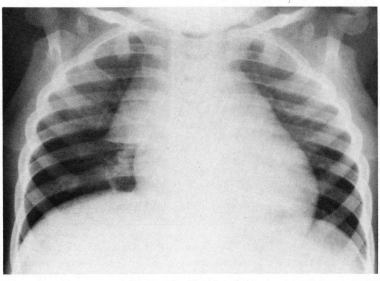

Figure 17. Thymic sail sign.

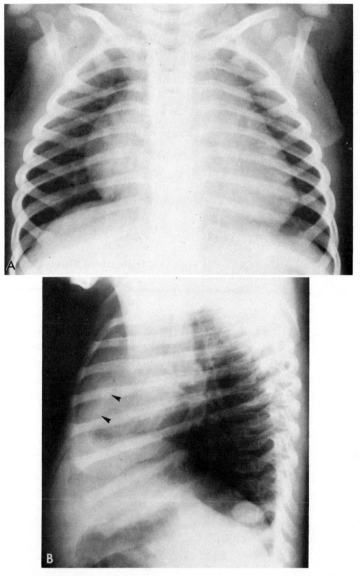

Figure 18. *A,* Apparent cardiomegaly on anteroposterior projection. *B,* The lateral view shows a normal retrocardiac space. The anterior density is caused by the thymus (*arrows*).

eases (Kirkpatrick and DiGeorge, 1968). Since thymic involution occurs with stress, its absence cannot usually be diagnosed with certainty on chest radiographs. Conversely, definite identification of thymic tissue may be helpful in assessment of immune disorders.

Middle Mediastinum

The heart and pericardium are the major components of the middle mediastinum. In infants, cardiac morphologic features are difficult to assess because of the thymus, which drapes over the anterior aspect of the pericardium. In addition, the heart is more transverse in position and the right cardiac border, which is formed by the right atrium, is relatively prominent. While the ratio of the transverse diameter of the heart to that of the thorax is usually given as 0.5 or less for the child, the measurements of Bakwin and Bakwin

(1935) indicate a mean cardiothoracic ratio of 0.53 to 0.57 during the first year of life. Considerable variation in these measurements occurs in normal infants and children. These variations are related to the phase of the respiratory and cardiac cycles during which the radiographic exposure is made as well as to the variable size of the thymus.

The arch of the azygos vein casts an oval shadow on frontal projection at the right tracheobronchial junction. It varies in size with posture, respiration and disease states involving right-sided heart function. It is, however, not consistently visible in infants and younger children, and according to Wishart (1972), it can be so variable that correlation of its width with pathologic states is uncertain.

Posterior Mediastinum

The posterior mediastinum should be assessed to detect neurogenic tumors, which displace the paravertebral pleural reflections. The left lateral border of the descending aorta may be clearly visible during childhood, but cannot usually be seen in the infant. Chest radiographs taken in the immediate newborn period often show a small mass to the left of the upper mediastinum. This shadow, which is due to the closing ductus arteriosus, has been termed the "ductus bump" by Berdon and coworkers (1965).

Pneumomediastinum

When alveolar rupture occurs, the extravasated gas traverses the pulmonary interstitium to enter the mediastinum (Macklin, 1939). On frontal projections, the air may be variably visible as an increased lucency adjacent to the heart borders. More often, however, the only direct evidence of pneumomediastinum is elevation of the thymic lobes away from the pericardium. This has been termed the spinaker-sail sign (Felson, 1969) (Fig. 15). Extension of air into the neck occurs more fre-

quently in infants than in older children. Occasionally, other mediastinal structures, such as the aortic arch, azygos vein, main pulmonary artery and superior vena cava, may also be outlined by mediastinal air (Fig. 16).

In the much less common pneumopericardium, gas completely surrounds the epicardium and will thus be visible in the pericardial sac between the central tendon of the diaphragm and inferior heart border, as well as within the pericardial reflections over the great vessels. In contrast to mediastinal emphysema, the thymus remains approximated to the pericardium.

Mediastinal Masses

Because of its extrapleural position, the surface of a mass that is adjacent to the lung is sharply defined. Its superior and inferior extremities tend to taper (Felson, 1969). Mediastinal masses can also be differentiated from lesions arising in the pulmonary parenchyma by the lack of an air bronchogram.

THE BRONCHI

The normal segmental bronchial anatomy is shown in Figures 11 and 12, pages 98 and 99, and in Figure 2, pages 110 to 114.

Air Bronchogram

This is perhaps the most revealing sign of pulmonary parenchymal disease in the radiologic armamentarium. The "air bronchogram" refers to the air-containing bronchi that become visible when the surrounding lung parenchyma is opacified because of alveolar consolidation or atelectasis (Fig. 19). Therefore, the "air bronchogram" indicates pulmonary parenchymal disease and is not seen in abnormalities of the pleura or in lesions arising in the mediastinum. For obvious reasons, the air bronchogram is not visible within solid parenchymal tumors and fluid-contain-

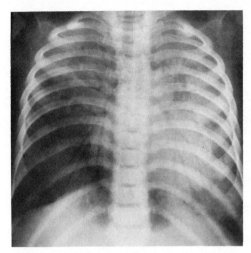

Figure 19. Bilateral, diffuse air bronchogram caused by *Pneumocystis carinii* pneumonia.

ings, which are most prominent in the lung bases, are thought to be due to bronchial wall thickening or "peribronchial infiltration" and are usually diagnosed as bronchitis or mild bronchopneumonia. However, the exact implications of these roentgen findings remain unclear.

Bronchiectasis

Bronchiectasis is associated with chronic pulmonary infection and is particularly severe in the lungs of patients with cystic fibrosis of the pancreas. Foreign body aspiration should also be considered as an etiologic agent in localized chronic pulmonary disease with bronchiectasis.

In chronic pneumonia (which frequently involves the right middle lobe), loss of lung volume may lead to secondary bronchial dilatation. A central bronchial obstruction need not be present. Bronchograms may demonstrate lack of normal tapering of bronchi and incomplete peripheral filling, but irreversible saccular bronchiectasis is rarely present.

ing pulmonary cysts. On the other hand, the mainstem and segmental bronchi can produce a normal "air bronchogram" because of their contiguity with other water density hilar structures and the normal thickness of their walls (Burko, 1962).

In the absence of major pulmonary disease, the bronchial lumens are sometimes outlined along a portion of their length or on cross section. These find-

In cystic fibrosis, bronchiectasis is eventually recognizable on plain films

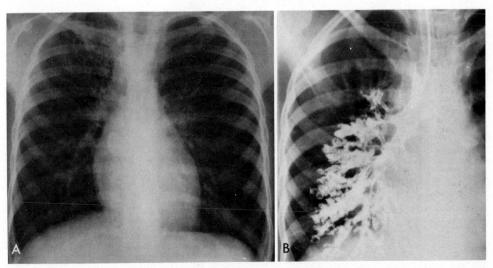

Figure 20. *A,* Bronchiectasis seems to be most marked in the right upper lobe of this patient with cystic fibrosis. *B,* On bronchography, extensive middle and lower lobe bronchiectasis becomes obvious. The upper lobe bronchi are incompletely filled.

because of either mucus filling of the dilated bronchi or peribronchial disease. On bronchography, the extent of bronchiectasis in these patients is often found to be surprisingly greater than was suspected on the plain films (Fig. 20).

Further abnormalities of the bronchial tree are discussed in the sections on lung volume (pp. 157 to 163).

THE HILA AND PULMONARY VESSELS

The right and left pulmonary arteries and the upper lobe veins are mainly responsible for the radiographic density of the hila. The major bronchi are projected as tubular lucencies. The lower lobe veins return to the left atrium below the hila. The bronchopulmonary lymph nodes are recognizable only if they enlarge. The right hilum, because of the configuration of the heart, may appear slightly more prominent than the left. Spurious differences in size of the hila can occur owing to

magnification when the chest is rotated. The left hilum is normally slightly higher than the right.

Assessment of Hilar Size

This is a largely subjective step in the evaluation of chest radiographs. The hila are decreased in size in cyanotic congenital heart disease, such as tetralogy of Fallot, and when there is hypoplasia or absence of a pulmonary artery. Enlargement of the pulmonary arteries is most commonly associated with left-to-right shunts. In the presence of a left-to-right shunt, Coussement and Gooding (1973) found that the diameter of the right descending pulmonary artery, as measured on frontal projections, was never less than that of the trachea.

Enlargement of the bronchopulmonary nodes imparts a lobular appearance to the border of the hilum that faces the lung. This is in contrast to the linear or slightly concave aspect presented by the pulmonary arteries. A well exposed, nonrotated lateral view is

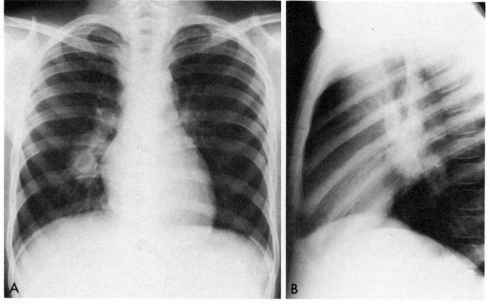

Figure 21. The enlargement of bronchopulmonary nodes in the right hilum (*A*) is well visualized on the lateral projection (*B*).

very helpful in the assessment of changes in size of the hila (Fig. 21).

The Pulmonary Vasculature

The pulmonary arteries and veins are responsible for the majority of the linear densities seen in the lungs. On plain chest radiographs and tomograms (Fletcher and Donner, 1968), the arteries and veins can be distinguished, since the arteries branch from the hilus segmentally with the bronchi and arch laterally and downward in a "weeping willow" pattern. The upper lobe veins course toward the heart in a position lateral to the arteries, and the lower lobe veins are nearly horizontal in their course to the left atrium.

Pulmonary Arteries

The size of the pulmonary arteries roughly correlates with the amount of flow. In a study by Schwarz and co-workers (1970), the presence of a left-to-right shunt was diagnosed with 100 per cent accuracy only when the pulmonary-systemic shunt ratio was greater than 2.2 to 1. Small shunts (Qp–Qs less than 1.4 to 1) were not appreciated in 45 to 58 per cent of cases. In assessing increased flow to the lungs, it is helpful to concentrate on the size of the arteries in the middle third of the lungs. In the lung periphery, a fine reticular pattern may be seen as the smaller arterial branches become visible owing to engorgement.

Pulmonary arterial hypertension is recognizable when there is an exaggerated discrepancy between the caliber of the central and peripheral pulmonary arteries. In children, these findings seem to be more useful in visualizing pulmonary vascular changes due to mitral valve disease than in the diagnosis of pulmonary hypertension due to a left-to-right shunt.

Decreased arterial flow associated with cyanotic congenital heart disease results in hyperlucent lungs with decreased vascular markings and frequently increased volume.

Bronchial Arteries

On plain films, the bronchial arteries are not visible at their point of origin from the descending aorta. Their intrapulmonary branches, however, may be recognized as fine, reticular densities in the central and basilar portions of the lungs of patients whose pulmonary arterial flow is reduced owing to cyanotic congenital heart disease.

Pulmonary Veins

The caliber of the pulmonary veins increases as they become engorged. They can be distinguished from pulmonary arteries by their somewhat tortuous course, which can be traced to the periphery of the lungs. Pulmonary veins can also be recognized as such by their lack of peripheral tapering and absence of artery-like branching, as well as by the more horizontal path of the lower lobe veins. An increase in pulmonary venous pressure is reflected by distention of veins in the upper lung zones due to spasm of the veins in the lung bases.

Pulmonary Edema

Leakage of fluid from the pulmonary microvascular bed will result in interstitial pulmonary edema. Edema occurs if the increased volume of fluid cannot be removed by the pulmonary lymphatics.

An early sign of fluid in the perivascular interstitial space is a loss of definition of the pulmonary veins. This sign is best appreciated in the middle third of the lungs and is probably more reliable than loss of definition of hila, or "hilar haze."

Interstitial edema is also manifested radiologically by Kerley "A" and "B" lines, which are caused by fluid in the interlobular septa (Heitzman and Ziter, 1966) (Fig. 22). The "A" lines are thin linear densities that tend to radiate upward from the hila. The "B" lines are the short horizontal linear densities seen in the lung periphery near the costophrenic angles. The latter are dif-

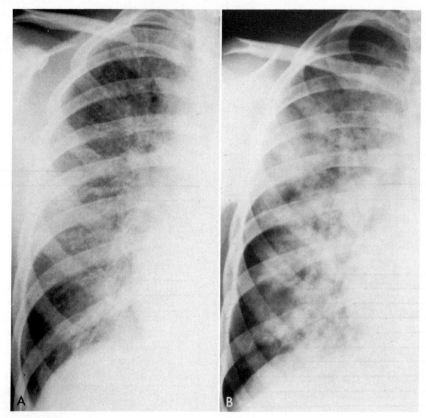

Figure 22. *A*, Reticular pattern with Kerley "A" and "B" lines in interstitial edema. *B*, At a later date, the same patient developed a "fluffy" coalescent pattern of alveolar edema.

ficult to resolve in the lungs of small infants, but similar horizontal lines may be seen in the retrosternal area on a well exposed lateral view. The fissures of the lungs become apparently thickened because of subpleural edema.

Alveolar edema, which is preceded by interstitial edema, fills the air spaces and produces ill-defined homogeneous shadows of water density, through which an air bronchogram may be visible. The classic picture of alveolar edema is one in which the medial aspects of both lungs are involved and the cortex is spared, producing a "bat's wing" appearance. However, variations are numerous, the prime example being the predominantly right-sided edema that may be related to differences in respiratory motion of the two lungs and the position of the patient. When there is underlying chronic lung disease, the patterns of pulmonary edema may be very atypical (Hublitz

and Shapiro, 1969). Radiologic signs of congestive heart failure are notoriously difficult to recognize in patients with late cystic fibrosis because of destruction of the pulmonary vascular bed as well as similar density patterns that have resulted from chronic pulmonary infection.

Pulmonary edema serves as a model for the study of other types of air space and interstitial disease to be discussed below.

PULMONARY CONSOLIDATION

Pneumonia is the chief cause of pulmonary consolidation* in children. The

---

*The term "consolidation" is used here, since it more accurately describes the pathologic changes in the lung parenchyma than the more popular designation "infiltration."

anatomic distribution of an inflammatory exudate is identical with that of a transudate due to pulmonary edema in that there is involvement of the air spaces and interstitium of the lung. Since cellular debris is of the same density as edema fluid, the radiographic appearance of pulmonary edema and pneumonia is similar and even indistinguishable.

While pulmonary infection involves both the air spaces and the interstitium, the shadows cast by the air space or alveolar consolidation usually predominate.

Alveolar (Air Space) Disease

Alveolar lesions are recognized by their ill-defined, fluffy margins, a tendency to coalesce, large areas of involvement and the presence of an air bronchogram (Felson, 1967). The air bronchogram is identical with that seen in alveolar pulmonary edema (Fig. 19). The "air alveologram" is another feature of pneumonia that imparts a mottled appearance because of numerous small lucencies cast by uninvolved groups of alveoli.

Pneumonia may be lobar or segmental in distribution, although many (probably most) pneumonias of childhood are nonsegmental. This can be explained by a tendency for the disease to spread circumferentially from lobule to lobule via intra-alveolar pores of Kohn (Fraser and Wortzman, 1959).

For the radiologist, an unnerving aspect of childhood pneumonia is its occasional presentation as a fairly large spherical density. If an air bronchogram is lacking, the specter of primary tumor or metastasis arises. With pneumonia, however, the edges are usually not as well defined as those of a parenchymal mass and it usually does not present a perfectly circular shadow on both anteroposterior and lateral views. Repeat radiographs a few days later usually reveal the true nature of the lesion (Fig. 23).

Localization of Disease

For purposes of physiotherapy, bronchoscopy and surgery, the exact localization of pulmonary densities becomes necessary. Although, as noted previously, disease may not be wholly con-

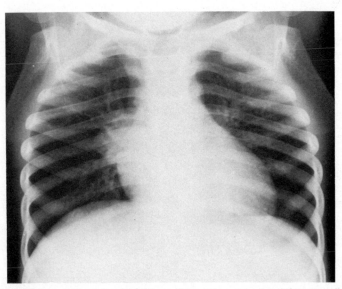

Figure 23. A round mass due to pneumonia is superimposed over the right hilum. The disease, which is in the superior segment of the right lower lobe, does not create a positive silhouette with the hilum or heart border because of its posterior location (compare with Fig. 24).

fined to a segment or even a lobe, when it does correspond to the anatomic distribution of the bronchial tree, its anatomic distribution can be determined see Fig. 2, pp. 110 to 114). It is helpful to localize pulmonary consolidation by contiguity with a fissure, e.g., consolidation limited on its inferior aspect by the minor fissure must involve the contiguous (anterior) segment of the upper lobe.

Silhouette Sign

A lengthy discussion of anatomic details is not within the scope of this chapter, but this would seem an appropriate place to discuss an important aid to diagnosis and localization—the "silhouette sign." This sign refers to the fact that the borders of contiguous structures of similar radiopacity will be obscured by one another. The concept

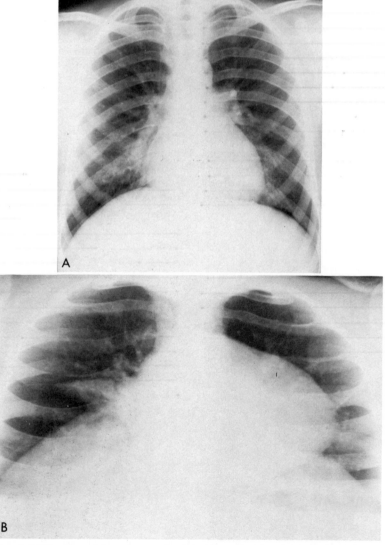

Figure 24. *A,* Obliteration of the right heart border indicates middle lobe disease. *B,* The anteroposterior lordotic view of the same patient shows a wedge-shaped atelectatic middle lobe.

can then be applied to a disease process that produces a water density when it is in contact with structures of similar density, such as the heart, aortic arch and superior surface of the diaphragm. A positive silhouette sign is present when there is loss of the borders of these structures (Felson and Felson, 1950). The silhouette sign is most frequently used for localization of disease to the right middle lobe and lingula, in which case the right and left heart borders, respectively, are obscured (Fig. 24). If disease is localized in the basilar segments of the lower lobes, there is obliteration of the adjacent diaphragmatic surfaces. The right upper mediastinal border may be lost owing to disease in the anterior segment of the right upper lobe, and the apicoposterior segment of the left upper lobe may mask the aortic knob.

Absence of a silhouette sign can also be helpful. For example, a lesion in the superior segment of a lower lobe is projected through the hilum and may be mistaken for perihilar pneumonia or hilar enlargement. Careful observation will reveal the borders of the hilum distinctly visible through the density, since this segment is separated from the more anterior hilum by normally aerated lung (Fig. 23).

The silhouette sign is occasionally falsely positive, since the right heart border may be obscured by a normal pulmonary artery or by the parasternal soft tissues of the anterior chest wall in patients with pectus excavatum.

Observer Errors

In general, there is a tendency toward overdiagnosis of pneumonia in the cardiophrenic area of the right lung. This is due to poor resolution of the numerous pulmonary vessels in this region, which can often be corrected by obtaining a well exposed anteroposterior supine view of the chest in maximum inspiration.

On the other hand, consolidations in the left lung behind the heart are often overlooked because of the large similar density of the ventricles. This fault in diagnosis is usually the combined product of underexposure of the chest film and lack of observer perception. Since these pneumonias involve the posterior aspects of the lung bases, they are revealed on a well positioned lateral view, which shows an apparent increase in density of the lower thoracic vertebrae just above the posterior cardiophrenic angle. The lower thoracic vertebrae normally appear more lucent than the upper because of the large volume of superimposed lung and absence of overlying axillary and scapular shadows. Therefore, an interruption of this sequence of densities, which might be termed a positive "spine sign," will indicate the presence of pulmonary disease (Fig. 25).

INTERSTITIAL DISEASE

As noted elsewhere, inflammatory disease of the lung usually involves the air spaces as well as the interstitium. Other disorders, such as sarcoid and histiocytosis X, are also predominantly interstitial. Interstitial pulmonary edema (Fig. 22 A) is a prime example of involvement of the perivascular interstitial space and interlobular septa. When the parenchymal or interalveolar interstitium is involved, a reticulonodular pattern is produced. A diffuse cloudy or "ground-glass" appearance of the lungs has also been attributed to involvement of the parenchymal interstitium. The term "honeycomb" lung, which is often associated with histiocytosis X, implies a reticular pattern in which small cysts are visible. Examples of interstitial disease are shown in Figures 26 to 28.

Radiologic interpretation of interstitial involvement is useful in determining the cause of chronic pulmonary disease. However, since a combination of interstitial and alveolar involvement is common in acute pneumonia, this ex-

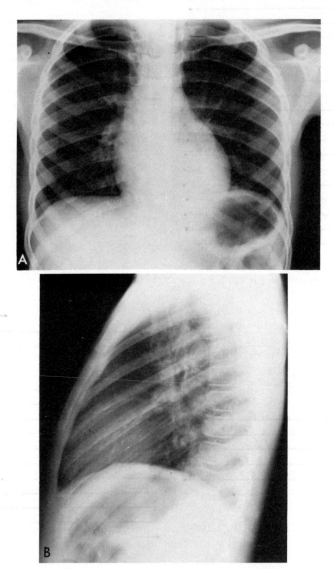

Figure 25. *A,* The left basilar pneumonia has created an increase in density behind the heart on the left. *B,* On lateral projection, the pneumonia is superimposed over the lower thoracic vertebrae.

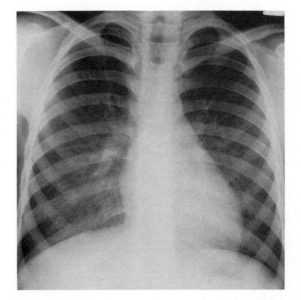

Figure 26. Bilateral "ground-glass" appearance of lungs due to interstitial disease associated with hypersensitivity reaction. There is no air bronchogram.

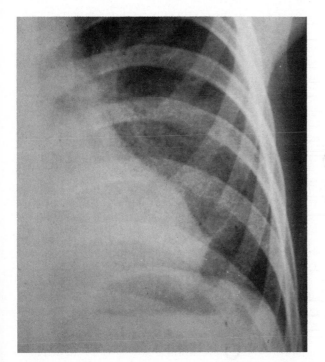

Figure 27. Reticular pattern, best seen in left lower lobe in patient with desquamative interstitial pneumonitis.

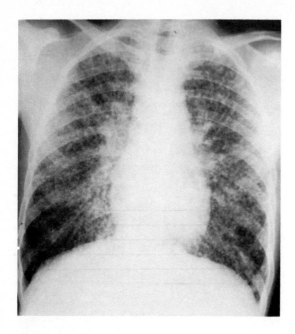

Figure 28.   Nodular interstitial pattern due to sarcoid.

ercise in pattern recognition is not usually helpful in differentiating viral and bacterial pneumonia.

DECREASED LUNG VOLUME

Atelectasis

Collapse of lung parenchyma occurs for two basic reasons: ① due to obstruction of an airway and resorption of gas from the alveolus, or ② secondary to compression by fluids or gas in the pleural space or by an intrathoracic mass. Atelectasis may involve varying amounts of lung parenchyma, depending on the size and numbers of airways that are occluded. Thus, atelectasis may involve an entire lung, one or more lobes, segments or subsegments.

Lobar collapse is identified by an increase in density of the involved lung and rearrangement of the position of the interlobar fissures. For example, the major fissures shift posteriorly when the lower lobes collapse (Fig. 12 B). Right upper lobe atelectasis causes the minor fissure to rotate upward and medially. The major fissure is retracted upward and anteriorly when the left upper lobe becomes atelectatic. Loss of volume of the middle lobe results in a laterally tapering wedge-shaped density bounded by the major and minor fissures, which can be elegantly demonstrated by means of an anteroposterior lordotic view (Fig. 24 B).

Lobar collapse may be incomplete. The degree of atelectasis is modified by the rate of resorption of gas from the alveolus, the chronicity of obstruction and the presence of pre-existing parenchymal disease. An air bronchogram will be seen as the alveoli collapse. Just as in pulmonary consolidation, a positive silhouette sign develops as the dense atelectatic lung parenchyma obliterates the margins of the adjacent mediastinal and diaphragmatic structures.

Lobar atelectasis also results in a number of recognizable secondary signs, which vary to some degree according to the site of involvement:

① narrowing of the intercostal spaces on the ipsilateral side;

② elevation of the hemidiaphragm adjacent to a lower lobe collapse;

③ upward displacement of the hilum in upper lobe atelectasis and downward displacement in lower lobe collapse;

④ shift of the cardiac silhouette or trachea toward the atelectatic lobe; ⑤ compensatory hyperinflation of uninvolved portions of lung or of the opposite lung.

The latter two indirect effects of lobar collapse require further comment. Tracheal shift may be detected clinically and radiologically when upper lobe atelectasis occurs in older children and adults. However, shift of the trachea alone is a less valuable sign in infants because of the natural redundancy of the trachea and its tendency to buckle to the right. Instead, when an upper lobe is atelectatic, the entire mediastinum appears to tilt toward the collapsed lobe. Furthermore, when there is reduction in volume of a lower lobe, shift of the heart toward the side of collapse occurs especially readily in infants because of the marked elasticity of the mediastinal structures.

Compensatory hyperinflation of uninvolved lobes of the same lung or of the opposite lung is recognized by hyperlucency and splaying of the affected pulmonary vessels. Actual herniation of lung across the upper mediastinum toward the affected hemithorax is common. Occasionally, confusion may arise between primary and compensatory emphysema. This will be discussed in the section on increased lung volume.

In terms of displacement of intrathoracic structures, atelectasis at the segmental or subsegmental level does not cause a significant change. Both are recognized by an increase in density of the involved lung parenchyma. Segmental collapse produces a wedge-shaped density, the apex of which is directed toward the hilum. Platelike areas of subsegmental atelectasis appear as short horizontal linear streaks above the diaphragmatic domes. These tend to occur in disorders in which there is diminished diaphragmatic motion and are not frequently seen in children.

Acute asthma is one example of disease in which multiple areas of segmental and subsegmental atelectasis occurs. The diffuse streaky densities that result may be incorrectly diagnosed as pneumonia. The proper diagnosis is usually clarified by follow-up films made a day or two after the acute attack. Two other situations in which diffuse atelectasis of both lungs occurs also deserve special mention.

The first is hyaline membrane disease, in which there is a deficiency of surfactant and, therefore, increased surface tension, leading to alveolar collapse (Avery and Mead, 1959). The classic reticulogranular pattern seen radiologically is produced by overdistention of small airways and some of the air spaces, in contrast to the densities produced by other areas of parenchymal collapse (Recavarren and coworkers, 1967) (Fig. 29). This pattern bears some resemblance to the "air alveologram" discussed on page 155. Homogeneous opacification of the lungs in hyaline membrane disease signifies even more extensive parenchymal atelectasis.

A second situation where massive and rapid collapse of both lungs can occur is when the alveoli contain high concentrations of inspired oxygen. Occlusion of the endotracheal tube of a newborn infant or a period of apnea will result in rapid resorption of oxygen at the alveolar-capillary level and consequent atelectasis of both lungs within minutes (Fletcher and Avery, 1973).

Atelectasis versus Dysgenesis

Congenital absence of a lung or lobe simulates atelectasis, and bronchography or angiography may be necessary for correct diagnosis. When the entire lung is absent, the hemithorax is completely opaque and is occupied by the mediastinum. The size of the hemithorax, however, may not be decreased as markedly as when massive atelectasis occurs. Hypoplasia of a lobe is accompanied by an increase in extrapleural alveolar tissue, which on lateral radiographs creates a substernal opacity extending from the thoracic inlet to the diaphragm (Felson, 1972).

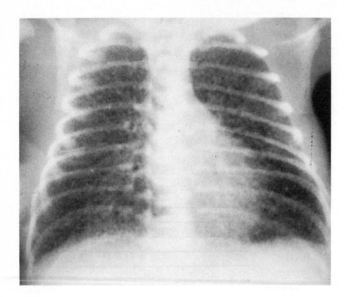

Figure 29. Reticulogranular pattern of hyaline membrane disease.

This opaque stripe is somewhat similar to that produced by collapse of the left upper lobe.

Pneumothorax and pneumomediastinum are indirect signs of pulmonary hypoplasia in newborn infants and are prevalent in infants born with renal malformations and Potter's syndrome (Stern and coworkers, 1972).

INCREASED LUNG VOLUME

An increase in volume of a lobe or lung is usually due to an increase in the amount of gas contained within the alveoli. Only occasionally is the lung increased in density as well as volume, as in the case of Klebsiella pneumonia, bronchial obstruction in the fetal lung and rare malformations and cysts.

Hyperaeration may be unrelated to primary pulmonary disease when it results from acidosis or is associated with cyanotic congenital heart disease. However, obstruction or spasm of small airways, as in emphysema or bronchiolitis, will cause diffuse bilateral pulmonary hyperaeration. Consideration of several disorders that cause a localized increase in lung volume is in order here.

Bronchial Foreign Body

Obstructive emphysema due to an inhaled foreign body results from a ball-valve mechanism by which the foreign body allows the passage of air distal to it but impedes its egress. The resultant voluminous lung or lobe produces a shift of the mediastinum to the opposite side. When these findings are present on routine chest radiographs, they do not present a diagnostic problem. However, when a patient presents with clinical features of airway obstruction and findings are minimal or absent on routine radiographs, expiration films and fluoroscopy are required. The important feature of this type of bronchial occlusion is the ability of the normal lung to partially deflate. On expiration, this causes the mediastinum to shift away from the obstructed side.

Congenital Lobar Emphysema

This disorder, which causes an increase in volume of a lobe, will also shift the mediastinum toward the unaffected side. This change, plus partial

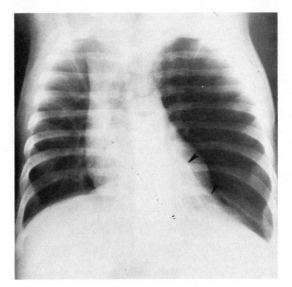

Figure 30. Lobar emphysema involving the left upper lobe, causing compression atelectasis of the left lower lobe (*arrows*) and producing marked shift of the mediastinum to the right.

compression atelectasis of the adjacent portions of the ipsileratal lung (Fig. 30), accounts for varying degrees of respiratory distress. The size of the emphysematous lobe is unchanged throughout the respiratory cycle.

Idiopathic Hyperlucent Lung (Swyer-James-Macleod Syndrome)

It seems appropriate to include this entity here, for although the involved lung is slightly smaller than normal, air is trapped within it. No central bronchial obstruction is present, but the peripheral bronchi are "pruned" because of pre-existing obliterative bronchiolitis. The hyperlucency is caused by overdistended alveoli and diminished pulmonary arterial flow (Cumming and coworkers, 1971). Despite the slight hypoplasia of the involved lung, the associated air-trapping causes shift of the mediastinum toward the contralateral side on expiration.

Compensatory Emphysema

On routine chest radiography, it may be difficult to differentiate between hyperaeration of a lobe or lung due to obstructive emphysema and overinflation due to compensatory emphysema asso-

ciated with atelectasis elsewhere. This can be resolved by fluoroscopy, since air is not trapped on expiration in an otherwise normal lung that is voluminous because of compensatory emphysema. Therefore, it will increase in density and decrease in volume on expiration.

GENERAL REFERENCES

Avery, M. E., and Fletcher, B. D.: *The Lung and its Disorders in the Newborn Infant.* Philadelphia, W. B. Saunders Company, 1974.

Felson, B.: *Chest Roentgenology.* Philadelphia, W. B. Saunders Company, 1973.

Fraser, R. G., and Paré, J. A. P.: *Diagnosis of Diseases of the Chest.* Philadelphia, W. B. Saunders Company, 1970.

Kaufmann, H. J. (Ed.): *Progress in Pediatric Radiology.* Vol. I. Respiratory Tract. Chicago, Year Book Medical Publishers, Inc., 1967.

Poznanski, A. K.: *Practical Approaches to Pediatric Radiology.* Chicago, Year Book Medical Publishers, Inc., 1976.

Singleton, E. B., and Wagner, M. L.: *Radiologic Atlas of Pulmonary Abnormalities in Children.* Philadelphia, W. B. Saunders Company, 1971.

REFERENCES

Alazraki, N. P., and Friedman, P. J.: Posterior mediastinal "pseudo-mass" of the newborn. *Am. J. Roentgenol., 116*:571, 1972.

Avery, M. E.: Bronchography: outmoded procedure? *Pediatrics, 46*:333, 1970.

Avery, M. E., and Mead, J.: Surface properties in

relation to atelectasis and hyaline membrane disease. *Am. J. Dis. Child.*, 97:517, 1959.

Bakwin, H., and Bakwin, R. M.: Body build in infants. VI. Growth of the cardiac silhouette and the thoraco-abdominal cavity. *Am. J. Dis. Child.*, 49:861, 1935.

Berdon, W. E., Baker,D. H., and James, L. S.: The ductus bump: a transient physiologic mass in chest roentgenograms of newborn infants. *Am. J. Roentgenol.*, 95:91, 1965.

Bernard, J., Sauvegrain, J., and Nahum, H.: Tomography of the lungs in infancy and childhood: techniques, indications and results. *Progr. Pediatr. Radiol.*, 1:59, 1967.

Burko, H.: Considerations in the roentgen diagnosis of pneumonia in children. *Am. J. Roentgenol.*, 88:555, 1962.

Caffey, J., and diLiberti, C.: Acute atrophy of the thymus induced by adrenocorticosteroids: observed roentgenographically in living human infants. *Am. J. Roentgenol.*, 82:530, 1959.

Caffey, J., and Silbey, R.: Regrowth and overgrowth of the thymus after atrophy induced by the oral administration of adrenocorticosteroids to human infants. *Pediatrics*, 26:762, 1960.

Capitanio, M. A., and Kirkpatrick, J. A.: Obstructions of the upper airway in children as reflected on the chest radiograph. *Radiology*, 107:159, 1973.

Coussement, A. M., and Gooding, C. A.: Objective radiographic assessment of pulmonary vascularity in children. *Radiology*, 109:649, 1973.

Cumming, G. R., MacPherson, R. I., and Chernick, V.: Unilateral hyperlucent lung syndrome in children. *J. Pediatr.*, 78:250, 1971.

Davis, L. A.: Verticle fissure line. *Am. J. Roentgenol.*, 84:451, 1960.

Davis, L. A.: Standard roentgen examinations in newborns, infants and children: techniques, "portable" films, immobilization devices and fluoroscopy. *Progr. Pediatr. Radiol.*, 1:3, 1967.

DeLevie, M., Nogrady, M. B., and Spence, L.: Acute laryngotracheobronchitis (croup): correlation of clinical severity with radiologic and virologic findings. *Ann. Radiol.*, 15:193, 1972.

Dunbar, J. S.: Upper respiratory tract obstruction in infants and children. *Am. J. Roentgenol.*, 109:227, 1970.

Dunbar, J. S., and Favreau, M.: Infrapulmonary pleural effusion with particular reference to its occurrence in nephrosis. *J. Can. Assoc. Radiol.*, 10:24, 1959.

Fellows, K. E., Stigol, L., Shuster, S., Khaw, K. T., and Shwachman, H.: Selective bronchial arteriography in patients with cystic fibrosis and massive hemoptysis. *Radiology*, 114:551, 1975.

Felson, B.: The roentgen diagnosis of disseminated pulmonary alveolar diseases. *Semin. Roentgenol.*, 2:3, 1967.

Felson, B.: The mediastinum. *Semin. Roentgenol.*, 4:41, 1969.

Felson, B.: Pulmonary agenesis and related anomalies. *Semin. Roentgenol.*, 7:17, 1972.

Felson, B., and Felson, H.: Localization of intrathoracic lesions by means of the postero-anterior roentgenogram: the silhouette sign. *Radiology*, 55:363, 1950.

Felson, B., and Palayew, M. J.: The two types of right aortic arch. *Radiology*, 81:745, 1963.

Fleischner, F. G.: Atypical arrangement of free pleural effusion. *Radiol. Clin. North Am.*, 1:347, 1963.

Fletcher, B. D., and Avery, M. E.: The effects of airway occlusion after oxygen breathing on the lungs of newborn infants: radiologic demonstration in the experimental animal. *Radiology*, 109:655, 1973.

Fletcher, B. D., and Donner, M. W.: The use of full-chest tomography in the roentgenographic evaluation of pulmonary embolism. *Dis. Chest*, 54:13, 1968.

Franken, E. A., Jr., Hurwitz, R. A., and Battersby, J. S.: Unequal aeration of the lungs in children: the use of pulmonary angiography. *Radiology*, 109:401, 1973.

Fraser, R. G., and Wortzman, G.: Acute pneumococcal lobar pneumonia: the significance of nonsegmental distribution. *J. Can. Assoc. Radiol.*, 10:37, 1959.

Gooding, C. A.: Pulmonary angiography. In Gyepes, M. T. (Ed.): *Angiography in Infants and Children.* New York, Grune & Stratton, 1974, p. 99.

Grünebaum, M.: The roentgenologic investigation of congenital subglottic stenosis. *Am. J. Roentgenol.*, 125:877, 1975.

Heitzman, E. R., and Ziter, F. M., Jr.: Acute interstitial pulmonary edema. *Am. J. Roentgenol.*, 98:291, 1966.

Hublitz, U. F., and Shapiro, J. H.: Atypical pulmonary patterns of congestive failure in chronic lung disease: the influence of pre-existing disease on the appearance and distribution of pulmonary edema. *Radiology*, 93:995, 1969.

Joseph, P. M., Berdon, W. E., Baker, D. H., Slovis, T. L., and Haller, J. O.: Upper airway obstruction in infants and small children: improved radiographic diagnosis by combining filtration, high kilovoltage and magnification. *Radiology*, 121:143, 1976.

Keats, T. E., and Smith, T. H.: Air esophagogram: a sign of poor respiratory excursion in the neonate. *Am. J. Roentgenol.*, 120:300, 1974.

Kemp, F. H., Morley, H. M. C., and Emrys-Roberts, E.: A sail-like triangular projection from the mediastinum: a radiographic appearance of the thymus gland. *Br. J. Radiol.*, 21:618, 1948.

Kirkpatrick, J. A., Jr., and DiGeorge, A. M.: Congenital absence of the thymus. *Am. J. Roentgenol.* 103:32, 1968.

Landing, B. H., Lawrence, T.-Y. K., Payne, V. C., Jr., and Wells, T. R.: Bronchial anatomy in syndromes with abnormal visceral situs, abnormal spleen and congenital heart disease. *Am. J. Cardiol.*, 28:456, 1971.

MacEwan, D. W., Dunbar, J. S., Smith, R. D., and Brown, B. St. J.: Pneumothorax in young infants — recognition and evaluation. *J. Can. Assoc. Radiol.*, 22:264, 1971.

Macklin, C. C.: Transport of air along sheaths of pulmonic blood vessels from alveoli to mediastinum: clinical implications. *Arch. Intern. Med.*, 64:913, 1939.

Margulis, A. R.: The lesions of radiobiology for diagnostic radiology. *Am. J. Roentgenol.*, 117:741, 1973.

Meine, F. J., Lorenzo, R. L., Lynch, P. F., Capitanio, M. A., and Kirkpatrick, J. A.: Pharyngeal distention associated with upper airway obstruction. *Radiology*, 3:395, 1974.

Mishkin, F. S., Wagner, H. N., Jr., and Tow, D. E.: Regional distribution of pulmonary arterial blood flow in acute asthma. *J.A.M.A.*, 203:1019, 1968.

Moskowitz, P. S., and Griscom, N. T.: The medial pneumothorax. *Radiology*, 120:143, 1976.

Mulvey, R. B.: The thymic "wave" sign. *Radiology*, 81:834, 1963.

Nadel, J. A., Wolfe, W. G., Graf, P. D., Youker, J. E., Zamel, N., Austin, J. H. M., Hinchcliffe, W. A., Greenspan, R. H., and Wright, R. R.: Powdered tantalum: a new contrast medium for roentgenographic examination of human airways. *N. Engl. J. Med.*, 283:281, 1970.

Neuhauser, E. B. D., Harris, G. B. C., and Berrett, A.: Roentgenographic features of neurenteric cysts. *Am. J. Roentgenol.*, 79:235, 1958.

Nice, C. M., Jr., Waring, W. W., Killelea, D. E., and Hurwitz, L.: Bronchography in infants and children: barium sulfate as a contrast agent. *Am. J. Roentgenol*, 91:564, 1964.

Pendarvis, B. C., and Swischuk, L. E.: Lung scanning in the assessment of respiratory disease in children. *Am. J. Roentgenol.*, 107:313, 1969.

Recavarren, S., Benton, C., and Gall, E. A.: The pathology of acute alveolar disease of the lung. *Semin. Roentgenol.*, 2:22, 1967.

Rudavsky, A. Z., Leonidas, J. C., and Abramson, A. L.: Lung scanning for the detection of endobronchial foreign bodies in infants and children. *Radiology*, 108:629, 1973.

Schwarz, E. D., Dorst, J. P., Kuhn, J. P., Rowe, R. D., and Varghese, P. J.: Reliability of roentgenographic evaluation of ventricular septal defects in children. *Johns Hopkins Med. J.*, 127:164, 1970.

Smith, P. C., Swischuk, L. E., and Fagan, C. J.: An elusive and often unsuspected cause of stridor or pneumonia (the esophageal foreign body). *Am. J. Roentgenol.*, 122:80, 1974.

Stern, L., Fletcher, B. D., Dunbar, J. S., Levant, M. N., and Fawcett, J. S.: Pneumothorax and pneumomediastinum associated with renal malformations in newborn infants. *Am. J. Roentgenol.*, 116:785, 1972.

Wesenberg, R. L., and Struble, R. A.: Selective bronchial catheterization and lavage in the newborn. *Radiology*, 105:397, 1972.

Wishart, D. L.: Normal azygos vein width in children. *Radiology*, 104:115, 1972.

Wittenborg, M. H., Gyepes, M. T., and Crocker, D.: Tracheal dynamics in infants with respiratory distress, stridor and collapsing trachea. *Radiology*, 88:653, 1967.

CHAPTER SIX

PULMONARY FUNCTION TESTING IN THE OFFICE AND CLINIC

Richard J. Lemen, M.D.

The diagnosis and management of patients with pulmonary disease have been improved by the recent introduction of pulmonary function tests. However, some pulmonary function tests are difficult to perform, especially for children, or require sophisticated equipment. The use of those tests is limited to relatively few patients in respiratory physiology laboratories. Simple tests that can be performed easily by children in the office or clinic would have considerable value to the pediatrician.

Two simple tests of pulmonary function, the volume-time (VT) and the flow-volume (FV) curves, are recorded during a maximal vital capacity maneuver and provide enough information correctly to diagnose or manage most patients with pulmonary disease. Most children more than five years of age can be taught to perform a maximal vital capacity maneuver with reliability. Methods of performing, evaluating and interpreting these tests in the office or clinic are the concern of this chapter. The objective data obtained from these tests enhance evaluation of patients in the general ways that are summarized in Table 1.

Special Considerations

It is more difficult to obtain meaningful results in children than it is in adults with any tests. Perhaps this problem explains the general lack of enthu-

siasm for testing pulmonary function in children. Children frequently are tested in busy, adult-oriented laboratories, by personnel inexperienced in testing children, and with equipment not intended for studies in children. Results obtained under these circumstances probably are not worthwhile. Some considerations that are important for optimal pulmonary function results in children are (1) trained personnel, (2) trained patients, (3) pleasant laboratory environment and (4) the selection of appropriate equipment.

The personality of the person who conducts the testing procedure is a very

TABLE 1. USES OF PULMONARY FUNCTION STUDIES IN CHILDREN

Clinical

Patient Management
  To follow the course of pulmonary disease
  To evaluate the response to therapy
  To regulate the duration and form of
    therapy

Diagnosis
  To characterize pulmonary diseases
    physiologically
  To quantitate disease severity
  To evaluate the risks of diagnostic or thera-
    peutic procedures
  To suggest disease etiology
  To indicate specific therapy

Research

  To study changes in lung function with age
  To investigate the long-term effects of acute
    and chronic factors on lung growth

166

important factor in the success of the study. This person must be patient, friendly and able to relate to children. The same person should study the child each time because the motivation technique that works best for that child must be used repeatedly. A capable office or clinic nurse can be easily trained to perform these tests as part of her usual routine.

Each child must be trained during a practice period to perform a maximal vital capacity maneuver with reliability. Before the child is connected to the spirometer, a slow inspiration with a one- to two-second breath-hold at full inflation is demonstrated by the technician and practiced by the child; then, full deflation is demonstrated and practiced. Next, the maximal vital capacity maneuver is practiced, beginning with a slow full inflation, then by a brief breath-hold and a sudden sustained maximal expiratory effort lasting at least three seconds. Instructions to the child may take this form: "Take a deep breath, more, more, more; Now *Blow!* more, more, more, squeeze, squeeze, squeeeeeze...." Young children can be taught this procedure by playing "make believe it's your birthday and you have to blow out all the candles with only one breath."

Most children learn to perform the maximal vital capacity maneuver reliably after four to five minutes of practice, but some, especially those less than six years old, may require longer practice periods. If the child is too sick or simply will not perform maximally, the procedure should be stopped and any results should be disregarded. On the other hand, the cooperative child who still has not mastered the procedure benefits from the experience, but the data should not be reported. Only results obtained from a maximal effort that is sustained for at least three seconds after a full inflation should be reported. Usually, children less than 10 years of age perform better if they are standing; on the other hand, it does not seem to matter if older children are standing or sitting during the proce-

dure. The level of cooperation and difficulties such as fatigue or coughing should be included in the report.

The laboratory environment must be pleasant and free of distractions. Most patients perform better if they are alone and at ease with the technician. Painful procedures such as injections or blood sampling in close proximity to the laboratory should be avoided during the testing procedure.

The selection of pulmonary function equipment should depend on the indices that are measured, which in turn depend on their purpose: patient management or diagnosis. Suggestions for those who plan to start pulmonary function testing in their office and clinic are summarized in Table 2. Management decisions in patients with moderate or severe pulmonary disease are improved by consideration of changes in the forced vital capacity (FVC), the forced expiratory volume in one second ($FEV_{1.0}$) and its ratio to FVC ($FEV_{1.0}/FVC$) and peak expiratory flow (PEF). Other indices are less useful in these patients, but may be of value early in the course of obstructive airways disease when only the peripheral airways are involved. Information obtained from the diagnostic tests (Table 2) allows accurate diagnosis of most patients; however, some patients require more extensive testing and they should be referred to a respiratory physiology laboratory.

There are no uniform guidelines for pulmonary function equipment for children. Volume and flow discrimination must be sufficient to measure children's smaller flows and volume within ± 5 per cent accuracy. Studies in our laboratory (Lemen and Wegmann, unpublished data) indicate that some normal children and many patients with pulmonary disease have significant amplitude content, defined as 5 per cent or more of the maximum amplitude, out to 15 cycles/second. The rigorous equipment specifications that are summarized in Table 3 must be met if all the flow and volume indices from the maximal vital capacity maneuver

TABLE 2. RECOMMENDATIONS FOR PULMONARY FUNCTION TESTS AND EQUIPMENT FOR OFFICE AND CLINIC STUDIES

Place	Purpose	Test	Index*	Time Required (min.)	Equipment
Office	Management decisions	Peak expiratory flow Forced expiratory vital capacity	PEF FVC $FEV_{1.0}$ $FEV_{1.0}/FVC$	2 3	Peak flow meter Mechanical dry wedge spirometer
Clinic	Management decisions	Forced expiratory flow-volume curve	FEF_{max} FVC $FEV_{1.0}$ $FEV_{1.0}/FVC$	3	Electrical dry wedge spirometer and a rapidly responding XY recorder; or electronic spirometer and a rapidly responding XY recorder
Clinic	Diagnosis	Forced expiratory and inspiratory flow volume curves (1) before and after bronchodilators and (2) breathing air and helium in 20% oxygen	FEF_{max} FVC $FEV_{1.0}$ $FEV_{1.0}/FVC$ $FEF_{25\%, 50\%, 75\%}$ $FIF_{50\%}$	20–30	Electrical dry wedge spirometer and a rapidly responding XY recorder

*PEF, peak expiratory flow; FVC, forced vital capacity; $FEV_{1.0}$, forced expiratory volume in 1.0 second; FEF_{max}, maximal forced expiratory flow; $FEF_{25\%, 50\%, 75\%}$, forced expiratory flow at 25, 50, and 75 per cent of expired vital capacity; $FIF_{50\%}$, forced inspiratory flow at 50 per cent of vital capacity.

are to be recorded with acceptable accuracy (± 5 per cent). However, this equipment is expensive and impractical for use in the office or clinic with only a few pulmonary patients.

Some indices of pulmonary function can be recorded with acceptable accuracy with relatively inexpensive equipment, but caution in their selection is

TABLE 3. RECOMMENDATIONS FOR PULMONARY FUNCTION EQUIPMENT

Static Calibration
Volume
  range: 0–6 L
  discrimination: 20 ml./mm.
  linearity: within ± 1%
Flow
  range: 0–8 L/sec
  discrimination: 40 ml./sec./mm.
  linearity: within ± 1%
Time
  range: 0–8 sec.
  discrimination: 0.05 sec./mm.
  activated timer
    threshold: 50 ml./sec.
    marker at 1.0 and 3.0 sec.

Dynamic Calibration
  inertia and resistance: low
  flat amplitude response (± 5%) to 15 Hz

needed. One should not be misled that no calibrations are needed because of the quoted accuracy of an instrument. Construction imperfections, damage, aging and other factors make calibration necessary initially and at regular intervals. Techniques of calibration should be explained in the equipment manual; otherwise, these techniques can be found in textbooks of respiratory physiology.

Portable mechanical wedge spirometers such as the McKesson Vitalor or the Vitalograph are suitable for patient management decisions in the office. These instruments record FVC and $FEV_{1.0}$ with reasonable accuracy but are probably too inaccurate to be used for other flow indices. One flow index, peak expiratory flow (PEF), can be measured separately in the office with a Wright Peak Flow Meter.

Electronic spirometers are more expensive than mechanical wedge spirometers are, but have been increasing in popularity because of several time-saving features. Some electronic spirometers, such as those that measure flow with turbinometers or thermistors and volume by integration, may be too inaccurate for both flow and volume. Models with only a digital display of data are unsatisfactory because visual inspection of the tracings is essential for quality. Electronic spirometers that measure flow with high quality pneumotachograph-transducer systems (e.g., model 473–3A, Hewlett-Packard) and a rapid pen recorder are very accurate.

There are several advantages to displaying the events of the maximal vital capacity maneuver as a flow-volume curve. Flow calculations during expiration and inspiration and qualitative estimates of reproducibility are made easily. Flow-volume curves breathing air can be easily compared with those breathing helium and oxygen. The standard spirometer in many clinics is a nonportable bell type water seal spirometer (e.g., 9.0L Collins, W. E. Collins). These systems are very suitable for recording volume-time curves but not flow-volume curves. Dry wedge spirometers with electrical flow and volume outputs (e.g., Med-Science Model 570) can be used in the clinic for recording both VT and FV curves. The versatility of this type of spirometer makes possible the recordings of the patient management and diagnostic indices listed in Table 2.

Technique

During a maximal vital capacity maneuver, expired volume-time (VT) curves are recorded as illustrated in Figure 1. A "good" expiratory curve starts with a steep slope that is nearly linear, then tails off, markedly, near end-expiration. A brief delay at the onset of full expiration as illustrated in Figure 1 is common. The problem of the determination of zero time is solved by extrapolating the steep initial portion of the curve to the maximal inspiratory line. The forced vital capacity (FVC), the maximum volume of expired air, is read directly from the tracings at ambient temperature and pressure saturated with water vapor (ATPS).

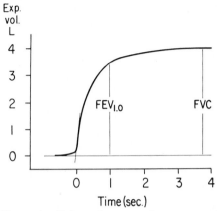

Figure 1. Volume-time curve for a 12-year-old normal boy. Zero time is determined by extrapolating the steepest part of the curve to the full inflation line. The forced expiratory volume in one second ($FEV_{1.0}$) and the forced vital capacity (FVC) are read directly from the tracing (ATPS) and converted to BTPS conditions.

The volume of gas expired from the lungs at body temperature, saturated with water vapor (BTPS), may be 8 to 10 per cent greater than the volume measured in a spirometer at room temperature. Thus, expired volume and airflow must be corrected from ATPS to BTPS conditions.

Two indices of flow are easily measured from the VT curve. The forced expiratory volume in one second ($FEV_{1.0}$) is the expired volume (BTPS) during the first second of a maximal expiratory effort (Fig. 1). The $FEV_{1.0}$ is usually expressed as its percentage of FVC to correct for size differences between patients. The determination of forced expiratory flow over the middle half of the FVC ($FEV_{25-75\%}$) is illustrated in Figure 2 *A, B* for a normal child and a patient with cystic fibrosis, respectively. A straight line, connecting points on the curve at 25 and 75 per cent of the FVC, is extended to intersect two vertical lines 1.0 second apart. The $FEF_{25-75\%}$ is the expired volume (BTPS) determined from the slope of the line in liters (ATPS) per second. It is possible to measure peak expiratory flow (PEF) by drawing a tangent to the steepest part of the VT curve, but this practice is not recommended because it

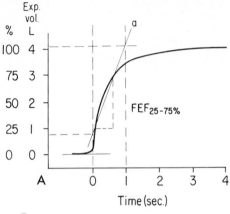

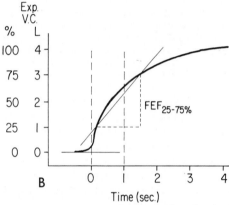

Figure 2. Volume-time curves for a normal child (*A*) and a child with obstructive airways disease (*B*). The average slope is determined by connecting points on the curve at 25 and 50 per cent expired vital capacity (*line a*). The $FEF_{25-75\%}$ in liters per second (ATPS) is read directly from the tracing by extending line a to intercept two vertical lines (*dashed*) 1.0 second apart.

expired vital capacity ($FEF_{25\%,\,50\%,\,75\%}$) and forced inspiratory flow at 50 per cent vital capacity ($FIF_{50\%}$) are read directly from the recordings (ATPS) and converted to BTPS. An automatic timer with time markers at 1.0 and 3.0 seconds permits calculations of the $FEV_{1.0}/FVC$ ratio and the approximate duration of expiration.

Maximal expiratory flow is linearly related to expired volume in normal subjects (Fig. 3 *A*) at all lung volumes more than 25 per cent below full inflation. Curvilinearity of this portion of the curve as illustrated in Figure 3*B* is associated with airway disease. A straight line drawn from the flow at 25

is too inaccurate. It is more accurate to measure PEF independently with a Wright Peak Flow Meter.

The flow-volume curve demonstrates instantaneous flow against lung volume during a maximal expiratory and inspiratory vital capacity maneuver. The maximal expiratory vital capacity maneuver is followed by a maximal inspiratory maneuver to full inflation. Typical FV curves for a normal child and a patient with mild obstructive airway disease are illustrated in Figure 3 *A*, *B*, respectively. Maximal forced expiratory flow (FEF_{max}), forced expiratory flow at 25, 50, and 75 per cent of

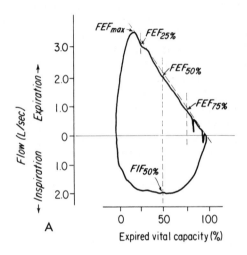

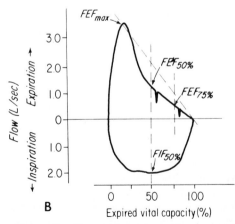

Figure 3. Flow-volume curves for a normal child (*A*) and a child with moderate obstructive airways disease (*B*). See text for explanation.

per cent expired VC to the end-expiratory point emphasizes the linearity or curvilinearity of the FV curve. The curvilinearity score, the ratio of the actual flow at 50 per cent expired VC to the flow predicted from the straight line, is a method of quantitating curvilinearity.

If patient effort and cooperation were maximal, the FEF_{max} and FVC of four to six FV curves should be reproducible within 5 per cent of their maximum. The FEF_{max} should be achieved rapidly with only 25 per cent or less of the VC expired from maximum inflation. Flow-volume curve performed while coughing repeatedly during expiration should achieve the same flows at lung volumes more than 25 per cent below full inflation as those curves performed normally.

Comparisons of flow-volume curves performed while breathing air or helium in 20 per cent oxygen (He/O_2) are useful to diagnose large and small airway obstruction. The child breathes the He/O_2 mixture for five to six minutes from a non-rebreathing system, and the maximal expiratory flow volume curve is performed while the child continues to breathe the He/O_2. The He/O_2 FV curve is compared with the air FV curve as illustrated in Figure 4 A, B for a normal child and one with mild obstructive airway disease, respectively. The ratio of flows achieved while breathing He/O_2 and air at 50 and 75 per cent of expired vital capacity and

the point of identical flow (PIF) are obtained as illustrated in Figure 4 A, B.

Interpretation

Many factors must be considered if pulmonary function tests are to reflect accurately the pathophysiologic features of pulmonary diseases. Patient effort, the lesion's anatomical location and its severity, and the sensitivity of each test to discriminate normal from abnormal function must be considered in the interpretation of the results.

Some tests depend on maximal effort from the patient; others do not. Figure 3 A illustrates the parts of the maximal vital capacity maneuver that are dependent or independent of effort. The effort-dependent tests are those tests that are measured at high lung volumes, the first 25 per cent of the expired vital capacity from full inflation, such as PEF or FEF_{max}, and are measured at all lung volumes during inspiration. The effort-independent tests are those tests that are measured at low lung volumes, the lower 75 per cent of the expired vital capacity. Expiratory flows such as the $FEF_{50\%}$ are not increased by more than moderate levels of effort; therefore, small differences in maximal effort between children have little influence on these results. Effort-independent tests are influenced more by the lung's static properties, dynamic compression of the airways, and the resistance of the peripheral airways

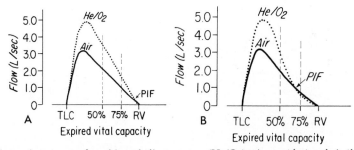

Figure 4. Flow-volume curves breathing a helium-oxygen (He/O_2) mixture (*dots*) and air (*heavy line*) for a normal child (*A*) and a child with mild peripheral airways obstruction (*B*). In *B*, the ratio of expiratory flow breathing He/O_2 to air at 50 and 75 per cent expired vital capacity is reduced, although the curvilinearity score in air is near normal. The point of identical flow (PIF) occurs at a higher lung volume in *B*.

than by small differences in maximal effort.

Obstruction of the central airways (larynx, trachea, and main stem bronchi) early in its course reduces expiratory flow at high lung volumes, and flows during inspiration; then, as the obstruction of these airways increases, expiratory flow is reduced at progressively lower lung volumes. The relationship of reduced inspiratory to expiratory flow at mid-vital capacity $FEF_{50\%}/FIF_{50\%}$ depends on the location of the lesion in the extrathoracic or intrathoracic central airways as illustrated in Figure 5. Since these flows are at least partly effort-dependent, evidence that the patient performed with maximal effort is essential to the interpretation of these results.

Increased resistance of airways peripheral to the central airways is the most common cause of reduced expiratory flow at low lung volumes as illustrated in Figure 3 B. The early detection of peripheral airways disease is increased by comparing FV curves obtained while the patient breathes air or a helium/oxygen (He/O_2) mixture. Convective acceleration and turbulent flow are decreased while breathing the less dense He/O_2 mixture; therefore, resistance in the central airways is reduced during maximal expiration owing to less pressure losses from turbulence and convective acceleration. Flow patterns in the peripheral airways

are laminar and independent of gas density. As a result of the relative importance of turbulence and convective acceleration to laminar flow pressure losses, expiratory flow is increased with the He/O_2 mixture as illustrated in Figure 4 A. As resistance of the peripheral airways increases as a result of disease, the lung volume at which flow becomes independent of density increases as illustrated in Figure 4 B, and the point of identical flow (PIF) occurs at higher lung volumes.

Effort dependence and effort independence also may influence how the results of each index of pulmonary function are reported. There is still a difference of opinion concerning what to report as the results, the "best" or the "average." The curves with the largest FVC and $FEV_{1.0}$ are commonly selected as the "best" results. The mean results of four to six measurements may be reported as the "average" results. The "best" seems valid for effort-dependent indices because it represents the patient's strongest effort. On the other hand, it can be argued that the "average" is more typical of the patient's usual performance and may be more appropriate for indices that are effort-independent. In addition, the interpretation of sequential studies in one individual requires an estimate of the within-individual variation of that index. In our laboratory, indices are reported from

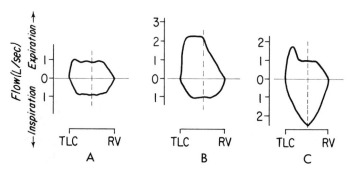

Figure 5. Maximal expiratory and inspiratory flow-volume curves (*A*) in fixed obstruction (e.g., postintubation tracheal stenosis) of the central airways (larynx, trachea, main stem bronchi). Variable obstruction of the extrathoracic (*B*) or intrathoracic (*C*) central airways produces flow patterns characteristic of dynamic changes in airway diameter during inspiration or expiration in these regions.

the "best" effort, and the "average" results are used to interpret sequential studies.

The discrimination of normal from abnormal pulmonary function results can be done in three ways: (1) by comparing a patient's results as a percentage (or standard deviation) from the mean predicted results for a normal population; (2) by considering the interrelationships of different pulmonary function indices; and (3) by considering their change with time.

The least discriminating method is to compare the results of each test with its predicted value for a normal population. The normal values used in our laboratory are summarized in Table 4. The large between-individual variability of each test is apparent from the large percentage of the mean predicted value that is equal to one standard deviation (SD). These differences can

be eliminated by expressing the results in SD from the mean predicted values; however, the power of the index to discriminate normal from abnormal results is still limited because a patient's position in the normal population before his illness is not known. For example, if a patient's normal FVC was + 1.95 SD, his disease process would have to reduce his FVC by 42 per cent before it would be clearly below the normal limit of −2.0 SD for predicted values. On the other hand, if a child's normal FVC was −1.95 SD, a small decrease in FVC owing to disease would result in clearly reduced values.

The relative sensitivity of each index to detect abnormalities varies considerably. Table 5 lists the indices in increasing sensitivity to detect disease of the peripheral airways. The FVC is reduced both in obstructive airways diseases (e.g., asthma and cystic fibrosis)

TABLE 4. SUMMARY OF NORMAL DATA FOR OUR LABORATORY

Index	Sex	Mean	% mean/SD
VOLUME-TIME CURVE*			
VC (ml.)	Males	$0.0044 \times$ Ht. (cm.)$^{2.67}$	13
	Females	$0.0033 \times$ Ht. (cm.)$^{2.72}$	13
$FEV_{1.0}/FVC$ %	Males and females	86	7
PF (L/sec.)	Males and females	$\dfrac{5.24 \times \text{Ht. (cm.)} - 425.57}{60}$	13
FEF_{25-75}% (L/sec.)	Males and females	$\dfrac{2.62 \times \text{Ht. (cm.)} - 207.7}{60}$	33
FLOW-VOLUME CURVE†			
FVC (ml.)	Males	$0.0597 \times$ Ht. (cm.) $- 5.8657$	14
	Females	$0.0482 \times$ Ht. (cm.) $- 4.5629$	11
FEF_{max} (L/sec.)	Males	$0.0993 \times$ Ht. (cm.) $- 8.815$	16
	Females	$0.0823 \times$ Ht. (cm.) $- 6.805$	12
FEF_{50}% (L/sec.)	Males	$0.0589 \times$ Ht. (cm.) $- 4.7800$	25
	Females	$0.0539 \times$ Ht. (cm.) $- 4.0180$	20
FEF_{75}% (L/sec.)	Males	$0.0286 \times$ Ht. (cm.) $- 2.3748$	30
	Females	$0.0289 \times$ Ht. (cm.) $- 2.2934$	27
FEF_{50}%/FIF_{50}%	Males and females	0.9	
HELIUM-OXYGEN AND AIRFLOW RATIOS‡		Mean $\pm$ SE	
Helium/airflow $\times$ 100			
at 50%		147 ± 4	
at 25% VC		144 ± 5	
PIF (% VC)		5 ± 1	
Curvilinearity score§		0	

*Normal data from Polgar and Promadhat.
†Normal data from Warwick (unpublished data).
‡Normal data from Fox, Bureau, Taussig, et al.
§Normal data from Landau, Taussig, et al.

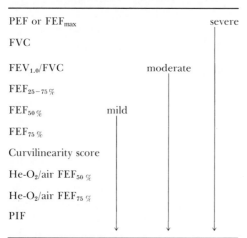

PEF or FEF_{max}		severe
FVC		
$FEV_{1.0}/FVC$	moderate	
$FEF_{25-75\%}$		
$FEF_{50\%}$	mild	
$FEF_{75\%}$		
Curvilinearity score		
He-O_2/air $FEF_{50\%}$		
He-O_2/air $FEF_{75\%}$		
PIF		

*Indices listed in increasing sensitivity.

and in restrictive diseases (e.g., pulmonary fibrosis and scoliosis). Distinction between obstructive and restrictive disease can be made by looking at indices of flow.

The $FEV_{1.0}/FVC$ ratio may be reduced in obstructive airways disease but is usually normal or above in restrictive diseases. Reductions of PEF and FEF_{max} are more sensitive than is the $FEV_{1.0}/FVC$ ratio to detect obstruction of the central airways, because part of the $FEV_{1.0}$ occurs over that part of the FVC that reflects peripheral airway function. The FEF_{max} and PEF usually are reduced in severe peripheral airways disease, but some of these patients may have normal PEF and FEF_{max} because of initially high flow transients that occur prior to airway closure. On the other hand, some of the $FEV_{1.0}$ reflects central airways function; therefore, the $FEV_{1.0}/FVC$ may be normal early in the course of diseases that affect either the central or peripheral airways. The $FEF_{25-75\%}$ measures the average flow over the middle half of the FVC and is less influenced by central airways disease than is the $FEV_{1.0}/FVC$ ratio. For this reason, the $FEF_{25-75\%}$ is more sensitive to peripheral airways function than the $FEV_{1.0}/$

FVC ratio is. Determination of the PIF and helium-oxygen to airflow ratios at 50 and 75 per cent expired vital capacity are currently the most sensitive tests for early detection of peripheral airways disease that are suitable for children in the office and clinic.

All of these indices are reduced to varying degrees as airway obstruction worsens. This fact has led us to view the severity of pulmonary diseases in a qualitative manner as shown in Table 5. The severity of a patient's disease is judged by how many and what tests are

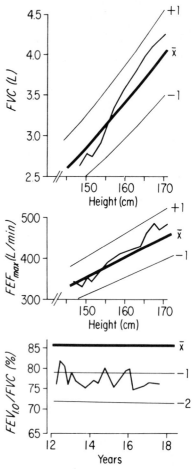

Figure 6. Sequential changes in FVC, PEF, and $FEV_{1.0}/FVC$ in a boy with mild but stable obstructive airways disease associated with cystic fibrosis. The variability of repeated measurement was less than the variability among individuals for the normal population (mean $\pm$ 2 SD). Changes in these variables of more than 1.0 SD for the population suggest a significant change in the patient's pulmonary function.

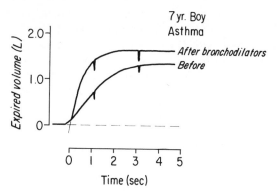

Figure 7. Volume-time curves before and after bronchodilator inhalation. The FVC and $FEV_{1.0}$/FVC are normal after the bronchodilator, suggesting airway smooth muscle construction was responsible for the reduced $FEV_{1.0}$ and FVC before bronchodilators.

abnormal (more than 2 SD below the predicted mean) without regard for the absolute value.

In our Section of Pulmonary Diseases, FVC, $FEV_{1.0}$ and FEF_{max} are measured in each child over age five years with each visit. We find that following these indices with time is more informative than on the single occasion because changes in pulmonary function (improved or worsening) are easier to detect than simply discriminating normal or abnormal. The within-individual variability of each patient for each test must be known in order to determine that a given test has changed significantly from a previous study. Studies in our laboratory (Lemen and Wegmann, unpublished data) suggest that the within-individual variation of these indices in normal subjects and patients with stable pulmonary disease is considerably less than the between-individual variation (Table 4). Children tend to "seek their own level" within the normal population and their results vary less than 1 SD with time as illustrated in Figure 6 for one patient with mild but stable obstructive pulmonary disease. We assume a significant change (improved or worsening) has occurred in our patients when a test result changes more than 1 SD for the whole population. This rule also applies to interpretations of a patient's responses to bronchodilators.

Figure 7 illustrates the VT curves of a seven-year-old boy with asthma before and after inhalation of nebulized isoproterenol. His FVC and

$FEV_{1.0}$/FVC increased by 1.2 SD and 5.4 SD, respectively, to normal values after isoproterenol inhalation. These findings suggest airway smooth muscle constriction was responsible for the reduced $FEV_{1.0}$/FVC and FVC; however, only the $FEV_{1.0}$/FVC was clearly abnormal before isoproterenol inhalation. His "reduced" FVC at − 1.5 SD for the normal population was apparent only by its "significant" increase to − 0.2 SD after isoproterenol inhalation.

A different response to isoproterenol inhalation is illustrated by the FV curves in Figure 8. In this nine-year-old-boy, isoproterenol inhalation increased his FVC and FEF_{max} signifi-

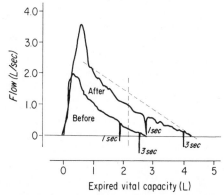

Figure 8. Flow-volume curves in an asthmatic 14-year-old boy. Inhalation of bronchodilators (*after*) resulted in an increase in FEF_{max} and flows at low volumes as illustrated by $FEF_{50\%}$ (*vertical dashed line*). Reduced flows after inhalation of bronchodilators are indicated by the curvilinearity of flows at low lung volume compared with their predicted flows (*diagonal dashed line*).

cantly by 3.8 and 4.4 SD, respectively. However, his $FEV_{1.0}$ increased less than his FVC did; thus, his $FEV_{1.0}/FVC$ ratio was reduced after the bronchodilator. His FVC and FEF_{max} were within normal predicted values (± 2 SD) after the bronchodilator, but flow at low lung volumes remained reduced as indicated by its curvilinearity and a curvilinearity score of 0.34. These results suggest that smooth muscle constriction of the peripheral airways was only partially relieved, or some other factor (e.g., airway mucus or edema) may have been responsible for these effects.

REFERENCES

Committee Recommendations: The assessment of ventilatory capacity. Statement of the Committees on Environmental Health and Respiratory Physiology, American College of Chest Physicians. *Chest, 67*:95, 1975.

Cotes, J. E.: *Lung Function: Assessment and Application in Medicine.* 3rd ed. Oxford, England, Blackwell Scientific Publications, 1975.

Despas, P. J., Leroux, M., and Macklem, P. T.: Site of airway obstruction in asthma as determined by measuring maximal expiratory flow breathing air and a helium-oxygen mixture. *J. Clin. Invest., 31*:3235, 1972.

Drew, C. D. M., and Hughes, D. T. D.: Characteristics of the Vitalograph spirometer. *Thorax, 24*:703, 1969.

Fitzgerald, M. X., Smith, A. A., and Gaensler, E. A.: Evaluation of "electronic" spirometers. *N. Engl. J. Med., 289*:1283, 1973.

Fox, W. W., Bureau, M. A., Taussig, L. M., Martin, R. R., and Beaudry, P. H.: Helium flow-volume curves in the detection of early small airways disease. Evaluation in cystic fibrosis children with mild pulmonary involvement. *Pediatrics, 54*:293, 1974.

Hyatt, R. E., and Black, L. F.: The flow-volume curve. A current perspective. *Am. Rev. Resp. Dis., 107*:191, 1973.

Kory, R. C., and Hamilton, L. H.: Evaluation of spirometers used in pulmonary function studies. *Am. Rev. Resp. Dis., 87*:228, 1963.

Kryger, M., Bode, F., Antic, R., and Anthonisen, N.: Diagnosis of obstruction of the upper and central airways. *Am. J. Med., 61*:85, 1976.

Landau, L. I., Taussig, L. M., Macklem, P. T., and Beaudry, P. H.: Contribution of inhomogeneity of lung units to the maximal expiratory flow-volume curve in children with asthma and cystic fibrosis. *Am. Rev. Resp. Dis., 111*:725, 1975.

Lemen, R.: Office pulmonary function testing in children. *Audio-Digest, Vol.* 21, December 23, 1975.

Levison, H., and Godfrey, S.: Cystic fibrosis. In Mangos, J., and Talamo, R. (Eds.): *Projections into the Future.* New York, Stratton Intercontinental Medical Book Corp., 1976, pp. 3–25.

Macklem, P. T.: Airway obstruction and collateral ventilation. *Physiol. Rev., 51*:368, 1971.

Mead, J.: Mechanical properties of lungs. *Physiol. Rev. 41*:281, 1961.

Mead, J., Turner, J. M., Macklem, P. T., and Little, J. B.: Significance of the relationship between lung recoil and maximum expiratory flow. *J. Appl. Physiol., 22*:95, 1967.

Miller, R. D., and Hyatt, R. E.: Evaluation of obstructing lesions of the trachea and larynx by flow-volume loops. *Am. Rev. Resp. Dis., 108*:475, 1973.

Polgar, G., and Promadhat, V.: *Pulmonary Function Testing in Children: Techniques and Standards.* Philadelphia, W. B. Saunders Company, 1971.

Stead, W. W., Wells, H. S., Gault, N. L., et al.: Inaccuracy of the conventional water-filled spirometer for recording rapid breathing. *J. Appl. Physiol., 14*:448, 1959.

Wang, C. S., Boyington, D. G., and Krumholz, R. A.: Comparison of spirometry measurements using McKesson Vitalor and Collins spirometer. *Dis. Chest, 55*:258, 1969.

Waring, W. W.: Pulmonary function testing in children. *Paediatrician, 1*:152, 1972–1973.

Wells, H. S., Stead, W. W., Rossing, T. D., et al.: Accuracy of an improved spirometer for recording of fast breathing. *J. Appl. Physiol., 14*:451, 1959.

Wever, A. M. J., Britton, M. G., and Hughes, D. D. T.: Evaluation of two spirometers—a comparative study of the Stead-Wells and the Vitalograph spirometers. *Chest, 70*:244, 1976.

Zapletal, A., Motoyama, E. K., Van De Woestijne, K. P., Hunt, V. R., and Bouhuys, A.: Maximal expiratory flow volume curves and airway conductance in children and adolescents. *J. Appl. Physiol., 26*:308, 1969.

CHAPTER SEVEN

AGE AS A FACTOR IN RESPIRATORY DISEASE

J. C. Hogg, M.D.

NORMAL LUNGS

In considering age as a factor in respiratory disease, it is useful to reflect on the nature of the tracheobronchial tree and the way in which the lung grows. Examination of a bronchogram (Fig. 1 *A*) clearly illustrates that the tracheobronchial tree is a highly branched system of tubes. Data from Horsfield and Cumming (1968) shown in Figure 1 *B* demonstrate the number of times an airway can divide along an axial pathway from the trachea to the lobular or alveolar branches. These data show that it is possible to reach the alveolar branches in as few as eight or as many as 24 divisions, depending on the pathway followed. The location of airways that are 2 mm. in internal diameter in adult lung was studied by Weibel (1963), who found that 2 mm. airways are located anywhere from the fourth to the fourteenth generation of branching (Fig. 1 *C*). Weibel also found in the same study that the total cross-sectional area of each generation increases rapidly and is especially large beyond the fourteenth generation, where airways are less than 2 mm. in diameter (Fig. 1 *D*). This means that the total cross-sectional area of the airways 2 mm. in diameter is much larger than that of more central airways, and the cross-sectional area continues to increase rapidly as the alveoli are approached.

In order to think about gas flow in a complicated system such as the tracheobronchial tree, it is useful to consider a simple model (Fig. 2). Figure 2 *A* shows a single tube branching into two daughter tubes, in which flow will depend on the driving pressure and resistance offered by the tubes. This effect on flow can be expressed either as resistance, which is the pressure drop divided by the flow, or as conductance, which is the flow divided by driving pressure. With a constant flow, the pressure drop per unit length ($\Delta P/\Delta L$) will be linear. In looking at this simple model, we can gain important insights into the nature of flow in the tracheobronchial tree by considering the factors that influence the relative conductance or resistance of the parent branch to that of the daughter branches. In this simple model under steady-state conditions, the flow through the parent branch is exactly the same as the sum of the flows through the two daughter branches. Under conditions in which the sum of the cross-sectional area of the two daughter branches is exactly the same as the cross-sectional area of the parent branch, it is possible to calculate that the pressure drop along the daughters will be greater than the pressure drop along the parent branch. Indeed, it can be calculated that the pressure drop along the daughters will be greater than that of the parent until the ratio of the cross-sectional area of the parent to the cross-sectional area of the daughters reaches the value of $1/\sqrt{2}$. In other words, the sum of the cross-sectional areas of the two daughters exceeds that of the parent by 41.4 per cent when the pressure drop is equal. However, when

177

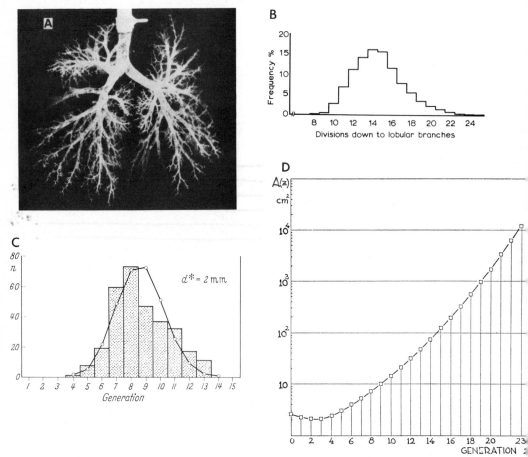

Figure 1. *A,* Normal adult bronchogram. *B,* Frequency distribution of the number of divisions from the trachea to the lobular branches or alveoli in normal lungs. This shows that alveoli can be reached in as few as eight divisions or as many as 24 divisions from the trachea, depending on the pathway followed. *C,* Frequency distribution of airways 2 mm. in diameter in adult lungs, where 2 mm. airways are most frequently found at generation eight but can be found from generations four to 14. *D,* Cross-sectional area at each of the generations in the tracheobronchial tree. Note that the cross-sectional area of the 2 mm. airways, i.e., from generation four to 14, is quite large in relation to the more central airways, such as the trachea and main stem bronchi. Also note that the airways beyond generation 14 are increasing rapidly in total cross-sectional area. (*B,* from Horsfield, K., and Cumming, G.: *J. Appl. Physiol., 24:*373, 1968. *C* and *D* from Weibel, E. R.: *Morphometry of the Human Lung.* Berlin, Springer-Verlag, 1963.)

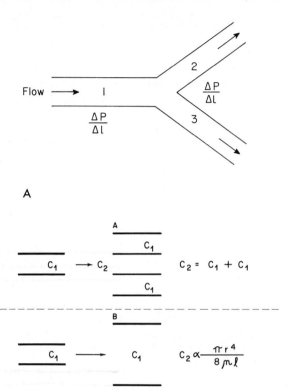

Figure 2. *A*, Model of a tube branching into two daughters. *B*, The relative effect of increasing the conductance (C) by increasing the number of existing tubes or increasing the size of the existing tubes. Note that increasing the number of tubes has the effect of increasing the conductance by the addition of tubes in parallel, that is, overall conductance is the sum of the individual conductances ($C_2 = C_1 + C_1$). By comparison, increasing the size of the tube has the effect of increasing the conductance in proportion to the radius to the fourth power ($C_2 \propto \dfrac{\pi r^4}{8\eta l}$; where r = radius, η = viscosity of the gas, and l = length of the tube).

When conductance through the daughter tubes is equal to that of the parent, then:

(1) $r^4_1 = r^4_{2a} + r^4_{2b}$

and

(2) $\dfrac{r^4_1}{r^4_{2a} + r^4_{2b}} = 1$

Since cross-sectional area is proportional to r^2, then

(3) $\dfrac{\sqrt{r^4_1}}{\sqrt{r^4_{2a} + r^4_{2b}}} = \dfrac{r^2_1}{\sqrt{r^4_{2a} + r^4_{2b}}} = 1$

(4) If the ratio of cross-sectional areas is:

$$\dfrac{r^2_1}{\sqrt{r^4_{2a}} + \sqrt{r^4_{2b}}} = \dfrac{1}{x}$$

and $r^4_1 = 1$ and $r^4_{2a} = r^4_{2b} = 0.5$, then substituting in (4):

$$\dfrac{1}{\sqrt{0.5} + \sqrt{0.5}} = \dfrac{1}{0.7 + 0.7} = \dfrac{1}{1.4} = \dfrac{1}{\sqrt{2}}$$

the cross-sectional area of the two daughters exceeds that of the parent by more than $1/\sqrt{2}$, the pressure drop along the daughters will be less than that along the parent. (See legend for Fig. 2 for calculations.)

Another important point when considering this simple model is a comparison of the relative effect of increasing the cross-sectional area of the daughter branches by either increasing the number of daughters or by increasing the size of the existing daughters. Figure 2 B demonstrates that increasing the number of daughter branches has a simple additive effect on conductance ($C_2 = C_1 + C_1$) because the effect is that of adding branches in parallel. Increasing the size of existing branches, on the other hand, has a much greater effect on conductance because under these conditions, conductance changes in proportion to the change in radius of the tube raised to the fourth power.

In applying these concepts to the tracheobronchial tree of the normal adult lung, the cross-sectional area of each succeeding generation increases markedly (approximately doubles) as the lung periphery is approached (Fig. 1 D). The conductance of each succeeding branch of airway increases steadily so that peripheral airways conductance is very large. This fact is illustrated by measurements made in adult human lungs; as shown in Figure 3, the conductance of airways smaller than 2 mm. in diameter is much greater than the conductance of airways larger than 2 mm. in adult lungs.

The arguments developed for adult lung do not apply to the child, since there are compelling reasons to believe that in the child's lung the total cross-sectional area of each generation increases at a slower rate as one approaches the periphery of the lung. This means that the conductance of small airways in children's lungs is disproportionately small when compared with adults. This simple anatomic fact has important consequences related to how the infant lung responds to acute airway disease and the type of anatomic

abnormality that develops with chronic airways disease. Data on the variation in conductance of peripheral and central airways as a function of age are shown in Figure 4, which is taken from a detailed study (Hogg and coworkers, 1970) on the distribution of airways conductance in normal lungs from children and adults who died of nonrespiratory disease. The ordinate shows the conductance corrected for size by expressing it per gram of lung tissue, and the abscissa shows the age of the subject. The graph shows that central airways conductance (the conductance of the airways from below the larynx to about the fifteenth generation of branching) changes very little with age. However, the conductance of small airways (i.e., those beyond the fifteenth generation) shows a dramatic change at about five years of age. Since careful studies have shown that the total number of airways is exactly the same for both adults and children (Bucher and Reid, 1961; Reid, 1967), this can only mean that the peripheral airways are disproportionately narrow in the early years of life. The reason for this disproportionate distribution of conductance between peripheral and cen-

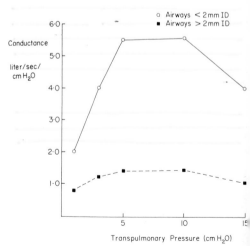

Figure 3. The mean conductance of airways less than 2 mm. in diameter and greater than 2 mm. in diameter in adult lungs. These data are calculated from the mean data of Hogg, Macklem and Thurlbeck (1968).

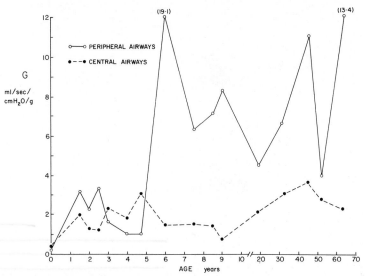

Figure 4. Comparison of peripheral and central airways conductance as a function of age in normal human lungs. The data are corrected for size by expressing the conductance as ml. seconds/gram of lung and for lung inflation by expressing all data at a transpulmonary pressure of 5 cm. H_2O. (Replotted from Hogg, Williams, Richardson, et al., 1970.)

tral airways must be related to the way in which the lung grows.

Several important points must be kept in mind in comparing the relationship of the conducting airways with the air spaces as a function of age. First, we know (Bucher and Reid, 1961; Reid, 1967) that the number of conducting airways is complete by about the first trimester of pregnancy, whereas the spaces that will contain air begin to change from a glandular to an alveolar pattern during the later part of gestation. It can be calculated from the data of Stigol and coworkers (1972) that the lungs of newborns (40 to 50 cm. body length) contain 2.45 ± 0.59 ml. of air per gram at total lung capacity, whereas children of about four years of age (90 to 110 cm. body length) have lungs that contain 6.00 ± 1.83 ml. of air per gram, and children of nine or ten years of age (130 to 140 cm. body length) have lungs that contain 8.11 ± 1.64 ml. of air per gram of tissue.

The nature of alveolar addition has been recently studied by Burri (1974), who showed that the air spaces developed septae that partitioned the alveo-lar ducts. Figure 5 *A*, which is from the study of Hislop and Reid (1974), shows that the air spaces have few septae at birth, more at two months, and many more at seven years. Precisely when growth by septal division (increase in alveolar number) stops and when growth by increasing the size of existing alveoli begins is less clear. Dunnill (1962) thought that the early growth in the lung was accomplished by the addition of new alveoli, whereas later growth was accomplished by growth in size of existing alveoli. Data shown in Table 1, on the other hand, suggest that the number of alveoli per terminal airway must increase markedly through the pubertal growth spurt. Nevertheless, there must be a period when the alveoli begin to grow in size as well as number, and because the alveoli completely surround airways (Fig. 5 *B*), it is likely that the conducting airways begin to change their size at this point. When this occurs, even though the increase in dimension of each individual airway is small, the effect on peripheral airways conductance will be large because, like

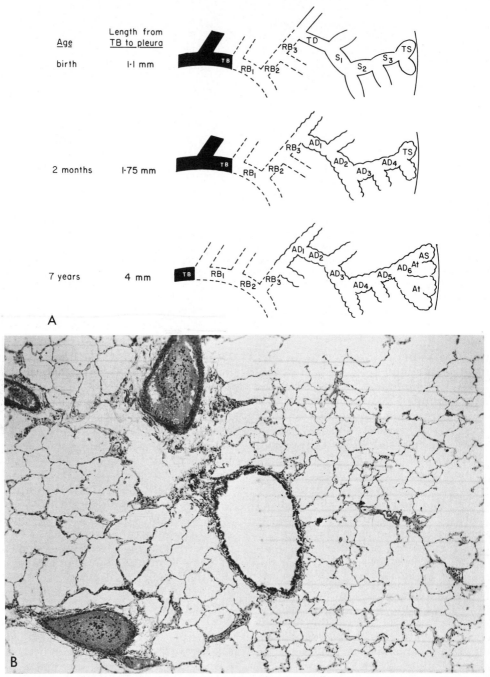

Figure 5. *A,* Diagram modified from Hislop and Reid (1974) showing that the lung grows initially by increasing the number of alveoli by the ingrowth of septae and formation of the alveolar ducts. (TB, terminal bronchiole; RB, respiratory bronchiole; AD, alveolar duct.) *B,* The peripheral conducting airways are completely surrounded by alveoli and cannot begin to change their dimensions until the dimensions of the surrounding alveoli begin to change.

TABLE 1.   RELATIONSHIP BETWEEN NUMBER OF ALVEOLI AND NUMBER OF TERMINAL AIRWAYS WITH AGE

Age (yrs.)	Body Length (cm.)	Body Weight (kg.)	Observed Lung Weight (gm.)	Number of Airways	Number of Alveoli/Airway
Newborn	47.0	3.0	38	8592	0.87×10^4
1.5	75.0	8.4	153	10332	1.67×10^4
2.0	82.0	11.9	308	14880	1.91×10^4
2.5	82.5	13.1	266	5270	3.68×10^4
3.0	98.0	15.0	190	9275	4.21×10^4
4.0	100.0	15.8	236	15400	1.85×10^4
4.75	98.0	13.0	144	7700	2.30×10^4
6.0	125.0	23.2	210	9128	3.32×10^4
7.5	108.0	18.2	213	5346	5.68×10^4
8.5	126.0	21.2	290	7824	3.96×10^4
9.0	122.0	25.0	305	14344	2.32×10^4
19	160	69	950	10764	35.6×10^4
31	150	59	600	7188	36.8×10^4
45	160	38	950	11595	34.6×10^4
52	180	77	1000	15600	33.4×10^4
63	162	68	1100	13284	36.6×10^4

the tube in Figure 2, the effect is magnified by the fourth power of the change in radius. To summarize, we can state that the conductance of the peripheral airways will be disproportionately small in the first few years of life when air space growth is occurring primarily by the addition of alveoli. Small changes in alveolar size and therefore peripheral airways size, which begin somewhat later, cause a marked increase in airways conductance.

Another important feature of lung growth that influences the nature of disease is the development of collateral pathways of ventilation. In the adult lung, the collateral pathways are well developed so that it is easy to ventilate the parenchyma beyond obstructed airways. The pores of Kohn (Macklin, 1936) provide pathways directly through alveolar walls; Lambert's canals (Lambert, 1957) provide pathways from bronchi to alveoli; and there may be an additional pathway connecting respiratory bronchioles to one another in some species (Martin, 1966). These collateral pathways, particularly the pores of Kohn, are known to increase both in number and in size with increasing age. This means that the very young subject is twice disadvantaged. First, his peripheral conducting airways are disproportionately narrow. Second, the pathways for the collateral ventilation are not well developed in the first few years of life, so that ventilation beyond obstructed units is much more difficult than it is for the adult.

DISEASED LUNGS

In considering pulmonary disease in the light of the previous discussion, it is useful to consider what may happen to the adult and child following exactly the same respiratory insult. In temperate climates like North America, it is a common occurrence for people to have an upper respiratory tract infection followed by a lower respiratory tract infection several times each year. Let us consider the relative importance of this on the child and on the adult. If we assume that the infection is capable of spreading along the entire tracheobronchial tree and does not affect one site more than another, one would expect a vastly different result in the adult than in the child. First of all, narrowing of the peripheral airways by infection

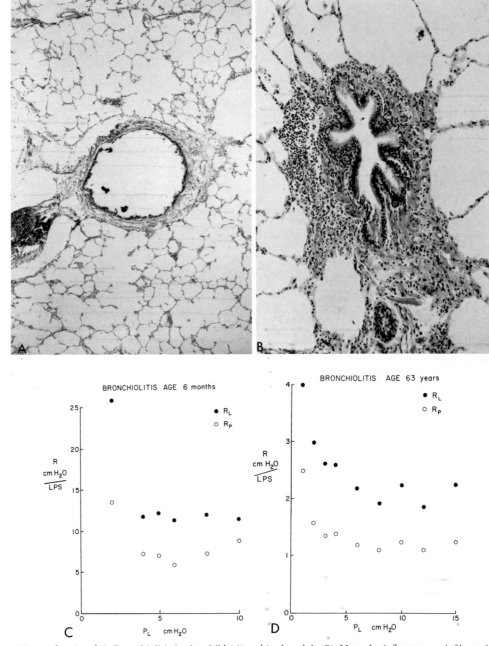

Figure 6. *A* and *B*, Bronchiolitis in the child (*A*) and in the adult (*B*). Note the inflammatory infiltrate in the walls of airways in both cases. *C* and *D*, Distribution of conductance in a child (*C*) and an adult (*D*) with bronchiolitis. The child died of bronchiolitis, while the adult had unrecognized bronchiolitis when death occurred from a cerebral hemorrhage.

would have a greater effect on peripheral airway conductance in the child than in the adult for the reasons outlined previously. This narrowing would also have a greater tendency to cause abnormal gas exchange in the child, since there would be less opportunity for collateral ventilation beyond the narrowed airways. Therefore, when inflammation occurs in the tracheobronchial tree of very young children, there is a tendency to call the disease bronchiolitis (High, 1957), even though it is likely that the whole tracheobronchial tree is involved. On the other hand, when adults acquire an upper respiratory tract infection followed by a lower respiratory tract infection, they have no difficulty with gas exchange because the cross-sectional area of the peripheral airways is very large and collateral ventilation is well developed. When airways become obstructed, adequate ventilation of the units beyond the obstruction is more easily achieved.

This can be illustrated by two patients, one adult and one child, both of whom had disease in the tracheobronchial tree involving peripheral airways. Figure 6 A and B shows the disease of the peripheral airways, which, if anything, is worse in the adult. The point of interest is that the child died a respiratory death due to "bronchiolitis," while the adult died suddenly of a cerebrovascular accident but happened to have "influenza with bronchitis" at the time of death. Figure 6 C and D shows the total airway resistance (R_L) and peripheral airway resistance (R_P) as a function of lung distending pressure (P_L). Note that bronchiolitis in the child is associated with a five- to sevenfold increase in both total and peripheral airway resistance as compared with the adult with bronchiolitis. This indicates that the same insult (i.e., a viral infection of the lower respiratory tract) has a much different effect on the young child, in whom it can cause death, than on the adult, in whom it was an incidental finding unrelated to the cause of death.

When we focus on the effect of repeated infections of the tracheobronchial tree, it can be shown from the published literature that bronchiectasis (Whitwell, 1952) and bronchitis and emphysema (Thurlbeck, 1968) have a very marked difference in age distribution. This is summarized in Figure 7, which shows the frequency distribution against age of four groups of patients reported in the literature; "bronchiolitis" apparently occurs very rarely after age three or four years, bronchiectasis is primarily a disease of young people, and bronchitis and emphysema are problems in a much older age group. However, we have already seen in Figure 6 that bronchiolitis does occur in adults but is difficult to recognize because adult airways have a very large conductance. We also know that bronchiectasis occurring either by itself or as a complication of fibrocystic disease (Fig. 8) is associated with severe disease in small airways, where narrowing and eventual obliteration lead to shortening of the bronchial tree and severe peripheral airways obstruction (Reid, 1950; Shwachman, 1967; Esterly and Oppenheimer, 1968). Finally, since organic disease of these same peripheral airways is the main site of obstruction in chronic bronchitis and emphysema (Hogg and coworkers, 1968), it is apparent that peripheral airways obstruction is a common factor in bronchiolitis, bronchiectasis, pulmonary complication of fibrocystic disease, and bronchitis and emphysema. This suggests that the disorder of anatomy varies because the insult to the airways occurred at a different age.

Indeed, in the light of the foregoing discussion of lung growth, it seems highly likely that repeated respiratory infections in young children would lead to atelectasis and infection, because peripheral airways are more easily obstructed and collateral ventilation beyond the obstruction is poorly developed. These two features, atelectasis and infection, are precisely those required to produce bronchiectasis experimentally; therefore, it seems likely

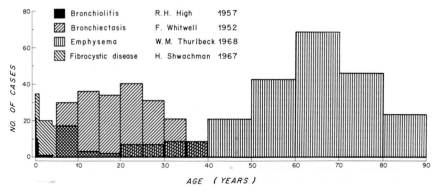

Figure 7. Age distribution of bronchiolitis, bronchiectasis, bronchitis and emphysema, and fibrocystic disease. Peripheral airway obstruction is a common factor of all these diseases. The stage of lung growth at the time of the insult may determine the type of abnormality that is produced.

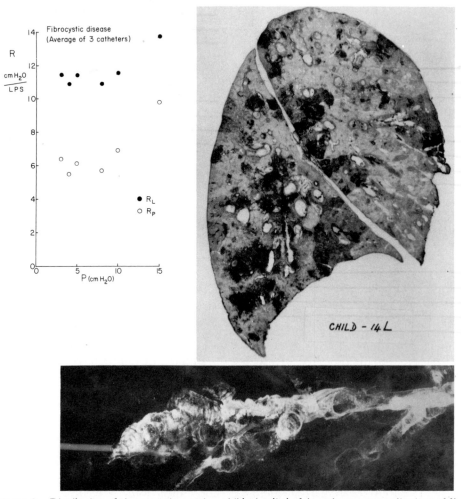

Figure 8. Distribution of airways resistance in a child who died of the pulmonary complications of fibrocystic disease, with the accompanying whole lung sections and bronchogram showing the marked bronchiectasis in this case. Peripheral airway resistance (R_p) accounts for about 50 per cent of total airway resistance (R_L).

that repeated infections from almost any source beginning in early childhood and carrying on through to the adult period would lead to chronic bronchiectasis. Thus, it is not surprising that the repeated pulmonary infections associated with cystic fibrosis result in the disorder of anatomy we call bronchiectasis (Fig. 8). On the other hand, repeated insults to the airways in an adult from irritants such as cigarette smoke could also lead to inflammation of peripheral airways. In this age group, any obstruction could easily be bypassed by ventilation of the parenchyma distal to the obstruction by collateral channels. However, the resulting mechanical stress to the alveolar wall might well be a factor leading to destruction of the alveolar wall and to the lesion we call emphysema.

In summary, it is useful to think of the process of lung growth when considering obstructive pulmonary disease. As we have seen, disease in peripheral conducting airways is a common feature in bronchiolitis, bronchiectasis, bronchitis and emphysema, and the pulmonary complications of fibrocystic disease. The hypothesis that a common insult such as peripheral airways inflammation might have a vastly differing effect, depending on the stage of lung growth at the time of the insult, seems reasonable. In the young child, peripheral airways are disproportionately narrow and the collateral ventilation pathways poorly developed. Disease of the small airway therefore results in "bronchiolitis." A similar insult in the adult might be called bronchitis because disease in the peripheral airways is difficult to detect. Repeated insults in the child might lead to atelectasis and bronchiectasis, whereas the same repeated insult in the adult might contribute to the breakdown of alveolar walls because of excessive use of collateral channels.

REFERENCES

Bucher, U., and Reid, L.: Development of the intersegmental bronchial tree: a pattern of branching and development of cartilage at various stages of intra-uterine life. *Thorax, 16*:207, 1961.

Burri, P. H.: Postnatal growth of the rat lung. III. Morphology. *Anat. Rec., 180*:77, 1974.

Dunnill, M. S.: Postnatal growth of the lung. *Thorax, 17*:329, 1962.

Esterley, J. R., and Oppenheimer, E. H.: Cystic fibrosis of the pancreas: structural changes in peripheral airways. *Thorax, 23*:670, 1968.

High, R. H.: Bronchiolitis. *Pediatr. Clin. North Am., 4*:183, 1957.

Hislop, A., and Reid, L.: Development of the acinus of the human lung. *Thorax, 29*:90, 1974.

Hogg, J. C., Macklem, P. T., and Thurlbeck, W. M.: Site and nature of airway obstruction in chronic obstructive lung disease. *N. Engl. J. Med., 278*:1355, 1968.

Hogg, J. C., Williams, J., Richardson, J. B., et al.: Age as a factor in the distribution of lower airway conductance and in the pathologic anatomy of obstructive lung disease. *N. Engl. J. Med., 282*:1283, 1970.

Horsfield, K., and Cumming, G.: The morphology of the bronchial tree in man. *J. Appl. Physiol., 24*:373, 1968.

Lambert, M. W.: Accessory bronchiolo-alveolar channels. *Anat. Rec., 127*:472, 1957.

Macklin, C. C.: Alveolar pores and their significance in the human lung. *Arch. Pathol., 21*:202, 1936.

Martin, H. B.: Respiratory bronchioles as the pathway for collateral ventilation. *J. Appl. Physiol., 21*:1443, 1966.

Reid, L. M.: Reduction in bronchial subdivisions in bronchiectasis. *Thorax, 5*:233, 1950.

Reid, L.: The embryology of the lung. In De Reuck, A. B. S., and Porter, R. (Eds.): *Development of the Lung.* (CIBA Foundation Symposium.) Boston, Little, Brown and Company, 1967, pp. 109–130.

Shwachman, H.: Cystic fibrosis. In Kendig, E. L., Jr.: *Disorders of the Respiratory Tract in Children.* Philadelphia, W. B. Saunders Company, 1967.

Stigol, L. C., Vawter, G. F., and Mead, J.: Studies on the elastic recoil of the lung in a pediatric population. *Am. Rev. Resp. Dis., 105*:552, 1972.

Thurlbeck, W. M.: *Chronic Obstructive Lung Disease.* Pathology Annual. New York, Appleton-Century-Crofts, 1968, pp. 367–368.

Weibel, E. R.: *Morphometry of the Human Lung.* Berlin, Springer-Verlag, 1963.

Whitwell, F.: A study of the pathology and pathogenesis of bronchiectasis. *Thorax, 7*:213, 1952.

SECTION II

INTENSIVE CARE OF
RESPIRATORY
DISORDERS

CHAPTER EIGHT

INTENSIVE CARE OF RESPIRATORY DISORDERS

Reynaldo D. Pagtakhan, M.D., and Victor Chernick, M.D.

Disorders of respiratory structure and function with consequent ventilatory failure remain a significant cause of morbidity and mortality in infancy and childhood. This chapter considers the pediatric patient who is in imminent or frank respiratory failure, classifies the disorder according to the predominant functional abnormality and discusses an intensive approach to therapy. Since a detailed presentation is beyond the scope of this chapter, a discussion of therapeutic principles is the main approach. Therapeutic advances have been made possible because of an increased understanding of the pathophysiology of respiratory disorders, the increasing availability of equipment that is appropriate for the pediatric patient and the ability to monitor the results of respiratory therapy, and, in particular, the facility to measure arterial blood gas tensions easily.

FUNCTIONAL CLASSIFICATION OF RESPIRATORY DISORDERS

Effective pulmonary exchange of oxygen and carbon dioxide requires clear airways, normal lungs and chest wall, and adequate pulmonary circulation. The integrity of the pulmonary system plus a normal respiratory control mechanism ensures adequate total alveolar ventilation and a proper relationship between ventilation and perfusion. The adequacy of gas exchange in the lungs is reflected in the tensions of oxygen and carbon dioxide in the arterial blood leaving the lung. This subject has been reviewed in great detail in Chapter 1.

Respiratory disorders may be classifed according to cause or to the dominant functional abnormality. The latter classification is utilized here because it forms the basis for a rational approach to intensive therapy of respiratory disorders. Three types of functional derangement may be delineated: (1) obstructive lung disease, (2) restrictive lung disease and (3) inefficient gas transfer (Table 1). This approach is purposely oversimplified, and it is well recognized that in many disease pro-

TABLE 1. FUNCTIONAL CLASSIFICATION OF RESPIRATORY DISORDERS

1) *Obstructive Lung Disease* (Increased resistance to airflow)
   Upper respiratory tract
   Lower respiratory tract

2) *Restrictive Lung Disease* (Impaired lung expansion)
   Loss of lung volume
   Decreased distensibility
   Chest wall disturbance

3) *Inefficient Gas Transfer* (Insufficient alveolar ventilation for carbon dioxide removal or impaired oxygenation of pulmonary capillary blood)
   Impaired respiratory control mechanism
   Diffusion defect

TABLE 2.   CAUSES OF OBSTRUCTIVE RESPIRATORY DISEASE

Site of Disturbance	Specific Disease Conditions	
	NEWBORN AND EARLY INFANCY	LATE INFANCY AND CHILDHOOD
Upper Airway		
Anomalies	Choanal atresia, Pierre-Robin syndrome, flabby epiglottis, laryngeal web, tracheal stenosis, vocal cord paralysis, tracheomalacia, vascular ring	Tracheal stenosis, vocal cord paralysis, vascular ring, laryngotracheomalacia
Aspiration	Meconium, mucus, vomitus	Foreign body, vomitus
Infection		Laryngotracheitis, diphtheria, epiglottitis, peritonsillar or retropharyngeal abscess
Tumors	Hemangioma, cystic hygroma, teratoma	Papilloma, hemangioma, lymphangioma, teratoma, hypertrophy of tonsils and adenoids
Allergic or reflex	Laryngospasm from local irritation (intubation) or tetany	Laryngospasm from local irritation (aspiration, intubation, drowning) or tetany, allergy
Lower Airway		
Anomalies	Bronchostenosis, bronchomalacia, lobar emphysema, aberrant vessels	Bronchostenosis, lobar emphysema, aberrant vessels
Aspiration	Amniotic contents, tracheoesophageal fistula, pharyngeal incoordination	Foreign body, vomitus, pharyngeal incoordination (Riley-Day syndrome), drowning
Infection	Pneumonia, pertussis	Bronchiolitis, pneumonia, tuberculosis (endobronchial, hilar adenopathy), cystic fibrosis
Tumors		Bronchogenic cyst, teratoma, atrial myxoma
Allergic or reflex		Bronchospasm (allergic or secondary to inhalation of noxious gases)

cesses all three types of functional derangement may be present. Inefficient gas transfer is most often secondary to restrictive or obstructive lung disease, thus leading to a mismatching of ventilation and perfusion of the lung. Inefficient gas transfer may also appear as a primary disorder, such as a diffusion defect or an impaired ventilatory control mechanism, leading to alveolar hypoventilation.

It is possible to classify all pulmonary disease conditions into their primary disturbance of function. Since most conditions affecting the respiratory system are different in the newborn period and early infancy from those in late infancy and childhood, it is useful to consider these separately. Tables 2, 3 and 4 contain illustrative causes of obstructive and restrictive lung disease

and disorders of inefficient gas exchange in infancy and childhood. The subsequent sections will deal with the recognition of respiratory failure and the principles of emergency care and continued management of both acute and chronic respiratory disorders.

RECOGNITION OF RESPIRATORY FAILURE

Respiratory disease may have an abrupt onset or may occur insidiously; respiratory failure, then, may occur as an emergency situation or may be preceded by gradual and progressive deterioration of respiratory function. Insufficient alveolar ventilation from any cause invariably results in hypoxemia and hypercapnia, which may contribute

TABLE 3. CAUSES OF RESTRICTIVE RESPIRATORY DISEASE

	Specific Disease Conditions	
Site of Disturbance	NEWBORN AND EARLY INFANCY	LATE INFANCY AND CHILDHOOD
Parenchymal		
Anomalies	Agenesis, hypoplasia, lobar emphysema, congenital cyst, pulmonary sequestration	Hypoplasia, congenital cyst, pulmonary sequestration
Atelectasis	Hyaline membrane disease	Thick secretions (postoperative)
Infection	Pneumonia	Pneumonia, cystic fibrosis, bronchiectasis, pleural effusion, pneumatocele
Alveolar rupture	Pneumothorax (spontaneous or iatrogenic)	Pneumothorax (trauma, asthma)
Others	Pulmonary hemorrhage, pulmonary edema, Wilson-Mikity syndrome	Pulmonary edema, lobectomy, chemical pneumonitis
Chest Wall		
Muscular	Diaphragmatic hernia, eventration, edema, Wilson-Mikity syndrome	Amyotonia congenita, poliomyelitis, diaphragmatic hernia, eventration, myasthenia gravis, muscular dystrophy, botulism
Skeletal malformations	Hemivertebrae, absent ribs, thoracic dystrophy	Kyphoscoliosis, hemivertebrae, absent ribs
Others	Abdominal distention	Obesity, flail chest

to further depression of ventilation and thereby culminate in frank respiratory failure and death. However, severe respiratory distress is not always associated with carbon dioxide retention, and hypoxemia may be present in the absence of clinically detectable cyanosis. Thus, precise assessment of ventilatory adequacy must be based on both clinical and laboratory studies. The clinical signs and laboratory findings associated with impending or frank respiratory failure are listed in Table 5. Approximate normal values for frequently used indices of cardiopulmonary function are shown in Table 6. Although estimation of arterial blood gases and pH is a necessary part of the assessment in

TABLE 4. CAUSES OF INEFFICIENT GAS TRANSFER

Site of Disturbance	Specific Disease Conditions
Pulmonary Diffusion Defect	
Increased diffusion path between alveoli and capillaries	Pulmonary edema, pulmonary fibrosis, collagen disorders, Pneumocystis carinii, sarcoidosis
Decreased alveolocapillary surface area	Pulmonary embolism, sarcoidosis, pulmonary hypertension, mitral stenosis, fibrosing alveolitis
Inadequate erythrocytes and hemoglobin	Anemia, hemorrhage
Respiratory Center Depression	
Increased cerebrospinal fluid pressure	Cerebral trauma (birth injuries), intracranial tumors, central nervous system infection (meningitis, encephalitis, sepsis)
Excess central nervous system depressant drugs	Maternal oversedation, overdosage with barbiturates or morphine
Excessive chemical changes in arterial blood	Severe asphyxia (hypercapnia, hypoxemia)
Toxic	Tetanus

TABLE 5. CRITERIA OF RESPIRATORY FAILURE

Clinical Signs

Respiratory
Tachypnea
Altered depth and pattern of
  respiration (deep, shallow,
  apnea, irregular)
Chest wall retractions
Flaring of alae nasi
Cyanosis
Decreased or absent breath
  sounds
Expiratory grunting
Wheezing and/or prolonged
  expiration

Cardiac
Bradycardia
Hypotension
Cardiac arrest

Cerebral
Restlessness
Irritability
Headache
Mental confusion
Seizures
Coma

Laboratory Findings

Hypoxemia (acute or chronic)
Hypercapnia (acute or chronic)
Acidosis (metabolic and/or respiratory)

order to provide precise information regarding gas exchange in the lung, these studies obviously are unimportant when one is faced with an emergency situation. Clinical judgment is paramount at this time, and the skilled physician or nurse must be able to assess the situation and initiate therapeutic measures within moments.

RESUSCITATION

Only minutes separate the onset of complete apnea from the ensuing ven-tricular fibrillation or asystole. No other clinical setting demands more immediate decision and organized action, and both physicians and nurses must be skilled in emergency procedures. The sequential steps in resuscitation are outlined in Table 7. Resuscitation equipment should be readily accessible and checked daily. A list of suggested equipment is presented in Table 8.

Regardless of the cause of respiratory arrest and the age of the patient, the following basic approach should not only result in increased survival but also prevent hypoxic brain damage. Appropriate modifications of this scheme may be made and will be dependent upon the presence of other members of the resuscitation team. The cardinal rule is to use the simplest readily available procedure.

External Cardiac Massage

Cessation of respiratory function can be tolerated a few minutes longer than cardiac standstill and absent cerebral circulation. Thus, the first step is to palpate the peripheral pulses and quickly check the heart beat. Absence of femoral or temporal pulse is sufficient indication to commence external cardiac massage at a rate of 100 to 120 times per minute in newborn infants and 60

TABLE 6. APPROXIMATE NORMAL VALUES

Parameter	Newborn Infant	Older Infant and Child
Respiratory frequency (breaths/minute)	40–60	20–30 (to 6 years)
		15–20 (above 6 years)
Tidal volume (ml./kg.)	5–6	7–8
Arterial blood	7.30–7.40	7.30–7.40 (to 2 years)
pH		7.35–7.45 (above 2 years)
P_{CO_2} (mm. Hg)	30–35	30–35 (to 2 years)
		35–45 (above 2 years)
Standard HCO_3^- (mEq./liter)	20–22	20–22 (to 2 years)
		22–24 (above 2 years)
P_{O_2} (mm. Hg)	60–90	80–100
Heart rate (beats/minute)	120–200	100–180 (to 3 years)
		70–150 (above 3 years)
Blood pressure (mm. Hg)		
Systolic	60–90	75–130 (to 3 years)
		90–140 (above 3 years)
Diastolic	30–60	45–90 (to 3 years)
		50–80 (above 3 years)

TABLE 7. PRINCIPLES OF RESUSCITATION

Cardiac Massage

Airway Patency
  Extension of the neck with upward traction on the mandible
  Clearing of the oropharynx with finger, bulb syringe, suction
  Oropharyngeal tube
  Orotracheal intubation with direct laryngoscopy
  Tracheotomy
  Bronchoscopy

Artificial Ventilation and Oxygenation
  Mouth-to-mouth, -nose or -tube
  Bag and mask
  Bag-to-tube

Pharmacologic Agents
  Narcotic antagonists
  Alkali
  Glucose
  Bronchodilators
  Osmotic diuretics
  Cardiac stimulants
  Antiarrhythmic agents

to 80 per minute in older children. Auscultation for the heart beat should be done quickly so that the onset of cardiac massage is not delayed.

Two essentials of effective and safe cardiac massage must be fulfilled: (1) the patient's spine must be supported during compression of the sternum, and (2) sternal pressure must be forceful but not traumatic. Sternal compression applied too vigorously may result in rib and sternal fractures, hepatic tears and ruptured stomach. Effective cardiac massage may be achieved in very small infants by joining the fingers of both hands behind the patient's back with both thumbs on the middle sternum. In larger infants, one hand is placed under the infant's back and the heel of the other hand on the middle sternum. In an older child, a firm board (1/2 inch thick plywood) is placed under the patient's spine and both hands are used to compress the junction between the middle and lower thirds of the sternum. Cardiac massage should be started and maintained for 5 to 10 seconds. By this time, measures

designed to ensure airway patency and artificial ventilation should be instituted. Cardiac compression should be interspersed with ventilation at a ratio of 1 breath for every 5 to 8 compressions. Signs of recovery include palpable peripheral pulse, return of pupils to normal size and the disappearance of mottling and cyanosis.

Airway Patency

Rapid restoration of airway patency is mandatory and has to be done almost

TABLE 8. EQUIPMENT ON A MOBILE RESUSCITATION CART

Suction apparatus (bulb syringe; 2-holed Rausch rubber catheters sizes 8, 10, 16, 18; De Lee glass trap; Cole endotracheal catheters)
Oropharyngeal airway (sizes 0, 00, 000, 1, 2, 3)
Breathing bag (Hope resuscitator; large and small)
Face mask (Rendell-Baker sizes 1, 2, 3, 4)
Laryngoscope (handles—2; straight and curved blades—Miller size 0, 1, Guedel size 1; Welch-Allyn plastic; spare batteries)
Endotracheal tube and connector (see Table 9)
Endotracheal adaptors (Bennett tracheostomy adapter set with elbow tube)
Magill forceps
Tracheotomy tray and tube
Bronchoscope (pediatric size)
Oxygen source and appropriately fitted nipples
Pharmacologic agents (Narcan, Isuprel, Adrenalin, calcium chloride, sodium bicarbonate, 50 per cent glucose, lidocaine, procainamide, digoxin, Valium, THAM, aminophylline, mannitol, urea)
Fluids (normal saline; 50 per cent dextrose in water) and administration set
Syringes (1-, 2-, 5-, 10-, 20- and 50-ml)
Needles (2-inch long gauge 16, 18, 20, 22; 3-inch long gauge 18–20)
Cardiac board (plywood 1/2-inch thick)
Cardiac synchronizer and DC-defibrillator
Cutdown and umbilical vessel catheterization trays
Adhesive tape (1 roll, 1/2 inch; 1 role, 1 inch)
Scissors
Stopwatch

Notes:
  1. Equipment must be checked daily against list posted on cart.
  2. Nursery and older child intensive care units and casualty area must have separate carts.
  3. The cart should be modified to meet the specific needs of the area serviced.
  4. There should also be on the cart a list of commonly used drugs and their stock concentration, recommended dose and common complications (see Table 10).

simultaneously with external cardiac massage. In the absence of obstruction by secretions or foreign material, airway patency can be achieved by extending the neck and pulling the mandible forward, thereby lifting the tongue from the posterior pharyngeal wall. Overextension of the neck must be avoided in small infants. One should always first check for obstructing material by spending a few seconds clearing the oropharynx with the finger, bulb syringe or suction tube. Once this is accomplished, an oropharyngeal tube should be inserted, thereby maintaining pharyngeal patency. Direct laryngoscopy and orotracheal intubation are essential when bag and mask breathing is ineffective because of an inadequate airway. Orotracheal tube sizes for the pediatric age group are listed in Table 9. Transparent polyvinylchloride endotracheal tubes that satisfy the armed forces standard implant tests and lightweight nylon connectors are recommended.

If an airway cannot be established in such conditions as severe epiglottitis, laryngospasm, trismus or laryngeal foreign body, an emergency tracheotomy must be performed. This may be rapidly achieved by percutaneous insertion of a 15-gauge needle into the trachea through the cricoid membrane. A single vertical slit just below the cricoid through two or three tracheal rings without removing a segment of cartilage is the next procedure of choice. Often, a bronchoscope may be inserted when tracheal intubation has failed, and this may be followed by a less hurried tracheostomy. Emergency bronchoscopy is indicated for the removal of an aspirated foreign body when it is lodged in a main-stem bronchus, but bronchoscopy is not an emergency when the foreign body is lodged in a more distal airway. Bronchoscopic removal of thick mucopurulent secretions is seldom an emergency. Large volumes of secretions may be removed by direct laryngoscopy and endotracheal suction. While exercising speed in initiating emergency treatment, the attending physician must always consider other causes of acute respiratory difficulty, such as a tension pneumothorax, which is promptly relieved by needle thoracentesis.

Artificial Ventilation and Oxygenation

Mouth-to-mouth, mouth-to-nose, or bag and mask ventilation of the lung should begin immediately after checking airway patency. A plastic oropharyngeal airway that prevents obstruction of the pharynx by the tongue should be inserted. Artificial respiration must be done cautiously with close

TABLE 9.   OROTRACHEAL TUBE SPECIFICATIONS FOR THE PEDIATRIC AGE GROUP

Age Group	French Size	Internal Diameter (mm.)	Length (cm.)	15-mm. Male Connector Size (mm. I.D.)
Newborn ($\leq$ 1.0 kg.)	11–12	2.5	10	3
Newborn ($\geq$ 1.0 kg.)	13–14	3.0	11	3
1–6 months	15–16	3.5	11	4
6–12 months	17–18	4.0	12	4
12–18 months	19–20	4.5	13	5
18–36 months	21–22	5.0	14	5
3–4 years	23–24	5.5	16	6
5–6 years	25	6.0	18	6
6–7 years	26	6.5	18	7
8–9 years	27–28	7.0	20	7
10–11 years	29–30	7.5	22	8
12–14 years	32–34	8.0	24	8

observation of chest and abdominal wall expansion, since excessive pressure may produce pneumothorax, pneumomediastinum or gastric distention. These complications are more apt to be encountered in newborn infants, who require no more than 15 to 20 ml. tidal volume, an amount that is approximately the volume of the adult mouth with cheeks distended with air.

There are several types of bag and mask arrangements that are in common use at the present time. The conventional anesthesia bag requires an inflow of oxygen or air to reinflate the bag; the other type is a self-inflation bag. Either is satisfactory, but generally the concentration of oxygen by the latter type is limited. Whenever feasible,

50 per cent oxygen or greater should be delivered. Bag and mask ventilation must also be done cautiously to prevent lung rupture. It is worthwhile noting that aspirated vomitus and secretions will be driven down the tracheobronchial tree during positive pressure ventilation; prior suctioning is therefore a most important initial step. In the newborn period, diaphragmatic hernia should be ruled out as the cause of acute respiratory distress, since positive pressure breathing may aggravate the situation by introducing air into the gastrointestinal tract. When an adequate upper airway cannot be established, tracheal intubation is required. A 15 mm. male tracheal tube connector should fit directly into the 5 mm. fe-

TABLE 10. PHARMACOLOGIC AGENTS USEFUL IN CARDIORESPIRATORY EMERGENCIES

Agents*	Stock Solution		Initial Intravenous Dose		
	Quantity Supplied (ML.)	Concentration per ML.	Per Kilogram	Maximum Dose	Remarks
Naloxone hydrochloride (Narcan)					
Neonatal	2	0.02 mg.	0.01 mg.	—	May repeat every 3 min. for 2 more doses.
Adult	1	0.40 mg.		0.40 mg.	
Sodium bicarbonate, 7.5%	50	0.9 mEq.	2–5 mEq.†	45 mEq.	May repeat every 10 to 15 min.
Tris(hydroxymethyl) aminomethane (THAM 0.3 M.)	1000	0.3 mEq.	2–5 mEq.	45 mEq.	May cause respiratory depression.
Aminophylline	10	25 mg.	5–7 mg.‡		Place in drip chamber and give over 15 to 20 min.
Epinephrine (Adrenalin 1:1000)	1	1 mg.	0.01–0.04 mg.‡	0.5 mg.	May repeat every 5 min.§
Isoproterenol hydrochloride (Isuprel 1:5000)	1	0.2 mg.	0.001–0.004 mg.†	0.04 mg.	Best given as a continuous infusion.§
Lidocaine, 2% (Xylocaine)	5	20 mg.	0.5–2 mg.	100 mg.	May repeat every 10 to 30 min.
Procainamide hydrochloride (Pronestyl)	10	100 mg.	4–8 mg.		Give over 5 min. with continuous ECG and BP monitoring. Repeat every 5 min.
Calcium chloride, 10%	10	100 mg.	15–30 mg.†	1 gm.	Maximum is 2 ml./min.
Calcium gluconate, 10%	10	100 mg.	15–30 mg.†	1 gm.	Repeat every 30 to 60 min. in infants and every 3 to 6 min. in older children.
Mannitol, 20% (Osmitrol)	500	200	0.5–1.5 gm.		Monitor heart rate. Give over a 1- to 3-hour period.
Urea, 30% (Urevert)	300	300	1.0–1.5 gm.		Give over 30-min. period.
Glucose, 50%	50	500	0.1–1.0 gm.		

*Agents are listed by generic names; common trade name is in parentheses.
†May also be given by intracardiac route.
‡Use lower dose (3 to 4 mg./kg.) if patient had prior aminophylline treatment.
§A solution with a concentration of 0.002 to 0.004 mg./ml. is used for continuous infusion. Adjust rate according to patient's response.

male fitting on the bag and mask apparatus.

Pharmacologic Agents

By this stage, an intravenous infusion should have been started in order to provide a route for drug, plasma expander or blood administration. Pharmacologic agents commonly used during the acute resuscitation phase are listed in Table 10. Naloxone hydrochloride (Narcan) is superior to levallorphan and nalorphine as a specific narcotic antagonist. It does not depress ventilation or aggravate respiratory depression. Maximal effect is seen two or three minutes after intravenous administration; it is delayed to 15 minutes after intramuscular or subcutaneous administration. In the immediate neonatal period, it is most often used to treat respiratory depression caused by placental transfer of narcotic analgesics administered to the mother. Failure to obtain improvement after two or three doses at five-minute intervals suggests that causes other than narcotic overdosage may be responsible for the patient's condition. Sodium bicarbonate is the agent of choice for the correction of metabolic acidosis and should be administered prior to the estimation of blood pH when there has been severe hypoxia. Tris(hydroxymethyl)aminomethane (THAM) has been used to correct metabolic acidosis, but may cause respiratory arrest and hypoglycemia; this drug has no advantage over sodium bicarbonate in terms of buffering capacity, but does circumvent the administration of large quantities of sodium ion. Glucose (50 per cent) is used in hypoglycemic shock. In status asthmaticus, a loading dose (e.g., 7 mg. per kilogram) of aminophylline diluted in three volumes of saline is given intravenously over 15 minutes for prompt optimal bronchodilation. Intravenous isoproterenol or salbutamol may be added, but moment-to-moment monitoring of the vital signs is mandatory. Mannitol, urea and dexamethasone have been successfully employed to reduce cerebral edema.

Cardiac stimulants, given by the intravenous or intracardiac route, are used in cardiac arrest or severe bradycardia. Epinephrine and isoproterenol increase cardiac output by increasing myocardial contractility and stroke volume. It should be noted that these agents may precipitate the onset of ventricular fibrillation, particularly in the hypoxic heart. Calcium chloride also increases myocardial contractility and may be effective when adrenergic drugs have failed. Atropine sulfate is indicated for the treatment of profound bradycardia, particularly when associated with premature ventricular contraction and hypotension, to improve cardiac output and reduce the chance of ventricular fibrillation. Dopamine increases cardiac output and dilates renal, mesenteric, coronary and cerebral vessels. It is an effective agent for shock in the adult but has not been extensively tested in children.

In contrast to adults, cardiac asystole occurs more frequently than fibrillation in children, and cardioversion is rarely required. When necessary, a DC-defibrillator should be used in the initial attempt at conversion of ventricular fibrillation. It is also indicated in tachycardia without palpable peripheral pulses and in those with apparent cardiac standstill, since it may sometimes be impossible in an emergency to be certain whether the heart is in a fine ventricular fibrillation or true asystole. Initial dose of defibrillator shock varies with the size of the child — 2 watt-second/kg. body weight for a child under 50 kg. (Table 11). Since the damage resulting from countershocks is directly proportional to the energy used, it is safer to commence with this dose and then double the dose if unsuccessful. Recurrent ventricular fibrillation is treated by lidocaine or procainamide, both of which decrease myocardial excitability and slow conduction. Lidocaine has a shorter duration of action than procainamide and appears to be

TABLE 11. INITIAL DOSE RANGE OF DEFIBRILLATOR SHOCK*

Weight (kg.)	Watts-second
<2.5	5
2.5–10	5–20
10–20	20–40
20–40	40–80
over 40	100

*Double this dose if unsuccessful.

less toxic. It is also effective in controlling multifocal premature ventricular beats and episodes of ventricular tachycardia.

RESUSCITATION OF THE NEWBORN INFANT

The newborn infant is able to tolerate asphyxia longer than the adult because of larger cardiac glycogen stores. In addition, it is likely that the neonatal brain is more efficient at anaerobic metabolism than that of older infants and children. Nonetheless, neurologic sequelae directly correlate with the duration of asphyxia, and resuscitation must therefore be as prompt as in older infants and children. Skilled personnel and special equipment are required because of the small size of the infant. The general approach to resuscitation is essentially the same in newborn infants as in older children, but asystole is rare and an ineffective cardiac output is usually corrected by adequate oxygenation. It is unusual, then, that cardiac stimulants are indicated in the newborn infant with respiratory failure, for such stimulants are rarely effective when bradycardia or a poor cardiac output fails to respond to artificial ventilation and oxygenation.

Since the newly born infant has a large surface area for heat loss, hypothermia is common unless the infant is immediately dried and an external heat source supplied. Since hypothermia increases the metabolic demand for oxygen, this may produce a critical situation in vital organs in the asphyxiated infant. An effective means of maintaining optimal body temperature of the infant in the delivery room is by the use of infrared heat lamps. During resuscitation of the critically ill newborn infant, care must be taken to avoid excessive heat loss.

IMMEDIATE POSTRESUSCITATION PHASE

Once the immediate crisis has passed and the acute problem has been resolved, the tracheal tube may be removed. The timing of this removal requires astute clinical judgment and is aided by assessment of blood gas tensions. Recovery of an adequate spontaneous ventilation following a period of respiratory arrest requires a minimum of three to four hours of continuous patient observation in order to recognize the development of posthypoxic complications such as hyperexcitability, fever, visual disturbances and seizures. It is good clinical practice to re-examine within two to four weeks any child discharged after an acute episode of apnea.

Most patients must remain in the hospital following successful resuscitation. Once the critical phase has passed, laboratory investigations are pursued as dictated by the historical information; chest roentgenogram is obtained and arterial blood gases and pH are determined. All of this information will aid in determining the need for further respiratory assistance, more laboratory investigations and a specific treatment regimen. Historical and laboratory data can now be assessed to determine the need for transfer to the intensive care unit of the hospital for continued management.

CONTINUING RESPIRATORY CARE

The general principles underlying an intensive approach to the management of severe respiratory disorders involve continuing efforts at ensuring airway patency, adequate gas exchange in the lung and institution of specific therapy (Table 12).

Maintenance of Airway Patency

In the intensive care unit, airway obstruction is most often caused by the retention of pulmonary secretions. An appreciation of this fact has resulted in the evolution of methods designed to aid the drainage of these secretions. In addition, airway obstruction may be caused by increased bronchomotor tone or mucosal edema, and therapy is also directed at increasing airway diameter.

DRAINAGE OF SECRETIONS. It is generally accepted that adequate hydration by the administration of oral or parenteral fluids is the optimal way to ensure that tracheobronchial secretions are thinned and are able to move easily out of the respiratory tract. Increasing the water vapor content of inspired air (humidification) will reduce respiratory water loss, but it should be recalled that full saturation at room temperature is only about 50 per cent saturation at body temperature. Under usual circumstances, the inspired air is fully humidified in the nose and upper airway. Dehydration of the lower respiratory tract is prone to occur during hyperventilation, during oxygen therapy or in patients with artificial airways in which the upper respiratory tract has been bypassed. Consequently, humidification is essential under these conditions to prevent drying of the lower respiratory tract mucosa and inspissation of mucus. Under these circumstances, the inspired air should be warmed and fully humidified.

Humidification is associated with the hazard of gram-negative infection, particularly Pseudomonas. Special precau-

TABLE 12. PRINCIPLES OF CONTINUING CARE OF RESPIRATORY DISORDERS

I. Maintenance of Airway Patency
  A. *Drainage of Tracheobronchial Secretions*
   1) Hydration of secretions
      Systemic fluid
      Humidification
      Aerosolized water (mist)
      Avoidance of drying agents
   2) Removal of secretions
      Coughing
      Suctioning (oropharyngeal, endotracheal)
      Chest pummeling and postural drainage
      Bronchoscopy
  B) *Optimal Airway Diameter*
      Bronchodilator medication
      Aerosolized
      Systemic (oral, intravenous)

II. Oxygenation
   Methods of Administration
      Face mask
      Tent
      Head box
      Incubator
   Indication and Precautions

Tracheal Airway
   Intubation
   Tracheostomy

Mechanical Ventilatory Support
   Criteria for Selection
   Types of Mechanical Ventilators
   Complications and their Management

Additional Therapy
   Medical
      Bronchodilators
      Steroids
      Antimicrobials
      Diuretics
      Digitalis
      Analgesics and narcotics
      Chest wall strapping
      Oxygen
      Transfusion
   Surgical
      Thoracentesis (air, fluid)
      Pleural drainage (air, fluid)
      Thoracotomy and direct repair
      Tonsillectomy and adenoidectomy

tions must be taken to ensure that the water reservoir remains sterile. In many intensive care units, it is recommended that the water reservoir and all tubing leading to the patient be changed every 24 hours. In the water reservoir of incubators, the addition of acetic acid has been shown to be effective in preventing the proliferation of gram-negative organisms.

Aerosolized water (mist) is commonly used to supply extra water to the respiratory tract, particularly in conditions such as croup, bronchitis, pneumonia and cystic fibrosis. The rationale for the use of mist for lower respiratory tract diseases has recently been questioned because of the evidence that most of the water droplets are filtered out of the nose and upper airway and are subsequently swallowed; only a minimal amount actually reaches the lung. Thus, the role of mist therapy in thinning secretions is in considerable doubt and is most likely inefficient in comparison with adequate humidification and systemic hydration. Hazards associated with mist include: infection, possible overhydration (particularly when ultrasonic nebulizers are used), and an unstable thermal environment.

In general, parasympatholytic drugs, such as atropine, and antihistamines must be avoided, since these agents dry respiratory mucus and interfere with proper drainage. For certain asthmatic children, atropine plays a beneficial role. It may act either by inhibiting production of cyclic GMP, thereby preventing smooth muscle contraction, or by abolishing reflex increase in airways resistance induced by cold air, dust inhalation, and the like.

Cough is the most effective method of removing secretions. Deep inspiration augments the normal widening of thoracic airways and triggers an effective cough. When the cough mechanism is depressed or inadequate, such as in the immediate postoperative period, oropharyngeal suction, which stimulates cough, must be done frequently. In the presence of endotracheal intubation or tracheostomy, the ability to cough is seriously impaired, and frequent direct suctioning is required. However, excessive suctioning may result in irritation of the tracheal mucosa and bleeding. Furthermore, suction catheters may damage respiratory mucosa unless there is a single end hole. The presence of side holes allows the respiratory mucosa to be sucked in and damaged if the end hole becomes occluded. Since the normal defense mechanisms of the respiratory tract have been bypassed, bacteria are easily introduced unless special precautions are taken. It is generally recommended that sterile catheters be used once and then discarded and that personnel wear sterile disposable gloves.

Secretions may be mobilized by chest pummeling and postural drainage; this technique is widely used in conditions associated with excessive secretions, such as pneumonia, bronchiectasis and cystic fibrosis. Proper positioning for maximal drainage by gravity depends on the site of the involved lobe and is discussed in detail elsewhere in this book (Chapter 4, Diagnostic and Therapeutic Procedures). Therapeutic bronchoscopy is indicated for the removal of an aspirated foreign body and is used less commonly for the removal of thick secretions.

B) OPTIMAL AIRWAY DIAMETER. In normal subjects, bronchodilator agents have been shown to decrease airway resistance, indicating the presence of smooth muscle tone in small airways. Thus, pharmacologic agents have been used extensively in respiratory disease to dilate small airways in the hope that secretions will be more effectively drained (Table 10). Bronchodilators may act by decreasing smooth muscle tone (beta adrenergic effect), by reducing mucosal congestion through vasoconstriction (alpha adrenergic effect) or by the exertion of a direct relaxant action on smooth muscle. The commonly used bronchodilators include isoproterenol, salbutamol, terbutaline (all β-adrenergic), epinephrine (α-adrenergic) and aminophylline (direct muscle relaxant). Salbutamol and terbutaline have more selective action on the β_2-adrenergic receptors in the bronchial wall, thus avoiding significant cardiac stimulation. In the acutely ill patient, adrenergic drugs are administered directly to the lungs as an aerosol; aminophylline is given intravenously. In addition to these treatment modalities, intravenous isoproterenol has proved a useful adjunct to the therapy of children with severe bronchospasm and respiratory failure. Presumably, the drug increases effective pulmonary blood flow, which in turn allows improvement in the metabolic function to the lung and an increase in perfusion with an associated lowering of the Pa_{CO_2}. It is mandatory that patients selected for this treatment be in the intensive care unit where continuous cardiac monitoring is done. Limitations of intravenous isoproterenol therapy include tachycardia above 200/per minute and arrhythmia. Salbutamol given intravenously does not have these limitations, but has not been extensively tested in children.

Proper administration of aerosolized isoproterenol or epinephrine requires a deep, slow inspiration; the subject should make a maximal exhalation, and aerosol should be delivered at the beginning of inspiration. The breath should be held for two or three seconds at the end of inspiration. When the patient cannot take a deep inspiration, the drug may be administered by an intermittent positive pressure device (IPPB). Aminophylline is a very effective bronchodilator when administered intravenously as a continuous infusion at a daily dose of 15 mg. per kilogram body weight. One-fourth of the daily dose is infused every six hours. In this dose we have not seen signs of intoxication (central nervous system stimulation) in infants and older children; however, toxic blood concentrations of aminophylline may be reached when it is administered by rectal suppository, since absorption via this route is unpredictable. It is ideal, when feasible, to monitor blood levels of aminophylline for a more effective and safe therapy. Serum concentration should be 10 to 20 micrograms per milliliter. Aminophylline has also been used in the treatment of apnea of prematurity but is still considered experimental. The premature infant may have insufficient hepatic enzymes to metabolize the drug, and measurement of blood levels is mandatory.

Steroids are effective in reducing bronchospasm in allergic disorders but are ineffective in the presence of infection, such as in bronchiolitis.

Increased Oxygen Tension in Inspired Gas

Once the resuscitation phase has passed, the optimal method for determining the necessity for increasing the inspired oxygen concentration is by the direct measurement of the arterial oxygen tension. Even in the absence of cyanosis, the presence of hypoxemia may be inferred by signs such as restlessness, confusion and coma. Under these circumstances, oxygen should be administered immediately, and blood gas tension measurements should be obtained as soon as feasible. It must be emphasized that cyanosis is a poor indicator of hypoxemia, since this sign depends on the concentration of hemoglobin. Cyanosis will be apparent only when there is about 5 grams per 100 ml. reduced hemoglobin in the capillaries. Thus, in the presence of anemia, cyanosis may be difficult to detect; in the presence of polycythemia, cyanosis may be evident even though the blood oxygen content is adequate for tissue demands. Cyanosis requires the administration of oxygen until blood gas tensions are measured. In the presence of a right-to-left cardiac shunt, oxygen will have little or no effect on arterial P_{CO_2}.

There are several methods of oxygen administration. Nasal catheters and cannulas are not usually tolerated by pediatric patients. Oxygen delivered via the oxygen inlet of an incubator is limited to a concentration of 40 per cent. When oxygen is delivered into a tent, the concentration varies, depending on leaks, but usually attains a concentration of 25 to 30 per cent. Face masks usually deliver a maximum of 40 per cent oxygen. Use of a head box allows attainment of a higher, more stable oxygen concentration, up to 95 to 100 per cent, and may be used in newborn infants and older children when such concentrations are required. Regardless of the technique used, it is essential that oxygen be heated and humidified by bubbling it through a heated nebulizer. In order to avoid damage to the lungs, oxygen administration should be discontinued as soon as possible as indicated by serial blood gas tension measurements. Reduction of inspired oxygen concentration must be done stepwise and cautiously. Both concentration and duration of oxygen therapy must be recorded accurately. A well calibrated oxygen analyzer must be used to check the inspired concentration at frequent intervals; this must be done at least every two hours. The necessity for closely monitoring arterial P_{O_2} in preterm newborn infants is related to both pulmonary oxygen toxicity and the danger of retrolental fibroplasia. In any patient, oxygen should be administered at the lowest concentration sufficient to maintain the arterial P_{O_2} between 60 and 80 mm. Hg and not exceeding 100 mm. Hg.

The administration of oxygen may cause further respiratory depression if there has been chronic respiratory failure and a loss of sensitivity to carbon dioxide. This situation is uncommon in the pediatric patient, but has been encountered in patients with cystic fibrosis.

Nasotracheal Intubation and Tracheostomy (Tracheal Airway)

Although it is technically more difficult than orotracheal intubation, nasotracheal intubation is the preferred route when an adequate upper airway must be maintained for more than 12 hours. This route facilitates oral and pharyngeal hygiene and provides a more stable fixation, which reduces the complication of tracheal erosion and the danger of accidental extubation. Satisfactory placement of the tube should be confirmed by auscultation

and roentgenogram. The tip of the tube should be at least 1 cm. above the carina. Infants and children less than 10 years of age never require cuffed tubes. In older children, the cuff should be inflated to the minimum volume sufficient to provide an adequate tracheal seal. The cuff should be deflated hourly for two to five minutes in order to minimize pressure necrosis.

In newborn infants, we have used nasotracheal tubes for as long as three weeks without complications. However, in older children, tracheostomy should be done if the tracheal airway is required beyond one week. Plastic polyvinylchloride tracheostomy tubes rather than metal ones are preferred by some physicians because they are simple to use and easily cleaned. However, the safety feature of an inner cannula in the metal tube is felt by some to be important. Cuffed tracheostomy tubes are seldom required.

Mechanical Ventilatory Support

SELECTION OF PATIENTS. The use of a mechanical ventilator is warranted for any patient whenever prolonged ventilatory support is needed to ensure effective clearance of carbon dioxide and to maintain sufficient tissue oxygenation. Respiratory insufficiency per se is not an indication for mechanical support; the degree and duration of respiratory failure determine the need for a mechanical aid to breathing. Table 13 lists the generally accepted selection criteria for mechanical ventilation without which a patient's survival is unlikely or serious neurologic sequelae might be anticipated. The major parameters evaluated include respiratory pattern, heart rate and degree of acidosis, hypercapnia and hypoxemia. It must be emphasized that clinical signs and laboratory findings complement each other. Two or more episodes of apnea with bradycardia or cardiac arrest in a newborn infant require immediate mechanical ventilatory support even in the absence of arterial blood pH and gas tensions analysis. In less acute circum-

TABLE 13. SELECTION CRITERIA FOR MECHANICAL VENTILATION

Parameter	Newborn Infant	Older Child
*Clinical**		
Respiratory pattern	Apnea	Apnea
Cardiac pattern	Bradycardia	Bradycardia
	Cardiac arrest	Cardiac arrest
Laboratory†		
Pao$_2$ (mm. Hg)	Less than 40	Less than 55 to 60
pHa	Less than 7.00	Less than 7.25
Paco$_2$ (mm. Hg)	Greater than 70 to 75	Greater than 60

*More than one episode of apnea with bradycardia or an episode of cardiac arrest is adequate indication for initiation of mechanical ventilation even in absence of blood gas data.

†While breathing 100 per cent O$_2$.

Note: Laboratory values less severe than those indicated above must be supplemented by clinical evidence of severity to warrant initiation of mechanical ventilation.

stances, the severity and duration of clinical signs and symptoms may indicate impending respiratory failure even in the presence of normal alveolar ventilation (P$_{CO_2}$). Under these circumstances, mechanical ventilation may be initiated in an attempt to avoid an acute crisis.

TYPES OF VENTILATORS. Ventilators can substitute for or assist a patient's respiratory effort. When used as a substitute (controller), the ventilator cycles automatically at fixed settings and totally controls ventilation. When used to assist (assistor), the patient's inspiratory effort triggers the mechanical inspiratory phase of the ventilators. When provision is made for both machine control and patient's participation (controller-assistor), the ventilator controls respiration as long as the patient's respiratory frequency is below a preselected rate and assists breathing when the patient's respiratory frequency rises above the selected rate. It must be noted that in small infants with weak respiratory efforts, the "assist" mode is usually unreliable.

Ventilators have also been classified as positive pressure and negative pressure machines, depending on how lung inflation is artifically achieved. The positive pressure machine inflates the lung by increasing airway pressure above atmospheric pressure; with a negative pressure ventilator, a subatmospheric pressure is created around the chest wall while airway pressure remains atmospheric. Either class of ventilators produces an intermittent *positive* transpulmonary pressure (airway pressure greater than pleural pressure), which is essential for lung inflation.

Ventilators differ according to their primary control of cycling mechanism. The three main types are (1) volume-cycled — when delivery of a fixed volume of gas terminates the inspiratory phase; (2) pressure-cycled — when attainment of a preselected pressure setting initiates the expiratory phase independent of the duration of inspiration; and (3) time-cycled — when inspiration and expiration are terminated by a preset cycle duration and gas flow rate. Overriding time cycling is used as a safety feature in the first two types to ensure intermittent pulmonary inflation. The three types have additional built-in safety features. Volume- and time-cycled machines are pressure-limited; pressure-cycled machines are flow rate — limited.

Table 14 lists the commonly used ventilators. The efficacy of a particular ventilator depends more on the skill and experience of the clinician than on the machine itself. Nonetheless, one type may best suit a particular age group under certain conditions. The volume-cycled (pressure-limited) machine is effective when airway resistance is markedly increased and lung compliance decreased, since even under these

TABLE 14. TYPES OF COMMONLY
USED MECHANICAL VENTILATORS*

Volume-cycled (Pressure-limited)*
　　Bennett MA-1
　　Bourns LS-104
　　Emerson Postoperative
　　Engstrom

Pressure-cycled (Flow rate–limited)†
　　Bennett PR-1 and PR-2
　　Bird Mark VII and VIII

Time-cycled (Pressure-limited)
　　Air Shields Isolette‡
　　East-Radcliffe
　　Air Shields
　　Baby Bird§

---

*Emerson postoperative and Engstrom venti-
lators are used as *controllers* only; all other types
listed have provision for independent patient
cycling (*assistor-controller*).

†Has overriding time cycling in addition to the
safety limit indicated.

‡Used as a negative pressure ventilator.

§Constant flow feature allows the use of intermittent mandatory ventilation (IMV).

---

circumstances the appropriate tidal volume will continue to be delivered.
However, a sudden increase in compliance may lead to lung rupture. Furthermore, it is difficult to detect leaks in
the system unless inspiratory pressure
is monitored. In contrast, use of the
pressure-cycled (flow rate–limited)
ventilator in the presence of leaks disturbs the attainment of the preset pressure and thereby alters the cycling pattern; this situation should alert the
intensive care unit staff. However, a
decrease in dynamic compliance, such
as that caused by accumulation of secretions, may be associated with a decrease in tidal volume. This situation
may go unrecognized, since the ventilator will continue to cycle at the preset
pressure.

Overriding time cycling is a safety
feature contained in most ventilators,
which ensures continued cycling should
other mechanisms fail. Primary time-
cycled (pressure-limited) machines deliver a tidal volume in the time allotted
to inspiration. Since this type usually
has a wide range of available flow rates,
it can accommodate changes in airway

resistance and lung compliance, but it
functions most effectively when airways
are relatively clear and lung compliance
is stable. The constant flow feature of
the Baby Bird allows the infant to
breath spontaneously even though a
very slow rate is set on the machine (so-
called intermittent mandatory ventilation).

A negative pressure ventilator, available commercially as a purely time-
cycled machine, has the advantage of
not requiring tracheal intubation. Except in the treatment of hyaline membrane disease in newborn infants, this
type of ventilator has not been used extensively in treating respiratory failure
associated with pulmonary disease.
However, in such infants, the ventilator
has not provided good control of alveolar ventilation; that is, it has not been
effective in lowering arterial P_{CO_2}.

It has recently been appreciated that
in conditions associated with low lung
volumes, such as hyaline membrane
disease, atelectasis and severe pneumonia (viral, Pneumocystis, meconium
aspiration), alveolar collapse may be
alleviated or prevented by the use
of a positive end-expiratory pressure
(PEEP). Alveolar pressure is not allowed
to return to zero (atmospheric pressure), but is held at 3 to 5 cm. H_2O
above atmospheric pressure during expiration. This technique increases the
efficiency of oxygen transfer in the
lung (reduces the alveolar-arterial oxygen tension difference), thereby facilitating adequate tissue oxygenation at
lower concentrations of inspired oxygen. The ability to oxygenate adequately at low inspired concentration of
oxygen is important in order to prevent
the toxic effect of oxygen on the lung.

The use of a constant positive transpulmonary pressure or continuous distending pressure (CDP) in spontaneously breathing infants has been
employed extensively in the treatment
of hyaline membrane disease. This has
been accomplished by several methods
without the necessity of resorting to artificial ventilation in severely ill infants
with adequate spontaneous alveolar

ventilation (arterial P_{CO_2} less than 70 mm. Hg). One method utilizes an endotracheal tube and bag system. The infant breathes into a rubber bag kept at a preset positive pressure. Carbon dioxide is washed out of the system by a high flow of gas, which leaks out at one end of the bag. The pressure in the bag is determined by the rate of gas inflow and by controlling the outflow with a screw clamp. Continuous positive airway pressure (CPAP) has also been applied to the upper airways using nasal prongs, a face mask or a sealed head box. Another approach uses the negative pressure ventilator in such a way as to provide a continuous subatmospheric chest wall pressure (CNP) while the infant breathes spontaneously. This method does not require endotracheal intubation, and leaves the facial area clear for nursing care; however, access to the body is difficult, and significant leaks may cool the infant. CPAP has also been used with varying success for the treatment of apnea of prematurity.

COMPLICATIONS. Complications of respirator therapy occur frequently, even with a highly skilled intensive care team, and personnel must be continually aware of the hazards associated with ventilatory support (Table 15). Aseptic technique is mandatory for tracheal airway care, since nosocomial infection constitutes a large and potentially preventable problem. Pseudomonas infection from contaminated water reservoirs can be prevented by careful attention to the source of water supply and by changing reservoirs and tubing frequently.

Endotracheal intubation interferes with the drainage of pulmonary secretions, and special attention must be paid to maintaining effective drainage by use of suctioning and chest physiotherapy. Tubes may cause other problems, such as local necrosis, and cuffed tubes must be deflated every hour. Malposition of the tube is frequent, and radiologic examination of the chest must be done to ensure proper placement.

TABLE 15. SOME COMPLICATIONS ASSOCIATED WITH MECHANICAL VENTILATION

Respiratory
Tracheal lesions (erosion, edema, stenosis, granuloma, obstruction, perforation)
Accidental endotracheal tube displacement (into main-stem bronchus, esophagus, hypopharynx) or actual extubation
Infection (tracheitis, pneumonitis)
Air leaks (pneumothorax, pneumomediastinum, interstitial emphysema)
Trapping of gas (hyperinflation)
Excessive secretions (atelectasis)
O_2 hazards (depression of ventilation, bronchopulmonary dysplasia)
Pulmonary hemorrhage

Circulatory
Impairment of venous return (decreased cardiac output and systemic hypotension)
O_2 hazard (retrolental fibroplasia, cerebral vasoconstriction)
Septicemia
Intracranial hemorrhage (intraventricular, subarachnoid)
Hyperventilation (decreased cerebral blood flow)

Metabolic
Increased work of breathing ("fighting" the ventilator)
Alkalosis (potassium depletion, excessive bicarbonate therapy)

Renal and Fluid Balance
Antidiuresis
Excess water in inspired gas

Equipment Malfunction (Mechanical)
Power source failure
Ventilator malfunction (leaks, valve dysfunction)
Improper humidification (overheating of inspired gas, inspiratory line condensation)
Improper tubing connections (kinked line, disconnection)

Use of a high concentration of inspired oxygen may be necessary to provide normal arterial oxygenation but must be accompanied by frequent analysis of arterial P_{O_2}. The premature infant is susceptible to retrolental fibroplasia, particularly if arterial P_{O_2} rises above 150 to 200 mm. Hg. Pulmonary fibrosis and necrosis of bronchiolar epithelium (bronchopulmonary dysplasia) are complications of the prolonged use of high concentration of oxygen in association with mechanical ventilation and may reflect a direct toxic action of oxygen on the lung. It is likely that this complication can be reduced in frequency if the use of inspired oxygen above 60 per cent is limited. Reduction of inspired oxygen below 60 per cent should be made as rapidly as possible. Careful monitoring of both inspired oxygen concentration and arterial P_{O_2} is mandatory. In newborn infants with hyaline membrane disease, the use of CPAP, CNP, and artificial ventilation with PEEP has reduced the prevalence of bronchopulmonary dysplasia, but artificial ventilation with PEEP has doubled the prevalence of lung rupture, including interstitial emphysema of the lung, pneumomediastinum and pneumothorax.

All ventilators increase pleural pressure relative to peripheral venous pressure; venous return to the heart may be impaired if excessive pressures are used. The expiratory phase should be longer than the inspiratory phase, and a time ratio of 2:1 or higher is generally recommended. If the patient is not breathing in rhythm with the ventilator ("fighting" the ventilator), the work of breathing may be increased, thereby leading to increased oxygen demands and carbon dioxide production. Under these circumstances, it is best to sedate the patient with morphine or diazepam or to paralyze him with curare or succinylcholine and to completely take over (control) respiration artificially.

The use of ultrasonic nebulizers to humidify inspired gas may be associated with a positive water balance via the respiratory tract, and this must be taken into account in calculating fluid requirements. Proper function of the ventilator requires frequent checks on tubing connection, valve operation, humidifier apparatus and the power source, whether pneumatic or electric. It should be emphasized that a clear understanding of the general principles of mechanical ventilation and the capabilities and limitations of the specific ventilator used is crucial in reducing the incidence of complications or preventing a fatality.

Additional Therapy

Intensive management of respiratory disorders often requires additional treatment, depending on the etiologic or pathophysiologic features of the problem. The additional therapy may be either medical or surgical in nature (Table 12).

MEDICAL THERAPY. The role of bronchodilator agents has been discussed earlier. The patient with status asthmaticus may be refractory to this drug until pH and blood gases are returned to normal. Steroids are effective, but there is often a delay of 12 to 24 hours. Steroids reduce the inflammatory response to inhaled or aspirated material and are particularly efficacious following the aspiration of gastric juice or hydrocarbons.

Appropriate antimicrobial treatment of infection requires culture and sensitivity studies of tracheal aspirate, sputum, blood, gastric aspirate or loculated fluid in the chest. Pending the results of these studies, one is justified in beginning broad-spectrum antibiotic coverage in a patient who is acutely ill with an undetermined infection. Once the culture results are available, the specific antibiotic coverage is continued.

Diuretics (e.g., furosemide, ethacrynic acid) and morphine are indicated in acute pulmonary edema. Morphine reduces venous return and thereby decreases pulmonary blood volume and pressures. Cardiac failure is treated with digoxin. Narcotic analgesics are also indicated in severe chest wall injury or with severe chest pain as in the immediate postoperative period. However, depression of ventilation and of the cough mechanism must be avoided; analgesics must, therefore, be given judiciously and are discontinued as soon as possible. Pain associated with the movement of small flail segments of the chest wall may be reduced by compression strapping with a sandbag. Rib fracture, however, should not be strapped, since this interferes with expansion of the lung and leads to accumulation of secretions.

Severe hemoptysis or hemothorax may require appropriate blood transfusion. Not infrequently, the anemia may be so severe as to impair tissue oxygenation, and supplemental oxygen becomes essential until blood volume is restored. When a pneumothorax is small, nonprogressive and mildly symptomatic, oxygen inhalation (100 per cent) is occasionally used to facilitate the absorption of air from the pleural cavity.

SURGICAL THERAPY. Certain chest conditions can be properly and definitively managed only by surgical intervention. Thus, a tension pneumothorax from any cause requires immediate aspiration of air. When air leakage continues, a chest tube should be placed through the second intercostal space in the midclavicular line and connected to an underwater seal. Suction may be required if the leak is large. The accumulation of liquid in the pleural space (e.g., blood) may also require tube drainage by placing the tube into the dependent part of the pleural space. If the fluid is purulent and thick, open chest evacuation may be necessary; this is followed by tube drainage. Control of persistent air leaks from the lung or unrelenting hemorrhage requires thoracotomy for direct repair or emergency resection. Although never an emergency, tonsillectomy and adenoidectomy provide a permanent cure of the pulmonary hypertension and respiratory failure occasionally associated with marked hypertrophy of the tonsils and adenoids.

MONITORING

Close observation of the acutely ill child is mandatory but is supplemented by other methods of monitoring the status of the patient. The availability of modern blood gas equipment that allows the measurement of arterial pH, P_{CO_2} and P_{O_2} on microsamples permits frequent assessment of these parameters. The need for continuous monitoring of the patient's status and the status of the equipment required for treatment has caused a remarkable growth in the availability of electronic devices. Associated with the use of such monitoring devices are certain hazards that are largely preventable.

Monitoring of Patient Status

Close observation of the seriously ill child requires (1) visual inspection of the color to estimate the level of arterial oxygen saturation, (2) observation of the diaphragmatic movement and the use of accessory muscles to gauge respiratory difficulty, and (3) auscultation of the thorax to determine tube placement and need for endotracheal suction. At the first sign of a change in status, arterial blood gas analysis must be done. These measurements may be required as frequently as every 30 minutes when the patient's condition is unstable; when the clinical picture appears stable, blood gas studies need be done only two or three times a day. In the newborn infant, an indwelling umbilical arterial catheter is used for sampling and also for infusion of fluid. The tip of the catheter should be below the level of the renal arteries. An arterialized capillary sample may suffice as an alternative, but P_{O_2} measurements are unreliable because they often do not reflect the arterial P_{O_2}. Continuous monitoring of arterial P_{O_2} (or saturation) and arterial P_{CO_2} may become feasible within the near future. Temperature, heart rate, ECG, blood pressure, respiratory rate and the concentration of inspired oxygen may be monitored intermittently. Continuous monitoring of these parameters is now feasible with modern electronic equipment. It is beyond the scope of this chapter to comment in detail about precise methods of monitoring or the efficacy or need for continuous monitoring of a patient or given parameter.

Each intensive care area should have its own specific guidelines, and these will vary with the age of the patient as well as with the personal preferences of the members of the intensive care team.

Monitoring of Equipment Function

Constant surveillance of the equipment used for treatment and monitoring is essential in order to avoid complications. Not infrequently, equipment malfunction (see Table 15) may go unrecognized and can compromise the patient's status beyond assistance. An audiovisual alarm is an appropriate method to signal any mechanical malfunction. Periodic checkup of the alarm system per se is essential.

To ensure adequate monitoring of both patient and equipment, a flow sheet record of clinical observation, laboratory findings and mechanical ventilatory adjustment is extremely useful.

Electrical Hazards and Safety Measures

A potentially lethal hazard of the use of multiple monitoring devices is electrocution of patient or personnel. The hazard is primarily introduced because of stray electric currents or a faulty grounding system. Stray electric currents may be present because of a gross fault in the equipment. Frequent and regular inspection of all electrically operated devices in the intensive care unit, even when not in use, is most important in detecting grossly faulty equipment.

A more subtle source of stray electric current exists in all electronic monitoring devices because of leaks of small amounts of current to the metal case of the instrument. All equipment used in the intensive care area should be supplied with a three-pronged plug that contains a special third ground wire connected to the instrument case. Thus, current leaking to the case is carried to ground. Even though these currents are small, they constitute a hazard if the current is allowed to flow

close to the heart, for example, via the umbilical artery catheter. As little as 20 microamperes (20×10^{-6} amperes) may cause ventricular fibrillation when applied directly to the heart, whereas it requires 5000 times this amount when the current is introduced externally.

Because of the subtle hazard of stray electric currents, special attention must be paid to grounding, frequent testing and personnel education. There should be a single effective ground consisting of a low-resistance wire that connects to all electric outlets in the unit. The use of the conduit for grounding is inadequate because the conduit is subject to mechanical damage or corrosion. Multiple pieces of equipment attached to the same patient must be grounded to a common point, such as a connection to a single bank of wall receptacles. This is necessary in order to avoid small amounts of current flowing from one ground point to another (ground loops).

Despite the use of a separate ground wire, breakage of ground connection frequently occurs inside the wall receptacle. Therefore, wall receptacles should be routinely tested for adequate ground connection. Equipment should also be routinely tested for leakage currents and other faults, since with passage of time there is gradual deterioration of electrical components and insulating material. Tests for leakage current should be carried out at the instrument case as well as at the site of application to the patient (e.g., electrodes). Existing hospital safety codes are inadequate for medical equipment, since they do not take into account the hazard of leakage current. Thus, before purchasing equipment, one must obtain the manufacturer's specifications with regard to leakage current. Despite this precaution, each piece of equipment should be tested by the hospital engineer before actual use with a patient.

Each member of the intensive care team must be trained in the correct use of equipment and should also be aware of the potential hazard of electrical

equipment. Consultation with a know-
ledgeable electrical engineer is advisable, since the situation in a particular
hospital is often complex and requires
expert advice.

SUMMARY

Intensive treatment of respiratory
disease in infancy and childhood
requires a clear understanding of the
pathophysiology of disease processes in
the younger age group and of the technological advances in respiratory care
equipment. This chapter contains a
classification of pediatric respiratory
disorders according to the predominant functional derangement and a
consideration of the recognition of imminent or frank respiratory failure.
The principles of emergency and continuing intensive care of respiratory
disorders have been discussed in depth.
Details regarding intensive care unit organization, structural design or equipment have been omitted. Therapeutic
advances have been accelerated over
the past decade because of the increasing skill of intensive care personnel as
well as an improvement in equipment.
In the final analysis, the success of such
a unit depends on the availablility of
physicians, nurses, respiratory technologists, physiotherapists and others

organized into a team with special ex-
pertise and dedication.

REFERENCES

Anthony, C. L., Crawford, E. W., and Morgan, B.
    C.: Management of cardiac and respiratory ar-
    rest in children. *Clin. Pediatr., 8*:647, 1969.
Avery, M. E., and Fletcher, B. D.: *The Lung and
    Its Disorders in the Newborn Infant.* 3rd Ed. Phila-
    delphia, W.B. Saunders Company, 1974.
Behrman, R. E., James, L. S., Klaus, M., Nelson,
    N., and Oliver, T.: Treatment of the asphyxi-
    ated newborn infant. *J. Pediatr., 74*:981, 1969.
Chernick, V.: Hyaline membrane disease: ther-
    apy with constant lung distending pressure. *N.
    Engl. J. Med., 289*:302, 1973.
Chernick, V., and Raber, M.: Electrical hazards
    in the newborn nursery. *J. Pediatr., 77*:143,
    1970.
Daily, W. J. R., and Smith, P. C.: Mechanical
    ventilation of the newborn infant. I and II.
    Curr. Probl. Pediatr., 1:1 (June) and *1*:1 (July),
    1971.
Egan, D. F.: *Fundamentals of Inhalation Therapy.* St.
    Louis, C. V. Mosby Company, 1969.
Gutgesell, H. P., Tacker, W., Geddes, L., Davis,
    J., Lie, J. T., and McNamara, D.: Energy dose
    for ventricular defibrillation in children. *Pedi-
    atrics, 58*:898, 1976.
Smith, R. M.: The critically ill child: respiratory
    arrest and its sequelae. *Pediatrics, 46*:108, 1970.
Standards for Cardiopulmonary Resuscitation
    and Emergency Cardiac Care. *J.A.M.A., 227*
    (Suppl.):833, 1974.
Stephenson, H. E., Jr. (Ed.): *Cardiac Arrest and
    Resuscitation.* 4th Ed. St. Louis, C.V. Mosby
    Company, 1974.
Todd, J. S. (Ed.): Symposium on Intensive Care
    Units. *Med. Clin. North Am.,* Vol. 55, September,
    1971.

SECTION III

RESPIRATORY DISORDERS IN THE NEWBORN

CHAPTER NINE

CONGENITAL MALFORMATIONS OF THE LOWER RESPIRATORY TRACT

Arnold M. Salzberg, M.D., and Frank E. Ehrlich, M.D.

PECTUS CARINATUM (PIGEON BREAST)

Pectus carinatum is an uncommon structural deformity of the sternum in which sternal protrusion occurs with or without unilateral or bilateral costal cartilage recession. The excavatum abnormality is four to seven times more common than this variety.

There are two basic types of deformity (Brodkin, 1953). The most common involves a lower chondrogladiolar prominence (oblique form). The other type has an upper chondromanubrial prominence with a depressed gladiolus (arcuate form). Uncommonly, there may also exist asymmetry with one-sided prominence. Males are much more often affected than females.

The surgical indications in the first two decades of life are mostly cosmetic and psychic.

The operative procedure consists of variously placed sternal osteotomies and chondrectomy of offending cartilages. Mortality and morbidity are very low, and the immediate and long-term results are satisfactory.

STERNAL CLEFTS (FISSURA STERNI CONGENITA)

A partial or total midline vertical split in the sternum represents a persistence of the embryonic separation of the two sternal cartilage bars, which have failed to unite (Hansen, 1919). Partial fissures are more common than total sternal fissures. Furthermore, the partial split is more commonly seen in the cranial part of the sternum. These can be associated with an ectopic but otherwise normal heart, or with ectopia cordis with intrinsic congenital cardiac disease. Sternal clefts may also accompany a more complex abnormality with pathologic apertures in the abdominal wall, diaphragm and pericardium and a herniated, malformed heart.

The midline defect is appreciated on physical examination. The paradoxical movement of the anterior chest wall and the subcutaneous cardiac dance are specific findings, and on occasion are the only indications for surgical intervention. More frequent indications for surgical correction may include cyanosis, dyspnea, tachycardia or recurrent respiratory infections, particularly in the newborn.

The unfused sternal bars of the flexible chest wall can be surgically apposed in the neonatal period. Sabiston (1958) has described a sound method of repair in the older infant by oblique mobilization of the costal cartilages. Autogenous cartilage has also been advocated in this situation. More recently, the advantages of opening the caudal bridge have been emphasized. Essentially, this creates a bifid sternum and allows a better closure of the sternal bars, especially when done at an early age, when the thoracic cavity is most malleable.

PECTUS EXCAVATUM (FUNNEL CHEST)

There are characteristic morphologic deformities in pectus excavatum that have been known since antiquity and that make the diagnosis fairly obvious on inspection. Physiologic implications and therapy are not quite so standardized.

The three anatomic segments of the sternum are not equally involved in pectus excavatum. The superior manubrium is normal. The sharp slope inward, toward the vertebral column, begins at the manubriogladiolar junction, and the depression is deepest at the gladiolar-xiphoid articulation. The depth of this concavity varies widely from a shallow excavation to near contact with the vertebral colum. The xiphoid or ensiform may then proceed outward, deviate laterally or become rotated. Deformities of the lower costal cartilages form an essential part of the malformation. From the costochondral junctions, the cartilages proceed away from the chest wall, then angulate sharply inward toward their sternal attachments and thus become abnormal in length and direction. The deformity may be asymmetrical, although the symmetrical ones are six times more common.

Etiologic concepts are legion, but can be distilled into a workable number. Both Brodkin (1953) and Chin (1957) have implicated a functional deficiency of the anterior diaphragm that, by default, allows the unopposed remaining diaphragm to distort a pliable sternum and costal cartilages. Respiratory obstruction cannot be frequently causative, but may aggravate an existing deformity by accentuating sternal retractions. Bowers has emphasized defective pectoral muscles, while Brown (1939) described a short central tendon running between the diaphragm and the sternum. These two factors are not consistently present. An interesting etiologic possibility is that of a primary, misdirected, excessive growth of cartilage that eventually drives the lower part of the sternum backward. Of course, simultaneous or sequential diaphragmatic weakness with cartilage overgrowth is also a possibility. Finally, failure of osteogenesis and chondrogenesis, rather than diaphragmatic maldevelopment, has been emphasized by Mullard (1967).

The degree of structural deformity at birth may be minimal or extensive and may remain stationary, progress or regress. With age, growth of the thorax in an anteroposterior direction is restricted, but lateral development is uninhibited, and the disparity in the different diameters becomes obvious. Functionally, in the newborn and the infant, the labile breast bone may move paradoxically, but this relents with fixation and rigidity, and a deeply concave pectus may move normally with respiration as the child becomes older.

The depth of the gladiolar-ensiform excavation influences the position and volume of the intrathoracic viscera. There is cardiac compression between the sternum and vertebrae or dislocation of the heart into the left hemithorax with encroachment on the space occupied by the left lung. The basis for pulmonary and cardiac dysfunction exists, and the right side of the heart appears especially vulnerable, but it is difficult to document physiologic aberrations precisely. Bates, Macklem and Christie (1971) concluded that no consistent data have been accumulated that would incriminate pectus excavatum as an etiologic factor in the production of chronic pulmonary disease.

Clinically, the deformity is apparent at or shortly after birth, but is not associated with symptoms at this time except for the occasional occurrence of paradoxical movement of the lower part of the sternum, which rarely produces respiratory distress. In the older infant or child there may be decreased exercise tolerance, chest pain, palpitations, repeated upper respiratory tract infections, wheezing, stridor and cough. The deformity, at times, is cosmetically objectionable and embarrassing to the child and his parents. These children are exposed to peer ridicule, will often not participate in outdoor activities and may become reticent and introspective. The psychologic impact may be the only or chief complaint but, in itself, can be crippling. On physical examination, the inward angle of the gladiolar-xiphoid junction in the infant may be exaggerated with inspiration, documenting the paradoxical movement. Obliteration of the deformity

should occur with expiration, and Chin (1957) felt that failure to do so was a sign of irreversibility. On further inspection, the anteroposterior diameter of the elongated chest is narrow compared with the lateral diameter. The round shoulders accentuate a dorsal kyphosis or kyphoscoliosis and protuberant abdomen (Fig. 1). The apical cardiac impulse is often shifted to the left and may be accompanied by a systolic murmur, which is usually innocent.

X-ray examination of the chest quantitatively confirms the clinical diagnosis. The mediastinum and the heart are squeezed to the left of the vertebral column. The chest is wide on the posteroanterior view, and narrow on lateral films (Fig. 2). A radiopaque marker on the skin of the sternal depression nicely delineates the curvature and the restricted area between the posterior breast bone and the anterior vertebral column. Bronchograms have shown left lower lobe bronchiectasis, but the correlation remains poor.

The electrocardiogram may record a complex variety of changes, including right axis deviation, which probably represents displacement and not intrinsic or concomitant heart disease. An increased venous pressure has been

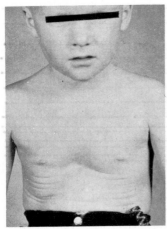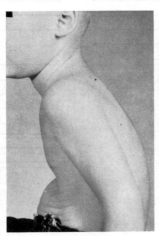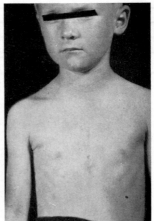

Figure 1. A moderate pectus excavatum in a four-year-old boy with rounded shoulders, kyphosis and protuberant abdomen. There is a reasonable cosmetic result one year after surgical correction.

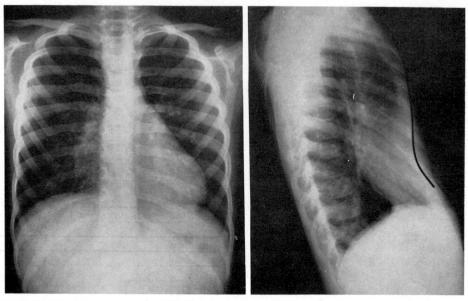

Figure 2.   Typical roentgenographic findings in a five-year-old boy with a pectus excavatum, demonstrating an absent right cardiac border and minimal deviation of the cardiac mass into the left hemithorax with angulation of the anterior ends of the middle and lower ribs. The chest is wide in the anteroposterior view and narrow in the lateral film. The lung fields are normal.

noted occasionally as a reflection of cor pulmonale and may be associated with a slight increase in right atrial pressure on cardiac catheterization. Pulmonary function studies have not demonstrated a consistent pattern. Often, vital capacity, maximal breathing capacity and total lung capacity are within the normal range, although Orzalesi and Cook (1965) have reported lower than mean predicted values in 12 children with pectus. Only four of these, however, had an abnormally low vital or maximal breathing capacity. It is of some interest that in five of the 12 patients studied before and after pectus correction, there was no significant improvement in pulmonary function. Ravitch and Matzen (1968), however, have recorded an 11-year-old girl with severe pectus and left lung agenesis whose pulmonary function improved after surgical repair. Welch (1958), too, has found a reduction in the vital and maximal breathing capacities in the lung volume in three of nine children so tested. The clinical and laboratory information, then, in the majority of patients is likely to exhibit a cosmetic deformity with variable psychologic implications,

vague cardiorespiratory symptoms and minimal objective evidence of heart-lung dysfunction. Later in life a few patients with severe pectus excavatum and chronic pulmonary sepsis in whom the chest wall becomes rigidly fixed are said to have an insidious decrease in pulmonary function and perhaps emphysema. For this small group, operative correction has been advised as a prophylactic measure. Certainly, however, the selection of patients on the basis of future invalidism is most difficult.

Additional indications for the surgical treatment of pectus excavatum might include children whose seriously depressed funnel chest is associated with measurable evidence of cardiopulmonary disease, or a cosmetic deformity with poor posture that is psychologically oppressive and cannot be otherwise handled. This approach would exclude the newborn and the infant from surgery, except for the rare neonate with uncontrollable paradoxical movement whose diaphragm might be separated from the sternum as suggested by Phillips (1960).

Meyer, in 1911, first attempted surgical correction of a pectus. The contemporary operative treatment for funnel chest was instigated by Brown (1939), who proposed the limited procedure of detaching or removing the xiphoid from the substernal ligament and diaphragm. Unfortunately, recurrence was frequent and stimulated the development of a host of more extensive thoracic wall operations. Basically, the deformity must be freed from all attachments, overcorrected and splinted. The technique popularized by Ravitch (1949) is preferred by many because it fulfills the technical principles simply, without cumbersome external or internal appliances. Stanford and his group (1972) utilized a molded Silastic subcutaneous implant for correction of pectus defects in patients with cosmetic indications only. This technique is not applicable to patients in whom growth is still a significant consideration, but may be useful in pectus excavatum complicated by unilateral absence of the pectoral muscles.

Postoperatively, exercise tolerance may increase, and growth and development may accelerate. Other associated symptoms have been relieved. In a few instances, improvement in cardiac and pulmonary function studies has been noted. The immediate cosmetic results are usually acceptable and tend to remain so for the first three years, especially if the correction is performed between three and eight years of age. Long-term follow-up studies are more divergent. Chin's clinic reported a 40 per cent recurrence after ten years, while Wada and Ikeda's (1972) group had a 3 per cent recurrence rate. Younger patients corrected by Ravitch's technique have a low recurrence rate. The operative morbidity and mortality are very reasonable.

CONGENITAL ABSENCE OF RIBS

This is an unusual bony deformity of the thoracic cage that is usually asso-

ciated with other muscular and orthopedic anomalies (Fig. 3). The defect frequently involves the highest and lowest ribs, and clinical repercussions are minimal. Conversely, when ribs in the midthoracic region are absent, lung function may be altered.

In 1895, Thomson suggested that perhaps the hand of the fetus, applying pressure on the chest wall, produced the defect, which may be unilateral or bilateral and usually extends from the sternum anteriorly to the posterior axillary line. Involvement of the second, third, fourth and fifth ribs would remove part of the origin of the pectoralis major muscle, and therefore absence of this muscle is a commonly associated defect; less common is breast agenesis on the same side. Hemivertebrae and kyphoscoliosis may be present.

The defect often produces no physiologic disturbance if the anomaly is single, small, and so localized that a lung hernia is not produced. If the second through the fifth ribs are absent

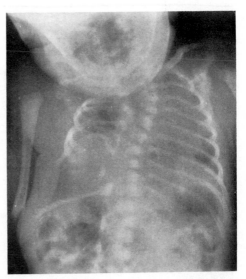

Figure 3. Anteroposterior x-ray film of the thorax demonstrates absent and deformed ribs on the right. Soft tissue changes, consistent with the loss of supporting structures, are also present. There is scoliosis with convexity to the left, and the heart is dislocated into the left hemithorax. Segmentation anomalies of the dorsal spine are also noted.

anteriorly, a large lung hernia may occur, and lack of chest wall support here can lead to dramatic paradoxical respirations. Kyphoscoliotic heart disease, with cor pulmonale and congestive heart failure, may complicate congenitally absent ribs.

Symptoms may vary from none to severe dyspnea secondary to paradoxical respiratory movements and mediastinal flutter. Relatively few infants, however, present with advanced respiratory distress, and less serious difficulties will gradually disappear as the lung protrusion diminishes with growth.

Therapy is based on the contribution of the rib defect to the clinical picture and is seldom required. When symptoms are severe enough to produce respiratory embarrassment, local pressure may stablilize the chest, although Rickham (1959) felt that an inappropriate bandage may worsen the distress. Certainly, if critical symptoms persist in spite of conservative chest wall support, homologous rib grafting should be done. On occasion, adolescent girls may require cosmetic breast surgery for an ipsilateral rudimentary breast.

CONGENITAL ANTERIOR DIAPHRAGMATIC HERNIA (MORGAGNI)

Morgagni hernias occur behind the sternum through defects in the diaphragm that are perhaps secondary to a developmental failure of the retrosternal segment of the septum transversum. The defect on the left is usually obliterated by pericardium; therefore, most of the hernias are on the right. Although these may be the most frequent tumors of the anterior inferior mediastinum in the pediatric age, they are the rarest type of congenital diaphragmatic hernia, accounting for one per 300 hernias. They are more common in females. More than half have a sac containing omentum or transverse colon. Those that do not contain bowel are the more difficult diagnostic problems.

Many infants and children with an anterior diaphragmatic defect are asymptomatic, and the hernia is found on incidental chest roentgenogram.

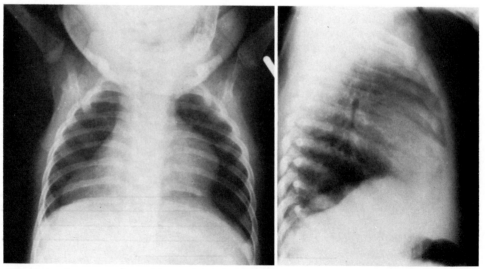

Figure 4. Anteroposterior and lateral films of the chest demonstrate a homogeneous shadow adjacent to the right heart border and diaphragm. The shadow is anterior in location with a smooth margin against the lung, as is seen with a Morgagni hernia. (Dr. M. B. Kodroff.)

Others may have abdominal complaints simulating gallbladder or peptic ulcer disease or constipation. A third group presents with chest symptoms of retroxiphoid pain, dyspnea and cough. Finally, acute findings with strangulation are said to occur in 10 per cent. Here, a succussion sound synchronous with the cardiac impulse may be diagnostic.

The diagnosis may be ultimately supported by roentgenograms showing a moderately dense tumor, usually at the right cardiophrenic angle in the posteroanterior film, and in the anterior mediastinum on the lateral view (Fig. 4). A barium enema may delineate a thoracic transverse colon and also demonstrate an elevated transverse colon if omentum is incarcerated. An omental hernia may be suggested by changes in angulation of the transverse colon with inspiration and expiration. Liver scan and arteriography can be used to define those hernias containing liver.

Abdominal herniorrhaphy is advised for most Morgagni hernias because of the possibility of incarceration or strangulation, although the thoracic approach has been advocated by Boyd (1961). Results are consistently satisfactory.

CONGENITAL DIAPHRAGMATIC HERNIA OF BOCHDALEK

Posterolateral diaphragmatic hernia through the pleuroperitoneal sinus is perhaps the most urgent of all neonatal thoracoabdominal emergencies. If the diagnosis is not immediate in otherwise normal neonates symptomatic in the first postnatal 24 hours, the mortality will be excessive.

The maldevelopment has been catalogued as frequently as one in 2200 to one in 3500 births, or about 8 per cent of major congenital anomalies, and is left-sided in 85 to 90 per cent of cases. At present, it may be outnumbered by hiatal hernia, but requires operative intervention as a lifesaving measure much more often. Concomitant defects that occur with some regularity are midgut malrotation, extralobar sequestration and congenital heart disease.

The hernia site between the chest and the abdomen results from a failure of closure of the pleuroperitoneal canal. The diaphragm is largely formed from the septum transversum and dorsal mesentery, which, at first, separates the thoracic systems from the abdominal organs. The defect in the posterolateral areas of the diaphragm is the last to close and is eventually bridged at the sixth to eighth week (20 mm. stage; 48 days) of fetal development by pleural and peritoneal membranes. Body wall mesoderm eventually insinuates between these membranes and becomes the diaphragmatic muscle. Early, arrested development in the region of the foramen of Bochdalek, prior to the presence of pleura and peritoneum, produces a hernia without a sac, and this is the most frequent anatomic situation. The left side is favored because diaphragmatic closure normally occurs here later than on the right. If the pleuroperitoneal membranes are formed without muscular development, a hernial sac for the Bochdalek defect has been created. Finally, aborted muscle ingrowth between the properly fashioned pleura and peritoneum may lead to a thin, fibrous tissue layer rather than substantial contractile muscle, and eventration results. Baffes (1962) has emphasized the role of an early return of the midgut (35 to 50 mm. stages; 55 to 65 days) from its umbilical domicile to the peritoneal cavity in the creation and maintenance of Bochdalek hernias.

The aperture in the posterolateral leaf of the diaphragm may vary in size from a small defect to absence or agenesis of the entire muscle, and this may occur bilaterally. Small and large bowel, stomach and spleen on the left and liver on the right have been found in the appropriate pleural cavity. In less than 10 per cent of the cases, a constricting hernia sac is present. Without this peritoneal or pleural investment, the herniated viscera may extend to the apex of the thorax. This migration of intraperitoneal structures is possible because of their insecure posterior peritoneal attachments, and is reflected in the reported 20 per cent incidence of simultaneous malrotation. As in omphalocele, the peritoneal cavity shrinks down to accommodate the remaining viscera.

Since the Bochdalek hernia has been present since early intrauterine life, compression of the ipsilateral lung may have occurred prior to the development of the lung buds (75 to 90 days); this process may also afflict the contralateral lung because of the severe mediastinal shift. The result of such compression is the development of bilateral pulmonary hypoplasia, more marked on the ipsilateral side, and deLorimier, Tierney and Parker (1967) have produced a similar chain of events in fetal lambs with surgically produced Bochdalek hernia. This is the major factor in the excessive mortality in the early neonate with or without operation. The combined lung weights in nonsurvivors are distinctly below the average similar weights for other stillborns of the same range of body weight. Actually, lung expansion and growth will occur in most survivors, but may take days or weeks, depending on the degree of pulmonary differentiation.

The pathophysiologic features are basically the same before and after operation. The hypoplastic lungs cannot adequately ventilate or oxygenate, thereby resulting in arterial oxygen desaturation, a mixed respiratory and metabolic acidosis and finally pulmonary hypertension. This is compounded by the abnormal pulmonary arterial tree, which has more muscle, is "stiffer" and is more likely to develop hypertension. Right to left intrapulmonary and ductal shunting is inevitable and increases venous admixture already produced by the ventilation-perfusion problem in the hypoplastic, collapsed lung. Ox-

ygenation and ventilation are worsened, and the cycle continues.

On examination of the newborn, immediate cardiorespiratory distress is striking and does not clear with pharyngotracheal toilet. Cyanosis, dyspnea, tachypnea and tachycardia are fairly constant. The involved hemithorax, usually the left, is relatively protuberant, and chest expansion is bilaterally uneven. Breath sounds are absent on the left, and percussion may be resonant. It is unusual to hear thoracic peristalsis. The apical cardiac impulse is dislocated to the right, and the abdomen is scaphoid.

The majority of patients with Bochdalek hernia have critical symptoms within the first 72 hours of life. After this, the history is likely to be marred by chronic respiratory and gastrointestinal ailments, and strangulation may occur.

Plain films of the chest in conventional views are almost always diagnostic, and the use of contrast material gives little constructive aid to the workup and introduces the danger of aspiration. The mediastinum is markedly displaced, and very little lung tissue on either side aerates properly. The diaphragmatic line on the affected side is difficult or impossible to visualize. Signet ring radiolucencies in the thorax suggestive of air-filled loops of bowel are contrasted with a distinct loss of normal gastrointestinal pattern within the abdomen (Fig. 5). If the hernia is right-sided, the liver alone may encroach on intrathoracic space, and liver scan may be necessary for diagnosis.

In preparing for the differential diagnosis, Moore (1957) has emphasized the triad of dyspnea, cyanosis and apparent dextrocardia. On x-ray film, the lesions simulate congenital cystic adenomatoid malformation, diffuse congenital pulmonary cysts and pneumatoceles. Neither of the latter two is particularly frequent in the immediate neonatal period, and an infectious background is often lacking. Moreover, with all three, the abdominal gastrointestinal configuration is normal. Other

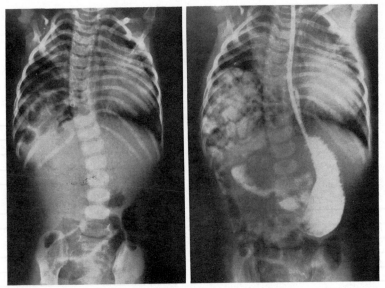

Figure 5. The plain anteroposterior thoracoabdominal radiograph shows a scoliosis of the spine and asymmetry of the chest with the left side larger. The heart and trachea are dislocated to the left. The dome of the left diaphragm is intact; the right cannot be seen. Multiple signet ring radiolucencies and mottled densities are noted in the lower half of the right hemithorax. The right lung is confined to the upper half of the hemithorax, and the peripheral left lung is hyperaerated. The normal gastrointestinal air pattern within the abdomen is absent.

Through the nasogastric tube, contrast material has been instilled and superfluously documents the finding of Bochdalek hernia, which is apparent in the plain film.

entities that can be separated with minimal difficulty are laryngotracheal obstruction, atelectasis, pneumothorax, true dextrocardia, congenital heart and cerebral disease, and lobar emphysema. It may be impossible, but is unnecessary, to separate Bochdalek hernia, eventration and phrenic nerve paralysis. The treatment in the presence of catastrophic symptoms is surgical in each instance.

Since a significant number of neonates with congenital posterolateral diaphragmatic hernias expire shortly after birth even with a correct, prompt diagnosis, proper emergency attention may enable the infant to survive the short preoperative interval. In this regard, effective, constant nasogastric suction may relieve or prevent the devastating intrathoracic gastrointestinal distention. Gentle positive pressure resuscitation must be done through an endotracheal tube to avoid forcing oxygen down the esophagus and further dilating the gastrointestinal tract. Overenthusiastic inflation of the lungs may produce unilateral or bilateral pneumothorax. The patient should be kept warm in order to reduce oxygen consumption. Serial blood gas and pH determinations must be obtained promptly, and vigorous treatment of the acidosis should be started in the preoperative period and continued throughout the operation.

Hedblom, in 1925, encouraged the emergency surgical approach for Bochdalek hernias by reporting a neonatal mortality rate of 75 per cent without operation. Today, under optimal conditions, the mortality with hernias repaired during the high-risk period of the first 24 hours of life is still 60 to 75 per cent, but it drops precipitously to less than 5 per cent after 72 hours of age.

It has been emphasized that operation should be done when the diagnosis is made, preceded by the shortest possible period of correct preoperative resuscitation, because a patient who is apparently well may become moribund within minutes and fail to respond.

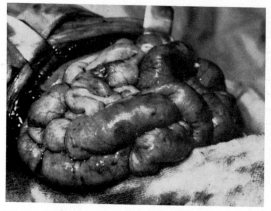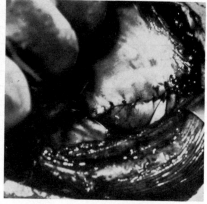

Figure 6. Small bowel extrudes through a low posterolateral right thoracotomy incision, relieving the pulmonary and mediastinal tamponade. After the hernial contents have been replaced within the abdomen, the diaphragmatic defect is closed in two layers.

The surgical incision may be made transthoracically or transperitoneally, and there are advocates for each (Fig. 6). A majority favors the abdominal route for neonatal hernias, and the transpleural approach for hernias repaired later than six months of age. If reduction of the viscera in the abdomen and a layered abdominal wall closure create prohibitive intra-abdominal pressures, additional space may be obtained by the creation of a ventral abdominal Silastic pouch or by just approximating the skin. A further extension of this latter concept has been proposed by Meeker and Snyder (1962), who suggest the construction of a gastrostomy and an intentional ventral hernia when the operation is done in the newborn. Ventral herniorrhaphy may be accomplished after one year of age.

Closure of the posterolateral defect is usually uncomplicated, although the absence of a hemidiaphragm may pose serious technical problems, which have been ingeniously handled by Teflon, Marlex and Ivalon grafts, pedicled abdominal or thoracic wall flaps, and liver. Extreme care should be taken to avoid adrenal injury during the operation, since adrenal damage may contribute to the mortality. An attempt should be made to visualize the lung on the involved side and the presence of a sac.

During the operation, the anesthesiologist cannot forcibly expand the ate-lectatic lung and, accordingly, must exert restraint in breathing for the patient in order to avoid pneumothorax, pneumomediastinum and a bronchopleural fistula. Postoperatively, the serial monitoring of blood gases and pH is continued through an indwelling arterial line, and titration is accomplished with expert assisted ventilation and metabolic support. The arterial line should be placed in the right radial artery to negate the effects of ductal shunting. An umbilical artery line can be employed if right to left shunting is minimal. Chest drainage is used without excessive negative pressure, and in those who survive, the lung will expand within a few days to several weeks. The insertion of a prophylactic chest tube on the contralateral side is gaining support, since pneumothorax is common and the associated mortality may be increased. Current investigational efforts are directed toward the pharmacologic control of pulmonary hypertension and the use of membrane oxygenators until lung maturation occurs.

CONGENITAL EVENTRATION OF THE DIAPHRAGM

Congenital eventration of all or part of one or both diaphragms follows the maldevelopment of diaphragmatic muscle and is commoner than acquired eventration secondary to phrenic nerve paralysis.

Embryologically, there is a complete or partial absence of muscular development in the septum transversum in the presence of normal pleura above and peritoneum below. These two membranes may be in direct juxtaposition or separated by only a thin fibrous sheath; usually, a small rim of muscle lies anteriorly between the pleuroperitoneal folds. Total eventration is said to be more frequent on the left, while a more localized or partial eventration is likely to be on the right side. The lesion has been found in the fetus, along with other local congenital anomalies, such as high renal ectopia and extralobar pulmonary sequestration.

Gross pathologic analysis demonstrates an absence or diminution of the diaphragmatic muscle, which becomes fibrous, thin and abnormally elevated. The phrenic nerve is smaller than normal; on microscopic examination, there is degeneration of the muscle, but not of the nerve.

Symptoms are produced by an extremely elevated diaphragm with minimal or no function, but usually without paradoxical movements compressing the ipsilateral lung. The resultant mediastinal shift and rotation then encroach on the opposite lung. Respiratory findings are compounded by elevation and angulation of the stomach and are exaggerated after eating or when in the Trendelenburg position.

The clinical picture may vary from an asymptomatic, elderly patient to an early neonatal death. It is not unusual to have respiratory distress of the order seen with a Bochdalek hernia, with dyspnea, tachypnea and cyanosis. Physical examination may demonstrate tracheal and cardiac shift, with dullness and absent breath sounds over the involved thorax, as well as a scaphoid upper abdomen and fullness in the region of the lower chest on the involved side. Gastrointestinal complaints of vomiting, flatulence and indigestion

or cough with bronchitis, and repeated pneumonia, may predominate in the older child.

Fluoroscopy and chest roentgenograms are essential to the diagnosis. The degree of diaphragmatic elevation is precisely documented by visualization of a definite, thin, unbroken arc above the abdominal viscera (Fig. 7). At first, diaphragmatic excursions may be properly synchronous, but minimal; later, perhaps, the diaphragm may move paradoxically and create mediastinal flutter. Atelectasis and mediastinal shift are seen.

The differential diagnosis includes: congenital posterolateral diaphragmatic hernia and phrenic nerve paralysis. If the congenital eventration moves paradoxically, it cannot be clinically separated from a hernia with a sac or a diaphragm elevated from nerve injury. In the usual Bochdalek hernia without a sac, however, the remaining diaphragm is difficult to see; when seen, it is located normally and not elevated. Other diagnoses that should be entertained are

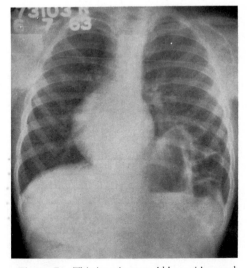

Figure 7. This is a six-year-old boy with a modest, asymptomatic eventration of the diaphragm whose x-ray film was taken during an infrequent respiratory infection. The heart is shifted to the right, and the right diaphragm is intact and at the proper level. The arc of the left diaphragm is elevated two interspaces above the right and surrounds gas-containing abdominal viscera.

various tumors and cysts, Morgagni hernia and perhaps pleural effusion. Barium studies and liver scan, separately or combined, can help in the differential diagnosis.

The course with congenital eventration is as unpredicatable as the symptoms are. Deaths have been reported in the untreated patient, and survival may be complicated by chronic pulmonary suppuration, diaphragmatic rupture, and ulcer and volvulus of the stomach. Usually, however, supportive treatment will suffice in the barely symptomatic infant. With dyspnea and cyanosis in the newborn, eventration should be handled by thoracotomy as urgently as is a Bochdalek hernia. With plication, which lowers the diaphragm, if the phrenic nerve is spared, mortality is low, respiratory distress is promptly abolished, and the immediate and long-term results are eminently satisfactory. The ipsilateral lung function may eventually approach normality. Goulston (1957) has demonstrated the efficacy of operation in older children with chronic gastric and respiratory complaints.

CONGENITAL HIATAL DIAPHRAGMATIC HERNIA

Recent literature emphasizes the frequency of hiatal hernias in the pediatric age group, especially during the first year. The extension of the stomach into the lower part of the chest occurs through an exaggerated crural defect that is usually congenital, but may be acquired by gastric expansion in an upward direction during excessive vomiting. This may explain some of the hiatal hernias associated with pyloric stenosis.

The majority of hiatal protrusions in infancy and childhood are sliding hernias in which the esophagogastric junction is above the crural level of the diaphragm. This particular anatomic configuration abolishes the acute esoph-agogastric angle and, with a wide crural ring, allows free gastric reflux, which produces the symptoms of the disease. The rarer paraesophageal hiatal hernia has a normal esophagogastric junction and crural aperture, the stomach herniating into the chest parallel to the esophagus, but separated from it by strands of diaphragmatic muscle. Incarceration may occur with this arrangement, but reflux is less likely.

Persistent bile-free vomiting, projectile or regurgitant, is found consistently. This may begin soon after birth or start at the third or fourth month, and simulates a late pyloric stenosis. The incessant vomiting may occur at night with aspiration and repeated bouts of pneumonia. Slow growth and development are often systemic manifestations of malnutrition, dehydration and chronic infection. Later, dysphagia from esophageal stricture and chronic pneumonitis with pulmonary fibrosis are seen. A peculiar contortion of the neck with hiatal hernia has been described.

Both hematemesis and melena can be confirmed by the clinical laboratory and are reflected in a blood loss anemia in about a third of patients. The barium swallow with cinefluoroscopy corroborates the diagnosis and the stricture formation, and plain chest films document the aspiration pneumonia (Fig. 8). Burford and Lischer (1956) have emphasized the role of esophagoscopy in detailing the esophagitis and stenosis.

The differential diagnosis in the newborn and the infant involves other entities that produce rumination, chronic, relentless vomiting with failure to thrive, actual malnutrition and depressed growth, repeated pneumonias, upper gastrointestinal tract bleeding, anemia and dysphagia.

In the majority of patients, the hernia is small and symptoms are not critical, although there is no correlation between size and symptoms. In this sizable group, conservative therapy consisting of the continuous upright position (at least 60 degrees), frequent,

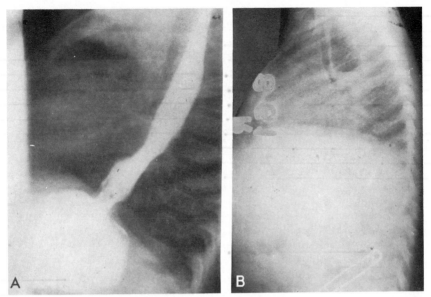

Figure 8.   A seven-month-old male infant with persistent bile-free vomiting, recurrent episodes of aspiration pneumonia and poor weight gain. *A,* The lateral esophagogram reveals minimal dilatation in the region of the middle third, with tapering and irritability of the distal portion of the esophagus. The presence of gastric mucosa above the diaphragm in a hiatal hernia is demonstrated. *B,* One month later, an air-fluid level is seen in the posterior mediastinum at the level of the carina with considerable dilatation of the proximal part of the esophagus, documenting the progression of the stricture secondary to the hiatal hernia. A transthoracic approach to this sliding hiatal hernia with repair and dilatation resulted in complete rehabilitation.

small, thickened feedings and antispasmodics will suffice. Conservative therapy should be exhausted (up to 10 weeks) before operative intervention is undertaken; 80 to 90 per cent of lesions will respond to conservative measures, usually within three to four weeks. Surgical repair, either thoracic or abdominal, is reserved for patients who fail to grow and develop normally, continue with bleeding, are developing a stricture and accordingly are considered medical failures. Hiatal herniorrhaphy can reverse this sequence of events by obliterating the hernial sac and reconstructing the normal esophagogastric junction and angle. The operation should occlude the patulous hiatus, anchor the esophagus below the diaphragm, and reinstate the acute gastroesophageal angle. While many still favor anterior gastropexy, the operation of choice may be the Nissen funduplication with crural suturing. This gives the lowest recurrence rate with an acceptable result. The morbidity and mortality following a technically satisfactory procedure are quite good, with relief of symptoms occurring in about 90 per cent or more of patients. The pylorus should always be evaluated for its role in the genesis of this problem. If any delay in gastric emptying is present or if the vagi are injured at surgery, a pyloroplasty or pyloromyotomy should be done.

CHYLOTHORAX

Pleural chylous effusion is a rare but important reason for neonatal respiratory distress because the prognosis is fairly optimistic with conservative therapy.

Chylothorax, which occurs later in infancy or childhood, follows accidental trauma, left thoracotomy (usually for congenital cardiovascular anomalies), mediastinal tumor and infection. In the newborn, the etiologic factors are less precise. It has been reported after repair of a Bochdalek hernia. The basic noniatrogenic defect probably involves a malformation of the mediastinal and pulmonary lymphatics, with failure of orderly fusion and the production of multiple lymphatic fistulas. This may explain the generalized sources of chylous fluid found at postmortem examination.

The remainder of the lymphatic system is usually normal, although widespread lymphangiomatous disease has been reported. Males are afflicted twice as often as females. The effusions are more common on the right.

A newborn may present with the usual stigmata of respiratory distress—dyspnea, tachypnea and cyanosis without evidence of sepsis. On physical examination, the mediastinum is displaced with unilateral dullness and diminished breath sounds, although bilaterality has been reported at least once. Chest roentgenograms demonstrate opacification, usually on the right, with verification of the mediastinal shift.

The respiratory problem, which is secondary to compression atelectasis and mediastinal shift, is promptly relieved by aspiration of clear pleural fluid, which turns opalescent only after milk has been digested. The withdrawal of pleural chyle, with a concentration of lipids greater than 400 mg. per 100 ml., establishes the diagnosis, of course, and thoracenteses are continued until the pleural cavity remains dry. Varying numbers of thoracenteses have been used to control the effusion, which usually has a protein content about 1 gm. per 100 ml. Ancillary help can be provided by a medium chain triglyceride, low fat, high protein, high caloric diet. Parenteral hyperalimentation should be used if diet has failed to reduce chyle production.

In some instances, the chylothorax has persisted in spite of multiple aspirations and intercostal tube drainage, and thoracotomy was performed. In one patient, operated on by Randolph and Gross (1957), ligation of the thoracic duct controlled the lymphatic extravasation. Pleurodesis with iodized talc may have a place. Today, with diet and hyperalimentation, operation should rarely be necessary.

Although the overall prognosis is favorable, death may occur from infection and malnutrition, and mortality rates have been reported as high as 25 per cent in some series.

TRACHEAL AGENESIS AND STENOSIS

Aplasia, atresia or agenesis of the trachea is a rare congenital anomaly that to date seems incompatible with life. It would seem to occur because of a malformation in the development of the laryngotracheal groove.

Basically, the defect consists of partial or more often complete absence of the trachea below the larynx or cricoid, main stem bronchi that join in the midline, and a bronchoesophageal or tracheoesophageal fistula in 80 per cent of cases. The lungs may show lobulation abnormalities or intrapulmonary hemorrhage.

Clinically, these patients have respiratory problems at birth and die within a few hours. In at least one instance, the diagnosis was suspected and confirmed, and reconstructive surgery ingeniously performed, with survival of the patient for six weeks. Intragastric oxygen at birth may prolong life if a fistula is present, and thus permit emergency surgical treatment. In Fonkalsrud's (1963) case, surgery consisted of division of the cervical esophagus with utilization of the proximal end as a salivary fistula and the distal stoma for the airway, division of the esophagus below the congenital esophagobronchial fistula and gastrostomy. To date, there has been no satisfactory surgically treated case with long-term survival. This may have to await further progress in transplantation or prosthetics.

Congenital stenosis of the trachea has been reported by Holinger (1957) as a fibrous stricture in the form of webs; these are usually located in the subglottic area or just above the carina, although diffuse involvement has also been recorded. Respiratory difficulty is characterized by stridor. The diagnosis may be suspected on plain lateral x-ray films of the neck and chest, and the stenosis confirmed by contrast tracheogram or tracheoscopy. Dilatation alone has not been particularly helpful, and tracheostomy may be necessary for acute respiratory problems. Successful transthoracic repair has been reported by Cantrell and Guild (1964). If possible, observation and conservative therapy should be exhausted, since growth at the stenotic area can eventuate in an adequate lumen. Othersen (1974) has recorded the use of intraluminal stenting with large-dose steroid injection into the stenotic area in a congenital subglottic stenosis.

TRACHEOMALACIA

In infancy, the tracheal lumen is largely maintained by tracheal cartilages. If cartilaginous rings are congenitally absent, small, malformed or too pliable, essential support is lacking, and such lack may lead to a functional tracheal stenosis and obstruction. This primary tracheomalacia is an unusual but usually benign form of respiratory distress in the newborn and the young infant, and must be distinguished from the secondary type produced by extrinsic compression from a vascular ring or mediastinal tumor. The same pathologic process may be localized to a bronchus with resultant congenital lobar emphysema.

Tracheal expansion and contraction occur with inspiration and expiration, respectively; these variations in airway size are minimized during sleep and shallow respiration, and are exaggerated by forceful breathing, as with crying. With incomplete structural support of the trachea, the normal luminal narrowing during expiration becomes exaggerated, and in severe instances the lumen may be small for inspiration.

Clinically, there may be wheezing, cough, stridor, dyspnea, tachypnea and cyanosis, and these are made worse by pulmonary sepsis and secretions. On physical examination, expiration is prolonged, and there may be emphysema, but there is no localization by auscultation except with secondary infection. Opisthotonos has been reported. The neck, the mouth and the pharynx are normal; ear cartilage may be absent. Chest roentgenograms are almost invariably done on inspiration, and the lungs may be exceptionally well aerated. Lateral films of the neck and chest taken during inspiration and, if possible, expiration may be helpful in the diagnosis.

The esophagogram is normal, but a contrast tracheogram done with cinefluorography in the lateral view may demonstrate the abnormal tracheal wall mobility. Laryngoscopy is normal down to the vocal cords, which, too, may be excessively soft; the combination of laryngotracheomalacia is not unusual. Careful bronchoscopy under local anesthesia with inspection of the entire trachea may show close approximation of the anterior and posterior tracheal walls near the carina at any phase of respiration, but most often during expiration. Passage of the bronchoscope to the carina is followed by less respiratory distress, since the flaccid area is splinted.

The differential diagnosis involves a vascular ring, mediastinal tumor, tracheal web, foreign body, and obstructive lesions of the upper airway. Unfortunately, the ultimate diagnosis of tracheomalacia must often be established by exclusion. The positive findings of excessive tracheal wall mobility and airway relief with the passage of the bronchoscope are at times arbitrary and inconclusive.

Treatment involves the control of infection and secretions by specific antibiotics and humidification. Conservative therapy should be persistent, since cartilaginous development will eventually support the airway, and this may be correlated with concomitant stiffening of the aural cartilages. Clinical improvement is definite in the majority of cases by six months of age, and spontaneous recovery in the remainder may be anticipated at one year. Tracheostomy has been used, but is rarely indicated.

VASCULAR RING

In 1945, Gross inaugurated the current surgical management of vascular ring anomalies, over 200 years after their morphologic description. Since then, documentation of this early contribution to cardiovascular surgery has been profuse.

Although numerous variations from the normal aortic arch development have been reported, only a few distinct patterns can produce extrinsic tracheal obstruction, and even these may be incidental findings without clinical correlation. The most likely types that compromise the trachea or esophagus, singly or together, are (1) right aortic arch with left ligamentum arteriosum or patent ductus arteriosus; (2) double aortic arch; (3) anomalous innominate or left carotid artery; and (4) aberrant right subclavian artery. The right aortic arch and double aortic arch account for the largest number.

(1) A right aortic arch represents a persistent right fourth brachial vessel, which normally disappears. If this artery, in front of the trachea, is combined with a ductus or a ligamentum arteriosum that runs behind the esophagus, circular incarceration of the trachea and esophagus has taken place, and symptoms may follow. This anomaly has been reported to be more common in males as opposed to the double aortic arch, which is allegedly more common in females.

(2) With double aortic arch, the ascending aorta bifurcates and sends one branch to the right of the trachea and esophagus and then posterior to the esophagus to help form the descending aorta after joining the second branch of the arch, which proceeded in front and to the left of the trachea. Again, a ring is fashioned, and there may be respiratory distress.

(3) Anomalous innominate or left carotid arteries may produce direct anterior pressure on the tracheal wall because of delayed or premature takeoff from the arch. Thus, the innominate origin from the arch is to the left of its normal source, while the left carotid arises to the right of its usual site. Both vessels must then run over the tracheal cartilages to reach their eventual destination, and in so doing may produce a pressure phenomenon.

(4) The aberrant right subclavian artery is most often asymptomatic, but may constrict the posterior esophageal wall and produce dysphagia as it courses from the descending aorta toward the right and behind the esophagus. It is not likely to produce respiratory symptoms.

The common denominator in these arch anomalies is compression and narrowing of the tracheoesophageal complex. Air exchange is impeded, especially expiration. There is interference with deglutition, and esophageal distention proximal to the area of obstruction may further constrict the narrowed trachea. Respiratory tract secretions are usually increased and poorly handled. Aspiration becomes almost inevitable.

The clinical findings begin early, usually in the first year of life, and are most acute with a double aortic arch; they usually begin later and are less acute with a right aortic arch associated with an encircling ligamentum or ductus, and are still less acute with anomalies that produce pressure only anteriorly, such as aberrant left carotid and innominate arteries.

Signs and symptoms frequently start in the nursery with raucous respirations, intercostal retraction, dyspnea and tachypnea. There is an invariable exacerbation of the respiratory problem with feedings, and cyanosis with coughing is likely at this time. On examination, the chest may be slightly emphysematous, expiration is prolonged, and stridor is apparent. Auscultation may demonstrate expiratory wheezing and rhonchi that are diffuse and sometimes transmitted. Opisthotonos has been emphasized, and neck flexion is not tolerated.

Plain x-ray films in the conventional views may show unusually well aerated lungs, migatory atelectasis, pneumonia, and sometimes a right aortic arch. Chest roentgenograms may fail, however, to explain the respiratory difficulty. On good lateral films, the trachea may be narrowed just above the carina. Contrast material in the esophagus will document various combinations of posterior or lateral indentations at the same level as the tracheal constriction (Fig. 9). A normal esophagogram will exclude a critically symptomatic vascular ring, and this becomes the funda-

mental diagnostic study. Endoscopy will confirm these findings, and compression of the posterior esophageal pulsatile bulge by the scope with loss of right radial pulse is diagnostic of an aberrant right subclavian artery. If respiratory distress is not critical, contrast material in the trachea will delineate the anterior tracheal wall compression. In the infant, this can be done without general anesthesia by direct tracheal instillation or by overflow from the hypopharynx.

The presence of a vascular ring can be proved by angiocardiography (Fig. 10). This demonstration in the presence of clinical symptoms and roentgenographic or endoscopic evidence of tracheoesophageal compression secures the diagnosis. In addition, contrast studies may facilitate the dissection and uncover other cardiovascular anomalies that were clinically unsuspected. This can be of particular significance with a right aortic arch, since there is a high incidence of associated intracardiac anomalies.

The differential diagnosis involves

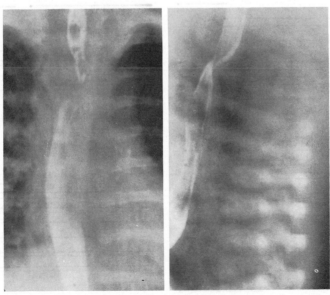

Figure 9.   A posteroanterior and lateral barium swallow demonstrates encirclement of the esophagus at the level of the aortic arch in a two-month-old infant with dyspnea and noisy respirations. There is narrowing of the lumen from extrinsic pressure with forward displacement, noted best in the lateral projection. The posteroanterior film shows minimal deviation to the left, with tapering of the esophagus proximal to a horizontal area of constriction.

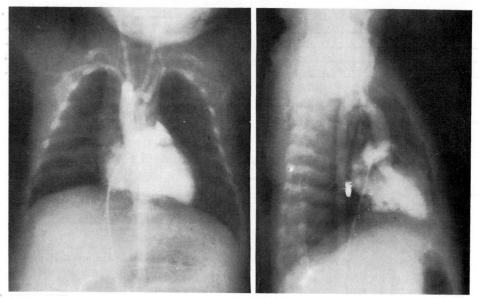

Figure 10. Selected posteroanterior and lateral films from a venous angiocardiogram, done by Dr. Page Mauck, through the right atrium, foramen ovale and left atrium demonstrates two separate, contrast-filled channels originating at the superior aspect of the ascending aorta. On the lateral view, the larger superior posterior arch and smaller inferior anterior limb fuse posteriorly at the origin of the descending aorta. In the two composite films, the innominate artery arises prior to the formation of the double arch, while the left-sided branches arise from the smaller anterior limb. In the frontal projection, the posterior arch has a short diagonal course to the left and downward before merging to form the descending aorta.

the clinical picture of respiratory distress, stridor and dysphagia. Cervical and hypopharyngeal obstruction can be ruled out by physical examination of the neck and the mouth and by laryngoscopy. Mediastinal tumors and most foreign bodies are excluded by the radiographs. This restricts the diagnostic possibilities to a vascular ring, tracheal stenosis, tracheoesophageal fistula without atresia, and tracheomalacia. The esophagogram is the next step in the orderly establishment of the diagnosis and begins to limit the possibilities.

After the diagnosis has been established, a short period of observation is useful, since only those patients with severe symptoms, recurrent respiratory infections, failure to thrive, dysphagia, and respiratory distress should be considered for surgery (Mustard, 1962). With prolonged hospitalization, however, a considerable mortality arises from the natural course of the disease, especially with a double aortic arch or right

arch–left ligamentum arteriosum. Death may be sudden, due to compression or sepsis, and may be secondary to pneumonia. In the severely symptomatic infant, tube feeding, frequent pharyngeal suction, specific antibiotic therapy, high humidity and controlled oxygen and temperature are indispensable in the preoperative period. Careful, direct tracheal aspiration may be appropriate at this time.

The surgical treatment for an offensive vascular ring is now fairly standard. In all cases, careful attention should be paid to the anatomy of the recurrent laryngeal nerve. With right aortic arch and a ligamentum arteriosum, division of the latter provides relief. A double aortic arch will require division of the smaller arch, usually the anterior one. The ligamentum or ductus should also be interrupted, and the remnant of the anterior arch sutured to the undersurface of the sternum without separation from the trachea (Fig. 11). Inspection and palpation

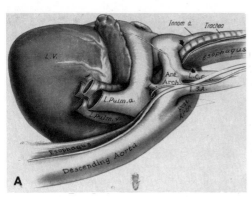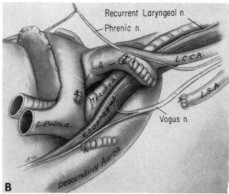

Figure 11. *A*, The operative findings through a left posterolateral fourth interspace incision confirm the presence of a double aortic arch. *B*, The left subclavian artery and ligamentum arteriosum were divided, and the smaller anterior arch was transected well to the left of the origin of the left common carotid artery. The remnant of the anterior arch may then be sutured to the undersurface of the sternum without being separated from the trachea.

of the lateral tracheal walls may reveal a cartilaginous deformity, which might alter the postoperative course.

Surgical intervention for an aberrant left carotid artery is rarely required. When indicated, it consists in displacement of the vessel rather than division. An innominate artery, usually but not always aberrant (Mustard and co-workers, 1969), may be a significant factor in producing varying degrees of tracheal obstruction by anterior tracheal compression. In severe cases, the diagnosis is suggested by a "reflex apneic" syndrome in the presence of other signs and symptoms of vascular ring and is confirmed by contrast esophagram, cinetracheography, endoscopy, and aortic angiography. The vast majority of patients can be treated medically, but about 10 per cent will need suspension of the innominate artery and base of the aorta to the sternum. This enlarges the tracheal lumen by drawing the anterior tracheal wall forward.

The immediate postoperative period after vascular ring surgery may be precarious because operative and anesthetic trauma may compromise the airway. Most complications occur in association with those cases having a double aortic arch. Attention should be paid to the possibility of malacia of the trachea or a main stem bronchus and its effect on postoperative respirations. Fortunately, tracheostomy is rarely required. The stridor usually disappears, and feedings are taken without choking or aspiration. Respirations are not affected by flexion or extension of the head, but the loud nature persists for a few months.

Operative results are uniformly good, and relief from the respiratory distress is predictable. Surgical mortality and morbidity rates are low.

TRACHEOESOPHAGEAL FISTULA WITHOUT ESOPHAGEAL ATRESIA

Instances of communication between the trachea and the esophagus with an otherwise normal esophagus occur in about 3 per cent of tracheoesophageal fistulas, and according to Schneider and Becker (1962), approximately 28 such infants are born each year in the United States. Although symptoms from this congenital abnormality are fairly gross, the diagnosis is usually delayed, and a considerable amount of respiratory morbidity is likely to result (Fig. 12). This is unfortunate, since babies with an H-type fistula have a

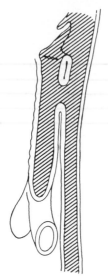

Figure 12. Diagram of tracheoesophageal fistula without esophageal atresia. The actual communication is much smaller than depicted.

lower incidence of anomalies and higher birth weight than newborns with other types of tracheoesophageal fistula.

The tracheoesophageal connection is almost always small, and the majority are found in the neck, from below the larynx to the thoracic inlet. With this arrangement, the lungs become, in essence, a diverticulum of the esophagus, and continuous and relentless pulmonary soiling is the basis for extensive pulmonary infection.

The diagnosis should be considered in the presence of recurrent pneumonitis without clear cause, or when bouts of coughing, choking or cyanosis follow the ingestion of fluids. There is no dysphagia, and solids may be swallowed and gavage feedings given without difficulty. On physical examination, gastric distention is prominent, especially after crying and coughing, as air is fed through the fistula into the esophagus and the stomach. The lung fields are noisy after liquid feedings, but clear before such feedings. The severity of symptoms may parallel the size of the fistula.

Plain chest roentgenograms often demonstrate the stigma of chronic pulmonary sepsis, especially in the right upper lobe. In addition, attempts should be made to visualize the fistula by x-ray examination or endoscopy. Utilization of the Storz scopes with the Hopkins telescopic lens system has made this approach extremely profitable. Esophagograms in the various prone positions may be fruitful, especially if cinefluoroscopy is used. With continuous recording of the contrast swallow, filling of the trachea through a fistula can be distinguished from overflow aspiration, and abnormal peristalsis of the esophagus distal to the fistula sometimes may be visualized. Several examinations may be necessary for radiographic diagnosis. Esophagoscopy and bronchoscopy are very likely to demonstrate the specific orifices, and dyes, such as methylene blue inserted into one lumen, may be recovered in the other lumen, especially if the esophagus distal to the fistula is occluded with a Foley catheter. This diagnosis may be difficult to substantiate, but repeated studies should be done until it is confirmed. Surgery should not be done without a definitive diagnostic study.

The differential diagnosis of this variant of tracheoesophageal fistula should include chronic bacterial pulmonary disease, chalasia, achalasia, hiatal hernia, cystic fibrosis, neurogenic dysphagia, vascular ring and agammaglobulinemia.

Operative division and suture of the fistula through a transcervical approach are very satisfactory in most instances. Very few must be handled transthoracically. The operative mortality rate is reasonable, and deaths are largely due to the crippling nature of the chronic pulmonary disease in patients whose diagnosis has not been prompt.

ESOPHAGEAL ATRESIA

The various types of esophageal atresia compose an important segment of those congenital abnormalities that produce respiratory distress in the newborn.

The commonest anatomic configuration of this primitive foregut anomaly, with an incidence of 85 per cent, is esophageal atresia with distal tracheoesophageal fistula. In perhaps 5 to 10 per cent of the cases of esophageal atresia, there is no fistula between the distal esophagus and the trachea (Fig. 13). Atresia with proximal tracheoesophageal fistula and tracheal fistula from both upper and lower esophageal pouches present infrequently.

The incidence of this anomaly has been variously recorded, but one in 3500 births is a reasonable census, and males predominate. At least 25 per cent are premature, and the same percentage have additional critical malformations, such as congenital heart disease, mongolism, hydronephrosis, duodenal atresia and tracheomalacia; 10 per cent of these babies will have an imperforate anus, and one-half will have vertebral anomalies.

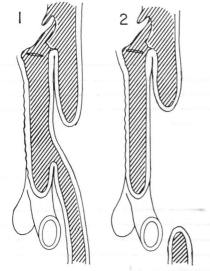

Figure 13. By far the commonest morphologic variation of esophageal atresia is proximal atresia with distal tracheoesophageal fistula (1). Much less frequent is proximal atresia without a tracheoesophageal fistula in which the distal part of the esophagus, seen diagrammatically, actually ends blindly just above the crura of the diaphragm (2).

Aberrations in the development of the primary, common respiratory-digestive anlage form the basis for this anomaly. Separation into the anterior pulmonary and posterior gut components by fusion of internal septa is incomplete and may explain the presence of communications or fistulas. A complete lack of septal ingrowth is associated with the more serious, related deformity of laryngotracheoesophageal cleft. The intrauterine interruption of the vascular supply to the esophagus, vascular anomalies with constriction, or the failure of intraluminal esophageal vacuolization may explain the atresia.

Gross pathologic information is useful in the diagnosis and management of this lesion. With the usual proximal atresia and distal fistula arrangement, the upper blind pouch is large and substantial, and usually ends about 8 cm. from the superior alveolar ridge in the region of the azygos vein. The arterial supply from the inferior thyroid artery is rich, runs in a vertical manner, and is difficult to interrupt. Conversely, the lower segment is small and flimsy and originates from the region of the distal posterior membranous trachea, carina or right main stem bronchus. Its arteries are distributed radially from the intercostals, and a small tracheal vessel may nourish the esophageal end of the tracheoesophageal fistula. Accordingly, ischemia and necrosis of the distal esophagus are constant hazards of the operative dissection. Congenital stenosis and a diaphragm-like atresia below the tracheoesophageal fistula in the distal esophagus have been reported.

The attachment of the lower part of the esophagus to the region of the bifurcation of the trachea places this segment in some juxtaposition to the upper pouch. Fortunately, in a fourth of such cases, the two muscle walls are in actual contact and anastomosis is relatively simple; in the remaining three-fourths, the anastomosis is more difficult because the segments are separated by a gap varying from 1 mm. to several centimeters. In the 5 to 10 per cent of atresias without fistula, the proximal esophagus is similar to its counterpart in the more usual variance, but the distal esophagus is actually a small gastric diverticulum that barely extends above the diaphragmatic crura and, of course, ends blindly. The two segments are widely separated and cannot be joined surgically in the immediate postnatal period.

The respiratory distress sustained by newborns with proximal atresia and distal fistula is instigated by three factors. Obviously, secretions that collect in the upper pouch may overflow into the trachea. Second, gastric juice refluxes through the tracheoesophageal fistula and floods the lungs. Finally, the fistula provides a convenient route for gastric distention, upward displacement of the diaphragm and critical interference with pulmonary function.

The clinical picture begins with a history of hydramnios in 25 per cent of the mothers. Profuse, bubbly, oral mucus appears early and almost continuously covers the baby's chin in spite of persistent oropharyngeal aspiration. Tachypnea and dyspnea soon follow, with intermittent episodes of choking and cyanosis. Regurgitation promptly occurs after the initial and subsequent feedings, and the aspiration explosively exacerbates the respiratory distress. This latter finding is exaggerated in the rare atresia with a proximal fistula, since the ingested liquid reaches the lungs directly through the fistula as well as by overflow of the proximal pouch. On further examination, the abdomen is protuberant, flatus is quickly and incessantly passed, and consolidation may be demonstrated in the region of the right upper lobe. If the abnormality is an atresia without a fistula, the incidence of maternal hydramnios may be higher, pulmonary consolidation may be lower, and the abdomen is scaphoid. Otherwise, the findings in these two groups are similar.

Thoracoabdominal roentgenograms in conventional views may show consolidation of the right upper lobe or more diffuse pneumonitis. Air in the gastrointestinal tract is seen with the usual atresia and distal fistula, although it is said that small fistulas may prevent air from leaking into the stomach. Conversely, large amounts of gastric air may suggest a large fistula, and therapy becomes more urgent because of the exaggerated respiratory distress. An airless abdomen is presumptive evidence of atresia without a distal fistula. On lateral thoracic x-ray films, the proximal atretic pouch may be delineated by air, but this is made clearer by the insertion of a small radiopaque urethral catheter under fluoroscopy. Coiling of a fairly stiff catheter at a level between the second and fourth thoracic vertebrae concludes the regional diagnostic exercise. Contrast material should not be necessary. When used, it should be restricted to a small amount (0.5 ml.) of water-soluble material. Gastrografin is especially irritating and should be avoided. The contrast material should be aspirated at the conclusion of the examination (Fig. 14). Delays in diagnosis could be avoided if orogastric catheterization follows pharyngeal suctioning in newborns, preferably with the same catheter.

These and other diagnostic studies are utilized to establish the presence of additional anomalies that may affect therapy. Thus, the mediastinal dissection can be more readily performed if a right-sided aortic arch has been noted preoperatively. Congenital heart, cerebral, gastrointestinal and neurologic anomalies must be considered and uncovered with some dispatch before the correct operative approach can be planned. Associated cardiovascular anomalies are particularly lethal.

The diagnosis of atresia with fistula should be strongly suspected, then, on the basis of maternal hydramnios, excessive mucus, respiratory distress and regurgitation. The suspicion is strengthened by the passage of a catheter into the esophagus that stops 6 to 8 cm. from the gums. The final confirmation is obtained by fluoroscopic examination.

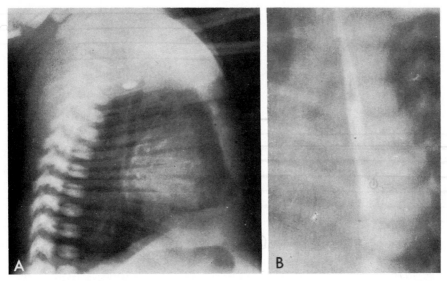

Figure 14. *A,* Lateral upright chest roentgenogram after instillation of 0.5 ml. of contrast material into the esophagus defines the atresia at the level of the fourth thoracic vertebra. There is gas in the stomach. *B,* A spot film three weeks after surgical repair demonstrates an adequate, undistorted lumen.

Preoperatively, the upper pouch is aspirated through an indwelling catheter. A semiupright position should be maintained during transportation or in the nursery Isolette to prevent or minimize gastric reflux through the fistula, although the Trendelenburg position has been advocated by some. High humidity and antibiotics are used to control pneumonia. Constant nursing of a high order should be started on admission and continued until the issue is no longer in doubt.

The operative management of isolated atresia without a fistula requires esophageal elongation and approximation of the blind ends by bouginage or an eventual reversed gastric tube or colon transplant, since the two ends of the esophagus are widely separated and cannot be anastomosed. The operation immediately after diagnosis is gastrostomy under local anesthesia. Contrast study through the stomach with the infant in sharp Trendelenburg position will outline the short, blind, distal esophageal stump. The proximal pouch is drained by a nasal sump type catheter, and the gastrostomy tube is used for feeding. Both pouches are then elongated toward each other by bouginage until sufficient proximity for an anastomosis is obtained. If this maneuver is not successful, a cervical esophagostomy is created to drain saliva, and esophageal replacement is anticipated at 18 months of age. The same steps can be followed when a large gap prevents anastomosis in the usual variety of atresia (Fig. 15).

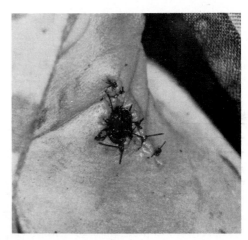

Figure 15. Proximal esophagostomy, or salivary fistula, in the right side of the neck of a newborn with esophageal atresia without fistula.

Several operative approaches are available for atresia with distal fistula. The ultimate decision is based on the degree of prematurity, presence of other anomalies, time of diagnosis, presence or absence of pneumonia, exact anatomic configuration of the lesion, and preference of the surgeon. Transpleural or extrapleural ligation of the fistula and end-to-end or end-to-side esophagoesophagostomy with or without gastrostomy are ideal and constitute the accepted approach in the full-term newborn with no serious anomalies or pneumonia. Varying degrees of prematurity, pneumonitis and concomitant abnormalities drastically alter mortality, so that staged procedures have assumed some popularity in certain clinics. Gastrostomy alone may be chosen as the primary, emergency step to decompress the fistula and control the pneumonia. To this can be added parenteral hyperalimentation or a duodenal feeding tube along with suction of the proximal esophageal pouch. Meeker and Snyder (1962), Randolph and coworkers (1968) and Touloukian and coworkers (1974) have individually suggested transabdominal gastric division and double gastrostomy for the critically affected premature infant. Feedings are instilled into the distal tube, decompression of the tracheoesophageal fistula is accomplished through the proximal tube, and the thorax is not molested. Under ideal circumstances, these arrangements are commensurate with improvement in the size and health of the patient in preparation for definitive surgery. If these temporizing measures are inadequate, extrapleural ligation of the fistula and fixation of the oversewn distal esophagus to the endothoracic fascia permits feeding while the upper pouch remains on continuous or intermittent suction. With good nursing care, this arrangement is compatible with growth and development, and the esophageal anastomosis may be accomplished at a time of election in a better-risk infant. If such nursing cannot be provided, aspiration pneumonia from the upper pouch is almost inevitable, and in these circumstances, the very premature infant had best be committed to a salivary fistula and esophageal substitute. This is less than ideal, but the mortality is a distinct improvement over that of primary repair in this group.

The acute postoperative period is critical and deserves maximum attention. The respiratory tract is especially vulnerable, and prophylaxis is the therapeutic goal. All the advantages of an Isolette are utilized. The pharynx must be carefully aspirated, without injury to the fresh anastomosis, to prevent aspiration and stimulate coughing. Feedings should be started on the second to fourth postoperative day with homeopathic amounts of glucose water and formula, initially administered by slow drip through the gastrostomy tube. Oral feedings are started with a 0.6 ml. medicine dropper; this minimal volume can be handled by the proximal esophagus and its anastomosis without overflow (Potts). This should be done after a barium swallow has verified a patent anastomosis without leaks.

Complications are legion, but the most catastrophic is disruption of the suture line and resultant empyema. The initial mortality from this can be lessened by an extrapleural operative approach, which would confine the contamination to an extrapleural plane. Definitive treatment consists of effective naso–upper esophageal pouch and gastric catheter drainage along with duodenal feeding or parenteral hyperalimentation. The brassy postoperative cough is usually temporary and not related to a recurrence of the fistula, which does occur in about 10 per cent of cases with a rather high mortality. This complication can be diagnosed nicely by esophagoscopy with the instillation of methylene blue through an endotracheal tube. Anastomotic strictures occur within three months in one-fourth of the survivors and are heralded by dysphagia, regurgitation, cough and recurrent pneumonia (Fig. 16). Treatment at first consists of dilatation, started on the basis of dysphagia corre-

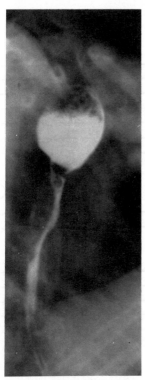

Figure 16. A barium swallow in a one-year-old male infant with dysphagia who was born with proximal esophageal atresia and distal tracheoesophageal fistula managed by ligation of the fistula and esophagoesophagostomy in one stage. This single film shows gross saccular dilatation of the proximal esophagus above an area of stricture at the level of the anastomosis. Several dilatations over a string provided an adequate lumen.

lated with changes on the roentgenogram. Resection has been advised for recalcitrant strictures, and perhaps should be combined with a gastric antireflux procedure. Postoperative pneumonia can also be instigated by faulty motility of the distal esophagus with reflux following operative vagus nerve damage.

The overall rate of survivors today with primary definitive operations from a generous aliquot of children's and general hospitals approaches 70 per cent; this is elevated to 90 per cent of full-term newborns who are otherwise normal. Primary anastomosis in small babies with severe pneumonia or anomalies carries a 60 to 70 per cent mortality rate, but this can be reversed with

operative staging. However, primary repair should not be denied a marginally small baby because of size alone.

CONGENITAL BRONCHIAL STENOSIS

Congenital stricture of the bronchus occurs predominantly in a main stem or middle lobe bronchus and can produce acute and chronic pulmonary infection (Swenson, 1962). Inflammatory scarring of the congenitally stenosed bronchus provides an ideal environment for distal suppuration, atelectasis and bronchiectasis.

Chest roentgenograms will demonstrate various stages of pneumonitis, atelectasis and perhaps compensatory emphysema.

Bronchoscopy and bronchography confirm the diagnosis.

Treatment consists of the resection of uncomplicated localized stenosis of main stem bronchi, with varying degrees of lung resection for more diffuse, complicated and distal lesions.

BRONCHOGENIC CYST

Congenital intrathoracic tumors of bronchogenic origin are found in the posterior or middle mediastinum, most often in its midthird, behind or close to the tracheobronchial tree and often attached to it by an obliterated or patent stalk. They account for less then 5 per cent of mediastinal masses in infants and children. These malformations are usually single, more frequent on the right, and associated with local bronchovascular anomalies, including a systemic pulmonary blood supply. A few bronchogenic cysts have been reported within the esophagus, pericardium and pulmonary parenchyma. In the latter location, the cysts may be multilocular.

Embryologically, respiratory tissue, at various stages of development, becomes pinched off and separated, and the eventual location and histologic features of the bronchogenic cyst depend partly on the time of this dislocation from the main respiratory body. Early partition from the foregut produces a cyst with some similarity to esophageal and gastroenteric duplications. Later cystic development from distal bronchoalveolar structures may simulate congenital pulmonary cysts.

The majority of bronchogenic cysts will be paratracheal, carinal, hilar or paraesophageal in location (Maier, 1948), between 2 and 10 cm. in diameter and unilocular, and have a substantial wall and contain mucus, pus or blood. On microscopic examination, there is a lining of ciliated columnar respiratory epithelium surrounded by disorganized muscle, cartilage and fibrous tissue.

There may be some difficulty, pathologically and clinically, in separating congenital bronchogenic cysts from acquired cysts and abscesses, especially in the older infant and the child. The presence of respiratory epithelium lining a cyst in embryos and newborns is considered evidence of a congenital abnormality. Unfortunately, secondary infection can obliterate this characteristic lining, and subsequent healing may occur with bronchial mucosa; the final histologic picture, then, is similar to an epithelialized, chronic lung abscess.

Clinical findings are based on (1) proximal tracheobronchial obstruction producing atelectasis or emphysema with respiratory distress, (2) moderate obstruction with distal pulmonary sepsis and (3) suppuration of the cyst by contamination through a tracheobronchial communication. This may be followed by slough of the respiratory epithelium and replacement by granulation tissue with chronic infection. Finally, (4) some cysts are asymptomatic and are diagnosed only by routine x-ray examination or x-ray films taken for some other reason.

Carinal cysts usually produce dramatic symptoms of respiratory obstruction in infancy, and the distress parallels the size of the cyst to the point of sudden death (Fig. 17). Cysts in other locations are more likely to become infected or lead to repeated pulmonary parenchymal infection in the older infant and the child. The clinical picture may mimic a lung abscess with fever, chest pain, wheezing, cough, dysphagia, hemoptysis, purulent sputum, and plain or push-up stridor.

The diagnosis may be suspected after x-ray examination of the chest by various techniques, although unfortu-

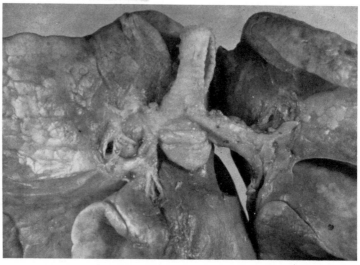

Figure 17.   Autopsy specimen of a carinal bronchogenic cyst.

nately, some infants with severe respiratory distress can have very subtle roentgenographic changes (Fig. 18). Fluoroscopic or cineradiographic visualization of ascent with swallowing is possible if a firm tracheal attachment is present. Displacement, separation and compression of the trachea and esophagus and elevation of the carina with flattening of the bronchial angle can also be seen at the same examination.

Chest roentgenograms can document these findings and demonstrate a solitary, smooth-walled, noncalcified tumor widening the mediastinum on one or both sides and sometimes associated with pneumonia, atelectasis or emphysema. With a tracheobronchial communication, a fluid level in a thickwalled cyst should arouse suspicion. Planigrams, bronchograms and endoscopy are occasionally helpful (Fig. 19).

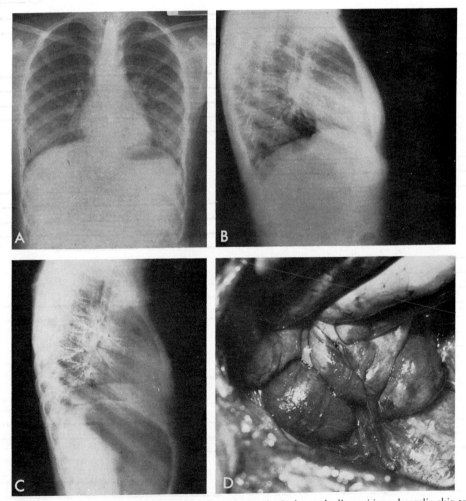

Figure 18.   A ten-year-old girl, exposed to tuberculosis, who had a markedly positive tuberculin skin test reaction. A mediastinal mass did not regress after six months of therapy in a sanatorium. *A, B,* The posteroanterior and lateral chest films show a normal cardiovascular silhouette. There is a mass posterior to the border of the right side of the heart with smooth margins, which covers almost two interspaces. The lateral film localizes the density to the area beneath the right hilus. The mass is denser than surrounding lung, but more radiolucent than the heart. The lung fields are otherwise not remarkable. *C,* A lateral bronchogram shows no filling of the middle lobe, with adequate filling elsewhere. *D,* At thoracotomy, a bilobed bronchogenic cyst, in the region of the inferior pulmonary vein and ligament, was resected.

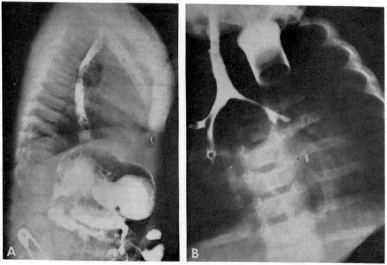

Figure 19. A two-month-old infant with intermittent, severe respiratory distress. *A*, A lateral film with a barium-filled esophagus demonstrates an irregular, smoothly marginated radiolucency in the midmediastinum at the level of the carina with slight narrowing of the esophagus at this level. *B*, The anteroposterior tracheo-bronchogram reveals widening of the tracheal bifurcation and narrowing of the left main stem bronchus by extrinsic pressure. Within the limbs of the two main stem bronchi is an area of radiolucency with smooth borders, compatible with an air-filled cyst under tension. A bronchogenic cyst attached to the left main stem bronchus was removed.

Low-lying mediastinal cysts or even those centrally located may be difficult to separate from a host of other mediastinal tumors. The differential diagnosis includes diaphragmatic hernia, tuberculosis, pyogenic lung abscess, sarcoidosis, emphysema, lymphoma, teratoma, hamartoma, mediastinal granuloma, metastatic lung tumors, sequestration, pneumatocele and pulmonary cysts.

Since a bronchogenic cyst may rupture into a bronchus or pleura, bleed profusely, become badly infected and produce sudden death, early diagnosis is imperative, and surgical intervention should be utilized, unless there is some serious contraindication, in order to establish a diagnosis and avoid annoying or catastrophic sequelae. The actual surgical exercise involves resection of the cyst alone or with various amounts of pulmonary tissue surrounding the cyst. Aberrant systemic arteries and bronchial anomalies can be troublesome. Morbidity and mortality following surgery are acceptable with few sequelae.

PULMONARY AGENESIS, APLASIA AND HYPOPLASIA

Varying degrees of absence of pulmonary tissue have been recorded in a number of instances. Bilateral pulmonary agenesis is a rare malformation that may occur with anencephalic monsters (Potter, 1952). Slightly more frequent is unilateral pulmonary agenesis, in which the trachea runs directly into the sole bronchus, with an absent carina. Pulmonary aplasia is the commonest variant and consists of a carina and main stem bronchial stump with an absent distal lung. Functionally, unilateral lung agenesis and aplasia are similar. Lobar agenesis and aplasia are rarer than complete absence of one lung and usually occur as a combination of the right upper and middle lobes. Finally, pulmonary hypoplasia has been described as a mass of poorly differentiated lung parenchyma connected to a malformed bronchus.

Embryologically, these malformations correspond to a failure of development of the respiratory system from the foregut. Arrest at the stage of the primitive lung bud produces bilateral pulmonary agenesis. The respiratory anlage at a later stage may develop only unilaterally and lead to lung agenesis. Lobar agenesis then becomes developmental arrest on one side in an older embryo. Finally, pulmonary hypoplasia may occur during the last trimester of pregnancy with failure of final alveolar differentiation. The high incidence (greater than 50 per cent) of associated cardiac, gastrointestinal, genitourinary and skeletal malformations, as well as frequent variations in the bronchopulmonary vasculature, lends support to generalized teratogenic factors.

Pathologically, the sole lung is larger than normal in pulmonary agenesis, and this enlargement is true hypertrophy and not emphysema. In addition, Lukas and coworkers (1953) have reported vascular changes secondary to hypertension in the residual lung, although others find no evidence that resting pulmonary artery hypertension or emphysema develops with a normal cardiovascular system.

The wide variation in clinical findings is explained only partially by the amount of involved pulmonary tissue, although obviously this is an important factor. About 50 per cent of the patients with unilateral pulmonary agenesis survive. Death, however, is usually related to the associated serious anomalies.

The history may include harsh breathing, dyspnea, tachypnea, repeated upper respiratory tract infections and respiratory distress, with cyanosis on exertion. Inspection of the chest does not suggest an absent lung, since the external appearance is normal. Herniation of the sole lung and massive mediastinal shift and rotation fill the empty hemithorax. In addition, there is flat percussion over a dislocated heart, which may suggest dextrocardia in the presence of a right-sided agenesis. Breath sounds from the herniated,

hypertrophied lung are heard on the side of the agenesis except in the axilla and the base. With lobar agenesis, respiratory symptoms and mediastinal displacement occur, but are more subtle.

X-ray films of the chest show a homogeneous density on the involved, agenetic side with mediastinal rotation and shift. Lung herniation can be seen beneath the sternum on lateral films. X-ray films of lobar agenesis may simply exhibit mediastinal shift. The electrocardiogram is useful in separating agenesis from dextrocardia, and pulmonary function studies demonstrate a reduction in vital capacity and exercise tolerance.

The diagnosis should be suspected when respiratory difficulty occurs with tracheal deviation in the presence of a symmetrical chest and the chest roentgenogram is suggestive of massive atelectasis and mediastinal shift. Body section roentgenograms may strengthen the possibility of pulmonary agenesis. The diagnosis is confirmed by bronchoscopy, which fails to demonstrate one major bronchus, and by bronchography, which documents this finding. With lobar aplasia, bronchograms are indispensable, since the pathologic changes may not be visible to the bronchoscopist. Angiography may demonstrate suspected cardiac anomalies and aberrant pulmonary vessels and has been used to diagnose the varying causes of unequal pulmonary aeration in children (Franken and coworkers, 1973).

It is difficult to separate atelectasis from pulmonary or lobar agenesis on clinical grounds. In the differential diagnosis, Schaffer and Avery (1971) suggest that the bilateral peripheral aerated lung rules out the diagnosis of unilateral pulmonary agenesis. Endoscopy and bronchography can settle the issue.

In reviewing the mortality from pulmonary agenesis, it is apparent that chronic dyspnea with cough and repeated respiratory infections are ominous prognostic signs; so indeed is a right-sided agenesis, in which the mortality is twice that of left-sided agenesis. This is probably related to a more severe mediastinal and cardiac displacement, with great vessel disturbances secondary to the greater mass of lung tissue on the right. A tracheobronchial foreign body may produce the initial symptoms, and at least three fatalities have been reported during attempts at endoscopic removal.

Pulmonary resection may be indicated in lobar agenesis if the lung parenchyma on the side of the agenesis is supplied by abnormal bronchi or arteries to which incapacitating symptoms can be ascribed (Adler, Herrmann and Jewett, 1958). For pulmonary agenesis, acute infections are treated conventionally; repeated infections may deserve continuous antibiotic therapy and postural drainage. Borja, Ransdell and Villa (1970) have emphasized the importance of conservative management, including the prevention of "spillage pneumonitis" from the agenetic stump in newborns.

CONGENITAL PNEUMATOCELE (PULMONARY HERNIA)

The presence of lung tissue outside the usual confines of an intact bony thorax is a most infrequent finding in the neonatal period. About 20 per cent of all lung hernias are congenital; the remainder follow trauma.

The usual site of a congenital pulmonary hernia is the cervical region because of the absence of the endothoracic fascia in this area. Hernias in the region of the axilla have also been reported. Conversely, acquired post-traumatic hernias will occur in the midthoracic region.

The infant is usually asymptomatic, although local tenderness and slight dyspnea have been observed. Examination may demonstrate a supraclavicular mass that will increase in size with crying.

Treatment is usually superfluous.

CONGENITAL PULMONARY CYSTS

Cooke and Blades (1952) have classified congenital cystic disease of the lung into a bronchogenic type, an alveolar type, and a combination of these types. The entire group is probably outnumbered by acquired cysts; nevertheless, it includes a substantial segment of salvageable infants and children with respiratory distress and suppuration. There is a relative absence of other anomalies; cystic disease elsewhere is rare, and the pulmonary cystic problem, whether single or multiple, is usually limited to one lobe.

Since cysts have been recorded in late embryos and newborns, an anomalous development of the bronchopulmonary system has been postulated at the stage of terminal bronchiolar or early alveolar formation. This may evolve by intrapulmonary alveolar dissociation or partial bronchiolar recanalization with stenosis. The distal alveolated pulmonary cyst is then formed on the basis of expiratory obstruction through an area of bronchiolar narrowing. These essential postuterine respiratory dynamics might explain the paucity of these cysts in embryos.

The usual gross pathologic specimen exhibits a single, multiloculated, unilobar, peripheral air-filled cyst with a tracheobronchial communication. Common variants include multiplicity of cysts, bilateral lung or segmental distribution and absence of bronchial communication. Pus may be present. On microscopic examination, the thin congenital cyst wall contains bits of smooth muscle and perhaps cartilage and is lined by columnar epithelium. With the exception of acute staphylococcal pneumatocele, which has an obvious acute infectious background, most acquired cysts have an inner lining of squamous epithelium and can be separated histologically from the congenital cysts. Unfortunately, contamination and inflammation may destroy these helpful criteria, so that an infected congenital cyst, acquired cyst and lung abscess may be indistinguishable pathologically and clinically.

The clinical pathogenesis derives from a cyst-airway connection, either directly or through the pores of Kohn, with free access on inspiration and obstruction during expiration. Under these circumstances, there is an acute or chronic distention of the cyst leading to progressive increase in intrathoracic tension, frequently in the neonatal period. Compression of the unilateral lung and of the diaphragm, mediastinal shift and contralateral atelectasis are the usual sequence of events. If cyst drainage is poor, suppuration develops.

In the newborn and the infant, clinical findings are usualy due to progressive tension as the congenital pulmonary cyst gradually distends with air. Tension pneumothorax can develop at this stage, either spontaneously or by needle aspiration. Respiratory and circulatory embarrassment is manifested by tachypnea, tachycardia, dyspnea, stridor, cyanosis, hyperresonance, absence of breath sounds, and displaced trachea and heart without history or signs of infection. By late infancy and childhood, infection is almost invariably present, and cough, fever and hemoptysis with repeated, localized episodes of pulmonary sepsis become more prominent as the cyst evolves into a lung abscess.

Although at times there is a startling lack of correlation between symptoms and roentgenographic findings, plain roentgenograms of the chest will corroborate the diagnosis and help in the differential diagnosis. The congenital pulmonary alveolar cyst may occupy the entire hemithorax and appear as a circular or oval, thin-walled, air-filled cavity containing faint strands of lung. Normally aerated or atelectatic lung may be present at the apex and the base, but not at the hilus. There is a mediastinal shift, the diaphragm is depressed, pneumonia is absent, the pleura is not thickened, and other areas of translucency may be seen (Fig. 20). A fluid level with the cyst is unusual. Bronchography may be useful.

It is difficult, perhaps impossible, to separate pulmonary cysts from lobar emphysema. Emphysematous respiratory distress may be more explosive, but this is not a substantial differential factor in the face of common roentgenographic findings. The treatment is similar. The pulmonary cysts of cystic fibrosis and Letterer-Siwe disease should be excluded by the absence of other manifestations of the disease. Diaphragmatic hernia may simulate multiple lung cysts, but the immediate neonatal appearance of the hernia is very suggestive. Barium contrast x-ray studies are useful in those cases where

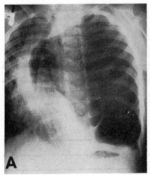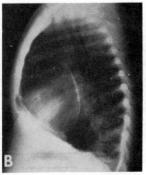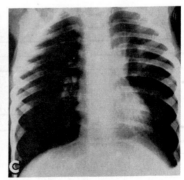

Figure 20. A 13-month-old infant with minimal respiratory distress. Posteroanterior and lateral chest films demonstrate gross hyperlucency of the left hemithorax. Frontal projection shows mediastinal displacement to the right. Pulmonary septal markings are noted within the area of hyperinflation. There is herniation of the left lung across the anterior mediastinum with flattening of the left diaphragm and widening of the left intercostal spaces. The right lung is compressed. C, After left upper lobe lobectomy, an overexposed x-ray film reveals good aeration bilaterally with return of the mediastinum toward the midline.

clinical presentation occurs later in the neonatal period. A staphylococcal pneumatocele may complicate a virulent pneumonia, and the changes in size and configuration of this type of acquired cyst may be volatile. Since spontaneous resolution here is expected, it would be a great error to confuse pneumatoceles with congenital cysts. An infected congenital cyst and encapsulated empyema may look alike; many chests have been drained with a diagnosis of empyema, but characteristically, unlike empyema, obliteration of the infected cyst does not occur in the presence of adequate dependent drainage. Angiography may be useful in separating congenital from postinfectious cysts. The respiratory distress will suggest pneumothorax, but there are no linear strands in or around the area of translucency, and a hilar shadow representing compressed lung is likely with pneumothorax.

The fate of congenital pulmonary cystic disease is rarely spontaneous regression. Left untreated or drained, pleural rupture with tension pneumothorax, infection with abscess, recurrent disabling bronchopneumonia, bronchopleural fistula, hemorrhage and expansion with suffocation may be encountered. Accordingly thoracotomy is advised in order to avoid these complications and the exceedingly poor prognosis associated with large, moderately symptomatic cysts. Elective lobectomy is the usual planned procedure, and every attempt should be made to conserve functioning pulmonary tissue (Fig. 21). Pneumonectomy for more generalized disease has been reported. At times, emergency resection must be done for the acute respiratory distress that threatens life. In this situation, needle aspiration and decompression of the tension cyst may be a worthwhile preparatory step on the way to the operative suite. Thoracentesis cannot be used definitively because pneumothorax and pleural soiling will follow.

The repeatedly infected lung cyst deserves systemic antibiotic therapy in the preoperative period, and resection should be done without prior drainage. At operation, Clatworthy (1960) suggests aspiration of a fluid-filled cyst in order to provide exposure and to prevent bronchotracheal spillage. Aberrant systemic arteries must be considered, especially for lower lobe cysts. Postoperative nursing should be carried out in an intensive care unit with appropriate equipment, and must be of the highest order.

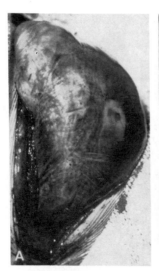 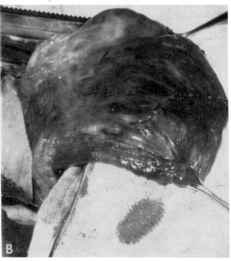

Figure 21. *A,* Extrusion of a left upper lobe pulmonary cyst, under tension, through an intercostal incision, with relief of respiratory distress that had become accentuated during the induction of anesthesia. *B,* The multiloculated cyst after deflation.

LOBAR EMPHYSEMA

Abnormal lobar distention can produce subtle or gross respiratory distress in an otherwise normal newborn or infant. Recognition of this entity is rewarding, since excisional therapy is fairly specific and the results are satisfactory.

The disease is usually unilobar and often confined to either an upper or middle lobe, but may be segmental, bilobar or bilateral or involve an entire lung. The left upper lobe is the most frequent site, followed by middle and right upper lobe. At least 10 per cent of patients have congenital heart disease, and a larger percentage have other anomalies.

Etiologic factors are profuse and, at times, specifically applicable; more often, the underlying mechanism is vague and escapes pathologic confirmation. Certainly, the emphysema secondary to a foreign body, tuberculosis, ECHO virus infection, mediastinal tumor, bronchial adenoma and stenosis is well established, but does not often produce the distinctive pattern of infantile lobar emphysema. In only half of the cases can an etiologic factor be found. The current favorite explanation for this form of lobar hyperaeration involves partial bronchial obstruction or intrinsic alveolar disease. The bronchial obstruction can be engendered by complete absence of cartilage, bronchomalacia, exuberant mucosal folds, extrinsic vascular and lymph node compression, bronchial distortion from an anterior mediastinal lung hernia and retained secretions. The common denominator hinders expiration by organic bronchial narrowing compounded by functional expiratory bronchial collapse. This valvular arrangement leads to a hugely overdistended, noncollapsible lobe with widespread alveolar emphysema and rupture and small subpleural blebs. The pulmonary arteries are normal in contradistinction to unilateral pseudoemphysema, in which small pulmo-nary arteries are normal in contradistinction to unilateral pseudoemphysema, in which small pulmonary arteries supply a normal or small emphysematous lobe. The report of the surgical pathologist, although confirming the emphysematous nature of the parenchymatous disease, is often disappointing in its etiologic parameters. Perhaps the majority of surgical specimens are resected distal to intrinsic intrabronchial disease, or extrinsic causative factors such as anomalous vessels are left undisturbed. Lincoln and coauthors (1971), however, have reported hypoplasia or absence of bronchial cartilaginous plates in 22 of 28 resected patients. Finally, Bolande and coworkers (1956) have suggested that alveolar fibrosis cannot handle normal expiration with the development of emphysema. Others have suggested that alveolar elasticity is abnormal. Leape and Longino (1964), in a substantial clinical contribution, postulate the etiologic combination of alveolar disease with bronchial obstruction.

The clinical profile is formed by a space-occupying emphysematous lobe producing ipsilateral lobar atelectasis and diaphragmatic compression, mediastinal shift and contralateral lung atelectasis. Decompression of the overdistended lobe into the atelectatic lobe is prevented by the immaturity and distortion of the pores of Kohn.

Progressive respiratory distress from birth to six months of age, but especially in the first month, will parallel the degree of emphysema. Cough, wheezing, dyspnea, tachypnea, tachycardia, stridor and intermittent cyanosis are aggravated with feeding. To this may be added retraction and bulging of the thorax, tracheal and cardiac shift, hyperresonant percussion and diminished breath sounds. There is no history of an antecedent infection.

Thoracic roentgenograms, in various positions, especially during expiration, must be obtained. On lateral view, a translucent anterior mediastinum is suggestive of lung herniation. Anteroposterior films will show a large hyper-lucent area containing vague lung and bronchovascular markings. The left upper lobe is most frequently involved. Adjacent lobes are compressed, the diaphragm is pushed downward, rib interspaces are wide, and the mediastinum is shifted into the opposite hemithorax with compression of the lung (Fig. 22). On fluoroscopy, the emphysematous segment remains constant in area, regardless of the phase of respiration. Air trapping can be confirmed by lateral decubitus films, since a normal dependent lung becomes relatively dense, whereas the lucency persists with emphysema. Bronchograms demonstrate incomplete distal filling of the affected bronchi. A pulmonary scan will show reduced perfusion of the affected parenchyma and may be helpful.

The differential diagnosis must exclude those lesions producing respiratory distress, but for which thoracotomy may not be indicated. Bronchoscopy can be utilized if a foreign body is a possibility, and may be warranted in children whose first symptoms occur after six months of age. Postpneumonic pneumatocele and bronchiolitis both have a septic background. Pulmonary cystic disease may be similar, but usually begins a little later in life. Fortunately, excision is proper for both. A tension pneumothorax will not have lung markings in the areas of radiolucency, and the nubbin of compressed lung in this condition is likely to be hilar rather than supradiaphragmatic or apical. Atelectasis with compensatory emphysema is not characterized by such pronounced respiratory distress. Pulmonary agenesis can be ruled out by bronchoscopy and bronchograms. Diaphragmatic hernia should not pose a problem, but can be separated by the use of contrast material.

Rarely, symptomatic infantile lobar emphysema will resolve spontaneously or with conservative therapy including bronchoscopy (Murray and coworkers, 1967; Eigen, Lemen and Waring, 1976). Such may be the case with obstruction secondary to a mucous plug. The usual course is relentlessly

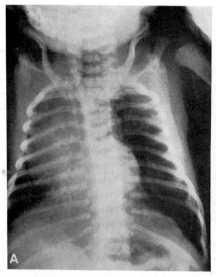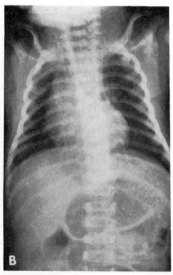

Figure 22. *A*, The anteroposterior chest roentgenogram of this newborn with respiratory distress demonstrates a shift of the mediastinum to the right with overinflation of the left lower lobe. There is depression of the left diaphragm, and the volume of the right lung is restricted. *B*, After left lower lobe lobectomy for lobar emphysema, the mediastinum has returned toward the midline, and the diaphragm is normally located. There is better aeration of the right lung and slight radiolucency of the upper lobe, which has expanded and filled the left hemithorax.

progressive toward tension emphysema. The prognosis without treatment, then, is exceedingly poor, and the mortality rate is high. Accordingly, excisional therapy, usually lobectomy but perhaps segmental resection (Lilly), should be done when the diagnosis is accompanied by symptoms. Only when the diagnosis is purely on a radiologic basis can thoracotomy be deferred.

Early age, concomitant congenital heart disease or severe respiratory symptoms should not contraindicate operation. Lobectomy has been done successfully within the first day of life, and simultaneous pulmonary and cardiovascular surgery has been done on several occasions. If the newborn is in extremis, thoracentesis can provide time for thoracotomy at the expense of a tension pneumothorax. This is its only role, and aspiration should not be used definitively. During the induction of anesthesia, vigorous positive pressure may inflate the emphysematous lobe and produce an extension of the respiratory distress. The emergency is over when the distended lobe herniates through the posterolateral thoracotomy incision with decompression of the thorax. There is no peculiar postoperative morbidity, and relief is immediate.

The operative mortality rate today is less than 5 per cent. Long-term follow-up shows normal growth and development, marred in rare instances by similar or less severe emphysema of other lobes with residual postoperative symptoms of pulmonary infection.

PULMONARY SEQUESTRATION

Pulmonary tissue that is embryonic and cystic, does not function, is isolated from normal functioning lung and is nourished by systemic arteries has been aptly called pulmonary sequestration. The intrapulmonary variant is contained within otherwise normal lung parenchyma. The less common extralobar sequestration is divorced from and accessory to the ipsilateral lung.

Fundamentally, pulmonary sequestration represents a malformation of the primitive respiratory and vascular systems in which fetal lung tissue is segregated from the main tracheobronchial apparatus and ultimately has its own systemic artery. The sequence and time of these embryologic events have aroused a great deal of curiosity. Pryce (1946) felt that persistent aberrant fetal pulmonary blood vessels exerted traction on a segment of an equally primitive lung bud that then split off from the parent lung. The arterial trauma during and after the actual detachment is thought to lead to cystic degeneration. Others propose a primary pulmonary separation soon after the foregut stage, with subsequent acquisition of a blood supply from the nearest and most convenient source, which happens to be the aorta. Smith, in 1956, suggested that sequestration was secondary to pulmonary artery deficiency and that the cysts followed systemic blood pressure flow after birth. Boyden (1958) concluded from the available data that the respiratory and vascular anomalies were unexplained, could not be related as to cause and occurred coincidentally. Halasz, Lindskog and Liebow (1961) postulated the presence of an additional, low, anterior foregut respiratory duplication with subsequent sequestration, but retention of the original aortic blood supply. The occasional association of esophagobronchial fistula with sequestration supports this contention. Finally, Yoneuda and coworkers found independent occurrences of the malformed lung and aberrant artery (Iwai and coworkers, 1973). They support the theory of an accessory bronchopulmonary bud arising from the foregut.

Both types of sequestration have certain similar pathologic characteristics as well as clear-cut differences. The pathologic tissue is largely fetal and profusely cystic, and contains disorganized, airless and nonpigmented alveoli, bronchi, cartilage, respiratory epithelium and a systemic artery. It is often secondarily infected, bronchiectatic or atelectatic, and is usually located in the region of the lower lobes (Figs. 23 and 24). The aberrant arteries may arise from the thoracic or abdominal aorta and, in the latter instance, pierce the diaphragm and run through the pulmonary ligament before reaching the sequestration. The elastic vessel walls may become atherosclerotic, and the lumen varies considerably in size.

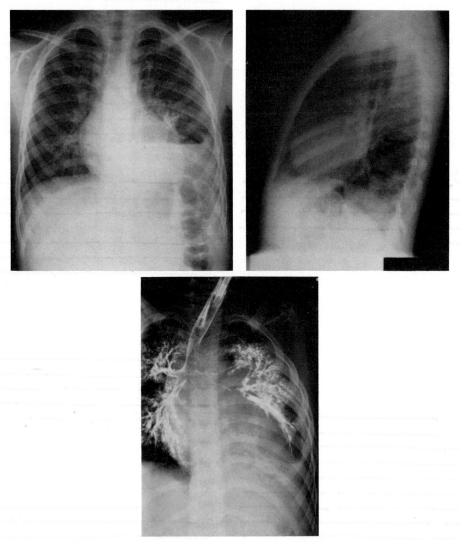

Figure 23. A five-year-old child with repeated upper respiratory infections for the past two years. On the posteroanterior projection there is a cystlike structure with an air-fluid level in the left lower lobe and minimal pleural fluid or thickening at the left base. Otherwise, the lungs are clear except for minimal residual contrast from previous bronchography. There is slight enlargement of the heart. The lateral view at a later date shows a cyst in the posterior aspect of the left lower lobe with a thin, well defined rim. No air-fluid level is seen. The bronchi of the left lower lobe are compressed and displaced anteriorly. The bilateral bronchogram in the frontal projection demonstrates a normal right bronchogram. The left bronchogram demonstrates elevation of the left main stem bronchus. There is elevation and lateral displacement of the lower lobe bronchi, which are partially filled and compressed. Consolidation in the left lower lobe is seen with a cystlike structure partially filled with fluid. (Dr. T. R. Howell.)

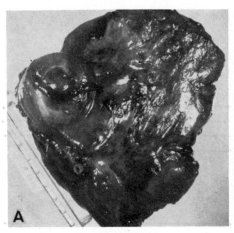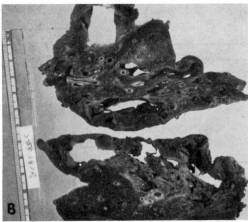

Figure 24. *A,* Gross external appearance of intralobar sequestration, left lower lobe, in an older child. Note aberrant systemic artery in lower left corner of specimen. *B,* Cross section of inflated, formalin-fixed specimen with multiple cysts, surrounded by compressed parenchyma. (Courtesy of Drs. James W. Brooks and Saul Kay, Medical College of Virginia.)

The intralobar sequestration is encircled by visceral pleura, and has no pleural separation from the rest of the lobe; it usually occurs in the lower lobes, although Clagett has reported the lesion in the upper lobes (Bruwer and coworkers, 1950). The remainder of the affected lobe and lung is normal, except that a small communication with the sequestration may have been maintained, reopened or created infection. A communication with the gastrointestinal tract is rare, and so are other anomalies. The systemic arteries are likely to be large, and the veins drain into the pulmonary system. Over half are diagnosed after adolescence, and symptoms in neonates and infants are infrequent.

Extralobar sequestration can occur from the thoracic inlet to the upper part of the abdomen, but characteristically is a left-sided (in over 90 per cent), ball-like pliable mass between the diaphragm and the lower lobe and outside the visceral pleura. Communications with the trachea, bronchi, esophagus, stomach and small bowel have been reported, but are rare. The systemic arteries are small, the venous drainage is likewise systemic through the azygos system, and other anomalies, principally congenital pleuroperitoneal hernias, are frequently concurrent. Over half are diagnosed before one year of age, and males are affected three to four times more often than females.

The basis for symptoms is infection through a fistula between the sequestration and either the airway or digestive tract. The congenital, pathologic tissue may be contaminated by contiguous pneumonitis or hematogenous localization with the formation of the primary or additional fistulas. Accordingly, the arresting clinical feature, especially with intralobar sequestration, is recurrent, persistent, progressive pulmonary sepsis in the form of pneumonitis or lung abscess, or both. This is manifested by weight loss, chills, fever, cough, hemoptysis and pyoptysis. Physical examination may elicit pathologic findings at the bases paravertebrally, and on several occasions a murmur has been noted. With extralobar sequestration, infection is less frequent, and the child may be asymptomatic and present with an intrathoracic mass.

Plain chest films will show a triangulated density in the region of the medial basal segment of a lower lobe, with displacement of the bronchovascular markings. Sometimes there is a dense linear projection toward the aorta. Body section radiography may amplify these findings. With abscess, of course, a fluid level may be present along with surrounding pneumonitis. The diagnosis is suggested by the restriction and localization of roentgenographic findings to the same area associated with repeated clinical episodes.

Bronchography is extremely helpful, since the sequestration will not fill with dye, but its periphery is outlined by bronchi that are filled. Aortography through the descending aorta will delineate the anomalous arterial supply and thus confirm the nature of the pulmonary density. This may also prove helpful at the time of surgery. At bronchoscopy, purulent secretions are absent from the main stem bronchi, even with pulmonary suppuration.

Extirpation is the only reasonable approach after the diagnosis has been established. Antibiotics must be used for the acute infection and should be given before and after operation. Intralobar sequestration is handled by lobectomy; segmental resection will not suffice, since the sequestration is not clearly demarcated. An extralobar sequestration can be removed without disturbing the remaining lobes, and the Bochdalek hernia can be repaired, if present. The only technical problem with either form of sequestration is the anomalous systemic artery or arteries, and exsanguination has followed their inadvertent division. The frequency of this vascular anomaly should be appreciated in all lower lobe lesions in infants and children exposed to thoracotomy.

Morbidity and mortality rates are exceedingly low if resection precedes repeated infections. Postoperative results are uniformly good.

CONGENITAL CYSTIC ADENOMATOID MALFORMATION OF THE LUNG

Cystic adenomatoid pulmonary hamartoma, first described by Chin and Tang in 1949, is a rare variant of congenital cystic disease and, like it, can produce respiratory difficulty by tension and infection.

Careful investigation of postmortem material by Kwittken and Reiner (1962) would seem to implicate a developmental "adenomatoid" overgrowth of pulmonary tissue in the region of the end bronchioles, with suppression of alveolar growth. On examination, this presents as a massive and fleshy unilobar enlargement, although bilobar and bilateral involvement has been described. On microscopic examination, cystic degeneration, excessive terminal bronchiolar tissue and areas of premature alveolar differentiation are interspersed with normal lung. Rosenkrantz and coworkers have suggested that the lesion is not a hamartoma but focal pulmonary dysplasia, since the cyst walls may contain skeletal muscle (Buntain and coworkers, 1974).

The basis for symptoms is the pulmonary replacement by the malformation, and compression of normal lung and mediastinum by the bulky size of the lesion and its enlarging cysts. Prematurity, hydramnios and anasarca, possibly secondary to caval compression or torsion, are frequently associated findings, and the presenting picture is respiratory distress soon after birth. Examination demonstrates mediastinal shift toward the opposite side in a newborn with associated dyspnea, tachypnea and perhaps cyanosis. Fairly specific radiologic findings, described by Craig, Kirkpatrick and Neuhauser (1956), include pulmonary densities with radiolucent areas and mediastinal shift to the opposite side (Fig. 25).

The differential diagnosis is essentially a radiologic one and includes the more usual forms of congenital and acquired cystic disease, lobar emphysema, and Bochdalek hernia.

The urgency for operation in the newborn parallels that for obstructive emphysema, and indeed the tension phenomenon in both is remarkably similar. Lobectomy has been curative in a number of instances, some of which have been reported in small prema-

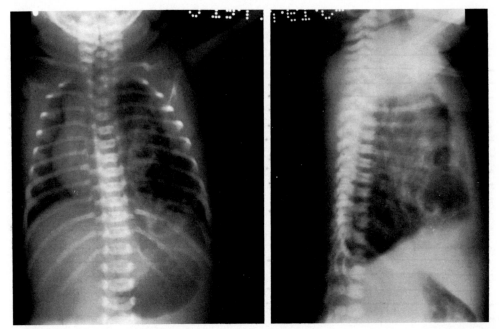

Figure 25. This 48-hour-old male infant had progressive respiratory distress since birth. Frontal and lateral projections demonstrate cardiac and mediastinal shift to the right. The right lung is clear, as is the apex of the left lung. In the remainder of the left lung there are multiple cystlike areas interspersed with linear and nodular consolidations. There is no pleural fluid or pneumothorax. The gastric air bubble is normally located. Left lower lobe lobectomy was done promptly and confirmed the preoperative diagnosis of cystic adenomatoid malformation. (Dr. T. R. Howell.)

tures soon after birth. Segmental resections should not be done, since the complication rate is excessive. Later in life, secondary infection, which is almost inevitable, constitutes an indication for thoracotomy.

CONGENITAL PULMONARY LYMPHANGIECTASIS

This unusual congenital dilatation of the pulmonary lymphatics produces severe respiratory distress in the newborn and is often associated with other crippling anomalies, such as congenital left heart disease, especially those producing obstruction to pulmonary venous flow. This may provide the basis for the persisting fetal pulmonary lymphatics.

Pathologically, according to Laurence (1955), there is diffuse overgrowth of the entire lymphatic system of both lungs, which become heavy, bulky and inelastic, with grossly prominent subpleural cystic lymphatics. It is quite unlike a localized lymphangioma and is not associated with chylothorax.

Symptomatically, there is immediate respiratory distress with dyspnea and cyanosis, which may be aggravated by a pneumothorax. X-ray films of the chest may show a diffuse, generalized mottling similar to hyaline membrane disease, along with emphysema in the remaining functioning lung (Carter and Vaughn, 1961). There may be some resemblance clinically to neonatal local hyperaeration (Wilson-Mikity syndrome), but differentiation can be accomplished.

Treatment is nonspecific, and the prognosis with diffuse involvement is hopeless.

PULMONARY ARTERIOVENOUS FISTULA

A congenital pulmonary arteriovenous fistula represents a direct intrapulmonary connection between pulmonary artery and vein without an intervening capillary bed. This cavernous arteriovenous aneurysm is the basis, then, for a right-to-left shunt, and is an uncommon cause of symptoms, including cyanosis, in the pediatric age group. Accordingly, the diagnosis is not often made in children in spite of its congenital nature. Bosher, in an exhaustive review in 1959, reported 17 patients under ten years of age, and Shumaker, in 1963, recorded 31 patients who were treated surgically between five months and 16 years of age. From this material it is apparent that the fistula occurs in the lower lobes in about 60 per cent of the instances, is single in 65 per cent and is unilateral in 75 per cent. Bilateral multiplicity is found in the remainder.

Etiologically, the pulmonary vascular malformation represents a failure of maturation of the fetal splanchnic bed in which arteriovenous communications may normally exclude the pulmonary capillaries. There may, however, be a widespread basic blood vessel abnormality, since familial hemorrhagic telangiectasis of the Osler-Weber-Rendu variety often occurs simultaneously.

On gross pathologic examination, the actual arteriovenous fistula is subpleural or hilar and may simulate a saccular, cavernous hemangioma because of its aneurysmal swelling. The fistula is fed by at least one afferent artery, usually pulmonic, less often bronchial, and is drained by several veins, almost always pulmonary. There are numerous communications between artery and vein in this tortuous, dilated wormlike vessel mass. On microscopic examination, the arteriovenous fistula is lined with vascular endothelium. Carcinomatous degeneration has been recorded by Hall (1935) and Wollstein (1931).

The clinical picture of this anomaly is created by an intrapulmonic right-to-left shunt in which unoxygenated pulmonary artery blood flows directly into the pulmonary veins and thence into the systemic circulation without gas exchange in the pulmonary capillaries. Although 50 per cent of the blood volume can be so rerouted in massive fistulization, Ellis has estimated that a 25 per cent shunt will produce diagnostic clinical findings.

Generalized telangiectasis, noted especially on the skin and mucous membranes, has been described in half of the patients with pulmonary arteriovenous fistula. Dyspnea, rubor, cyanosis, clubbing of the fingers and toes, hemoptysis, epistaxis, exercise intolerance and hemorrhagic conjunctiva are common complaints. On physical examination, a thrill may be felt, and a systolic or continuous murmur and bruit may be heard over the shunt, especially during inspiration. The heart is normal to auscultation. The blood pressure, pulse, venous pressure, electrocardiogram and cardiac output are within normal variations.

Clinical pathologic and radiologic studies are essential for the final diagnosis. Polycythemia in the range of 7 to 10 million red blood cells, 18 to 25 gm. of hemoglobin and a hematocrit level of 60 to 80 per cent are fairly standard. The arterial oxygen saturation is consistently low, drops lower with exercise, and will rise, but not to normal, with 100 per cent oxygen.

Routine chest films in various views demonstrate one or more homogeneous, noncalcified pulmonary densities with irregular, fairly sharp peripheral margins, confluent with the ipsilateral hilus. Body section roentgenograms may bring out the vascular nature of the tissue between the peripheral lesion and the hilus. The tumor may pulsate at fluoroscopy, decrease in size during the Valsalva maneuver, and become larger with the Müller test. Venous cineangiography with full chest films can delineate the offending fistula accurately and uncover smaller fistulas that were not hitherto suspected (Fig. 26). Pressure studies may record a normal systolic but low diastolic pulmonary artery pressure.

Cyanotic cardiac anomalies are excluded in the differential diagnosis by the presence of a lung tumor and the absence of various murmurs and aberrations in pulse, blood pressure, venous pressure, cardiac output, heart size configuration and electrocardiogram, all of which are normal in pulmonary arteriovenous fistula.

Complications during the natural history of the untreated disease are formidable. Exsanguination from a massive spontaneous hemothorax or hemoptysis can occur. Any localized infection may initiate septicemia and brain abscess, and polycythemia can

lead to embolic and thrombotic phenomena. The prognosis is obviously more serious and less manageable with widespread bilateral shunts or diffuse hereditary telangiectasis.

Excisional therapy should be done in symptomatic infants and children with localized disease, especially when accompanied by hereditary telangiectasis. In 31 pediatric patients there has been one operative death, and the morbidity rate is equally low. The results have been eminently satisfactory and have stimulated a more aggressive surgical approach toward the isolated pulmonary arteriovenous aneurysm with minimal or no symptoms and the more widely distributed fistulas with gross symptoms. Several experienced observers have commented on the clinical improvement following excision of the major dominant pulmonary fistula even

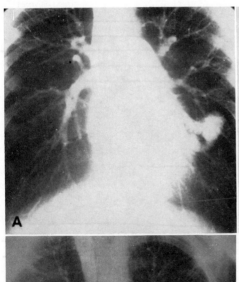

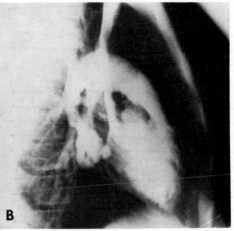

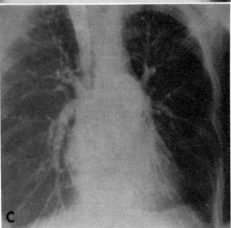

Figure 26. This was a virtually asymptomatic 15-year-old male with a family history of hereditary telangiectasia for three generations whose plain chest film showed a vague shadow in the left lower lung field. *A, B,* Preoperative posteroanterior and lateral angiocardiograms demonstrated a large pulmonary arteriovenous aneurysm in the anterior basal segment of the left lower lobe. A segmental resection was performed with total excision of the arteriovenous fistula. *C,* Postoperative posteroanterior angiocardiogram revealed no evidence of any arteriovenous communication in either lung. (Courtesy of Dr. Thomas N. P. Johns, Johnston-Willis Hospital, Richmond, Virginia.)

though smaller diffuse fistulas remain unmolested.

Lobectomy has been the procedure of choice in the majority of children. Unfortunately, normal pulmonary parenchyma was sacrificed because the dissection was not limited to the actual borders of the pathologic tissue. Since multiple shunts are often of paramount importance, postoperative results parallel the conservation of functioning lung. Accordingly, Bosher and then Murdock and, more recently, Björk have described the technique and practicality of local excision in a bloodless field in preference to segmental resection or lobectomy.

REFERENCES

Pectus Carinatum; Sternal Clefts; Pectus Excavatum

Adkins, P. C.: Pectus excavatum. *Am. Surg.,* 24:571, 1958.

Adkins, P. C., and Gwathmey, O.: Pectus excavatum: an appraisal of surgical treatment. *J. Thorac. Surg.,* 36:714, 1958.

Ashmore, P. G.: Management of some deformities of the thoracic cage in children. *Can. J. Surg.,* 6:430, 1963.

Avery, M. E., and Fletcher, B. D.: *The Lung and Its Disorders in the Newborn Infant.* 3rd Ed. Philadelphia, W. B. Saunders Company, 1974, p. 172.

Bates, D. V., Macklem, P. T., and Christie, R. V.: *Respiratory Function in Disease, An Introduction to the Integrated Study of the Lung.* 2nd. Ed. Philadelphia, W. B. Saunders Company, 1971, p. 243.

Becker, J. M., and Schneider, K. M.: Indications for the surgical treatment of pectus excavatum. *J.A.M.A.,* 180:22, 1962.

Bigger, I. A.: The treatment of pectus excavatum or funnel chest. *Am. Surg.,* 18:1071, 1952.

Billig, D. M., and Immordino, P. A.: Congenital upper sternal cleft: a case with successful surgical repair. *J. Pediatr. Surg.,* 5:257, 1970.

Brodkin, A. H., Jr.: Pectus excavatum: surgical indications and time of operation. *Pediatrics,* 11:582, 1953.

Brodkin, H. A.: Pigeon breast–congenital chondrosternal prominence. *Arch. Surg.,* 77:261, 1958.

Brown, A. L.: Pectus excavatum (funnel chest). *J. Thorac. Surg.,* 9:164, 1939.

Brown, A. L., and Cook, O.: Cardiorespiratory studies in pre- and postoperative funnel chest (pectus excavatum). *Dis. Chest,* 20:378, 1951.

Brown, J. J. M.: The thoracic wall. In Brown, H. H. M. (Ed.): *Surgery of Childhood.* Baltimore, Williams & Wilkins Company, 1963, p. 790.

Cantrell, J. R., Haller, J. A., and Ravitch, M. M.: The syndrome of congenital defects involving the abdominal wall, sternum, diaphragm, pericardium, and heart. *Surg. Gynecol. Obstet.,* 107:602, 1958.

Chin, E. F.: Surgery of funnel chest and congenital sternal prominence. *Br. J. Surg.,* 44:360, 1957.

Chin, E. F., and Adler, R. H.: Surgical treatment of pectus excavatum (funnel chest). *Br. Med. J.,* 1:1064, 1954.

Eijgelaar, A., and Butel, J. H.: Congenital cleft sternum. *Thorax,* 25:490, 1970.

Fink, A., Rivin, A., and Murray, J. F.: Cardiopulmonary effects of funnel chest. *Arch. Intern. Med.,* 108:427, 1961.

Flavell, G.: *An Introduction to Chest Surgery.* London, Oxford University Press, 1957, p.66.

Gross, R. E.: *The Surgery of Infancy and Childhood, Its Principles and Techniques.* Philadelphia, W. B. Saunders Company, 1953, p. 57.

Groves, L. K.: Deformities of the anterior chest wall. *Cleveland Clin. Q.,* 30:55, 1963.

Haller, J. A., Jr., Peters, G. N., Mazur, D., and White, J. J.: Pectus excavatum: a 20-year surgical experience. *J. Thorac. Cardiovasc. Surg.,* 60:375, 1970.

Hanlon, C. R.: Surgical treatment of funnel chest (pectus excavatum). *Am. Surg.,* 22:408, 1956.

Hansen, F. N.: The ontogeny and phylogeny of the sternum. *Am. J. Anat.,* 26:41, 1919.

Hansen, J. L., and Jacoby, O.: Pulmonary function in pectus excavatum deformity. *Acta Chir. Scand.,* 111:25, 1956.

Hay, W., and Dodsley, J.: *Deformity.* London, 1754, pp. 4, 20.

Howard, R.: Funnel chest: its effect on cardiac function. *Arch. Dis. Child.,* 34:5, 1959.

Howard, R. N.: Funnel chest: report of a series of one hundred cases. *Med. J. Aust.,* 2:1092, 1955.

Humphreys, G. H., and Connolly, J. E.: The surgical technique for the correction of pectus excavatum. *J. Thorac. Cardiovasc. Surg.,* 40:194, 1960.

Jackson, J. L., and others: Pectus excavatum. *Am. J. Surg.,* 98:664, 1959.

Jensen, N. K., Schmidt, W. R., and Garamella, J. J.: Funnel chest: a new corrective operation. *J. Thorac. Cardiovasc. Surg.,* 43:731, 1962.

Jensen, N. K., Schmidt, W. R., Garamella, J. J., and Lynch, M. F.: Pectus excavatum and carinatum: the how, when, and why of surgical correction. *J. Pediatr. Surg.,* 5:4, 1970.

Jewett, T. C., Butsch, W. L., and Hug, H. R.: Congenital bifid sternum. *Pediatr. Surg.,* 52:932, 1962.

Keshishian, J. M., and Cox, P. A.: Management of recurrent pectus excavatum. *J. Thorac. Cardiovasc. Surg.,* 54:740, 1967.

Kondraisin, M. I.: Congenital funnel chest in children. *Pediatrica,* 42:56, 1963.

Koop, E. C.: The management of pectus excavatum. *Surg. Clin. North Am.,* 36:1627, 1956.

Lam, C. R., and Brinkman, G. L.: Indications

and results in the surgical treatment of pectus excavatum. *Arch. Surg., 78*:322, 1959.

Lam, C. R., and Taber, R. E.: Surgical treatment of pectus carinatum. *Arch. Surg., 103*:191, 1971.

Lester, C. W.: Funnel chest and allied deformities of thoracic cage. *J. Thorac. Surg., 19*:507, 1950.

Lester, C. W.: Funnel chest: its cause, effects, and treatment. *J. Pediatr., 37*:224, 1950.

Lester, C. W.: Pigeon breast. *Ann. Surg., 137*:482, 1953.

Lester, C. W.: Pigeon breast, funnel chest, and other congenital deformities of chest. *J.A.M.A., 156*:1063, 1954.

Lester, C. W.: The etiology and pathogenesis of funnel chest, pigeon breast, and related deformities of the anterior chest wall. *J. Thorac. Surg., 34*:1, 1957.

Lester, C. W.: Funnel chest, the status 360 years after its first description. *Arch. Pediatr., 75*:493, 1958.

Lester, C. W.: Pectus carinatum, pigeon breast and related deformities of the sternum and costal cartilages. *Arch. Pediatr.*, October, 1960, p. 399.

Lester, C. W.: Surgical treatment of protrusion deformities of the sternum and costal cartilages (pectus carinatum, pigeon breast). *Ann. Surg., 153*:441, 1961.

Lindsey, E. S., and Harris, J. A.: Congenital and acquired chest deformities in children. *South. Med. J., 63*:875, 1970.

Lindskog, G. E., and Felton, W. L., II: Considerations in the surgical treatment of pectus excavatum. *Ann. Surg., 142*:654, 1955.

Lindskog, G. E., Liebow, A. A., and Glenn, W. W. L.: *Thoracic and Cardiovascular Surgery with Related Pathology*. New York, Appleton-Century-Crofts, Inc., 1962, p. 31.

Logan, W. D., Jr., and others: Ectopic cordis: report of a case and discussion of surgical management. *Surgery, 57*:898, 1965.

Meyer, L. (1911): Cited by Ochsner, A., and DeBakey, M. E.: Chonechondrosternon. Report of a case and review of the literature. *J. Thorac. Surg., 8*:469, 1939.

Moghissi, K.: Long-term results of surgical correction pectus excavatum and sternal prominence. *Thorax, 19*:350, 1964.

Mullard, K.: Observations on the aetiology of pectus excavatum and other chest deformities, and a method of recording them. *Br. J. Surg., 54*:115, 1967.

Orzalesi, M. M., and Cook, C. D.: Pulmonary function in children with pectus excavatum. *J. Pediatr., 66*:898, 1965.

Paltia, V., Parkkulainen, K. V., and Sulamaa, M.: Indications for surgery in funnel chest. *Ann. Pediatr. Fenniae, 5*:183, 1959.

Peters, R. M., and Johnson, G., Jr.: Stabilization of pectus deformity with wire strut. *J. Thorac. Cardiovasc. Surg., 47*:814, 1964.

Phillips, W. L.: Pectus excavatum. *S. Afr. Med. J., 34*:6, 1960.

Pilcher, R. S.: Trachea, bronchi, lungs and pleura. In Brown, J. J. M. (Ed.): *Surgery of Childhood*. Baltimore, Williams & Wilkins Company, 1963, p. 664.

Polgar, G., and Koop, C. E.: Pulmonary function in pectus excavatum. *Pediatrics, 32*:209, 1963.

Potts, W. J.: *The Surgeon and the Child*. Philadelphia, W. B. Saunders Company, 1964, p. 79.

Ramsay, B. H.: Transplantation of the rectus abdominis muscle in the surgical correction of a pectus carinatum deformity with associated parasternal depressions. *Surg. Gynecol. Obstet., 116*:507, 1963.

Ravitch, M. M.: Operative treatment of pectus excavatum. *Ann. Surg., 129*:429, 1949.

Ravitch, M. M.: Pectus excavatum and heart failure. *Surgery, 30*:178, 1951.

Ravitch, M. M.: Operation for correction of pectus excavatum. *Surg. Gynecol. Obstet., 106*:618, 1958.

Ravitch, M. M.: Operative correction of pectus carinatum (pigeon breast). *Ann. Surg., 151*:705, 1960.

Ravitch, M. M.: Operative treatment of congenital deformities of the chest. *Am. J. Surg., 101*:588, 1961.

Ravitch, M. M.: Congenital deformities of the chest wall. In Benson, C. D., and others (Eds.): *Pediatric Surgery*. Vol. 1. Chicago, Year Book Medical Publishers, Inc., 1962, p. 235.

Ravitch, M. M.: Technical problems in the operative correction of pectus excavatum. *Ann. Surg., 162*:29, 1965.

Ravitch, M. M.: Disorders of the sternum and the thoracic wall. *In* Sabiston, D. C., Jr., and Spencer, F. C.: *Gibbon's Surgery of the Chest*. 3rd Ed. Philadelphia, W. B. Saunders Company, 1976, p. 324.

Ravitch, M. M., and Matzen, R. N.: Pulmonary insufficiency in pectus excavatum associated with left pulmonary agenesis, congenital clubbed feet and ectromelia. *Dis. Chest, 54*:58, 1968.

Rehbein, F., and Wernicke, H. H.: The operative treatment of the funnel chest. *Arch. Dis. Child., 32*:5, 1957.

Robicsek, F., and others: The surgical treatment of chondrosternal prominence (pectus carinatum). *J. Thorac. Cardiovasc. Surg., 45*:691, 1963.

Robicsek, F., and others: Technical considerations in the surgical management of pectus excavatum and carinatum. *Ann. Thorac. Surg., 18*:549, 1974.

Roccaforte, D. S., Mehnert, J. J., and Peniche, A.: Repair of bifid sternum with autogenous cartilage. *Ann. Surg., 149*:448, 1959.

Sabiston, D. C.: The surgical management of congenital bifid sternum with partial ectopia cordis. *J. Thorac. Surg., 23*:118, 1958.

Sanger, P. W., Robicsek, F., and Taylor, F. H.: Surgical management of anterior chest deformities: a new technique and report of 153 operations without a death. *Surgery, 48*:510, 1960.

Sanger, P. W., Taylor, F. H., and Robicsek, F.: Deformities of the anterior wall of the chest. *Surg. Gynecol. Obstet., 116*:515, 1963.

Schaub, F., and Wegmann, T.: Elektrokardiographische Veranderungen bei Trichterbrust. *Cardiologia, 24*:39, 1954.

Stanford, W., and others: Silastic implants for correction of pectus excavatum. *Ann. Thorac. Surg., 13*:529, 1972.

Swenson, O.: *Pediatric Surgery.* 2nd Ed. New York, Appleton-Century-Crofts, Inc., 1962, p. 119.

Van Buchem, F. S. P., and Nieveen, J.: Findings with funnel chest. *Acta Med. Scand., 174*:657, 1963.

Wachtel, F. W., Ravitch, M. M., and Grishman, A.: Relation of pectus excavatum to heart disease. *Am. Heart J., 52*:121, 1956.

Wada, J., and Ikeda, K.: Clinical experience with 306 funnel chest operations. *Int. Surg., 57*:707, 1972.

Welch, K. J.: Satisfactory surgical correction of pectus excavatum deformity in childhood. *J. Thorac. Surg., 36*:697, 1958.

Welch, K. J., and Vos, A.: Surgical correction of pectus carinatum (pigeon breast). *J. Pediatr. Surg., 8*:659, 1973.

Wichern, W. A., Jr., and Lester, C. W.: Funnel chest. *Arch. Surg., 84*:170, 1962.

Congenital Absence of Ribs

Aschner, B. B., Kaizer, M. N., and Small, A. R.: Flaring of ribs associated with other skeletal anomalies. *Conn. Med. J., 19*:383, 1955.

Brown, J. J. M.: The thoracic wall. In Brown, J. J. M. (Ed.): *Surgery of Childhood.* Baltimore, Williams & Wilkins Company, 1964, p. 789.

Fishmann, A. P., Turino, G. M., and Bergofsky, E. H.: Disorders of respiration and circulation in subjects with deformities of thorax. *Mod. Concepts Cardiovasc. Dis., 27*:449, 1958.

Flavell, G.: *An Introduction to Chest Surgery.* London, Oxford University Press, 1957, p. 65.

Goodman, H. I.: Hernia of lung. *J. Thorac. Surg., 2*:368, 1933.

Lindsey, E. S., and Harris, J. A.: Congenital and acquired chest deformities in children. *S. Med. J., 63*:875, 1970.

Ravitch, M. M.: The operative treatment of congenital deformities of the chest. *Am. J. Surg., 101*:588, 1961.

Ravitch, M. M.: The chest wall. In Genson, C. D., and others (Eds.): *Pediatric Surgery.* Vol. 1. Chicago, Year Book Medical Publishers, Inc., 1962, p. 245.

Ravitch, M. M.: Disorders of the sternum and the thoracic wall. *In* Sabiston, D. C., Jr., and Spencer, F. C.: *Gibbon's Surgery of the Chest.* 3rd Ed. Philadelphia, W. B. Saunders Company, 1976, p. 324.

Rickham, P. P.: Lung hernia secondary to congenital absence of ribs. *Arch. Dis. Child., 34*:14, 1959.

Swenson, I.: *Pediatric Surgery.* 2nd Ed. New York, Appleton-Century-Crofts, Inc., 1962, p. 118.

Thomson, J.: *Teratologia.* Vol. 2. Edinburgh, W. Green and Sons, 1895, p. 1.

Congenital Anterior Diaphragmatic Hernia (Morgagni); Congenital Diaphragmatic Hernia of Bochdalek

Avery, M. E., and Fletcher, B. D.: *The Lung and Its Disorders in the Newborn Infant.* 3rd Ed. Philadelphia, W. B. Saunders Company, 1974, p. 164.

Baffes, T. G.: Diaphragmatic hernia. In Benson, C. D., and others (Eds.): *Pediatric Surgery,* Vol. 1. Chicago, Year Book Medical Publishers, Inc., 1962, p. 251.

Baran, E. M., Houston, H. E., Lynn, H. B., and O'Connell, E. J.: Foramen of Morgagni hernias in children. *Surgery, 62*:1076, 1967.

Belsey, R.: The surgery of the diaphragm. In Brown, J. J. M. (Ed.): *Surgery of Childhood.* Baltimore, Williams & Wilkins Company, 1963, pp. 758, 780.

Benjamin, H. B.: Agenesis of the left hemidiaphragm. *J. Thorac. Surg., 46*:265, 1963.

Bentley, G., and Lister, J.: Retrosternal hernia. *Surgery, 57*:567, 1965.

Boix-Ochoa, J., Peguero, G., Seijo, G., Natal, A., and Canals, J.: Acid-base balance and blood gases in prognosis and therapy of congenital diaphragmatic hernia. *J. Pediatr. Surg., 9*:49, 1974.

Boles, E. T., Jr., Schiller, M., and Weinberger, M.: Improved management of neonates with congenital diaphragmatic hernias. *Arch. Surg., 103*:344, 1971.

Bowers, V. M., Jr., McElin, T. W., and Dorsey, M. M.: Diaphragmatic hernia in the newborn: diagnostic responsibility of the obstetrician. *Obstet. Gynecol., 6*:262, 1955.

Boyd, D. P.: Diaphragmatic hernia of the foramen of Morgagni. *Surg. Clin. North Am., 41*:839, 1961.

Butler, N., and Claireaux, A. E.: Congenital diaphragmatic hernia as a cause of perinatal mortality. *Lancet, 1*:659, 1962.

Campanale, R. P., and Rowland, R. H.: Hypoplasia of the lung associated with congenital diaphragmatic hernia. *Ann. Surg., 142*:176, 1955.

Carter, R. E. B., Waterson, D. J., and Aberdeen, E.: Diaphragmatic hernia in infancy. Lancet, *1*:656, 1962.

Cerilli, G. J.: Foramen of Bochdalek hernia. *Ann. Surg., 159*:385, 1964.

Chatrath, R. R., ElShafie, M., and Jones, R. S.: Fate of hypoplastic lungs after repair of congenital diaphragmatic hernia. *Arch. Dis. Child., 46*:633, 1971.

Comer, T. P., Schmalhorst, W. R., and Arbegast, N. R.: Foramen of Morgagni hernia diagnosed by liver scan. *Chest, 63*:1036, 1973.

Cook, R. C. M., and Beckwith, J. B.: Adrenal injury during repair of diaphragmatic hernia in infants. *Surgery, 69*:251, 1971.

deLorimier, A. A., Tierney, D. F., and Parker, H. R.: Hypoplastic lung in fetal lambs with surgically produced congenital diaphragmatic hernia. *Surgery, 62*:12, 1967.

Filler, R. M., Randolph, J. G., and Gross, R. E.: Esophageal hiatus hernia in infants and children. *J. Thorac. Surg., 47*:551, 1964.

Fitchett, C. W., and Tavarex, V.: Bilateral congenital diaphragmatic herniation. *Surgery, 57*:305, 1965.

Flavell, G.: *An Introduction to Chest Surgery.* London, Oxford University Press, 1957, p. 231.

Gans, S. L., and Hackworth, L. E.: Respiratory obstructions of surgical import. *Pediatr. Clin. North Am.,* 6:1023, 1959.

Gross, R. E.: *The Surgery of Infancy and Childhood, Its Principles and Techniques.* Philadelphia, W. B. Saunders Company, 1953, p. 428.

Hajdu, N. H., and Sidhva, J. N.: Parasternal diaphragmatic hernia through the foramen of Morgagni. *Br. J. Radiol.,* July 1955, p. 428.

Harrington, S. W.: Various types of diaphragmatic hernia treated surgically; report of 430 cases. *Surg. Gynecol. Obstet.,* 86:735, 1948.

Haupt, G. L., and Myers, R. N.: Polyvinyl formalized (Ivalon) sponge in the repair of diaphragmatic hernia. *Arch. Surg.,* 80:103; 613, 1960.

Hedblom, C. A.: Diaphragmatic hernia. *J.A.M.A.,* 85:947, 1925.

Hermann, R. E., and Barber, D. H.: Congenital diaphragmatic hernia in the child beyond infancy. *Cleveland Clin. Q.,* 30:73, 1963.

Holcomb, G. W., Jr.: A new technique for repair of congenital diaphragmatic hernia with absence of the left hemidiaphragm. *Surgery,* 51:534, 1962.

Hope, J. W., and Koop, C. E.: Differential diagnosis of mediastinal masses. *Pediatr. Clin. North Am.,* 6:379, 1959.

Jemerin, E. E.: Diaphragmatic hernia through foramen of Morgagni. *J. Mount Sinai Hosp. (N. Y.),* 30:415, 1963.

Johnson, D. G., Deaner, R. M., and Koop, C. E.: Diaphragmatic hernia in infancy: factors affecting the mortality rate. *Surgery,* 62:1082, 1967.

Keith, A.: *Human Embryology and Morphology.* London, Edward Arnold, 1948.

Kelly, K. A., and Bassett, D. L.: An anatomic reappraisal of the hernia of Morgagni. *Surgery,* 55:495, 1964.

Kenigsberg, K., and Gwinn, J. L.: The retained sac in repair of posterolateral diaphragmatic hernia in the newborn. *Surgery,* 57:894, 1965.

Kiesewetter, W. B., Gutierrez, I. Z., and Sieber, W. K.: Diaphragmatic hernia in infants under one year of age. *Arch., Surg.,* 83:561, 1961.

Kinsbourne, M.: Hiatus hernia with contortions of the neck. *Lancet,* 1:1058, 1964.

Kitagawa, M., Hislop, A., Boyden, E. A., and Reid, L.: Lung hypoplasia in congenital diaphragmatic hernia. *Br. J. Surg.,* 58:342, 1971.

Ladd, W. E., and Gross, E. R.: *Abdominal Surgery of Infancy and Childhood.* Philadelphia, W. B. Saunders Company, 1941.

Lewis, M. A. H., and Young, D. G.: Ventilatory problems with congenital diaphragmatic hernia. *Anaesthesia,* 24:571, 1969.

McNamara, J. J., Eraklis, A. J., and Gross, R. E.: Congenital posterolateral diaphragmatic hernia in the newborn. *J. Thorac. Cardiovasc. Surg.,* 55:55, 1968.

Meeker, I. A., Jr., and Snyder, W. H., Jr.: Surgical management of diaphragmatic defects in the newborn, a report of twenty infants each less than one week old. *Am. J. Surg.,* 104:196, 1962.

Moore, T. C., and others: Congenital posterolateral diaphragmatic hernia in the newborn. *Surg. Gynecol. Obstet.,* 104:675, 1957.

Murdock, A. I., Burrington, J. B., and Swyer, P. R.: Alveolar to arterial oxygen tension difference and venous admixture in newly born infants with congenital diaphragmatic herniation through the foramen of Bochdalek. *Biol. Neonate,* 17:161, 1971.

Murphy, D. R., and Owen, H. F.: Respiratory emergencies in the newborn. *Am. J. Surg.,* 101:58, 1961.

Neville, W. E., and Clowes, G. H. A., Jr.: Congenital absence of hemidiaphragm and use of a lobe of liver in its surgical correction. *Arch. Surg.,* 69:282, 1954.

Nixon, H. H., and O'Donnell, B.: *The Essentials of Pediatric Surgery.* London, William Heinemann, Ltd., 1961, p. 36.

Osebold, W. R., and Soper, R. T.: Congenital posterolateral diaphragmatic hernia past infancy. *Am. J. Surg.,* 131:748, 1976.

Polk, H. C., and Burford, T. H.: Hiatal hernia in infancy and childhood. *Surgery,* 54:521, 1963.

Potts, W. J.: *The Surgeon and the Child.* Philadelphia. W. B. Saunders Company, 1959, p. 64.

Raphaely, R. C., and Downes, J. J.: Congenital diaphragmatic hernia: prediction of survival. *J. Pediatr. Surg.,* 8:815, 1973.

Richardson, W. R.: Thoracic emergencies in the newborn infant. *Am. J. Surg.,* 105:524, 1963.

Riker, W. L.: Congenital diaphragmatic hernia. *Arch. Surg.,* 69:291, 1954.

Rosenkrantz, J. G., and Cotton, E. K.: Replacement of left hemidiaphragm by a pedicled abdominal muscular flap. *J. Thorac. Cardiovasc. Surg.,* 48:912, 1964.

Sabga, G. A., Neville, W. E., and Del Guercio, L. R. M.: Anomalies of the lung associated with congenital diaphragmatic hernia. *Surgery,* 50:547, 1961.

Schuster, S. R.: The recognition and management of diaphragmatic hernias in infancy and childhood. *Q. Rev. Pediatr.,* 15:171, 1960.

Shaffer, J. O.: Prosthesis for agenesis of the diaphragm. *J.A.M.A.,* June 15, 1964, p. 168.

Simpson, J. S.: Ventral silon pouch: method of repairing congenital diaphragmatic hernias in neonates without increasing intra-abdominal pressure. *Surgery,* 66:798, 1969.

Snyder, W. H., and Greany, E. M.: Congenital diaphragmatic hernia: 77 consecutive cases. *Surgery,* 57:576, 1965.

Starrett, R. W., and deLorimier, A. A.: Congenital diaphragmatic hernia in lambs: hemodynamic and ventilatory changes with breathing. *J. Pediatr. Surg.,* 10:575, 1975.

Sulamaa, M., and Viitanen, I.: Congenital diaphragmatic hernia and relaxation. *Acta Chir. Scand.,* 124:288, 1962.

Thomsen, G.: Diaphragmatic hernia in the newborn, incidence of neonatal fatalities. *Acta Chir. Scand., 283*(Suppl.):267, 1961.

White, M., and Dennison, W. M.: *Surgery in Infancy and Childhood, A. Handbook for Medical Students and General Practitioners.* Edinburgh, E. & S. Livingstone, Ltd., 1958, p. 300.

Congenital Eventration of the Diaphragm

Arnheim, E. E.: Congenital eventration of the diaphragm in infancy. *Surgery*, 35:809, 1954.

Avery, M. E, and Fletcher, B. D.: *The Lung and Its Disorders in the Newborn Infant.* 3rd Ed. Philadelphia, W. B. Saunders Company, 1974, p. 160.

Baffes, T. C.: Diaphragmatic hernia. In Benson, C. D., and others (Eds.): *Pediatric Surgery.* Vol. 1. Chicago, Year Book Medical Publishers, Inc., 1962. p. 259.

Belsey, R.: The surgery of the diaphragm. In Brown, J. J. M. (Ed.): *Surgery of Childhood.* Baltimore, Williams & Wilkins Company, 1963, p. 786.

Bisgard, J. D.: Congenital eventration of diaphragm. *J. Thorac. Surg.*, 16:484, 1947.

Chin, E. F., and Lynn, R. B.: Surgery of eventration of the diaphragm. *J. Thorac. Surg.*, 32:6, 1956.

Firestone, F. N., and Taybi, H.: Bilateral diaphragmatic eventration: demonstration by pneumoperitoneography. *Surgery,* 62:954, 1967.

Flavell, G.: *An Introduction to Chest Surgery,* London, Oxford University Press, 1957, p. 233.

Gans, S. L., and Hackworth. L. E.: Respiratory obstructions of surgical import. *Pediatr. Clin. North Am.*, 6:1023, 1959.

Goulston, E.: Eventration of the diaphragm. *Arch. Dis. Child.*, 32:9, 1957.

Laxdal, O. E., McDougall, H., and Mellin, G. W.: Congenital eventration of the diaphragm. *N. Engl. J. Med.*, 250:401, 1954.

Lindskog, G. E., Liebow, A. A., and Glenn, W. W. L.: *Thoracic and Cardiovascular Surgery with Related Pathology.* New York, Appleton-Century-Crofts, Inc., 1962, p. 546.

Michelson, E.: Eventration of the diaphragm. *Surgery,* 49:410, 1961.

Pomerantz, M.: The diaphragm. *In* Sabiston, D. C., Jr., and Spencer, F. C.: *Gibbon's Surgery of the Chest.* 3rd Ed. Philadelphia, W. B. Saunders Company, 1976, p. 788.

Schaffer, A. J., and Avery, M. E.: *Diseases of the Newborn.* 3rd Ed. Philadelphia, W. B. Saunders Company, 1971, p. 138.

Thomas, T. V.: Nonparalytic eventration of the diaphragm. *J. Thorac. Cardiovasc. Surg.*, 55:586, 1968.

Thomas, T. V.: Eventration of the diaphragm. *Ann. Thorac. Surg.*, 10:180, 1970.

Congenital Hiatal Diaphragmatic Hernia

Avery, M. E., and Fletcher, B. D.: *The Lung and Its Disorders in the Newborn Infant.* 3rd Ed. Philadelphia, W. B. Saunders Company, 1974, p. 164.

Blattner, R. J.: Hiatal hernia. *J. Pediatr.*, 72:424, 1968.

Boles, E. T., and Izant, R. J., Jr.: Spontaneous chylothorax in the neonatal period. *Am. J. Surg.*, 99:870, 1960.

Burford, T. H., and Lischer, C. E.: Treatment of short esophageal hernia with esophagitis by Finney pyloroplasty. *Ann. Surg.*, 144:647, 1956.

Cahill, J. L., Aberdeen, E., and Waterston, D. J.: Results of surgical treatment of esophageal hiatal hernia in infancy and childhood. *Surgery,* 66:597, 1969.

Herbst, J., Friedland, G. W., and Zboralske, F. F.: Hiatal hernia and "rumination" in infants and children. *J. Pediatr.*, 78:261, 1971.

Jewett, T. C., Jr., and Waterston, D. J.: Surgical management of hiatal hernia in children. *J. Pediatr. Surg.*, 10:757, 1975.

Kamal, I., and Guiney, E. J.: The treatment of hiatus hernia in children by anterior gastropexy. *J. Pediatr. Surg.*, 7:641, 1972.

Lilly, J. R., and Randolph, J. G.: Hiatal hernia and gastroesophageal reflux in infants and children. *J. Thorac. Cardiovasc. Surg.*, 55:42, 1968.

Monereo, J., Cortes, L., and Blesa, E.: Peptic esophageal stenosis in children. *J. Pediatr. Surg.*, 8:475, 1973.

Prinsen, J. E.: Hiatus hernia in infants and children: a long-term follow-up of medical therapy. *J. Pediatr. Surg.*, 10:97, 1975.

Rohatgi, M., Shandling, B., and Stephens, C. A.: Hiatal hernia in infants and children: results of surgical treatment. *Surgery,* 69:456, 1971.

Chylothorax

Avery, M. E., and Fletcher, B. D.: *The Lung and Its Disorders in the Newborn Infant.* 3rd Ed. Philadelphia, W. B. Saunders Company, 1974, p. 263.

Boles, E. T., and Izant, R. J., Jr.: Spontaneous chylothorax in the neonatal period. *Am. J. Surg.*, 99:870, 1960.

Chernick, V., and Reed, M. H.: Pneumothorax and chylothorax in the neonatal period. *J. Pediatr.*, 76:624, 1970.

Eichenwald, H. F., and McCracken, G. H., Jr.: Chylothorax. In Vaughan, V. C., III, and McKay, R. J. (Eds.): *Nelson Textbook of Pediatrics.* 10th Ed. Philadelphia, W. B. Saunders Company, 1975, p. 998.

Forbes, G. B.: Chylothorax in infancy. *J. Pediatr.*, 25:191, 1944.

Gingell, J. C.: Treatment of chylothorax by producing pleurodesis using iodized talc. *Thorax,* 20:261, 1965.

Higgins, C. B., and Mulder, D. G.: Chylothorax after surgery for congenital heart disease. *J. Thorac. Cardiovasc. Surg.*, 61:411, 1971.

Maier, H. C.: The pleura. In Sabiston, D. C., and Spencer, F. C. (Eds.): *Gibbon's Surgery of the Chest.* 3rd Ed. Philadelphia, W. B. Saunders Company, 1976, p. 370.

Morphis, L. G., Arcinue, E. L., and Krause, J. R.: Generalized lymphangioma in infancy with chylothorax. *Pediatrics,* 46:566, 1970.

Perry, R. E., Hodgman, J., and Cass, A. B.: Pleural effusion in the neonatal period. *J. Pediatr.*, 62:838, 1963.

Randolph, J. G., and Gross, R. E.: Congenital chylothorax. *Arch. Surg.*, 74:405, 1957.

Ravitch, M. M.: Chylothorax. In Benson, C. D., and others (Eds.): *Pediatric Surgery.* Vol. 1.

Chicago, Year Book Medical Publishers, Inc., p. 353.

Schaffer, A. J., and Avery, M. E.: *Diseases of the Newborn.* 3rd Ed. Philadelphia, W. B. Saunders Company, 1971, p. 168.

Wiener, E. S., Owens, L., and Salzberg, A. M.: Chylothorax after Bochdalek herniorrhaphy in a neonate. *J. Thorac. Cardiovasc. Surg.,* 65:200, 1973.

Williams, K. R., and Burford, T. H.: The management of chylothorax. *Ann. Surg.,* 160:131, 1964.

Tracheal Agenesis and Stenosis

Bigler, J. A., and others: Tracheotomy in infancy. *Pediatrics,* 13:476, 1954.

Cantrell, J. R., and Guild, H. G.: Congenital stenosis of the trachea. *Am. J. Surg.,* 108:297, 1964.

Fonkalsrud, E. W., Martell, R. R., and Maloney, J. V.: Surgical treatment of tracheal agenesis. *J. Thorac. Cardiovasc. Surg.,* 45:520, 1963.

Holinger, P. H.: The infant with respiratory stridor. *Pediatr. Clin. North Am.,* 2:403, 1955.

Holinger, P. H., and Johnston, K. C.: Clinical aspects of congenital anomalies of the trachea and bronchi. *Dis. Chest,* 31:613, 1957.

Holinger, P. H., and others: Congenital malformations of the trachea, bronchi and lung. *Ann. Otol.,* 61:1159, 1952.

Hopkinson, J. M.: Congenital absence of the trachea. *J. Pathol.,* 107:63, 1972.

Joshi, V. V.: Tracheal agenesis. *Am. J. Dis. Child.,* 117:341, 1969.

Ochsner, J. L., and LeJeune, F. E., Jr.: Tracheal and esophageal obstructions in infants. *South. Med.,* 57:1340, 1964.

Oliver, P., and others: Tracheotomy in children. *N. Engl. J. Med.,* 267:631, 1962.

Othersen, H. B., Jr.: The technique of intraluminal stenting and steroid administration in the treatment of tracheal stenosis in children. *J. Pediatr. Surg.,* 9:683, 1974.

Rubin, L. R., and others: Elective tracheostomy in infants and children. *Am. J. Surg.,* 98:880, 1959.

Witzleben, C. L.: Aplasia of the trachea. *Pediatrics,* 32:31, 1963.

Tracheomalacia

Cox, W. L., and Shaw, R. R.: Congenital chondromalacia of the trachea. *J. Thorac. Cardiovasc. Surg.,* 49:1033, 1965.

Burford, T. H., and Ferguson, T. B.: Congenital lesions of the lungs and emphysema. In Sabiston, D. C., and Spencer, F. C. (Eds.): *Gibbon's Surgery of the Chest.* 3rd ed. Philadelphia, W. B. Saunders Company, 1976, p. 611.

Holinger, P. H., and Johnston, K. C.: The infant with respiratory stridor. *Pediatr. Clin. North Am.,* 2:403, 1955.

Holinger, P. H., and others: Congenital malformations of the trachea, bronchi, and lung. *Ann. Otol.,* 61:1159, 1952.

Levin, S. J., Scherer, R. A., and Adler, P.: Cause of wheezing in infancy. *Ann. Allergy,* 22:20, 1964.

Lynch, J. I.: Bronchomalacia in children. Considerations governing medical vs. surgical treatment. *Clin. Pediatr.,* 9:279, 1970.

Ochsner, J. L., and LeJeune, F. E., Jr.: Tracheal and esophageal obstruction in infants. *South. Med. J.,* 57:1333, 1964.

Vascular Ring

Abreu, A. L., Surgery of the heart and great vessels. In Brown, J. J. M. (Ed.): *Surgery of Childhood.* Baltimore, Williams & Wilkins Company, 1963, p. 705.

Avery, M. E., and Fletcher, B. D.: *The Lung and Its Disorders in the Newborn Infant.* 3rd Ed. Philadelphia, W. B. Saunders Company, 1974, p. 115.

Bahnson, H. T.: The aorta. *In* Sabiston, D. C., Jr., and Spencer, F. C.: *Gibbon's Surgery of the Chest.* 3rd Ed. Philadelphia, W. B. Saunders Company, 1976, p. 878.

Bernatz, P. E., Lewis, D. R., and Edwards, J. E.: Division of the posterior arch of a double aortic arch for relief of tracheal and esophageal obstruction. *Proc. Staff Meet. Mayo Clin.,* 34:173, 1959.

Blumenthal, S., and Ravitch, M. M.: Seminar on aortic vascular rings and other anomalies of the aortic arch. *Pediatrics,* 20:896, 1957.

Boyle, W. F., and Shaw, C. C.: Right-sided aortic arch. *N. Engl. J. Med.,* 256:392, 1957.

Cartwright, R. S., and Bauersfield, S. R.: Thoracic aortography in infants and children. *Ann. Surg.,* 150:266, 1959.

De Bord, R. A.: Double aortic arch in infancy. *Ann. Surg.,* 161:479, 1965.

Eklof, O., Ekstrom, G., Eriksson, B. O., Michaelsson, M., Stephensen, O., Soderlund, S., Thoren, C. and Wallgren, G.: Arterial anomalies causing compression of the trachea and/or the oesophagus. *Acta Paediatr. Scand.,* 60:81, 1971.

Fineberg, C., and Stofman, H. C.: Tracheal compression caused by an anomalous innominate artery arising from a brachiocephalic trunk. *J. Thorac. Surg.,* 37:214, 1959.

Gans, S. L., and Hackworth, L. E.: Respiratory obstructions of surgical import. *Pediatr. Clin. North Am.,* 6:1023, 1959.

Griswold, H. E., and Young, M. D.: Double aortic arch: report of 2 cases and review of the literature. *Pediatrics,* 4:751, 1949.

Gross, R. E.: *The Surgery of Infancy and Childhood: Its Principles and Techniques.* Philadelphia, W. B. Saunders Company, 1953, pp. 806, 913.

Gross, R. E.: Thoracic surgery for infants. *J. Thorac. Cardiovasc. Surg.,* 48:152, 1964.

Gross, R. E.: *An Atlas of Children's Surgery.* Philadelphia, W. B. Saunders Company, 1970, p. 132.

Gross, R. E., and Neuhauser, E. B. D.: Compression of trachea or esophagus by vascular anomalies; surgical therapy in 40 cases. *Pediatrics,* 7:69, 1951.

Gross, R. E., and Ware, P. F.: The surgical significance of aortic arch anomalies. *Surg. Gynecol., Obstet., 83*:435, 1946.

Haller, J. A., Jr., Peters, G. N., White, J. J., and Dorst, J. P.: Selection for operative correction of symptomatic tracheal compression from an aberrant innominate artery in infants. (Unpublished paper.)

Holinger, P. H., and Johnston, K. C.: The infant with respiratory stridor. *Pediatr. Clin. North Am., 2*:403, 1955.

Holinger, P. H., and others: Congenital malformations of the trachea, bronchi and lung. *Ann. Otol., 61*:1159, 1952.

Lasher, E. P.: Types of tracheal and esophageal constriction due to arterial anomalies of the aortic arch, with suggestions as to treatment. *Am. J. Surg., 96*:228, 1958.

Lindskog, G. E., Liebow, A. A., and Glenn, W. W. L.: *Thoracic and Cardiovascular Surgery, with Related Pathology.* New York. Appleton-Century-Crofts, Inc., 1962, p. 750.

Mahoney, E. B., and Manning, J. A.: Aortic arch; congenital abnormalities. *Pediatr. Digest*, March 1965.

Moes, C. A. F., Izukawa, T., and Trusler, G. A.: Innominate artery compression of the trachea. *Arch. Otolaryngol., 101*:733, 1975.

Mustard, W. T.: Vascular rings compressing the esophagus and trachea. In Benson, C. D., and others (Eds.): *Pediatric Surgery.* Vol. 1. Chicago, Year Book Medical Publishers, Inc., 1962, p. 427.

Mustard, W. T., Bayliss, C. E., Fearon, B., Pelton, D., and Trusler, G. A.: Tracheal compression by the innominate artery in children. *Ann. Thorac. Surg., 8*:312, 1969.

Nikaidoh, H., Riker, W. L., and Idriss, F. S.: Surgical management of "vascular rings." *Arch. Surg., 105*:327, 1972.

Nixon, H. H., and O'Donnell, B.: *The Essentials of Paediatric Surgery.* London, William Heinemann, Ltd., 1961, p. 40.

Ochsner, J. L., and LeJeune, F. E., Jr.: Tracheal and esophageal obstruction in infants. *South. Med. J., 57*:1333, 1964.

Park, C. D., Waldhausen, J. A., Friedman, S., Aberdeen, E., and Johnson, J.: Tracheal compression by the great arteries in the mediastinum. *Arch. Surg., 103*:626, 1971.

Richardson, D. W.: Thoracic emergencies in the newborn infant. *Am. J. Surg., 105*:524, 1963.

Riker, W. L., and Potts, W. J.: Cardiac lesions amenable to surgery: current status. *Pediatr. Clin. North Am., 6*:1055, 1959.

Schaffer, A. J., and Avery, M. E.: *Diseases of the Newborn.* 3rd Ed. Philadelphia, W. B. Saunders Company, 1971.

Swenson, O.: *Pediatric Surgery.* 2nd Ed. New York, Appleton-Century-Crofts, Inc., 1962, p. 202.

Vaughan, V. C., III, and McKay, R. J. (Eds.): *Nelson Textbook of Pediatrics.* 3rd Ed. Philadelphia, W. B. Saunders Company, 1975.

Wychulis, A. R., Kincaid, O. W., Weidman, W.

H., and Danielson, G. K.: Congenital vascular ring: surgical considerations and results of operation. *Mayo Clin. Proc., 46*:182, 1971.

Tracheoesophageal Fistula without Esophageal Atresia; Esophageal Atresia

Abrahamson, J., and Shandling, B.: Esophageal atresia in the underweight baby: a challenge. *J. Pediatr. Surg., 7*:608, 1972.

Ashcraft, K. W., and Holder, T. M.: The story of esophageal atresia and tracheoesophageal fistula. *Surgery, 65*:332, 1969.

Avery, M. E., and Fletcher, B. D.: *The Lung and Its Disorders in the Newborn Infant.* 3rd Ed. Philadelphia, W. B. Saunders Company, 1974, p. 134.

Baker, D. C., Flood, C. A., and Ferrer, J. M., Jr.: Postoperative esophageal stenosis. *Ann. Otol., 63*:1082, 1954.

Battersby, J. S., Jolly, W. W., and Fess, S. W.: Esophageal atresia: a comprehensive study of 210 patients. *Bull. Soc. Int. Chir.,* No. 5/6, 1971, p. 415.

Bedard, P., Girvan, D. P., and Shandling, B.: Congenital H-type tracheoesophageal fistula. *J. Pediatr. Surg., 9*:663, 1974.

Blumberg, J. B.: Laryngotracheoesophageal cleft, the embryologic implications: review of the literature. *Surgery, 57*:559, 1965.

Burford, T. H., and Ferguson, T. B.: Congenital lesions of the lungs and emphysema. In Sabiston, D. C., and Spencer, F. C. (Eds.): *Gibbon's Surgery of the Chest.* 3rd Ed. Philadelphia, W. B. Saunders Company, 1976, p. 611.

Burgess, J. N., Carlson, H. C., and Ellis, F. H., Jr.: Esophageal function after successful repair of esophageal atresia and tracheoesophageal fistula. *J. Thorac. Cardiovasc. Surg., 56*:667, 1968.

Cohen, S. J.: Unusual types of esophageal atresia and tracheoesophageal fistulae. *Clin. Pediatr., 4*:271, 1965.

Cohen, S. R.: The diagnosis and surgical management of congenital tracheoesophageal fistula without atresia of the esophagus. *Ann Otol. Rhinol. Laryngol., 79*:1101, 1970.

Comming, W. A.: Esophageal atresia and tracheoesophageal fistula. *Radiol. Clin. North Am., 13*:277, 1975.

DeBoar, A., and Potts, W. J.: Congenital atresia of the esophagus with tracheoesophageal fistula. *Surg. Gynecol. Obstet., 104*:475, 1957.

Desjardins, H. G., Stephens, C. A., and Moes, C. A. F.: Results of surgical treatment of congenital tracheoesophageal fistula, with a note on cine-fluorographic findings. *Ann. Surg., 100*:14, 1964.

Dudgeon, D. L., Morrison, C. W., and Woolley, M. M.: Congenital proximal tracheoesophageal fistula. *J. Pediatr. Surg., 7*:614, 1972.

Eraklis, A. J., and Gross, R. E.: Esophageal atresia — management following an anastomotic leak. *Surgery, 60*:919, 1966.

Falletta, G. P.: Recommunication on repair of congenital tracheoesophageal fistula. *Arch. Surg., 88*:779, 1964.

Ferguson, C. C.: Management of infants with esophageal atresia and tracheoesophageal fistula. *Ann. Surg., 172*:750, 1970.

Flavell, G.: *The Oesophagus.* London, Butterworth, 1963, pp. 20, 24.

Franklin, R. H.: The Oesophagus. In Brown, J. J. M. (Ed.): *Surgery of Childhood.* Baltimore, Williams & Wilkins Company, 1963, pp. 747, 754.

Gans, S. O., and Hackworth, L. E.: Respiratory obstructions of surgical import. *Pediatr. Clin. North Am., 6*:1023, 1959.

Goldenberg, I. S.: An unusual variation of congenital tracheoesophageal fistula. *J. Thorac. Cardiovasc., Surg., 40*:114, 1960.

Gross, R. E.: *The Surgery of Infancy and Childhood, Its Principles and Techniques.* Philadelphia, W. B. Saunders Company, 1953, p. 77.

Groves, L. K.: Surgical treatment of esophageal atresia and tracheoesophageal fistula in the infant. *Cleveland Clin. Q., 25*:227, 1958.

Haight, C.: Congenital tracheoesophageal fistula without esophageal atresia. *J. Thorac. Surg., 17*:600, 1948.

Haight, C.: The management of congenital esophageal atresia and tracheoesophageal fistula. *Surg. Clin. North Am., 41*:1281, 1961.

Haight, C.: The esophagus. In Benson, C. D., and others (Eds.): *Pediatric Surgery.* Vol. 1. Chicago, Year Book Medical Publishers, Inc., 1962, p. 266.

Hays, D. M.: An analysis of the mortality in esophageal atresia. *Am. J. Dis. Child., 103*:765, 1962.

Hays, D. M.: Esophageal atresia: current management. *Pediatr. Digest,* April 1965.

Hays, D. M., and Snyder, W. H.: Results of conventional operative procedures for esophageal atresia in premature infants. *Am. J. Surg., 106*:19, 1963.

Heimlich, H. J.: Peptic esophagitis with stricture treated by reconstruction of the esophagus with a reversed gastric tube. *Surg. Gynecol. Obstet., 114*:673, 1962.

Helmsworth, J. A., and Pryles, C. V.: Congenital tracheoesophageal fistula without esophageal atresia. *J. Pediatr., 38*:610, 1951.

Herwig, J., and Ogura, J.: Congenital tracheoesophageal fistula without esophageal atresia. *J. Pediatr., 47*:298, 1955.

Holder, T. M.: Transpleural versus retropleural approach for repair of tracheoesophageal fistula. *Surg. Clin. North Am., 44*:1433, 1964.

Holder, T. M.: Thoracic surgery in infants. In Sabiston, D. C., and Spencer, D. C. (Eds.): *Gibbon's Surgery of the Chest.* 3rd ed. Philadelphia, W. B. Saunders Company, 1976, p. 294.

Holder, T. M., and Ashcraft, K. W.: Esophageal atresia and tracheoesophageal fistula. *Ann. Thorac. Surg., 9*:445, 1970.

Holder, T. M., and Gross, R. E.: Temporary gastrostomy in pediatric surgery. *Pediatrics, 26*:37, 1960.

Holder, T. M., McDonald, V. G., and Woolley, M. W.: The premature or critically ill infant with esophageal atresia: increased success with

a staged approach. *J. Thorac. Cardiovasc. Surg., 44*:344, 1962.

Holder, T. M., and others: Esophageal atresia and tracheoesophageal fistula. *Pediatrics, 34*:542, 1964.

Holinger, P. H., Brown, W. T., and Maurizi, D. G.: Endoscopic Aspects of postsurgical management of congenital esophageal atresia and tracheoesophageal fistula. *J. Thorac. Cardiovasc. Surg., 49*:22, 1965.

Holinger, P. H., and others: Congenital malformations of trachea, bronchi and lung. *Ann. Otol., 61*:1159, 1952.

Howard, R., and Meyers, N. A.: Esophageal atresia — a technic for elongating the upper pouch. *Surgery, 58*:725, 1965.

Humphreys, G. H., Hogg, B. M., and Ferrer, J.: Congenital atresia of esophagus. *J. Thorac. Surg., 32*:332, 1956.

Johnson, P. W.: Elongation of the upper segment in esophageal atresia. Report of a case. *Surgery, 58*:741, 1965.

Kafrouni, G., Baick, C. H., and Wooley, M. M.: Recurrent tracheoesophageal fistula: a diagnostic problem. *Surgery, 68*:889, 1970.

Kappelman, M. M., Dorst, J., Haller, J. A., and Stambler, A.: H-type tracheoesophageal fistula. *Am. J. Dis. Child., 118*:568, 1969.

Karlan, M., Thompson, J., and Clatworthy, H. W.: Congenital atresia of the esophagus with tracheoesophageal fistula and duodenal atresia. *Surgery, 41*:544, 1957.

Killen, D. A., and Greenlee, H. B.: Transcervical repair of H-type congenital tracheoesophageal fistula: review of the literature. *Ann. Surg., 162*:145, 1965.

Koop, C. E.: Atresia of the esophagus: technical considerations in surgical management. *Surg. Clin. North Am., 42*:1387, 1962.

Koop, C. E., Kiesewetter, W. B., and Johnson, J.: Treatment of atresia of the esophagus by the transpleural approach. *Surg. Gynecol. Obstet., 98*:687, 1954.

Lafer, D. J., and Boley, S. J.: Primary repair in esophageal atresia with elongation of the lower segment. *J. Pediatr. Surg., 1*:585, 1966.

Leix, F., and Schwab, C. E.: End-to-side operative technic for esophageal atresia with tracheoesophageal fistula. *Am. J. Surg., 118*:225, 1969.

Lindskog, G. E., Liebow, A. A., and Glenn, W. W. L.: *Thoracic and Cardiovascular Surgery with Related Pathology.* New York, Appleton-Century-Crofts, Inc., 1962, p. 481.

Lloyd, J. R., and Clatworthy, H. W.: Hydramnios as an aid to early diagnosis of congenital obstruction of the alimentary tract: a study of the maternal and fetal factors. *Pediatrics, 21*:903, 1958.

Lynn, H. B., and Divia, L. A.: Tracheoesophageal fistula without atresia of the esophagus. *Surg. Clin. North Am., 41*:871, 1961.

Mahour, G. H., Woolley, M. M., and Gwinn, J. L.: Elongation of the upper pouch and delayed anatomic reconstruction in esophageal atresia. *J. Pediatr. Surg., 9*:373, 1974.

Martin, L. W., and Hogg, S. P.: Esophageal atresia and tracheoesophageal fistula. *Am. J. Dis. Child.*, 99:828, 1960.

Meeker, I. G., and Snyder, W. H.: Gastrostomy for the newborn surgical patient. *Arch. Dis. Child.*, 37:159, 1962.

Mellins, R. B., and Blumenthal, S.: Cardiovascular anomalies and esophageal atresia. *Am. J. Dis. Child.*, 107:160, 1964.

Moncrief, J. A., and Randolph, J. G.: Congenital tracheoesophageal fistula without atresia of the esophagus—a method for diagnosis and surgical correction. *J. Thorac. Cardiovasc. Surg.*, 51:434, 1966.

Morse, G. W., Anderson, E. V., and Arenson, N.: Congenital tracheoesophageal fistula without esophageal atresia: an improved method of demonstration. *Am. Surg.*, 24:112, 1958.

Murphy, D. R., and Owen, H. F.: Respiratory emergencies in the newborn. *Am. J. Surg.*, 101:581, 1961.

Nixon, H. H., and O'Donnell, B.: *The Essentials of Pediatric Surgery.* London, William Heinemann, Ltd., 1961, p. 32.

Pieretti, R., Shandling, B., and Stephens, C. A.: Resistant esophageal stenosis associated with reflux after repair of esophageal atresia: a therapeutic approach. *J. Pediatr. Surg.*, 9:355, 1974.

Randolph, J. G., Tunnell, W. P., and Lilly, J. R.: Gastric division in the critically ill infant with esophageal atresia and tracheoesophageal fistula. *Surgery*, 63:496, 1968.

Redo, S. F.: Congenital esophageal atresia and tracheoesophageal fistula. Fifteen-year experience. *N. Y. State J. Med.*, November 1975, p. 2372.

Rehbein, F., and Yanagiswa, F.: Complications after operation for oesophageal atresia. *Arch. Dis. Child.*, February 1959, p. 24.

Reploge, R. L.: Esophageal atresia: plastic sump catheter for drainage of the proximal pouch. *Surgery*, 54:296, 1963.

Richardson, W. R.: Thoracic emergencies in the newborn infant. *Am. J. Surg.*, 105:524, 1963.

Rigg, W., Jr.: Congenital tracheoesophageal fistula without esophageal atresia. *South. Med. J.*, 62:135, 1969.

Sandegard, E.: The treatment of oesophageal atresia. *Arch. Dis. Child.*, 32:475, 1957.

Schaffer, A. J., and Avery, M. E.: *Diseases of the Newborn.* 3rd Ed. Philadelphia, W. B. Saunders Company, 1971.

Schneider, K. M., and Becker, J. M.: The "H-type" tracheoesophageal fistula in infants and children. *Surgery*, 51:677, 1962.

Schultz, L. R., and Clatworthy, H. W.: Esophageal strictures after anastomosis in esophageal atresia. *Arch. Surg.*, 87:136, 1963.

Schwartz, S. I., and Dale, W. A.: Unusual tracheoesophageal fistula with membranous obstruction of the esophagus and postoperative hypertrophic pyloric stenosis. *Ann. Surg.*, 142:1002, 1955.

Shaw, R. R., Paulson, D. L., and Siebel, E. K.: Congenital atresia of the esophagus with tracheoesophageal fistula, treatment of surgical complication. *Ann. Surg.*, 142:204, 1955.

Stephens, C. A., Mustard, W. T., and Simpson, J. S.: Congenital atresia of the esophagus with tracheoesophageal fistula. *Surg. Clin. North Am.*, 36:1465, 1956.

Swenson, O.: *Pediatric Surgery.* 2nd Ed. New York, Appleton-Century-Crofts, Inc., 1962, p. 155.

Swenson, O., and others: Repair and complications of esophageal atresia and tracheoesophageal fistula. *N. Engl. J. Med.*, 267:960, 1962.

Touloukian, R. H., and Stinson, K. K.: Temporary gastric partition: a model for staged repair of esophageal atresia with fistula. *Ann. Surg.*, 171:184, 1970.

Touloukian, R. J., Pickett, L. K., Spackman, T., and Biancani, P.: Repair of esophageal atresia by end-to-side anastomosis and ligation of the tracheoesophageal fistula: a critical review of 18 cases. *J. Pediatr. Surg.*, 9:305, 1974.

Tuqan, N. A.: Annular stricture of the esophagus distal to congenital tracheoesophageal fistula. *Surgery*, 52:394, 1962.

Waterston, D. J., Bonham-Carter, R. E., and Aberdeen, E.: Congenital tracheoesophageal atresia. *Lancet*, 2:55, 1963.

Yahr, W. Z., Azzoni, A. A., and Santulli, T. V.: Congenital atresia of the esophagus with tracheoesophageal fistula: an unusual variant. *Surgery*, 52:937, 1962.

Young, D. G.: Successful primary anastomosis in oesophageal atresia after reduction of a long gap between the blind ends by bouginage of the upper pouch. *Br. J. Surg.*, 54:321, 1967.

Zachary, R. B., and Emery, J. L.: Failure of separation of larynx and trachea from the esophagus: persistent esophagotrachea. *Surgery*, 49:525, 1961.

Congenital Bronchial Stenosis

Chang, N., Hertzler, J. H., Gregg, R. H., Lofti, M. W., and Brough, A. J.: Congenital stenosis of the right mainstem bronchus. *Pediatrics*, 41:739, 1968.

Holinger, P. H., and others: Congenital malformations of the trachea, bronchi and lung. *Ann. Otol.*, 61:1159, 1952.

Swenson, O.: *Pediatric Surgery.* 2nd Ed. New York, Appleton-Century-Crofts, Inc., 1962, p. 123.

Bronchogenic Cyst

Ackerman, L. V.: Personal communication cited in Gibbon, J. H., Jr. (Ed.): *Surgery of the Chest.* 2nd Ed. Philadelphia, W. B. Saunders Company, 1969, p. 321.

Alshabkhoun, S., Starkey, G. W., and Asnes, R. A.: Bronchogenic cysts of the mediastinum in infancy. *Ann. Thorac. Surg.*, 4:532, 1967.

Bressler, S., and Wiener, D.: Bronchogenic cyst associated with an anomalous pulmonary artery arising from the thoracic aorta. *Surgery*, 35:815, 1954.

Bruwer, A., Clagett, O. T., and McDonald, J. R.: Anomalous arteries to the lung associated with congenital pulmonary abnormality. *J. Thorac. Surg., 19*:957, 1950.

Culiner, M. M., and Grimes, O. F.: Localized emphysema in association with bronchial cysts or mucoceles. *J. Thorac. Cardiovasc. Surg., 41*:306, 1961.

Burford, T. H., and Ferguson, T. B.: Congenital lesions of the lungs and emphysema. *In* Sabiston, D. C., and Spencer, F. C. (Eds.): *Gibbon's Surgery of the Chest.* 3rd Ed. Philadelphia, W. B. Saunders Company, 1976, p. 611.

Dabbs, C. H., Peirce, E. C., and Rawson, F. L.: Intrapericardial interatrial teratoma (bronchogenic cyst). *N. Engl. J. Med., 256*:541, 1957.

Desforges, G.: Primitive foregut cysts. *Ann. Thorac. Surg., 4*:574, 1967.

Eraklis, A. J., Griscom, N. T., and McGovern, J. B.: Bronchogenic cysts of the mediastinum in infancy. *N. Engl. J. Med., 281*:1150, 1969.

Flavell, G.: *An Introduction to Chest Surgery.* London, Oxford University Press, 1957, p. 126.

Gans, S. L., and Hackworth, L. R.: Respiratory obstructions of surgical import. *Pediatr. Clin. North Am., 6*:1023, 1959.

Gerami, S., Richardson, R., Harrington, B., and Pate, J. W.: Obstructive emphysema due to mediastinal bronchogenic cysts in infancy. *J. Thorac. Cardiovasc. Surg., 58*:432, 1969.

Greenfield, L. J., and Howe, J. S.: Bronchial adenoma within the wall of a bronchogenic cyst. *J. Thorac. Cardiovasc. Surg., 49*:398, 1965.

Gross, R. E.: *The Surgery of Infancy and Childhood, Its Principles and Techniques.* Philadelphia, W. B. Saunders Company, 1962, p. 780.

Hope, J. W., and Koop, C. E.: Differential diagnosis of mediastinal masses. *Pediatr. Clin. North Am., 6*:379, 1959.

Jones, P.: Developmental defects in lungs. *Thorax, 10*:205, 1955.

Kirwan, W. O., Walbaum, P. R., and McCormack, R. J. M.: Cystic intrathoracic derivatives of the foregut and their complications. *Thorax, 28*:424, 1973.

Leigh, T. F., and Weens, H. S.: *The Mediastinum.* Springfield, Illinois, Charles C Thomas, 1959, p. 136.

Lindskog, G. E., Liebow, A. A., and Glenn, W. W. L.: *Thoracic and Cardiovascular Surgery, with Related Pathology.* New York, Appleton-Century-Crofts, Inc., 1962, p. 452.

Maier, H. C.: Bronchogenic cysts of the mediastinum. *Ann. Surg., 127*:476, 1948.

Moersch, H. J., and Clagett, O. T.: Pulmonary cysts. *J. Thorac. Surg., 16*:179, 1947.

Opsahl, T., and Berman, E. J.: Bronchogenic mediastinal cysts in infants: case reports and review of literature. *Pediatrics, 30*:372, 1962.

Pilcher, R. S.: Trachea, bronchi, lungs and pleura. In Brown, J. J. M. (Ed.): *Surgery of Childhood.* Baltimore, Williams & Wilkins Company, 1963, p. 667.

Pontius, R. G.: Bronchial obstruction of congenital origin. *Am. J. Surg., 106*:8, 1963.

Potts, W. J.: *The Surgeon and the Child.* Philadelphia, W. B. Saunders Company, 1964, p. 71.

Schaffer, A. J., and Avery, M. E.: *Diseases of the Newborn.* 3rd Ed. Philadelphia, W. B. Saunders Company, 1971, p. 159.

Schlumberger, H. G.: Tumors of the mediastinum. In *Atlas of Tumor Pathology.* Fascicle 18. Washington, D.C., Armed Forces Institute of Pathology, 1951.

Swenson, O.: *Pediatric Surgery,* 2nd Ed. New York, Appleton-Century-Crofts, Inc., 1962, p. 124.

Trossman, C. M.: Push-up stridor caused by a bronchogenic cyst. *Am. J. Dis. Child., 107*:293, 1964.

Webb, W. R., and Burford, T. H.: Studies of the re-expanded lung after prolonged atelectasis. *Arch. Surg., 66*:801, 1953.

Weisel, W , Claudon, D. B., and Darin, J. C.: Tracheal adenoma in juxtaposition with a mediastinal bronchogenic cyst. *J. Thorac. Surg., 37*:687, 1959.

Pulmonary Agenesis, Aplasia and Hypoplasia

Adler, R. H., Herrmann, J. W., and Jewett, T. C.: Lobar agenesis of the lung. *Ann. Surg., 147*:267, 1958.

Avery, M. E., and Fletcher, B. D.: *The Lung and Its Disorders in the Newborn Infant.* 3rd Ed. Philadelphia, W. B. Saunders Company, 1974, p. 153.

Booth, J. B., and Berry, C. L.: Unilateral pulmonary agenesis. *Arch. Dis. Child., 42*:361, 1967.

Borja, A. R., Ransdell, H. T., and Villa, S.: Congenital developmental arrest of the lung. *Ann. Thorac. Surg., 10*:317, 1970.

Brunner, S., and Nissen, E.: Agenesis of the lung. *Am. Rev. Resp. Dis., 87*:103, 1963.

Burford, T. H., and Ferguson, T. B.: Congenital lesions of the lungs and emphysema. In Sabiston, D. C., and Spencer, F. C. (Eds.): *Gibbon's Surgery of the Chest.* 3rd Ed. Philadelphia, W. B. Saunders Company, 1976, p. 611.

Claireaux, A. E., and Ferreira, H. P.: Bilateral pulmonary agenesis. *Arch. Dis. Child., 33*:364, 1958.

Ferguson, C. F.: Interesting bronchopulmonary problems of early life. *Laryngoscope, 80*:1347, part 2, 1970.

Franken, E. A., Jr., Hurwitz, R. A., and Battersby, J. S.: Unequal aeration of the lungs in children. The use of pulmonary angiography. *Radiology, 109*:401, 1973.

Harris, G. B. C.: The newborn with respiratory distress: some roentgenographic features. *Radiol. Clin. North Am., 1*:499, 1963.

Holinger, P. H., and others: Congenital malformations of the trachea, bronchi, and lung. *Ann. Otol., 61*:1159, 1952.

Landing, B. H.: Anomalies of the respiratory tract. *Pediatr. Clin. North Am., 4*:73, 1957.

Lindskog, G. E., Liebow, A. A., and Glenn, W. W. L.: *Thoracic Cardiovascular Surgery, with Related Pathology.* New York, Appleton-Century-Crofts, Inc., 1962, p. 103.

Lukas, D. S., Dotter, C. T., and Steinberg, I.: Agenesis of the lung and patent ductus arteriosus with reversal of flow. *N. Engl. J. Med., 249*:107, 1953.

Maltz, D. L., and Nadas, A. S.: Agenesis of the lung. *Pediatrics, 42*:175, 1968.

Martinez-Jimenez, M., and others: Agenesis of the lung with patent ductus arteriosus treated surgically. *J. Thorac. Cardiovasc. Surg., 50*:59, 1965.

Minetto, E., Galli, E., and Boglione, G.: Agenesia, aplasia, hypoplasia pulmonare. *Minerva Med., 49*:4635, 1958.

Morison, J. E.: *Foetal and Neonatal Pathology.* London, Butterworth & Company, 1952.

Morton, D. R., Klassen, K. P., and Baxter, E. H.: Lobar agenesis of the lung. *J. Thorac. Surg., 20*:665, 1950.

Oyamada, A., Gasul, B. M., and Holinger, P. H.: Agenesis of the lung. Report of a case with review of all previously reported cases. *Am. J. Dis. Child., 85*:182, 1953.

Pilcher, R. S.: Trachea, bronchi, lungs, and pleura. In Brown, J. J. M. (Ed.): *Surgery of Childhood.* Baltimore, Williams & Wilkins Company, 1963, p. 665.

Potter, E. L.: *Pathology of the Fetus and the Newborn.* Chicago, Year Book Publishers, Inc., 1952, p. 261.

Ravitch, M. M.: Agenesis of the lung. In Benson, C. D., and others (Eds.): *Pediatric Surgery.* Vol. 1. Chicago, Year Book Medical Publishers, Inc., 1962, p. 346.

Schaffer, A. J., and Avery, M. E.: *Diseases of the Newborn.* 3rd Ed. Philadelphia, W. B. Saunders Company, 1971, p. 124.

Spencer, H.: *Pathology of the Lung.* New York, Macmillan Company, 1962, p. 27.

Tuynman, P. E., and Gardner, L. W.: Bilateral aplasia of lung. *Arch. Pathol., 54*:306, 1952.

Waddell, J. A., Simon, G., and Reid, L.: Bronchial atresia of the left upper lobe. *Thorax, 20*:214, 1965.

Congenital Pneumatocele (Pulmonary Hernia)

Goodman, H. I.: Hernia of lung. *J. Thorac. Surg., 2*:368, 1933.

Lindskog, G. E., Liebow, A. A., and Glenn, W. W. L.: *Thoracic and Cardiovascular Surgery, with Related Pathology.* New York, Appleton-Century-Crofts, Inc., 1962, p. 51.

Ravitch, M. M.: Disorders of the sternum and the thoracic wall. *In* Sabiston, D. C., Jr., and Spencer, F. C.: *Gibbon's Surgery of the Chest.* 3rd Ed. Philadelphia, W. B. Saunders Company, 1976, p. 324.

Rickman, P. P.: Lung hernia secondary to congenital absence of ribs. *Arch. Dis. Child., 34*:14, 1959.

Congenital Pulmonary Cysts

Avery, M. E., and Fletcher, B. D.: *The Lung and Its Disorders in the Newborn Infant.* 3rd Ed. Philadelphia, W. B. Saunders Company, 1974, p. 144.

Bowden, K. M.: Congenital cystic disease of lung. *Med. J. Aust., 2*:311, 1948.

Boyden, E. A.: Bronchogenic cysts and the theory of intralobar sequestration: new embryologic data. *J. Thorac. Surg., 35*:604, 1958.

Burford, T. H., and Ferguson, T. B.: Congenital lesions of the lungs and emphysema. In Sabiston, D. C., and Spencer, F. C. (Eds.): *Gibbon's Surgery of the Chest.* 3rd Ed. Philadelphia, W. B. Saunders Company, 1976, p. 611.

Caffey, J.: On the natural regression of pulmonary cysts during early infancy. *Pediatrics, 11*:48, 1953.

Clatworthy, H. W., Jr.: Intrathoracic tumors and cysts. In Ariel, I. M., and Pack, G. T. (Eds.): *Cancer and Allied Diseases of Infancy and Childhood.* Boston, Little, Brown & Company, 1960, p. 143.

Cooke, F. N., and Blades, B.: Cystic disease of the lungs. *J. Thorac. Surg., 23*:546, 1952.

Crawford, T. J., and Cahill, J. L.: The surgical treatment of pulmonary cystic disorders in infancy and childhood. *J. Pediatr. Surg., 6*:251, 1971.

Dickson, J. A., Clagett, O. T., and McDonald, J. R.: Cystic disease of the lung and its relation to bronchiectatic cavities: a study of 22 cases. *J. Thorac. Surg., 15*:196, 1946.

Donald, J. G., and Donald, J. W.: Congenital cysts of the lung. *Ann. Surg., 141*:944, 1955.

Egan, R. W., Jewett, T. C., and Macmanus, J. E.: Congenital lesions of the thorax in infancy demanding early surgical treatment. *Arch. Surg., 77*:584, 1958.

Gans, S. L., and Hackworth, L. E.: Respiratory obstructions of surgical import. *Pediatr. Clin. North Am., 6*:1023, 1959.

Gilbert, J. W., and Myers, R. T.: Intrathoracic tension phenomena in the neonatal period and infancy. *Arch. Surg., 76*:402, 1958.

Grimes, O. F., and Farber, S. M.: Air cysts of the lung. *Surg. Gynecol. Obstet., 113*:720, 1961.

Gross, R.: Congenital cystic disease: successful pneumonectomy in a three week old baby. *Ann. Surg., 123*:229, 1946.

Guest, J. L., and others: Pulmonary parenchymal air space abnormalities. *Ann. Thorac. Surg., 1*:102, 1965.

Herrmann, J. W., Jewett, T. C., and Galletti, G.: Bronchogenic cysts in infants and children. *J. Thorac. Surg., 37*:242, 1957.

Holinger, P. H., and others: Congenital malformations of trachea, bronchi, and lung. *Ann. Otol., 61*:1159, 1952.

Jones, J. C., Almond, C. H., Snyder, H. M., and Meyer, B. W.: Congenital pulmonary cysts in infants and children. *Ann. Thorac. Surg., 3*:297, 1967.

Landing, B. H.: Anomalies of the respiratory tract. *Pediatr. Clin. North Am., 4*:73, 1957.

Lichtenstein, H.: Congenital multiple cysts of the lung. *Dis. Chest, 24*:646, 1953.

Lindskog, G. E., Liebow, A. A., and Glenn, W. W. L.: *Thoracic and Cardiovascular Surgery, with Related Pathology.* New York, Appleton-Century-Crofts, Inc., 1962, p. 104.

Maier, H. C.: The pleura. In Sabiston, D. C., and Spencer, F. C. (Eds.): *Gibbon's Surgery of the Chest*. 3rd Ed. Philadelphia, W. B. Saunders Company, 1976, p. 370.

Minnis, J. F., Jr.: Congenital cystic disease of the lung in infancy. *J. Thorac. Cardiovasc. Surg., 43*:262, 1962.

Murphy, D. R., and Owen, H. F.: Respiratory emergencies in the newborn. *Am. J. Surg.*, May 1961, p. 581.

Nixon, H. H., and O'Donnell, B.: *The Essentials of Pediatric Surgery*. London, William Heinemann, Ltd., 1961, p. 38.

Opsahl, T., and Berman, E. J.: Bronchogenic mediastinal cysts in infants. *Pediatrics, 30*:372, 1962.

Potts, W. J.: *The Surgeon and the Child*. Philadelphia, W. B. Saunders Company, 1964, p. 68.

Potts, W. J., and Riker, W. L.: Differentiation of congenital cysts of lung and those following staphylococcal pneumonia. *Arch. Surg., 61*:684, 1950.

Pryce, D. M.: Lining of healed but persistent abscess cavities in lung with epithelium of ciliated columnar type. *J. Pathol. Bacteriol., 60*:259, 1948.

Ravitch, M. M.: Congenital cystic disease of the lung. In Benson, C. D., and others (Eds.): *Pediatric Surgery*. Vol. 1. Chicago, Year Book Medical Publishers, Inc., 1962. p. 355.

Ravitch, M. M., and Hardy, J. B.: Congenital cystic disease of lung in infants and children. *Arch. Surg., 59*:1, 1949.

Riker, W. L.: Lung cysts and pneumothorax in infants and children. *Surg. Clin. North Am., 36*:1613, 1956.

Schaffer, A. J., and Avery, M. E.: *Diseases of the Newborn*. 3rd Ed. Philadelphia, W. B. Saunders Company, 1971, p. 149.

Slim, M. S., and Melhem, R. E.: Congenital pulmonary air cysts. *Arch. Surg., 88*:923, 1964.

Spandler, B. P.: Pathogenesis and treatment of pulmonary tension cavities. *Am. Rev. Tuberc. Pulmon. Dis., 76*:370, 1957.

Spencer, H.: *Pathology of the Lung (Excluding Pulmonary Tuberculosis)*. New York, Macmillan Company, 1962, pp. 40, 45.

Swan, H., and Aragon, G. E.: Surgical treatment of pulmonary cysts in infancy. *Pediatrics, 14*:651, 1954.

Swenson, O.: *Pediatric Surgery*. 2nd Ed. New York, Macmillan Company, 1962, p. 120.

Szots, I., and Jakab, T.: Indications for urgent operation in pulmonary tension disorders in childhood. *Arch. Dis. Child., 39*:172, 1964.

Vanhoutte, J. J., and Miller, K. E.: Angiographic contribution to the determination of the etiology of some pulmonary cysts of infancy. *Am. J. Roentgenol. Radium Ther. Nucl. Med., 108*:569, 1970.

Woods, F. M.: Cystic diseases of the lung. *J. Int. Coll. Surg., 19*:568, 1953.

Lobar Emphysema

Avery, M. E., and Fletcher, B. D.: *The Lung and Its Disorders in the Newborn Infant*. 3rd Ed. Philadelphia, W. B. Saunders Company, 1974, p. 125.

Backman, A., Parkkulaimen, K. V., and Sulammaa, M.: Pulmonary tension emergencies in infants. *Ann. Paediatr. Fenn., 5*:172, 1959.

Baker, D.: Chronic pulmonary disease in infants and children. *Radiol. Clin. North Am., 1*:519, 1963.

Bates, D. V., Macklem, P. T., and Christie, R. V.: *Respiratory Function in Disease, an Introduction to the Integrated Study of the Lung*. 2nd Ed. Philadelphia. W. B. Saunders Company, 1971, p. 215.

Binet, J. P., Nezelof, C., and Fredet, J.: Five cases of lobar emphysema in infancy; importance of bronchial malformation and value of postoperative steroid therapy. *Dis. Chest, 41*:126, 1962.

Bolande, R. R., Schneider, A. F., and Boggs, J. D.: Infantile lobar emphysema, an etiological concept. *Arch. Pathol., 61*:289, 1956.

Burford, T. H., and Ferguson, T. B.: Congenital lesions of the lung and emphysema. In Sabiston, D. C., and Spencer, F. C. (Eds.): *Gibbon's Surgery of the Chest*. 3rd Ed. Philadelphia, W. B. Saunders Company, 1976, p. 611.

Burman, S. O., and Kent, E. M.: Bronchiolar emphysema (cirrhosis of the lung). *J. Thorac. Cardiovasc. Surg., 43*:253, 1962.

Butterfield, J., and others: Cystic emphysema in premature infants, report of an outbreak with the isolation of type 19 ECHO virus in one case. *N. Engl. J. Med., 268*:18, 1963.

Campbell, D., Bauer, A. J., and Hewlett, T. H.: Congenital localized emphysema. *J. Thorac. Cardiovasc. Surg., 41*:575, 1961.

Egan, R. W., Jewett, T. C., and Macmanus, J. E.: Congenital lesions of the thorax in infancy demanding early surgical treatment. *Arch. Surg., 77*:584, 1968.

Ehrenhaft, J. L., and Taber, R. E.: Progressive infantile emphysema, a surgical emergency. *Surgery, 34*:412, 1953.

Eigen, H., Lemen, R. J., and Waring, W. W.: Congenital lobar emphysema: long-term evaluation of surgically and conservatively treated children. *Am. Rev. Resp. Dis., 113*:823, 1976.

Fischer, H. W., Potts, W. J., and Holinger, P. H.: Lobar emphysema in infants and children. *J. Pediatr., 41*:403, 1952.

Fischer, H. W., Lucido, J. L., and Lynxwiler, C. P.: Lobar emphysema. *J.A.M.A., 166*:340, 1958.

Floyd, F. W., and others: Bilateral congenital lobar emphysema surgically corrected. *Pediatrics, 31*:87, 1963.

Gans, S. L., and Hackworth, L. E.: Respiratory obstructions of surgical import. *Pediatr. Clin. North Am., 6*:1023, 1959.

Hendren, W. H., and McKee, D. M.: Lobar emphysema of infancy. *J. Pediatr. Surg., 1*:24, 1966.

Henry, W.: Localized pulmonary hypertrophic emphysema. *J. Thorac. Surg., 27*:197, 1954.

Jewett, T. C., Jr., and Adler, R. H.: Localized pulmonary emphysema of infancy. *Surgery, 43*:1958.

Jones, J. C., and others: Lobar emphysema and congenital heart disease in infancy. *J. Thorac. Cardiovasc. Surg.*, 49:1, 1965.

Kanphuys, E. H. M.: Congenital lobar emphysema. *Arch. Chir. Neerl.*, 14:93, 1962.

Kennedy, J. H., and Rothman, B. F.: The surgical treatment of congenital lobar emphysema. *Surg. Gynecol. Obstet.*, 121:253, 1965.

Korngold, H. W., and Baker, J. M.: Nonsurgical treatment of unilobar obstructive emphysema of the newborn. *Pediatrics*, 14:296, 1954.

Kress, M. B., and Finkelstein, A. H.: Giant bullous emphysema occurring in tuberculosis in childhood. *Pediatrics*, 30:269, 1962.

Kruse, R. L., and Lynn, H. B.: Lobar emphysema in infants. *Mayo Clin. Proc.*, 44:525, 1969.

Landing, B. H.: Anomalies of the respiratory tract. *Pediatr. Clin. North Am.*, 4:73, 1957.

Leape, L. L., and Longino, L. A.: Infantile lobar emphysema. *Pediatrics*, 34:246, 1964.

Leape, L. L., Ching, N., and Holder, T. M.: Lobar emphysema and patent ductus arteriosus. *Pediatrics*, 46:97, 1970.

Lewis, J. E., and Potts, W. J.: Obstructive emphysema with a defect of the anterior mediastinum. *J. Thorac. Surg.*, 21:438, 1959.

Lincoln, J. C. R., Stark, J., Subramanian, S., Aberdeen, E., Bonham-Carter, R. E., Berry, C. L., and Waterston, D. J.: Congenital lobar emphysema. *Ann. Surg.*, 173:55, 1971.

Lindskog, G. E., Liebow, A. A., and Glenn, W. W. L.: *Thoracic and Cardiovascular Surgery, with Related Pathology.* New York. Appleton-Century-Crofts, Inc., 1962, p. 357.

Mauney, F. M., Jr. and Sabiston, D. C., Jr.: The role of pulmonary scanning in the diagnosis of congential lobar emphysema. *Am. Surg.*, 36:20, 1970.

May, R. L., Meese, E. H., and Timmes, J. J.: Congenital lobar emphysema: case report of bilateral involvement. *J. Thorac. Cardiovasc. Surg.*, 48:850, 1964.

Mercer, R. D., Hawk, W. A., and Karakjian, G.: Massive lobar emphysema in infants: diagnosis and treatment. *Cleveland Clin. Q.*, 28:270, 1961.

Moore, T. C.: Chondroectodermal dysplasia (Ellis–Van Creveld syndrome) with bronchial malformation and neonatal tension lobar emphysema. *J. Thorac. Cardiovasc. Surg.*, 46:1, 1963.

Murphy, D. R., and Owen, H. F.: Respiratory emergencies in the newborn. *Am. J. Surg.*, 101:581, 1961.

Murray, G. F.: Congenital lobar emphysema. *Surg. Gynecol. Obstet.*, 124:611, 1967.

Murray, G. F., Talbert, J. L., and Haller, J. A., Jr.: Obstructive lobar emphysema of the newborn infant—documentation of the "mucus plug syndrome" with successful treatment by bronchotomy. *J. Thorac. Cardiovasc. Surg.*, 53:886, 1967.

Myers, N. A.: Congenital lobar emphysema. *Aust. N. Z. J. Surg.*, 30:32, 1960.

Nelson, T. Y.: Tension emphysema in infants. *Arch. Dis. Child.*, 32:38, 1957.

Nelson, T. Y., and Reye, D.: Tension emphysema: a surgical emergency in infants. *Med. J. Aust.*, August 28, 1954, p. 342.

Nixon, H. H., and O'Donnell, B.: *The Essentials of Pediatric Surgery.* London, William Heinemann, Ltd., 1961, p. 40.

Overstreet, R. M.: Emphysema of a portion of the lung in the early months of life. *J. Dis. Child.*, 57:861, 1939.

Pierce, W. S., deParedes, C. G., Friedman, S., and Waldhausen, J. A.: Concomitant congenital heart disease and lobar emphysema in infants: incidence, diagnosis, and operative management. *Ann. Surg.*, 172:951, 1970.

Potts, W. J.: *The Surgeon and the Child.* Philadelphia, W. B. Saunders Company, 1959, p. 70.

Raynor, C. C., Capp, M. P., and Sealy, W. C.: Lobar emphysema of infancy. *Ann. Thorac. Surg.*, 4:374, 1967.

Riker, W. L.: Neonatal respiratory distress. In Benson, C. D., and others (Eds.): *Pediatric Surgery.* Vol. 1. Chicago, Year Book Medical Publishers, Inc., 1962, p. 352.

Robertson, R., and James, E. S.: Congenital lobar emphysema. *Pediatrics*, 8:795, 1951.

Schaffer, A. J., and Avery, M. E.: *Diseases of the Newborn.* 3rd Ed. Philadelphia, W. B. Saunders Company, 1971, p. 80.

Spencer, H.: *Pathology of the Lung (Excluding Pulmonary Tuberculosis).* New York, Macmillan Company, 1962, p. 408.

Thomson, J., and Forfar, J. O.: Regional obstructive emphysema in infancy. *Arch. Dis. Child.*, 33:97, 1958.

Urban, A. E., Stark, J., and Waterston, D. J.: Congenital lobar emphysema. *Thoraxchirurgie*, 23:255, 1975.

Vaughan, V. C., III, and McKay, R. J.: *Nelson Textbook of Pediatrics.* 10th Ed. Philadelphia, W. B. Saunders Company, 1975, p. 989.

White, M., and Dennison, W. M.: *Surgery in Infancy and Childhood, a Handbook for Medical Students and General Practitioners.* Edinburgh, E.&S. Livingstone, Ltd., 1958, p. 304.

Williams, H., and Campbell, P.: Generalized bronchiectasis associated with deficiency of cartilage in the bronchial tree. *Arch. Dis. Child.*, 35:182, 1960.

Wiseman, D. H.: Unilateral pseudoemphysema—a case report. *Pediatrics*, 35:300, 1965.

Zatzkin, H. R., Cole, P. M., and Bronsther, B.: Congenital hypertrophic lobar emphysema. *Surgery*, 52:505, 1962.

Pulmonary Sequestration

Asp, K., and others: Sequestrations in children. *Ann. Paediatr. Fenn.*, 9:270, 1963.

Avery, M. E., and Fletcher, B. D.: *The Lung and Its Disorders in the Newborn Infant.* 3rd Ed. Philadelphia, W. B. Saunders Company, 1974, p. 156.

Boyden, E. A.: *Segmental Anatomy of the Lungs.* New York, McGraw-Hill Book Company, Inc., 1955.

Boyden, E. A.: Bronchogenic cysts and the theory of intralobar sequestration: new embryologic data. *J. Thorac. Surg.*, 35:604, 1958.

Breton, A., and others: Pulmonary sequestration: aortographic diagnosis and pathogenic discussion. *Arch. Franc. Pediatr.*, 16:751, 1959.

Britton, R. C., Weston, J. T., and Landing, B. H.: Plastic injection techniques in pediatric pathology, with particular reference to roentgenographic analysis of injected specimens. *Bull. Int. A. M. Mus.*, 31:124, 1950.

Bruwer, A., Clagett, O. T., and McDonald, J. R.: Anomalous arteries to the lung associated with congenital pulmonary abnormality. *J. Thorac. Surg.*, 19:957, 1950.

Buntain, W. L., Isaacs, H., Jr., Payne, V. C., Jr., Lindesmith, G. G., and Rosenkrantz, J. G.: Lobar emphysema, cystic adenomatoid malformation, pulmonary sequestration, and bronchogenic cysts in infancy and childhood: a clinical group. *J. Pediatr. Surg.*, 9:85, 1974.

Burford, T. H., and Ferguson, T. B.: Congenital lesions of the lungs and emphysema. In Sabiston, D. C., and Spencer, F. C. (Eds.): *Gibbon's Surgery of the Chest*. 3rd Ed. Philadelphia, W. B. Saunders Company, 1976, p. 611.

Bryon, N. D., Campbell, D. C., and Hood, R. H.: Lower accessory lung. *J. Thorac. Cardiovasc. Surg.*, 47:605, 1964.

Carter, R.: Pulmonary sequestration. *Ann. Thorac. Surg.*, 7:68, 1969.

Claman, M. A., and Ehrenhaft, J. L.: Bronchopulmonary sequestration. *J. Thorac. Cardiovasc. Surg.*, 39:531, 1960.

DeBakey, M., Arey, J. B., and Brunazzi, R.: Successful removal of lower accessory lung. *J. Thorac. Surg.*, 19:304, 1950.

Demos, N. J., and Teresi, A.: Congenital lung malformations. A unified concept and a case report. *J. Thorac. Cardiovasc. Surg.*, 70:260, 1975.

Elliott, G. B., and others: Thoracic sequestration cysts of fetal bronchogenic and esophageal origin. *Can. J. Surg.*, 4:522, 1961.

Ellis, F. H., McGoon, D. C., and Kincaid, O. W.: Congenital vascular malformations of the lungs. *Med. Clin. North Am.*, 48:1069, 1964.

Flavell, G.: *An Introduction to Chest Surgery*. London, Oxford University Press, 1957, p. 129.

Gallagher, P. G., Lynch, J. P., and Christian, H. J.: Intralobar bronchopulmonary sequestration of the lung. *N. Engl. J. Med.*, 257:643, 1957.

Gans, S. L., and Potts, W. J.: Anomalous lobe of lung arising from the esophagus. *J. Thorac. Surg.*, 21:313, 1951.

Gerald, F. P., and Lyons, H. A.: Anomalous artery in intralobar bronchopulmonary sequestration. *N. Engl. J. Med.*, 259:662, 1958.

Halasz, N. A., Lindskog, G. E., and Liebow, A. A.: Esophagobronchial fistula and bronchopulmonary sequestration. *Ann. Surg.*, 155:215, 1961.

Hutchin, P.: Congenital cystic disease of the lung. *Rev. Surg.*, March–April 1971, p. 79.

Iwai, K., Shindo, G., Hajikano, H., Tajima, H., Morimoto, M., Kosuda, T., and Yoneuda, R.: Intralobar pulmonary sequestration, with special reference to developmental pathology. *Am. Rev. Resp. Dis.*, 107:911, 1973.

Kafka, B., and Becco, V.: Simultaneous intra- and extrapulmonary sequestration. *Arch. Dis. Child.*, 35:51, 1960.

Kergin, F. G.: Congenital cystic disease of lung associated with anomalous arteries. *J. Thorac. Surg.*, 23:55, 1952.

Kilman, J. W., and others: Pulmonary sequestration. *Arch. Surg.*, 90:648, 1965.

Landing, B. H.: Anomalies of the respiratory tract. *Pediatr. Clin. North Am.*, 4:73, 1957.

Landing, B. H., and Wells, T. R.: Tracheobronchial anomalies in children. *Perspect. Pediatr. Pathol.*, 1:1, 1973.

Lindskog, G. E., Liebow, A. A., and Glenn, W. W. L.: *Thoracic and Cardiovascular Surgery, with Related Pathology*. New York, Appleton-Century-Crofts, Inc., 1962, p. 195.

Mannix, E. P., and Haight, C.: Anomalous pulmonary arteries and cystic disease of the lung. *Medicine*, 34:193, 1955.

Muller, H.: Inaugural Dissertation, University of Halle; quoted by Ramsey, J. N., and Reiman, D. L.: Bronchial adenomas arising in mucous glands. *Am. J. Pathol.* 29:339, 1953.

Pierce, W. S., deParedes, C. G., Raphaely, R. C., and Waldhausen, J. A.: Pulmonary resection in infants younger than one year of age. *J. Thorac. Cardiovasc. Surg.*, 61:875, 1971.

Pryce, D. M.: Lower accessory pulmonary artery with intralobar sequestration of lung. *J. Pathol. Bacteriol.*, 58:457, 1946.

Pryce, D. M., Sellors, T. H., and Blair, L. G.: Intralobar sequestration of lung associated with an abnormal pulmonary artery. *Br. J. Surg.*, 35:18, 1947.

Quinlan, J. J., Shaffer, V. D., and Hiltz, J. E.: Intralobar pulmonary sequestration. *Can. J. Surg.*, 6:418, 1963.

Ravitch, M. M.: Congenital cystic disease of the lung. In Benson, C. D., and others (Eds.): *Pediatric Surgery*. Vol. 1. Chicago, Year Book Medical Publishers, Inc., 1962, p. 360.

Simopoulos, A. P.: Intralobar bronchopulmonary sequestration in children: diagnosis by intrathoracic aortography. *Am. J. Dis. Child.*, 97:796, 1959.

Smith, R. A.: A theory of the origin of intralobar sequestration of lung. *Thorax*, 11:10, 1956.

Smith, R. A.: Some controversial aspects of intralobar sequestration of the lung. *Surg. Gynecol. Obstet.*, 114:57, 1962.

Solit, R. W.: The effect of intralobar pulmonary sequestration on cardiac output. *J. Thorac. Cardiovasc. Surg.*, 49:844, 1965.

Song, Y. S.: Lower pulmonary aberrant lobe. *South. Med. J.*, 49:1137, 1956.

Spencer, H.: *Pathology of the Lung (Excluding Pulmonary Tuberculosis)*. New York, Macmillan Company, 1962, p. 32.

Sperling, D. R., and Finck, E. J.: Intralobar bronchopulmonary sequestration. Association with a murmur over the back in a child. *Am. J. Dis. Child.*, 115:362, 1968.

Symbas, P. N., Hatcher, C. R., Jr., Abbott, O. A., and Logan, W. D., Jr.: An appraisal of pulmonary sequestration: special emphasis on unusual manifestations. *Am. Rev. Resp. Dis.*, 99:406, 1969.

Talalak, P.: Pulmonary sequestration. *Arch. Dis. Child.*, 35:57, 1960.

Turk, L. N., III, and Lindskog, G. E.: The importance of angiographic diagnosis in intralobar pulmonary sequestration. *J. Thorac. Cardiovasc. Surg.*, 41:299, 1961.

Van Rens, T. J. G.: Intralobar sequestration of lung: review of its possible origin and report on five cases. *Arch. Chir. Neerl.*, 14:63, 1962.

Waddell, W. R.: Organoid differentiation of fetal lung; histologic study of differentiation of mammalian fetal lung in utero and in transplants. *Arch. Pathol.*, 47:277, 1949.

Witten, D. M., Clagett, O. T., and Hiltz, J. E.: Intralobar pulmonary sequestration involving the upper lobes. *J. Thorac. Cardiovasc. Surg.*, 43:523, 1962.

Congenital Cystic Adenomatoid Malformation of the Lung

Avery, M. E., and Fletcher, B. D.: *The Lung and Its Disorders in the Newborn Infant.* 3rd Ed. Philadelphia, W. B. Saunders Company, 1974, p. 148.

Bain, G. O.: Congenital adenomatoid malformation of the lung. *Dis. Chest*, 36:430, 1959.

Belanger, R., Lafleche, L. R., and Picard, J. L.: Congenital cystic adenomatoid malformation of the lung. *Thorax*, 19:1, 1964.

Breckenridge, R. L., Rehermann, R. L., and Gibson, E. T.: Congenital cystic adenomatoid malformation of the lung. *J. Pediatr.*, 67:863, 1965.

Buntain, W. L., Isaacs, H., Jr., Payne, V. C., Jr., Lindesmith, G. G., and Rosenkrantz, J. G.: Lobar emphysema, cystic adenomatoid malformation, pulmonary sequestration, and bronchogenic cysts in infancy and childhood: a clinical group. *J. Pediatr. Surg.*, 9:85, 1974.

Chin, K. Y., and Tang, M. Y.: Congenital adenomatoid malformation of one lobe of a lung with general anasarca. *Arch. Pathol.*, 48:311, 1949.

Craig, J. M., Kirkpatrick, J., and Neuhauser, E. B. D.: Congenital cystic adenomatoid malformation of the lung in infants. *Am. J. Roentgenol.*, 76:516, 1956.

Demos, N. J., and Teresi, A.: Congenital lung malformations. A unified concept and a case report. *J. Thorac. Cardiovasc. Surg.*, 70:260, 1975.

Halloran, L. G., Silverberg, S. G., and Salzberg, A. M.: Congenital cystic adenomatoid malformation of the lung: a surgical emergency. *Arch. Surg.*, 104:715, 1972.

Holder, T. M., and Christy, M. G.: Cystic adenomatoid malformation of the lung. *J. Thorac. Cardiovasc. Surg.*, 47:590, 1964.

Hutchin, P.: Congenital cystic disease of the lung. *Rev. Surg.*, March–April 1971, p. 79.

Kwittken, J., and Reiner, L.: Congenital cystic adenomatoid malformation of the lung. *Pediatrics*, 30:759, 1962.

Landing, B. H.: Anomalies of the respiratory tract. *Pediatr. Clin. North Am.*, 4:73, 1957.

Landing, B. H., and Wells, T. R.: Tracheobronchial anomalies in children. *Perspect. Pediatr. Pathol.*, 1:1, 1973.

Merenstein, G. B.: Congenital cystic adenomatoid malformation of the lung. Report of a case and review of the literature. *Am. J. Dis. Child.*, 118:772, 1969.

Pierce, W. S., deParedes, C. G., Raphaely, R. C., and Waldhausen, J. A.: Pulmonary resection in infants younger than one year of age. *J. Thorac. Cardiovasc. Surg.*, 61:875, 1971.

Congenital Pulmonary Lymphangiectasis

Avery, M. E., and Fletcher, B. D.: *The Lung and Its Disorders in the Newborn Infant.* 3rd Ed. Philadelphia, W. B. Saunders Company, 1974, 149.

Brown, M. D., and Reidbord, H. E.: Congenital pulmonary lymphangiectasis. *Am. J. Dis. Child.*, 114:654, 1967.

Carter, R. W., and Vaughn, H. M.: Congenital pulmonary lymphangiectasis. *Am. J. Roentgenol.*, 86:576, 1961.

Fronstein, M. H., Hooper, G. S., Besse, B. E., and Ferreri, S.: Congenital pulmonary cystic lymphangiectasis. *Am. J. Dis. Child.*, 114:330, 1967.

Javett, S. N., Webster, I., and Braudo, J. L.: Congenital dilatation of the pulmonary lymphatics. *Pediatrics*, 31:416, 1963.

Landing, B. H.: Anomalies of the respiratory tract. *Pediatr. Clin. North Am.*, 4:73, 1957.

Laurence, K. M.: Congenital pulmonary cystic lymphangiectasis. *J. Pathol. Bacteriol.*, 70:325, 1955.

Laurence, K. M.: Congenital pulmonary lymphangiectasis. *J. Clin. Pathol.*, 12:62, 1959.

Laurence, K. M.: Personal communication; cited in Spencer, H.: *Pathology of the Lung.* New York, Macmillan Company, 1962, p. 58.

Rywlin, A. M., and Fojaco, R. M.: Congenital pulmonary lymphangiectasis associated with a blind common pulmonary vein. *Pediatrics*, 41:931, 1968.

Spencer, H.: *Pathology of the Lung (Excluding Pulmonary Tuberculosis).* New York, Macmillan Company, 1962, p. 58.

Pulmonary Arteriovenous Fistula

Björk, V. O.: Local extirpation of multiple bilateral pulmonary arteriovenous aneurysms. *J. Thorac. Cardiovasc. Surg.*, 53:293, 1967.

Bosher, L. H., Jr., Blake, D. A., and Byrd, B. R.: An analysis of the pathologic anatomy of pulmonary arteriovenous aneurysms, with particular reference to the applicability of local excision. *Surgery*, 45:91, 1959.

Burford, T. H., and Ferguson, T. B.: Congenital Lesions of the lung and emphysema. *In* Sabiston, D. C., Jr., and Spencer, F. C.: *Gibbon's Surgery of the Chest.* 3rd Ed. Philadelphia, W. B. Saunders Company, 1976, p. 611.

Charbon, B. C., Adams, W. F., and Carlson, R. F.: Surgical treatment of multiple arteriovenous fistulas in the right lung in a patient having undergone a left pneumonectomy seven years earlier for the same disease. *J. Thorac. Surg.,* 23:188, 1952.

Clatworthy, H. W., Jr.: Intrathoracic tumors and cysts. *In* Ariel, I. M., and Pack, G. T. (Eds.): *Cancer and Allied Diseases of Infancy and Childhood.* Boston. Little, Brown, and Company, 1960, p. 149.

Dargeon, H. W.: *Tumors of Childhood, a Clinical Disease.* New York, Paul B. Hoeber, Inc., 1964.

Goldman, A.: Pulmonary arteriovenous fistula with secondary polycythemia occurring in two brothers. *J. Lab. Clin. Med.,* 32:330, 1947.

Goldman, A.: Arteriovenous fistula of the lung: its hereditary and clinical aspects. *Am. Rev. Tuberc.,* 57:266, 1948.

Gomes, M. R., Bernatz, P. E., and Dines, D. E.: Pulmonary arteriovenous fistulas. *Ann. Thorac. Surg.,* 7:582, 1969.

Hall, E. M.: Malignant hemangioma of the lung with multiple metastasis. *Am. J. Pathol., 11*:343, 1935.

Hodgson, C. H., and Kaye, R. I.: Pulmonary arteriovenous fistula and hereditary hemorrhagic telangiectasia. *Dis. Chest, 43*:449, 1963.

Hope, J. W., and Koop, C. E.: Differential diagnosis of mediastinal masses. *Pediatr. Clin. North Am., 6*:379, 1959.

Husson, G. S., and Wyatt, T. C.: Primary pulmonary obliterative vascular disease in infants and young children. *Pediatrics, 23*:493, 1959.

Klassen, K.: Personal communication to H. W. Clatworthy, Jr. *In* Ariel, I. M., and Pack, G. T. (Eds.): *Cancer and Allied Diseases of Infancy and Childhood.* Boston, Little, Brown and Company, 1960, p. 149.

Landing, B. H.: Anomalies of the Respiratory Tract. *Pediatr. Clin. North Am.,* 4:73, 1957.

Lansdowne, M.: Discussion of paper by A. Goldman: *J. Lab. Clin Med., 32*:330, 1947.

Lindgren, E.: Roentgen diagnosis of arteriovenous aneurysm of the lung. *Acta Radiol.,* 27:586, 1946.

Lindskog, G. E., Liebow, A. A., and Glenn, W. W. L.: *Thoracic and Cardiovascular Surgery, with Related Pathology.* New York. Appleton-Century-Crofts, Inc., 1962, p. 110.

Maier, H. C., and others: Arteriovenous fistula of the lung. *J. Thorac. Surg.,* 17:13, 1948.

Michael, P.: *Tumors of Infancy and Childhood.* Philadelphia, J. B. Lippincott Company, 1964, p. 252.

Mitchell, F. N.: Pulmonary arteriovenous telangiectasis. *South. Med. J., 47*:1157, 1954.

Moyer, J. H., and Ackerman, A. J.: Hereditary hemorrhagic telangiectasis associated with pulmonary arteriovenous fistula in two members of a family. *Ann. Intern. Med.,* 29:775, 1948.

Murdock, C. E.: Pulmonary arteriovenous fistulectomy. *Arch. Surg., 86*:44, 1962.

Muri, J.: Arterio-venous aneurysm of the lung. *Dis. Chest, 24*:49, 1953.

Ravitch, M. M.: Anomalies of the pulmonary vessels. *In* Benson, C. D., and others (Eds.): *Pediatric Surgery.* Vol. 1. Chicago, Year Book Medical Publishers, Inc., 1962, pp. 361, 363.

Seaman, W. B., and Goldman, A.: Roentgen Aspects of pulmonary arteriovenous fistula. *Arch. Intern. Med., 89*:70, 1952.

Shefts, L.: Discussion of Paper by H. C. Maier, et al.

Shumaker, H. B., Jr., and Waldhausen, J. A.: Pulmonary arteriovenous fistulas in children. *Ann. Surg., 158*:713, 1963.

Sweet, R. H.: Discussion of Paper by H. C. Maier, et al.

Taber, R. E., and Ehrenhaft, J. L.: Arteriovenous fistulae and arterial aneurysms of the pulmonary arterial tree. *Arch. Surg., 73*:567, 1965.

Vaughan, V. C., and McKay, R. J.: *Nelson Textbook of Pediatrics.* 10th Ed. Philadelphia, W. B. Saunders Company, 1975.

Weiss, D. L., and Czeredarczuk, O.: Rupture of an angiomatous malformation of the pleura in a newborn infant. *Am. J. Dis. Child., 96*:370, 1958.

Wollstein, M.: Malignant hemangioma of the lung with multiple visceral foci. *Arch. Pathol., 12*:562, 1931.

General References

Arey, L. B.: *Developmental Anatomy, a Textbook and Laboratory Manual of Embryology.* 7th Ed. Philadelphia. W. B. Saunders Company, 1965.

Avery, M. E., and Fletcher, B. D.: *The Lung and Its Disorders in the Newborn Infant.* 3rd Ed. Philadelphia, W. B. Saunders Company, 1974.

Bates, D. V., Macklem, P. T., and Christie, R. V.: *Respiratory Function in Disease, an Introduction to the Integrated Study of the Lung.* 2nd Ed. Philadelphia, W. B. Saunders Company, 1971.

Brown, J. J. M. (Ed.): *Surgery of Childhood.* Baltimore, Williams & Wilkins Company, 1963.

Buntain, W. L., Isaacs, H., Jr., Payne, V. C., Jr., Lindesmith, G. G., and Rosenkrantz, J. C.: Lobar emphysema, cystic adenomatoid malformation, pulmonary sequestration, and bronchogenic cyst in infancy and childhood: a clinical group. *J. Pediatr. Surg.,* 9:85, 1974.

Comroe, J. H., Jr., and others: *The Lung, Clinical Physiology and Pulmonary Function Tests.* 2nd Ed. Chicago, Year Book Medical Publishers, Inc., 1962.

Demos, N. J., and Teresi, A.: Congenital lung malformations. A unified concept and a case report. *J. Thorac. Cardiovasc. Surg., 70*:260, 1975.

Flavell, G.: *An Introduction to Chest Surgery.* London, Oxford University Press, 1957.

Flavell, G.: *The Oesophagus.* London, Butterworth, 1963.

Gross, R. E.: *Surgery of Infancy and Childhood. Its Principles and Techniques.* Philadelphia, W. B. Saunders Company, 1953.

Gross, R. E.: *An Atlas of Children's Surgery.* Philadelphia, W. B. Saunders Company, 1970.

Hamilton, W. J., Boyd, J. D., and Mossman, H.

W.: *Human Embryology (Prenatal Development of Form and Function).* 2nd Ed. Cambridge, W. Heffer & Sons, Ltd., 1952.

Hutchin, P.: Congenital cystic disease of the lung. *Rev. Surg.,* March–April 1971, p. 79.

Landing, B. H., and Wells, T. R.: Tracheobronchial anomalies in children. *Perspect. Pediatr. Pathol., 1*:1, 1973.

Leigh, T. F., and Weens, H. S.: *The Mediastinum.* ·Springfield, Illinois, Charles C Thomas, 1959.

Lindskog, G. E., Liebow, A. A., and Glenn, W. W. L.: *Thoracic and Cardiovascular Surgery, with Related Pathology.* New York, Appleton-Century-Crofts, Inc., 1962.

Mustard, W. T., and others (Eds.): *Pediatric Surgery* 2nd Ed. Vol. 1. Chicago, Year Book Medical Publishers, Inc., 1969.

Nixon, H. H., and O'Donnell, B.: *The Essentials of Pediatric Surgery.* London, William Heinemann, Ltd., 1961.

Patten, B. M.: *Human Embryology.* 2nd Ed. New York, McGraw-Hill Book Company, Inc., 1953.

Pierce, W. S., deParedes, C. G., Raphaely, R. C., and Waldhausen, J. A.: Pulmonary resection in infants younger than one year of age. *J. Thorac. Cardiovasc. Surg., 61*:875, 1971.

Potts, W. J.: *The Surgeon and the Child.* Philadelphia, W. B. Saunders Company, 1959.

Rickham, P. P., and Johnston, J. H.: *Neonatal Surgery.* New York, Appleton-Century-Crofts, Inc., 1969.

Sabiston, D. C., and Spencer, F. C. (Eds.): *Gibbon's Surgery of the Chest.* 3rd Ed. Philadelphia, W. B. Saunders Company, 1976.

Schaffer, A. J., and Avery, M. E.: *Diseases of the Newborn.* 3rd Ed. Philadelphia, W. B. Saunders Company, 1971.

Spencer, H.: *Pathology of the Lung (Excluding Pulmonary Tuberculosis).* New York, Macmillan Company, 1962.

Swenson, O.: *Pediatric Surgery.* 3rd Ed. Vol. 1. New York, Appleton-Century-Crofts, Inc., 1969.

Vaughan, V. C., III, and McKay, R. J.: *Nelson Textbook of Pediatrics.* 10th Ed. Philadelphia, W. B. Saunders Company, 1975.

White, M., and Dennison, W. M.: *Surgery in Infancy and Childhood, a Handbook for Medical Students and General Practitioners.* Edinburgh, E.&S. Livingstone, Ltd., 1958.

CHAPTER TEN

RESPIRATORY DISORDERS IN THE NEWBORN

Mildred T. Stahlman, M.D.

The importance of abnormalities in respiration in the newborn cannot be overemphasized. Abnormalities of pulmonary ventilation, whether from intrinsic or extrinsic causes, are associated with most of the morbidity and mortality of newborn babies. During the past two decades, a great deal of clinical interest and investigative effort has gone into studies of pulmonary function in both normal and abnormal circumstances, and vigorous attempts are being made to recognize, understand and, if possible, correct abnormalities with rational therapy. This chapter, although not attempting to be all-inclusive, will deal with a number of these conditions in the hope that pediatricians dealing with newborns will be encouraged to assume a more vigorous approach toward the investigation and therapy of respiratory problems in small infants.

An understanding of intrauterine and intrapartum events is vital in the diagnosis of neonatal respiratory distress, and good communication between obstetrician and pediatrician is clearly in the baby's best interest.

EVALUATION OF THE INFANT WITH RESPIRATORY DIFFICULTY

A history of maternal polyhydramnios suggests the possibility of upper gastrointestinal obstruction, such as esophageal atresia associated with a tracheoesophageal fistula. A premature baby of a mother who has had previous premature babies with respiratory distress suggests hyaline membrane disease, as does a maternal history of diabetes or a nonelective cesarean section. The latter especially seems to be true if maternal bleeding has been the indication for section. A history of fetal bradycardia or tachycardia suggests intrauterine distress. This may be associated with the passage of meconium, respiratory depression at birth and subsequent respiratory problems associated with meconium aspiration pneumonia. This becomes even more likely if the pregnancy is abnormally prolonged. The amount and timing of maternal analgesia, sedation and anesthesia are important considerations in the differential diagnosis of respiratory depression, asphyxia and brain hemorrhage. Prolonged and difficult labor, especially if umbilical cord compression is suspected, is often associated with asphyxia, with both metabolic and respiratory acidosis, shock and occasionally pulmonary edema. A history of being the smaller of premature twins might suggest hypoglycemia, while the possibility of baby-to-baby transfusion with either hypervolemia or hypovolemia should be kept in mind. A maternal setup for Rh, ABO or other rare blood factor incompatibility should alert the physician to the possibility of cardiac failure associated with severe anemia as a cause of respiratory distress. A difficult

271

manipulative delivery suggests brain hemorrhage, and so might a maternal bleeding diathesis, such as idiopathic thrombocytopenic purpura. Maternal ingestion of iodides can produce thyroid enlargement in the newborn sufficient to embarrass respiration, and reserpine given to the mother can cause enough edema of the nasal mucosa of the newborn to produce severe difficulties in breathing. A history of premature rupture of the membranes, especially if associated with signs of infection in the mother or foul-smelling amniotic fluid, arouses suspicion of intrauterine bacterial sepsis with pneumonia. A history of respiratory depression at birth necessitating positive pressure resuscitation alerts one to the possibility of pneumothorax or pneumomediastinum as a cause of subsequent respiratory embarrassment.

A complete physical examination is often delayed or only sketchily done in distressed babies, especially in small prematures. Most such babies will be housed in incubators, which present a noisy environment and a barrier to careful evaluation of physical signs. Nevertheless, inspection usually provides the most valuable information. Such findings as meconium staining or peeling skin on a thin baby bring to mind the likelihood of meconium aspiration pneumonia; a flat abdomen suggests diaphragmatic hernia. Inspection of the respiratory pattern may suggest the difference between central nervous system disease, mechanical obstruction to the airway, intrinsic pulmonary pathologic changes and congenital cardiac disease.

The presence or absence of visible cyanosis can be a deceptive physical sign in the newborn. Many normal newborn babies have venous stasis with cyanosis of the hands and feet for several hours after birth. Because most normal babies are polycythemic by adult standards and appear plethoric, the same number of grams of unsaturated hemoglobin that produces visible cyanosis indicating serious disease in an adult may be associated with mild disorders or even with normal transitional circulation of the newborn. In contrast, a cold baby may appear to have his hemoglobin fully saturated with oxygen in the presence of a lowered arterial oxygen tension by virtue of the shift to the left of the oxygen dissociation curve for hemoglobin that is associated with hypothermia. The normal newborn has a small functioning right-to-left shunt through the foramen ovale for several days, and anatomic closure does not occur for several weeks. Therefore, hard crying, breath-holding, or straining with defecation or urination associated with a Valsalva maneuver may increase the functional shunting manyfold and produce transient, visible cyanosis. On the other hand, a newborn who has bled excessively or who is anemic from hemolytic disease may be in serious respiratory distress and even have a high percentage of his arterial blood unsaturated without showing visible cyanosis because of profound anemia. One of the most characteristic features of severe metabolic acidosis, which may accompany hyaline membrane disease and many other severe respiratory or circulatory disturbances, is the extreme peripheral vasoconstriction that accompanies a very low blood pH and may mask the degree of hemoglobin unsaturation. Such babies are ashen gray rather than blue, and if unheeded this becomes a poor prognostic sign.

As a part of a routine physical examination of a baby in respiratory difficulties, it is advisable to pass a large-bore catheter into the stomach, introducing air while auscultating over the left upper quadrant in order to identify an intact upper gastrointestinal tract. The stomach is then emptied as completely as possible by suction. Such material as meconium or maternal blood can be identified, and in the case of suspected amnionitis, the contents may be cultured and examined directly for the presence of polymorphonuclear leukocytes and bacteria.

Physical examination of the chest in a newborn can be deceptive as to the degree and type of disease inside. Crepitation of air over the upper part of the sternum in the neck or signs of venous distention in the head and neck are good indications of mediastinal emphysema, but they are frequently absent even though "air block" exists. Inequality of breath sounds — loud on one side, diminished or absent on the other, and interpreted as a sign of pneumothorax — often points to the wrong side of involvement. Rhonchi are frequently heard in newborns with many types of respiratory embarrassment; however, after the oropharynx has been suctioned free of secretions and debris, fine rales are relatively rare, even in the face of widespread parenchymal involvement. When fine rales do occur, they are of significance and are usually associated with bacterial pneumonia. Moist rales are usually heard with pulmonary hemorrhage or frank pulmonary edema, but occur late as a sign of cardiac failure in a newborn. "Poor air entry" is a description of the early auscultatory findings in hyaline membrane disease and is replaced by scratchy, sandpaper to-and-fro sounds late in the disease as the prognosis becomes poorer. Inspiratory stridor points to partial obstruction in the upper airway, from the oropharynx through the trachea, whereas wheezing respiratory sounds are usually associated with bronchial or bronchiolar obstructive disease, which may be localized or widespread. Expiratory grunt is frequently associated with hyaline membrane disease, but may also occur with meconium aspiration pneumonia, bacterial pneumonia and other causes of severe respiratory distress.

Cardiac murmurs may be difficult to assess in the newborn in respiratory distress. Many murmurs, later clearly audible and associated with congenital cardiac defects, may be inapparent in the newborn because of altered relations in pressure, flow and resistance associated with the transitional circulation. Although the ductus arteriosus is open and may be shunting large amounts of blood for a period of hours, even in the term or premature newborn, and for many days in distressed infants, murmurs are rarely heard in the first two days after birth. Their appearance is usually also associated with a rising systemic and falling pulmonary arterial pressure; at first they are systolic in time. Only occasionally are typical continuous diamond-shaped murmurs heard with the ductus in an otherwise normal neonate, and when they occur, they usually persist. Continuous ductal murmurs frequently appear, however, in the very immature infant or the hyaline membrane disease infant on day three or four, often associated with the appearance of moist rales and a roentgenographic picture of pulmonary edema.

Persistent tachycardia over 160 per minute or bradycardia less than 100 per minute may be present with hypoxia from any cause, and both are frequently relieved by adequate oxygenation. In contrast to the adult, tachycardia may be absent as a physical sign and a clue to severe hemorrhage in the newborn. Bradycardia may also signal hyperkalemia.

An easily palpable liver in respiratory distress may mean many things, ranging from frank cardiac failure to extramedullary hematopoiesis associated with hemolytic disease, liver involvement with cytomegalic inclusion disease, bacterial sepsis or parasites, or emphysema associated with a flattened diaphragm.

Edema may be equally difficult to evaluate. The ability to pit edema requires that the subcutaneous fluid collection be shifted under extrinsic pressure. In the case of the newborn whose skin and subcutaneous tissues are stretched tightly for the first time, pitting may be difficult to demonstrate. Nevertheless, a surprisingly large percentage of baby's body weight may be inapparent edema fluid, most readily diagnosed by observing the shiny, smooth aspect of the skin, especially that of the palms and soles, and the flabby fold of swollen skin along the posterior axillary line, visible when a baby is lying supine. In contrast to this type of generalized edema most frequently seen in premature infants, and most severe in those with hyaline membrane disease, is the anasarca of the hydropic baby, who is more obviously edematous and frequently also shows frank ascites associated with his severe anemia. This also is in striking contrast to the postmature baby, who is a good candidate for meconium aspiration pneumonia and shows dry, cracking and peeling integument, but frequently has definite pitting edema of the dorsa of the hands and feet.

Every baby with a respiratory distress that persists or is of any severity deserves a roentgenologic examination. Anteroposterior and lateral portable films can be made with good radiologic technique in an incubator with minimal disturbance to the infant if the x-ray technicians and nurses are properly oriented as to the positioning and x-ray settings required. Although several clinical entities can produce the same shadows in the lung fields, many others are specific, such as pneumothorax, diaphragmatic hernia and bullous emphysema. Other radiographic pictures, not so specific, must be classified as "compatible with" by the radiologist, and the most likely diagnosis is ascribed by the clinician, who has the advantage of a history and physical examination. In the case of specific difficult diagnoses, such as an "H" type of tracheoesophageal fistula or occult diaphragmatic hernia behind the heart, special roentgenographic techniques using contrast media may aid in the correct diagnosis.

The electrocardiogram is a useful tool in the monitoring and management of many newborns with respiratory difficulties, but only rarely is it of diagnostic aid. Some types of congenital cardiac defects, such as endocardial fibroelastosis or tricuspid atresia, may have a highly suggestive electrocardiogram, with abnormal preponderance of the left side of the heart for a newborn.

In the case of conduction defects and arrhythmias, the electrocardiogram is pathognomonic. It is rarely a helpful prognosticator in hyaline membrane disease, except as a valuable index of serum hyperkalemia. The prolonged atrioventricular conduction associated with hyperkalemia in these infants demands prompt and specific treatment.

Arterial blood gas and pH measurements are of tremendous help in differentiating different types of physiologic impairment associated with respiratory distress of varied causes, and repeated measurements are useful both in prognosticating the outcome and in directing therapy.

Many more elaborate tests of pulmonary function have been devised for the newborn, usually as an adaptation from techniques applicable to adults. In research laboratories under trained supervision, these can actually pinpoint and quantitate the specific types of physiologic and biochemical abnormalities present in distressed babies. Many of these techniques have recently been summarized. Most clinicians who treat distressed newborns have only their eyes, ears and hands, a roentgenogram and electrocardiogram, and perhaps a pH and arterial oxygen tension to help them in their diagnosis and to direct their therapy. Fortunately, each will have his own brain for a computer, and if the data are programmed correctly, great accuracy can be achieved and, with experience, correct correlations can be made.

EFFECTS OF A TRANSITIONAL CIRCULATION ON NEONATAL RESPIRATORY DISTRESS

After birth, with the separation of the infant from the placenta (which has served as the fetal lung) and with the onset of respiration, a period of time exists during which the neonatal circulatory pattern undergoes profound adjustments. Normally, with the onset of breathing, pulmonary blood flow is increased manyfold as a consequence of mechanical lung expansion and of progressively better oxygenation to the lung, both of which reduce the pulmonary vascular resistance. This occurs concomitantly with a rise in total systemic vascular resistance consequent to the removal of the large placental runoff. The net effect of these changes is to lower the pulmonary arterial pressure at the same time that the systemic pressure is increased and to reverse the pressure gradient across the ductus arteriosus. A bidirectional ductus arteriosus shunt occurs for a short period, and during this time the systemic venous return still exceeds that from the pulmonary veins, and a right-to-left shunt through the foramen ovale persists. As these changes in systemic and pulmonary vascular resistance progress, the shunt through the ductus becomes totally left-to-right, increasing the amount of pulmonary venous return to the left atrium. This acts to close the foramen ovale valve, which lies on the left side of the atrial septum. As better oxygenation occurs with better pulmonary perfusion, the ductus arteriosus, which is sensitive to oxygen tension, begins to constrict, and shunting through the ductus is progressively diminished and functionally ceases in the normal term infant about 24 hours after birth.

The principal differences between the circulation of the newborn and that of an older child or adult are (1) the presence of an anatomically open ductus arteriosus capable of shunting blood in two directions, either into or away from the lungs; and (2) an unsealed foramen ovale valve, which can readily be forced open to allow right-to-left shunting at times when the pressure gradient is in the direction of the inferior vena cava to the left atrium. There is evidence to suggest that the intact valve may be so stretched by an engorged left atrium as to allow left-to-right shunting at the atrial level. Whether the unconstricted ductus will allow right-to-left, left-to-right or bidirectional shunting to occur (and, if so, its magnitude and timing) is largely dependent upon the differential pressure gradient between the aorta and the pulmonary artery and on the relative resistances of the systemic and pulmonary circulations. Shunting between the atria, on the other hand, seems to be largely dependent upon their different elasticity characteristics. Therefore, situations that either increase pulmonary resistance or lower systemic resistance, or both, will promote resumption of the fetal direction of shunting through both the foramen ovale and the ductus arteriosus.

Pulmonary disease that itself leads to hypoxia and pulmonary arterial hypertension may thus promote extrapulmonary right-to-left shunting and the maintenance of an unconstricted ductus, resulting in further hypoxemia and the establishment of a vicious cycle.

Many types of pulmonary disease in the newborn are associated with this type of circulatory maladjustment, especially if inadequate pulmonary oxygenation is present from the moment of birth. Among the more common types of pathologic processes are hyaline membrane disease and intrauterine aspiration pneumonia. Birth asphyxia leading to shock and systemic hypotension or drug depression producing hypoventilation can also be associated with similar maladjustment in the transitional circulation and persistence of the right-to-left direction of fetal shunts. Shock, whether from perinatal blood loss, from trauma, from endotoxemia associated with sepsis or of central origin, will promote persistent fetal circulatory patterns in the early neonatal period when pulmonary vascular resistance is normally high. In these instances, even minor degrees of pulmonary involvement in processes impeding oxygenation may tip the balance of pulmonary versus systemic resistance. Pharmacologic approaches toward reversing persistent fetal circulatory patterns should be preceded by careful assessment of the underlying precipitation process involved, and management of such things as depleted blood volume, acidosis or infection should be carried out before resorting to potent vasodilators. The importance of early and adequate pulmonary oxygenation is stressed in situations in which pulmonary hypoxia produces further hypoxemia from extrapulmonary shunting, since oxygenation can lower pulmonary resistance, raise aortic pressure, decrease right-to-left shunting through both the foramen ovale and the ductus arteriosus, and promote ductus closure.

RESPIRATORY DEPRESSION, ASPHYXIA AND RESUSCITATION

Of the many functions that the placenta serves the fetus in utero, that of gas exchange is almost the only one which must be assumed by the infant immediately upon delivery. Infants may survive for hours or days with renal agenesis, atresia of the gut, many extreme forms of cardiac malformations and even anencephaly; but he must breathe or die. It is still unclear what factor or combination of factors is important in the initiation of normal respiration by the newly delivered baby. It is possible that the infant in utero lacks the stimuli that induce normal extrauterine respiration, so that the normal circulation on both sides of the placenta maintains fetal blood pH, carbon dioxide tension and oxygen tension at levels incapable of stimulating respiration in utero. In addition, the environmental temperature is stable, and most tactile and painful stimuli are absent. At delivery, the separation from maternal blood gas regulation, the abrupt environmental temperature change, the tactile and frequently the painful stimuli and the rising level of chemical stimuli all may summate to induce respiration. We now know from studies on intrauterine lambs and from continuous ultrasonography in human fetuses that movements of the chest wall stimulating respiratory movements occur as parturition approaches, and that gasping or cessation of the normal "breathing" may signify fetal distress. This type of normal activity may be reflex in origin, and probably implies an intact and reactive nervous system.

In the United States, by far the commonest causes of neonatal respiratory depression of some degree are maternal analgesia or anesthesia. All the general anesthetics are capable of depressing respiration to some degree, depending upon the depth of anesthesia. Many of the commonly used analgesics, such as Demerol or the barbiturates, are capable of producing respiratory depression. The amount given, the timing in relation to delivery, the maturity of the infant and his state of well-being in utero all may have a profound effect upon the degree to which they depress a given infant.

If an infant already in some jeopardy in utero because of a compromised placental circulation that impairs his ability to initiate breathing is further sedated, even lightly, by an inhalation anesthetic that requires pulmonary ventilation for its elimination, the additive effect of moderate asphyxia and mild anesthesia may be enough to suppress breathing completely. Likewise, if drugs that are normally conjugated in the liver and, in utero, are metabolized by the mother's liver happen to be in high concentration in a premature baby's circulation at the moment of birth, and if his liver is partially or completely deficient in the enzymes necessary for such a conjugation owing to immaturity or impaired liver function associated with intrauterine insult, the infant may remain sedated for many hours. Most babies, fortunately, are in an excellent metabolic state in utero, are mature at birth, and tolerate even large amounts of maternal sedation surprisingly well. It is the baby already in jeopardy in utero who requires the most careful judgment in maternal sedation.

Serial studies of the newborn infant's arterial blood immediately after birth have shown that many vigorous infants who have high Apgar scores and who initiate and maintain respiration in a normal fashion may have extremely low aortic oxygen levels at the moment of birth, associated with varying degrees of hypercapnia and lowered pH. Despite prompt respiration and rising arterial oxygen levels, metabolic acidosis continues to develop for several minutes, gradually being corrected over the first hour after birth in the normal infant. It is now clear from these studies, and from those in which blood from the fetal scalp was sampled during labor, that cord blood at delivery reflects changes in the functional relations between mother and fetus during delivery and does not reflect the normal intrauterine state. Serial studies of pH and blood gases of maternal and fetal blood, carried out for many days and using techniques of intrauterine catheterization in sheep which allow a minimum of disturbance of either ewe or fetus, have shown normal levels of carbon dioxide tension and high oxygen saturation prior to the onset of labor.

Animal experiments have shown rapid changes in pH and blood gases during acute postdelivery asphyxia, the oxygen content of arterial blood falling to zero in $2\frac{1}{2}$ minutes, the carbon dioxide tension rising at a rate of approximately 10 mm. Hg per minute, and the pH dropping initially at about 0.1 pH unit per minute. The rapidity with which these changes occur indicates that the period of intrapartum asphyxia of the normal newborn infant must have been very brief.

Carefully controlled studies of asphyxia in newborn monkeys have shown some important considerations relating to resuscitation of the newborn infant. Studies have shown that the longer artificial ventilation is delayed after asphyxia leading to prolonged apnea, the more time will be required for the resuscitation of the infant.

Initial resuscitation can usually be carried out on a mild to moderately asphyxiated infant by prompt aspiration of nose and oropharynx with a bulb syringe, followed by bag and mask ventilation with oxygen. A proper fit of the mask to the infant's face, the maintenance of the infant's chin without neck flexion with a small roll beneath the neck, and pressures adequate to demonstrate chest wall rise and audible breath sounds are essential for adequate ventilation. If profound asphyxia is present, or if there is any deterioration during bagging, prompt introduction of an endotracheal tube under direct laryngeal visualization followed by suction and immediate ventilation is indicated.

The severely asphyxiated infant who requires more than a few minutes of positive pressure to initiate respiration will almost certainly have bradycardia and will be in profound shock. External cardiac massage is indicated once the lungs are expanded. This can readily be applied to the newborn infant with two fingers compressing the chest just to the left of the sternum. Massage should be applied at a rate of 100 to 120 times a minute, and interrupted every five seconds to permit several full inflations of the lung.

The beneficial effects of intravenous buffers and glucose in asphyxiated animals suggest that their use in severely asphyxiated human newborns may be a helpful adjunct to other resuscitative procedures, and such seems to be the case. If buffers such as THAM [tris(hydroxymethyl)aminomethane] or sodium bicarbonate are to be used, it is desirable to be able to monitor the blood pH and to regulate the dosage accordingly.

Evidence seems clear in animals that the length of asphyxia before resuscitative and supportive measures are begun is critical for the development of brain damage. In the newborn infant, knowledge of the extent and length of intrauterine asphyxia is frequently inaccessible. The use of serial estriol determinations, ultrasonographic evidence of fetal growth retardation, fetal scalp pH monitoring during labor, and fetal heart rate patterns in response to uterine contractions are helpful in anticipating and assessing perinatal distress. Until better techniques are developed that allow a more accurate assessment of the fetal state in utero and during delivery, the prevention of neurologic damage incident to birth asphyxia must be based upon these assessments, and prevention, if possible, by prompt and vigorous measures directed toward physiologic and biochemical correction of the degree of asphyxia present at birth.

INTRAUTERINE ASPIRATION PNEUMONIA (MASSIVE ASPIRATION SYNDROME, MECONIUM ASPIRATION PNEUMONIA)

The presence of meconium staining of the amniotic fluid and fetus should alert the physician to the possibility of several adverse conditions in the neonate. If the meconium staining is fresh, as indicated by its dark green color, it is indicative of recent, probably intrapartum interruption in oxygen supply to the fetus, such as cord compression. In many infants, such an event is transient and nonrecurrent, especially if promptly recognized and treated, and the fetus, although acutely asphyxiated in utero, may recover completely by the time of delivery. However, if the insult has been profound, repetitive or continuous up until the time of delivery, the infant may show profound asphyxia and shock at birth, with severe respiratory depression, bradycardia and flaccidity requiring the most vigorous resuscitative efforts and supportive treatment. In addition to birth asphyxia, such an infant may also have begun to gasp before delivery, thereby sucking large amounts of particulate meconium into his respiratory tree,

which on gasping or positive pressure resuscitation become more distally displaced. This meconium may plug the tracheobronchial tree initially, or may cause later respiratory distress referred to as meconium aspiration pneumonia.

In other infants, the amniotic fluid, skin, cord and nails are not green, but yellow-stained. This is indicative of some more remote and perhaps chronic insult to the fetus, since it is almost always associated with other signs of placental dysfunction. These signs include evidence of intrauterine weight loss, with flabby, loose folds of skin, especially about the buttocks and thighs, drawn and pinched facies, loss of vernix, dry, cracking and peeling skin, sparse subcutaneous tissue, and a tendency toward hypoglycemia. The intrauterine passage of meconium is rare in normally grown infants of less than 36 weeks' gestation despite evidence of asphyxia, and yellow staining most frequently occurs in postmature infants. Peeling of the integument, which may be extensive in utero, when associated with asphyxia of such magnitude as to produce intrauterine gasping, allows the aspiration and, indeed, bronchial and alveolar impaction of sheets of squamous cells, mixed with vernix, meconium and other amniotic debris (Fig. 1). At birth, it may be impossible to remove such debris adequately by suction. Severe respiratory distress results. (It should be stated that normal amniotic fluid is not thought to be harmful to the lung; it is rapidly absorbed by the pulmonary lymphatics.) After initial resuscitation, which is frequently necessary because of central nervous system depression, these babies usually exhibit a strong respiratory effort with deep retraction of the costal margins, loud grunting and appreciable cyanosis. A chest roentgenogram usually shows patchy and irregular gross densities and radiolucencies, indicative of the inequality of aeration of various portions of the lung (Fig. 2). Intercostal spaces may bulge outward, and the diaphragmatic leaves become flattened by the patchy areas of overdistention pro-

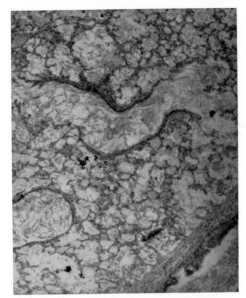

Figure 1. Photomicrograph of the lung of a postmature infant dying with intrauterine aspiration pneumonia, showing sheets of squamous cells packed into all air passages and scattered meconium pigment.

distress for several days, requiring only supportive oxygen therapy and perhaps initial intravenous buffering of a lowered pH. The severely ill infants, however, usually require a continuous high oxygen environment, repeated buffering of pH, and some form of ventilatory assistance for several days. Persistent fetal circulatory patterns are common in these severely ill babies, as demonstrated by a significant difference in oxygenation of blood from the right brachial or temporal artery and the aorta distal to the ductus arteriosus. With profound hypoxia unresponsive to other measures, demonstrable persistent right-to-left ductal shunting may respond to careful administration of pulmonary vasodilators. Even with vigorous treatment the mortality rate is high, and neurologic residua are common in survivors. The need for new modes of adequate intrauterine assessment is again empha-

duced by the ball-valve airway obstruction. Pneumothorax is a frequent complication of such partial obstruction. Even mildly symptomatic infants may have highly abnormal chest roentgenograms.

High carbon dioxide tension in arterial blood reflects the degree of pulmonary involvement, and the low oxygen tension reflects the degree of both intrapulmonary and extrapulmonary right-to-left shunting as well as probable diffusion impairment within the lung. The lowered arterial pH reflects the degree of respiratory acidosis, but this is frequently accompanied by a profound metabolic acidosis, especially if there are signs of prolonged intrauterine distress. Seizures and other evidences of neurologic involvement are common. The use of barbiturates and other analeptic drugs that depress the respiratory center is contraindicated unless ventilation is assisted. Dilantin is the drug of choice for the control of neonatal seizures.

Many of these babies may run a course of moderate clinical respiratory

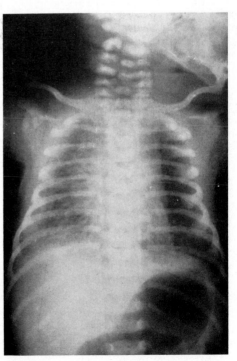

Figure 2. Anteroposterior roentgenogram of the chest of a postmature infant with severe intrauterine aspiration pneumonia, showing coarse mottling of the right lung field and emphysema of the left lung.

sized by this small but profoundly affected group of babies.

Aspiration of regurgitated feedings is a fairly common occurrence in newborn infants, especially prematures, and such aspirates are capable of causing acute respiratory symptoms and subsequent pneumonia. Such aspiration, if massive and overwhelming, and especially if it consists of large milk curds, may prove immediately fatal to a small, weak premature by occluding the airway completely. Most infants, however, if promptly and adequately suctioned, will recover. Occasionally, subsequent to an aspiration episode, an infant will exhibit signs of respiratory distress consisting of tachypnea, fever and rales. X-ray examination of the chest may show patchy or streaky perihilar densities. Supportive therapy is frequently all that is necessary, although prophylactic antibiotics may be given to prevent secondary bacterial pneumonia. Gradual improvement usually occurs over a three- to four-day period.

EMPHYSEMA, PNEUMOTHORAX AND PNEUMOMEDIASTINUM (AIR BLOCK)

The term "emphysema" implies that some portion of the lung is overdistended with air. Simple emphysema may occur as a compensatory mechanism for filling the chest cavity in conditions in which portions of the lung lose volume, such as lobar atelectasis or pulmonary agenesis. Unaffected portions of the lung then become overdistended simply by the negative pressure within the thorax, inducing them to fill the extra space and lessen the excessive negative intrapleural pressure created by the loss of lung volume. In a number of locations in the newborn's lung, air can be found to collect abnormally. Such collections may occur spontaneously in otherwise apparently normal lungs from iatrogenic cause or as a complication of intrinsic pulmonary disease.

Interstitial emphysema is the accumulation of air in interstitial tissue after rupture of alveoli. This air may then dissect along sheaths of blood vessels and bronchi and progress back along their course into the mediastinum, forming multiple blebs of widely varying size between the heart and the anterior chest wall. Since the interstitial space is in direct communication with the rich perivascular and peribronchial lymphatics, diffuse interstitial air may accumulate in these lymphatic channels and greatly disturb fluid homeostasis of the lung. If dissection occurs toward the periphery of the lung, subpleural blebs will be formed, probably in subpleural lymphatics. These are capable of easy rupture into the pleural space, producing pneumothorax.

Iatrogenic interstitial emphysema, pneumothorax or pneumomediastinum can occur in a normal lung with the injudicious use of unmonitored positive pressure resuscitation, frequently applied by an airtight mask without a clear airway. Both the magnitude and the duration of the application of pressure must be taken into account in order to avoid rupture of alveoli, since "safe" pressures may be harmful if applied over a too prolonged period of time. In the case of iatrogenic rupture, symptoms and signs of distress may be present from the onset of respiration at birth. Since respiratory symptoms may be present because of underlying pulmonary disease, such as meconium aspiration, which necessitated the resuscitative efforts, every baby with persistent respiratory symptoms following positive pressure resuscitation deserves anteroposterior and lateral x-ray examination of the chest (Fig. 3). The introduction of lateral roentgenograms of the infant's chest taken with the infant positioned on his back and shot through from the side have allowed the identification of collections of pleural air that compress the mediastinal contents and heart posteriorly and that

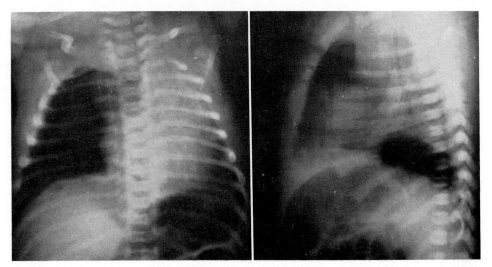

Figure 3. Anteroposterior and lateral chest roentgenograms of a postmature infant two hours after birth, showing a right tension pneumothorax following resuscitation.

might appear insignificant in amount in a film taken with the infant placed on his side or on an anteroposterior film.

Since pneumothorax or pneumomediastinum can also occur spontaneously as a complication of pulmonary disease, such as bacterial pneumonia, especially staphylococcal, or in the course of severe hyaline membrane disease, repeat x-ray examination is likewise indicated when during the course of such a disease process a sudden deterioration occurs or if respiratory symptoms fail to subside concomitant with other signs of clinical improvement. Pneumothorax or pneumomediastinum may significantly complicate the course of severe hyaline membrane disease, since a lung deficient of surfactant, once completely collapsed, is difficult to re-expand, and diffuse interstitial air dissection may have preceded rupture into the pleural cavity. A small pneumothorax or pneumomediastinum not associated with increasing tension may go unnoticed, or may be diagnosed only incidentally on the chest roentgenogram. On those occasions when the air accumulation is large, and especially when under progressively increasing tension, respiratory distress may be so severe as to constitute an emergency necessitating immediate relief.

The baby with a large tension pneumothorax or pneumomediastinum is in acute respiratory embarrassment. Vigorous respiratory efforts are maintained as long as central nervous system integrity lasts. Cyanosis is usually marked, and grunting may occur on expiration. The baby frequently lies with head drawn back, using all the accessory muscles of respiration. The chest shows a rather square and bulging appearance, with shoulders drawn back.

In the case of pneumomediastinum, crepitus may occur under the sternum as air dissects into the suprasternal notch and up the neck. Distention appears in the neck veins if cardiac compression and impedance of systemic venous filling occur. Auscultation may be misleading as to the location of the air, but the heart can be shifted to either side by pneumothorax, or heart sounds muffled by overlying air accumulation. In the case of pneumothorax, x-ray films of the chest will establish the proper location of the air collection. An anteroposterior film alone may be inadequate in the case of a modest-sized pneumomediastinum, since only a faint translucency around the heart shadow appears, but a lateral film will confirm its presence. In cases of large accumu-

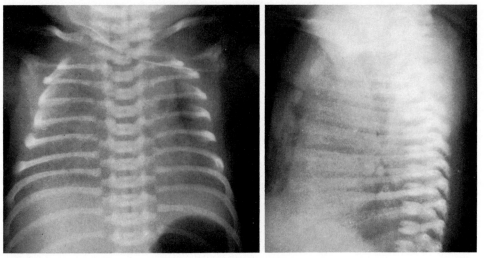

Figure 4.   Anteroposterior and lateral chest roentgenograms of an infant with severe hyaline membrane disease taken five hours after birth, showing reticulogranular pattern with a thin rim of mediastinal air seen just to the left of the cardiac border on the anteroposterior view and between the heart and sternum on the lateral view.

lations of air in the anterior part of the mediastinum, the chest roentgenogram will show the air bulging out on both sides of the heart, tempting needle aspiration (Figs. 4 and 5). This, however, is usually a futile procedure, since the air is not collected in a single large pocket, but in multiple blebs of varying sizes. Tapping with a needle frequently results in a pneumothorax without relief of the mediastinal pressure. Small and moderate-sized accumulations of mediastinal air, if not life-threatening, can safely be left alone and watched closely by repeated chest roentgenograms for progression or resolution. Such babies may require supportive measures, such as added oxygen, and

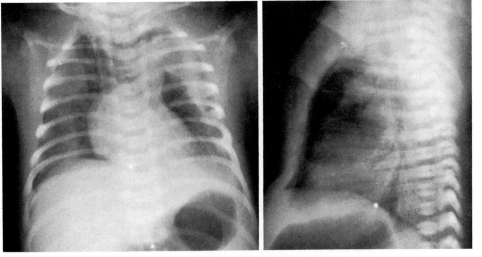

Figure 5.   The same infant as in Figure 4, 35 hours after birth, showing progression of the pneumomediastinum with a large accumulation of air seen surrounding the heart shadow on the anteroposterior view and posterior compression of the heart on the lateral view. A small rim of pneumothorax is seen on the right. This infant was not resuscitated, and the pneumomediastinum was presumed to be spontaneous.

deserve alert and constant nursing care. Massive collections of air in the mediastinum that produce severe cardiac and respiratory symptoms and appear to be life-threatening may be treated by incision of the jugular notch and blunt dissection into the anterior part of the mediastinum. Air blebs are ruptured, and a drain is left in the mediastinal space when the neck wound is closed.

The treatment of choice of a collection of intrapleural air is largely dependent upon its size and whether there exists a tension pneumothorax that reaccumulates after evacuation. Small pneumothoraces may be associated with little or no respiratory distress and may be left untreated and observed clinically and roentgenologically. Most will clear spontaneously. A large accumulation of air, however, sufficient to produce respiratory symptoms, should be removed. If it is apparent that a tension pneumothorax exists, a large-bore catheter with multiple holes near the end is introduced into the anterior chest, connected to an underwater trap, and connected to 10 to 12 cm. of water, negative pressure. Experience has shown that in newborns continuous negative pressure is necessary to prevent the reaccumulation of air and to keep the lung expanded. As long as air bubbles through the trap with respiration, the system is left unchanged. When bubbling ceases and an x-ray film indicates that insignificant amounts of pleural air remain, the tube can first be clamped for a period of hours, the chest re-evaluated, and if air has still not reaccumulated, the tube removed. In rare instances, air continues to accumulate for many days, and in such cases surgical closure of a rent in the lung may be necessary. Infants with chest tubes or repeated pleural aspirations may be placed on wide-spectrum antibiotics, since the opportunities for infection are great. Oxygen, assisted ventilation, careful nursing and other supportive measures such as intravenous fluid therapy during the acute course may be lifesaving.

HYALINE MEMBRANE DISEASE

The respiratory distress syndrome of prematurity, or clinical hyaline membrane disease, is the commonest single cause of severe respiratory symptoms in the newborn. It is associated with approximately 30 per cent of all neonatal deaths, with 50 to 70 per cent of all deaths in premature infants, and is thought to account for approximately 25,000 deaths per year in the United States alone. It is felt to occur exclusively in prematurely born infants. Even though some babies with the disease have birth weights greater than the arbitrary level of 2500 gm., they have other evidences of immaturity, including low gestational age and absence of palpable breast tissue. Babies of diabetic mothers have an especially high incidence; although many of these infants are large at birth, premature delivery is common. Infants born by cesarean section are also thought to be especially likely to have hyaline membrane disease, although evidence suggests that the degree of immaturity of the sectioned baby is a more important factor than the section itself. There are also many suggestions that the indication for the section has great influence on the incidence of the disease; hyaline membrane disease is 13 times as common when the indication is maternal bleeding than when the cesarean section is an elective one. There are many other suggestions that conditions occurring in late pregnancy or incident to delivery that might be expected to compromise the oxygen supply to the fetus, such as maternal bleeding and hypotension and birth asphyxia if associated with premature birth, may be important in the pathogenesis.

There seems to be ample evidence that the baby who will subsequently show signs and symptoms of hyaline membrane disease will, on close observation, show some abnormality in respiration at birth, leading to the strong suspicion that the stage is set by intrauterine or intrapartum fetal insult.

These babies frequently have low Apgar scores at birth and require stimulation or resuscitative efforts to establish sustained respiration. The smaller prematures, particularly, may show depression of the central nervous system far beyond that which their maternal analgesic dosage would suggest. Whether this phenomenon is related to the lack of ability to metabolize even light sedation on the part of a baby already in jeopardy in utero, or to a central depression that may be part of the disease process itself, it is a poor prognostic sign.

As soon as respiration is established, an audible expiratory grunt usually appears, along with some degree of labored respiration. In mildly affected babies, grunting may quickly disappear as soon as they are placed in an oxygen-enriched atmosphere, but the respiratory pattern usually continues to show tachypnea of 80 to 100 per minute with rapid, shallow breathing, frequently punctuated by irregularities such as cogwheel inspiration. The more severely affected baby will continue to grunt or cry on expiration despite oxygen supplementation. Although the respiratory rate usually increases with warming and oxygenation in the first few hours of life to 70 to 80 per minute, persistent rates above 100 per minute are not as common as they are in more mildly affected infants. Severely ill babies also show inspiratory retraction of the sternum and lower costal margin, often associated with paradoxical bulging of the abdomen below the diaphragm, creating a seesaw motion and a pseudopectus deformity (Fig. 6). Retraction may be greater and more obvious in smaller babies with weaker chest walls. It is rarely deep in the more mildly affected babies. On auscultation, there is only "poor air entry," rales of any kind being rare in the early stage of the disease. Tachycardia above 160 per minute is common in most distressed babies until they have been well oxygenated. It is often striking to observe the disappearance of audible grunting, even in severely ill babies,

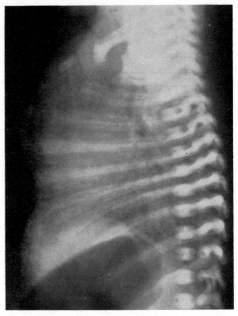

Figure 6. Lateral chest roentgenogram of a premature infant made 48 hours after birth, showing the pseudopectus deformity of the chest and air bronchogram associated with severe hyaline membrane disease.

and the subsidence of tachycardia when they are given adequate oxygen concentrations to breathe. Edema is common in these infants, being most obvious in the dorsa of the hands and feet, the shiny, full palms and soles, the puffy eyes and the full skin fold in the posterior axillary line of a supine infant. Flaccidity with poor muscle tone and joint relaxation is also characteristic, and the baby assumes a supine frog-leg position with ease.

The roentgenogram is usually characteristic in severe disease, even in the first few hours after birth, but may be only suggestive in more mildly affected infants and become characteristic only if the infant's status worsens. The film of the lung fields shows a diffuse, fine granularity throughout, which, if not prominent, is best distinguished with a bright light (Fig. 7). There is no evidence of gross lobar or lobular atelectasis; the diaphragms are low, and the ribs horizontal. Heavy, diffuse granularity is characteristic of the severe dis-

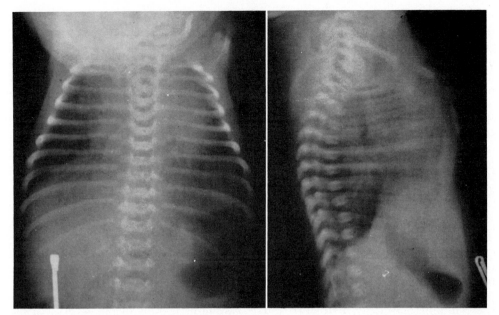

Figure 7. Anteroposterior and lateral chest roentgenograms taken at one hour after birth of a 1701 gm. infant in moderately severe respiratory distress due to hyaline membrane disease. They show a diffuse, fine reticulogranular pattern throughout the lung fields and air bronchogram extending into the periphery of the lung fields.

ease (Fig. 8). An air bronchogram extending into the fine radicals can usually be clearly seen. The heart may appear enlarged, especially the first days of life, and this is often best substantiated by subsequent diminution in size on serial x-ray films. The lateral film may demonstrate the extent of

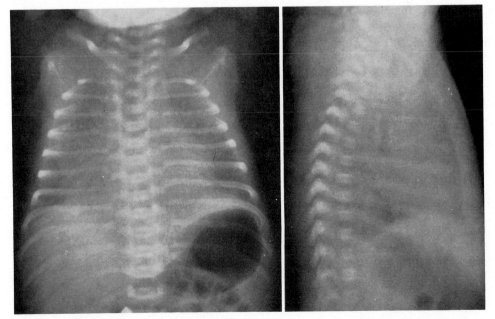

Figure 8. Anteroposterior and lateral roentgenograms of the chest of an 1162 gm. infant taken two hours after birth, showing the generalized reticulogranular pattern of severe hyaline membrane disease.

sternal retraction or air in the mediastinum, which occasionally occurs in the course of the disease. A thymus is usually prominent.

Although some infants, especially the near-term prematures affected, may have a less severe course than others, clinical hyaline membrane disease should be differentiated from other types of respiratory distress in premature infants because of its different natural history and different prognosis. Many asphyxiated prematures will demonstrate a clinical and roentgenographic picture soon after birth difficult to distinguish from hyaline membrane disease, but with prompt and vigorous treatment, including oxygen, buffers, the use of low levels of constant distending airway pressure and diuretics, these infants may clear their apparent excess pulmonary fluid and improve rapidly, both clinically and roentgenologically.

The infant with hyaline membrane disease, however, continues to require oxygen, constant distending airway pressure, even ventilatory assistance, and supportive measures for two to three days before spontaneous recovery begins to occur. This does not imply a lack of response to therapy such as CPAP, but a necessity to maintain it for continued stability of the lung until the infant's own surfactant production can be reestablished. Severely ill babies show a very low arterial oxygen tension on room air; although initially it may be raised above 100 mm. Hg on high oxygen inhalation, as the disease progresses this no longer becomes possible. Oxygenation becomes progressively more difficult in babies who are going to die, and a persistent level of oxygen tension below 40 mm. Hg with 100 per cent oxygen inhalation is an ominous sign. The arterial pH in severely ill babies is also low, usually below 7.25, reflecting both respiratory and metabolic acidosis in most instances. The pH, however, can usually be regulated to near-normal levels by the repeated use of intravenous buffers such as sodium bicarbonate, except in moribund babies.

The arterial carbon dioxide tension is frequently elevated above 45 mm. Hg, but only in the depressed babies, in those with cerebral hemorrhage, or in those who are deteriorating is it above 70 mm. Hg. Blood lactic acid levels indicating metabolic acidosis become elevated above 50 mg. per 100 ml. only in the most severely ill babies; levels of this magnitude are considered poor prognostic signs. Blood lactic acid seems to reflect tissue hypoxia associated with poor perfusion rather than anoxemia itself. Serum potassium may rise to dangerously high levels, especially in very small infants, those with occult hemorrhage, and those who have been allowed to undergo hypothermia. Serum protein levels are frequently low, but reflect the size of the baby more closely than they do the severity of the disease. Serum calcium levels are frequently low, but rarely produce symptomatic tetany. The blood urea nitrogen and phosphorus levels may be elevated, reflecting a catabolic state, but do not add to the prognostic outlook.

Physiologic measurements of pulmonary function on these infants have shown abnormally low compliance, i.e., a markedly negative intrathoracic pressure necessary to move a normal volume of air. Total ventilation may be greatly increased, but alveolar ventilation is decreased, producing an increased ratio of dead space to tidal volume and an elevated arterial carbon dioxide tension. Abnormal ventilation-to-perfusion ratios exist within the lung, contributing to both the lowered arterial oxygen tension and elevated arterial carbon dioxide tension.

Studies of lungs of infants dying with hyaline membrane disease have shown abnormalities in pressure-volume curves, with such low volumes on the deflation curve when low pressures are reached as to indicate a lack of alveolar stability on end-expiration. The maintenance of alveolar stability sufficient for a normal functional residual capacity to exist is due to the presence of a surface-active phospholipid complex, known as surfactant, lining the alveolar walls. This material is produced by alveolar type II cells, which store it and release it in response to a variety of stimuli. The more immature the infant, the less likely he is to have a mature mechanism for surfactant production, and also the more limited is the surface area for gas diffusion in extrauterine life. As lung maturation progresses, there is functional differentiation of type II cells and the development of true alveoli where alveolar walls are made up of capillaries lined with type I epithelium differentiated for gas diffusion. Both factors contribute to the decreased susceptibility of the more mature infant to hyaline membrane disease. However, the infant whose lung is still in a transitional stage of maturation of both the surfactant system and the pulmonary vascular bed is especially susceptible to intrauterine, intrapartum, or immediate postpartum insult where type II cells are functionally and anatomically destroyed. Their regeneration along with the lysis and phagocytosis of the membrane material contributes to the time-table of improvement during the natural history of this disease entity.

Studies of the cardiovascular system have shown moderate systemic hypotension, which can usually be improved by high oxygen inhalation or by the infusion of buffers or whole blood. Many of these infants have a low red cell volume, which should be replaced. Aortic pressure, however, usually increases over the first few days of life except in those babies who will subsequently die. The ductus arteriosus is open, the direction and magnitude of the shunt depending on the pressures and resistances in the systemic and pulmonary arterial systems. Many severely ill infants initially show transient bidirectional shunting through the ductus arteriosus and large right-to-left shunts through the foramen ovale. These right-to-left shunts will usually diminish in size, since adequate oxygenation and pH normalization are associated with increasing left-to-right ductus shunting, increased systemic pressure and pulse

pressure and increasing arterial oxygen tension. This suggests that pulmonary oxygenation is capable of lowering pulmonary arterial pressure and resistance, thereby decreasing the degree of hypoxemia by decreasing right-to-left shunting through the ductus and foramen ovale. Significant left-to-right shunts are common with all degrees of severity in distressed infants who are in an increased oxygen environment. Small to moderate-sized right-to-left shunts through the foramen ovale are also common in babies who do not have extremely large left-to-right shunts through the ductus arteriosus capable of raising left atrial pressure high enough to close the foramen valve.

In infants over 34 weeks of gestation who are improving on the third or fourth day of life, ductus murmurs are frequently heard transiently, but signs of cardiac failure are rare and functional closure is usually apparent within several days. In infants of less than 34 weeks of gestation, however, and especially in those of less than 32 weeks of gestation, the appearance of a symptomatic left-to-right shunt on the third or fourth day of life is extremely common. As oxygenation improves with improving lung function and pulmonary vascular resistance falls, a large left-to-right shunt may lead to tachycardia, tachypnea and increasing oxygen dependence, the appearance of rales and increasing precordial activity, cardiomegaly and pulmonary plethora on roentgenogram, and eventually hepatomegaly and peripheral edema. With vigorous medical management of cardiac failure, including digitalis, diuretics, CPAP and normal oxygenation, most infants without complications will survive. Ductal closure will usually proceed at 34 to 36 postconceptual weeks. Medical management requires the most meticulous physician and nursing attention to details. At the present time, the relative merits of surgical closure or pharmacologic closure with inhibitors of prostaglandin synthesis are being explored.

The severely ill infant may continue

to grunt loudly, although grunting may disappear with high oxygen inhalation, buffering, and the use of CPAP. Deep retraction, however, persists for 48 to 72 hours without CPAP, and in very severely ill babies for many days to weeks. These babies are frequently both clinically and biochemically worse in their second 24 hours of life than in their first, with falling arterial oxygen tensions despite high oxygen inhalation and repeated decline in arterial pH after satisfactory initial pH buffering, indicating progressive worsening of their disease. Scratchy, sandpaper breath sounds are frequently audible. It is at this time that respiratory failure most often begins to be apparent, with physical exhaustion of the baby, and a gradual lessening of the respiratory rate and effort unaccompanied by clinical or biochemical improvement. Irregular respiration may be followed by periods of apnea and bradycardia, ashen cyanosis appears, and death occurs if ventilatory assistance is not given. Constant and experienced nursing and physician attendance is necessary throughout, since respiratory failure demands immediate management. Most severely ill infants will benefit from maintaining their alveolar stability and preserving a normal functional residual capacity with the early and judicious use of CPAP. The level should be carefully matched to the need of the infant, since levels higher than needed may lead to air dissection and pneumothorax, large dead space ventilation, and eventually diminished pulmonary blood flow.

Pressures should not only be raised carefully with worsening disease, but also lowered promptly with improvement, if adverse effects are to be avoided. Lower levels of inspired oxygen can usually be used if CPAP is effective. If ventilatory assistance is also necessary, PEEP can often be a useful adjunct to successful management. Many babies, though clinically and biochemically severely ill, if supported, especially with adequate CPAP, will be able to survive this second 24 hours without ventilatory assistance and grad-

ually begin to show improvement by the third to fourth day. Brief episodes of apnea, frequently associated with excessive mucus, are common during this period, and during this time constant and expert nursing attention is mandatory. Diuresis also occurs on about the third to fourth day in these infants with loss of edema. They gradually become more alert, develop better muscular tone, begin to show hunger, and will suck a pacifier. Small oral feedings can usually be begun by the fourth day of life. As arterial oxygen tension rises, CPAP pressures can be decreased and environmental oxygen concentrations can be gradually diminished, and weaning to room air is usually completed by the fourth or fifth day, occasionally later in the sickest infants. Jaundice is common in the third to seventh day, frequently of alarming degree, being most severe in the most immature babies and in those with suspected occult hemorrhage.

Babies who do not fit into this pattern almost invariably have other complicating factors modifying their course. One of the commonest of these complications is cerebral hemorrhage. Frank tonic and clonic seizures are rarely seen in prematures, although extensor spasms frequently occur.

The time of the occurrence of large intraventricular hemorrhage frequently found at autopsy in severely ill infants is usually in the second 24 hours after birth. In such instances, the extreme severity of the disease is probably associated with the pathogenesis of the hemorrhage, and death is a frequent outcome.

Extremely small immature babies may also show an atypical course, physical exhaustion playing a role in their early respiratory failure. Persistent hypothermia and profound metabolic acidosis are common. These complications may contribute to their high mortality rate in the face of moderately severe respiratory symptoms.

Secondary infection, especially pneumonia with gram-negative saprophytic infection such as with pseudomonas or a klebsiella, has been a cause of late death in some series of babies with hyaline membrane disease, usually related to chronic endotracheal intubation.

The postmortem findings in those babies who die are usually characteristic. The heart, when visualized in situ, is dilated, and the right atrium and venae cavae are engorged with blood. The liver is also usually large and congested. The lungs are full, solid, airless, dark purplish-red and liver-like in consistency. Pressure-volume curves on excised lungs have shown abnormally low alveolar stability at low deflation pressures. Measurements of surface tension on film from lung homogenates show abnormal surface properties. This suggests that in babies who die the normal amount of alveolar lining layer surfactant necessary for maintaining normal lung stability is either absent or inactivated in some way. The ductus arteriosus is usually unconstricted in babies dying in the first three days of life. Cerebral hemorrhage, especially intraventricular hemorrhage, has been a common finding at autopsy.

Microscopic sections of the lungs of babies dying early in the disease, before 18 hours, may show a high degree of constriction of the small arterioles adjacent to alveolar ducts and respiratory bronchioles, with beginning sloughing of the epithelium of these air sacs, protein-containing material in their lumens and a moderate degree of alveolar atelectasis. Scanty, patchy or ill-formed membranes that appear to be made up of sloughed cell debris in a protein-containing matrix may be seen lining some of the dilated respiratory bronchioles and alveolar ducts (Fig. 9). The longer the baby has survived before death, the more well formed and homogeneous these membranes appear, and the less apparent are the cellular components. Also, the arteriolar constriction becomes less apparent with time, the alveolar atelectasis more profound, and the dilatation of alveolar ducts more striking by contrast. In babies who have been kept alive for

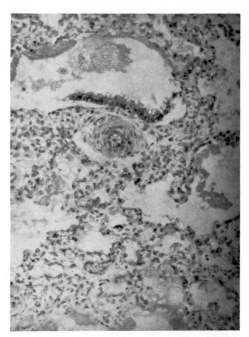

Figure 9. Photomicrograph of the lung of a premature infant dying 16 hours after birth, showing arteriolar constriction with sloughing epithelium of a respiratory bronchiole adjacent, and early hyaline membrane formation.

many days by mechanical ventilation and who have subsequently died, atelectasis may remain profound, the membranes are only partially resolved and new type II alveolar cells appear to invade the membranes and reline denuded alveolar walls.

Other babies showing the typical clinical picture of hyaline membrane disease who have died from unrelated causes at seven to ten days have shown re-expanding alveoli and varying degrees of resolution of the membranes as relining of denuded airways with new migrating alveolar type II cells progressed.

Any approach to therapy in a disease process whose cause is in question, but whose pathogenesis is becoming more and more clear-cut, must rely on the correction of those biochemical or physiologic abnormalities that can be demonstrated at any particular stage of development of the disease. If hypoxia is present, normal oxygenation should be attempted; if metabolic acidosis is present, buffers such as sodium bicarbonate or THAM should be useful; if cardiac failure is in evidence, digitalis is indicated; or if hyperkalemia develops, the serum potassium level may be lowered with intravenous administration of glucose and insulin. If alveolar volume is collapsing on end-expiration, the use of CPAP to maintain it is indicated. In the face of respiratory failure, ventilatory assistance is mandatory and may, indeed, be lifesaving.

If a high pulmonary vascular resistance exists, maintaining the fetal pattern of circulation with right-to-left shunting through the ductus arteriosus and foramen ovale, it may be partially or perhaps completely relieved by high oxygen inhalation and correction of the pH and blood volume toward normal, especially if these measures are applied early in the disease. Whether other pharmacologic means, such as Priscoline, are necessary or desirable must be evaluated in individual cases. Obviously, one would like to restore lung compliance to normal, but methods so far used have not proved satisfactory. The value of continuous physician supervision and expert individual nursing care cannot be ignored in the overall therapy of any small or sick newborn. This is especially true in babies with severe respiratory distress whose status may change from moment to moment and who may require a rapid change of therapeutic approach or just immediate suction of the oropharynx. Nurses experienced in making detailed and frequent observations on distressed infants and capable of acting on them with judgment have proved to be invaluable helpers in the overall management of the disease.

The ultimate goal in therapy is obviously prevention. There is increasingly convincing evidence that the use of steroids at the appropriate time in gestation, before complete alveolization of the lung has occurred and when the surfactant system is in the process of development, may be capable of inducing lung maturation within a relatively short interval sufficient to reduce the susceptibility to hyaline membrane disease appreciably. Their use in the fetus with threatened delivery at a time of high susceptibility seems warranted if contraindications, such as maternal pre-eclampsia or evidence of growth retardation, do not exist. The unknown risks must be weighed against the possible advantages in each case, since steroids act not upon the lung alone, but also on many other organ systems. However, we must continue to ask for the best obstetric care possible, the most judicious conduct of labor and delivery of pregnancies at risk, prompt and adequate resuscitation of the newborn when indicated, and continuity of care and responsibility between the delivery room and the nursery. From this point on, rational therapy must be based on the findings in a particular baby at the time the therapy is contemplated, since what may be good or necessary at one time may be harmful at another. Methods for assessing the fetus in utero are at present only rudimentary, and future progress in this important field will probably depend largely upon their development.

TYPE II RESPIRATORY DISTRESS SYNDROME

Among the various kinds of respiratory distress in the newborn, a group of infants present with many clinical, radiologic and physiologic similarities, and it is believed that they share a similar cause for their respiratory distress. They resemble infants with clinical hyaline membrane disease (CHMD) in many of its aspects, but have certain distinguishing features, a different natural history, and a far more sanguine prognosis. This disorder has been referred to as respiratory distress syndrome type II, transient tachypnea of the newborn or neonatal disseminated atelectasis by various authors.

By history, these infants show many of the maternal antecedents of infants with CHMD, such as cesarean section, bleeding, prolapsed cord or diabetes. The use of analgesics such as Demerol is prominent in the labor records. Most are less than 3000 grams birth weight and most are under 38 weeks of gestational age. Physical evidence of some degree of immaturity is present in all. If one excludes the infants of diabetic mothers, they are of appropriate size for gestational age, as are infants with CHMD. They do not show clinical evidence of chronic placental insufficiency as displayed by intrauterine weight loss, loss of vernix, or meconium staining of cord and nails.

Respiratory distress in the form of tachypnea, loud grunting on expiration, and flaring of alae nasi is present early after birth. The degree of intercostal and infracostal retraction and the use of accessory muscles of respiration vary from infant to infant, but are present to some extent in all. Cyanosis in room air frequently occurs. Most show grunting during the first hours after birth, and retraction for about 24 hours. However, a few infants are symptomatic for as long as 96 hours. Tachypnea is always present by six hours of age, and extremely high rates of respiration are common. Tachypnea, lasting seven to eight days, is usually the last sign of respiratory disease to disappear in some infants despite other signs of well-being.

The roentgenogram findings after six hours of postnatal life are impressively different from those of CHMD. They show some degree of diffuse overexpansion of both lung fields as evidenced by increased radiolucency, increased anteroposterior diameter on lateral film, flattening or depression of the diaphragm, and bulging of the interspaces. Occasionally, herniation of one lung across the upper mediastinum is also seen. This overexpansion remains in most follow-up films during the first week of life.

Heavy central bronchovascular markings extending out from the hilum are common in the first few days. Pulmonary infiltrates, usually quite patchy in distribution, occasionally occur. The typical generalized diffuse reticulogranular pattern of hyaline membrane disease is not seen. The lobar fissure between the right upper and right middle lobes is frequently visualized in early films, and a lateral rim of pleural fluid is occasionally found.

Another striking difference between these infants and those with CHMD is their ability to be hyperoxygenated in a 100 per cent oxygen environment throughout the course of their disease. This is a reflection of their small physiologic right-to-left intrapulmonary shunts and the absence of significant shunting through the foramen ovale. This group of infants can be well oxygenated at all times, but most show an aortic Po_2 that increases with time up to 30 hours, rather than a decreasing one as in CHMD.

Many have a significantly lowered pH, elevated base deficit or Pa_{co_2} above 40 mm. Hg early in the course of the disease, suggesting that both metabolic and respiratory acidosis accompanying birth asphyxia are common. However, many infants are able to correct their own acid-base balance toward normal with time. Although respiratory symptoms persist, compensation is usually adequate. Neither the systemic hypotension nor significant shunting through the ductus arteriosus or foramen ovale in either direction, as seen in CHMD, appears in these infants.

The most striking historical facts are those of frequent maternal heavy sedation and mild asphyxia at birth in relatively immature infants. The clinical and radiologic findings strongly suggest lower airway obstruction with a ball-valve effect and overdistention peripherally. This could be brought about by failure to clear the airway adequately of mucus and other accumulated debris before the onset of respiration, which frequently happens in cesarean section deliveries and in infants who are either mildly asphyxiated or oversedated. The infant moderately depressed from whatever cause, even if adequately suctioned initially, has depressed gag, swallow and cough reflexes, and may pool secretions in the hypopharynx or tracheobronchial tree for many hours after birth. Delayed absorption of fetal lung fluid has also been implicated.

It is suggested that in some instances this might be a preventable disease. The avoidance of overuse of analgesics that are depressant to the central nervous system seems important in infants, especially immature infants, and especially in those pregnancies where the infants in utero could be anticipated to be in jeopardy. Attention to details of resuscitation at delivery and careful nursing of such infants might minimize the disease process. The maintenance of adequate oxygenation without risking the danger of overoxygenation becomes a therapeutic problem and justifies aortic catheterization in infants with persistent respiratory disease and oxygen dependence. Skin electrode monitoring may obviate this need. Buffering of the metabolic acidosis with enough sodium bicarbonate solution to raise the infant's buffer capacity by 5 mEq. per liter of body water would seem desirable even in the absence of pH measurements. Repeated use of buffers is rarely, if ever, necessary. The administration of calories in the form of glucose solution parenterally over the acute stage of the disease is advisable, since infants with respiratory rates above 80 do not have time to hold their breath and suck. Oral feedings may be initiated cautiously as symptoms subside.

The importance of recognizing these infants as a distinct entity would seem to be principally in the differentiation from CHMD and the avoidance of overzealous treatment.

INFECTIONS OF THE LUNG

Bacteria may be introduced into the newborn's lung by aspiration of infected material, such as the intrauterine aspiration of amniotic contents in the presence of amnionitis or the intrapartum aspiration of maternal fecal material; by contamination during the birth process; by contamination from hospital personnel, such as occurs in some cases of neonatal staphylococcal pneumonia; or as a complication of a more generalized process, such as sepsis.

Intrauterine bacterial pneumonia occurs almost exclusively in those infants whose mothers' membranes have been ruptured for more than 12 hours before delivery. In these instances, the mother may show signs of infection such as fever and abdominal tenderness, and the amniotic fluid may be noticeably foul and purulent at the time of delivery. Overt signs of amnionitis may be absent, however.

An infant born after prolonged rupture of the membranes should have cultures taken from the nasopharynx, blood and skin before bathing. Aspiration of the stomach contents and microscopic examination for the presence of excessive numbers of polymorphonuclear leukocytes and especially for the identification of intracellular bacteria may be helpful in the early diagnosis of babies at high risk from intrauterine infection. In the absence of symptoms in either mother or child, prophylactic administration of antibiotics to the infant may be withheld until cultures are positive or symptoms of infection develop. If contamination of the baby's respiratory tract has been recent or occurred intrapartum, pneumonia may be only one of the manifestations of generalized sepsis, which may include meningitis, hepatic and renal abscesses, osteomyelitis and other localizations of blood stream dissemination.

In the past, organisms that most frequently infected the infant in his intrauterine environment were gram-negative rods of the colon bacillus group, Proteus organisms and *Pseudomonas aeruginosa*. Many of these organisms are considered to be saprophytes or nonpathogenic "normal flora" in other circumstances, but they are capable of rapidly fatal disease in the newborn infant.

In recent years, group B hemolytic

streptococci have emerged as the principal cause of neonatal pneumonia. This organism rarely causes symptoms in the mother. The infant may be contaminated intrapartum, not as the result of prolonged rupture of membranes or amnionitis, but simply by passage through the birth canal. Many of these infants are at term and show no symptoms of infection in the early hours after birth. By six to 12 hours of life, however, the infant may suddenly and rapidly show signs and symptoms of profound pulmonary involvement and cardiovascular collapse suggestive of endotoxemic shock. The roentgenogram usually shows patchy involvement, which progresses rapidly, and pleural fluid, especially on the right, is common. Metabolic acidosis, tachypnea, tachycardia and poor peripheral perfusion are common, with hypotensive collapse in severe cases. Disseminated intravascular coagulopathy with bleeding may be seen. Meningitis may be present as a severe component of the disease. In immature infants, the differential diagnosis with hyaline membrane disease is often difficult. Indeed, they may be coexistent. The mortality rate is high, and early suspicion and initiation of adequate antibiotic therapy is mandatory if infants are to survive. Many more infants will show surface contamination with group B streptococci than become symptomatic, and unknown factors in host susceptibility may well play a role in their selection.

Babies with intrauterine gram-negative pneumonia are usually severely ill from birth and may have respiratory distress indistinguishable from clinical hyaline membrane disease. Rales may appear with more regularity, but otherwise the infants retract and grunt, and have cyanosis and air hunger similar to other infants in severe respiratory distress. Fever may be absent or of low grade and may be replaced by hypothermia. The early roentgenogram appearance of the lung may likewise be difficult to distinguish from the generalized reticulogranular pattern seen in hyaline membrane disease (Fig. 10). Later roentgenograms may resemble

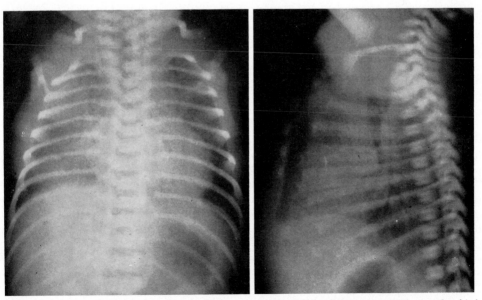

Figure 10.   Anteroposterior and lateral roentgenograms of the chest of an infant 12 hours after birth, showing diffuse granularity throughout both lung fields. This mother's membranes had been ruptured more than 24 hours before delivery, and *Pseudomonas aeruginosa* was cultured from both blood and lung of the infant.

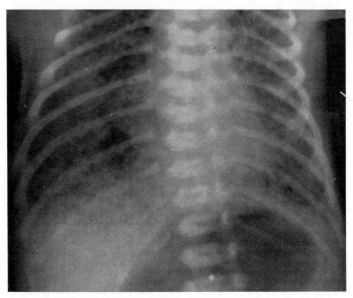

Figure 11. Anteroposterior roentgenogram of the chest of an infant 60 hours after birth whose blood culture grew out *E. coli* and from whose lung *E. coli* and *Pseudomonas aeruginosa* were cultured at autopsy. The x-ray film shows coarse, diffuse infiltration throughout both lung fields.

diffuse bronchopneumonia or show early abscess formation (Fig. 11). Respiratory and metabolic acidosis and anoxemia are found on arterial blood gas analysis. Other systemic signs of infection may be apparent if more generalized infection is present and if the infant survives for several days after birth. Among these are opisthotonos and seizures in the case of meningitis, or an umbilical cord with a reddened base and oozing foul-smelling purulent material. Disseminated intravascular coagulation may also be present.

Widespread pneumonia, especially if the blood culture is positive, is a frequently fatal disease and demands prompt and vigorous specific treatment if the infant is to survive. After initial cultures of the amniotic fluid, skin, nasopharynx and blood have been taken, administration of broad-spectrum antibiotics capable of dealing effectively with the most likely organisms should be started promptly. A lumbar puncture may yield an organism that may be promptly identified on smear and Gram stain. Sensitivity to the drugs used may be evaluated when cultures become positive, and changed as indi-

cated. Supportive care in the form of oxygen, buffers and careful nursing are frequently indicated, and ventilatory assistance may be necessary in the face of respiratory failure.

If a newborn infant shows signs and symptoms compatible with bacterial pneumonia several days after birth, the likelihood of a gram-negative organism as the etiologic agent is lessened, and staphylococcal and group A streptococcal pneumonia occur with increased frequency as nosocomial infections. Infants exposed to hemolytic streptococci may contract impetigo neonatorum, frequently associated with omphalitis and blood stream dissemination. Group A streptococcal pneumonia rarely occurs in the absence of sepsis. This type of infection can rapidly spread throughout a nursery, and early isolation precautions, specific bacteriologic indication and prompt antibiotic therapy are advisable. Signs and symptoms of pulmonary involvement and roentgenographic evidence of pulmonary infiltration, which appears frequently as bronchopneumonia, are usually accompanied or preceded by the appearance of oozing omphalitis or skin blebs filled

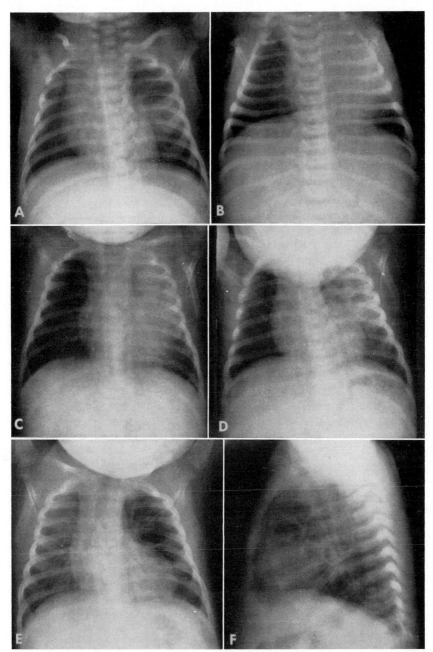

Figure 12. *A,* Anteroposterior roentgenogram of the chest of a three-week-old infant admitted with symptoms of fever and tachypnea whose nasopharyngeal cultures grew out phage type 80–81 staphylococci. Pneumonic infiltrate is seen in the left midlung field. *B,* Anteroposterior roentgenogram of the chest of the same infant one day later, showing progression of the infiltrate. *C,* Anteroposterior roentgenogram of the chest one day later, showing beginning resolution of the infiltrate. *D,* Anteroposterior roentgenogram of the chest one day later, showing further resolution of the pneumonia. *E,* Anteroposterior roentgenogram of the chest of the same infant 13 days later, showing multiple pneumatoceles in the left upper lung field. *F,* Lateral roentgenogram of the chest the same day as in *C,* showing the location of the pneumatoceles. These cleared without treatment.

with thin purulent material from which organisms may readily be cultured.

Staphylococcal infection in the newborn may likewise take many presenting forms, only one of which is pneumonia. Infants may harbor pathogenic staphylococci in their nasopharynx for many weeks without symptoms, only to present with acute pneumonia later. Omphalitis and skin infection in the form of impetigo neonatorum or "scalded skin syndrome" are likewise common, but pulmonary involvement frequently follows only a carrier state. Such infants are acutely and seriously ill, show severe respiratory symptoms with or without the appearance of rales, and have a tendency to bleb formation in the lung, which may rupture and produce sudden pneumothorax. A chest roentgenogram shows the patchy, mottled appearance of areas of infiltration; emphysema and pleural fluid or air collection are common (Fig. 12). Pneumatoceles frequently appear suddenly. Prompt and vigorous antibiotic therapy based on organism sensitivity is indicated. If enough pleural fluid has accumulated to compress functioning lung tissue and produce added respiratory symptoms, thoracentesis is indicated. Surgical drainage may be necessary for encapsulated pus or chronic abscess formation. Pneumatoceles can usually be treated conservatively.

Other bacterial organisms occasionally infect the newborn's lung and must be specifically identified by culture; specific treatment is based on sensitivity studies.

Adenovirus has occasionally been identified in lungs of newborns dying with a widespread cell-destructive pneumonia, and there is reason to believe that it may have been contracted from personnel handling the infants.

Other viral agents, such as the parainfluenza group, have rarely been identified in neonatal pneumonia, but their role even in these instances is somewhat questionable. Pneumonic involvement may also occur with cytomegalic inclusion disease. Spirochetal pneumonia may occur with congenital syphilis, but

is a rare disease in this country at present. Intrauterine infection with Toxoplasma organisms may also occur, and, rarely, widespread and fatal pneumonia results. Other protozoan organisms, such as *Pneumocystis carinii,* may occasionally be found, but in this country their occurrence is rare.

PULMONARY HEMORRHAGE

The occurrence of some extravasated blood in the lungs of newborn infants at autopsy is common, but, to date, the mechanism of its appearance in many instances is unclear. Even in circumstances in which a generalized bleeding diathesis occurs in a newborn with bleeding from many sites, a specific cause is often lacking. Pulmonary hemorrhage as an isolated occurrence is rare, but may appear suddenly from several days of age to several weeks, especially in premature infants, and may be rapidly fatal. More commonly, it is found as a complication of other underlying diseases, such as bacterial pneumonia, sepsis, hemolytic disease of the newborn, kernicterus, and central nervous system hemorrhage. A baby may have respiratory distress and bloody tracheal fluid from birth, or at several days of age may bleed with no premonitory signs. The sudden appearance of blood in the mouth and nose accompanied by extreme respiratory distress, often shock and rapid respiratory failure in a previously asymptomatic infant is a distressing and frustrating occurrence. Immediate blood transfusion may combat shock, and ventilatory assistance and CPAP may tide the baby over the acute episode. Broad-spectrum antibiotics are indicated if any suspicion of sepsis is present. Many, but not all, of these infants have changes in their blood-clotting mechanisms consistent with the diagnosis of disseminated intravascular coagulation (DIC) with consumptive coagulopathy. This is thought to be an intermediary mechanism of disease, rather than a primary one.

Shock, whether from severe asphyxia, from trauma, from hypovolemia, from endotoxemia with sepsis, or cardiogenic or neurogenic, is the most frequent common denominator of DIC. The treatment of the infant bleeding with DIC should include partial exchange transfusion with fresh heparinized blood. The maintenance of heparinization may depend on subsequent events.

In recent years, as more and more very immature infants below 1200 grams are surviving, the occurrence of acute pulmonary hemorrhage frequently has been recognized as associated with the development of a large left-to-right ductus shunt. With the fall in pulmonary vascular resistance, the presence of an unconstricted ductus arteriosus places an acute strain on the pulmonary vascular bed, and pulmonary capillary engorgement followed by rupture is increasingly seen. It is possible CPAP can prevent this event in some instances. Much more needs to be known about the factors controlling the newborn's pulmonary vascular bed.

CONGENITAL LOBAR EMPHYSEMA

Although the term "congenital lobar emphysema" implies prenatal origin (see Chapter 9, Congenital Malformations of the Lower Respiratory Tract), many instances of this entity are almost certainly acquired and have no primary congenital abnormality of the lung involved in their origin. As the name implies, overdistention of one or more lobes occurs, frequently the right upper or right middle lobe, because either intrinsic or extrinsic partial obstruction interferes with deflation of this particular area. Deficiency of the bronchial cartilage involving only one lobe may occur, and this, by failing to supply stability during expiration, produces overdistention of the parenchyma of the

lung aerated by that bronchus. Partial intraluminal obstruction with associated lobar emphysema may occur as the result of aspirated foreign material; extraluminal compression producing partial obstruction may be associated with a large variety of pulmonary and mediastinal masses, such as bronchogenic cysts, teratomas of the anterior mediastinum, and neuroblastomas and cysts of the posterior mediastinum. Emphysema of the right lower lobe has also been seen in association with congenital cardiac disease in a newborn when high pressure in the pulmonary artery produced by a ventricular septal defect resulted in a greatly dilated pulmonary artery, which, in the presence of a right aortic arch, was responsible for the partial bronchial obstruction.

In some instances, what has appeared to be lobar emphysema has developed following diffuse air dissection in infants with hyaline membrane disease. Gradual enlargement of the individual lobe over a three- to four-week period, associated with increasing symptoms of respiratory embarrassment, have necessitated surgical removal. Large, dilated perivascular and peribronchial lymphatics have been present in addition to distended alveoli, and large, sometimes multinucleated or ciliated cells may appear lining these false air spaces. This suggests the persistence of dissected interstitial air in lymphatics with attempts to "alveolize" them. If only one lobe has been involved in the process, surgical removal has been curative.

Regardless of the demonstrable cause or lack of it, symptoms are similar. Wheezing occurs, in some instances from birth, in others only after weeks or months. The degree of respiratory distress depends largely upon compression of normally functioning lung by the overdistended lobe. Herniation of the affected lobe across the mediastinum may occur, the heart may be displaced, and the unaffected lobe, unless lung markings are seen, cannot easily be distinguished from a lung cyst

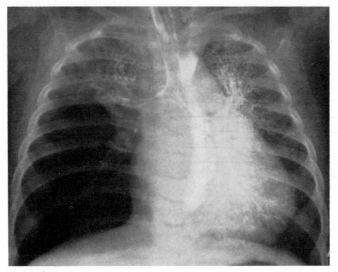

Figure 13. Bronchogram and esophagogram on an infant with lobar emphysema of the right lower lobe due to congenital heart disease. The infant had a right aortic arch and a large interventricular septal defect with pulmonary hypertension producing enough distention to compress the right lower lobe bronchus between the aorta and the pulmonary artery.

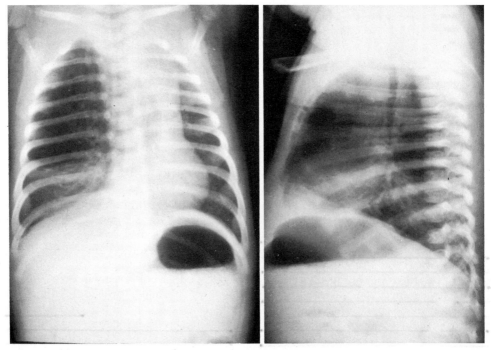

Figure 14. Anteroposterior and lateral films on a week-old infant with severe respiratory symptoms, showing lobar emphysema of the right upper lobe and compression of the right middle and lower lobes. No cause for the overdistention of the right upper lobe was found at operation.

(Figs. 13 and 14). Cardiac displacement or atelectasis may be confirmed by x-ray study.

Treatment is dependent upon the severity of the respiratory difficulties. If severe respiratory distress and cyanosis are present, prompt bronchoscopy should be performed in order to remove any intraluminal obstruction. In most cases, however, surgical removal of the affected lobe will be necessary to provide relief. Asymptomatic babies may be watched for progression of the process, since some spontaneously regress.

LUNG CYSTS AND PNEUMATOCELES

Considerable controversy exists concerning the classification of lung cysts in small infants. (See Chapter 9.) Most agree, however, that true congenital cysts are rare in the newborn, and that most lesions formerly thought to be cysts were, in fact, pneumatoceles, probably resulting from staphylococcal pneumonia. Lung cysts lined with ciliated columnar epithelium do exist, but their congenital origin is in doubt.

Bronchogenic cysts may occur in the lumen of a major bronchus, partially occluding it and producing lobar emphysema distally or completely occluding it with atelectasis. If present in the mediastinum, they may not be readily visible on routine x-ray films of the chest, but bronchography will help to identify their location. Wheezing, stridor and frequent bouts of infection are common.

A more common location for congenital cysts is in the periphery of the lung, where they may or may not communicate with bronchi. They may be single or multiple and contain cartilage and elastic tissue in their walls.

If symptomatic, congenital lung cysts should be surgically removed; they may constitute a surgical emergency. If asymptomatic, particularly if there is question of their differentiation from pneumatoceles, they may be followed clinically and roentgenologically, and operation can be delayed until some future time after the infant has attained somatic growth.

Pneumatoceles, often of large size, occur with considerable frequency during the course of staphylococcal pneumonia in infancy. They occasionally occur with pneumonia associated with other organisms. Characteristic are their frequent change in size and their complete regression. Symptoms of lung compression are common, but if pneumatoceles are not infected and pus-containing, or are not life-threatening because of size or location, conservative management is advisable. The importance of the different natural histories of congenital and acquired lung cysts in infancy is stressed, since unnecessary major surgery can be avoided in many instances.

AGENESIS AND HYPOPLASIA OF THE LUNGS

Complete agenesis of both lungs, a single lobe or a single lung may occur. (See Chapter 9.) Agenesis of a single lung is more frequent and may be associated with other anomalies. The left lung is more apt to be absent than the right. The remaining lung and mediastinal structures shift into the empty cavity and fill both sides of the chest (Fig. 15). The trachea will be deviated toward the affected side, and evidence of dullness and diminished breath sounds are usually found. As the remaining lung herniates to the affected side, these latter signs may disappear. The existing lung is thought to be hypertrophied rather than emphysematous, and cyanosis will not exist, since no pulmonary vessels perfuse the affected side. No treatment is possible.

Hypoplasia of an entire lung or of a portion of it is usually associated with other congenital anomalies. With diaphragmatic hernias in which abdom-

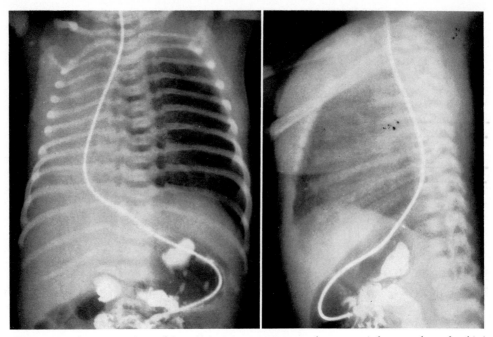

Figure 15. Anteroposterior and lateral chest roentgenograms taken on an infant two days after birth, showing agenesis of the right lung. A catheter is in the esophagus.

inal contents enter the chest cavity during intrauterine life, hypoplasia of the lung on the affected side may result, presumably from interference with lung growth. Pulmonary hypoplasia sometimes accompanies renal agenesis, or Potter's syndrome. These infants have a characteristic facies with epicanthal folds, flattened nose and low-set ears. Rarely, a single hypoplastic lung will exist with systemic arterial blood supply and venous drainage into the inferior vena cava.

CONGENITAL DIAPHRAGMATIC HERNIA

A potentially correctable cause of neonatal respiratory distress is herniation of abdominal viscera into the chest cavity through a defect in the diaphragm. The most frequent site of herniation is the foramen of Bochdalek, situated in the posterior aspect of the diaphragm. The next most common site is the foramen of Morgagni just behind the sternum. The proportion of left-sided herniation is considerably more than on the right side, and both hollow and solid viscera may enter the chest. (See Chapter 9.)

Symptoms may be present from birth or may appear in the first days of life, or the defect may remain completely asymptomatic. Very early symptoms are related to the compression of pulmonary tissue by the herniated viscera. If parts of the gastrointestinal tract are herniated, vomiting may result, and signs of intestinal obstruction may appear as the lumen fills with gas and fluid.

Physical signs will depend upon the amount and consistency of herniated abdominal contents. In the case of solid viscera, dullness will be present over the affected side, whereas if dilated loops of bowel fill the chest, hyperresonance may result. Bowel sounds may be heard over the chest on auscultation, and the abdomen is characteristically

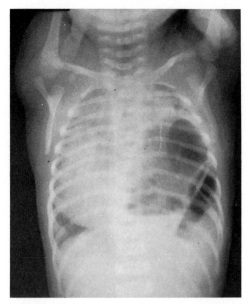

Figure 16. Anteroposterior roentgenogram of the chest of a newborn infant in severe respiratory distress, showing a diaphragmatic hernia through the foramen of Bochdalek with abdominal contents in the left chest cavity and displacement of the heart to the right.

flattened. X-ray examination will usually be diagnostic, especially if gut is present (Fig. 16). The introduction of contrast medium in the bowel will confirm the diagnosis, but is seldom necessary or advisable.

The treatment is immediate surgical replacement of abdominal viscera. The hazards of sudden death with delayed operation are considerable. Even with successful surgery, oxygenation is often difficult to manage postoperatively, and mortality in such instances is high.

VASCULAR RINGS

A great number of variations occur in the embryologic development of the paired aortic arches, and some of them produce partial obstruction to the tracheobronchial tree. (See Chapter 9.) The most common anomalies found to be associated with such symptoms are double aortic arch, right aortic arch with ligamentum arteriosum, anomalous innominate artery, anomalous left common carotid artery and aberrant subclavian artery. Although many of these anomalies may not completely encircle the trachea and the esophagus, each may be capable of partially occluding them because of relatively fixed relations with other structures. Stridor, wheezing respiration and occasionally severe respiratory distress with cyanotic episodes, especially when the head is flexed, are characteristic of these infants. They tend to lie with the neck hyperextended, a position that presumably allows less restriction of the airway. Partial obstruction of the esophagus is frequently manifested by inability to swallow ingested foods, especially solids, without regurgitation; aspiration pneumonia is a frequent complication. Newborn babies are rarely severely symptomatic, but symptoms appear to become worse in the first few months of life. Diagnosis of the degree of obstruction can be made by x-ray studies during instillation of contrast medium in the esophagus. The exact nature of the vascular anomaly may be elucidated by angiography if the obstruction is not ligamentous in part. Surgical correction of symptomatic lesions should be done early, since the point of tracheal compression may fail to develop properly, and tracheal stenosis may remain. Asymptomatic lesions may be ignored.

ESOPHAGEAL ATRESIA AND TRACHEOESOPHAGEAL FISTULA

Both esophageal atresia and tracheoesophageal fistula occur rarely as separate entities, but their occurrence in various combinations is frequent. The various possibilities are (1) esophageal atresia alone; (2) tracheoesophageal fistula alone; or (3) esophageal atresia with (a) upper fistula, (b) lower fistula or (c) double fistula. Type 3b accounts for 90 per cent of all defects of this sort seen. (See Chapter 9.)

The diagnosis is frequently first suspected when an alert nurse reports that a newborn infant has excessive mucus and cannot handle his secretions adequately. Suction will provide temporary relief, but secretions continue to accumulate and overflow, usually resulting in aspiration and respiratory distress. Feedings will likewise be regurgitated and frequently aspirated, and the chest becomes filled with rhonchi and coarse rales. In those infants in whom only esophageal atresia alone exists, the abdomen will remain flat, but if there is a fistula to the lower esophageal segment with or without esophageal atresia, the abdomen usually becomes distended with air, especially if the respiratory effort is great. The diagnosis can be made in those cases with esophageal atresia by gently attempting to insert a catheter into the stomach and introducing air through it while listening with a stethoscope over the left upper quadrant of the abdomen. If no sound of air entry into the stomach is heard, esophageal atresia is likely. A catheter curling in a blind pouch and thought to be in the stomach may be misleading.

X-ray film of the esophagus using a contrast will confirm the presence of a blind pouch of esophagus and occasionally demonstrate the fistula as well (Fig. 17). In the case of a fistula without esophageal atresia, the diagnosis may be difficult even after repeated x-ray examination. In such a case, cinefluorography with both trachea and esophagus simultaneously filled with contrast medium may be necessary (Fig. 18). Prompt surgical correction is indicated if aspiration pneumonia, if not already present, is inevitable, and secondary infection is common. Even small prematures have survived with corrective surgery and careful postoperative management. The infant should be kept partially upright prior to surgery, since regurgitation of proteolytic enzymes and acid from the gastrointestinal tract

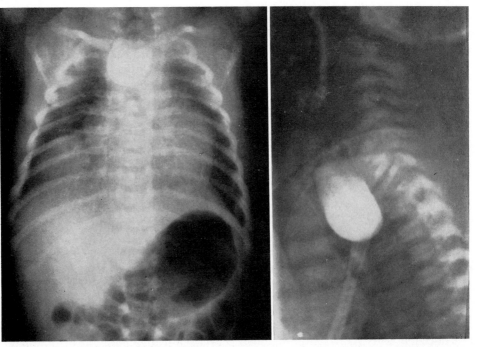

Figure 17. Anteroposterior and lateral films of an infant with a type 3b tracheoesophageal fistula, showing the contrast-filled blind esophageal pouch and secondary aspiration pneumonia.

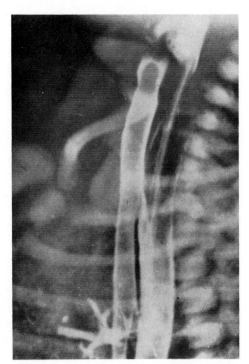

Figure 18. Simultaneous tracheal and esophageal filling with Lipiodol in an infant with an H type of tracheoesophageal fistula, demonstrating the communication.

into the lung causes a very tissue-destructive pneumonia, and a constant suction catheter should be kept in the blind pouch.

MICROGNATHIA WITH GLOSSOPTOSIS

Congenital hypoplasia of the mandible occurs with several of the so-called first arch defects, such as the Treacher Collins syndrome and the Pierre Robin syndrome, or it may occur as an isolated lesion.

When micrognathia is severe and coupled with glossoptosis, intermittent episodes of dyspnea and cyanosis can occur, especially in association with the supine position. The tongue falls backward over the glottis, effectively obstructing the airway, and the harder the infant struggles, the more firmly the tongue is sucked against the air passage. Aspiration of feedings associated with inability to suck properly is also common. The immediate treatment is to place the infant in the prone position so that the tongue falls forward, establish an airway, and as soon as is feasible suture the tongue to the soft tissue of the floor of the mouth, including the lower gum margin. This effectively prevents cyanotic attacks and allows the infant to feed properly; it can be loosened when the infant grows older and the mandible develops.

CHOANAL ATRESIA

Acute respiratory distress may present at birth if the nasal passages have failed to perforate and either bony or membranous obstruction remains. Such obstruction may be unilateral or bilateral. If it is unilateral, the infant may be symptomless, but if bilateral, mouth-breathing is obligatory. Such infants usually have episodic bouts of acute respiratory symptoms, most often associated with feeding when mouth-breathing becomes intermittent. Choking spells and aspiration of feedings are frequent. The diagnosis, suspected when no air enters the chest with the mouth held closed, can be confirmed by inability to pass a small catheter through the nose into the nasopharynx and by failure to hear breath sounds on auscultation over the nares. Radiopaque material can be instilled into the anterior nasal cavity with the patient supine, and lateral films will demonstrate the point of obstruction. Tube feedings and an oral airway should be instituted as soon as the diagnosis is made.

Early surgical correction is usually advised in the case of bilateral obstruction, since aspiration pneumonia and respiratory acidosis are almost inevitable complications. This consists of perforation of the obstruction and introduction of obturators followed by dilatation through either transnasal or transpalatal routes.

Surgical correction of unilateral choanal atresia can be deferred until a future elective time.

NONPULMONARY CAUSES OF RESPIRATORY SYMPTOMS IN THE NEWBORN

CENTRAL NERVOUS SYSTEM HEMORRHAGE

There are several locations for bleeding into the central nervous system in the newborn that may give rise to respiratory symptoms. *Subdural hematomas* frequently occur in large infants, associated with a long and difficult labor or manipulative delivery, and are thought to be traumatic in origin. They usually present with focal or generalized signs of central nervous system irritation, such as tonic or clonic seizures, nystagmus or extensor spasms, and, except for apneic attacks of cyanosis associated with seizures, rarely present with respiratory symptoms.

In contrast, both *intraventricular hemorrhage* and widespread *subarachnoid hemorrhage* may present a difficult differential diagnosis with other forms of respiratory distress in the newborn, partly because they are most commonly seen in premature infants who may have asphyxia or hyaline membrane disease, or in dysmature infants with signs of intrauterine aspiration pneumonia. Both types of hemorrhage are said to be due to anoxia and shock. In many instances in which large intraventricular hemorrhages are found at autopsy, there seems to be a clear-cut history of the onset of central nervous system symptoms on the second or third day of life. Hematologic findings consistent with the diagnosis of disseminated intravascular coagulation consumptive coagulopathy have been shown in many of these infants; this is thought to be secondary to the underlying disease. Others seem to have defects in the second stage of clotting.

Irregular and periodic respiration followed by apneic attacks is frequent. Occasionally, however, hyperventilation occurs without roentgenographic signs of pulmonary disease, usually accompanied by a mottled, ashen gray cyanosis, shocklike picture and metabolic acidosis indicative of vascular collapse. Extensor spasms are common, and frank seizures may occur. As in other cases of central nervous system symptoms in the newborn where the lung is also involved, drugs that depress respiration are contraindicated unless ventilation is adequately controlled, and Dilantin is the drug of choice for the control of seizures. The carbon dioxide tension in the arterial blood in the absence of respiratory failure is low as a reflection of the extrapulmonary origin of the hyperventilation, and arterial oxygen unsaturation, if present, can usually be relieved by high oxygen inhalation in the absence of apnea or if ventilation is supported. Complete and sudden respiratory failure frequently occurs, but this may be modified by ventilatory assistance. If the infant with massive cerebral hemorrhage survives for several hours, a fall in hematocrit value from the level at birth, jaundice of more than expected degree for the state of prematurity, and hyperkalemia may be evidence of the amount of blood loss from the intravascular pool and subsequent extravascular blood destruction. Prolonged apneic attacks may lessen over several days to weeks if the infant survives, but the incidence of hydrocephalus and residual neurologic impairment is high.

When cerebral hemorrhage is an accompaniment of such pulmonary conditions as hyaline membrane disease or intrauterine aspiration pneumonia, the diagnosis is difficult and the prognosis grave. Infants who because of pulmonary disease desperately need to hyperventilate to survive do not tolerate central depression of their respiratory stimuli, such as frequently occurs with cerebral hemorrhage.

Understanding of the etiologic mechanisms of production, prevention and management of cerebral hemorrhage in the newborn currently presents one of the most challenging fields of our ignorance.

CONGENITAL CARDIAC DISEASE

PULMONARY EDEMA AND CARDIAC FAILURE

Relatively few congenital cardiac malformations present with acute respiratory symptoms in the neonatal period. Infants with many of the varieties of cyanotic congenital cardiac defects that have severe cyanosis and acute dyspneic episodes associated with diminished pulmonary blood flow later in life are free from such symptoms in early infancy because of the persistence of the ductus arteriosus as a left-to-right shunt. Its persistence promotes the return of adequate amounts of oxygenated blood to the left atrium. Some of the most common cardiac anomalies to present with pulmonary symptoms in the neonatal period are aortic atresia with hypoplasia of the left side of the heart, postductal coarctation of the aorta and fibroelastosis. All these may present with moist rales, frank pulmonary edema and roentgenographic evidence of pulmonary vascular congestion (Fig. 19).

The most commonly seen cardiac failure in the newborn at the present time is that associated with persistence of a patent ductus arteriosus in infants of very low birth weight, both with and without hyaline membrane disease (see p. 287). Half of those infants of less than 1200 grams birth weight who do not have any primary pulmonary disease except a very immature lung will have a symptomatic patent ductus arteriosus. By the third or fourth day of life, these infants begin to have recurrent episodes of apnea, concomitant with the appearance of a typical ductus murmur, rales, dyspnea and tachycardia. Increased precordial hyperactivity with cardiomegaly and pulmonary plethora on roentgenogram follow, and eventually liver enlargement and systemic edema appear. Most infants can be

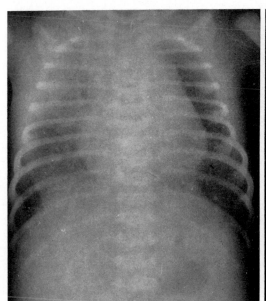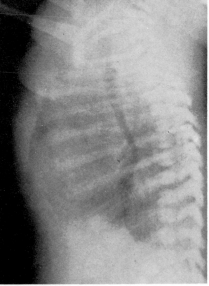

Figure 19. Anteroposterior and lateral chest films of an infant with aortic atresia and hypoplastic left ventricle, showing pulmonary venous engorgement and pulmonary edema.

successfully managed with low levels of nasal CPAP, digitalis, diuretics, low levels of oxygen and careful nursing care. Some may require assisted ventilation as well. The risks and advantages of early surgical or pharmacologic closure are being evaluated. Most ducts will close spontaneously by 34 to 36 postconceptual weeks, but the management of the infant with a large left-to-right ductus shunt requires meticulous care on the part of all concerned.

A much more subtle and gradually developing variety of heart failure is that associated with a persistently patent ductus arteriosus with a large left-to-right shunt in a more mature infant. Frequently, there is a history of respiratory distress in the neonatal period indistinguishable from classic hyaline membrane disease. Such an infant, often a moderate-sized premature, may be without any audible murmur for the first one or two weeks of life. When present, the murmur may initially be only systolic in timing. It usually becomes more typical and continuous as time goes on and the infant grows, expanding his blood volume and adjusting his pulmonary resistance to extrauterine life. The subtle and insidious onset of tachypnea and tachycardia is observable on the infant's graphic record, and dyspnea and fatigue associated with feedings appear. A rapid weight gain may be seen concomitant with clinical signs of edema. Such an infant usually responds well to digitalization, diuretics and, if symptoms are severe, added oxygen and CPAP. Most such infants can be tided over without surgery at this age; if followed up, the majority are found to lose their murmur several months later. An occasional infant will have a persistent murmur with or without symptoms of intractable failure. In the presence of intractable failure, prompt surgical closure of the ductus is indicated.

The occurrence of transient pulmonary congestion and cardiac dilatation associated with birth asphyxia has been described. Serial chest roentgenograms strongly suggest that such is the case, and frank and sudden pulmonary edema can also be seen early in the course of severe hyaline membrane disease. It seems likely to be due to intrapartum asphyxial damage to the heart when followed by high oxygen therapy of severe hyaline membrane disease, leading to a rapid fall in pulmonary vascular resistance. This, when associated with an unconstricted ductus arteriosus, can rapidly flood the lungs and, in the face of a weakened myocardium, allow left atrial pressure to rise; pulmonary vascular congestion and occasionally frank alveolar edema result. The low oncotic pressure of plasma in premature infants with low serum proteins would favor this.

Most episodes of pulmonary congestion associated with asphyxia clear as the infant regains acid-base balance and the myocardium improves. Infants with hyaline membrane disease in whom frank pulmonary edema occurs in the first few hours after birth usually run a course typical of severe and often fatal disease.

Acute pulmonary edema in the newborn from whatever cause should be treated with CPAP, positive pressure ventilation for respiratory failure, oxygenation, correction of acid-base disturbance, diuresis and rapid digitalization if heart failure is present.

PAROXYSMAL ATRIAL TACHYCARDIA

Paroxysmal atrial tachycardia can occur in the neonatal period and has even been diagnosed in utero with the fetal electrocardiogram. Most small infants with paroxysmal atrial tachycardia fall into a similar clinical picture. In most cases in this age group, no etiologic factors are found. The majority are males. These acutely ill infants frequently present with the picture similar to that of pneumonia or septicemia. They are ashen gray with clammy, cold skin and shocklike appearance. Respiration is rapid and labored, and rales are usually heard. The heart is frequently enlarged and the rate so rapid as to be difficult to count. The liver is usually easily palpable, and the peripheral and periorbital edema is apparent. The electrocardiogram shows a fixed rate, usually greater than 200 per minute, and P waves are rarely identifiable. The QRS complex is normal, resembling that of the ventricular complex with a sinus rhythm, in contrast to that of ventricular tachycardia.

Vagal stimulation by unilateral carotid sinus pressure may be tried, but is only rarely effective in reverting the arrhythmia in small infants in congestive failure. Digitalis is considered to be the drug of choice at this age. Digoxin may be given over a 12- to 18-hour period in a dosage of 45 to 60 micrograms per kilogram intramuscularly in three divided doses, with a maintenance dosage of one-eighth the digitalizing dose twice daily thereafter. Only rarely is it necessary to resort to Prostigmin, quinidine or procainamide, the latter two finding their principal use in paroxysmal ventricular tachycardia.

The change in clinical status in a small, desperately ill infant following digitalization is usually dramatic. The color improves, restlessness and cough disappear, and within 24 hours the baby begins to diurese. The heart size and liver size return to normal within a few days. Prophylactic digitalization should be continued for at least one month after reversion to a normal rhythm, at which time cessation can be attempted. If the supraventricular tachycardia recurs, digitalis should be resumed for an additional six months. The prognosis for small infants is usually good, since there is usually no evidence of underlying heart disease.

PULMONARY SYMPTOMS ASSOCIATED WITH HEMOLYTIC DISEASE, ACUTE HYPERVOLEMIA AND HYPOVOLEMIA

Infants born with severe hemolytic disease of the newborn may present with acute respiratory symptoms from a number of causes. In the case of massive hemolysis associated with hydrops fetalis, the anasarca is considered to be a manifestation of intrauterine heart failure due to extreme anemia, combined with hypoalbuminemia. Such infants may, indeed, present in heart failure, the immediate treatment of which is exchange transfusion. Exchange transfusions should be small and frequent, and they should be performed in such a way as to avoid such further hemodynamic alterations. Often, leaving an excess of blood is beneficial in the most profoundly affected infants, since they may have hypovolemia rather than hypervolemia. Indeed, leaving a deficit in blood volume at the end of the exchange may precipitate shock. In addition to anemia, many of these severely ill and dyspneic infants have profound metabolic acidosis associated with tissue hypoxia, with arterial pH levels below 7.0. Careful addition of buffers such as THAM to the exchange blood and thereafter will rapidly improve the acid-base balance and help restore the circulatory status toward normal, since shock accompanies such low levels of pH.

An additional cause of respiratory symptoms in the newborn with hemolytic disease may be massive ascites, which, by elevating the diaphragm, severely limits ventilation. If such is apparent, abdominal paracentesis is indicated, care being taken to avoid the enlarged liver and spleen.

In the case of acute blood loss in the neonate, respiratory symptoms and tachycardia may be disarmingly absent until complete cardiovascular collapse supervenes. The treatment is immediate replacement of blood loss and search for its source, which may be obscure. The presence of fetal hemoglobin in the maternal blood may demonstrate intrauterine bleeding into the maternal circulation. Intrapartum hypovolemia may also result from umbilical cord occlusion, which compresses the umbilical vein but leaves the arteries filling the placenta, or cesarean section, where the infant is lifted higher than umbilical venous pressure at the time of cord clamping. Transient tachypnea and a poor peripheral circulation may be apparent until blood volume is restored to normal. Other occult hemorrhage, such as intraventricular, from splenic rupture or from ulceration of the gastrointestinal tract, may occur in the neonatal period and be extremely difficult to diagnose or to localize. A falling hematocrit may alert the physician to the event.

Hypervolemia may occur as a baby-to-baby transfusion in twins, or simply as a temporary overloading of the circulation with placental blood if the infant cries or gasps vigorously before the cord is clamped. Mild to moderate respiratory symptoms may result; the tachypnea and tachycardia usually subside in a matter of hours as blood volume adjustments occur. If persistent symptoms of acute hypervolemia of this variety occur, or if hyperviscosity is present with an extremely high hematocrit, a partial exchange transfusion may be indicated.

NEUROMUSCULAR WEAKNESS AS A CAUSE OF NEONATAL RESPIRATORY DISTRESS

Unilateral *paralysis of the vocal cords* in the newborn infant is most frequently seen on the left side, presumably from injury to the recurrent laryngeal nerve at the time of birth. Bilateral paralysis is much less common and is thought to be central in origin. Symptoms are hoarseness and stridor, which may persist for several years. Laryngoscopy should be done to identify the lesion and to rule out other causes of stridor. In extreme cases, a tracheostomy may be necessary.

Phrenic nerve paralysis also may occur at birth as the result of a difficult delivery. It is frequently associated with brachial nerve palsy, although it may occur as an isolated lesion. The right diaphragm is more often affected than the left. Symptoms, if present, consist of cyanosis, dyspnea and a feeble cry. Fluoroscopic examinations for diaphragmatic motion confirm the diagnosis. Complications arise if the atelectatic lung becomes infected, and may result in death. Plication of the diphragm may be necessary in severe cases.

Weakness of the muscles of respiration, including the intercostals and the diaphragm in congenital myasthenia gravis, amyotonia congenita and poliomyelitis of the newborn, may result in severe hypoventilation and its consequences. Myasthenia may be transient if the infant is born to a myasthenic mother, or persistent if born to a normal mother. Symptoms in the former may not appear until several days after birth. In either case, they consist of weakness, feeble cry and poor ability to suck and swallow. Ptosis is occasionally seen. A therapeutic trial with Tensilon (edrophonium chloride), 0.1 ml. subcutaneously, will confirm the diagnosis if improvement in strength occurs in 10 to 15 minutes.

Amyotonia congenita is a rare familial disease characterized by generalized and progressive skeletal muscle weakness, with sphincter tone and with sensation intact. Involvement of the intercostal muscles and diaphragm leads to retraction and hypoventilation. No treatment is known.

Intrauterine and neonatal infection with *poliomyelitis* virus can likewise affect the muscles of respiration as well as other muscle groups. Central respiratory paralysis is also possible. Those infants with respiratory muscle involvement, if it is not permanent, might presumably be carried by ventilatory assistance, as are those with neonatal tetanus, but so far none has been reported.

The prognosis of neonatal *tetanus*, once considered an almost uniformly fatal disease from respiratory failure, has recently been significantly improved by the successful use of ventilatory assistance combined with curare, antitoxin and careful nursing care. Although a rare disease in the United States, it is extremely common in certain parts of the world where obstetric practices may include deliberate contamination of the umbilical cord stump by material that is frequently spore-containing. In some instances it is contracted at the time of circumcision. The incubation period is usually short, and the infant begins to have tetanic seizures frequently associated with apnea. These become more severe and more prolonged, and the infant usually dies if ventilation is unassisted, despite other therapeutic measures. Positive pressure ventilation through either a tracheostomy or endotracheal tube combined with curarization has relieved cyanosis and hypoventilation, since the lung is normally compliant if not secondarily infected. Tracheostomies in small infants may become difficult to remove. If successful removal is accomplished after several months, residual deformity of the trachea may be left as a complication.

ASSISTED VENTILATION IN NEONATAL LUNG DISORDERS

Although there were sporadic attempts to carry out assisted ventilation in small infants for many years, usually without much success, widespread interest in its use dates to the early 1960s. Following the successful demonstration by Smythe and Bull (1959) that a modified adult ventilator could be used to manage infants with severe neonatal tetanus, other adult ventilators have been modified for use in small subjects, and a number have been specifically designed for this purpose.

The array of machines available at the present time is impressive, but each has its specific limitations. The choice begins with simple devices, such as a bag and mask, which often can be used quite successfully in newborn resuscita-

tion and in the treatment of brief apnea attacks in small immature infants without pulmonary disease. An endotracheal tube can be substituted for the mask to ensure delivery of gas into the respiratory tract at a given pressure, utilizing either a bag or an infant anesthesia machine that has one-way ventilatory valves and a CO_2 absorber in the system. This is also manually operated, but can be used successfully for many hours in a wide variety of newborn pulmonary conditions. A number of types of automatically cycled systems are available, some of which can be set to be triggered by the inspiratory effort of the infant himself. This gives considerable versatility, since they can be used either for ventilatory control or only as assistance. These automatically cycled machines are of several different types. Some have an automatic inspiratory cutoff when a given pressure is reached; others discontinue when the preset volume is attained. Some have limitations of rate and ratio of inspiration to expiration, and some are extremely flexible in their capabilities with continuous flow of gas throughout the respiratory cycle. One machine uses the principle of creating a negative pressure around the thorax during inspiration; the head is maintained at atmospheric pressure so that air is sucked into the lung rather than pushed into it, as an augmentation of normal breathing. All of these types of assisted ventilation have considerable limitations, and their failure is usually dependent on their being expected to perform tasks of which they are mechanically incapable. Their success depends largely upon the pulmonary mechanism of the disorder for which they are being used and the skill, dedication and familiarity of the personnel who are responsible for their use.

The easiest type of assisted ventilation is that carried out on a normal lung, such as during anesthesia for neonatal surgery. Low pressures can be used to achieve normal alveolar volumes. Likewise, one can use normal concentrations of ventilating gases and achieve satisfactory blood gas levels.

The problem of ventilating an essentially normal lung becomes more complicated with long-term management, such as is usually needed with neonatal tetanus in which three to four weeks of assistance may be necessary, accompanied by all of the inherent hazards of prolonged intubation or tracheotomy in the small infant. The small, very immature infant with apneic attacks may also become a major problem, not because his lung cannot be ventilated with ease, since it usually can, but because the apnea often appears to be of reflex origin and, when severe, is frequently associated with signs of cardiovascular collapse. A bag and mask with ambient gas concentrations will usually suffice for attacks of short duration, but more profound attacks, especially if associated with hypotension and bradycardia, will require more vigorous resuscitation. CPAP at low levels, with or without ventilation at a slow rate, may be helpful. Some infants who have these repeated profound attacks will not survive despite vigorous management, and usually demonstrate intracranial hemorrhage at autopsy. Which is the cause and which is the effect, the apnea or the hemorrhage, is still an important unanswered question.

The use of assisted ventilation in infants with primary pulmonary disorders has somewhat different requirements than it does in those conditions in which the lung is not primarily at fault. If pulmonary compliance is impaired, as it is in hyaline membrane disease, in which there is progressive tendency for alveolar collapse at normal end-expiratory pressures, higher inspiratory pressure may be necessary to achieve normal alveolar volumes; or in the case of negative pressure respirators, a more negative inspiratory pressure is necessary. This may be the limiting factor in the effectiveness of the ventilatory assistance in these circumstances, since rupture of those alveoli left with open airways is likely to occur as they are overdistended with either a fixed volume or increasing pressure. The result may be interstitial emphysema, which may dissect back into the mediastinum as pneumomediastinum or peripherally as a unilateral or bilateral pneumothorax. These are extremely serious complications, especially in the face of poor lung compliance, since the re-expansion of a completely collapsed lung with impaired compliance may be difficult, and diffuse interstitial air greatly impairs lung function. Not only must one risk the hazards of increased pressure, either positive or negative, with the intrinsic pulmonary disease associated with poor compliance, but oxygen concentrations considerably above ambient level must be used because of increasing intrapulmonary right-to-left shunting and the persistence of extrapulmonary shunting through fetal pathways.

The introduction by Gregory and coworkers (1970) of the use of end-expiratory pressure in infants with poor compliance has a sound physiologic basis, since alveolar collapse occurs at the lower pressures of the expiratory limb of the pressure-volume loop. The maintenance of a low positive end-expiratory pressure would tend to maintain a functional residual volume during expiration and improve the distribution of alveolar air, achieving a better ventilation-to-perfusion ratio. This is essentially what the expiratory grunt of the distressed newborn infant does with forced expiration against a partially closed glottis. The demonstration that adequate oxygenation is more readily achieved with this technique at lower inspired oxygen concentrations attests to its usefulness. Its limitations are based on its ability to produce an abnormally high functional residual capacity with CO_2 retention, the limitation of pulmonary capillary blood flow in a lung with normal compliance, and the possible complication of diffuse interstitial emphysema, often leading to pneumothorax when it is overzealously employed, especially when combined with positive pressure ventilation. The use of nasal CPAP allows an automatic safety valve of opening the mouth, and is quite satisfactory in many infants requiring CPAP alone.

Those machines designed to control ventilation, whether with pressure or volume limitation, are most useful in the extremely ill infant who can no longer maintain his own ventilatory effort. This is especially true in those infants less than 1500 grams in weight. In addition, the management of the infant's nursing care, exclusive of his ventilation, can more readily be carried out when the infant is in an Isolette or open bed than when he is in a body tank. Oral feedings can be begun early through an indwelling catheter that is inserted into the stomach or jejunum and attached to an open syringe barrel hung from the top of the Isolette. This allows regurgitation up the tube into the reservoir and avoids overfeeding and overdistention. Oral feedings can be supplemented with parenteral fluids containing calories. Such things as portable roentgenograms are more easily obtained, and umbilical catheters are more readily managed. The negative pressure respirator has one great advantage — that of not requiring an endotracheal tube. It is generally agreed that the infant with severe pulmonary disease cannot be successfully carried on a mask for prolonged periods of time, regardless of the type of machine to which it is attached. The negative pressure machine is likewise somewhat limited in the extremely ill infant with profound pulmonary disease, since its success depends on its use as a ventilatory assist rather than as a ventilatory control. When the profoundly ill infant ceases to make his own respiratory efforts synchronously with the negative pressure respirator, the stomach may have an easier distensibility than the lung if pulmonary compliance is impaired sufficiently. The respirator then serves no useful purpose as far as pulmonary function is concerned. Such infants must be intubated and put on another type of ventilator.

An orogastric tube may be inserted into the stomach and connected onto continuous low suction pressure of 8 to 9 cm. H_2O for abdominal distention. This will usually keep the stomach satisfactorily deflated in an infant who is still making respiratory efforts with the respirator or who is on CPAP alone. Care must be taken to avoid hypokalemia from loss through suction.

In addition to hyaline membrane disease, other types of pulmonary diseases in the newborn have been successfully managed with assisted ventilation; their limitation of use is usually related to the severity of the underlying disease process, such as intrauterine pneumonia. Severe meconium aspiration pneumonia has been successfully ventilated, but pneumothorax has been a frequent complication because of plugging of the airways with meconium and ball-valve obstruction, leading to easy overdistention of some alveoli.

The complications of the use of assisted ventilation in small infants are myriad. Some of these, such as rupture of alveoli with the production of interstitial emphysema, pneumomediastinum or pneumothorax, have already been mentioned and are dealt with in detail elsewhere. The complication of excessively high inspiratory pressure or the maintenance of too high an end-expiratory pressure may compromise pulmonary capillary blood flow. The problems of maintaining an adequate pulmonary toilet through a small endotracheal tube are serious ones and require meticulous care if obstruction with secretions or cellular debris is not to occur. Strict aseptic technique must be maintained in the handling of tracheal lavage and suction. All tubing, nebulizers, and similar pieces of equipment that are used in the ventilatory system should be changed every 24 hours, and must be gas-sterilized and degassed before replacement to avoid such saprophytic bacterial contamination as that with *Pseudomonas aeruginosa*. Endotracheal cultures should be done repeatedly in order to detect secondary pulmonary infection as early as possible. All fluids used in the nebulizer system should likewise be changed at least every 24 hours. Inspired oxygen concentrations should be kept at a minimum for acceptable blood oxygen levels, since direct oxygen toxicity to the newborn lung may become a problem after its prolonged use.

In some instances, ventilation of the lung is more readily accomplished than is satisfactory oxygenation, and hypocapnia may develop. Since cerebral blood flow is compromised at low levels of arterial P_{CO_2}, it may be desirable to add 3 to 5 per cent CO_2 to the inspired gas mixture or to increase the dead space of the ventilatory system to maintain a normal arterial CO_2.

Because of the many risks incurred with all types of effective assisted ventilation, every effort should be made to wean the infant from the respirator at the first possible moment. Since the natural history of hyaline membrane disease is one of increasingly poor compliance and oxygen dependency for the first 48 to 72 hours after birth, this is the time when assisted ventilation is likely to be the most beneficial; the beginning of weaning should be possible by 72 to 96 hours after birth. If, by this time, it is impossible to see improvement in an infant's own ability to ventilate and oxygenate, one begins to suspect some secondary process is assuming dominance; this may be central depression from intracranial hemorrhage or prior severe hypoxia with shock, secondary infection, severe interstitial emphysema, atelectasis of major portions of the lung from obstruction of the airway or severe electrolyte imbalance, especially hypokalemia with muscle weakness or the appearance of pulmonary edema secondary to a large left-to-right ductal shunt.

The criterion for instituting some level of CPAP in hyaline membrane disease is usually a Pa_{O_2} of less than 50 mm. Hg in more than 50 per cent O_2.

The criteria for using assisted ventilation have varied from one intensive care unit to another; the indications are usually based on an inability to satisfactorily oxygenate an infant above 50 mm. Hg in 95 to 100 per cent inspired oxygen concentrations after CPAP, the appearance of unresponsive apnea, and other combinations of prognostic signs, such as acidemia or hypercapnia. However, regardless of the varied types of apparatus chosen, or the combinations of criteria used in patient selection, survival results of ventilated infants with hyaline membrane disease have been largely dependent upon birth weight. Survival now approaches 80 per cent in infants above 1000 grams birth weight, and 90 to 100 per cent by 2000 grams.

Future efforts should be aimed at salvaging more of these infants in the very low birth weight groups.

REFERENCES

Adamsons, K., Jr., Berhman, R., Dawes, G. S., James, L. S., and Koford, C.: Resuscitation by positive pressure ventilation and tris-hydromethyl-aminomethane of rhesus monkeys asphyxiated at birth. *J. Pediatr.*, 65:807, 1964.

Avery, M. E.: *The Lung and Its Disorders in the Newborn Infant.* Philadelphia, W. B. Saunders Company, 1974, pp. 40–54.

Avery, M. E., Gatewood, O. G., and Brumley, G.: Transient tachypnea of the newborn. *Am. J. Dis. Child.*, 3:380, 1966.

Beinfield, H. H.: Ways and means to reduce infant mortality due to suffocation, importance of choanal atresia. *J.A.M.A.*, 170:647, 1959.

Boss, J. H., and Craig, J. M.: Reparative phenomena in lungs of neonates with hyaline membranes. *Pediatrics*, 29:890, 1962.

Burnard, E. D., and James, L. S.: Atrial pressures and cardiac size in newborn infants: relationships, with degree of birth asphyxia and size of placental transfusion. *J. Pediatr.*, 62:815, 1963.

Chun, J., and others: The pulmonary hypoperfusion syndrome. *Pediatrics*, 35:733, 1965.

Cohen, M. M., Weintraub, D. H., and Lilienfeld, A. M.: The relationship of pulmonary hyaline membrane to certain factors in pregnancy and delivery. *Pediatrics*, 26:42, 1960.

Diament, H., and Kinnman, J.: Congenital choanal atresia. Report of a clinical series with special references to early symptoms and therapy. *Acta Paediatr.*, 52:106, 1963.

Edwards, J.: Malformations of the aortic arch system manifested as "vascular rings." *Lab. Invest.*, 2:56, 1950.

Faxelius, G., Raye, J., Gutberlet, R., Swanstrom, S., Tsiantos, A., Victorin, L., Dolanski, E., Dehan, M., Dyer, N., Lindstrom, D., Brill, A. B., and Stahlman, M.: Red cell volume measurements and acute blood loss in high-risk newborn infants. *J. Pediatr.*, 90:273, 1977.

Gregory, G. A., Kitterman, J. A., Phibbs, R. H., Tooley, W. H., and Hamilton, W. K.: Continuous positive airway pressure with spontaneous respiration: a new method of increasing arterial oxygenation in the respiratory distress syndrome. *Pediatr. Res.*, 4:469, 1970.

James, L. S.: Acidosis of newborn and its relation to birth asphyxia. *Acta Paediatr.*, 49(Suppl. 122):17, 1960.

James, L. S., and Adamsons, K., Jr.: Respiratory physiology of the fetus and newborn. *N. Engl. J. Med.*, 271:1352; 1403, 1964.

James, L. S., Weisbrot, J. M., Prince, C. E., Holaday, D. A., and Apgar, V.: Acid-base status of human infants in relation to birth asphyxia and onset of respiration. *J. Pediatr.*, 52:379, 1958.

Kirschner, P. A., and Strauss, L.: Pulmonary interstitial emphysema in the new infant. Precursors and sequelae. *Dis. Chest*, 46:417, 1964.

Kottler, R. E., Malan, A. E., and Heese, H. deV.: Respiratory distress syndrome in the newborn. *S. Afr. J. Radiol.*, 2:36, 1964.

Liggins, G. C.: Prenatal glucocorticoid treatment. Prevention of respiratory distress syndrome. *Ross Conference on Pediatric Research*. Lung Maturation and the Prevention of Hyaline Membrane Disease. December, 1975.

Nadas, A. S.: *Pediatric Cardiology*. 2nd Ed. Philadelphia, W. B. Saunders Company, 1973, p. 23.

Prod'ham, L. S., Levison, H. L., Cherry, R. B., and Smith, C. A.: Adjustment of ventilation, intrapulmonary gas exchange and acid-base balance during the first day of life. *Pediatrics*, 35:662, 1965.

Saling, E.: Mikroblutuntersuchungen am Feten: Klinischer Einsatz und erste Ergebinisse. *Fortschr. Geburtshilfe Gynaekol.*, 162:56, 1964.

Smythe, P. M.: Studies of neonatal tetanus and on pulmonary compliance of the totally relaxed infant. *Br. Med. J.*, 1:565, 1965.

Smythe, P. M., and Bull, A.: Treatment of tetanus neonatorum with intermittent positive pressure respirator. *Br. Med. J.*, 2:107, 1959.

Stahlman, M. T.: Treatment of cardiovascular disorders of the newborn. *Pediatr. Clin. North Am.*, 11:377, 1964.

Stahlman, M. T., Malan, A., Shepard, F., Blankenship, W., Young, W., and James, G.: Negative pressure assisted ventilation in infants with hyaline membrane disease. *J. Pediatr.*, 76:174, 1970.

Swyer, P. R.: Results of artificial ventilation. *Biol. Neonate*, 16:148, 1970.

Tsiantos, A., Victorin, L., Relier, J. P., Dyer, N., Sundell, H., Brill, A. B., and Stahlman, M.: Intercranial hemorrhage in the prematurely born infant: timing of clots and evaluation of clinical signs and symptoms. *J. Pediatr.*, 85:854, 1974.

Usher, R., McLean, F., and Maughan, G. M.: Respiratory distress syndrome in infants delivered by cesarean section. *Am. J. Obstet. Gynecol.*, 88:806, 1964.

CHAPTER ELEVEN

BRONCHOPULMONARY DYSPLASIA

BARRY V. KIRKPATRICK, M.D., and WILLIAM E. LAUPUS, M.D.

Neonatal intensive care and refined techniques in mechanical ventilation have reduced the high mortality associated with neonatal respiratory distress syndrome (hyaline membrane disease). With increase in survival, there has been the recognition of a progressive disease of the lung parenchyma and airways called bronchopulmonary dysplasia (BPD). The first concise report by Northway and coworkers in 1967 attempted to correlate the clinical, histologic and radiographic stages of this illness in infants surviving hyaline membrane disease after mechanical ventilation. Northway divided BPD into four stages. Each stage was not a definite entity unto itself, but served only as a marker of progression. A great amount of overlap occurred between each stage.

The Four Stages of Bronchopulmonary Dysplasia

Stage I (two to three days) — period of acute respiratory distress;

Stage II (four to ten days) — period of regeneration;

Stage III (ten to 30 days) — period of transition to chronic disease;

Stage IV (beyond one month) — period of chronic disease.

Even after 10 years of clinical recognition, the exact cause (if indeed there is only one etiologic agent) still eludes investigators. Oxygen therapy in elevated concentrations, intermittent positive pressure ventilation, delay in healing of the premature lung following hyaline membrane disease, endotracheal intubation, poor tracheal toilet of ventilated infants, lack of humidification of inspired gases, and the presence of a patent ductus arteriosus are but a few conditions associated with or implicated in the development of bronchopulmonary dysplasia. Predisposing conditions producing lung injury and subsequent BPD are variable, since treatment modalities often are not the same from institution to institution, or from patient to patient within any one institution, or indeed from hour to hour in any one patient.

MECHANICAL VENTILATION

Positive Pressure Ventilation Versus Negative Pressure Ventilation

Chronic pulmonary disease has been recognized in infants surviving hyaline membrane disease after either intermittent positive pressure ventilation (IPPV) or transthoracic negative pressure ventilation (NPV). Controlled studies comparing these two treatment modalities are absent. At some neonatal centers, negative pressure ventilation is used frequently, and the incidence of BPD is reported to be low. However, since the majority of NP ventilators commercially available operate most effectively with infants over 1500 gm., many series reporting the results of NP ventilation are limited to larger and therefore more mature infants. It is difficult to compare the incidence of BPD after IPPV with that following NPV because patient populations are not the same. Newer modifications of negative pressure ventilation can now accommodate infants of a much smaller size. The effectiveness of this modification in improving survival rates and altering the incidence of BPD is still unknown.

Damage to the pulmonary tree after IPPV has been documented by Stocks and Godfrey (1976). Serial measurements of lung function were made in three groups of infants requiring mechanical ventilation (IPPV), or CPAP with added O_2, or O_2 alone. Only the group requiring IPPV had an increase in airway resistance (R_{aw}) at seven months of age (p value $< .0005$), while other parameters of lung function (thoracic gas volume, tidal volume, frequency and compliance) were similar in all groups. Even though these patients did not have BPD clinically, lung damage was attributed to the mechanical effects of IPPV.

Similar measurements of R_{aw} in NPV patients are not available, though several investigators have reported long-term pulmonary function abnormalities in NPV survivors.

The question of the effects of IPPV without supplemental O_2 must also be raised. DeLemos and coworkers (1969) failed to produce lung damage in newborn lambs from IPPV without added oxygen. Similar human studies are not available, but one can speculate that the combined effects of IPPV with O_2 can produce pulmonary damage.

Pressure-Limited Versus Volume Ventilators

Within our own nursery, we have not been able to correlate the development of BPD to the type of positive pressure ventilator used. BPD occurred with equal frequency (13 per cent) in infants surviving hyaline membrane disease regardless of whether a volume-limited or pressure-limited positive pressure ventilator was employed.

Newer techniques in IPPV, such as low flow rates, reversed inspiratory to expiratory ratio (e.g., I:E of 2:1), low respiratory rates and the use of intermittent mandatory ventilation (IMV), may further reduce the damage thought to be imparted by IPPV. Long-term studies with adequate follow-up utilizing these new treatment modalities are needed, and these techniques require further evaluation.

Oxygen Toxicity

Oxygen has long been recognized as toxic to the lung of humans and lower animals. Mammalian lung exposed to oxygen at 100 per cent concentration will show evidence of toxic effects within a few hours. Oxygen exposure in various concentrations produces histologically diffuse microhemorrhagic changes in lung capillaries as well as altered ciliary action, inhibition of pulmonary development (in growing animals), pulmonary edema, and an increase of surface tension as measured in lung extracts of some species. The effects of elevated oxygen exposure to surfactant production in human neonates are still unclear. Premature infants may be particularly vulnerable to the toxic effects of oxygen owing to their low levels of a recently reported substance, superoxide dismutase (SOD). SOD may be effective in catalyzing dismutation of the oxygen-free radical that is thought to cause pulmonary damage. Additionally, DNA synthesis within the lung has been shown to be inhibited by oxygen exposure.

Damage by oxygen is due to its direct effect on lung tissue and is not related to the level of arterial oxygen tension. In ventilated infants, oxygen concentration and/or duration of oxygen exposure correlates poorly with the degree of BPD seen. Our own experience confirms the inconsistency of BPD to O_2 concentration and length of exposure.

Histologic changes in the lung of neonates exposed to high concentrations of O_2 delivered in hoods or in conjunction with negative pressure ventilation are less pronounced than those alterations seen following O_2 and IPPV. Oxygen alone, therefore, is probably not responsible for BPD.

Patent Ductus Arteriosus

It is unclear whether a persistent patent ductus arteriosus is a causative agent in the development of BPD or is reflective of altered pulmonary compliance and blood flow. It has been shown that an opened ductus arteriosus often accompanies severe respiratory distress in the preterm infant and that it may be a significant contributing factor to the duration of the infant's respiratory failure and subsequent need for mechanical ventilation. In our own experience, 80 per cent of BPD patients have an opened ductus arteriosus during the early stages (I to III). Recently there has been a trend for early closure of the ductus arteriosus. The effects of this procedure in altering the incidence of BPD is unknown.

Air Block

There is a strong association between the development of an acute air block, especially pulmonary interstitial emphysema, and the later recognition of bronchopulmonary dysplasia. While an air block itself does not seem to have direct causative effect, it often reflects the reduced lung compliance of the patient. Low lung compliance is directly related to the severity of the initial disease necessitating mechanical ventilation. Since the patient with poor lung compliance often requires higher inspiratory pressure or increased tidal volume to achieve adequate ventilation, injury to the lung is more likely to occur, and the incidence of BPD can be expected to increase. One-third of our BPD patients had either pulmonary interstitial emphysema or other acute air block.

Other Factors

HEALING PROCESS OF HYALINE MEMBRANE DISEASE. Northway and others thought that BPD could be an accentuation of the normal healing process of hyaline membrane disease following treatment with oxygen and mechanical ventilation. However, clinical, radiographic and histologic evidence of BPD has been documented in infants who never had HMD but needed mechanical ventilation. Also, BPD has been reported in infants who recovered from HMD, but later suffered some catastrophic event (CNS hemorrhage, septic shock) that required mechanical ventilation.

Infants mechanically ventilated for problems other than HMD may, therefore, be at risk for BPD. It would seem that HMD is not a necessary precursor for the development of bronchopulmonary changes.

GESTATIONAL AGE. More than one study has discounted the gestational age of the patient as a factor in BPD development. In our series of 33 BPD patients, 77 per cent were 32 weeks of gestation or less by Dubowitz's clinical assessment, and 84 per cent had a birth weight of less than 1500 gm. Experience with this group of patients would suggest that BPD is more frequent in the smaller and more premature infant.

Endotracheal Intubation, Humidification and Tracheal Toilet Problems

These three procedures have been incriminated in the development of BPD. It is difficult to remove them from the list of etiologic agents, since they are intimately involved in the management of the infant with respiratory distress syndrome receiving positive pressure ventilation.

Endotracheal tubes do cause upper airway damage. We have seen only one case of BPD out of 47 infants (<2000 gm.) treated with endotracheal intubation for delivery of CPAP. It would seem unlikely, therefore, that endotracheal intubation per se causes BPD.

Poor humidification and poor techniques in tracheal toilet have also been associated with BPD. Our routine for caring for an endotracheal tube is the same for the mechanically ventilated infant as for the infant receiving endotracheal tube CPAP. The incidence of BPD in these two treatment modalities is 13 per cent, versus 2 per cent in our nursery. With good nursing management of the intubated patient, serious damage to the lungs and airways can be minimized.

Summary of Etiologic Factors

With multiple insults occurring to the lung of the mechanically ventilated premature infant, it is probable that no one factor is responsible for BPD. IPPV and oxygen exposure appear to be major factors. Poor airway care, low lung compliance with acute air block, and prolonged mechanical ventilation may add additional injury to the lung. These insults are more pronounced in the premature infant who is 32 weeks of gestation or less and weighing less than 1500 gm.

CLINICAL–RADIO-GRAPHIC–HISTOLOGIC CORRELATION

The four stages of BPD as originally discussed by Northway can be expanded to provide a better clinical understanding (see Fig. 1), since not every patient with hyaline membrane disease develops BPD, and not every patient with BPD becomes severely oxygen-dependent with chronic pulmonary damage.

Stage I (Acute respiratory distress—two to three days)

Tachypnea, cyanosis in room air, retractions and grunting mark this phase clinically. Roentgenograms are characteristic of acute respiratory distress syndrome; underinflation, air bronchograms and a ground-glass appearance within the lung parenchyma are seen (Fig. 2). Histologic findings in the lung include atelectasis, interstitial thickening, hyaline membrane organization in the alveolar ducts and necrosis of bronchiolar mucosa.

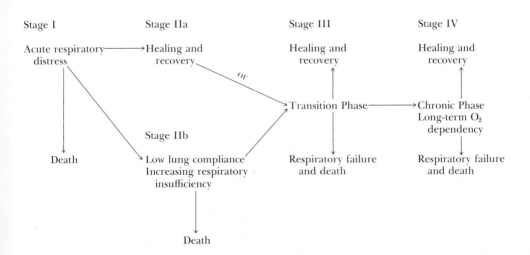

Figure 1. Progression of bronchopulmonary dysplasia. (Modified from a suggestion by V. V. Joshi, M.D., unpublished data.)

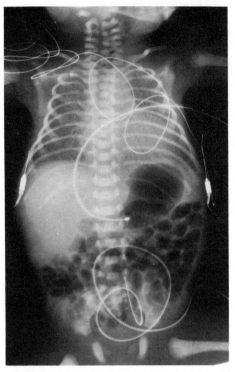

Figure 2. Early hyaline membrane disease with characteristic air bronchograms and hypoinflation (Stage I).

Stage IIa (Recovery phase)

Over a period of approximately three to ten days, the infant's respiratory condition stabilizes; some patients slowly improve, while others fail to do so and progress to Stage III. Those who are recovering from the acute phase require reductions in $F_{I_{O_2}}$, minute ventilation, and positive end-expiratory pressure. They eventually are weaned from a ventilator to a hood with supplemental oxygen, and then to room air. During this phase, the radiograph improves. The lung becomes more normally inflated and there is marked reduction of atelectasis. Histologic specimens obtained at this time are usually from patients who have died from causes other than respiratory failure and show the repair of bronchial mucosa and a reduction of atelectasis. Squamous metaplasia and deposition of necrotic mucosal cells into the small bronchi are constant findings.

Stage IIb

Rather than improve, these patients display a drop in lung compliance and become more difficult to ventilate. Minute ventilation and oxygen requirements increase. Pulmonary interstitial emphysema or other air blocks, such as pneumothorax or pneumomediastinum, may develop. Severe respiratory failure, pulmonary hemorrhage and CNS hemorrhage often cause the patient's demise at this point.

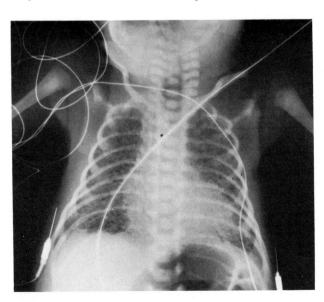

Figure 3. Pulmonary interstitial emphysema. Air dissected into the interstitium of the lung gives this radiograph a characteristic bubbly appearance.

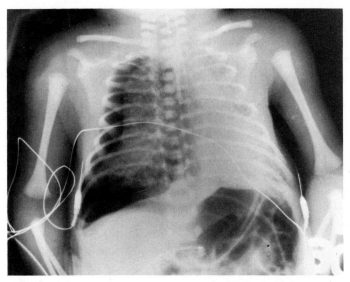

Figure 4. Tension pneumothorax following pulmonary interstitial emphysema. Note the mediastinal shift with compression of the left lung. The right lung remains partially expanded by a supporting network of interstitial air (Stage IIb).

Radiographs may show "white out" or complete opacification of both lung fields. Air bronchograms are typical, and air block (especially pulmonary interstitial emphysema or pneumothorax) is common (Figs. 3 and 4).

At autopsy, the lungs of these patients are stiff and have scattered areas of emphysema, atelectasis and severe necrosis with cellular debris within the terminal airways. Pneumonia and/or some degree of an inflammatory response may also be present.

Stage III (Transition phase)

Patients who reach this stage either are oxygen-dependent (from IIa) or have survived Stage IIb and still require mechanical ventilation. During Stage III they are often stable in their oxygen demands or ventilatory support

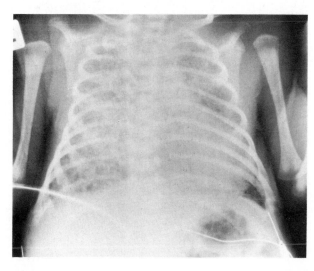

Figure 5. By Stage III, alternating areas of alveolar collapse and focal emphysema give the lung a cystic appearance.

and can either slowly improve or develop progressive respiratory failure. Blood gases in Stage III patients reflect hypoventilation (Pa_{O_2} 50 to 70 torr) and some degree of desaturation. Those who improve will slowly decrease the need for supplemental oxygen, though some degree of desaturation may continue for a long period of time.

Radiographs are quite characteristic (Fig. 5). The cystic appearance of the lung parenchyma is due to alternate areas of focal hyperaeration, consolidation and fibrosis of supporting structures within the lung.

Histologically, the predominantly necrotic phase has now been replaced by healing or metaplastic changes. Extensive bronchial and bronchiolar mucosal metaplasia and hyperplasia are seen. Alveolar emphysema and coalescence in spherical groupings with atelectasis of surrounding alveoli, interstitial edema and course focal thickening of basement membranes are features of this stage.

Stage IV (Chronic phase)

Patients in the chronic phase either are stable or may develop progressive respiratory failure and die. Pa_{CO_2} levels may reach over 100 torr despite mechanical ventilation. Often, some degree of right-sided heart failure and pulmonary hypertension are present. Fluid retention, progressive cardiac failure and general deterioration make these patients very difficult to treat effectively.

Those infants who are long-term oxygen-dependent need many months to resolve their disease. We have had patients in oxygen for longer than one year; in some centers, patients have been treated who required oxygen for over 20 months.

Reported survival rates for BPD (Stages III and IV) range from 30 to 50 per cent. Obviously, many infants at Stage I or II are not recognized clinically and are not included in these figures. Respiratory failure, progressive cor pulmonale or catastrophic events such as sepsis or a CNS hemorrhage are causes for most late BPD deaths.

At Stage IV, those patients with progressive respiratory failure have radiographs with massive amounts of fibrosis and striking areas of consolidation. The patients who are stable or improving have roentgenograms that are not as severe. Scattered areas of atelectasis with hyperexpansion and generally radiolucent films are typical (Fig. 6). These findings will remain for a long period of time.

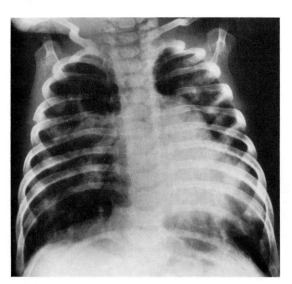

Figure 6. Hyperexpansion, air trapping and several areas of consolidation are characteristic of Stage IV.

The lungs of infants dying at this time show massive amounts of fibrosis and progressive destruction of the alveoli and airways from Stage III. Lung biopsies from living, improving patients show continuation of the reparative process. Focal alveolar emphysema, hypertrophy of peribronchiolar smooth muscle, perimucosal fibrosis, mucosal metaplasia and vascular abnormalities consistent with pulmonary hypertension make up the histologic characteristics of the lung at this stage. As the patient improves, the amount of lung with a more normal architecture increases in relation to areas of damage. Some degree of abnormality may continue for several years.

PATIENT MANAGEMENT

For the pediatrician treating the infant with hyaline membrane disease, there is no question that supplemental oxygen and mechanical ventilation, when indicated, are accepted forms of therapy and cannot be withheld despite the possibility of producing lung injury.

The treatment of BPD requires patience on the part of the pediatrician, the nursing staff and, most of all, the family. Tincture of time, plus good supportive care, is indicated. Oxygen, while toxic, must be used to prevent hypoxemia. Blood gases should be monitored, and the F_{IO_2} must be regulated to maintain the Pa_{O_2} at 50 to 60 torr.

Good nutrition is essential, and adequate calories with sufficient protein for growth must be given intravenously and/or orally. The cardiac status must be monitored, and evidence of volume overload and cardiac failure treated promptly with fluid restriction and diuretics. Digoxin has limited use.

Good nursing care is essential. Careful attention must be given to positioning (semi-Fowler appears best), chest physiotherapy, suctioning the upper airway and observation for increased amounts of tachypnea and/or cyanosis.

Respiratory tract infections, considered mild in most infants, may be critical in these fragile patients. Fever, tachypnea, cough, increased difficulty in breathing and more pronounced rales often accompany an acute infection. Frank respiratory failure may occur; mechanical ventilation and other support may be necessary. This type of setback can be overcome and must be explained in detail to the family.

Since many of these infants will be hospitalized for a prolonged period of time, an effective, multidisciplined program must be created to meet the emotional and developmental needs of the baby. Physical therapists, occupational therapists and the nursing staff should be integrated along with the parents into an organized program of tactile, visual and auditory stimulation. Play periods, cuddling, reading and talk periods, using soothing tones, should be as much a part of the day-by-day routine and are as important as nursing care, nutrition and the physician's rounds. Parents should be involved in caring for their hospitalized infant so that they will develop a strong emotional bond to the infant and be able to look after his needs effectively after he is discharged to the home. Careful instructions should be given to the parents in regard to the baby's general health care needs, including nutrition and immunizations. While the baby has been hospitalized, the parents can learn about his normal breathing patterns (frequency, rhythm, degree of retractions) and normal coloration (usually some degree of cyanosis) so that they can develop a "feel" for what is "normal" for their child. Once discharged, the infant should be seen by a competent pediatrician periodically for well infant care and acutely for any upper or lower respiratory tract infections or whenever there has been an acute change in respiratory or cardiovascular status.

Good follow-up care should include a complete history since the last examination, detailing any evidence of acute respiratory embarrassment or cyanosis, and a complete dietary history. During the physical examination, somatic growth parameters, including head circumference, length and weight, should be logged on an appropriate growth chart. Developmental assessment utilizing a standard test, such as a Denver Developmental Test, can be helpful in evaluating the infant's developmental milestones.

During the physical examination, moderate tachypnea (60 to 80/min.) in an undisturbed infant is not unusual. Some retractions may also be noted. Bilateral rales are common and may be present for several months. Cardiomegaly, bounding pulses and hepatomegaly often are present in varing degrees for the better part of the first year of life. As the patient becomes older, these findings become less pronounced, but may be exacerbated during an acute febrile illness. A barrel-shaped chest with increased anteroposterior diameter is not unusual and may persist for many months.

Once discharged, the BPD patient will often have the following problems:

1. Increased number of hospitalizations for pulmonary disorders, including pneumonia, bronchiolitis and bronchitis. Often these children present with upper respiratory tract illnesses that initially appear to be benign; however, they may rapidly progress into respiratory embarrassment with more tachypnea and cyanosis and require hospitalization. Supportive care including oxygen, intravenous fluids and physiotherapy seems to be of some use. Antibiotics may or may not be helpful, depending on the cause of the infection, although it is sometimes difficult for the pediatrician to withhold antibiotics because of the patient's marginal respiratory reserve. Opportunistic organisms, such as *Staphylococcus aureus* or gram-negative organisms, may further complicate treatment.

2. Many of these patients have hyperexpansion of the thorax and some degree of tachypnea over a period of several months after being discharged from the newborn intensive care nurseries. Cyanosis during crying or other stressful times is common. Even at rest, tachypnea may be frightening to parents and must be explained as a possible problem prior to the patient's discharge. Rales are common, and occasionally frank wheezing has been found on physical examination. Physicians unfamiliar with BPD should be aware of these findings.

3. Chest films usually lag several weeks to many months behind the clinical status of the patient, and may continue to show general hyperexpansion with areas of atelectasis, consolidation and localized emphysema. Parents and referring physicians should be informed that the chest film may not be related to the current clinical condition of the patient. Inexperienced physicians may overread these films, and diagnoses such as pneumonia, congenital lobar emphysema or foreign body aspiration may be made incorrectly. Chest films must be interpreted on the basis of the patient's medical history and previous radiographic studies.

4. Pulmonary function. Once an infant has progressed to the stage of clinical and radiographic findings of BPD, pulmonary function studies will be abnormal. Low lung compliance with an increased lung volume has been found by Bryan and coworkers (1973). Stahlman and coworkers (1973) report several post–hyaline membrane disease ventilator patients (IPPV- and NPV-treated) with restrictive or obstructive pulmonary function patterns. By five years of age, exercise intolerance is rare, and cyanosis is no longer seen.

With current techniques, BPD will continue to be a problem for survivors of mechanical ventilation. Improved methods for ventilatory support that will reduce damage to the lung should be sought. In addition, a better understanding of the mechanisms of pulmonary cellular damage and repair is needed. Research into these areas may prevent or reduce the severity of BPD in the future.

Finally, for all concerned with the BPD patient, it is important to remember that the lung is a dynamic organ that will continue to grow for several years. Once the patient is no longer oxygen-dependent, there is an excellent chance for recovery. Since the disease has been recognized only recently, long-term studies in adults have not been done. From our management of BPD patients from infancy to early childhood, we have been impressed with how many critically ill infants can slowly improve to a condition of near-normal health.

REFERENCES

Autor, A. P., Frank, L., and Roberts, R. J.: Developmental characteristics of pulmonary superoxide dismutase: relationship to idiopathic respiratory distress syndrome. *Pediatr. Res.*, 10:154, 1976.

Berg, T. G., Pegtakham, R. D., Reed, M. H., Langston, C., and Chernick, V.: Bronchopulmonary dysplasia and lung rupture in hyaline membrane disease: influence of continuous distending pressure. *Pediatrics*, 55:51, 1975.

Boat, T. F., Klunerman, J. I., Fanaroff, A. A., and Matthews, L.: Toxic effects of oxygen on cultured human neonatal respiratory epithelium. *Pediatr. Res.*, 7:607, 1973.

Borrerjee, C. K., Girling, D. J., and Wigglesworth, J. S.: Pulmonary fibroplasia in newborn babies treated with oxygen and artificial ventilation. *Arch. Dis. Child.*, 47:509, 1972.

Bryan, M. H., Hardie, M. J., Reilly, B. J., and Swyer, P. R.: Pulmonary function studies during the first year of life in infants recovering from the respiratory distress syndrome. *Pediatrics*, 52:169, 1973.

deLemos, R., Wolfsdorf, J., Nochman, R., et al.: Lung injury from oxygen in lambs: the role of artificial ventilation. *Anesthesiology*, 30:609, 1969.

Hakanson, D. O., Coshore, W. J., Gauvin, N. E., and Stern, L.: The negative-pressure respirator: an improved design. *Pediatrics*, 56:601, 1975.

Harrod, J. R., L'Heureux, P., Wangensteen, O. D., and Hunt, C. E.: Long-term follow-up of severe respiratory distress syndrome treated with IPPB. *J. Pediatr.*, 84:277, 1974.

Hawker, J. M., Reynolds, E. O. R., and Taghizadeh, A.: Pulmonary surface tension and pathological changes in infants dying after respira-

tory treatment for severe hyaline membrane disease. *Lancet*, 2:75, 1967.

Johnson, J. D., Malachowski, N. C., Grobstein, R., et al.: Prognosis of children surviving with the aid of mechanical ventilation in the newborn period. *J. Pediatr.*, 84:272, 1974.

Joshi, V. V., Mandavia, S. G., Stern, L., and Wigglesworth, T. W.: Acute lesions induced by endotracheal intubation. *Am. J. Dis. Child.*, 124:646, 1972.

Kirkpatrick, B. V., and Mueller, D. G.: Respiratory distress syndrome in the newborn: three years experience. *Va. Med. Mon.* (in press).

Lamarre, A., Linsao, L., Reilly, B. J., et al.: Residual pulmonary abnormalities in survivors of the idiopathic respiratory distress syndrome. *Am. Rev. Resp. Dis.*, 108:56, 1973.

Maylan, F., Kramer, S. K., Todres, I. D., and Shannon, D. C.: Bronchopulmonary dysplasia and mechanical ventilation. Abstract. *Pediatr. Res.*, 10:465, 1976.

Northway, W. H., Rosan, R. C., and Porter, D. Y.: Pulmonary disease following respiratory therapy of hyaline membrane disease: bronchopulmonary dysplasia. *N. Engl. J. Med.*, 276:357, 1967.

Outerbridge, E. W., Nogrady, M. D., Beaudry, P. H., and Stern, L.: Idiopathic respiratory distress syndrome. *Am. J. Dis. Child.*, 123:99, 1972.

Philip, A. G. S.: Oxygen plus pressure plus time: the etiology of bronchopulmonary dysplasia. *Pediatrics*, 55:44, 1975.

Pusey, V. A., Macpherson, R. I., and Chernick, V.: Pulmonary fibrosis following prolonged artificial ventilation of newborn infants. *Can. Med. Assoc. J.*, 100:451, 1967.

Rhodes, P. G., Hall, R. T., and Leonidas, J. C.: Chronic pulmonary disease in neonates with assisted ventilation. *Pediatrics*, 55:788, 1975.

Shepard, F. M., Johnston, R. B., Katte, E. C., et al.: Residual pulmonary findings in clinical hyaline membrane disease. *N. Engl. J. Med.*, 279:1063, 1968.

Stahlman, M. T., Hedvall, G., Dolanski, E., et al.: A six-year follow-up of clinical hyaline membrane disease. *Pediatr. Clin. North Am.*, 20:433, 1973.

Stahlman, M. T., Malon, A. F., Shepard, F. M., et al.: Negative pressure assisted ventilation in infants with hyaline membrane disease. *J. Pediatr.*, 76:174, 1970.

Stern, L.: The use and misuse of oxygen in the newborn infant. *Pediatr. Clin. North Am.*, 20:447, 1973.

Stern, L., Ramos, A. D., Outerbridge, E. W., and Beaudry, P. H.: Negative pressure artificial respiration: use in treatment of respiratory failure of the neonate. *Can. Med. Assoc. J.*, 102:595, 1970.

Stocks, J., and Godfrey, S.: The role of artificial ventilation, oxygen, and CPAP in the pathogenesis of lung damage in neonates: assessment by serial measurements of lung function. *Pediatrics*, 57:352, 1976.

CHAPTER TWELVE

CHRONIC RESPIRATORY DISTRESS IN THE PREMATURE INFANT (WILSON-MIKITY SYNDROME)

Victor G. Mikity, M.D.

The syndrome of chronic respiratory distress in the premature infant was first reported in 1960 from the premature center of the Los Angeles County–University of Southern California Medical Center. The most striking component of the syndrome was the very distinctive chest radiograph seen in all the infants. Since the initial report, cases have been reported from around the world. The increased incidence in the past 16 years may be attributable to the fact that chest radiographs are taken on all premature infants with respiratory distress.

Clinical Manifestations

All the infants were immature babies with birth weight ranging from 820 to 2,440 grams. The maternal history revealed no consistent or characteristic pattern other than premature labor and birth. The majority of infants were moderately to severely depressed at birth. Transient respiratory distress, which cleared in 12 to 48 hours after birth, was present in 11 of 34 infants studied. The chest radiograph taken during the period of early distress in these infants was normal, and a definitive diagnosis of the cause of the respiratory distress could not be established. Three infants developed acute respiratory distress syndrome, with grunting and retractions that cleared in 72 hours, and had the characteristic chest radiograph of hyaline membrane disease. Symptoms and the chest radiograph cleared spontaneously in these three infants, and they were well before the onset of symptoms of chronic respiratory distress.

Onset of symptoms was mild and frequently intermittent, making the time of onset difficult to determine accurately. The most frequent onset symptoms were transient cyanosis, hyperpnea and retractions. Apneic spells appeared at the onset in only five instances, but apnea was frequently encountered later in the course of the disease. Cough was present in four patients. The infants' disease followed a pattern of increasing severity of respiratory symptoms, lasting from two to six weeks after onset. This was followed by a period of most severe respiratory symptoms lasting a few days to several weeks. Rales, which were usually absent in the early stage of the syndrome, frequently appeared at this time. Signs and symptoms then slowly decreased during the following weeks to months. Hyperpnea and substernal and intercostal retraction were the last physical findings to disappear. The illness was most severe in the least mature infants. The three infants with gestation age greater than 34 weeks had mild symptoms of relatively short duration.

Twelve of the 34 infants died (ten at the age of 18 to 86 days) during the period of severe respiratory distress. In 22 surviving infants, the abnormal respiratory signs cleared completely in three to 24 months. Six of the survivors had mental retardation with varying degrees of neurologic impairment. The oldest survivor in our series is now 15 years of age, is asymptomatic, and appears to be in good health.

Laboratory studies were mainly negative. Extensive cultures for bacteria and fungi were negative or grew normal flora. Studies for the presence of virus in fresh lung tissue were taken at biopsy and were negative. Serologic tests for syphilis and respiratory virus were negative. Routine blood studies and urinalysis were normal. Determination of trypsin and chymotrypsin of stool was normal, and early electrocardiograms were normal.

The treatment of the infant varied, and this was influenced by changes in nursery routines and by the increasing knowledge of the nature of the syndrome. The majority of children were given antibiotics for suspected interstitial pneumonia early in the course of their illness; however, five infants did not receive antibiotics while in the nursery. The majority of infants received supplemental oxygen during the first days of life because of transient respiratory distress; however, three infants were given no supplemental oxygen at any time. An additional six infants received oxygen for less than 24 hours, until symptoms had been present several days. Four received supplemental oxygen for the first time after chronic symptoms were present. The more severely ill infants received supplemental oxygen in concentrations of 30 to 45 per cent for periods of several weeks because of persistent retraction and cyanosis.

Radiologic Findings

The radiologic findings in chronic respiratory distress of premature in-fants can be divided into two separate stages. The first stage of the syndrome appears in the chest radiograph taken from one day to six weeks of age. The findings show a striking similarity in all cases. In this group of patients there was a bilateral, coarse, streaky infiltrate with small cystic areas throughout all lobes of the lungs. The cystic areas varied in size from 1 to 4 mm. Their walls were surprisingly well defined, measuring 0.5 to 1 mm. in thickness. The cardiovascular silhouette and pulmonary vascularity were normal (Figs. 1 and 2). The film was characteristic of a diffuse interstitial infiltration. Changes characteristic of the second stage appeared from one to five and one-half months. The cystic foci at the bases appeared to enlarge and coalesce (Fig. 2). Eventually, the lower lobes became overexpanded and hyperlucent with some flattening of the diaphragm. This is consistent with some degree of air trapping. The upper lobes showed bilateral, residual, strandlike infiltrates. These changes slowly resolved during periods varying from three months to two years. The pulmonary overexpansion and hyperlucency were the last ab-

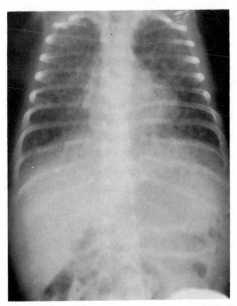

Figure 1. Diffuse interstitial infiltrate with small cystic areas that are diffusely spread through all five lobes. These represent focal areas of hyperaeration.

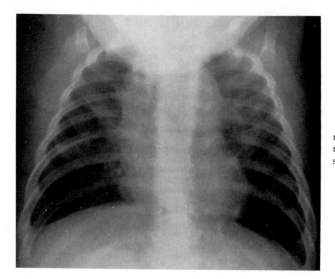

Figure 2. Basal emphysema with residual changes in the upper lobe that represent residual areas of interstitial changes.

normalities to disappear. There were no residual changes in the lung or pleura, and the chest radiograph was completely normal in the patients who survived. Chest radiographs taken at varying intervals following clearing, up to 11 years, have all remained normal.

Pathologic Findings

Eleven lung biopsies were performed on ten infants. On microscopic examination, in both biopsy and autopsy, the lung fields in the first stage of the syndrome showed areas of collapse, with approximation of alveolar septae and foci of hyperinflation. These areas suggest residual foci of immature lungs, with thickened intra-alveolar septae and adjacent areas of hyperaeration. The degree of the immaturity was usually proportionate to the weight of the infant at the time of biopsy or autopsy. Interstitial tissue of fetal mesenchymal types, associated with cuboidalization and poor septal vascularization, was prominent in the lower weight infants. In those of higher weights, or in the older age groups, the alveolar structure approached the mature appearance seen in term infants. The lungs in the second stage showed hyperinflation only.

Discussion

One of the most striking features of the syndrome is its occurrence in immature infants. One case, however, has been described in a term infant of 39 weeks gestational age, and it has been reported by Grossman and coworkers (1965). The average birth weight in our series was 1280 grams, the majority of cases occurring in the 1000- to 1500-gram birth weight range. The incidence in premature infants at the premature center is one to 450. The male is most susceptible; twice as many males as females develop this syndrome.

The maternal history details were not specific. The maternal age and parity showed a wide range, and no consistent pattern could be determined.

The clinical history, the radiographs and the pathologic findings all followed a predictable course that could be divided into two stages. The insidious onset of respiratory symptoms, following a period of relative normality, was characteristic. The early radiographic change usually preceded the onset of clinical symptoms. The lungs in the second stage showed hyperinflation with upper lobe segmental atelectasis.

The most likely pathogenesis of the syndrome is considered to be an abnormal air distribution in the lungs and a disturbance in the ventilation-perfusion ratio, secondary to the characteristics of an immature lung.

Wilson-Mikity syndrome should not be confused with bronchopulmonary dysplasia, a disease associated with respirator therapy and oxygen toxicity. The pathologic findings of the two diseases are completely different (see Chapter 11, Bronchopulmonary Dysplasia).

REFERENCES

Aherne, W. A., Cross, K. W., Hey, E. N., and Lewis, S. R.: Lung function and pathology in a premature infant with chronic pulmonary insufficiency (Wilson-Mikity snydrome). *Pediatrics,* *40*:962, 1967.

Baghdassarian, O. M., Avery, M. E., and Neuhauser, E. B. D.: A form of pulmonary insufficiency in premature infants. *Am. J. Roentgenol.,* *89*:1020, 1963.

Bucci, G., Iannaccone, G., Scalamandre. A., Savignoni, P. G., and Mendicini, M.: Observations on the Wilson-Mikity syndrome. *Ann. Paediatr.,* *206*:135, 1966.

Burnard, E. D., Grattan-Smith, P., Picton-Warlow, C. G., and Grauaug. A.: Pulmonary insufficiency in prematurity. *Aust. Paediatr. J.,* *1*:12, 1965.

Butterfield, J., Moscovici, C., Berry, C., and Kempe, C. H.: Cystic emphysema in premature infants. *N. Engl. J. Med., 268*:18, 1963.

Grossman, H., Berdon, W. E., Mizrahi, A., and Baker, D. H.: Neonatal focal hyperaeration of the lungs (Wilson-Mikity syndrome). *Radiology, 85*:409, 1965.

Mikity, V. G., Hodgman, J. E., and Tatter, D.: The radiological findings in delayed pulmonary maturation in premature infants. *Progr. Pediatr. Radiol., 1*:149, 1967.

Swyer, P. R., Delivoria-Papadopoulos, M., Levinson, H., Reilly, B. J., and Balis, H. U.: The pulmonary syndrome of Wilson and Mikity. *Pediatrics, 36*:374, 1965.

Wilson, M. G., and Mikity, V. G.: A new form of respiratory disease in premature infants. *J. Dis. Child., 99*:489, 1960.

SECTION IV

INFECTIONS OF THE RESPIRATORY TRACT

CHAPTER THIRTEEN

ANTIMICROBIAL THERAPY

JEROME O. KLEIN, M.D.

Effective antimicrobial agents are now available for eradication of most microorganisms (with the exception of viruses) responsible for pulmonary infections in children. These drugs can be classified into three groups:

① The penicillins—penicillin G, penicillinase-resistant penicillins, ampicillin and amoxicillin, and carbenicillin. These are the drugs of choice for gram-positive cocci and gram-negative cocci (Neisseria meningitidis) and coccobacilli (Hemophilus influenzae).

② Alternatives to penicillin for the allergic patient—cephalosporins, erythromycin, lincomycin and clindamycin, tetracyclines, sulfonamides and the combination trimethoprim-sulfamethoxazole, and vancomycin. Some of these drugs are also used for treatment of disease due to various nonbacterial organisms, including mycoplasmas, chlamydiae, rickettsiae and protozoa (Pneumocystis carinii).

③ Antibiotics effective against gram-negative enteric bacteria—the aminoglycosides (streptomycin, kanamycin, gentamicin, tobramycin and amikacin), chloramphenicol and the polymyxins.

In this section, consideration is given to the properties that govern use of these drugs: in vitro efficacy, absorption and excretion, adverse side-effects and toxicity, and selected aspects of administration. Antibiotics of value in treating disease due to fungi and mycobacteria are discussed in the chapters dealing with those pathogens.

THE PENICILLINS

Penicillin G

Penicillin G approaches the ideal antibiotic in combining maximal bactericidal activity with absence of toxicity. It is the drug of choice for treatment of respiratory infections caused by Streptococcus pneumoniae, non-penicillinase-producing strains of Staphylococcus aureus, groups A and B beta-hemolytic streptococci, anaerobic streptococci, oropharyngeal strains of Bacteroides fragilis, and organisms less commonly associated with pulmonary disease such as Corynebacterium diphtheriae, Neisseria meningitidis, Bacillus anthracis and Pasteurella multocida. It is remarkable that no strains of S. pneumoniae or groups A or B beta-hemolytic streptococci resistant to penicillin G have emerged during the more than 30 years since this antibiotic has been in use. In contrast, many strains of S. aureus are resistant to penicillin G, and initial therapy for significant pulmonary disease believed to be due to this organism must include a penicillinase-resistant penicillin.

Several oral and parenteral forms of penicillin G are available. The choice of parenteral preparation of this antibiotic is based on the pattern of absorption. Aqueous (soluble) penicillin G produces high peak levels of antibacterial activity in serum within 30 minutes after intramuscular (IM) administration but is rapidly excreted, and most activity is

331

dissipated within two to four hours. If given by the intravenous (IV) route, the peak is higher and earlier, and the duration of antibacterial activity in serum is shorter (approximately two hours).

Procaine penicillin G (IM) produces lower levels of serum antibacterial activity (approximately 10 to 30 per cent of the level achieved by the same dose of the aqueous form); however, the activity remains in the serum for six to 12 hours.

Benzathine penicillin G (IM) is a repository preparation providing low (approximately 1 to 2 per cent of the level achieved by the same dose of the aqueous form) but prolonged levels of antibacterial activity measurable in serum for 14 days or more.

Oral preparations (PO) of buffered penicillin G and phenoxymethyl penicillin (penicillin V) are absorbed well from the gastrointestinal tract; the peak level of serum activity of penicillin V (PO) is approximately 40 per cent, and that of buffered penicillin G (PO) is approximately 20 per cent of the level achieved by the same dose of aqueous penicillin G administered IM.

The oral preparations can be used for patients with minor respiratory infections or during convalescence from severe disease when parenteral therapy is no longer required. Children who appear severely ill initially, who have significant underlying disease, or who have complications (empyema, abscess) require the higher serum and tissue antibacterial activity provided by a parenteral form of penicillin G.

Aqueous penicillin G (IM or IV) is used for severe or complicated pneumonia. The doses in such cases should be given at frequent intervals, usually every four hours, until the infection has been brought under control. The peak level of serum activity following procaine penicillin (IM) is lower than the level provided by a comparable oral dose of penicillin V. Therefore, IM administration of procaine penicillin should be reserved for the patient who cannot tolerate oral penicillins because of vomiting or diarrhea, the comatose patient, or the patient who requires the

consistency and reliability of a parenteral preparation although the disease is not severe enough to warrant frequent doses of aqueous penicillin G (IM or IV).* Benzathine penicillin G (IM) is appropriate only for highly sensitive organisms in tissues that are well vascularized so that the drug can diffuse readily to the site of infection. Although this preparation has been effective in some cases of uncomplicated pneumonia due to *S. pneumoniae*, the level of antibacterial activity in serum and tissues is low, and clinical and bacteriologic failure is frequent when benzathine penicillin G is used.

Penicillinase-resistant Penicillins

The vast majority of strains of *S. aureus* that cause disease in hospitalized patients are resistant to penicillin G, and the number of strains of resistant staphylococci in patients who have community-acquired disease is increasing rapidly. Thus, at present, the penicillinase-resistant penicillins are the drugs of choice for initial management of the patient with staphylococcal disease. A list of available preparations and their in vitro activity against some gram-positive cocci is presented in Table 1.

Methicillin was the first penicillinase-resistant penicillin to be introduced, and it proved effective for severe staphylococcal disease. However, it is available only in parenteral form. Oxacillin and nafcillin, which were introduced later, are available in both parenteral and oral preparations and have greater in vitro activity against gram-positive cocci. Cloxacillin and dicloxacillin are available only in oral forms and are absorbed more efficiently from the gastrointestinal tract than are the other oral drugs. Although differences exist among these five penicillins in protein-binding properties, degradation by penicillinase, and in vitro antistaphyloccal activity, all five drugs are effective in treatment of staphylo-

---

*See Chapter 18, page 385, for a somewhat different approach.

TABLE 1. THE PENICILLINASE-RESISTANT PENICILLINS

Generic Name (Trade Name)	Available Forms		Minimum Inhibitory Concentration μg./ml. (median)		
	PAREN-TERAL	ORAL	Staph. aureus*	STREP. GROUP A	S. pneumoniae
Methicillin (Staphcillin, Celbenin)	+	−	3.1	0.2	0.2
Nafcillin (Unipen)	+	+	0.6	0.04	0.02
Oxacillin (Prostaphlin, Bactocill)	+	+	1.6	0.04	0.1
Cloxacillin (Tegopen)	−	+	0.8	0.04	0.2
Dicloxacillin (Dynapen, Pathocil, Veracillin)	−	+	0.15	0.02	0.05

*Penicillinase producers.

coccal disease, and clinical studies have shown them to be comparable when used in an appropriate dosage schedule. In addition, all but methicillin have proved to be effective against infections due to S. pneumoniae and beta-hemolytic streptococci, although penicillin G should still be considered the drug of choice for these infections.

A significant proportion of staphylococci isolated from patients in Western Europe have been reported to be resistant to methicillin and other penicillinase-resistant penicillins and cephalosporins. In contrast, the incidence of such strains in the United States remains low (approximately 1 per cent in recent reports). Nevertheless, bacterial resistance must be considered as a possible cause of therapeutic failure whenever a patient with staphylococcal disease who is receiving an adequate amount of a penicillinase-resistant penicillin does not respond appropriately. Gentamicin or vancomycin is usually effective for these methicillin-resistant strains of staphylococci.

Ampicillin and Amoxicillin

Ampicillin and amoxicillin are effective in vitro against a wide spectrum of bacteria: S. pneumoniae, beta-hemolytic streptococci, non-penicillinase-producing strains of S. aureus, oropharyngeal strains of anaerobic bacteria, N. meningitidis and non-penicillinase-producing strains of Hemophilus influenzae and of some gram-negative enteric bacilli, including Escherichia coli and Proteus mirabilis.

Ampicillin is available for oral or parenteral administration; amoxicillin is available in oral form only. Amoxicillin provides levels of activity in serum that are higher and more prolonged than those achieved with equivalent doses of ampicillin. An additional advantage of amoxicillin is that absorption is not altered when the antibiotic is administered with food, whereas absorption of ampicillin is decreased significantly when it is given with food.

Because it is effective against both S. pneumoniae and H. influenzae, the major pathogens in pulmonary infections in pre-school age children, ampicillin has been used widely for respiratory infections in this age group. In recent years, however, ampicillin-resistant strains of both nontypable and type b H. influenzae have been reported throughout the United States and Western Europe. This resistance appears to be a new phenomenon; few resistant strains were detected before 1972. Resistance to ampicillin is attributable to production of a penicillinase that hydrolyzes ampicillin, penicillin G and V, and, to a lesser extent, carbenicillin. At present, children with documented or suspected severe infection (including sepsis, meningitis or pneumonia) due to H. influenzae should receive chloramphenicol as part of initial management. The antimicrobial regimen should be reevaluated when the results of cultures and antimicrobial tests are available. Ampicillin continues to be the antibiotic of choice for children with mild to moderately severe pneumonia that may be due to

H. influenzae. But the physician must obtain results of antibiotic susceptibility tests when *H. influenzae* is isolated from the sputum, blood or other significant body fluid or secretion, and must follow the patient's clinical course to be certain that the response to the antibiotic is satisfactory.

Carbenicillin

This semisynthetic penicillin has a unique spectrum of activity; it is efficacious against gram-positive cocci, *H. influenzae,* and some gram-negative enteric bacilli resistant to other penicillins. The last group includes Enterobacter species, *Pseudomonas aeruginosa,* and most strains of proteus (including *P. mirabilis* and indole-positive species). The value of carbenicillin in systemic infection appears to be limited by the relatively high serum concentrations of drug required for inhibition of sensitive organisms, but this deficiency is overcome, in part, by the low toxicity of the drug even when it is given in large intravenous doses. A combination of carbenicillin and gentamicin provides broad coverage and synergistic activity against some gram-negative enteric bacilli. The two drugs have been used effectively in treatment of serious infections due to *P. aeruginosa* in patients with compromised defense mechanisms.

An oral preparation, indanyl carbenicillin, is available; however, low levels of serum activity preclude its use for infections of the respiratory tract. Indanyl carbenicillin produces urinary concentrations sufficient for treatment of some urinary tract infections due to bacteria that are resistant to other available oral antimicrobial agents.

Toxicity and Sensitization

The penicillins have no dose-related toxicity unless excessively large doses are used. Penicillins do have an epileptogenic potential; regimens of 60 million or more units per day or very rapid intravenous injection of 5 million or more units in adults have resulted in seizures. This reaction does not occur with smaller dosage schedules in adults unless the patient is in renal failure or has some underlying focal brain lesion. Nephritis and bone marrow depression have been reported in a few cases after methicillin therapy, but this finding is rare and does not warrant any change in consideration of the drug for the patient with serious staphylococcal disease. Thrombocytopenia with purpura due to drug-induced platelet aggregation has been noted after use of carbenicillin and penicillin G.

The major concern with use of penicillin is not toxicity but sensitization. Acute anaphylactic reactions are infrequent (approximately one per 20 thousand courses), but a significant number of fatalities occur each year because such a large number of individuals are treated with this antibiotic. The physician must identify the patient who will subsequently react to penicillin and avoid use of the drug in that patient. Serologic assays for detection of antibodies to penicillin are not of proven value in identification of patients who will have an immediate life-threatening reaction. Antigens used for skin-testing have been unreliable because of false-negative reactions (inability to detect the patient who will subsequently react to penicillin). In addition, some patients have had an anaphylactic reaction from the small amount of antigen administered. New skin-test antigens, including penicilloyl polylysine and the minor determinant mixture (containing benzyl penicillin and its metabolic breakdown products) have been investigated by Levine and associates. These materials show considerable promise but require further documentation of their safety, sensitivity and specificity. At present, the physician must rely on the patient's history of an adverse reaction after administration of a penicillin. If the reaction appears to be related to the administration of a penicillin, the drug should be avoided for minor infections. If a life-threatening infection should occur and penicillin is clearly the optimal drug, as in the case of overwhelming pneumonia due to *S. pneumoniae*, the physician may choose to administer the drug under carefully controlled conditions; a small dose may be injected initially in an extremity and followed by increasing doses given every 30 minutes. Epinephrine, a tourniquet and a tracheotomy set should be available in the event of a severe reaction during the testing period. All penicillins are cross-reactive in regard to sensitization, and allergy to any one implies sensitization to all.

ANTIMICROBIAL AGENTS USED AS ALTERNATIVES TO PENICILLINS

The Cephalosporins

The cephalosporins (Table 2) are among the antimicrobial agents that may be used as alternatives to penicillins for therapy of patients allergic to penicillin. The cephalosporins have a broad range of activity that encompasses gram-positive cocci (including penicillinase-producing *S. aureus*) and some gram-negative enteric bacilli. At present, seven cephalosporins are available in the United States, and several are undergoing clinical trials. The drugs of this group differ from each other in absorption, distribution and excretion, and, to a lesser extent, in toxicity and antibacterial spectrum.

Of the oral preparations, cephalexin and cephradine are absorbed well from the gastrointestinal tract, and food does not alter absorption significantly. Cephaloglycin is absorbed less well, and levels of activity in serum are inadequate for treatment of respiratory infections; the drug should be reserved for use in patients with susceptible infections of the urinary tract.

Cephalothin, cephaloridine, cefazolin, cephapirin and cephradine are available for parenteral administration. These drugs may be administered by either intramuscular or intravenous routes. Pain is significant, however, after intramuscular injection of cephalo-

TABLE 2. CURRENTLY AVAILABLE CEPHALOSPORINS*

Generic Name	Trade Name	Route of Administration	
		PO	IM, IV
Cephalothin	Keflin	−	+
Cephaloridine	Loridine	−	+
Cefazolin	Ancef, Kefzol	−	+
Cephapirin	Cefadyl	−	+
Cephradine	Velosef, Anspor	+	+
Cephalexin	Keflex	+	−
Cephaloglycin	Kafocin	+	−

*May 1977.

thin and cephapirin; thus, the intravenous route is preferable for these preparations. Cefazolin produces the highest peak level of activity and has the longest half-life in serum; cephapirin and cephalothin have lower levels of activity and shorter half-life in serum; the serum activity of cephaloridine and cephapirin is intermediate.

The cephalosporins appear to be safe for use in children. A few reports of toxicity have appeared: some adult patients with underlying kidney disease who received large doses of cephaloridine developed renal tubular necrosis; nephrotoxicity occurred in patients who received both cephalothin and gentamicin, but the basis for the toxicity remains uncertain. The cephalosporins may produce allergic reactions similar to those caused by penicillins, and there is cross-sensitization among the various cephalosporins. Allergic reactions may occur in patients who have histories of sensitivity to penicillin; most such patients, however, have received cephalosporins without incident. The antigenic relationship of the penicillins and the cephalosporins is still uncertain, and caution should be used when a cephalosporin is administered to a patient with a known allergy to penicillin.

Cephalosporins are of value for treatment of pulmonary infections due to gram-positive cocci in children with a known or ambiguous history of allergy to penicillin. Since the activity of cephalosporins for *H. influenzae* is variable, these drugs should be used with caution if this organism is a known or suspected cause of the infection. Some gram-negative enteric bacilli that are resistant to multiple antibiotics may be sensitive to one or more cephalosporins, but many gram-negative enteric bacilli are resistant to these drugs. Therefore, the cephalosporins should not be used alone for initial therapy of pulmonary infections that may be due to gram-negative enteric bacilli; rather, they should be used when antibiotic susceptibility tests indicate that the cephalosporins are uniquely effective for the causative organism.

Erythromycin

Erythromycin is effective in vitro against gram-positive cocci of importance in respiratory infections, i.e., S. pneumoniae, beta-hemolytic streptococci, and penicillinase- and non-penicillinase-producing S. aureus. In addition, the drug is highly active against Mycoplasma pneumoniae, Corynebacterium diphtheriae and Bordetella pertussis. Erythromycin is not uniformly active against H. influenzae.

Several preparations are available for oral administration. These include erythromycin base, erythromycin stearate (a salt), erythromycin ethylsuccinate (an ester), and erythromycin estolate (the salt of an ester). Erythromycin base is unstable at the low pH of the stomach; thus, absorption of this compound taken orally is incomplete. The other forms are absorbed better from the gastrointestinal tract, but since the base is the only compound with antibacterial activity, the other preparations must be hydrolyzed to the base in the body. The estolate provides the highest serum concentrations, but there is still controversy about which of the preparations provides the most biologically active drug at the site of infection.

Two preparations are available for intravenous administration, the glucoheptonate and the lactobionate. Intramuscular administration of these forms is painful and should be avoided.

With the exception of the estolate, the available preparations of erythromycin are well tolerated and are not toxic. The estolate may give rise to a cholestatic jaundice that is believed to be a hypersensitivity reaction. Since this syndrome has not been observed with other forms of erythromycin, the ester is thought to be responsible for the hepatotoxicity. The jaundice has been noticed in patients who receive the drug for more than 14 days. Jaundice disappears when the administration of the drug is stopped. Few cases have been reported in children. At present, potential hepatotoxicity does not appear to be a contraindication to use of the estolate in children. Nevertheless, physicians using this preparation should limit duration of therapy to 10 days and should be alert for signs of liver involvement.

Erythromycin is an effective alternative to penicillin for treatment of pulmonary infections due to S. pneumoniae or beta-hemolytic streptococci. The drug is also effective for mild to moderate infections due to S. aureus. The patients with allergy to penicillin and severe S. aureus infection requiring high dosages of parenteral drug are better treated with a cephalosporin. If H. influenzae is believed to be the cause of the respiratory infection, erythromycin is inadequate for initial therapy. Erythromycin is effective in alleviating the signs and symptoms of respiratory disease due to M. pneumoniae, although the organism usually is not cleared from the upper respiratory tract. Erythromycin eradicates B. pertussis from the nasopharynx and is used to reduce the period of infectivity of patients with B. pertussis infection. The drug is also used as prophylaxis for persons in intimate contact with such patients. It is less certain that erythromycin alters the clinical course of pertussis.

Lincomycin and Clindamycin

Both lincomycin and clindamycin are effective in vitro against gram-positive cocci, but are inactive against *H. influenzae*, *N. meningitidis* and gram-negative enteric bacilli. Clindamycin is also active against some anaerobic bacteria, including penicillin-resistant Bacteroides species. Clindamycin provides higher levels of activity in serum than does lincomycin, and in contrast to lincomycin, its absorption through the intestines is not decreased when the drug is taken in close temporal relation to meals.

Diarrhea and pseudomembranous enterocolitis may follow use of clindamycin; however, most cases of such adverse reactions have been in elderly patients, those with severe illness, or those receiving several antibiotics. The drug has been well tolerated in children; diarrhea has not been a common side-effect, and there are few reports of enterocolitis. These two antibiotics may be considered as alternatives to penicillin for the allergic patient with streptococcal, pneumococcal or sensitive staphylococcal infections. Most pulmonary infections due to anaerobic organisms in the respiratory tract are sensitive to penicillin G, but some strains may be sensitive only to clindamycin.

The Tetracyclines

The tetracyclines are effective against a broad range of microorganisms, including gram-positive cocci, some gram-negative enteric bacilli, *M. pneumoniae*, rickettsiae, chlamydiae and *B. pertussis*. Caution must be used in consideration of the tetracyclines as alternatives to penicillin for the allergic patient; a significant proportion of group A streptococci and some strains of *S. pneumoniae* are resistant to tetracycline.

Seven tetracycline compounds are available for oral administration in the United States: tetracycline, chlortetracycline, oxytetracycline, demethylchlortetracycline, methacycline, doxycycline and minocycline. Tetracycline, chlortetracycline, doxycycline and minocycline are also available for intravenous administration. With few exceptions, there are only minor differences in the in vitro activity of the different preparations, although minocycline may be effective for some strains of *S. aureus* resistant to other tetracyclines.

Tetracyclines are deposited in teeth during the early stages of calcification, and dental staining occurs. A relationship between total dose and visible staining has been established. Discoloration of the teeth has been seen in babies of mothers who received tetracycline after the sixth month of pregnancy. The permanent teeth are stained if the drug is administered after six months and before six years of age.

There are few indications for tetracycline in young children with respiratory infection; other effective antimicrobial agents are available for almost all infections against which tetracycline might be used. Therefore, the use of tetracycline in children should be avoided unless there is a specific indication. The Committee of the Food and Drug Administration that oversees usage of antibiotics recently recommended removal of tetracycline drops for use in children and also recommended stronger label warnings on pediatric uses of the syrup.

The Sulfonamides

Sulfapyridine, discovered in 1938, was the first antimicrobial agent to be effective for therapy of pneumococcal pneumonia. Prontosil, described in 1935 by Domagk, had earlier been demonstrated to be effective against infections due to hemolytic streptococci. Soon after, however, resistance to the sulfonamides appeared in both the streptococcus and the pneumococcus. Today, applicability of sulfonamides for respiratory infection is limited; they are the drugs of choice only for treatment of pulmonary infection due to Nocardia. The sulfonamides are effective for upper respiratory infections (such as otitis media) due to *H. influenzae* and for bacteremia and focal disease (including meningitis) due to susceptible strains of *N. meningococcus*. These drugs should not be considered as alternatives to penicillin for treatment of infections due to *S. pneumoniae*, beta-hemolytic streptococci or *S. aureus*.

Trimethoprim-sulfamethoxazole

Trimethoprim-sulfamethoxazole (TMP-SMZ) is a new antimicrobial combination with significant activity against a broad spectrum of gram-positive and gram-negative pathogens. The mixture is absorbed well from the gastrointestinal tract; a parenteral preparation is not available for use at this time. Now (May 1977) in the United States, usage of TMP-SMZ for respiratory infections is limited to treatment of disease due to *Pneumocystis carinii*. Preliminary studies suggest that this combination will also be useful for treatment of respiratory infections due to *S. pneumoniae* and *H. influenzae*, but not for those due to beta-hemolytic streptococci.

Vancomycin

Vancomycin is a parenterally administered antibiotic whose spectrum of activity is limited to gram-positive organisms. It is administered only by the intravenous route because intramuscular injection causes pain and tissue necrosis. Ototoxicity may result from high concentrations of vancomycin in serum. The principal use of vancomycin is treatment of serious staphylococcal disease where the organism is resistant to the penicillinase-resistant penicillins and cephalosporins.

DRUGS EFFECTIVE AGAINST INFECTIONS DUE TO GRAM-NEGATIVE BACILLI

The Aminoglycosides

The aminoglycosides of current therapeutic importance include streptomycin, kanamycin, gentamicin, tobramycin and amikacin. The in vitro activity of these antibiotics against gram-negative enteric bacilli varies and must be defined for each institution on the basis of current results of sensitivity tests. At the Boston City Hospital (Boston, Massachusetts), the sensitivity pattern for 1976 (Table 3) indicates that streptomycin would be ineffective against a significant proportion of infections caused by this group of bacteria, whereas kanamycin, gentamicin and tobramycin are active against most isolates of *E. coli*, Enterobacter, Klebsiella, and Proteus. At present, gentamicin and tobramycin are the most active of the aminoglycosides against these organisms, and also the only drugs active against *P. aeruginosa*. Tobramycin is active against some strains of *P. aeruginosa* resistant to gentamicin. Amikacin was not tested routinely in the Boston City Hospital laboratory during this period.

TABLE 3. PERCENTAGES OF SELECTED BACTERIAL ISOLATES (2192 STRAINS) RESISTANT TO THE INDICATED ANTIBIOTICS (BOSTON CITY HOSPITAL, 1976)

Antibiotic	E. coli	Proteus mirabilis	Proteus (other)	Klebsiella	Entero-bacter species	Pseudomonas aeruginosa
Streptomycin	68	36	52	72	69	96
Kanamycin	22	19	23	43	36	98
Gentamicin	3	4	8	19	11	39
Tobramycin	7	3	15	20	8	8
Polymyxin	1	87	96	2	2	2
Chloramphenicol	7	20	31	23	14	93
Tetracycline	40	95	48	39	40	96
Ampicillin	31	19	79	92	79	99
Carbenicillin	33	19	31	95	45	14
Cephalothin	27	22	85	22	89	99

The spectrum of activity for this new aminoglycoside is similar to that of gentamicin and tobramycin but there is little cross-resistance, and so some gram-negative enteric bacilli resistant to gentamicin or tobramycin may be sensitive to amikacin.

All of the aminoglycosides may produce renal injury and damage to the eighth nerve in the form of impaired hearing or diminished vestibular function. Eighth nerve damage appears to be dose-related, although it has followed the use of relatively small doses, especially in patients with renal failure. Toxicity has not been a problem in children with normal kidney function who were treated with aminoglycosides in currently recommended dosage schedules.

Thus, if there is reason to suspect pulmonary infection due to gram-negative enteric bacteria (as in the case of pneumonia in newborn infants or in immunocompromised patients), the most effective aminoglycoside should be used. The physician must inspect, on a regular basis, the data provided by the hospital laboratory for current antibiotic susceptibility patterns. At present, gentamicin is used at the Boston City Hospital for initial therapy of patients with respiratory infection that may be due to gram-negative enteric bacilli. Tobramycin and amikacin are reserved for use in infections that would be uniquely sensitive to these drugs. The initial regimen is reevaluated when the results of cultures and susceptibility tests are available.

Chloramphenicol

Chloramphenicol is active against a broad range of gram-positive and gram-negative bacteria, chlamydiae and rickettsiae. The oral preparation is absorbed well; only the intravenous route should be used for parenteral administration, since lower levels of serum activity follow intramuscular use.

Concern for the infrequent but severe effect of chloramphenicol on bone marrow has limited the role of this antibiotic. Aplastic anemia is an idiosyncratic reaction that occurs in approximately one in 20,000 courses of administration of the drug. With few exceptions, aplastic anemia has followed use of the oral preparation. A dose-related anemia characterized by decreased reticulocyte count, increased concentrations of iron in serum, and vacuolization of erythroid and myeloid precursors in bone marrow may also occur, but ceases when the drug is discontinued.

Chloramphenicol should be used in the treatment of severe respiratory infections that are due to ampicillin-resistant *H. influenzae,* and in the treatment of pneumonia due to gram-negative enteric bacilli in the rare cases where chloramphenicol is the only effective agent.

The Polymyxins

Polymyxin and colistin are effective in vitro against a broad spectrum of gram-negative enteric bacilli, including *P. aeruginosa.* These drugs do not diffuse well across biologic membranes and are most effective when they come into direct contact with the causative agent, as in urinary tract infections or when applied topically. The polymyxins are less effective in pneumonia, and usually fail to eradicate suppurative foci or other tissue infections.

IMPORTANT ASPECTS OF ADMINISTRATION OF ANTIBIOTICS

Dosage Schedules in Newborn Infants (Table 4)

Dosage schedules for parenteral antibiotics used in treatment of serious infections (including pneumonia) in newborn infants (up to 28 days of age) are given in Table 4. Gestational age and postnatal age are important factors in the clinical pharmacology of antibiotics during the first month of life; enzyme systems involved in the detoxification of drugs such as chloramphenicol may be deficient in the premature infant.

TABLE 4. DAILY DOSAGE SCHEDULES FOR ANTIBIOTICS OF VALUE IN TREATING BACTERIAL PNEUMONIAS IN NEWBORN INFANTS

Drug, Generic (Trade)	Route	Dosage/kg./24 Hours	
		<7 Days of Age	7 to 28 Days of Age
Penicillin G, crystalline (numerous)	IV, IM	50,000–100,000 units in 2 doses	100,000–200,000 units in 3 doses
Penicillinase-resistant penicillins			
Methicillin (Staphcillin, Celbenin)	IV, IM	50–100 mg. in 2 doses	100–200 mg. in 3 doses
Oxacillin (Prostaphlin, Bactocill)	IV, IM	50–100 mg. in 2 doses	100–200 mg. in 3 doses
Nafcillin (Unipen)	IM*	50–100 mg. in 2 doses	100–200 mg. in 3 doses
Broad-spectrum penicillins			
Ampicillin (numerous)	IV, IM	100 mg. in 2 doses	200 mg. in 3 doses
Carbenicillin (Geopen, Pyopen)	IV, IM	200–300 mg. in 4 doses	400 mg. in 4 doses
Aminoglycosides			
Kanamycin (Kantrex)	IV†, IM	15 mg. in 2 doses	15 mg. in 2 doses
Gentamicin (Garamycin)	IV†, IM	6 mg. in 2 doses	7.5 mg. in 3 doses
Tobramycin (Nebcin)	IV†, IM	4 mg. in 2 doses	5 mg. in 3 doses
Amikacin (Amikin)	IV†, IM	15 mg. in 2 doses	15 mg. in 2 doses
Chloramphenicol (Chloromycetin)	IV	Premature—25 mg. in 2 doses Term—25 mg. in 2 doses	Premature—25 mg. in 2 doses Term—50 mg. in 2 doses

*No clinical experience available for use intravenously in newborn infants.

†Intravenous administration over 30 to 60 minutes.

Rapidly maturing renal function requires alteration of dosage schedules after the first week of life so that antimicrobial activity of drugs excreted mainly by the kidney will be maintained in serum and tissues. Thus, different dosage schedules for the penicillins and some aminoglycosides are recommended for infants six days of age or younger and for infants one to four weeks of age.

Dosage Schedules in Infants and Children (Table 5)

These dosage schedules are classified for use in children with mild to moderate disease and in those with severe diseases. In general, the higher dosage schedules are used for more severe infections, those due to less susceptible organisms, and those located in areas of the body where diffusion of the antimicrobial agent is limited.

Dosage Schedules in Children with Renal Insufficiency

The kidney is the major organ of excretion for most antimicrobial agents, including the penicillins, aminoglycosides, polymyxins and tetracyclines (with the exception of doxycycline). Impaired excretion may result in high and possibly toxic concentrations of the drug in the blood and tissues if alterations in the dosage schedule are not considered.

Agents requiring adjustment of dosage include the aminoglycosides, tetracyclines (with the exception of doxycycline) and polymyxins.

Agents requiring adjustment of dosage only when renal failure is severe include the penicillins, cephalosporins and clindamycin.

Agents that do not require adjustment of the dosage schedule in renal impairment include erythromycin, chloramphenicol and doxycycline.

The dosage schedules may be altered by increasing the interval between doses or by decreasing individual doses. In most cases, the first dose can be given in the usual amount and the interval between subsequent doses lengthened. Various systems and "rules of thumb" have been developed to guide the physician. Formulas for adjustment of the dosages of gentamicin and kanamycin are based on derivation of the half-life from the serum level of creatinine. These data have been developed from studies of adults with renal impairment, and pediatricians must be cautious in adapting the formulas for use in children. Bioassays of antimicrobial activity in serum are now available in many hospital laboratories and should be used when aminoglycosides are administered to children with renal insufficiency. Serum specimens should be obtained at the time of the anticipated peak level (approximately one hour for aminoglycosides) and of the trough level (just before administration of the next dose) on the first day. Samples should be obtained again on subsequent days to ensure that a safe and effective dosage schedule is being used.

Food Interference with the Absorption of Some Oral Antibiotics

The intestinal absorption of some antibiotics is significantly decreased when the drugs are ingested with food (Table 6). Absorption of other antibiotics is only slightly affected by food. Antibiotics whose absorption is hindered by coadministration of food should be taken at least one hour before or two hours after meals.

Some Considerations in Administration of Parenteral Preparations

The availability of oral antimicrobial agents is of value in treatment of mild pulmonary disease. Most oral antibiotics vary in their absorption, however, and because higher serum levels of antibacterial activity are achieved by parenteral routes, the latter are preferable for moderately severe and severe infections. Only parenteral antibiotics should be used in the newborn infant with systemic infection.

Unless the patient is in shock or suf-

TABLE 5. DAILY DOSAGE SCHEDULES FOR ANTIBIOTICS OF VALUE IN TREATING BACTERIAL PNEUMONIAS IN PEDIATRIC PATIENTS BEYOND THE NEWBORN PERIOD

Drug, Generic (Trade)	Route	Dosage/kg./24 Hours	
		MILD-MODERATE INFECTIONS	SEVERE INFECTIONS
Penicillin G, crystalline (numerous)	IV, IM	25,000–50,000 units in 4 doses	100,000–300,000 units in 4–6 doses
Penicillin G, procaine (numerous)	IM	25,000–50,000 units in 1–2 doses	Inappropriate
Penicillin G, potassium (numerous)	PO	25,000–50,000 units in 4 doses	Inappropriate
Phenoxymethyl penicillin (numerous)	PO	25,000–50,000 units in 4 doses	Inappropriate
Penicillinase-resistant penicillins:			
Methicillin (Staphcillin, Celbenin)	IV, IM	100–200 mg. in 4 doses	200–300 mg. in 4–6 doses
Oxacillin (Prostaphlin, Bactocill)	IV, IM	50–100 mg. in 4 doses	100–200 mg. in 4–6 doses
	PO	50–100 mg. in 4 doses	Inappropriate
Nafcillin (Unipen)	IV, IM	50–100 mg. in 4 doses	100–200 mg. in 4–6 doses
	PO	50–100 mg. in 4 doses	Inappropriate
Cloxacillin (Tegopen)	PO	25–50 mg. in 4 doses	Inappropriate
Dicloxacillin (Dynapen, Pathocil, Veracillin)	PO	12.5–25 mg. in 4 doses	Inappropriate
Broad-spectrum penicillins:			
Ampicillin (numerous)	IV, IM	50–100 mg. in 4 doses	200–400 mg. in 4 doses
	PO	50–100 mg. in 4 doses	Inappropriate
Amoxicillin (Amoxil, Larotid, Polymox)	PO	20–40 mg. in 3 doses	Inappropriate
Carbenicillin (Geopen, Pyopen)	IV, IM	100–200 mg. in 4 doses	400–600 mg. in 4–6 doses
Cephalosporins:			
Cephalothin (Keflin)	IV, IM	40–80 mg. in 4 doses	100–150 mg. in 4–6 doses
Cephazolin (Kefzol, Ancef)	IV, IM	50 mg. in 4 doses	50–100 mg. in 4 doses
Cephalexin (Keflex)	PO	25–50 mg. in 4 doses	Inappropriate
Erythromycin:			
Erythromycin glucoheptonate (Ilotycin, IV)	IV	Inappropriate	20–50 mg.
Erythromycin lactobionate (Erythrocin, IV)			
Erythromycin base (Ilotycin, E-mycin)	PO	20–50 mg. in 3–4 doses	Inappropriate
Erythromycin ethylsuccinate (Pediamycin, Erythrocin)			
Erythromycin stearate (Erythrocin)			
Erythromycin estolate (Ilosone)			
Lincomycin (Lincocin)	IV, IM	10 mg. in 2 doses	20 mg. in 2 doses
Clindamycin (Cleocin)	IV, IM	10–25 mg. in 4 doses	25–40 mg. in 4 doses
	PO	8–16 mg. in 4 doses	Inappropriate
Aminoglycosides:			
Streptomycin (numerous)	IM	Inappropriate	20–40 mg. in 3 doses
Kanamycin (Kantrex)	IV, IM	Inappropriate	15 mg. in 2–3 doses
Gentamicin (Garamycin)	IV, IM	Inappropriate	5–7 mg. in 3 doses
Tobramycin (Nebcin)	IV, IM	Inappropriate	3–5 mg. in 3 doses
Amikacin (Amikin)	IV, IM	Inappropriate	15 mg. in 2–3 doses

TABLE 5. DAILY DOSAGE SCHEDULES FOR ANTIBIOTICS OF VALUE IN TREATING BACTERIAL PNEUMONIAS IN PEDIATRIC PATIENTS BEYOND THE NEWBORN PERIOD (*Continued*)

| Drug, Generic (Trade) | Route | Dosage/kg./24 Hours | |
		MILD-MODERATE INFECTIONS	SEVERE INFECTIONS
Polymyxins:			
Polymyxin B (Aerosporin)	IM	Inappropriate	25,000–40,000 units in 4 doses
Colistin sodium colistimethate (Coly-Mycin M)	IM	Inappropriate	2.5–5 mg. in 4 doses
Tetracycline (numerous)	IV	Inappropriate	10–20 mg. in 2 doses
	PO	20–40 mg. in 4 doses	Inappropriate
Chloramphenicol (Chloromycetin)	IV	Inappropriate	50–100 mg. in 3–4 doses
	PO	Inappropriate	50–100 mg. in 3–4 doses
Vancomycin (Vancocin)	IV	Inappropriate	40 mg. in 4 doses
Sulfonamides:			
Sulfadiazine	IV, SC	Inappropriate	120 mg. in 4 doses
Sulfisoxazole (Gantrisin)	IV, SC	Inappropriate	120 mg. in 4 doses
	PO	120 mg. in 4 doses	Inappropriate

fers from a bleeding diathesis, there is little or no therapeutic advantage for intravenous as opposed to intramuscular administration of the antibiotic. If prolonged parenteral therapy is anticipated, however, the pain on injection and the small muscle mass of the young child preclude the intramuscular route and make intravenous therapy preferable. Chloramphenicol, the tetracyclines and erythromycin should be given by the intravenous rather than the intramuscular route. Chloramphenicol is poorly absorbed from intramuscular sites. The intramuscular injection of tetracyclines and erythromycin causes local irritation and pain.

Penicillins may be administered by the "push" (intermittent) method of intravenous therapy, in which the drug is administered in five to 15 minutes and which produces high serum levels of antibacterial activity of short duration. The "steady drip" method produces a sustained low level of activity. There are no data to indicate a clinical advantage of one method over the other. Rapid administration (less than five minutes) of large intravenous doses of penicillins should be avoided because of possible central nervous system effects.

The antibacterial activity of some penicillins deteriorates if they are kept in solution at room temperature for a long period of time. Therefore, it is good practice to administer fresh solutions of the penicillin every six to eight

TABLE 6. EFFECT OF FOOD ON ABSORPTION OF SELECTED ORAL ANTIBIOTICS

Major Decrease	Minimal or No Decrease
Unbuffered penicillin G	Buffered penicillin G
Ampicillin	Penicillin V
	Amoxicillin
Penicillinase-resistant penicillins: oxacillin, nafcillin, cloxacillin and dicloxacillin	Cephalosporins: cephalexin, cephradine
Lincomycin	Clindamycin
Tetracyclines	Chloramphenicol
	Erythromycin

hours when the steady drip method is used.

The aminoglycosides (kanamycin, gentamicin, tobramycin and amikacin) may be administered intravenously over a period of 30 to 60 minutes. Because of possible eighth nerve toxicity at very high blood or tissue levels, these drugs should not be given by the "push" method.

Use of Probenecid with Penicillins

Probenecid increases the peak and duration of penicillin activity in the serum. The drug is used as an adjunct to penicillin therapy when high levels are necessary. Although this combination is not usually appropriate when parenteral penicillin is given to a child with pulmonary disease, probenecid may be of value in increasing levels of penicillin in serum and pleural effusions when oral treatment with penicillin is necessary. Probenecid is used most frequently when a prolonged course of therapy is necessary and there are no more sites to insert needles for intravenous administration. Oral penicillin alone or a combination of oral penicillin with one or two intramuscular doses each day plus one of probenecid may provide adequate levels to complete a course of therapy. The dose of probenecid is 10 milligrams per kilogram every six hours (adult dose, 500 mg. every six hours).

Direct Instillation of Antimicrobial Agents

Direct instillation of antimicrobial agents into various body fluids may be of value when diffusion of the drug to the site of infection is inadequate. Antibiotics diffuse well into the pleural space after parenteral administration, but intrapleural instillation should be considered when the empyema fluid is loculated by fibrous bands. If a chest tube is in place, antibiotics are instilled following irrigation through the tube. In susceptible infection, aqueous crystalline penicillin G (10,000 to 60,000 units), ampicillin (10 to 50 mg.), or a penicillinase-resistant penicillin or ce-

phalosporin (10 to 50 mg.) may be injected into the chest tube in 10 ml. of 0.85 per cent NaCl or sterile water. The clamp is maintained for one hour and then released for drainage. The instillations should be repeated three to four times during each day that the tube remains in place. If thoracenteses are done, antibiotic is introduced after the pleural fluid is aspirated.

WHAT TO LOOK FOR WHEN ANTIMICROBIAL THERAPY FAILS

If the patient does not respond appropriately to therapy with antimicrobial agents or subsequently has a relapse or recurrence of infection, the physician must review the illness to determine the reasons for failure. Variables affecting the outcome of antimicrobial therapy, including characteristics of the disease, the host, the drug and the microorganism, should be reevaluated. A list of factors responsible for or contributing to failure of antimicrobial agents is given in Table 7.

Disease Factors

The use of antibiotics for viral infection or incorrect choice of drugs for bacterial disease are major factors in apparent lack of response.

Failure to consider the role of drainage of a suppurative focus, such as empyema fluid, may result in persistent fever and toxicity.

Organisms may remain sequestered in undetected or inaccessible loci and cause a recurrence of disease after therapy is discontinued. The patient with pulmonary disease may have infections at other sites that require special management. Identification of the focus and drainage or more prolonged or different therapy may be necessary to effect a cure.

Host Factors

Patients whose normal humoral or cellular defense mechanisms are com-

TABLE 7. FACTORS CONTRIBUTING TO FAILURE OF ANTIMICROBIAL AGENTS IN PULMONARY INFECTION

Disease-related
Antibiotic inappropriate for disease
Ancillary therapy not instituted
Sequestered focus of infection (undetected or inaccessible)

Host-related
Defect in immune response to infection
Anatomic defect
Foreign body

Drug-related
Inadequate compliance
Improper dosage schedule—route, dose or duration
Inadequate diffusion to site of infection
Incompatibility of mixed drugs for oral or parenteral route
Deterioration of drug on storage

Organism-related
Protoplast formation
"Persisters"
Acquired resistance to antimicrobial agent
Superinfection with resistant bacteria

promised by congenital or acquired disease or immunosuppressive medications suffer from frequent infections, often of the respiratory tract. Bactericidal antibiotics are usually necessary in treating infection in these patients, since bacteriostatic agents depend on normal phagocytic and immunologic mechanisms to eradicate the infection.

Anatomic defects, congenital or traumatic, often result in infections and recurrence or relapse following apparently successful antimicrobial therapy. Thus, the patient with tracheoesophageal fistula or sequestration of segments of lung may pose a difficult problem in eradication of local infection.

A foreign body, such as an aspirated particle, may serve as a nidus for a persisting pulmonary infection.

Drug Factors

The most frequent drug-related factor in failure of antibiotic therapy is inadequate compliance—the patient did not take the medicine as prescribed. Before embarking on expensive and time-consuming tests to determine the basis for failure, the physician must be assured that the patient took the medication as instructed.

Other drug-related factors include poor choice of route of administration, inappropriate dosage schedule, and inadequate duration of therapy. For the most part, physicians must rely on empirically derived dosage schedules to provide assured results with minimal risk in terms of clinical failure or toxicity of the drug. Since recommendations change as new information is presented, the physician must be alert to the need to modify dosage schedules.

Incompatibility of intravenously administered drugs may result in physical or chemical changes and possible alteration of antibacterial activity. Whenever possible, each intravenous drug should be administered separately.

Some antimicrobial agents deteriorate on prolonged storage. Adherence to expiration dates recommended by the manufacturer safeguards against inadequate potency of the drug.

Diffusion of the drug to the site of infection may be inadequate. Some drugs, such as polymyxin, diffuse poorly across biologic membranes and would be expected to be ineffective for treatment of pulmonary abscesses or other suppurative foci.

Bacterial Factors

Factors directly related to the interaction of drugs and infecting organism include persistence of infection due to formation of protoplasts or of ill-defined "persisters" at the site of infection.

Development of resistance may be important in infection due to gram-negative enteric bacilli and in tuberculosis, but does not appear to be of clinical concern in staphylococcal disease treated with penicillinase-resistant penicillins (although resistance may develop if erythromycin alone is used).

Superinfection with new organisms

resistant to previously administered antibiotics is a particular problem in the patient with defective immune mechanisms or chronic respiratory infection.

Selected reviews are listed in the references for the reader who is interested in further information about the usage of antimicrobial agents for treatment of children with pulmonary infections.

REFERENCES

The Penicillins

Jacobson, J. A., McCormick, J. B., Hayes, P., et al.: Epidemiologic characteristics of infections caused by ampicillin-resistant *Hemophilus influenzae*. *Pediatrics*, 58:388, 1976.

Katz, S. L.: Ampicillin-resistant *Hemophilus influenzae* type b. A status report. *Pediatrics*, 55:145, 1975.

Kirby, W. M. M.: Chairman of Symposium: Symposium on carbenicillin. A clinical profile. *J. Infect. Dis.*, 122(Suppl.):S1, 1970.

Klein, J. O.: Shifts in microbial sensitivity: implications for pediatrics. *Hosp. Pract.*, May 1975, p. 81.

Klein, J. O., and Finland, M.: The new penicillins. *N. Engl. J. Med.*, 269:1019; 1074; 1128, 1963.

Levin, S., and Harris, A. A.: Principles of combination therapy. *Bull. N.Y. Acad. Med.*, 51:1020, 1975.

Levine, B. B.: Immunologic mechanisms of penicillin allergy. A haptenic model system for the study of allergic diseases of man. *N. Engl. J. Med.*, 275:1115, 1966.

Mann, C. H. (Consult. Ed.): Comparative assessment of the broad-spectrum penicillins and other antibiotics. *N.Y. Acad. Sci.*, 145:207, 1967.

McCracken, G. H., Jr., and Eichenwald, H. F.: Antimicrobial therapy: therapeutic recommendations and a review of newer drugs. I. Therapy of infectious conditions. *J. Pediatr.*, 85:297, 1974. II. The clinical pharmacology of the newer antimicrobial agents. *J. Pediatr.*, 85:451, 1974.

Smith, A. L.: Antibiotics and invasive *Hemophilus influenzae*. *N. Engl. J. Med.*, 294:1329, 1976.

Antimicrobial Agents Used as Alternatives to Penicillins

Braun, P.: Hepatotoxicity of erythromycin. *J. Infect. Dis.*, 119:300, 1969.

Dillon, H. C., and Derrick, C. W.: Clinical experience with clindamycin hydrochloride. I. Treatment of streptococcal and mixed streptococcal-staphylococcal skin infections. *Pediatrics*, 55:205, 1975.

Finland, M., and Kass, E. H. (General Chairmen and Guest Editors): Trimethoprim-sulfamethoxazole. *J. Infect. Dis.*, 128(Suppl.):S425, 1973.

Genot, M. T., Golan, H. P., Porter, P. J., et al.: Effect of administration of tetracycline in pregnancy on the primary dentition of the offspring. *J. Oral Med.*, 25:75, 1970.

Ginsburg, C. M., and Eichenwald, H. F.: Erythromycin. A review of its uses in pediatric practice. *J. Pediatr.*, 89:872, 1976.

Grossman, E. R., Walchek, A., Freedman, H., et al.: Tetracyclines and permanent teeth. The relation between dose and tooth color. *Pediatrics*, 47:567, 1971.

Keusch, G. T., and Present, D. H.: Summary of workshop on clindamycin colitis. *J. Infect. Dis.*, 133:578, 1976.

Louria, D. B., Kaminsk, T., and Buchman, J.: Vancomycin in severe staphylococcal infections. *Arch. Intern. Med.*, 107:225, 1961.

Moellering, R. C., and Swartz, M. N.: The newer cephalosporins. *N. Engl. J. Med.*, 294:24, 1976.

Swartzberg, J. E., Maresca, R. M., and Remington, J. S.: Gastrointestinal side effects associated with clindamycin. *Arch. Intern. Med.*, 136:876, 1976.

Yaffe, S. J.: Chairman for the Committee on Drugs. Requiem for tetracyclines. *Pediatrics*, 55:142, 1975.

Drugs Effective Against Infections Due to Gram-Negative Bacilli

Finland, M., and Hewitt, W. L. (Guest Editors): Second International Symposium on gentamicin, an aminoglycoside antibiotic. *J. Infect. Dis.*, 124(Suppl.):S1, 1971.

Finland, M., and Neu, H. C. (Guest Editors): Symposium of the Ninth International Congress of Chemotherapy in London, England: Tobramycin. *J. Infect. Dis.*, 134(Suppl.):S1, 1976.

Finland, M., Brumfitt, W., and Kass, E. H. (Guest Editors): Advances in aminoglycoside therapy: amikacin. *J. Infect. Dis.*, 134(Suppl.):S235, 1976.

Scott, J. L., Finegold, S. M., Belkin, G. A., et al.: A controlled double-blind study of the hematologic toxicity of chloramphenicol. *N. Engl. J. Med.*, 272:1137, 1965.

Whitelock, O-V. St. (Editor-in-Chief): The basic and clinical research of the new antibiotic, kanamycin. *Ann. N.Y. Acad. Sci.*, 76:17, 1958.

Important Aspects of Administration of Antibiotics

Kunin, C. M.: Antibiotic usage in patients with renal impairment. *Hosp. Pract.*, January 1972, p. 141.

McCracken, G. H.: Clinical pharmacology of antibacterial agents. In Remington, J. S., and Klein, J. O. (Eds.): *Infectious Diseases of the Fetus and Newborn Infant*. Philadelphia, W. B. Saunders Company, 1976, p. 1020.

Wallerstein, R. O., Condit, P. K., Kasper, C. K., et al.: Statewide study of chloramphenicol therapy and fatal aplastic anemia. *J.A.M.A.*, 208:2045, 1969.

Weinstein, L., and Dalton, A. C.: Host determinants of response to antimicrobial agents. *N. Engl. J. Med.*, 279:467, 1968.

CHAPTER FOURTEEN

TONSILLITIS AND ADENOIDITIS (THE TONSIL AND ADENOID PROBLEM)

William A. Howard, M.D.

The palatine and pharyngeal tonsils are part of a mass of lymphoid tissue encircling the nasal and oral pharynx known as Waldeyer's ring. Acute infections and conditions involving these tissues are among the most common afflictions of childhood. While involvement of pharyngeal and tonsillar tissues may be the initial manifestation of some systemic infections, this discussion is concerned with primary disease in this area, including both pharyngitis and tonsillitis. In addition, interest is centered on the possibility of chronic and persistent tonsil and adenoid involvement and the desirability or necessity of surgical removal of these structures as a method of treatment.

Pathogenesis

The lymphoid tissue of Waldeyer's ring undergoes physiologic hypertrophy and hyperplasia, usually greatest between two and five years of age, in response to infections in this general area. Whether or not this lymphoid tissue is a constituent of the bursal system of immunity, such hyperplasia is associated with an increase in lymphocytes in these tissues and with increased immunologic activity of the host in response to specific infections. T and B lymphocytes are present in large numbers, with B cells predominating.

All immunoglobulin classes are represented, with a predominance of B cells bearing surface immunoglobulins of the IgA and IgE types. Infections of the tonsils and adenoids are most prevalent during these early years, and as increasing resistance to infection develops, the frequency and severity of respiratory infections diminish rapidly, usually with a corresponding decrease in the size of the lymphoid mass. Under the stress of acute infection, tonsils and adenoids may undergo rapid enlargement, but as infection subsides, they generally return to their former state. One should not judge the tonsil by viewing it only under the stress of acute infection.

Clinical Manifestations

ACUTE INFECTIONS. Acute pharyngotonsillitis refers to all of the acute infections involving the pharynx and tonsils, regardless of cause. The frequency and severity of illnesses and complications are more likely to be related to the etiologic agent than to the presence or absence of the tonsils. The majority of acute infections in the pharyngeal area—perhaps as much as 80 per cent or more—are of viral origin, except during epidemics of streptococcal infection. Among the more common viral isolates are the adenoviruses, coxsackieviruses, influenza and parainfluenza viruses, and the respiratory syncytial virus. Experience at the Children's Hospital National Medical Center suggests that while respiratory syncytial virus is most often associated with significant respiratory tract illness, adenoviruses are more apt to be isolated from acute pharyngeal infections. With the exception of the virus causing infectious mononucleosis, other viral agents are rare. The clinical picture of these viral infections may be indistinguishable from bacterial involvement in the same area.

The Group A beta-hemolytic streptococcus is by far the most common infecting bacterial agent, but may account for no more than 10 to 15 per cent of the cases of pharyngotonsillitis. In epidemics, this number may increase significantly. Other infectious agents, such as *Hemophilus influenzae,* pneumococci and staphylococci, may be demonstrated by throat culture, but they are usually opportunistic organisms proliferating during a bout of viral pharyngitis and are not the cause of a significant number of primary infections. Diphtheria may produce an exudate when involving the pharynx, but it is a gratifyingly rare infection in these days of emphasis on routine immunizations.

Clinical Features. Several schemes have been devised to indicate the relative severity of pharyngeal infections, based largely on the appearance of the throat and tonsils, the presence of exudate, the presence or absence of cervical lymphadenitis and the degree of systemic reaction to the infection.. Regardless of appearance, it is difficult to differentiate streptococcal infections from other bacterial and viral causes by other than culture methods. The presence of fever, malaise and headache and the appearance of tender, swollen cervical lymph nodes may increase the likelihood of streptococcal involvement, and thus will tempt the clinician to initiate some form of therapy while waiting for culture results.

Viral pharyngitis may be ushered in by systemic symptoms of fever, malaise, headache, loss of appetite and perhaps sore throat of moderate severity. The pharyngeal symptoms and signs may appear 24 hours or more after the onset of illness. The degree of involvement of the pharynx may vary from mild redness and irritation to severe exudative pharyngotonsillitis, or nodular and ulcerative lesions of the soft palate, the tonsillar pillars and the posterior pharyngeal wall. Swollen, red and bleeding gums may also be encountered. Cervical lymph nodes may be enlarged, but generally are firmer and less tender than in streptococcal infections. The duration of infection is variable, from one to seven days. Leukocyte counts are of little help in indicating the etiologic agent, and diagnosis must usually wait upon the report of a negative throat culture. A specific viral agent may be isolated if appropriate laboratory facilities are available. Serial determinations of antibody titers may also indicate infection with a specific viral agent.

Streptococcal pharyngitis is usually more sudden in onset; acute systemic symptoms include headache, nausea, vomiting, fever and abdominal pain. The visible signs of pharyngeal involvement will appear early, with varying degrees of redness and often a petechial rash on the soft palate. The tonsils, if present, are enlarged and reddened, with surface injection, but may or may not show any exudate, regardless of the stage of the disease in which the examination is made.

Initial streptococcal infections involving the pharynx and tonsils may be somewhat less severe, more prolonged, and less well localized when compared with subsequent infections. Later infections are more acute and more localized, and exhibit more characteristic systemic symptoms, apparently as a result of immunologic alterations in both humoral and cell-mediated immune responses to the primary infection, such as may occur with pneumococcal infections.

The occasional appearance of a generalized rash may encourage the diagnosis of scarlet fever, whereas at other times the rash is blotchy and irregular. There seems little reason to consider such manifestations as anything more than complications of streptococcal infections that will respond to treatment of the primary infection. The development of either rheumatic fever or acute glomerulonephritis is considered to be a late response to infection, again mediated by altered host reaction. The classic picture of "streptococcosis" as originally described by Powers and Boisvert (1944) is seldom seen now, probably because of early and vigorous antibiotic therapy.

Differential Diagnosis. Differentiation of streptococcal pharyngitis from viral infections in the same area is apt to be difficult on clinical grounds alone. The exudates of diphtheria and infectious mononucleosis may be indistinguishable, and systemic symptoms may be similar. In the latter case, the diagnosis may be suggested by a slower onset, a more prolonged course, and the presence of other cases in the school or neighborhood. Herpangina may be recognized by the presence of papular, vesicular and ulcerative lesions on the soft palate, tonsillar pillars, and posterior pharyngeal wall. Rarely, one may see acute tonsillitis and cervical lymphadenitis as an early manifestation of leukemia or agranulocytosis, accompanied by petechial hemorrhages in the oropharynx and bruising in the skin. Throat cultures are essential when the diagnosis is in doubt; if the exudate is difficult to remove, or leaves residual bleeding areas when removed, a specific search for *Corynebacterium diphtheriae* is indicated.

Complications. Complications are unusual with viral infections unless there is some underlying disease process. Rashes are common with streptococcal infections, and in addition to scarlet fever may include erythema multiforme and erythema nodosum. Local extension of the disease may result in peritonsillar abscess and may also produce involvement of the sinuses, the middle ear, the mastoids and the meninges. Rheumatic fever and acute glomerulonephritis may occur as late complications and must be watched for after the acute infection has subsided. No specific M type has been associated with rheumatic fever, but M type 12 and 49 are known to be nephritogenic. Mesenteric adenitis mimicking the signs and symptoms of acute appendicitis may occur with any acute pharyngitis, regardless of its course.

Treatment. Viral pharyngitis will ordinarily require only symptomatic therapy. Positive cultures of *Hemophilus influenzae*, pneumococci or staphylococci may occur as complications of viral infections or as primary infections, but in any case should be treated with appropriate antibiotics. When streptococcal infection is suspected and a throat culture is taken, subsequent management may vary with the severity of the symptoms and the attitude of the physician. For the ill child with fever and systemic manifestations, it may be desirable to begin treatment while waiting for the results of the culture, since more rapid resolution of symptoms can be expected if a streptococcal infection is treated early. From the point of view of the patient and the parent, early control of symptoms is welcome, and treatment may be discontinued if the culture is negative. In milder cases it may be appropriate to defer treatment for the 12 to 24 hours required to obtain the culture results. When the culture is positive, oral administration of 400,000 units of penicillin three times daily for a 10-day period is entirely adequate if one can be assured of patient compliance; otherwise, a single injection of 600,000 to 1,200,000 units of benzathine penicillin is indicated. If penicillin is contraindicated, erythromycin is an acceptable substitute. Dosage for this drug is 10 to 20 mg./kg./day in divided doses for the 10-day period. Symptomatic therapy includes bed rest, extra fluids, acetaminophen for pain, warm saline gargles or irrigations, and foods as tolerated. Prevention of the development of rheumatic fever is assured in most instances if penicillin therapy is begun within four to six days after onset. Prevention of acute glomerulonephritis with any regimen of treatment is much less certain.

CHRONIC INFECTIONS. Chronic infection in the tonsils and adenoids may be associated with a variety of clinical manifestations. There may be recurrent bouts of acute infection manifested by a sore throat or a more or less continuous low-grade involvement, with or without fever. Some degree of cervical adenitis is often present, and there may be a history of recurring middle ear infections, with or without some degree of hearing loss. Mouth breathing may occur as a result of adenoid enlargement, and a heavy, fetid breath may be noted in the morning. Though less common than formerly, peritonsillar and retropharyngeal abscesses may develop adjacent to the chronically infected tonsil or adenoid.

A variety of other symptoms have been ascribed to diseased tonsils and adenoids, including fatigue, loss of appetite, failure to gain weight, so-called growing pains, difficulty in swallowing, chronic cough, frequent upper respiratory tract infections, postnasal drip, clearing of the throat and many others.

Physical findings generally relate to the size of the tonsils, which may be large or small, and of the adenoids, which are usually enlarged. The chronically infected tonsil cannot be diagnosed by a single, simple inspection, and usually a careful chronologic history is essential for a proper evaluation of the nature and degree of infection present. Additional findings will include varying degrees of cervical adenitis, nasal obstruction, occasional hearing loss, and not infrequently a collection of serous fluid behind the tympanic membrane, the so-called serous otitis media. When nasal obstruction has been present for a considerable

period of time, there may be a thoracic deformity, usually a simple funnel chest of varying depth, involving the lower portion of the sternum, the xiphoid and the neighboring rib cartilages. Some depression also may be noted at the level of attachment of the diaphragm. Malocclusion of varying degree, associated with enlarged adenoids and nasal obstruction, may help in producing what is termed the adenoid facies.

Many of these signs and symptoms can be produced by other causes, the most common of which is allergic involvement of the upper respiratory tract. It should be emphasized again that a careful history is most important in making a decision about the removal of tonsils and adenoids.

Indications for Adenotonsillectomy

Based upon an abundance of available evidence, a few salient facts may be noted.

Although a more conservative attitude has developed toward adenotonsillectomy, the operation is still extremely common, and probably is performed much too frequently.

The wide variation in the reported incidence of adenotonsillectomy in different groups rated according to age, geographic location, socioeconomic status, medical insurance and educational levels is such that one cannot escape the conclusion that the operation must at times be performed for reasons other than those purely medical.

Indications for operation vary greatly, emphasizing the lack of understanding of the basic function of this lymphoid tissue and the consequences of its early removal.

It is extremely difficult to assess the results of adenotonsillectomy because of the wide variety of indications for its performance and the lack of long-term follow-up by those who perform the operation, and because it is usually done at an age when gradual but spontaneous improvement in response to exposure to infection is to be expected.

Adenotonsillectomy is not without danger, 200 to 300 deaths being reported each year from this elective procedure.

Tonsillectomized persons are neither more nor less susceptible to streptococcal infections, nor is the clinical course of streptococcal disease modified. There is also no effect on the development of rheumatic fever or rheumatic valvular heart disease. Streptococcal infections are less readily recognized in tonsillectomized children, who may thereby escape adequate treatment.

The degree of antibody response in the nasopharynx to orally administered polio vaccine appears to be significantly higher when the vaccine is administered to children with intact tonsils. Also, pre-existing levels of local antibody may fall sharply after tonsillectomy, and may persist at these levels for several months. These observations may provide an explanation for the observed epidemiologic relationship between tonsillectomy and bulbar and paralytic poliomyelitis, and would suggest that the recently tonsillectomized child may still be more susceptible to natural infection with poliovirus.

With due consideration of the foregoing discussion, it is possible to give a brief résumé of the various situations that have been considered indications for adenotonsillectomy.

1) PERITONSILLAR ABSCESS. Once this complication has been diagnosed, there is fairly general agreement that a second attack should not be risked, and that adenotonsillectomy should be done as soon as feasible.

2) RECURRENT TONSILLITIS. Recent acute tonsillar infections, with fever, cervical adenitis and possibly otitis media, may constitute a sound indication for operation, especially if there is persistent evidence of chronic involvement between acute attacks. There exists the possibility, however, that such attacks represent new infections with differing etiologic agents, and that they constitute an immunologic experience that might occur regardless of the presence or absence of the tonsils. In spite of its failure to modify streptococcal disease, operative removal should be considered when tonsillitis is due to proved recurrent streptococcal infections.

RECURRENT "COLDS." Recurrent upper respiratory tract infections resembling the common cold generally are not controlled by adenotonsillectomy, and operation is not recommended.

3) RECURRENT OTITIS MEDIA. If ear infections are frequent, and there is any evidence of *hearing loss*, adenoidectomy alone should be considered the operation of choice. Removal of the tonsils should not be done at the same time unless there are specific indications.

4) HYPERTROPHIED TONSILS. Tonsillar enlargement alone, especially under the age of five to six years, is seldom if ever sufficient indication for operation. An exception to this may be when tonsils are so large as to affect swallowing and breathing, as suggested by the increasing number of reports of cor pulmonale resulting from tonsillar hypertrophy and airway obstruction.

ADENOID ENLARGEMENT. If adenoid enlargement is sufficient to cause noisy mouth-breathing, snoring, and persistent low-grade nasal congestion and discharge, removal of the adenoids is considered proper, provided one can be assured that the symptoms are not produced by allergic involvement in the same area.

CERVICAL ADENITIS. Chronic infection in the cervical lymph nodes, with frequent acute flare-ups, are fundamentally an indication of persistent infection in the pharyngeal area. Depending on the appearance of the tonsils and the degree of infection present, cervical adenitis may then constitute a valid indication for tonsillectomy.

5) (6) *Heart failure due to UA obstruction*

In considering the indications for adenotonsillectomy, it becomes apparent that there will be many instances in which removal of the adenoids may be the only surgical procedure indicated, and that results may be more satisfactory and much less disturbing if tonsillectomy is avoided. Also, in making a decision about operation, the possibility of an allergic cause of the signs and symptoms must be considered. Nasal obstruction, frequent upper respiratory tract involvement resembling "colds," serous otitis media, enlargement of tonsils and adenoids and diminished hearing may all appear on the basis of nasal allergy. Adenotonsillectomy may be indicated in the allergic child as well, but the indications for operation should be *at least* as stringent as those for the nonallergic child, if not more so. It is the consensus among pediatric allergists that adenotonsillectomy should not be undertaken in the allergic child until there has been a period of definitive treatment of the underlying allergy and adequate treatment of any accompanying infection. After three to six months of such treatment, the indications for operation may have lessened a great deal or may even have disappeared entirely. Removal of tonsils and adenoids in a child with untreated nasal allergy may be followed by the development of bronchial allergic symptoms.

Complications

Complications from adenotonsillectomy are relatively infrequent, with the exception of postoperative hemorrhage. Blood loss occasionally may be sufficient to warrant replacement by transfusion. Pneumonia, lung abscess, atelectasis and septicemia have occurred. As indicated earlier, death may occur, usually as a result of cardiac arrest, hemorrhage or infection. The psychologic reaction to the trauma of hospitalization and operation should not be overlooked.

Results from Adenotonsillectomy

Although the incidence of epidemic respiratory infections is not altered by the removal of the tonsils and adenoids, there may be a decrease in the number and severity of throat infections and in the amount of fever that accompanies them. Obstructive symptoms may be relieved, especially by adenoidectomy, but relief from recurrent otitis media is variable. There is generally a gradual disappearance of cervical adenopathy, and bouts of acute adenitis are decreased or absent. There may be gain in weight and apparent benefit to general health and appetite, but multiple factors may be involved in this evident improvement. It is unwise to promise too much as a result of adenotonsillectomy.

REFERENCES

Bakwin, H.: The tonsil-adenoidectomy enigma. *J. Pediatr., 52*:339, 1958.

Bluestone, C. D. (Chairman): Workshop on tonsillectomy and adenoidectomy. *Ann. Otol. Rhinol. Laryngol., 84*(Suppl. 18):1, 1975.

Canby, J. P.: Acquired fibrinogenemia. An unusual cause of post-tonsillectomy and adenoidectomy hemorrhage. *J.A.M.A., 183*:282, 1963.

Chamovitz, R., Rammelkamp, C. H., Jr., Wannamaker, L. W., and Denny, W. F., Jr.: The effect of tonsillectomy on the incidence of streptococcal disease and its complications. *Pediatrics, 26*:355, 1960.

Chobot, R.: Infectious aspects of asthma in children. In Prigal, S.: *Fundamentals of Modern Allergy.* New York, McGraw-Hill Book Company, Inc., 1960.

Clein, N.: Influence of tonsillectomy and adenoidectomy on children, with special reference to the allergic implications. *Ann. Allergy, 10*:568, 1952.

Gellis, S. L.: Personal communication to the author.

Howard, W. A.: Childhood complications of respiratory allergies. *Clin. Proc. Child. Hosp., D.C., 8*:210, 1952.

Howard, W. A.: Diagnosis and treatment of nasal obstruction in children. *Postgrad. Med., 21*:136, 1957.

Lelong, M.: Asthma et amygdalectomie. *Lille Med., 9*:77, 1964.

Ogra, P. L.: Effect of tonsillectomy and adenoidectomy on nasopharyngeal antibody response to poliovirus. *N. Engl. J. Med., 284*:59, 1971.

Powers, G. F., and Boisvert, P. L.: Age as a factor in streptococcosis. *J. Pediatr., 25*:481, 1944.

Ravenholt, R. T.: Poliomyelitic paralysis and tonsillectomy reconsidered. *Am. J. Dis. Child., 103*:658, 1962.

Reid, J. N., and Donaldson, J. A.: The indications for tonsillectomy and adenoidectomy. *Otolaryngol. Clin. North Am., 3*:339, 1970.

Sherman, W. B., and Kessler, W. R.: *Allergy in Pediatric Practice.* St. Louis, C. V. Mosby Company, 1957.

Sobel, G.: Adenotonsillectomy in the allergic child. In Prigal, S.: *Fundamentals of Modern Allergy.* New York, McGraw-Hill Book Company, Inc., 1960.

CHAPTER FIFTEEN

CROUP (EPIGLOTTITIS; LARYNGITIS; LARYNGO-TRACHEOBRONCHITIS)

Henry G. Cramblett, M.D.

Croup is a syndrome in which there is inspiratory stridor, cough and hoarseness due to varying degrees of laryngeal obstruction. The obstruction in infectious croup is due to inflammatory edema and spasm. In this chapter, infections involving the epiglottis, the vocal cords or the subglottic area will be considered together.

Incidence and Etiology

The true incidence of croup is difficult to determine. Undoubtedly this syndrome is responsible for a significant number of emergency calls to the physician, particularly at night. From an etiologic standpoint, croup is due to a virus in at least 85 per cent of cases. To date, the parainfluenza viruses have been recovered from patients with croup more commonly than any other virus or group of viruses. Hemophilus influenzae type b is responsible for the majority of cases of bacterial croup. Ordinarily, Hemophilus influenzae causes epiglottitis, but may involve other areas of the larynx, or the infection may extend into the tracheobronchial tree. With present immunization procedures Corynebacterium diphtheriae is a rare cause of croup, but this possibility must be kept in mind in dealing with a non-immunized patient. It is extremely doubtful if pneumococci, streptococci or staphylococci play a significant role in the causation of croup. In most carefully controlled studies the incidence of recovery of these potential pathogens is little greater in patients with croup than with similarly matched controls who do not have croup.

As far as the cause of viral croup is concerned, it has become increasingly apparent that the importance of any given virus in the origin of croup will vary from season to season, from year to year and from geographic area to geographic area. In early studies, Rabe (1948) showed that no more than 14.7 per cent of patients had disease as a result of infection with bacteria, with the inference that the remainder were caused by viruses. Table 1 summarizes the results of three different etiologic studies of viral croup. It is apparent

TABLE 1. ETIOLOGY OF NONBACTERIAL CROUP

Virus	Per Cent Reported		
	McLean (1963)	Parrott (1963)	Cramblett (1960)
Adenovirus		9	4
Influenza (A + B)	1.5	8	6
Parainfluenza 1	30	21	8
Parainfluenza 2	0.5	8	6
Parainfluenza 3	4	10	14
Respiratory syncytial		8	
ECHO viruses	0.2		10
Coxsackie viruses			2
No virus recovered	64	36	50

TABLE 2. ETIOLOGIC CLASSIFICATION OF CROUP SYNDROME

Infectious
  Bacterial
    Hemophilus influenzae type b
    Corynebacterium diphtheriae
  Viral
    Parainfluenza viruses, types 1, 2, 3
    Adenoviruses
    Influenza viruses
    Enteroviruses
    Respiratory syncytial virus
    Measles virus
    "Spasmodic" (directly or indirectly due to
      viral infection)
Mechanical
  Foreign body
  Secondary to surgical procedure
  Extrinsic mass
Allergic (angioneurotic edema)

---

from the table that the parainfluenza viruses are the most important ones yet recovered from patients with this disease. Yet, as additional studies are performed and virologic techniques are improved, it is possible that this picture will change. Overall, using present diagnostic techniques, it is possible to recover viruses from as many as 65 per cent of the patients with croup.

Since croup is a syndrome of multiple causes, it is well to remember that not all cases of laryngeal obstruction are due to infection. A summary of the causes of croup in children is contained in Table 2.

Anatomy of the Larynx

Knowledge of the anatomy of the larynx and contiguous structures is necessary for the understanding of the pathogenesis, diagnosis and treatment of children with croup.

The larynx is an organ consisting of a framework of several cartilages that are connected by synovial joints and held together by means of ligaments, membranes, muscles and mucosal lining (Figs. 1 and 2). The intrinsic and extrinsic musculature operates on the cartilages, bringing about changes in the relative positions of the vocal cords and producing differing degrees of tension in these folds. The lining of the mucous membrane is arranged in characteristic folds, which aid in phonation.

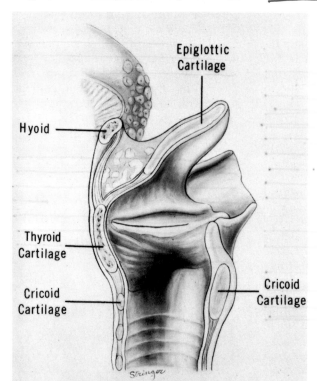

Epiglottic Cartilage

Hyoid

Thyroid Cartilage

Cricoid Cartilage

Cricoid Cartilage

Stringer

Figure 1. Sagittal view of the larynx showing normal anatomic relationships.

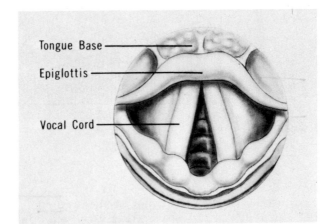

Tongue Base

Epiglottis

Vocal Cord

Figure 2. Superior view of the larynx showing normal anatomic relationships.

The thyroid cartilage is the largest and most important structure in the cartilaginous framework and encloses the larynx anteriorly and laterally. The cricoid cartilage, shaped like a signet ring, lies directly below the thyroid cartilage and forms a complete ring around the larynx below the vocal cord. The arytenoid cartilages are superimposed on the lamina of the cricoid cartilage and lie side by side posteriorly. The pair of corniculate cartilages surmounts the apex of each arytenoid cartilage. The cuneiform cartilages occupy a space in the aryepiglottic fold and are just anterior to the arytenoid and corniculate cartilages. The epiglottis contains the remaining cartilage of the larynx; this cartilage arches diagonally upward and backward from the anterior part of the thyroid cartilage to which it is attached by the thyroepiglottic ligament. This cartilage is also attached by a ligament to the hyoid bone, and the position of the epiglottis is largely determined by movements of the hyoid bone and the thyroid cartilage.

The cavity of the larynx is divided into three parts by two horizontal folds of mucous membranes that project medially from each lateral wall of the cavity. The upper pair of folds are the ventricular folds (false cords). The lower, more prominent pair are the vocal folds (true cords).

The mucous membrane that lines the larynx is continuous above with that of the pharynx and below with that of the trachea. Over the posterior (laryngeal) surface of the epiglottis, it is closely adherent; elsewhere, above the level of the vocal folds, it is loosely attached. Over the vocal folds the mucous membrane is very thin and tightly adherent.

The anatomic differences between the larynx of the infant or young child and the adult explain the reason why croup is principally a disease of children. The laryngeal airway is relatively smaller in the younger age groups in both diameter and surface area. Further, the mucous membrane is more loosely attached and there is greater vascularity. The glottis is smaller and more rapidly compromised by inflammatory edema and spasm.

Pathogenesis of and Predisposition to Croup

Patients with viral croup may have a preceding infection of the upper respiratory passages with primary involvement of the mucous membranes of the nose. After three to four days, the infection may progress to the area of the larynx where the true cords and subglottic structures become inflamed and edematous. Associated with viral croup, especially in those children with so-called spasmodic croup, there is an additional element of spasm that contributes to the laryngeal obstruction. In the past "spasmodic croup" was classified separately from infectious croup, but there are now data indicating that this form of the disease results directly or

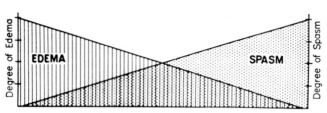

Figure 3. A schematic representation of the pathogenesis of croup. (From Cramblett, H. G.: Croup—present day concept. *Pediatrics,* 25:1071, 1960.)

indirectly from virus infection. Figure 3 is a diagrammatic presentation of the fact that edema and spasm may be present in varying degrees in infectious croup.

In infections due to *Hemophilus influenzae* type b, the primary site of inflammation is the epiglottis, which becomes enlarged because of inflammatory edema. This is a serious disease (see Diagnosis, p. 358). Inflammation may spread to involve the remainder of the supraglottic as well as the subglottic area. With *Hemophilus influenzae* infections the inflammation commonly extends downward into the respiratory tract, involving the trachea and bronchi. If this occurs, the prognosis is worse.

In croup due to *Corynebacterium diphtheriae*, it is usual to have inflammation and infection of the upper respiratory tract, including pharyngitis and rhinitis, preceding the signs and symptoms of laryngeal inflammation. There is usually "membrane" formation in the pharynx, or even in and around the larynx, which may give rise to complete, sudden obstruction if it becomes dislodged from the mucous membrane surface.

Regardless of the direct precipitating cause of croup, a number of factors are of importance in predisposing an individual child to the development of the syndrome. Even though some of these factors are poorly understood, they are worthy of consideration.

Age is an important factor. The majority of patients with viral croup are between the ages of three months and three years at the time when viral respiratory tract illnesses are most common. Hemophilus influenzal and diphtheritic croup occurs most commonly in children between the ages of two and 12 years.

The incidence of croup is higher among males than among females. Even in children with postoperative or traumatic croup, the same sex incidence prevails. There is no obvious explanation for this.

Most cases of croup occur during the cold season of the year. This is in all probability a reflection of the increased incidence of all respiratory tract infections during this period.

All the factors thus far mentioned that predispose to croup are those which have been statistically proved by the analysis of large series of cases. In addition to these, it has frequently been postulated that there are certain "endogenous factors" that predispose a given child to croup. Evidence for this includes the fact that croup tends to be recurrent in a child who has had one episode. Further, recent virologic studies reveal that all the viruses that have been associated with croup cause other types of clinical disease. There has been no one virus yet identified that causes only croup. The question why one child suffers croup as the result of a particular viral infection while another child has only a minor upper respiratory tract infection or involvement of the lower tracheobronchial tree without laryngeal involvement is still unanswered.

It has been postulated that an "anatomically defective larynx" or "immaturity" of the larynx may be a factor.

There is no evidence to suggest that these are important considerations. What constitutes the host factor in the pathogenesis of croup is unknown, but the concept must be accepted.

Evidence that "allergic" factors predispose to the development of croup is inconclusive. In one study, the family history of allergic disorders in children with croup and in a group of randomly selected children were analyzed. There was no difference. Among children with allergic diseases, there does not appear to be an increased incidence of croup.

Clinical Manifestations

The clinical manifestations of croup are mainly due to obstruction of the laryngeal airway and accordingly are the same, irrespective of the etiologic agent. Soon after the onset of cough and hoarseness, the child will exhibit inspiratory stridor. Retraction of the supraclavicular spaces, sternum, epigastrium and intercostal spaces occurs to a degree that is dependent upon the amount of compromise of the airway. Careful observation of the patient will enable the physician to localize the site of the obstruction. The patient is apprehensive and agitated until he becomes quiet; this is due to exhaustion. Any environmental distraction increases the restlessness. Intermittent cyanosis may occur.

Acute Epiglottitis

Acute epiglottitis is one of the pediatric medical emergencies that must be recognized early and treated energetically if a fatal outcome is to be avoided. The fatality rate is quoted at 8 to 12 per cent of patients with acute epiglottitis who are seen in the hospital. In the classic form of the disease, the patient, who is usually between two and 12 years of age, suddenly develops fever, inspiratory stridor and progressive intoxication. There is usually no preceding hoarseness and the voice is described as being muffled. Characteristically, the signs and symptoms of laryngeal obstruction due to inflammation of the epiglottis develop rapidly. The children appear quite anxious, are seriously ill, manifest air hunger, and are febrile. The rapidity of the progression of the disease is such that a physician is consulted within eight to 12 hours of the onset of symptoms. The interval from the onset of symptoms to death has been recorded as being as short as four to six hours. In our experience, in a series of 34 patients, the interval from the onset of illness to hospital admission was as follows: one to six hours—eight patients; six to 12 hours—four patients; 12 to 24 hours—11 patients; 24 to 48 hours—11 patients. The patients almost invariably show a leukocytosis accompanied by an increase of polymorphonuclear cells. The inflammatory process may extend to involve the tracheobronchial tree and may eventuate in pneumonia.

Acute Laryngitis;
Acute Laryngotracheitis;
Acute Laryngotracheobronchitis

For the purposes of this discussion, all three syndromes will be considered jointly, since all may be caused by the same viruses. From a practical standpoint, the only reason for differentiation is for purposes of prognosis.

Viral croup usually occurs between the ages of six months and three years. Invariably, there is a preceding history of upper respiratory tract infection consisting of rhinorrhea, coryza and fever. After two or three days and often quite suddenly, the child develops croup, with inspiratory stridor and a harsh, barking cough. At the time croup develops, more often than not, the child is afebrile. Because of difficulty in breathing, the children are apprehensive and restless, but they do not show the same degree of intoxication as children with *Hemophilus influenzae* epiglottitis. In viral croup, the obstruction is due to inflammatory swelling of the subglottic tissues and impingement upon the airway below the level of the glottis, coupled with spasm of the vocal cords. As an extension of the inflammatory process, tracheobronchitis may occur.

Laryngeal Diphtheria

In croup due to *Corynebacterium diphtheriae*, there is usually a preceding upper respiratory tract infection of three to four days' duration before the onset of symptoms of croup. A frequent sign in children with diphtheria is a serosanguineous nasal discharge. In addition, a membrane may be present in the posterior pharynx. The symptoms of croup usually develop slowly. Signs of severe obstruction may occur suddenly, however, if the membrane becomes dislodged and obstructs the laryngeal airway. The patients appear quite toxic.

Diagnosis

The diagnosis of *Hemophilus influenzae* type b epiglottitis may be established by observing a fiery red, swollen, edematous epiglottis on physical examination. It is to be stressed that before the patient is manipulated, and especially before efforts are made to visualize the epiglottis, the observer must be prepared to establish an airway either by intubation, tracheostomy or the placing of a large-caliber needle through the skin into the lumen of the trachea. The addition of the trauma of the examination to the patient's apprehension and the compromised airway may be enough to cause complete respiratory tract obstruction. Thus, although the diagnosis can be easily established by physical examination, this procedure is not one to be undertaken without due caution. In the establishment of an etiologic diagnosis, blood cultures are positive as often as are nasopharyngeal cultures or cultures taken directly from the epiglottis. A peripheral leukocyte count will show an increase in the total count with a preponderance of polymorphonuclear cells.

Although the larynx may be the sole site of infection in infections due to *Corynebacterium diphtheriae*, it is more often secondary to primary involvement of the pharynx. Otherwise, the clinical manifestations of disease are due to laryngeal obstruction and toxemia. The bacteriologic diagnosis can be made by recovery of *Corynebacterium diphtheriae* on Löffler's or tellurite medium. In specially equipped laboratories, fluorescent microscopy may be utilized for a more rapid diagnosis.

In diphtheritic croup, the presence of a serosanguineous nasal discharge and a membrane in the absence of a history of immunization against diphtheria are suggestive of the diagnosis.

In viral croup, the diagnosis is most often made by exclusion of infections due to *Corynebacterium diphtheriae* and *Hemophilus influenzae* type b. The child who has "spasmodic croup" or is afebrile most certainly has a virus infection. On the other hand, if the course of disease is not fulminating but the child is febrile, there is a marginal possibility that the disease is caused by *Hemophilus influenzae* type b. When available, throat washings for inoculation into tissue culture may provide an etiologic viral diagnosis. The parainfluenza viruses grow in monkey kidney cell cultures, where their presence is most easily recognized by hemadsorption of guinea pig erythrocytes. Influenza viruses may be similarly grown, or an alternate method is inoculation of the patient's secretions into embryonated hens' eggs. Adenoviruses and respiratory syncytial virus may be grown in continuous cell cultures. The enteroviruses grow well and produce cytopathic effects in many cell cultures.

Prognosis

The necessity for tracheostomy and the prognosis of croup vary according to the involvement of the various anatomic structures. In Rabe's series, 0.6

per cent of the cases with laryngitis required a tracheostomy, whereas 16.3 per cent of those with laryngotracheitis required this procedure. The important statistic is that 47 per cent of those with laryngotracheobronchitis had need for the establishment of an adequate airway by tracheostomy. In another series of patients with epiglottitis, 43 per cent of the patients required tracheostomy. In this same series, 12 per cent of the patients were dead on arrival at the hospital or died after admission.

In our own experience, 59 per cent of patients with epiglottitis required an artificial airway.

Treatment

Because patients with croup are severely ill enough to be hospitalized, it is important that they be handled with a minimum of activity in order not to aggravate their respiratory distress. The patient should be placed immediately in an atmosphere with high humidity and oxygen. The oxygen will help alleviate anxiety, apprehension and increased respiratory efforts. All diagnostic and nursing procedures should be kept to a minimum. Under no circumstances should a sleeping child with croup be awakened. In order to decrease apprehension and restlessness, it is helpful at times to sedate the patient cautiously. The same caution should be exercised in the administration of sedatives to these patients as that which is observed in any patient with respiratory difficulties. Phenobarbital may be used in a dosage of 6 mg. per kilogram of body weight per 24 hours in three or four divided doses.

In order that the child be minimally disturbed, it is advisable to administer fluids intravenously. This obviates the frequent arousal of the child, which may result in the exaggeration of symptoms. Intravenous fluids also ensure adequate hydration. Intermittent positive pressure breathing (IPPB) with aerosolized 2 per cent racemic epinephrine hydrochloride has been utilized for relief of obstructive signs and symptoms in infectious croup. While relief may be dramatic in some patients, others do not receive similar beneficial effects. The patient who does not receive relief on the first administration should not be subjected to repeated attempts with this mode of therapy. The patient who has had response to IPPB with epinephrine aerosol should be observed for rebound following therapy.

In those instances in which spasm of the larynx is more prominent than edema, administration of syrup of ipecac may produce prompt relief of symptoms. It is assumed that ipecac has a relaxing effect upon the larynx by means of a vagal response. Ipecac is given in subemetic doses, but frequently the full therapeutic effect of the drug is not achieved without vomiting. The usual dose is 1 drop per month of age up to two years. Children two years of age or older may be given 1 ml. per year of age. Any infant or child who receives ipecac should be closely observed in the hour following its administration to prevent aspiration of gastric contents in case emesis does occur. If symptoms subside, one can assume that the croup is at least partially caused by spasm, and valuable information is thus obtained without resort to laryngoscopy. If there is no response and the patient does not vomit, the same dosage may be repeated. Caution should be exercised to be certain that fluid extract of ipecac is not erroneously substituted for syrup of ipecac. The former is 14 to 20 times as potent as the latter and may cause serious toxic effects.

The value of adrenocorticosteroids in the treatment of croup continues to be debated. As is so often the case in disease syndromes of naturally variable course and outcome, there are no definitive studies establishing conclusively the value of, lack of value of, or danger of the use of steroids in this disease. There is the suggestion in hospitalized patients that, at most, steroids reduce the duration of obstructive signs and symptoms but do not decrease the length of hospitalization. Consequently, this author does not advocate the use of steroids in the therapy of croup.

In the patient with *Hemophilus influenzae* type b croup, the treatment of choice in the past has been ampicillin. However, with the emergence of strains of *Hemophilus influenzae* resistant to ampicillin, and since epiglottitis is a life-threatening infection, chloramphenicol may be used as effective initial therapy. Combination therapy with ampicillin and chloramphenicol has also been recommended as initial therapy on the basis that once sensitivities are determined, one or the other of the two antibiotics could be discontinued. Since the combination per se does not have a greater antibacterial activity than either drug alone, and since the danger of exposure to chloramphenicol will have already occurred, it seems preferable to use single drug therapy. Ampicillin should be administered intravenously in a dose of 200 mg. per kilogram of body weight per 24 hours in six divided doses. Chloramphenicol is administered intravenously in a dose of 50 to 100 mg. per kilogram of body weight per 24 hours in four divided doses (total daily adult dose is 2 to 4 gm.). In patients with infections due to *Corynebacterium diphtheriae*, the immediate therapy is the administration of antitoxin followed by the use of penicillin or erythromycin.

The decision as to the need for tracheostomy or intubation must always be based on the individual circumstances. If the signs and symptoms of laryngeal obstruction increase in spite of the aforementioned measures, the procedure will be necessary. Extension of the inflammatory process down into the tracheobronchial tree may likewise provide an indication if secretions are excessive. Careful timing of the procedure is important. Therefore, it is desirable to have an otolaryngologist see the patient as soon as possible after admission so that he may follow the progress of the disease carefully. Because of the sequelae and the difficulty in management, tracheostomy in infants is avoided whenever possible. As an emergency procedure, intubation with the insertion of an airway or the placing of a large-bore needle (14 gauge or greater) through the skin into the lumen of the trachea may be lifesaving and may provide an opportunity for a carefully performed tracheostomy later.

REFERENCES

Berenberg, W., and Kevy, S.: Acute epiglottitis in childhood: serious emergency, readily recognized at bedside. *N. Engl. J. Med., 258*:870, 1958.

Cramblett, H. G.: Croup—present day concept. *Pediatrics, 25*:1071, 1960.

James, J. A.: Dexamethasone in croup. *Am. J. Dis. Child., 117*:511, 1969.

Jordon, W. S., Graves, C. L., and Elwyn, R. A.: New therapy for postintubation laryngeal edema and tracheitis in children. *J.A.M.A., 212*:585, 1970.

McLean, D. M., Bach, R. D., Larke, R. P. B., and McHaughton, G. A.: Myxoviruses associated with acute laryngotracheobronchitis in Toronto, 1962–1963. *Can. Med. Assoc. J., 89*:1257, 1963.

Parrott, R. H.: Viral respiratory tract illnesses in children. *Bull. N. Y. Acad. Med., 39*:629, 1963.

Rabe, E. F.: Infectious croup. I. Etiology. *Pediatrics, 2*:225, 1948.

Sell, S. H. W.: The clinical importance of *Hemophilus influenzae* infections in children. *Pediatr. Clin. North Am., 17*:415, 1970.

Taussig, L. M., Castro, O., Beaudry, P. H., Fox, W. W., and Bureau, M.: Treatment of laryngotracheobronchitis (croup). *Am. J. Dis. Child., 129*:790, 1975.

Turner, J. A.: Present-day aspects of acute laryngotracheitis. *Can. Med. Assoc. J., 70*:401, 1954.

CHAPTER SIXTEEN

BRONCHITIS

J. A. Peter Turner, M.D.

The word "bronchitis" is common in medical terminology and implies inflammation of the bronchial mucosa. Its main clinical characteristic is cough with or without an increase in bronchial secretions. The disease is seldom a specific entity and usually occurs in association with similar involvement in other airways. Thus we find ourselves using such semantic combinations as sinobronchitis, laryngotracheobronchitis, asthmatic or asthmatoid bronchitis, bronchiolitis, capillary bronchitis, and so on.

Airways diseases, including bronchitis, are more pronounced in infants and young children because of the following peculiarities of lung structure that relate to age and to the growing state:

① All airways are present at birth. Lung growth during infancy and early childhood involves the addition of air spaces. Diseases involving the respiratory system exhibit a significant airways component in the young.

② Airway size is proportional to age. Therefore, mucosal edema or secretions produce more obstruction in a given airway in the younger subject.

③ With increasing age there is a decreasing tendency for airways to collapse. Even in the healthy state, it is possible that some lung units are closed throughout part of the tidal volume in the very young. This tendency increases the severity of symptoms and the degree to which gas exchange is impaired in the infant and young child with bronchial involvement.

④ The younger the subject is, the more apparent is dynamic compression of intrathoracic airways during expiration. With a reduction of airway caliber, for example due to inflammation and edema, there is an even greater tendency to obstruction of flow during expiration.

For the above reasons, involvement of the bronchi produces relatively more symptoms and offers a higher likelihood of complication in the young child in contrast to involvement in the older child and adult.

The changes associated with the clinical picture of bronchitis in childhood are similar to those of bronchiolitis in young infants. The differences in terminology relate to the clinical expression of disease created by the size of the airway involved. In the infant, because of small airway size and other factors noted above, there is a greater tendency for obstruction and impaired gas exchange in the presence of inflammatory edema and mucus secretion. Bronchiolitis will be dealt with in detail in the following chapter. The use of the adjectives "asthmatic" and "asthmatoid" relates to the commonly associated phenomena of expiratory prolongation and wheeze. In the young child and infant, this symptom is due not so much to constriction of smooth muscle as to the physiologic narrowing of the bronchi on expiration in airways compromised by edema of the bronchial mucosa and increased secretions.

Treatment of bronchitis is important because the condition imposes potential complications. The commonest of these is segmental obstruction due to mucus plugging. The right middle lobe and lingula are frequently involved, probably because of their anatomic nature. Subsequent atelectasis may ultimately result in bronchiectasis. Partial obstruction of the bronchus may occasionally produce air trapping with interstitial emphysema, pneumomediastinum or pneumothorax. There is increasing concern that recurrent bronchitis in childhood may presage the syndrome of chronic bronchitis in adults.

In considering the diseases in which inflammation of the bronchi plays a significant role, the following classifications will be used:

1. Infection: viral; bacterial; fungal agents.
2. Chemical factors.
3. Allergic factors.

Infection

VIRAL INFECTION. Acute bronchitis closely follows the pattern of upper respiratory tract infection in children. Since the majority of such infections are viral in origin, involvement of the bronchial tree by viral agents is proportionate. Epidemiologic studies have shown that such infections occur both seasonally and in epidemic pattern. The common agents isolated are the influenzas, the paramyxoviruses, the respiratory syncytial virus and the adenoviruses. Measles is a specific paramyxovirus infection that produces an inflammatory reaction of the tracheobronchial tree associated with cough during the acute stage of the illness.

Since the mortality rates in such diseases are low, material for pathologic study is scanty. One may assume from the few studies available that there is catarrhal inflammation of the bronchial mucosa together with stringy mucus only scantily mixed with leukocytes. In most instances such a reaction is self-limited. Clearing is associated with a reduction in the inflammatory reaction and with thinning of mucus, which may then be raised by ciliary activity and cough.

Clinical signs vary with the age of the child. As indicated previously, infection with viral agents may be responsible for the clinical picture of bronchiolitis in young infants. In the older infant and child, cough with variable wheezing is the most common expression of the infection. In the early stage the cough may be associated with coryza, but ultimately it progresses to a nonproductive hacking type of cough so familiar to the clinician. Although pyrexia may occur in association with the illness, normal temperature or only a low-grade fever may be present. Variable crepitations are heard on auscultation, depending on the size of the airways involved. These are usually coarse and inconstant and change with coughing.

The treatment of viral bronchitis depends largely on cough control. Although there are innumerable antitussive preparations commercially available, unfortunately the majority of these contain a combination of expectorant, sedative and antihistaminic agents in the same mixture. Cough control is based on two general principles. First, if secretions of the tracheobronchial tree are thin, then physiologic ciliary action may take place with beneficial results. Second, effective sedation may depress the cough reflex designed to clear the airway of the small child. The resulting inhibition of mucus clearance may result in bronchial obstruction. Expectorant therapy is therefore desirable. Humidification of inspired air is beneficial both in reducing inflammatory edema and in liquefying bronchial secretions. Steam, although a ready source of moisture, is not preferred in the treatment of bronchial disease. The droplet size from an ordinary steam kettle is too large to reach beyond the upper respiratory tract passages. Also, heat from steam may lead to drying of secretions. Cold moisture is preferable whenever possible, from a vaporizer producing a droplet 0.5 to 0.3 micron in size. In the hospitalized patient, mask inhalations of nebulized solutions may be effective in conjunction with physiotherapy to the chest to aid in the raising of secretions. Adequate hydration of the patient is of equal importance in maintaining thin bronchial mucus. This may be achieved by increasing oral fluid intake or, if necessary, by parenteral fluid therapy.

BACTERIAL INFECTION. The older medical literature contains many references to acute suppurative bronchitis in childhood. A number of these cases were undoubtedly due to unrecognized cystic fibrosis. Primary bacterial invasion of the healthy bronchial mucosa is extremely rare. Such agents manifest their effect only when there is some significant derangement of the normal bronchial defenses. An exception to this rule is Bordetella pertussis, which causes a specific primary bacterial infection of the superficial bronchial tissues. The organism produces an acute inflammatory reaction of the tracheobronchial mucosa together with secretion of viscid mucus and ciliary dysfunction. These, in turn, are responsible for the characteristic paroxysmal cough of pertussis, which has a nocturnal predilection and which may persist for weeks. Although the course of pertussis may be modified by prior vaccination, it is quite possible for the infection to be acquired after such immunization.

Primary tuberculosis in childhood may produce a specific endobronchitis resulting from the extrusion of infected caseous material from contiguous lymph nodes through the bronchial wall. This disease will be dealt with more fully in the chapter on tuberculosis (Chapter 46), but it should be noted here that tuberculous infection of the bronchi may produce cough together with radiologic evidence of segmental obstructive phenomena distal to the area of involvement. Under these circumstances, a Mantoux test may be an important diagnostic clue.

Other bacterial agents may colonize the bronchus. This is particularly the case if there is underlying derangement of the mucociliary apparatus. Such derangement may result from a preceding viral infection. Hemophilus influenzae, Staphylococcus, Diplococcus pneumoniae and streptococcus are commonly recovered from sputum or from bronchoscopic aspirate. Staphylococcus and the Pseudomonas species are frequently encountered in cystic fibrosis.

Recovery of bacterial agents from the bronchial tree is not necessarily an indication of invasion by such infection. It is therefore questionable whether antibiotic therapy is indicated. As a general rule, if the patient is febrile and if there is polymorphonuclear leukocytosis, appropriate antibiotic therapy may be employed. Ancillary treatment by inspired moist air and hydration is once again important because of the secretion component. For pertussis specifically, cough sedation is indicated. Dihydrocodeinone preparations are useful for that infection.

It is tempting to speculate about the relationship between viral and bacterial bronchial infection and underlying disturbances of immune mechanisms. In particular, there is no good evidence that secretory IgA, which is normally present in bronchial secretions, plays a role in the pathogenesis of bronchitis per se.

FUNGAL INFECTION. Fungi rarely produce bronchial disease in children. Monilia may invade the bronchial mucosa as secondary spread from oropharyngeal thrush. This may occur in the neonate, in infants and children who are terminal from other underlying conditions, or in those who are receiving immunosuppressive therapy. Bronchopulmonary aspergillosis as a significant entity is discussed in adult literature. The implications of recovery of Aspergillus from bronchial secretions in childhood are questionable, even in those patients whose symptoms would suggest allergic phenomena. The mycoses involving the respiratory tract are dealt with in detail in Chapter 50.

Chemical Factors

There is a growing interest in air pollution with regard to both chronic and acute chest disease in humans. The relationship of known pollutants to specific pulmonary disease has been studied mainly in the adult population. However, a recent study of children exposed to high ambient levels of NO_2 has demonstrated an increased incidence of bronchitis in those children. Further experimental work in animals has revealed a relationship between increased levels of NO_2 and facilitation of influenzal viral infection. This is presumably due to inhibition of alveolar macrophage interferon. Air pollution in the form of personal cigarette smoking or exposure to cigarette smoke in the home is a matter of increasing concern. Although most of the collected data have been concerned with the adult population, there is growing realization that children suffer the same effects from these environmental factors. With evidence of increasing smoking habits of young children, we must consider the possibility of cigarette smoke irritation as a cause of chronic cough or as a contributory factor to recurrent respiratory illness with bronchitis in childhood.

Inhalation of smoke from a burning building is responsible for acute bronchial edema with or without the added feature of heat damage. In severe cases, there are other factors to be considered, such as noxious gas inhalation together with pulmonary edema. In lesser exposures, however, there may be only bronchial irritation present. There is a difference of opinion, under those circumstances, as to the use of steroid therapy together with broad-spectrum antibiotic coverage. If such treatment is considered, it should be utilized over a short period of time rather than as a prolonged course.

Aspiration of feeding or stomach contents should be considered as a possible cause of recurrent bronchitis in early childhood. Anatomic malformations of the trachea and esophagus may be present, or there may be an underlying neurologic disorder producing esophageal dyskinesia or gastroesophageal reflux. Appropriate radiologic studies, including esophagram, may be necessary to elucidate the underlying problem.

Environmental exposures to such pulmonary irritants as moldy hay, asbestos fibers and the like are usually considered to be occupational hazards and are most frequently associated with frank pulmonary disease. In rare instances, however, the initial exposure to such factors may produce only bronchial irritation without lung involvement and may resemble an attack of asthmatoid bronchitis or constrictive bronchiolitis. Such a clinical picture has been reported in childhood.

Allergic Factors

Atopy is a common underlying factor in recurrent bronchitis. In the young child, the early manifestation of an allergic disorder may be the demonstration of recurrent cough with increased secretions as an exaggerated response to each upper respiratory tract infection. There may or may not be associated expiratory prolongation, which when present is responsible for the frequent use of the qualifying terms "asthmatic" and "asthmatoid."

The pathogenesis of this phenomenon is obscure, but it probably relates to underlying hypersensitivity of the bronchial mucosa. With the trigger of upper respiratory tract infection, there is produced a degree of edema or secretions, or both, sufficient to cause symptoms of bronchitis. Follow-up studies of such patients have revealed an incidence of asthma in later childhood significantly higher than that expected in the general population. These cases may sometimes be identified by high IgE levels with or without eosinophilia.

The common complication of this condition in the young child is that of mucus plugging as noted previously. Although the right middle lobe and lingula are frequently affected, any lung segment may be involved. It is not unusual to observe an individual child with this condition who demonstrates recurrent multisegmental pulmonary involvement, usually transient, over a period of months.

The management of these children involves recognition of the underlying problem. Examination of nasal mucous smears or bronchoscopic aspirate for eosinophils provides suggestive evidence of atopy. Increased serum levels of IgE may be helpful. Diagnostic allergy skin tests may be carried out after such tests become valid, between two and three years of age. Environmental control or hyposensitization procedures, or both, may be considered.

If underlying allergic problems are suspected, the use of bronchodilators may be helpful in therapy in addition to those measures already noted under other forms of bronchitis. Theophylline, in appropriate doses, is particularly useful in the older child, but may not be helpful in the young infant with this problem. Similarly, the administration of beta-adrenergic stimulants is more effective in the older child.

The younger the child is, the more troublesome are the symptoms of recurrent bronchitis on the basis of underlying allergy. There is a tendency, as the child grows older, for such symptoms to lessen in severity. Such an improvement may be simply related to increase in airway size and thus less compromise during an acute episode. These observations are in keeping with the evidence that asthma tends to improve with age as well. (See Chapter 41.)

REFERENCES

Anderson, D. O.: Smoking and respiratory disease. *Am. J. Health, 54*:1856, 1964.

Balchum, O. J., Felton, J. S., Jamison, J. N., Gaines, R. S., Clarke, D. R., Owan, T., and the Industrial Health Committee, the Tuberculosis and Health Association of Los Angeles County: A survey for chronic respiratory disease in an industrial city. *Am. Rev. Resp. Dis., 86*:675, 1962.

Bryan, A. C., Mansell, A., and Levison, H.: Development of the mechanical properties of the respiratory system. In L'Enfant, C.: *Lung Biology in Health and Disease.* New York, Marcel Dekker Inc. (in press).

Eisen, A. H., and Bacal, H. L.: The relationship of acute bronchiolitis to bronchial asthma, a 4 to 14 year follow-up. *Pediatrics, 31*:859, 1963.

Feingold, B. F.: Infection in bronchial allergic disease: bronchial asthma, allergic bronchitis, asthmatic bronchitis. *Pediatr. Clin. North Am., 6*:709, 1959.

Forbes, J. A., Bennett, N. M., and Gray, N. J.: Epidemic bronchiolitis caused by a respiratory syncytial virus; clinical aspects. *Med. J. Aust., 2*:933, 1961.

Foucard, T. A.: A follow-up study of children with asthmatoid bronchitis. *Acta Paediatr. Scand., 63*:129, 1974.

Garrow, D. H., and Taylor, C. E. D.: An investigation of acute respiratory disease in children admitted to hospital in the south west metropolitan region. *Arch. Dis. Child., 37*:392, 1962.

High, R. H.: Bronchiolitis (acute asthmatic bronchitis, acute capillary bronchitis). *Pediatr. Clin. North Am., 4*:183, 1957.

Holland, W. W., and Elliott, A.: Cigarette smoking, respiratory symptoms and anti-smoking propaganda. *Lancet, 1*:41, 1968.

Laurenzi, G. A.: Acute bronchial inflammation and infection. In Baum, G. L.: *Textbook of Pulmonary Diseases.* 2nd Ed. Boston, Little, Brown & Company, 1974, pp. 115–162.

Lewis, F. A., Rae, M. L., Lehman, N. I., and Ferris, A. A.: A syncytial virus associated with epidemic disease of the lower respiratory tract in infants and young children. *Med. J. Aust., 2*:932, 1961.

Lincoln, E. M., and Sewell, E. M.: *Tuberculosis in Childhood.* New York, McGraw-Hill Book Company, Inc., 1963.

Linhartova, A., and Chung, W.: Bronchopulmonary moniliasis in the newborn, *J. Clin. Pathol., 16*:56, 1963.

MacLean, D. M., Bach, R. D., Larke, R. P. B., and McNaghton, G. A.: Myxoviruses associated with acute laryngotracheobronchitis in Toronto 1962–1963. *Can. Med. Assoc. J., 89*:1257, 1963.

Mellins, R. B., and Park, S.: Respiratory complications of smoke inhalation in victims of fires. *J. Pediatr., 87*:1, 1975.

Morison, J. B., Medovy, H., and MacDonell, G. T.: Health education and cigarette smoking; a report on a 3-year program in the Winnipeg School Division, 1960–1963. *Can. Med. Assoc. J., 91*:49, 1964.

Mork, T.: International comparisons of the prevalence of chronic bronchitis. *Proc. R. Soc. Med., 57*:975, 1964.

Mortensen, E.: Follow-up on children with asthmatic bronchitis with a view of the prognosis. *Acta Paediatr. (Stockholm), 140*(Suppl.):122, 1963.

Olson, E. T.: Occurrence of silo-fillers' disease in children. *J. Pediatr., 64*:724, 1964.

Olson, L. C.: Pertussis. *Medicine, 54*:527, 1975.

Parrott, R. H., Kim, H. W., Vargosko, A. J., and Chanok, R. M.: Serious respiratory tract illness as a result of Asian influenza and influenza infections in children. *J. Pediatr., 61*:205, 1962.

Pearlman, M. E., Finklea, J. F., Creason, J. P.,

Shy, C. M., Young, M. M., and Horton, R. J. M.: Nitrogen dioxide and lower respiratory illness. *Pediatrics, 47*:391, 1971.

Reid, D. D.: Air pollution as a cause of chronic bronchitis. *Proc. R. Soc. Med., 57*:965, 1964.

Reid, D. D.: The beginnings of bronchitis. *Proc. R. Soc. Med., 62*:311, 1969.

Robbins, S. L.: *Pathology.* 3rd Ed. Philadelphia, W. B. Saunders Company, 1967.

Seal, R. M. E., Thomas, G. O., and Griffiths, J. J.: Farmer's lung. *Proc. R. Soc. Med., 56*:271, 1963.

Speer, F. (Ed.): *The Allergic Child.* New York, Harper & Row, 1963.

Valand, S. B., Acton, J. D., and Myrvik, Q. N.: Nitrogen dioxide inhibition of viral induced resistance in alveolar monocytes. *Arch. Environ. Health, 20*:303, 1970.

Williams, A.: Bronchitis, asthma and emphysema in childhood. *Med. J. Aust., 1*:781, 1957.

Williams, S.: Aetiology and diagnosis of bronchial asthma, bronchitis and emphysema in children. *Med. J. Aust., 1*:782, 1957.

CHAPTER SEVENTEEN

BRONCHIOLITIS

MARY ELLEN B. WOHL, M.D.

Bronchiolitis means inflammation of the bronchioles. In the child under two years of age, the term is applied to a clinical syndrome characterized by rapid respiration, chest retractions and wheezing.

Clinical Presentation

Bronchiolitis is one of the major causes of hospital admission in infants under the age of one year; most commonly, it affects infants under the age of six months (Gardner, 1973; Kim and coworkers, 1973; Parrott and coworkers, 1973). There appears to be a preponderance of male infants among those sick enough to require hospitalization. Characteristically, the infant develops mild rhinorrhea and cough and sometimes low-grade fever. Within one or two days, this is followed by the onset of rapid respiration, chest retractions and wheezing. The infant may be irritable, feed poorly and vomit (Reilly and coworkers, 1961; Heycock and Noble, 1962; Wright and Beem, 1965; Gardner, 1973; Hall and coworkers, 1976).

On physical examination, the respiratory rate is increased, often to rates above 50 or 60 breaths per minute. The pulse rate is usually increased, and body temperature may be normal or elevated as high as 41° C. Mild conjunctivitis or otitis is observed in some patients, and pharyngitis in about one-half (Reilly and coworkers, 1961; Gardner, 1973). Chest retractions are present. Prolonged expirations are frequently found, but breath sounds may be normal. Rhonchi and wheezes or rales are usually heard throughout the lungs. Respiratory distress may prevent adequate oral fluid intake and cause dehydration. Cyanosis is detectable in only a minority of the infants, but severe abnormalities of gas exchange can develop in the absence of cyanosis. Increased respiratory rate is a more sensitive indicator of impaired gas exchange, and rates of 60 breaths per minute or higher are associated with reduction of arterial oxygen tension and elevation of carbon dioxide tension (Reynolds, 1963a, b).

The radiographic manifestations (Rice and Loda, 1966; W. Simpson and coworkers, 1974) of bronchiolitis are nonspecific and include diffuse hyperinflation of the lungs with flattening of the diaphragms, prominence of the retrosternal space and bulging of the intercostal spaces (Fig. 1). Patchy or peribronchial infiltrates suggestive of interstitial pneumonia occur in the majority of infants. Pleural thickening and fluid are rarely observed and, when present, are minimal. Some infants with illness severe enough to require hospitalization have normal chest roentgenograms.

Etiology

In 1957, Chanock and Finberg isolated the respiratory syncytial (RS) virus from two infants with lower respiratory tract disease. Beem and coworkers in 1960 found this virus, originally isolated from the chimpanzee and termed the "chimpanzee coryza agent," in 31 of 95 infants under two years of age with acute lower respiratory tract disease. Subsequently, RS virus has been found to be the etiologic agent in

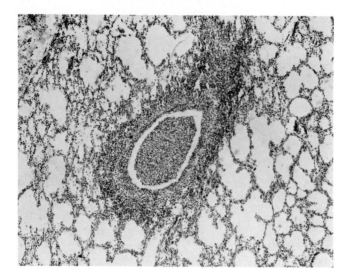

Figure 1. Histologic section of a bronchiole from an infant dying with acute bronchiolitis. The respiratory syncytial virus was grown from necropsy specimens. Peribronchiolar lymphoid infiltration and plugging of the lumen with exudate and cell debris can be seen. The surrounding alveoli are little affected. (Courtesy of Dr. W. Aherne.)

the majority of infants with bronchiolitis (Cradock-Watson and coworkers, 1971; Brandt and colleagues, 1973; Gardner, 1973; Kim and coworkers, 1973; McClelland and associates, 1961; Parrott and colleagues, 1973). Other viruses (Becroft, 1971; Cradock-Watson and coworkers, 1971; Glezen and Denny, 1973; Zollar and coworkers, 1973), primarily adenovirus, parainfluenza virus types I and III, enterovirus and influenza virus, have been associated with bronchiolitis in smaller numbers of cases. Particularly severe bronchiolitis associated with adenovirus infections has been observed in native (Indian, Eskimo, Métis) Canadian children (Morrell and coworkers, 1975).

Epidemics of RS virus disease occur between October and June, last approximately five months and follow a characteristic pattern of alternating short (7 to 12 months) and long (13 to 16 months) intervals between epidemic peaks (Brandt and coworkers, 1973; Glezen and Denny, 1973; Kim and coworkers, 1973). Adults as well as children are infected, but only infants develop the clinical syndrome of bronchiolitis (Parrott and coworkers, 1973; Hall and colleagues, 1976). In large urban populations, the peak age incidence of RS bronchiolitis is at two months (Parrott and coworkers, 1973);

in more rural settings, RS-associated bronchiolitis is observed up to the age of two years (Glezen and Denny, 1973). Although the incidence of RS infections appears to be the same in males and females, severe bronchiolitis is more likely to occur in male infants.

Epidemiologic studies of RS virus indicate that during an epidemic all age groups have appreciable attack rates, ranging from 29 per cent in infants to 17 per cent in adults (Hall and coworkers, 1976). Almost all infected individuals develop symptoms, particularly nasal congestion and cough. The virus is usually introduced into a family by an older child. The virus continues to be shed for an average of nine days in children under one year of age, but in some infants virus is shed for as long as 36 days (Hall and coworkers, 1975a). High titers of virus may remain present in nasal washings despite clinical improvement. In infants with bronchiolitis, there appears to be no correlation between severity of illness and amount of virus shed, although infants with RS viral pneumonia shed less virus than those with bronchiolitis (Hall and coworkers, 1975a). These and other observations indicate that factors other than the cytolytic effect of viral replication in the airways may be responsible for bronchiolitis in young infants.

Infants who had received a killed RS virus vaccine developed high levels of complement-fixing and neutralizing antibody to RS virus (Chanock and coworkers, 1970). Yet in an epidemic of RS infection, their disease was more severe than that in control infants. Severe bronchiolitis occurs in young infants in whom maternally acquired antibody might be highest. These observations suggest that the presence of antibody contributes to the production of disease. The hypothesis has been put forth that antigen-antibody complexes toxic to cells are formed (an Arthus or type III immune response in the classification of Gell and Coombs) (Chanock and coworkers, 1970). The observation that older infants with no evidence of antibody acquire typical RS bronchiolitis does not support this hypothesis (Parrott and coworkers, 1973).

The vaccinated infants also had evidence of specific cell-mediated immunity (delayed hypersensitivity) to RS virus (Kim and coworkers, 1976), and this, coupled with the observation that there are accumulations of lymphocytes around peripheral airways in infants with bronchiolitis, has led to the speculation that a type IV or cell-mediated immune response contributes to the production of disease.

The relative paucity of virus in the airways of infants with bronchiolitis examined at autopsy contrasted with the large quantities of virus present in the lungs of infants dying of RS pneumonia has led to the suggestion that a small amount of virus might trigger a type I immune response with the subsequent release of mediator substances (Gardner and coworkers, 1970). As yet, there is no evidence as to whether infants who acquire the disease have specific IgE antibodies to RS virus, which could combine with viral antigen to produce a type I immune response. Previous exposure to RS virus may be important in the pathogenesis of bronchiolitis. An epidemic of RS virus in two Arctic communities geographically isolated and so presumably without prior exposure to RS virus produced

cases of severe pneumonia but no bronchiolitis, whereas another epidemic of RS virus in an Arctic community near a military installation produced cases of bronchiolitis (Morrell and coworkers, 1975).

The relative rate of maturation of various components of the immune system may influence the type of disease produced by RS virus. The presence of secretory IgA antibody to RS virus on the nasal mucosa conveys some degree of protection, and the relative delay in the development of this system may be related to the occurrence of disease. However, specific IgA antibody is present in secretions of some infants with bronchiolitis.

Anatomic differences between the lungs of young infants and older children may contribute to the severity of bronchiolitis in infants. Resistance of peripheral airways is a larger part of overall airway resistance in infants than in adults. In the normal adult, the resistance of peripheral airways has little influence on the distribution of ventilation. This may not be true in infants. One may further speculate that a given amount of cellular debris and edema produces a greater degree of obstruction in the infant's small peripheral airways than in the older child's larger peripheral airways. The absence of effective collateral ventilation in the infant may contribute to the development of patchy atelectasis and the abnormalities of gas exchange. Smooth muscle exists in the periphery of the infant's lung as it does in the older child so that the infant's airways may respond to mediator substances if these are released. Finally, there are changes in the cell composition of the lung and in the composition of mucus that may contribute, in as yet undefined ways, to the reduction in the incidence and severity of bronchiolitis with increasing age.

Pathology

The initial abnormalities of the lower respiratory tract in RS virus bronchiolitis are necrosis of the respiratory

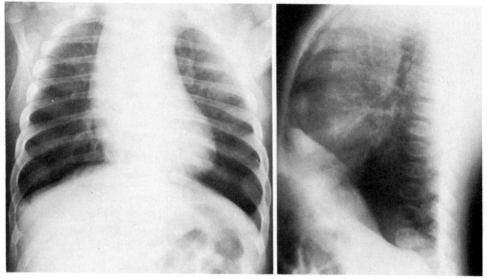

Figure 2.   Chest radiograph of an infant with the clinical syndrome of acute bronchiolitis.

epithelium and destruction of ciliated epithelial cells, followed by peribronchiolar infiltration with lymphocytes. The submucosa becomes edematous, but there is no destruction of collagen or elastic tissue (Fig. 2). Cellular debris and fibrin form plugs within the bronchioles. In most cases the alveoli are normal, except those immediately adjacent to the inflamed bronchioles. Occasionally there is more extensive alveolar involvement, and the increased cellularity of the subepithelial tissue of the bronchi and bronchioles extends to distant intra-alveolar walls. In such cases, edema fluid may accumulate within alveoli (McLean, 1956; Aherne and coworkers, 1970).

In addition to these changes, RS virus may cause severe pneumonia with extensive destruction of respiratory epithelium, necrosis of lung parenchyma and formation of hyaline membranes, similar to the pneumonia that occurs in adenovirus and parainfluenza type III infections (Aherne and coworkers, 1970).

Recovery from acute bronchiolitis begins with regeneration of the bronchiolar epithelium after three or four days, but cilia do not appear until much later, probably about 15 days. Mucous plugs are removed by macrophages (Aherne and coworkers, 1970).

Pathophysiology

As a result of the edema of the airway wall and the accumulation of mucus and of cellular debris, and perhaps even as a result of muscle spasm, many peripheral airways are narrowed and some are partially and others totally occluded. The patchy distribution and variable degree of obstruction produce atelectasis in some areas of the lung and overdistention in others.

The mechanics of respiration is abnormal (Krieger, 1964; Phelan and coworkers, 1968a; Wohl and coworkers, 1969). The infant breathes at a high lung volume, and resting end-expiratory lung volume (functional residual capacity) is approximately twice normal. Dynamic compliance is decreased, in part because the infant is breathing at a higher lung volume and hence on a stiffer portion of the volume-pressure curve of the lung, and in part because of the uneven distribution of resistances within the lung. Airway resistance is increased, although to a variable extent. Most studies have shown the greater increase to be on expiration, which is compatible with lower airway obstruction; the data in one study, however, suggest a substantial upper airway (above the level of the carina) component to the obstruction. The decrease in compliance and increase in resistance result in a substantial increase in the work of breathing.

Serious alterations in gas exchange occur as a result of the airway obstruction and patchy distribution of atelectasis (Reynolds, 1963a; Downes and coworkers, 1968; H. Simpson and coworkers, 1974). Arterial hypoxemia develops as the result of mismatching of pulmonary ventilation and perfusion ($\dot{V}/\dot{Q}$ abnormality), with continued perfusion of underventilated units and overventilation of poorly perfused units. The evidence that $\dot{V}/\dot{Q}$ abnormalities usually account for the hypoxemia comes from the observation that the hypoxemia can be corrected by the administration of 40 per cent oxygen (Reynolds, 1963a). The tension of carbon dioxide in arterial blood is variable. In some instances it is low and in others it is normal or only slightly elevated. However, in young infants in particular, some degree of carbon dioxide retention is noted sometime in the course of the disease. The likely mechanisms are severe mismatching of ventilation and perfusion and hypoventilation secondary to the markedly increased work of breathing. Blood pH is variable. Some infants exhibit a mild respiratory alkalosis. More commonly, metabolic acidosis is observed. The causes of this are complex. Poor caloric and fluid intake and the administration of salicylate may contribute to the ketoacidoses in infants. Finally, carbon dioxide retention can produce acute respiratory acidosis.

Diagnosis

The diagnosis of acute viral bronchiolitis is suggested by the clinical presentation, the age of the child and the presence of an epidemic of RS virus in the community. Routine laboratory tests are not specific. Chest roentgenograms, as noted previously, may be normal or may show peribronchial thickening, patchy atelectasis, segmental collapse or hyperinflation. The white blood cell count ranges from 5000 to 24,000 cells per mm.[3] In those patients with elevated white blood cell counts, there is a preponderance of polymorphonuclear leukocytes and band forms. A determination of hemoglobin level is not useful diagnostically but is helpful in assessing the effects of a decrease in arterial oxygen tensions.

Other causes of chest retraction and airway obstruction need to be excluded by careful physical and radiographic examination (Wright and Beem, 1965). These include obstruction of the nasopharynx by hypertrophied adenoids or a retropharyngeal abscess; laryngeal obstruction caused by abnormalities of the larynx, croup or a foreign body; or lobar emphysema. Occasionally, the hyperpnea of metabolic disorders such as salicylate poisoning may mask as bronchiolitis. Measurements of arterial blood gas tensions, pH, salicylate level (if the history is positive for salicylate administration) and serum electrolytes aid in making the proper diagnosis. Congestive heart failure secondary to a congenital malformation or viral myocarditis may present with clinical findings very similar to those of bronchiolitis, and a palpable liver and spleen found frequently in infants with bronchiolitis may contribute to the confusion. A past history of normal growth and development and the absence of a cardiac murmur assist in the diagnosis. Cardiac size should be evaluated on chest roentgenogram, and in case of doubt, an electrocardiogram should be obtained. However, infants with cardiac disease often develop congestive heart failure during viral infections, and the two conditions may coexist.

Certainty of diagnosis requires the use of immunofluorescent or virus isolation techniques, and these should be made more widely available. Immuno-fluorescent techniques applied to nasal aspirates have led to the diagnosis of RS in 78 per cent of infants hospitalized with bronchiolitis; results are available within 24 hours (Cradock-Watson and coworkers, 1971). Improved methods of obtaining nasal washings and bedside inoculation of the specimen provide equally high rates of virus identification (Hall and Douglas, 1975); results are available within four days. The increasing availability of such techniques should lead to a specific diagnosis in a large proportion of cases.

Treatment

At the present time, there is no specific therapy for the viral infection that is the cause of most cases of bronchiolitis or for the airway obstruction that results. The major aims of treatment are to support the infant, to detect possible complications and to protect other infants in the environment.

Since the virus is shed for days following the onset of the illness (Hall and coworkers, 1975a) and hospital-acquired infection is common (Hall and coworkers, 1975b), most infants should be nursed in isolation or, at the least, in surroundings where careful attention is given to handwashing and the prevention of child-to-child contact. Infants who are moderately or severely ill should be in a unit where they can be carefully observed with the aid of monitoring devices. The increased availability of monitors of respiratory and heart rates makes it possible to respond immediately if apnea, slowing of respiratory rate or increasing heart rate occur.

The major consequence of the airway obstruction and concomitant maldistribution of ventilation and perfusion is hypoxemia. Oxygen should be administered to infants with all but the mildest illnesses. Any techniques familiar to the nursing personnel may be used, provided that the oxygen is humidified and the flow rate of gas through the device is sufficient to prevent accumula-

tion of carbon dioxide. The inspired oxygen concentration must be monitored frequently. Concentrations of 35 to 40 per cent have been found to correct the arterial hypoxemia in most, but not all, infants (Reynolds, 1963a; H. Simpson and coworkers, 1974). The administration of oxygen to infants with carbon dioxide retention (arterial partial pressures of carbon dioxide up to 69 torr) has not been associated with increased carbon dioxide retention (H. Simpson and coworkers, 1974). In infants with no history of chronic obstructive pulmonary disease, oxygen can be safely administered without fear of significantly depressing respiration by blunting the hypoxic drive. However, a growing number of infants of very low birth weight are surviving respiratory distress syndrome of the newborn to be left with bronchopulmonary dysplasia of variable severity. Acute viral bronchiolitis may present a special problem in such infants, since some of them have chronic compensated carbon dioxide retention. Further impairment of gas exchange may make them severely hypoxemic, but the administration of increased concentrations of inspired oxygen may be associated with further carbon dioxide retention because hypoxemia may be their major respiratory stimulus. Frequent measurement of arterial gas tensions is required in these infants.

Mist has not proved beneficial to any appreciable degree, since little water reaches the lower respiratory tract to liquefy secretion.

With fever, chilling or shivering, oxygen consumption is increased. Small infants should be nursed in incubators or under radiant warmers; care should be taken that temperature is controlled in oxygen tents or other devices used for the administration of oxygen.

The routine administration of antibiotics has not been shown to influence the course of bronchiolitis (Field and coworkers, 1966), and there is little rationale for their use. The limited availability of rapid diagnostic techniques to identify RS or other viruses, the uncertainty about the cause of the disease in small, acutely ill infants, and the concern that viral infection may predispose to secondary bacterial invasion are arguments used to justify the administration of antibiotics. In the desperately ill child, in the situation where there is more than the usual uncertainty about a viral rather than a bacterial etiology of the disease, and in the infant whose condition suddenly deteriorates, antibiotics are generally administered. Ampicillin is often the chosen drug. The diversity of bacterial organisms reported in cases of concurrent viral and bacterial infection (Zoller and coworkers, 1973) makes it imperative that tracheal secretions be examined by Gram stain of smears and by culture. Blood cultures should probably be obtained from all infants at the time of hospitalization and from any infant who is deteriorating and to whom antibiotics are to be given.

The role of bronchodilators remains controversial. The relative importance of mechanical obstruction secondary to edema, accumulated secretions and cellular debris and of potentially reversible smooth muscle contraction is unknown. Measurements of pulmonary resistance have been used to evaluate the effect of a sympathomimetic drug administered by aerosol, but consistent responses have not been obtained (Phelan and Williams, 1969). The variability and insensitivity of resistance measurements and the variable dose delivered make interpretation of these results difficult. Studies evaluating the use of the theophylline compounds or newer atropine derivatives in the treatment of bronchiolitis are not available. Atropine-like agents, phosphodiesterase inhibitors (theophylline compounds) and beta adrenergic stimulants may yet prove to benefit selected patients. At present, there is no indication to include them as part of standard therapy.

Initial studies of the treatment of bronchiolitis with corticosteroids suggested that these drugs might favorably influence mortality and morbidity. However, large controlled studies have failed to demonstrate any significant clinical effect (Leer and coworkers, 1969). In particular, infants with a family history of allergy responded no differently from infants without such family history.

On admission to hospital, some infants are dehydrated because of poor fluid intake and have mild metabolic acidosis. Intravenous fluids should be given with care. It may be speculated that in the presence of the large, negative intrapleural pressures required to overcome the airway obstruction, added demands are made upon the left ventricle. Furthermore, the negative intrathoracic pressures are probably transmitted to the interstitium surrounding the fluid-exchanging vessels, enhancing fluid accumulation in the lung. The uneven distribution of the airway obstruction may result in amplification of these negative pressures, further enhancing fluid accumulation. The details of these mechanisms are discussed in the chapter on pulmonary edema.

Course and Complications

Although they may appear extremely ill on admission to the hospital, most infants, given adequate supportive care, are clinically improved within three to four days (Heycock and Noble, 1962). By two weeks from the height of the illness, the respiratory rate is normal, and arterial oxygen and carbon dioxide tensions are within the normal range in most infants (Reynolds, 1963b). Radiographic abnormalities have generally cleared by nine days from admission (Rice and Loda, 1966).

However, the clinical course may be prolonged (Heycock and Noble, 1962). Approximately 20 per cent of infants have a protracted course with persistent wheezing and hyperinflation of chest, evidence of continued airway obstruction on physiologic studies (Phelan and coworkers, 1968a; Wohl and coworkers, 1969) and persistent abnormalities of gas exchange (Reynolds, 1963b). These abnormalities may persist for many months. In addition, some infants with proved RS bronchiolitis go on to develop lobar collapse (Rice and Loda, 1966). The cause of this is unknown, but the radiographic abnormality may persist for several weeks or longer.

The frequency with which bacterial infection is superimposed upon RS or other viral bronchiolitis is difficult to ascertain. In one study (Sell, 1960), *Hemophilus influenzae* was cultured from the nasopharynx of the majority of infants with bronchiolitis, but the relationship of this finding to the illness is far from clear. It is possible, but not proved, that bacterial invasion of the blood stream may occur more readily following the cellular disruption in the airways in bronchiolitis. Pneumonia associated with a variety of bacterial organisms cultured from the blood has been reported in a small group of infants (Zoller and coworkers, 1973).

Sudden clinical deterioration followed by apnea has been reported from several centers (Downes and coworkers, 1968; Phelan and coworkers, 1968b; H. Simpson and coworkers, 1974). This has occurred in infants in whom frequent monitoring of arterial gases did not indicate that progressive carbon dioxide retention was the cause of the apnea. At present, the cause of apnea remains unexplained, but upper airway obstruction may be a contributing factor.

Estimates of the number of infants who develop severe respiratory failure and require assisted ventilation vary, but approximately one-quarter of all infants and young children hospitalized with lower respiratory tract disease are sufficiently ill to require serial measurements of blood gas tensions, and approximately 3 per cent require assisted ventilation (H. Simpson and coworkers, 1974). Useful clinical criteria are decreased or absent breath sounds on inspiration, severe inspiratory retractions, cyanosis in 40 per cent oxygen, and decreased or absent response to pain. These criteria, in conjunction with an arterial carbon dioxide tension above 65 or 70 torr, may be considered indications for intubation and mechanical ventilation.

Pneumothorax and pneumomediastinum are rare complications of acute viral bronchiolitis, but have been reported particularly in those infants placed on mechanical ventilators.

Relationship to Asthma

Numerous observations have been made of the high incidence (30 to 50 per cent) of asthma developing subsequently in children who had bronchiolitis during infancy (Wittig and Glaser, 1959; Eisen and Bacal, 1963; Simon and Jordan, 1967). Bronchiolitis occurring in a nonepidemic setting had been considered by some to be closely related to asthma and unrelated to viral infection. Elevated levels of IgE are associated with atopic disease and with asthma (Polmar and coworkers, 1972). The relationship of nonepidemic or non-RS viral bronchiolitis to asthma was strengthened by the significantly greater incidence of elevated serum IgE levels in patients with bronchiolitis occurring during non-RS epidemic months than in those with bronchiolitis occurring during an RS virus epidemic. Recent work, however, suggests that those children with presumed non-RS virus bronchiolitis and high serum IgE levels may have infections caused by parainfluenza virus, since infants with proved parainfluenza virus bronchiolitis have elevated levels of IgE (Sieber and coworkers, 1976).

There is a strong association between proved RS virus bronchiolitis and the subsequent development of asthma. More than half of the children studied two to seven years following proved RS virus bronchiolitis have recurrent episodes of wheezing characteristic of asthma. However, it is highly speculative whether infection with a virus such as parainfluenza virus contributes to the induction of atopy, and whether, because of hyperreactivity of the airways, the manifestations of RS virus infections are worse in those infants who will subsequently become asthmatic.

Long-term Sequelae

In some infants, lung function studies remain abnormal for months following bronchiolitis. However, until recently it was believed that no residual effects of the disease persist into late childhood, except for a greater than expected incidence of asthma. Recent studies of 15 asymptomatic older children who had been hospitalized for bronchiolitis under the age of 18 months indicate that long-term sequelae other than asthma do exist. Ten children had abnormal arterial oxygen tensions, and detailed studies of lung mechanics showed the persistence of abnormalities in the small airways (Kattan and coworkers, 1976).

BRONCHIOLITIS OBLITERANS

A chronic form of bronchiolitis, bronchiolitis obliterans, has been described in infants and young children following infections with adenovirus (Lang and coworkers, 1969; Becroft, 1971; Cumming and coworkers, 1971; Strieder and Nash, 1975). The initial clinical presentation does not differ from acute bronchiolitis caused by the RS virus except that rhinorrhea is not a prominent feature and evidence for bronchopneumonia is more common. The infant becomes ill with cough and fever and goes on to develop dyspnea and wheezing. On physical examination, wheezes and rales are heard. The radiographic features are initially nonspecific and consist of peribronchial thickening and increased interstitial markings with areas of patchy bronchopneumonia. Collapse and consolidation of segments or lobes are common.

Characteristically, the clinical and radiographic features of the disease wax and wane for several weeks or months, with recurrent episodes of atelectasis, pneumonia and wheezing. Recovery assessed clinically may be complete, but approximately 60 per cent of children with documented adenovirus pneumonia or bronchiolitis go on to develop evidence of chronic pulmonary disease. Persistent atelectasis (particularly of the right upper lobe in young children and of the left lower lobe in the older child), bronchiectasis, recurrent pneumonias, generalized hyperinflation and increased pulmonary markings on chest radiographs, and the development of the unilateral hyperlucent lung syndrome are among the reported long-term complications of adenovirus infection, particularly types 7 and 21.

Little is known about host factors that predispose to this unusual form of bronchiolitis. Maternal antibody may be protective, since the disease characteristically occurs in infants older than six months. In Canada it is seen more frequently in the Indian population, and in New Zealand in Polynesian children, suggesting that racial or socioeconomic factors may be important.

In lungs examined histologically, abnormalities of large- and medium-sized bronchi range from hypertrophy and piling up of the bronchial epithelium to cellular infiltration of the wall extending to the peribronchial space, with destruction and disorganization of the muscle and elastic tissue of the wall. Fibrosis of the wall and surrounding areas occurs. The most striking changes occur in the small bronchi and bronchioles. Here, the mucosa is destroyed and the lumen is filled with fibrous tissue. Typically, the terminal bronchioles are occluded, and the distal respiratory bronchioles are dilated. The vessels are narrowed and areas of overdistention, atelectasis and fibrosis occur within the alveolar region of the lung.

Bronchograms reveal marked pruning of the bronchial tree, and pulmonary angiograms reveal decreased vasculature in the involved lung. These findings may be localized, as in those children who develop unilateral hyperlucent lung sundrome, or may be more diffuse.

These sequelae of adenovirus infections should be considered in the diagnostic evaluation of children who develop recurrent infections and fixed airway obstruction following what may be presumed to be severe viral bronchiolitis and pneumonia. There are few data to support the association of bronchiolitis obliterans with RS virus infection, and bronchiolitis obliterans should not be considered a complication of RS virus bronchiolitis.

REFERENCES

Aherne, W., Bird, T., Court, S. D. M., Gardner, P. S., and McQuillin, J.: Pathological changes in virus infections of the lower respiratory tract in children. *J. Clin. Pathol.*, 23:7, 1970.

Becroft, D. M. O.: Bronchiolitis obliterans, bronchiectasis, and other sequelae of adenovirus type 21 infection in young children. *J. Clin. Pathol.*, 24:72, 1971.

Beem, M., Wright, F. H., Hamre, D., Egerer, R., and Oehme, M.: Association of the chimpanzee coryza agent with acute respiratory disease in children. *N. Engl. J. Med.*, 263:523, 1960.

Brandt, C. D., Kim, H. W., Arrobio, J. O., Jeffries, B. C., Wood, S. C., Chanock, R. M., and Parrott, R. H.: Epidemiology of respiratory synctial virus infection in Washington, D. C. III. Composite analysis of eleven consecutive yearly epidemics. *Am. J. Epidemiol.*, 98:355, 1973.

Chanock, R., and Finberg, L.: Recovery from infants with respiratory illness of a virus related to chimpanzee coryza agent (CCA). II. Epidemiologic aspects of infection in infants and young children. *Am. J. Hyg.*, 66:291, 1957.

Chanock, R. M., Kapikian, A. Z., Mills, J., Kim, H. W., and Parrott, R. H.: Influence of immunological factors in respiratory synctial virus disease of the lower respiratory tract. *Arch. Environ. Health*, 21:347, 1970.

Cradock-Watson, J. E., McQuillin, J., and Gardner, P. S.: Rapid diagnosis of respiratory syncytial virus infection in children by the immunofluorescent technique. *J. Clin. Pathol.*, 24:308, 1971.

Cumming, G. R., Macpherson, R. I., and Chernick, V.: Unilateral hyperlucent lung syndrome in children. *J. Pediatr.*, 78:250, 1971.

Downes, J. J., Wood, D. W., Striker, T. W., and Haddad, C.: Acute respiratory failure in infants with bronchiolitis. *Anesthesiology*, 29:426, 1968.

Eisen, A. H., and Bacal, H. L.: The relationship of acute bronchiolitis to bronchial asthma—a 4- to 14-year follow-up. *Pediatrics*, 31:859, 1963.

Field, C. M. B., Connally, J. H., Murtagh, G., Slattery, C. M., and Turkington, E. E.: Antibiotic treatment of epidemic bronchiolitis—a double-blind trial. *Br. Med. J.*, 1:83, 1966.

Gardner, P. S.: Respiratory syncytial virus infections. *Postgrad. Med. J.*, 49:788, 1973.

Gardner, P. S., McQuillin, J., and Court, S. D. M.: Speculation of pathogenesis in death from respiratory syncytial virus infection. *Br. Med. J.*, 1:327, 1970.

Glezen, W. P., and Denny, F. W.: Epidemiology of acute lower respiratory disease in children. *N. Engl. J. Med.*, 288:498, 1973.

Hall, C. B., and Douglas, R. G.: Clinically useful method for the isolation of respiratory syncytial virus. *J. Infect. Dis.*, 131:1, 1075.

Hall, C. B., Douglas, R. G., and Geiman, J. M.: Quantitative shedding patterns of respiratory syncytial virus in infants. *J. Infect. Dis.*, 132:151, 1975a.

Hall, C. B., Douglas, R. G., Geiman, J. M., and Messner, M. K.: Nosocomial respiratory syncytial virus infections. *N. Engl. J. Med.*, 293:1343, 1975b.

Hall, C. B., Geiman, J. M., Biggar, R., Kotok, D. I., Hogan, P. M., and Douglas, R. G.: Respiratory syncytial virus infections within families. *N. Engl. J. Med.*, 294:414, 1976.

Heycock, J. B., and Noble, T. C.: 1,230 cases of acute bronchiolitis in infancy. *Br. Med. J.*, 2:879, 1962.

Kattan, M., Keens, T., Lapierre, J. G., Levinson, H., and Reilly, B. J.: Pulmonary function abnormalities in symptom-free children 10 years after bronchiolitis. *Pediatr. Res.*, 10:457, 1976.

Kim, H. W., Arrobio, J. O., Brandt, C. D., Jeffries, B. C., Pyles, G., Reid, J. L., Chanock, R. M., and Parrott, R. H.: Epidemiology of respiratory syncytial virus infection in Washington, D. C. I. Importance of the virus in different respiratory tract disease syndromes and temporal distribution of infection. *Am. J. Epidemiol.*, 98:216, 1973.

Kim, H. W., Leikin, S. L., Arrobio, J., Brandt, C. D., Chanock, R. M., and Parrott, R. H.: Cell-mediated immunity to respiratory syncytial virus induced by inactivated vaccine or by infection. *Pediatr. Res.*, 10:75, 1976.

Krieger, I.: Mechanics of respiration in bronchiolitis. *Pediatrics*, 33:45, 1964.

Lang, W. R., Howden, C. W., Laws, J., and Burton, J. F.: Bronchopneumonia with serious sequelae in children with evidence of adenovirus type 21 infection. *Br. Med. J.*, 1:73, 1969.

Leer, J. A., Green, J. L., Heimlick, E. M., Hyde, J. S., Moffet, H. L., Young, G. A., and Barron, B. A.: Corticosteroid treatment in bronchiolitis. A controlled, collaborative study in 297 infants and children. *Am. J. Dis. Child.*, 117:495, 1969.

McClelland, L., Hilleman, M. R., Hamparian, V. V., Ketler, A., Reilly, C. M., Cornfield, D., and Stokes, J.: Studies of acute respiratory illnesses caused by respiratory syncytial virus. *N. Engl. J. Med.*, *264*:1169, 1961.

McLean, K. H.: The pathology of acute bronchiolitis—a study of its evolution. I. The exudative phase. *Australas. Ann. Med.*, *5*:254, 1956.

Morrell, R. E., Marks, M. I., Champlin, R., and Spence, L.: An outbreak of severe pneumonia due to respiratory syncytial virus in isolated arctic populations. *Am. J. Epidemiol.*, *101*:231, 1975.

Parrott, R. H., Kim, H. W., Arrobio, J. O., Hodes, D. S., Murphy, B. R., Brandt, C. D., Camargo, E., and Chanock, R. M.: Epidemiology of respiratory syncytial virus infection in Washington, D.C. II. Infection and disease with respect to age, immunologic status, race and sex. *Am. J. Epidemiol.*, *98*:289, 1973.

Phelan, P. D., and Williams, H. E.: Sympathomimetic drugs in acute viral bronchiolitis. Their effect on pulmonary resistance. *Pediatrics*, *44*:493, 1969.

Phelan, P. D., Williams, H. E., and Freeman, M.: The disturbances of ventilation in acute viral bronchiolitis. *Aust. Paediatr. J.*, *4*:96, 1968a.

Phelan, P. D., Williams, H. E., Stocks, J. G., and Freeman, M.: Artificial ventilation in the management of respiratory insufficiency in acute bronchiolitis. *Aust. Paediatr. J.*, *4*:223, 1968b.

Polmar, S. H., Robinson, L. D., and Minnefor, A. B.: Immunoglobulin E in bronchiolitis. *Pediatrics*, *50*:279, 1972.

Reilly, C. M., Stokes, J., McClelland, L., Cornfield, D., Hamparian, V. V., Ketler, A., and Hilleman, M. R.: Studies of acute respiratory illnesses caused by respiratory syncytial virus. 3. Clinical and laboratory findings. *N. Engl. J. Med.*, *264*:1176, 1961.

Reynolds, E. O. R.: The effect of breathing 40 percent oxygen on the arterial blood gas tensions of babies with bronchiolitis. *J. Pediatr.*, *63*:1135, 1963a.

Reynolds, E. O. R.: Recovery from bronchiolitis as judged by arterial blood gas tension measurements. *J. Pediatr.*, *63*:1182, 1963b.

Rice, R. P., and Loda, F.: A roentgenographic analysis of respiratory syncytial virus pneumonia in infants. *Radiology*, *87*:1021, 1966.

Rooney, J. C., and Williams, H. E.: The relationship between proved viral bronchiolitis and subsequent wheezing. *J. Pediatr.*, *79*:744, 1971.

Ross, C. A. C., Pinkerton, I. W., and Assaad, F. A.: Pathogenesis of respiratory syncytial virus diseases in infancy. *Arch. Dis. Child.*, *46*:702, 1971.

Sell, S. H. W.: Some observations on acute bronchiolitis in infants. *Am. J. Dis. Child.*, *100*:31, 1960.

Sieber, O. F., Riggin, R., Ryckman, D., and Fulginiti, V. A.: Elevation of serum immunoglobulin E (IgE) levels in infants with lower respiratory tract infections (LRTI) caused by parainfluenza viruses (PV). *Am. Rev. Resp. Dis.*, *113*:39, 1976.

Simon, G., and Jordan, W. S.: Infections and allergic aspects of bronchiolitis. *J. Pediatr.*, *70*:533, 1967.

Simpson, H., Matthew, D. J., Inglis, J. M., and George, E. L.: Virological findings and blood gas tensions in acute lower respiratory tract infections in children. *Br. Med. J.*, *2*:629, 1974.

Simpson, W., Hacking, P. M., Court, S. D. M., and Gardner, P. S.: The radiological findings in respiratory syncytial virus infection in children. II. The correlation of radiological categories with clinical and virological findings. *Pediatr. Radiol.*, *2*:155, 1974.

Strieder, D. J., and Nash, G.: Case records of the Massachusetts General Hospital. *N. Engl. J. Med.*, *292*:634, 1975.

Wittig, H. J., Cranford, N. J., and Glaser, J.: The relationship between bronchiolitis and childhood asthma. *J. Allergy*, *30*:20, 1959.

Wohl, M. E. B., Stigol, L. C., and Mead, J.: Resistance of the total respiratory system in healthy infants and infants with bronchiolitis. *Pediatrics*, *43*:495, 1969.

Workshop on bronchiolitis, June 28–29, 1976. Sponsored by the National Heart, Lung and Blood Institute, Division of Lung Diseases, National Institutes of Health. Pediatr. Res., *11*: 209, 1977.

Wright, F. H., and Beem, M. O.: Diagnosis and treatment: management of acute viral bronchiolitis in infancy. *Pediatrics*, *35*:334, 1965.

Zollar, L. M., Krause, H. E., and Mufson, M. A.: Microbiologic studies on young infants with lower respiratory tract disease. *Am. J. Dis. Child.*, *126*:56, 1973.

CHAPTER EIGHTEEN

BACTERIAL PNEUMONIAS: GRAM-POSITIVE

Margaret H. D. Smith, M.D.

GENERAL CONSIDERATIONS

The past century has seen a fantastic and still ongoing development in our understanding of infectious agents and infected hosts, an understanding that has been further enhanced by the proliferation of antimicrobial agents in recent decades. The availability of more precise methods of diagnosis and treatment, in turn, has alerted us to the fact that there are many more varieties of infection than could have been identified even 20 years ago, and that types of infection vary from place to place and from year to year for reasons that are not always clear. Pneumonia is a case in point: pneumococcal, staphylococcal and tuberculous pneumonias have decreased in prevalence; pneumonias due to meningococcus, beta hemolytic streptococcus group B, gram-negative bacteria, anaerobic bacteria, mycoplasma, chlamydia and viruses are increasingly recognized. The clustering of very ill infants and children in intensive care units, the tremendous use of respiratory therapy equipment and the large numbers of immunodepressed and immunosuppressed hosts have promoted the appearance and nosocomial spread of pneumonia-causing organisms unknown in an earlier era when pneumonia was almost always community-acquired. Thus, pneumonias present a kaleidoscopic picture that could not have been anticipated, particularly for the pediatrician who is increasingly assuming responsibility for the care of adolescents in whom pneu-

monia takes on many features of the disease as seen in the adult.

This chapter will present, in a general discussion, features common to many or all kinds of pneumonias, including the role of viruses in pathogenesis, diagnostic procedures, metabolic disturbances and therapy.

Role of Viruses in Pathogenesis

The airway is normally sterile from the trachea down to the terminal lung units. Sterility is ensured by a complex set of lung defense mechanisms recently reviewed in detail by Newhouse and coworkers. Evidence is increasing that at least in the case of most bacterial pneumonias that arise by inhalation (as opposed to the hematogenous route), viruses may enhance the susceptibility of the lower respiratory tract to infection in at least four ways: (1) viral infection increases secretions and thereby promotes aspiration of bacteria-laden fluid into the lung; (2) it may decrease ciliary activity, which in turn diminishes the capacity of the lung to clear bacteria from the respiratory tract; (3) it may decrease phagocytosis and bactericidal activity of alveolar macrophages; and (4) it may reduce the immune response.

Diagnostic Procedures

Recent years have seen increasing dissatisfaction with the use of throat cultures for determination of the etiologic agent in pneumonia. While the older literature presented abundant evidence that the results of well taken

378

nasopharyngeal cultures correlated well with blood cultures and autopsy findings, they have somehow fallen into disuse. Throat cultures do *not* correlate well, and sputum is difficult to obtain even in young adolescents — hence the interest in new procedures such as countercurrent immunoelectrophoresis, lung tap and transtracheal aspiration.

Countercurrent immunoelectrophoresis (CIE) permits detection of specific bacterial polysaccharide antigens in body fluids such as serum, urine, pleural fluid and spinal fluid (in meningitis). The procedure can be carried out expeditiously, and antisera are available for *Streptococcus pneumoniae* (both pooled and monotypic), *Hemophilus influenzae* type b, *Neisseria meningitidis* and Pseudomonas. The amount of antigen present is roughly proportional to the severity of the disease, and antigen is not detectable in individuals who are merely carriers of respiratory pathogens. This technique deserves widespread use.

Diagnostic lung puncture should be seriously considered in the case of any severely ill child with pneumonia in whom a prompt and correct diagnosis is essential; in a child who has responded poorly to therapy; or in a child with some underlying problem, such as leukemia, sickle cell disease or known immunodeficiency, in whom treatment is apt to be difficult, even with a definite etiologic diagnosis. Lung tap may be carried out with a thoracentesis needle; care should be taken to enter a heavily consolidated area and not a hyperaerated one, in which case pneumothorax is a likely complication.

Percutaneous transtracheal aspiration has yielded reliable information on the cause of pulmonary infection in adults, but has been little used in children because of the dangers of complications unless general anesthesia is used.

Metabolic Disturbances

Low blood sodium levels have long been observed to occur in patients with pneumonia, particularly at the outset of the disease. Hyponatremia is accompanied by hypo-osmolality of the serum, high urinary sodium level, normal serum potassium and normal renal and adrenal function. This clinical picture, relatively well studied in adults but poorly studied in children, is probably responsible for the convulsions that occur not uncommonly in pneumonia in children. The cause may be increased antidiuretic hormone (ADH) secretion due to reduced intrathoracic blood volume, or possibly to the production of an ADH-like substance by the damaged lung tissue.

Therapy

Hospitalization is often advisable, at least during the first two or three days of illness, to facilitate diagnostic laboratory procedures, the parenteral administration of drugs and, if needed, fluid and inhalation therapy.

Antimicrobial therapy has become ever more complex with the changing patterns of antimicrobial resistance of the microorganisms, development of new antimicrobial agents and greater understanding of their synergistic and antagonistic potential, and better knowledge of drug incompatibilities in general. Protein binding and beta-lactamase resistance need to be carefully considered in the case of the penicillins and cephalosporins. In the treatment of pneumonias due to gram-negative organisms in particular, advantage should be taken of the ability of penicillins (e.g., methicillin, carbenicillin) to damage the microbial cell wall, thereby facilitating the penetration and enhancing the effectiveness of gentamicin given concurrently. Penetration of antimicrobial agents into bronchial secretions seems likely to be quite important in lower respiratory infections, but it has been studied inadequately in adults and little, if at all, in children with acute infections. A comparative study in adults of ampicillin, cephalothin and gentamicin shows ampicillin to yield a tracheobronchopulmonary exudate level equal to only 10 per cent of the serum, cephalothin 25 per cent and gentamicin 40 per cent. Doubtless, considerable advances will be made in the near future to clarify our understanding of the principles of antimicrobial therapy in respiratory infections.

Supportive therapy includes administration of humidified oxygen whenever indicated by cyanosis, restlessness or unsatisfactory oxygenation on blood gas determination. In patients who are unable to ventilate adequately because of pleuritic pain or carbon dioxide narcosis, assisted ventilation may be lifesaving. Occasionally, the administration of one or two doses of codeine or Demerol for patients with severe pleuritic pain or intractable hacking cough promotes sleep and better oxygenation. Rapid digitalization may be indicated to relieve cardiac failure. Abdominal distention, a result of partial paralytic ileus, can be serious; oxygen administration, a semi-sitting position, a nasogastric tube, a rectal tube, and heat applied to the abdomen usually help. With impending convulsions, hyponatremia should be looked for; if present together with other signs of inappropriate ADH response, fluids should be restricted and the use of hypertonic saline immediately considered. Measures to lower body temperature should be resorted to only to relieve cardiac strain or to prevent convulsions; then, a tepid alcohol sponge to reduce the temperature no more than two or three degrees Fahrenheit may be beneficial.

PNEUMOCOCCAL PNEUMONIA

Bacteriology and Immunity

The pneumococcus *(Streptococcus pneumoniae)* is a gram-positive coccus that grows readily in fresh meat infusion broth with added peptone, especially under reduced oxygen tension or in the presence of a reducing agent such as cysteine or thioglycollic acid; the addition of blood to the medium increases viability, probably by providing catalase to destroy the hydrogen peroxide that otherwise accumulates. Filter paper disks containing bile or optochin serve as a useful presumptive means of identifying pneumococci; dropped onto a blood agar plate streaked with a culture of *viridans* streptococci, they will selectively inhibit the growth of pneumococcus, but not of other similar streptococci.

Immunologic classification of pneumococci into some 80 types depends on the production by all virulent strains of complex type-specific polysaccharide antigens, which can be identified by the use of type-specific antiserums.* In children, types 1, 6, 14, 18, 19 and 23 account for 60 to 70 per cent of pneumococcal infections, according to recent studies by Austrian (1975).

Resistance to pneumococcal infection seems to be determined both by nonspecific factors, such as the mucus secretions and ciliary action of the intact respiratory mucous membranes, a lively cough reflex and phagocytosis, as well as by type-specific humoral antibodies that facilitate phagocytosis by combining with capsular polysaccharide.

Antipneumococcal antibody is present predominantly in the IgG and IgA fraction; both type- and group-specific antipneumococcal antibodies appear in human colostrum, often to a high titer. IgA group-specific antibodies have also been detected in the saliva of some individuals. Patients with pneumonia develop increased levels of IgM and IgG during convalescence.

Antipneumococcal immunity varies with age. The pneumococcidal power of whole defibrinated blood as well as the level of mouse protective antibodies is high during the first month of the newborn infant's life, owing to passive transfer of maternal antibody; rare or absent between one and 15 months, antibodies rise to a peak titer in late adolescence.

---

*Available from the Statens Seruminstitut, Copenhagen, Denmark.

Epidemiology

Healthy carriage of one or up to five types of pneumococcus simultaneously is observed in 9 to 19 per cent of the normal human population as compared with 50 to 70 per cent 40 years ago. Abundant evidence, however, attests to the contagiousness of pneumococcal pneumonia. Lobar pneumonia due to the same type in twins, transmission from mothers to newborn infants, outbreaks of pneumococcal pneumonia within families as well as spread to contacts outside the family, and both explosive and endemic pneumococcal infections in orphanages, schools and dormitories have all been described. Children appear to be relatively more susceptible than adults, as shown by a higher attack rate among children under four years of age. Seasonal variations are well known and appear to be similar in both adults and children, with March the month of peak incidence. Since seasonal variations in the virulence of the pneumococcus seem unlikely, crowding and antecedent viral infections are probably the determining factors in precipitating overt disease. The pneumonia death rate is higher in years of high influenza virus activity.

Pathology and Pathogenesis

Pneumococcal pneumonia can be readily produced experimentally in rats and dogs by promoting aspiration of infected upper respiratory tract secretions through anesthesia, or narcosis with drugs such as morphine or alcohol. Viral infections, which greatly increase the volume of nasopharyngeal secretions, are probably frequently accompanied by aspiration. If aspiration is indeed such an important factor in pneumococcal pneumonia, then the straightness of the right main stem bronchus may account for the greater frequency of right-sided pneumonia, and for the more frequent involvement of the right upper lobe in small infants who spend most of the time recumbent. Cardiac failure, nephrosis and inhalation of smoke or kerosene promote fluid accumulation in the bronchioles and alveoli and probably predispose to pneumonia in the same way.

The characteristic lung lesion in pneumococcal pneumonia, whether localized ("lobar pneumonia") or disseminated ("bronchopneumonia"), consists of an outpouring of edema fluid into the alveoli; enormous numbers of leukocytes and some erythrocytes follow, pack the alveoli, and ingest the bacteria ("surface phagocytosis"); opsonizing antibodies, detectable several days after the onset of infection, hasten phagocytosis, but are not a necessary prerequisite. Later, macrophages reach the site and remove cellular and bacterial debris. In the meantime, however, the process may have extended further within the same segment or lobe, or may have been spread by infected bronchial fluid to another part of the chest. The pulmonary lymphatics are probably involved early in the process; the lymphatics and the thoracic duct probably serve as the route by which pneumococci reach the blood stream in some 10 to 25 per cent of patients with pneumococcal pneumonia. The lymphatics are probably also the route of spread to the visceral pleura, which is frequently involved, reacting with an outpouring of edema fluid, followed by fibrin deposition which in some cases is exuberant. The effusion may be sterile; or, if bacteria are present, leukocytes and macrophages follow. Tissue necrosis is not a feature of uncomplicated pneumococcal pneumonia; hence, rapid and complete resolution is the rule, unless the pneumonia is superimposed on an underlying lesion such as an aspirated foreign body, or is accompanied by atelectasis or by a massive fibrinous pleurisy in which bacteria are trapped and protected from the action of phagocytes, antibodies and antibacterial drugs.

As lung tissue becomes consolidated, both vital capacity and lung compliance decrease, and blood flows in part through consolidated areas where it is not oxygenated. All of these factors, plus coughing if present, increase the work of breathing and the work of the heart. Even in the parts of the lung that are not directly involved in the pneumonic process, there appears to be an increase in lung rigidity. Often, also, respiration is impeded by pleuritic pain. The result is falling arterial oxygen saturation and rising carbon dioxide tension together with a heavy load on the heart.

Clinical Features

The onset of pneumonia in infants and children is usually preceded by a relatively mild upper respiratory tract infection of some days' duration, and occasionally by a purulent unilateral conjunctival discharge in which pneumococci can be demonstrated, or by otitis media.

In *infants,* pneumonia is often ushered in by an abrupt rise in temperature to 103 to 105° F. and a generalized convulsion, accompanied in some cases by vomiting or diarrhea. Restlessness, apprehension, flaring of the alae nasi, rapid, shallow, grunting breathing, abdominal distention, slight circumoral cyanosis, tachycardia with a pulse rate of 160 per minute or more, and splinting of one side of the chest are all characteristic of the full-blown picture of pneumonia. Cough is frequently absent. Percussion is rarely helpful because the lesions are often patchy in distribution, and the chest is small. Auscultatory findings may be misleading: on auscultation, suppression of breath sounds is frequently detectable, but the showers of fine rales characteristic of early pneumonia in older patients are not to be relied on. The breath sounds are often exaggerated on the healthy side and so bronchial in quality as to suggest tubular breathing; hence, *inspection* is greatly important in determining the affected side. Even over the area of dullness in an infant with empyema, the breath sounds are not, however, always suppressed, because of the relatively small size of the chest, the inevitable thinness

of the layer of fluid and the short path of transmission for the breath sounds. When dullness to percussion is readily detectable in an infant, pleural effusion or empyema should be suspected. Abdominal distention is frequent and, when severe, is a poor prognostic sign; moreover, it may be impossible to ascertain the presence of peritonitis. Enlargement of the liver is important to assess, since this is usually the earliest sign of cardiac failure; but it is also often difficult to differentiate clinically between actual enlargement of the liver and downward displacement of the liver due to splinting of the diaphragm. If the liver edge is palpable more than three fingerbreadths or so below the right costal margin, and if the heart rate exceeds 160, or if a gallop rhythm or embryocardia is present, it is wise to assume that cardiac failure is complicating the pneumonia. Stiffness of the neck often accompanies pneumonia in infants; lumbar puncture is then mandatory to differentiate meningismus (normal spinal fluid under increased pressure) from very early meningitis (clear spinal fluid that on culture, however, yields pneumococcus) or from overt pneumococcal meningitis.

Older children display a clinical picture more like that associated with pneumonia in the adult. The initial phase, with headache, fever, malaise and possibly gastrointestinal symptoms, is followed within a few hours by high fever, often drowsiness interrupted by periods of restlessness, hacking, shallow cough and maybe delirium. The facies is anxious and lined and may be flushed, often with a tinge of circumoral cyanosis and dry lips. Rarely the cheek on the side of the pneumonia lesion is markedly flushed and the homolateral pupil dilated.

The older child often complains of chest pain and lies on the affected side in bed, with the knees drawn up. Chest findings, even in older children, are not quite like those characteristic of classic lobar pneumonia in adults; suppression of breath sounds over the affected area, often with no perceptible change on percussion, and few if any fine rales characterize the initial stage in children. Later, during resolution, rales are often readily heard. A friction rub is rare in children. Chest pain, when present, is sometimes referred to the abdomen. If the right leaf of the diaphragm is involved, acute appendicitis may be suspected; sometimes the prostration, high fever and abdominal tenderness may simulate the picture of acute liver abscess. Subdiaphragmatic abscess, which occasionally comes in question in adults under such circumstances, is so exceedingly rare in children that it can almost be disregarded. Although the spleen is usually enlarged at autopsy in fatal cases, it is rarely palpable in children with acute pneumococcal infections. Rashes sometimes occur—transient patches of erythema, or a few uriticarial wheals, or a usually rather sparse petechial eruption. Herpes simplex, frequent in adults, is not seen in children. Jaundice, osteomyelitis, prolongation of the coagulation time, decrease in the circulating platelets during the acute illness and urinary chloride retention have all been observed in children.

The entire clinical course of pneumococcal pneumonia has undergone a great change since the widespread use of antimicrobial drugs. The initial diagnosis is often rendered difficult by the fact that the patient has received some drugs before the diagnosis of pneumococcal pneumonia is seriously entertained, but the dose may have been insufficient or the duration of treatment too short for cure. Once the diagnosis is suspected and effective treatment instituted, an abrupt drop in the temperature usually ensues within a few hours, with concomitant improvement in the patient's appearance. Only under exceptional circumstances (e.g., remoteness from medical care) would a patient nowadays run the five- to ten-day febrile course, usually with high sustained fever, characteristic of untreated pneumococcal pneumonia, whether localized or disseminated.

Laboratory investigation usually reveals a leukocytosis of 18,000 to 40,000 cells with a shift to the left. White blood cell counts of less than 10,000 per cubic millimeter are a poor prognostic sign. A slight anemia is often present, especially during convalescence, as well as transient albuminuria.

Roentgenographic Appearance

Complete lobar consolidation is not common in infants and children. The distribution of the pneumonic consolidation is more often "patchy bronchopneumonia." The bronchi and the interstitial tissues are not involved, nor are the hilar lymph nodes usually notably enlarged. The pleura, however, frequently is involved, although the pleural lesions are often obscured early in the disease by the shadows of the alveolar consolidation. Although the lung lesions often clear within a week or so, roentgenographic improvement usually lags behind clinical improvement, and the residual pleural changes may persist for weeks. Lateral as well as frontal projections are essential for a proper understanding of the pathologic process (Fig. 1). *Most important of all is for the physician to be sure that a technically satisfactory pair of films, obtained during convalescence, is clear;* i.e., that the patient is not discharged from follow-up with some underlying process such as atelectasis, foreign body or tuberculosis.

Diagnosis

The diagnosis is suspected on the basis of characteristic history, clinical picture and initial roentgenographic findings. It is confirmed by the recovery of the etiologic agent from the blood stream or, rarely, from empyema fluid. Isolation of pneumococci from the nasopharynx by culture, particularly if present in large numbers, is suggestive evidence. Direct smear of the nasopharynx or throat for recognition of the causative organism has been found very useful in adults and is probably so in children, but has not been

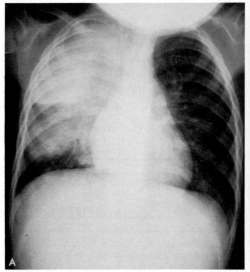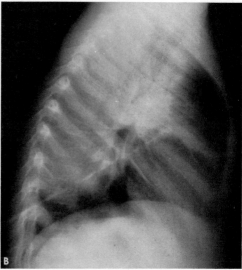

Figure 1. Pneumococcal lobar pneumonia in a four-year-old boy. Consolidation of right upper lobe and of superior segment of right lower lobe. *A,* Frontal view. *B,* Right lateral view.

widely used. The CIE technique, if available, should be used on serum and urine.

The correct diagnosis is substantiated in retrospect by the prompt response to antimicrobial drugs and complete roentgenographic clearing of the pneumonic process.

The differential diagnosis of pneumococcal pneumonia includes, first and foremost, pneumonia due to other infectious agents such as *Hemophilus influenzae, Klebsiella pneumoniae, Staphylococcus aureus,* streptococcus, *Mycoplasma pneumoniae* and the respiratory viruses. Acute pneumonia with splenomegaly should suggest the possibility of ornithosis or psittacosis, or of tuberculosis, particularly if the hilar lymph nodes are definitely enlarged. Endothoracic tuberculosis in children predisposes to secondary infection with respiratory pathogens, and it may be the latter that brings the patient to medical attention. Other underlying pulmonary lesions upon which pneumococcal pneumonia may be superimposed are atelectasis due to foreign body aspiration, bronchiectasis and fungal infections. If abdominal pain is pronounced, the differential diagnosis may include acute appendicitis or liver abscess. With se-

vere prostration and abdominal distention, acute peritonitis must be considered. In infants with convulsions or stiffness of the neck, meningitis may be present, either alone or in combination with pneumonia.

Management

The pneumococcus is sensitive to most of the commonly used *antimicrobial agents,* and particularly so to penicillin G, which is the drug of choice. The pneumococcus is, in fact, so sensitive to penicillin that the optimum dosage schedule is difficult to define. The effective dose is probably much smaller than that ordinarily used today; moreover, the interval between injections can probably be much longer. Injection of 25,000 to 50,000 units per kilogram of body weight per 24 hours, divided into four doses, of aqueous crystalline penicillin G intravenously or intramuscularly is recommended for the very sickest patients, followed by intramuscular procaine penicillin in a dose of 600,000 units daily. For patients who are not critically ill, aqueous procaine penicillin administered as above and, in addition, benzathine penicillin G in a dose of 600,000 units give a serum penicillin level that is bactericidal for pneumococcus for ten days without the drawbacks of frequent parenteral injections. Oral penicillin preparations, while frequently effective, are not always satisfactorily absorbed and probably should not be used.* Ampicillin is used in the treatment of pneumonia, particularly in young children, because it is effective in *H. influenzae* infections as well as in pneumococcal infections; however, the poor diffusion of ampicillin across the blood-bronchopulmonary barrier suggests the advisability of high dosage. Similarly, erythromycin in a dose of 50 to 100 mg. per kg. of body weight per day is effective against *H. influenzae* and most pneumococci, although erythromycin-resistant strains of the latter organism have been described. For this reason, erythromycin should be used for the treatment of pneumococcal pneumonia only in patients allergic to the penicillins.

Antimicrobial therapy should be continued for two to three days after defervescence and ?until clearing is present on the roentgenogram. Radiologic clearing, while rapid, may not be complete before two weeks and need not be complete before antimicrobial therapy is stopped. If pneumonia is complicated by otitis media, drug therapy must be considerably prolonged.

Complications

Otitis media, sinusitis (particularly ethmoiditis) and purulent *conjunctivitis* are apt to occur in association with pneumonia and usually clear simultaneously. *Empyema*, which formerly occurred in about 5 per cent of children with pneumococcal pneumonia, is now rarely seen; commonest during the second and third years of life, it should be treated in the same manner as staphylococcal empyema (see pp. 395, 484) and usually responds well. *Meningitis* should be considered in any patient

seriously ill with pneumonia, at any stage of the disease. Since meningitis requires much more intensive and prolonged therapy than pneumonia alone, lumbar puncture should be performed whenever stiffness of the neck, convulsions or other neurologic signs are present or whenever fever, irritability or leukocytosis persists. *Atelectasis* sometimes occurs with pneumonia, particularly in infants, and is due no doubt to plugging of a small bronchus by purulent secretion; it is best treated during the acute phase of the illness by appropriate postural drainage, physiotherapy and humidification of inspired air or oxygen, and should clear within a few days. If it persists, bronchoscopic aspiration is indicated and possible presence of a foreign body should be considered. Pneumococcal *pyarthrosis* and *osteomyelitis* formerly occurred in young children as complications of pneumonia, but in recent years have rarely been manifest in pneumococcal infections.

Fulminant pneumococcal septicemia and pneumococcal meningitis have been described repeatedly both in nonsplenectomized patients with hemoglobinopathies such as hemoglobin SS disease, CS disease and thalassemia and in patients splenectomized for any reason whatsoever. Common both to splenectomized patients and those with hemoglobinopathies is a marked and probably critical decrease in the mass of functional reticuloendothelial tissue, resulting in inadequate removal of bacteria from the blood stream. Although patients with fulminant septicemia rarely live to develop pneumonic consolidation, those with sickle cell disease are known to be particularly prone to all forms of pneumococcal infection including pneumonia.

Persons of any age with *sickle cell anemia* are prone to develop pneumonia, most often due to pneumococcus, often due to *Mycoplasma pneumoniae,* and sometimes due to other bacteria. Barrett-Connor (1971) has estimated the risk of a patient with sickle cell anemia developing pneumonia at 195.6 per

---

*See Chapter 13, page 332, for a somewhat different approach.

1000 patient years, as compared with 0.6 for the black population at large. Children under the age of three with sickle cell anemia have an attack rate of about 20 per cent, a major cause of hospitalization and death in this age group. Not only is the mechanism for removing blood-borne bacteria in these individuals inadequate, but opsonizing activity for pneumococci has been found deficient in the serum, related apparently to an abnormality in complement activation.

In the individual case, infarction may be impossible to differentiate from pneumonia without special radiologic techniques. However, infarction tends to be more common in adults, whereas pneumonia occurs much more commonly in young children. Also, infarction tends to involve a lower lobe, whereas pneumococcal infection tends to involve the upper and midlung areas. Because of the potential seriousness of pneumococcal infections in these patients, their frequency, the occurrence of fulminant pneumococcal sepsis and the tendency to slow resolution of pneumonias, prophylactic administration of oral penicillin on a regular basis is advocated by some. Polyvalent pneumococcal vaccines will, it is hoped, soon be available.

Prognosis

Although the death rate prior to chemotherapy was estimated at 20 to 30 per cent in infants, it was never high in older children and is now very much below 5 per cent.

Permanent sequelae of uncomplicated pneumococcal pneumonia do not occur. Delayed clinical or radiologic clearing is usually due to some underlying problem, such as a foreign body, tuberculosis, fungal infection, malignancy or infarct; to a mistaken diagnosis of pneumococcal pneumonia in which the patient is actually suffering from staphylococcal pneumonia; or to secondary superinfection.

MENINGOCOCCAL PNEUMONIA

Primary meningococcal pneumonia is increasingly being recognized in adolescents and adults, and one suspects that it must likewise occur in children. *Neisseria meningitidis*, if appropriately sought, can be found in increased numbers in secretions from patients with any viral infection. In three adolescent patients with pneumonia due to *N. meningitidis* group Y, Irwin and co-workers (1975) demonstrated good evidence of recent adenovirus or influenza virus infection. Bacteremia is rarely demonstrated, and inhalational spread is thought likely. There seems to be no distinctive clinical feature to suggest this etiologic agent. It can occur as a nosocomial infection, for example, in patients receiving clindamycin and gentamicin, to which it is resistant.

STREPTOCOCCAL PNEUMONIA

Due to Group A Beta Hemolytic Streptococcus

Infections due to the group A streptococci decreased strikingly in the 1940s and early 1950s; now they are on the increase again, but it is not clear whether the greater number of cases is due to the population increase or to some change in the characteristics of the microorganism itself. The incidence of streptococcal pneumonia is very difficult to evaluate. A 1942 report on 4849 cases of streptococcal disease seen in the pediatric service at the New Haven Hospital mentions 15 patients with empyema, but only one with "pneumonia." On the other hand, the Children's Medical Center in Boston admitted 93 patients with pneumonia between June 1958 and June 1959; 11 cases were attributed to the beta hemolytic streptococcus on the basis of positive cultures from nose, throat, pleural fluid or blood.

Streptococcal pneumonia, more often than other bacterial pneumonias, seems to complicate viral infections such as influenza, measles, chickenpox and rubella, or bacterial infections such as pertussis or pneumococcal pneumonia; or it may accompany other streptococcal illnesses such as pharyngitis or scarlet fever.

The salient pathologic changes comprise necrosis of the mucosa of the tracheobronchial passages with formation of ragged ulcers, thickened bronchioles filled with exudate, and patchy hemorrhagic interstitial bronchopneumonia, often symmetric, with extensive involvement of lymphatic channels both toward the draining lymph nodes and toward the pleural surfaces. Owing presumably to the production of streptokinase by group A streptococci, streptococcal exudates have a low fibrin content as compared with pneumococcal exudates; the very liquid consistency of streptococcal exudate is further assured by the deoxyribonucleases produced by these organisms.

The *clinical features* of streptococcal pneumonia are extremely variable. The onset may be sudden and accompanied by chills and pleuritic pain, or the disease may start as an insidious exacerbation of an underlying process, with gradual rise in fever and intensification of cough. A scarlatiniform rash or purpuric lesions of the extremities are rarely present. Empyema accompanied the pneumonia in six of 11 children reported by Kevy and Lowe (1961), and 16 of 55 patients of all ages described by Keefer and associates (1941). The white blood cell count varies in reported cases from 7000 to 59,000 per cubic milliliter. Bacteremia occurs in perhaps 10 per cent of the patients, mainly in the severely ill ones.

The *roentgenologic picture* (Fig. 2) closely resembles that seen in pneumonia due to *Mycoplasma pneumoniae* or *Staphylococcus aureus;* even the pneumatoceles described in the latter are occasionally found. Enlargement of the hilar lymph nodes can be striking, especially in young children, a feature that is not shared with pneumococcal pneumonia.

Diagnosis is established by the recovery of the beta hemolytic streptococcus

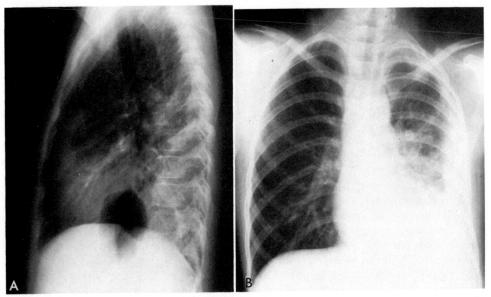

Figure 2. Pneumonia and accompanying empyema due to beta hemolytic streptococcus, group A.

group A from nose and throat cultures, from empyema fluid if present, or occasionally from the blood. Useful in retrospect, or as an adjunct, is a rise in the antistreptolysin-O titer; it does not, however, occur so regularly in the very young child as in the older one.

The mainstay of *treatment* is aqueous penicillin G administered parenterally at first, with rather prolonged oral administration during convalescence to prevent relapse. Erythromycin, clindamycin and the cephalosporins are all satisfactory alternative drugs for patients who are sensitive to penicillin.

Due to Group B Beta Hemolytic Streptococcus

Since 1971, group B beta hemolytic streptococcal infection has become increasingly important as a cause of mortality and serious morbidity among neonates, and has in many centers displaced gram-negative rods as the foremost pathogen in this age group.

Group B streptococcal infection occurs either in newborns less than five days old as an intrapartum infection, or in neonates up to six weeks of age. As an intrapartum infection, it is associated with maternal predisposing factors, such as prolonged rupture of membranes, maternal infection and low birth weight; approximately one-third of these infections are due to type I strains, one-third to type II strains, and one-third to type III strains. Occurring in neonates up to six weeks of age, the infection is due almost exclusively to type III strains, presenting most often as meningitis and probably in many cases due to nosocomial infection.

Neither in the "early onset" group nor in the "late onset" group is pneumonia the commonest clinical manifestation. However, in "early onset" disease particularly, extensive pulmonary changes are noted. Ablow and coworkers (1976) found that four out of eight fatal cases of group B infection displayed radiographic and clinical features compatible with neonatal pneumonia. The problem in these patients is to distinguish group B pneumonia from respiratory distress syndrome. In the individual case, greater likelihood of group B infection is suggested by the presence of prolonged rupture of the membranes in the mother, gram-positive cocci in the gastric aspirate, apnea and shock in the first 24 hours of life and lower peak inspiratory pressures on a volume-cycled respirator. The radiographic features of respiratory distress syndrome usually cannot be differentiated from group B streptococcal infection.

Clinical findings are those of a fulminant infection with apnea, hypoxia and hypercapnia. The mortality is very high; at autopsy, the pulmonary lesions may be patchy or extensive, often with many cocci on bacterial stains, but little inflammatory reaction. Empyema has been reported at least once.

Treatment should certainly include large doses of penicillin, to which all strains are sensitive. Since penicillin-aminoglycoside synergism has been demonstrated for streptococcus group D, it would be logical to add gentamicin, streptomycin or kanamycin. Numerous recurrences of infection have been reported after successful treatment, perhaps due to reinfection, and prolonged treatment seems warranted.

STAPHYLOCOCCAL PNEUMONIA

Bacteriology and Immunity

Staphylococcus aureus and *Staphylococcus epidermidis* are the two species which constitute a genus within the family of Micrococcaceae. Although mucoid, encapsulated strains have been described, they are rare, and encapsulation seems unrelated to pathogenicity. Able to grow readily on conventional culture media, *Staphylococcus aureus* frequently produces clear hemolysis on media containing blood. L-forms have been described; of practical importance may be the fact that these forms can develop in the presence of high concentrations of the penicillins; on the other hand, they tend to be more sensitive than the parent forms to erythromycin and clindamycin.

Typing of *Staphylococcus aureus* has been attempted by serologic differentiation of strains; unfortunately, because of the multiplicity of antigens produced and their overlap, this approach to classification has proved disappointing. Identification is usually by "bacteriophage typing," in which susceptibility to a standard set of four groups of lytic phages (each group containing one to nine phages), plus two "miscellaneous" ungrouped phages, is determined. Determination of antimicrobial sensitivity patterns may be a useful epidemiologic adjunct to phage typing.

Coagulase formation characterizes almost all pathogenic strains of *Staphylococcus aureus,* whereas nonpathogenic strains rarely display this property. Free staphylocoagulase interacts with a "coagulase-reacting factor" present in plasma to produce an active principle similar to thrombin. Coagulase-reacting factor levels are notably lower in children than in adults, and lower also in certain disease states such as viral pneumonia and infectious hepatitis. Several antigenically distinct coagulases have been described. Anticoagulases are found in the serums of children recovering from staphylococcal infections, as well as in monkeys after experimental infection. Active immunization with coagulase has been thought to confer some protection against staphylococcal disease in rabbits, but the role of coagulases and anticoagulases in human infection is far from clear. Other substances isolated from staphylococci include at least three hemolysins; also a "lethal toxin" and an enterotoxin; and leukocytotoxic substances, hyaluronidase and staphylokinase. Many strains produce penicillinase, an enzyme that opens the beta-lactam ring of the penicillin molecule; penicillinase production is increased not only by the presence of the penicillin substrate, but also by exposure to some of the synthetic penicillins. Relative resistance to phagocytosis characterizes many strains of *Staphylococcus aureus;* many, if phagocytized, survive long periods of time within leukocytes, protected from antimicrobial drugs and possible immune substances within the surrounding body fluids. In this respect, their behavior differs markedly from that of pneumococcus and *Klebsiella pneumoniae.* Although it is difficult to define the antistaphylococcal antibodies responsible for immunity, the falling incidence of staphylococcal pneumonia and sepsis with increasing age certainly suggests that immunity is important; in most reported series of staphylococcal pneumonia and empyema in children, some 30 per cent occur in infants three months of age or less, and 60 to 70 per cent in children under one year. Not only the incidence, but also the relative mortality, is much higher in infants.

Epidemiology and Pathogenesis

Staphylococcal infections, epidemic in the latter part of the nineteenth century and again in the 1950s, particularly in newborn nurseries and in older individuals in contact with newborns, have once more diminished in relative importance for reasons entirely unknown.

Transmission can be by the air-borne route or by direct personal contact, especially by the hands of personnel. Respiratory viruses seem to favor transmission of *Staphylococcus aureus,* and seem also to precipitate overt disease; epidemics of influenza in particular have long been associated with staphylococcal pneumonia.

Staphylococcal pneumonia can occur as a primary "bronchogenic" infection of the upper respiratory tract, seemingly alone, although it is not clear how often it is really concomitant with a viral infection. Staphylococcal pneumonia can also complicate measles, chickenpox or cystic fibrosis. In 15 to 20 per cent of cases, septic lung lesions arise secondary to staphylococcal infection elsewhere in the body.

There are few descriptions of the pathologic findings in staphylococcal pneumonias in children. MacGregor (1936) studied ten cases in the prechemotherapy era. Characteristic were "one or more areas of massive consolidation, sharply defined, intensely hemorrhagic." There was a "strong tendency to suppuration, especially in the bronchi, where the walls were destroyed." Grumbach and Blondet (1956) studied an infant who died after several weeks of penicillin treatment and found bullous cavities lined with a thick, pearly, connective tissue membrane; they demonstrated a tiny bronchial fistula plugged with mucus, and epithelialization of the interior of the communicating cavity. Elsewhere, a bronchus opened widely into the bullous cavity through a necrotic stoma. They postulated the development of a necrotic staphylococcal lesion, characteristic of staphylococcal lesions wherever they occur in the body, which either disappears by healing, with development of a bulla in the area left vacant, or by a tearing of the weakened area by the neighboring elastic traction of the normal lung. That some bullae collapse and heal rapidly, whereas others remain distended for long periods of time, may depend on whether or not epithelialization of the cavity takes place from the adjacent bronchus. Brown and associates (1963) believed that the annular or elliptical shadows often seen in staphylococcal pneumonia are "small Staph. abscesses and that the cystic spaces are the same lesions in their natural course of cavitation, thinning and ultimate disappearance." Hay (1960), however, suggested that these lesions are septic infarcts and that the annular lesions are due to cyst formation from "obstructive emphysema."

Experimental staphylococcal pneumonia of the "secondary" type, produced in rabbits by intravenous injection of *Staphylococcus aureus* cultures from patients, was studied by Herbenval and Debry (1956). Here, the fundamental lesion is a microbial arterial embolus, which may develop as a "cuff" near an arteriole and may rupture because of pressure changes in the surrounding air, with an implosion of pus into the surrounding tissues. It may bear no relation to a bronchus, or if the lesion should arise adjacent to a bronchus, there may be bronchial necrosis; there may be infarction of a blood vessel.

The importance of widespread, nonsuppurative vascular lesions described in staphylococcal septicemia should not be overlooked. Consisting of focal hemorrhages, fibrin thrombi in blood vessels, infarction with arterial or venous occlusion and renal cortical necrosis, they undoubtedly account in large part for the shock and prostration seen especially in older children.

In summary, the available data from human and experimental sources suggest that *Staphylococcus aureus*, whether it reaches the lung through the tracheobronchial tree or by way of the blood stream, gives rise to typical lesions either in the bronchial wall (in which case plugging of the bronchus by pus may occur, or evacuation of the abscess into the bronchus, or a bronchial fistula into the lung), or in a blood vessel (with subsequent infarction or implosion of the abscess into lung tissue), or in the lung tissue itself. The characteristic bullous lesions, pneumatoceles or abscesses that have been evacuated into the bronchus are kept open by the pus and fibrin plastered over their walls, and later by epithelialization from the bronchus. Pneumothorax and pyothorax probably result from rupture of necrotic lesions near the pleura. Widespread vascular lesions, when they occur, may account for the extreme degree of shock and prostration.

Clinical Features

The clinical features of staphylococcal pneumonia are as variable as the foregoing discussion would suggest. Sometimes there is no evidence of predisposing disease, staphylococcal or other; sometimes the pneumonia is secondary to skin lesions, osteomyelitis, mucoviscidosis, hypogammaglobulinemia or treatment with immunosuppressive drugs. At the onset, a mild upper respiratory tract infection may lead to a clinical picture typical of pneumonia, with fever, cough and rapid, grunting respirations; or the course may be fulminating, with prostration, cyanosis, dyspnea, shock and excessively high temperature. In the 329 cases reported by Rebhan and Edwards (1960) from the Hospital for Sick Children in Toronto, 13 per cent had symptoms for only one day, 50 per cent for four days, and the remainder for up to six weeks; fever was the commonest symptom, followed by cough, dyspnea, evidence of upper respiratory tract infection, anorexia, grunting, irritability and vomiting. Physical findings are often misleading, especially in the smaller infants, in whom the breath sounds may be well heard even in the presence of a massive pyopneumothorax. Mediastinal shift may be noted, or it may be absent despite a large pleural effusion. Tachypnea and cyanosis may be striking and may seem disproportionate to the meager physical signs and roentgenographic changes noted early in the disease. Abdominal distention is often pronounced, and the liver is palpable below the costal margin, owing either to true engorgement of the liver itself or to its downward displacement. The leukocyte count in a series of 24 patients reported by Pryles (1968) varied from 2800 to 72,700 cells, averaging 24,100 per cubic milliliter; polymorphonuclear cells predominated in all but one patient. Anemia often develops rapidly. Bacteremia was present in 41 per cent of Forbes and Emerson's (1957) patients under two years of age and in 20 per cent of the older children. Pyopneumothorax may develop abruptly, with acute respiratory difficulty, shift of the mediastinum toward the opposite side, cyanosis and prostration; aspirations of air and pus by syringe may be lifesaving. The disease almost always runs a long and stormy course, the duration of hospitalization averaging a month or more.

Roentgenographic Appearance

The admission roentgenogram in Rebhan and Edwards' (1960) series of 329 patients disclosed involvement of the right lung alone in 65 per cent, and of both lungs in 17 per cent. There was infiltration in 83 per cent, pleural effusion in 55 per cent, pneumothorax in 21 per cent and abscess or pneumatocele formation in 13 per cent. Characteristic is the rapid change in appearance of the lesions at the start of illness; often minimal at first, even in an extremely ill child, they progress from small, focal infiltrative lesions with faint mottling or haziness of the parenchyma to patchy consolidation to pneumatocele formation to empyema or pneumothorax, all within a few hours. Pneumatoceles, true abscesses and loculated areas of pyopneumothorax may be indistinguishable from each other. Pneumothorax may arise spontaneously from rupture of a small subpleural lesion, or it may follow a diagnostic thoracentesis; it may be self-limited, or, arising from a larger area of necrosis in the visceral pleura that constitutes a bronchopleural fistula, it may steadily increase in size and constitute a so-called tension pneumothorax with great shift of the mediastinum (Figs. 3 and 4). This picture is seen particularly in early infancy, and sudden death may result. Although at the onset of the illness the patient often appears much sicker than the chest roentgenogram alone would lead one to expect, clinical improvement usually precedes roentgenographic clearing by many days or even weeks. The pneumatoceles in particular may persist as thin-walled asymptomatic "cysts" for several months.

Diagnosis

Staphylococcal pneumonia is a likely possibility in every infant under one year of age with pneumonia, and particularly in those under three months. Prostration, cyanosis and respiratory

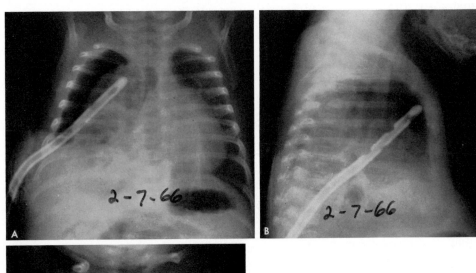

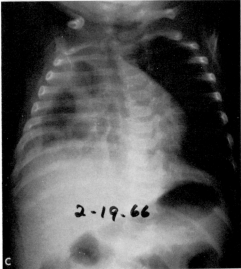

Figure 3. Staphylococcal pneumonia. *A,* Frontal view. Tube with waterseal drainage in place for six days. Persistent bronchopleural fistula and pneumothorax. "Swiss cheese" appearance of the basal segments of the right lower lobe due to pneumatoceles. *B,* Right lateral view. *C,* Diminished volume of entire right hemithorax, hyperaeration of the left lung, persistent pneumatoceles and pleural thickening. Patient clinically well, receiving orally antistaphylococcal drugs only.

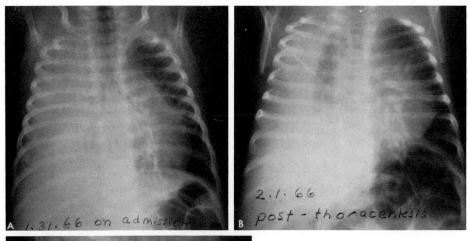

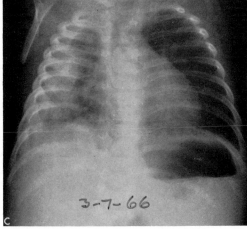

Figure 4. Staphylococcal pneumonia and empyema in a six-week-old infant, with mediastinum displaced to the left (*A*). Clinical signs of heart failure and respiratory arrest. *B*, Twelve hours later after removal of 200 ml. of purulent fluid with immediate dramatic benefit. *C*, At discharge. Further clearing of pneumonic and pleuritic lesions and disappearance of pneumatoceles.

difficulty with minimal roentgenographic changes; lower respiratory tract infection with total involvement of one hemithorax; pneumonia with pneumatocele or abscess formation, or pyopneumothorax are all typical pictures of staphylococcal pulmonary disease. In an older child with abrupt onset of prostration, shock, tachypnea and a temperature of 106° F. or over, staphylococcal pneumonia should be considered in the differential diagnosis (along with meningococcal bacteremia and Shigella infection). Severe cases of staphylococcal pneumonia and sepsis have been seen in adolescents with increasing frequency. Empyema that on thoracentesis yields pinkish or anchovy-colored pus is usually staphylococcal in origin, although the pus may be whitish or yellow. The presence of cystic fibrosis or of foci of staphylococcal infection elsewhere in the patient or his family may provide a useful clue to diagnosis.

To be considered in the differential diagnosis are pneumonia due to pneumococcus, *Hemophilus influenzae* (particularly in small children) or *Klebsiella pneumoniae;* progressive primary tuberculosis with cavity formation; aspiration of nonradiopaque foreign body with subsequent abscess formation; and diaphragmatic hernia with loops of bowel in the thorax.

The diagnosis can be immediately, albeit tentatively, confirmed by demonstrating clusters of gram-positive cocci in the pleural fluid obtained on thoracentesis, if fluid is present. Final diagnosis is established by isolating coagulase-positive *Staphylococcus aureus* from the blood, empyema fluid or lung puncture. Suitable specimens should be obtained and cultured immediately, before administration of antimicrobial drugs is begun. Determination of the sensitivity of the organism to *all* potentially useful antistaphylococcal drugs is an essential part of the initial bacteriologic diagnosis. Isolation of coagulase-positive *Staphylococcus aureus* in pure culture from the nasopharynx is highly suggestive evidence, as is also the presence of single or multiple abscesses or pneumatoceles on the roentgenogram of a tuberculin-negative child. Lung puncture or bronchoscopic aspiration is sometimes useful in confirming the diagnosis.

Management

Hospitalization is mandatory whenever staphylococcal pneumonia is seriously considered. Only in the hospital can the proper bacterial cultures of nasopharynx, throat and blood be obtained and studied for sensitivity to antimicrobial agents; and only the hospital is equipped to deal with the abrupt occurrence of bronchopleural fistula and the need for prolonged parenteral drug administration.

Antimicrobial therapy must be instituted immediately after cultures have been obtained. Numerous practical and theoretical considerations enter into the choice of the antimicrobial regimen: diffusibility of the drugs in tissues, serum binding, drug antagonism, persistence of staphylococci in leukocytes, microbial resistance and cross resistance, and possible importance of L-forms. Since it is in fact impossible to conduct controlled experiments on all these factors in human beings, there are inevitably almost as many recommended treatment schedules as there are treatment centers. Large doses of one or more of the penicillins are the backbone of treatment. A successful initial regimen in our experience has included aqueous penicillin G (50,000 units per kilogram of body weight per 24 hours, divided into four to six "stat" intravenous doses); methicillin (100 to 150 mg. per kilogram of body weight per 24 hours, also divided into four to six "stat" intravenous doses) (remember that methicillin solution is very labile and should be freshly prepared every eight hours!); and a third drug, usually erythromycin or clindamycin, which is administered parenterally at first, later orally. Nafcillin, cloxacillin, dicloxacillin and oxacillin are all effective antistaphylococcal drugs, but serum binding is greater than for methicillin. As soon as the pattern of the infecting organism is known, either penicillin G or methicillin is dropped, and the "third drug" is changed if need be. The cephalosporins, kanamycin, gentamicin and chloramphenicol are all useful antistaphylococcal agents that may be given, depending on special circumstances. Administration of at least two drugs effective by different mechanisms (i.e., a cell wall inhibitor, such as a penicillin or cephalosporin, plus a protein inhibitor, such as erythromycin) should be continued until the patient has been afebrile for a week, with oral administration of the "third drug" continued for at least two further weeks. Methicillin has been a very satisfactory drug for some years in the treatment of staphylococcal pneumonia, but methicillin-resistant strains have made their appearance; moreover, nephritis has been reported as a complication, particularly of prolonged administration.

Intrapleural administration of antimicrobial agents has never been shown to be beneficial.

Supportive therapy. The question of whether or not to use steroids has been discussed by Oleson and Quaade (1961), who observed that pneumothorax accompanied staphylococcal pneumonia in four of 19 adult patients treated *with* steroids, but occurred in none of the 26 patients who did not receive such drugs in addition to antimicrobial therapy. No satisfactory data are available with respect to children. Severe shock, however, accompanying acute staphylococcal pneumonia and sepsis should probably be treated with large amounts of intravenous plasma and hydrocortisone, perhaps also with chlorpromazine or dibenzyline, according to the best evidence available today.

SURGICAL CONSIDERATIONS. Shift of the mediastinum may supervene abruptly, owing to development of a tension pneumothorax, in which case removal of air by syringe may be lifesaving; or it may develop slowly, owing to collection of fluid or pus in the pleural cavity, in which case thoracen-

tesis should be performed; occasionally, shift of the mediastinum may be due to a large pneumatocele. In any of these situations, insertion of a chest tube combined with water-seal drainage often precipitates almost unbelievable improvement within minutes of insertion of the tube. The tube should be left in place, never clamped, and on continuous gentle suction (8 to 10 ml. of water) until bubbling and purulent discharge have ceased. Then it should be withdrawn a short distance each day. If in doubt, it is better to remove the tube rather than to leave it too long in situ, where it may serve as a foreign body and as a portal of entry for secondary bacterial invasion. Sometimes, while one tube is in place, a new lesion will appear (e.g., pneumatocele), requiring placement of a second or even a third tube; each lesion and each tube should be handled separately. Daily roentgenograms, including both posteroanterior and lateral views, are indispensable during the early phase of the illness in assuring that the tube (or tubes) is properly located and not kinked. Should the tube stop draining satisfactorily early in the course of illness, gentle irrigation with sterile saline may restore patency.

Resection of pneumatoceles and decortication are rarely, if ever, indicated, even though pneumatoceles or fibrothorax may persist for many months before clearing.

Prognosis

Although the reported mortality rate has varied considerably from one series to another, the deaths in well managed groups of patients at present probably do not exceed 10 per cent. The younger the patient, the graver the outlook. Long-term follow-up studies are few. Three or four years after a bout of staphylococcal pneumonia, resolution is almost always complete, with the disappearance of pneumatoceles and no apparent residual bronchiectasis. Hoffman, however, who carried out bronchograms on ten infants who recovered from staphylococcal empyema, demonstrated "minimal to moderate segmental dilatations" in one, whereas among seven older children he found one with gross bronchiectasis and two with minimal lesions.

REFERENCES

General Considerations

Glasgow, L.: Interaction of viruses and bacteria in host-parasite relations. *N. Engl. J. Med.,* *287*:42, 1972.

Hoeprich, P. D.: Etiologic diagnosis of lower respiratory tract infections. *Calif. Med.,* *112*:1, 1976.

Kilman, J. W., Clatworthy, H. W., Hering, J., Reiner, C. B., and Klassen, K. P.: Open pulmonary biopsy compared with needle biopsy in infants and children. *J. Pediatr. Surg.,* *9*:347, 1974.

Klein, J. O., and Gellis, S. S.: Diagnostic needle aspiration in pediatric practice. *Pediatr. Clin. North Am.,* *18*:219, 1971.

Lepow, M. L., Balassanian, N., Emmerick, J., Roberts, R. B., Rosenthal, M. S., and Wolinsky, E.: Interrelationships of viral, mycoplasmal, and bacterial agents in uncomplicated pneumonia. *Am. Rev. Resp. Dis.,* *97*:533, 1968.

Michaels, R. H., and Pozviak, C. S.: Countercurrent immunoelectrophoresis for the diagnosis of pneumococcal pneumonia in children. *J. Pediatr.,* *88*:72, 1976.

Mor, J., Ben-Galim, E., and Abrahamov, A.: Inappropriate antidiuretic hormone secretion in an infant with severe pneumonia. *Am. J. Dis. Child.,* *129*:133, 1975.

Newhouse, M., Sanchis, J., and Bienenstock, J.: Lung defense mechanisms. N. Engl. J. Med., *295*:990, 1045, 1976.

Rosenfeld, R. G., and Reid, M. J.: Letter: Inappropriate antidiuretic hormone secretion. *Am. J. Dis. Child.,* *129*:1105, 1975.

Selwyn, S.: Rational choice of penicillins and cephalosporins based on parallel in-vitro and in-vivo tests. *Lancet,* *2*:616, 1976.

Swartz, M. N.: Pneumonias: usual and unusual etiologies. *Ala. J. Med. Sci.,* *12*:369, 1975.

Wong, G. A., Peirce, T. H., Goldstein, E., and Hoeprich, P. D.: Penetration of antimicrobial agents into bronchial secretions. *Am. J. Med.,* *59*:219, 1975.

Pneumococcal Pneumonia

Austrian, R.: Letter: Pneumococcal vaccines. *J.A.M.A.,* *231*:345, 1975.

Barrett-Connor, E.: Acute pulmonary disease and sickle cell anemia. *Am. Rev. Resp. Dis.,* *104*:159, 1971.

Finland, M.: Recent advances in epidemiology of pneumococcal infections. *Medicine,* *21*:307, 1942.

Foy, H. M., Wentworth, B., Kenney, G. E.,

Kloeck, J. M., and Grayston, J. T.: Pneumococcal isolations from patients with pneumonia and control subjects in a prepaid medical care group. *Am. Rev. Resp. Dis.,* *111*:595, 1975.

Fraser, R. G., and Wortzman, G.: Acute pneumococcal lobar pneumonia: the significance of non-segmental lobar distribution. *J. Can. Assoc. Radiol.,* *10*:37, 1959.

Honig, G. R.: Sickling syndromes in children. *Adv. Pediatr.,* *23*:271, 1976.

Kabins, S. A., and Lerner, C.: Fulminant pneumococcemia and sickle cell anemia. *J.A.M.A.,* *211*:467, 1970.

Schonell, M. E.: Immunoglobulin levels in pneumonia. *Clin. Exp. Immunol.,* *8*:63, 1971.

Schulkind, M. L., Ellis, E. F., and Smith, R. T.: Effect of antibody upon clearance of I[125] labeled pneumococci by the spleen and the liver. *Pediatr. Res.,* *1*:178, 1967.

Whitaker, A. W.: Infection and the spleen: association between hyposplenism, pneumococcal sepsis and disseminated intravascular coagulation. *Med. J. Aust.,* *1*:1213, 1969.

Winkelstein, J. A., and Drachman, R. H.: Deficiency of pneumococcal serum opsonizing activity in sickle cell disease. *N. Engl. J. Med.,* *279*:459, 1968.

Wood, W. B.: Pneumococcal pneumonia. In Beeson, P. B., and McDermott, W. (Eds.): *Textbook of Medicine.* 13th Ed. Philadelphia, W. B. Saunders Company, 1971.

Meningococcal Pneumonia

Barnes, R. V., Dopp, A. C., Gelberg, H. J., and Silva, J., Jr.: *Neisseria meningitidis:* a cause of nosocomial pneumonia. *Am. Rev. Resp. Dis.,* *111*:229, 1975.

Galpin, J. E., Chow, A. N., Yoshikawa, T. T., and Guze, L. B.: Meningococcal pneumonia. *Am. J. Med. Sci.,* *269*:247, 1975.

Irwin, R. S., Woelk, W. K., and Condon, W. L., III: Primary meningococcal pneumonia. *Ann. Intern. Med.,* *82*:493, 1975.

Streptococcal Pneumonia

Ablow, R. C., Driscoll, S. E., Effmann, E. L., Gross, I., Jolles, C. J., Uauy, R., and Warshaw, J. B.: Comparison of early-onset group B streptococcal neonatal infection and the respiratory-distress syndrome of the newborn. *N. Engl. J. Med.,* *294*:65, 1976.

Anthony, B. F., and Concepcion, N. F.: Group B streptococcus in a general hospital. *J. Infect. Dis.,* *132*:561, 1975.

Broughton, D. D., Mitchell, W. C., Grossman, M., Hadley, W. K., and Cohen, M. S.: Recurrence of group B streptococcal infection. *J. Pediatr.,* *89*:183, 1976.

Katzenstein, A.-L., Davis, C., and Braude, A.: Pulmonary changes in neonatal sepsis due to group B beta-hemolytic *Streptococcus. J. Infect. Dis.,* *133*:430, 1976.

Keefer, C. S., Rantz, A., and Rammelkamp, C. H.: Hemolytic streptococcal pneumonia and empyema: a study of 55 cases with special reference to treatment. *Ann. Intern. Med.,* *14*:1533, 1941.

Kevy, S. V., and Lowe, B. A.: Streptococcal pneumonia and empyema in childhood. *N. Engl. J. Med., 264*:738, 1961.

Quirante, J., Cebellos, R., and Cassady, G.: Group B beta-hemolytic streptococcal infection in the newborn. I. Early onset infection. *Am. J. Dis. Child., 128*:659, 1974.

Steere, A. C., Aber, R. C., Warford, L. R., Murphy, K. E., Feeley, J. C., Hayes, P. S., Wilkinson, H. W., and Facklam, R. R.: Possible nosocomial transmission of group B streptococci in a newborn nursery. *J. Pediatr., 87*:784, 1975.

Staphylococcal Pneumonia

Brown, M., Buechner, H. A., Ziskind, M., and Weill, H.: Septicemic (pyemic) abscesses of the lung. *Transactions of the 22nd Research Conference in Pulmonary Diseases*, 1963.

Disney, M. E., Wolff, J., and Wood, B. S. B.: Staphylococcal pneumonia in infants. *Lancet, 1*:767, 1956.

Fisher, J. H., and Swenson, O.: Surgical complications of staphylococcic pneumonia. *Pediatrics, 20*:835, 1957.

Forbes, G. B., and Emerson, G. L.: Staphylococcal pneumonia and empyema. *Pediatr. Clin. North Am., 4*:215, 1957.

Gilbert, D. N., and Sanford, J. P.: Methicillin, critical appraisal after a decade of experience. *Med. Clin. North Am., 54*:1113, 1970.

Grumbach, R., and Blondet, P. L.: Etude anatomique d'une pneumopathie bulleuse extensive staphylococcique. *Presse Med., 64*:542, 1956.

Hay, D. R.: Pulmonary manifestations of staphylococcal pyemia. *Thorax, 15*:82, 1960.

Hendren, W. H., III, and Haggerty, R. J.: Staphylococcal pneumonia in infancy and childhood. *J.A.M.A., 168*:6, 1958.

Herbenval, R., and Debry, G.: Le poumon staphylococcique experimental. *Presse Med., 64*:542, 1956.

Hoffman, E.: Empyema in childhood. Thorax, *16*:128, 1961.

Huxtable, K. A., Tucker, A. S., and Wedgewood, R. J.: Staphylococcal pneumonia in childhood. *Am. J. Dis. Child., 108*:262, 1964.

MacGregor, A. R.: Staphylococcal pneumonia. *Arch. Dis. Child., 11*:195, 1936.

Mansbach, T. W., and Cho, C. T.: Pneumonia and pleural effusion: association with influenza A virus and *Staphylococcus aureus. Am. J. Dis. Child., 130*:1005, 1976.

Oleson, K. H., and Quaade, F.: Pneumothorax accompanying staphylococcic pneumonia in patients treated without steroids. *Lancet, 1*:535, 1961.

Pryles, C. V.: Antimicrobial therapy in staphylococcic disease of children. *Pediatr. Clin. North Am., 15*:167, 1968.

Ravenholt, R. T., and Ravenholt, O. H.: Staphylococcal infections in the hospital and community: hospital environment and staphylococcal disease. *Am. J. Public Health, 48*:3, 1958.

Rebhan, A. W., and Edwards, H. E.: Staphylococcal pneumonia, review of 329 cases. *Can. Med. Assoc. J., 82*:513, 1960.

Sabath, L. D., Garner, C., Wilcox C., and Finland, M.: Susceptibility of *Staphylococcus aureus* and *Staphylococcus epidermidis* to 65 antibiotics. *Antimicrob. Agents Chemother., 9*:962, 1976.

Shulman, S. T., and Ayoub, E. M.: Severe staphylococcal sepsis in adolescents. *Pediatrics, 58*:59, 1976.

Verwey, W. F., Williams, H. R., Jr., and Karslow, C.: Penetration of chemotherapeutic agents into tissues. In Hobby, E. L. (Ed.): *Antimicrobial Agents and Chemotherapy*. 1965, p. 1016.

CHAPTER NINETEEN

BACTERIAL PNEUMONIAS: GRAM-NEGATIVE

MARGARET H. D. SMITH, M.D.

PNEUMONIA DUE TO HEMOPHILUS INFLUENZAE

Nonencapsulated, so-called rough strains of *H. influenzae* are frequently present in the upper respiratory tract of normal persons, but appear to be of low pathogenicity. What relation they bear to the more pathogenic encapsulated strains a through f, and particularly to type b, which is responsible for almost all cases of frank Hemophilus infection, is not clear. A synergistic action between certain respiratory viruses and members of the Hemophilus group has been partially substantiated by the experiments of several investigators. Clinical observations during epidemics of influenza also suggest that simultaneous infection with *H. influenzae* and influenza virus may be more serious than infection with either alone.

Recent observations suggest that disease due to *H. influenzae* may be on the increase both in newborns and in older infants, and that this increase may possibly be associated with lower levels of circulating anti–*H. influenzae* antibody in the adult population. The precise incidence of *H. influenzae* pneumonia relative to other types of pneumonia is impossible to ascertain accurately; Honig and coworkers (1973) reviewed the literature, as well as their own experience, and estimated one in 2316, one in 900, and one in 833, in different series.

The pneumonia produced by *H. influenzae* may be either focal ("lobar pneumonia") or disseminated ("bronchopneumonia"). Microscopic examination of the lungs in fatal cases has shown circumscribed areas of consolidation, consisting mainly of polymorphonuclear leukocytes, with destruction of bronchial and bronchiolar epithelium, interstitial pneumonitis and hemorrhagic edema. The degree of edema produced by *H. influenzae* is often striking and is typified by acute epiglottitis and acute bronchiolitis caused by this organism. Neither on the basis of anatomic changes nor by roentgenogram or clinical picture, however, can *H. influenzae* pneumonia be differentiated with certainty from pneumococcal pneumonia. Some observers believe that the onset of *H. influenzae* pneumonia is apt to be more insidious; characteristic in the experience of others is a diffuse bronchopneumonia, accompanied by bronchiolitis and displaying on roentgenogram a "shaggy" appearance (Fig. 1). Pneumatoceles have also been seen in pneumonia due to *H. influenzae*. Infants are more often affected than older children, and seem more prone to bacteremia, empyema and concomitant pyarthrosis than older patients are, or than are infants in the same age group with pneumococcal pneumonia. Adults with *H. influenzae* pneumonia are said to display "apple green" sputum; discharge from sinuses and bronchi in older children with *H. influenzae* infection may also be green, but this is not a reliable diagnostic point. Prolonged, pertussis-like cough sometimes accompanies the disease. Leukocytosis is almost invariably striking (18,000 to 70,000 cells), with relative or even abso-

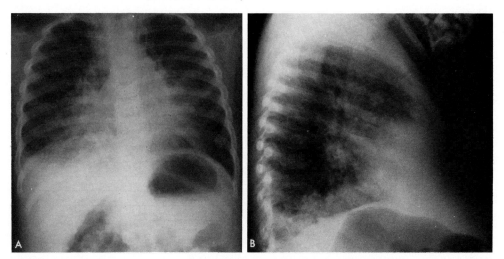

Figure 1. Pneumonia due to *Hemophilus influenzae*. *A*, Frontal view. Lobar consolidation of right lobe with overlying localized pleuritis (or small pleural effusion); also bronchitis and patchy bronchopneumonia. *B*, Right lateral view.

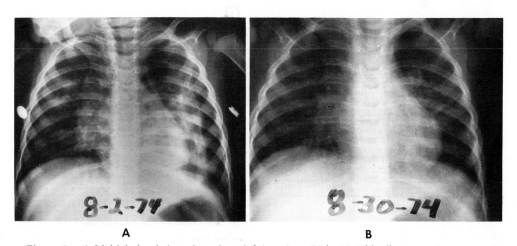

A   B

Figure 2. *A*, Multiple loculations throughout left lung in a child with *Klebsiella pneumoniae* pneumonia, *B*, followed by healing 4 weeks later.

lute lymphocytosis. The other features of the disease do not differ from those described under Pneumococcal Pneumonia (Chapter 18).

Diagnosis is established by finding *H. influenzae* in the blood culture or in the empyema fluid, if present. Very suggestive is the isolation of a near-pure culture of *H. influenzae* from the nasopharynx. Countercurrent immuno-electrophoresis is a relatively new technique that can be carried out with *H. influenzae* type b antiserum on blood, urine and, in appropriate cases, pleural or pericardial fluid; when available, it affords a quick and precise diagnosis.

Management includes the administration of appropriate antimicrobial drugs, including both ampicillin in large doses, i.e., more than 200 mg., because of the poor passage of ampicillin across the blood-bronchopulmonary barrier (see General Considerations, Chapter 18, p. 378), and chloramphenicol simultaneously because of the widespread occurrence of ampicillin-resistant strains of this organism. Initial treatment should be parenteral until clinical improvement, when oral preparations may be used for some five to seven days longer. Supportive therapy and the treatment of empyema are as described for Pneumococcal and Staphylococcal Pneumonia (pp. 380 and 388).

AEROBIC GRAM-NEGATIVE BACILLARY PNEUMONIA

Pneumonia due to aerobic gram-negative bacilli has become increasingly common in the past decade. While the increase has perhaps been more striking among adults, it has affected children also. Some of these pneumonias are "primary," occurring in patients with previously normal lungs; others are "secondary" to resolving primary pneumonia, occurring particularly as nosocomial infections. Several factors are undoubtedly at work:

1 The increasing number of children who are in fact "*compromised hosts*," surviving much longer than they did years ago because of modern methods of medical care. This group includes premature infants; children with cystic fibrosis; children with congenital anomalies of many kinds, especially cardiac and pulmonary; children with congenital immunodeficiencies or sickle cell anemia; children with malignancies and other conditions for which they are receiving immunosuppressive drugs, particularly while they are leukopenic;

2 The proliferation of *intensive care units*, where there is a dense population of patients at high risk, not only with some of the problems mentioned above, but also with shock or aspiration from various causes. Crowding and the type of care administered facilitate transmission of pathogens such as Pseudomonas, which are present in all hospitals but not in homes;

3 The close association that children suffering from the problems listed above must inevitably have with *doctors' offices* and medical outpatient departments, an experience that also exposes them to gram-negative pathogens rarely encountered by healthy children;

4 The widespread use of *antimicrobial drugs*, which upset the natural ecologic balance: only 2 per cent of normal individuals harbor gram-negative bacilli in the oropharynx, but this percentage rises sharply with administration of the usual antimicrobial agents.

The gram-negative bacilli involved are classified in two families: 1 the Enterobacteriaceae, which include Erwinia, Escherichia, the Klebsiella-Enterobacter-Serratia group, the Proteus-Providence group, and also others of lesser importance in pulmonary disease; and 2 the Pseudomonadaceae, including Acetobacter (formerly called Mima and Herellea), Moraxella, Alcaligenes, Flavobacterium, Aeromonas and Pseudomonas. Since these organisms differ widely both in pathogenictiy and in antimicrobial susceptibility, precise identification is useful; furthermore, correct speciation facilitates epidemiologic studies when these are indicated. The local hospital laboratory should be encouraged to send isolates to the State Health Department Laboratory, which can in turn rely upon the diagnostic laboratories of the Center for Disease Control in Atlanta as needed.

The *clinical picture* produced by the different gram-negative rods helps only slightly to identify the pathogen. *Klebsiella* pneumonia is well recognized in adults, occurring particularly in older people and in diabetics. In infants, its epidemic occurrence has been described in nurseries for prematures and newborns. The presence of copious, thick mucous secretion is suggestive. Cystic changes in the lung on roentgenogram, due to areas of necrosis like those which characterize staphylococcal pneumonia, are seldom reported, but they do occur in infants and adolescents, as in adults (Fig. 2). Bacteremia, empyema and residual pleural thickening have all been seen in association with Klebsiella pneumonia.

Pseudomonas pneumonia, due to *P. pyocyanea*, *P. cepacia* and other pseudomonads, occurs in general as a nosocomial infection in children hospitalized for serious underlying disease, particularly patients with cystic fibrosis or those under treatment for leukemia. Typical petechial and purpuric lesions, or tender areas of cellulitis in the perineal area, sometimes precede or accompany the pneumonia and suggest the diagnosis, as do also jaundice, enteritis and meningitis. Many of these patients are leukopenic from cytotoxic drugs. The very high mortality rate in Pseudomonas pneumonia treated with antimicrobial therapy alone (seven of eight patients under 15 years of age in Pennington's [1973] series), particularly in leukopenic patients, led to the trial, first in a dog model, then in patients, of compatible granulocyte transfusions as an adjunct to antimicrobial therapy. The results are encouraging.

Serratia marcescens is isolated most commonly from the urinary tract, rarely from the respiratory tract. The pneumonia that it produces is apt to be milder and more insidious in onset than are Klebsiella and Pseudomonas pneumonias.

E. coli, while responsible for 15 per cent of the fatalities in leukemic children, is not often a cause of pneumonia. Usually the organism is recovered from the blood stream, and the pulmonary lesions, if present, are a late manifestation.

The *diagnosis* of pneumonia in patients with underlying disease should be made as quickly and specifically as possible. Smears and cultures of the throat, if they show marked preponderance of gram-negative rods, suggest that these in fact play an etiologic role. Several throat cultures and blood cultures should be obtained at short intervals. In cooperative older children, transtracheal cultures should be considered. Lung puncture should not be too long deferred if the diagnosis cannot be established by simpler means.

Antimicrobial therapy, to be effective, depends on the results of identification and antimicrobial sensitivity of the organism. While awaiting the laboratory results, it is useful to know that at present (1976) the combination of carbenicillin and gentamicin is synergistic and effective against 70 per cent of *Pseudomonas aeruginosa* strains, and cephalothin and carbenicillin are effective against 70 to 80 per cent of *E. coli*, Klebsiella and Proteus strains, whereas *Serratia marcescens* infections are usually responsive to chloramphenicol and gentamicin. Amikacin is often effective against organisms resistant to gentamicin. All of these drugs should be used in maximal doses, since they do not pass well into bronchial secretions.

A useful way to *monitor therapy* is to maintain in subculture the original organism isolated from the patient, and daily test the bactericidal acitivity of the patient's serum against his own organism. A bactericidal serum dilution of at least 1:8 is usually considered to yield optimal clinical results.

Compatible *granulocyte transfusions*

(see above) should be considered for leukopenic patients with Pseudomonas infection.

In patients with abscess formation, as seen particularly in Klebsiella infections, transbronchial catheter drainage under fluoroscopic control has been found extremely beneficial in several cases.

REFERENCES

Pneumonia due to Hemophilus influenzae

Buddingh, G. J.: Bacterial dynamics in combined infection. A study of the population dynamics of strains of Hemophilus influenzae type b in combined infection with influenza C virus in embryonated eggs. Am. J. Pathol., 43:407, 1963.

Donald, W. D., and Coker, J. W.: Role of Hemophilus influenzae in respiratory infections of premature infants. Am. J. Dis. Child., 94:272, 1957.

Graber, C. D., Gershanik, J. J., Leukoff, A. H., and Westphal, W.: Changing pattern of neonatal susceptibility to H. influenzae. J. Pediatr., 78:948, 1971.

Honig, P. J., Pasquariello, P. S., Jr., and Stool, S. E.: H. influenzae pneumonia in infants and children. J. Pediatr., 83:215, 1973.

Jacobson, J. A., McCormick, J. B., Hayes, P., Thornsberry, C, and Kirvin, L.: Epidemiologic characteristics of infections caused by Ampicillin-resistant Hemophilus influenzae. Pediatrics, 58:388, 1976.

Michaels, R. H., Poziviak, C. S., Stonebraker, F. E., and Norden, C. W.: Factors affecting pharyngeal Haemophilus influenzae Type b colonization rates in children. J. Clin. Microbiol., 4:413, 1976.

Nyhan, W. L., Rectanus, D. R., and Fousek, M. D.: Hemophilus influenzae type b pneumonia. Pediatrics, 16:31, 1955.

Riley, H. D., Jr., and Bracken, E. C.: Empyema due to Hemophilus influenzae in infants and children. Am. J. Dis. Child., 110:24, 1965.

Sell, S. H. W., and Shapiro, H. L.: Interstitial pneumonitis induced by experimental infection with Hemophilus influenzae. Am. J. Dis. Child., 100:16, 1960.

Tillotson, J. R., and Lerner, A. M.: Hemophilus influenzae bronchopneumonia in adults. Arch. Intern. Med., 121:429, 1968.

Vinik, M., Altman, D. H., and Parks, R. E.: Experience with Hemophilus influenzae pneumonia. Radiology, 86:701, 1966.

Wald, E. R., and Levine, M. M.: Frequency of detection of Hemophilus influenzae type b capsular polysaccharide in infants and children with pneumonia. Pediatrics, 57:267, 1976.

Walker, S. H.: Respiratory manifestations of systemic Hemophilus influenzae infection. J. Pediatr., 62:386, 1963.

Aerobic Gram-Negative Bacillary Pneumonia

Crane, L. R., and Lerner, A. M.: Gram-negative pneumonia in hospitalized patients. Postgrad. Med., 58:85, 1975.

Dale, D. C., Reynolds, H. Y., Pennington, J. E., Elin, R. J., and Herzig, G. P.: Experimental Pseudomonas pneumonia in leucopenic dogs: comparison of therapy with antibiotics and granulocyte transfusions. Blood, 47:869, 1976.

Davis, J. T., Folte, E., and Blakemore, W. S.: Serratia marcescens: a pathogen of increasing clinical importance. J.A.M.A., 214:2190, 1970.

Groff, D. B., and Marquis, J.: Treatment of lung abscess by transbronchial catheter drainage. Radiology, 107:61, 1973.

Hughes, W. T., Feldman, S., and Cox, F.: Infectious diseases in children with cancer. Pediatr. Clin. North Am., 21:583, 1974.

Klastersky, J., Daneau, D., Swings, G., and Weerts, D.: Antibacterial activity in serum and urine as a therapeutic guide in bacterial infections. J. Infect. Dis., 129:187, 1974.

Marks, M. I., Prentice, R., Swarson, R., Cotton, E., and Eickhoff, T. C.: Carbenicillin and gentamicin: pharmacologic studies in patients with cystic fibrosis and Pseudomonas pulmonary infection. J. Pediatr., 79:822, 1971.

Meltz, D. J., and Grieco, M. H.: Characteristics of Serratia marcescens pneumonia. Arch. Intern. Med., 132:359, 1973.

Meyer, R. D., Lewis, R. P., Carmalt, E. D., and Finegold, S. M.: Amikacin therapy for serious gram-negative bacillary infections. Ann. Intern. Med., 83:70, 1975.

Pennington, J. E., Reynolds, H. Y., and Carbone, P. P.: Pseudomonas pneumonia: a retrospective study of 36 cases. Am. J. Med., 55:155, 1973.

Pierce, A. K., and Sanford, J. P.: Aerobic bacillary gram-negative pneumonias. Am. Rev. Resp. Dis., 110:647, 1974.

Sieber, O. F., and Fulginiti, V. A.: Pseudomonas cepacia pneumonia in a child with chronic granulomatous disease and selective IgA deficiency. Acta Paediatr. Scand., 65:519, 1976.

Stevens, R. M., Teres, D., Skillman, J. J., and Feingold, D. S.: Pneumonia in an intensive care unit. Arch. Intern. Med., 134:106, 1974.

Thaler, M. M.: Klebsiella-Aerobacter pneumonia in infants. Pediatrics, 30:206, 1962.

Waldvogel, F. A., et al.: In Klastersky, J. (Ed.): Clinical Use of Combination of Antibiotics. New York, John Wiley and Sons, 1975, pp. 90–108.

CHAPTER TWENTY

PNEUMOCYSTIS CARINII PNEUMONITIS

WALTER T. HUGHES, M.D.

Pneumocystis carinii pneumonitis is a unique infection of humans and lower animals with an unyielding penchant for the debilitated and immunodeficient host. Unlike other opportunistic infections of the compromised patient, this disease process and the causative agent remain confined to the lungs even in fatal cases. *P. carinii* was recognized as a cause of interstitial plasma cell pneumonitis of premature and marasmic infants in Europe during and following World War II, where the disease occurred in epidemic form. The first case of *P. carinii* pneumonitis in the United States was reported only 20 years ago. In contrast to the epidemic, infantile form in Europe, the American cases have been sporadic and have occurred in children and adults with some underlying disease. While the infantile form has become less prevalent over the past 15 years, the sporadic form in the United States has progressively increased in frequency. It is likely that more extensive use of immunosuppressive therapy and advances in medicine that have extended the longevity of patients with impaired resistance to infection account for the increasing prevalence of the infection.

Predisposing Factors

Underlying diseases related to the provocation of *P. carinii* pneumonitis have included: lymphoproliferative malignancies, solid tumors, congenital immune deficiency disorders, organ transplant recipients, Waldenström's macroglobulinemia, rheumatoid arthritis, rheumatic fever, Henoch-Schönlein purpura, thrombotic thrombocytopenic purpura, hemophilia, aplastic anemia, hemolytic anemia, Wiskott-Aldrich syndrome, nephrosis, hypoproteinemia and protein-calorie malnutrition; it has also occurred with some chronic infectious diseases such as tuberculosis, cryptococcosis and congenital rubella. It has been encountered in Vietnamese refugee children and rarely in otherwise healthy individuals.

The incidence of *P. carinii* pneumonitis has been related directly to the intensity of immunosuppressive therapy. Careful surveillance for two and a half years of a group of children with acute lymphocytic leukemia randomized in a prospective study to receive gradations of chemotherapy agents showed the incidence of this infection to be 5.0 per cent in those receiving only one drug for maintenance therapy; on the other hand, in those receiving four anticancer drugs, 22 per cent had *P. carinii* pneumonia. When mediastinal irradiation was added to intensive chemotherapy, the incidence of the pneumonitis was 36 per cent (Hughes and coworkers, 1975b).

Clinical Features

SIGNS AND SYMPTOMS. Two somewhat different clinical patterns may be recognized with *P. carinii* pneumonitis. Since one pattern has been predominant in premature and debilitated infants, it will be referred to as the "in-fantile" type.

In the infantile type the onset is usually slow, with nonspecific signs such as poor feeding and restlessness. Tachypnea and a peculiar cyanosis about the mouth and under the eyes may be the first signs of pulmonary involvement. Coryza, cough and fever are usually not present, and rales are rarely heard. Within one to two weeks, the respiratory distress has become severe, with marked tachypnea, flaring of nasal alae, sternal retraction and cyanosis. Sudden attacks of coughing may occur. Usually the duration of the illness is four to six weeks, and 25 to 50 per cent of cases will end fatally if untreated (Gajdusek, 1957). Infants between three and six months of age are most frequently affected.

The second type is encountered primarily in the immunosuppressed child and adult. Abrupt onset and fever are characteristic features here, in contrast to the infantile type. Other signs and symptoms are listed in Figure 1. The absence of rales is a usual feature. The natural course of the disease is one of a rapidly progressive course ending fatally in almost all the cases.

It should be kept in mind that either of the clinical types may occur in infants, children or adults and that patterns described have only general application. A fulminating, rapidly fatal course may occur in infants, and a subtle but progressive course may sometimes be encountered in adults and children.

ROENTGENOGRAM. The chest roentgenogram, with rare exception, depicts bilateral diffuse alveolar disease. The hilar areas are involved initially, with spread to the periphery. The infantile form shows interstitial infiltrate with hyperexpanded lung fields, whereas alveolar disease characterizes the other type (Fig. 2).

ACID-BASE AND BLOOD GAS PROFILE. Hypoxia with quite low arterial oxygen tension (Pa_{O_2}) almost always occurs; carbon dioxide retention is rarely present, and the arterial pH is usually increased. Concomitant with a decrease in Pa_{O_2} there is an increase in alveolar-arterial gradient and intrapulmonary right-to-left shunt.

NONSPECIFIC LABORATORY TESTS (HUGHES, 1975). The white blood cell count is usually unaffected by the infection. Although eosinophilia has been

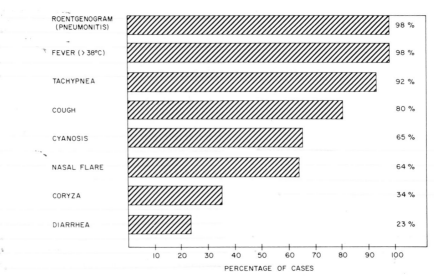

Figure 1. Clinical profile of 100 children with *P. carinii* pneumonitis and childhood malignancies admitted to St. Jude Children's Research Hospital. The diagnosis was made by lung aspirate, biopsy or autopsy studies. Bars indicate the percentage of patients with the respective abnormality at the time of admission.

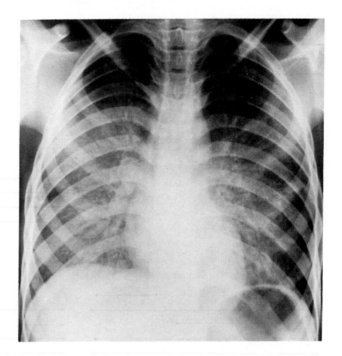

Figure 2. Chest roentgenogram showing evidence of moderately severe *P. carinii* pneumonitis. The pattern is one of diffuse alveolar disease with bilateral distribution. The superior portions of the upper lobes are usually the least involved, and the perihilar areas are the most frequently affected sites. Air bronchograms are discernible.

reported with *P. carinii* pneumonitis in sex-linked agammaglobulinemia, this response is the exception rather than the rule.

The serum immunoglobulin levels may be normal or decreased, depending on the type of primary disease. In the infantile form of the infection, the low immunoglobulin levels usually reached at the third to fourth month of age are believed to precondition the infant to intra-alveolar proliferation of *P. carinii*. When severe protein-calorie malnutrition is the predisposing condition, serum albumin values may be low.

Pathology

In fatal cases of *P. carinii* pneumonitis the lungs are diffusely involved, heavy and noncompliant and have the consistency and coloration of liver.

The histopathologic features of the infantile epidemic type differ from those of children and adults who are immunosuppressed (Dutz and co-workers, 1973). In the infantile form there is extensive involvement of the alveolar septae with plasma cell and lymphocyte infiltration. The septae may be five to 20 times the normal thickness. Up to three-fourths of the entire lung space is occupied by the distended septae. The alveolar spaces are also heavily infiltrated with organisms. In milder cases, often clinically undetected, *P. carinii* organisms are found in subpleural posterior alveoli with minimal focal interstitial plasma cell response.

In the immunoincompetent child and adult, the disease process is predominantly in the alveolar spaces with considerably less involvement of the alveolar septae than that seen in infants. The histopathologic features have been correlated with the extent of clinical disease (Price and Hughes, 1974). In "Stage I," isolated organisms are found adjacent to the alveolar wall or in the cytoplasm of the macrophage with no inflammatory response. These patients have no clinical evidence of the disease. In "Stage II" there is desquamation of alveolar cells containing organisms into the alveolar lumen with increasing numbers of organisms and minimal or no inflammatory response in alveolar septae. These patients may or may not have clinical evidence of pneumonitis. With "Stage III," extensive reactive and

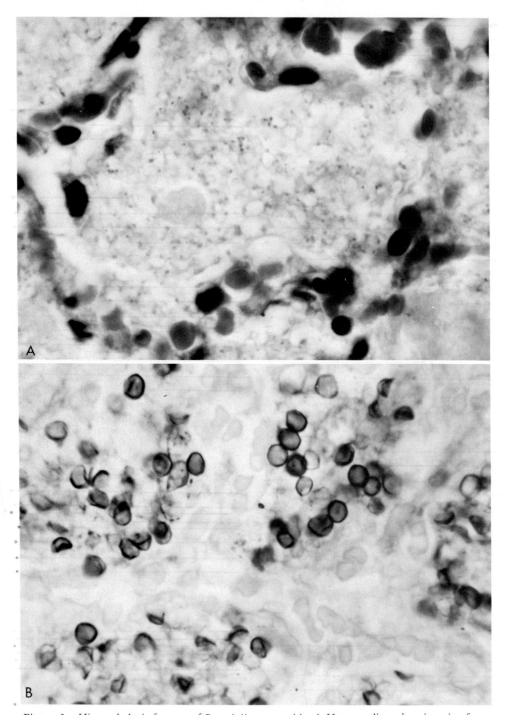

Figure 3. Histopathologic features of *P. carinii* pneumonitis. *A*, Hematoxylin and eosin stain of extensively infected (Stage III) lung. *P. carinii* organisms do not stain with H and E; therefore, the alveolar spaces appear to be filled with a pinkish "foamy proteinaceous" material. The alveolar septae are widened because of interstitial edema and lymphocytic infiltration. (Original magnification × 1180.) *B*, Gomori's methenamine-silver nitrate stain of the same lung section as *A*. *P. carinii* organisms fill the alveolar spaces. Only the cyst forms are stained. Cysts are 4 to 6 microns in diameter, brownish black, round, oval, and cup-shaped; two "nucleoid" parenthesis-like bodies may be seen in some of the organisms. (Original magnification × 1180.)

desquamative alveolopathy is found with large numbers of organisms within the alveolar cellular desquamate, and there is also extensive alveolar septal thickening with mononuclear inflammatory cells (Fig. 3). In this category all patients have clinical manifestations of pneumonitis.

CHARACTERISTICS OF THE ORGANISM. The taxonomy of *P. carinii* has not been established. The organism exists in three developmental forms, which represent stages in the life cycle. The largest form is at least 4 to 6 microns in diameter. This "cyst" form is rounded or crescent-shaped and possesses a thick cell wall. The cyst wall is readily impregnated with Gomori's methenamine silver nitrate (Fig. 4 *A*) or toluidine blue O stains (Fig. 4 *B*), but does not take up polychrome stains such as Giemsa, Wright or polychrome methylene blue reagents. However, these latter stains identify the intracystic structures referred to as "sporozoites" (Fig. 4 *C*). Up to eight sporozoites are found in mature cysts. These round, sickle-shaped or pleomorphic intracystic forms measure 1 to 2 microns in diameter. The extracystic forms are termed "trophozoites." These cells vary greatly in size and measure from 2 to 4 microns in diameter. The cytoplasm is bluish and bounded by an indefinite cell membrane. The nuclei are small and usually located eccentrically.

Little is known about the macromolecular structure of *P. carinii;* however, some histochemical studies have shown the cyst wall to consist of mucopolysaccharides, lipoproteins and chitinic acid.

Recently, *P. carinii* has been propagated in vitro in embryonic chick epithelial lung cell cultures (Pifer and Hughes, 1975). Here something has been learned of the reproductive cycle. The trophozoite attaches to but does not penetrate the host cell. While joined by microtubules, the parasite enlarges, then detaches and develops into a mature cyst. The method of cell replication has not been determined. Excystment occurs through breaks in

the cyst wall through which the sporozoites are expelled to become trophozoites (Fig. 4 *D*).

Diagnosis

For a definitive diagnosis, *P. carinii* must be demonstrated in lung tissue or fluid derived from the lung or lower respiratory tract.

Several approaches have been taken to obtain specimens for diagnosis (Hughes, 1975). Tracheal aspirates have been a reliable source of *P. carinii* organisms in infants with interstitial plasma cell pneumonia. This procedure has been less reliable for older children and adults.

Sputum, pharyngeal smears and gastric aspirates may only occasionally contain the organisms and cannot be depended upon to exclude the diagnosis.

Endobronchial brush biopsy has been used successfully in adults, but its use has been limited in children with *P. carinii* pneumonitis. Although adequate specimens may be obtained by percutaneous needle biopsy of the lung, this procedure is frequently followed by complications of pneumothorax and hemoptysis. Transbronchial lung biopsy may be utilized by the skillful operator. The standard surgical open-lung biopsy is the most dependable method for the diagnosis of this infection. It has the advantage of providing a specimen that reveals the histologic characteristics of the disease process, and the presence of a concomitant infection of another cause may be recognized. General anesthesia and endotracheal intubation are disadvantages.

Percutaneous needle aspiration of the lung provides a specimen that contains identifiable organisms in 85 per cent of cases. When this procedure is repeated in suspicious cases with nondiagnostic initial aspirates, the diagnosis can be made in over 90 per cent of the cases. However, pneumothorax is a complication frequently following this procedure as well as the other invasive techniques.

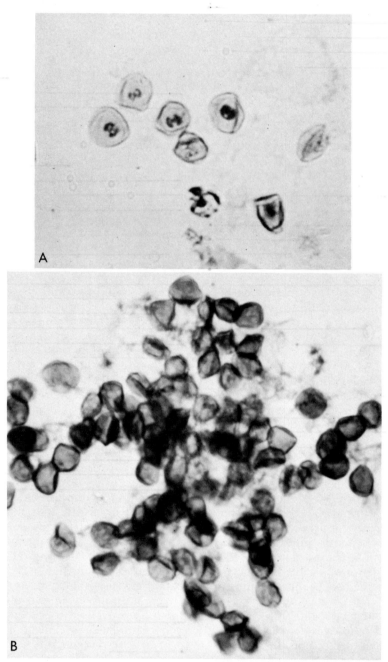

Figure 4. Specimens obtained by percutaneous transthoracic needle aspiration of the lung showing *P. carinii* stained by different methods. *A*, Gomori's methenamine–silver nitrate stain reveals the cysts as brownish black rounded and sometimes folded structures. The parenthesis-like "nucleoid" bodies are seen in some cysts and represent components of the cell wall. The intracystic sporozoites and extracystic trophozoite are not stained. (Original magnification × 1780.) *B*, Toluidine blue O stain depicts the same features as the Gomori stain, except cysts stain violet to lavender in color. (Original magnification × 1180.)

Legend continued on next page

Several staining techniques have been used to identify *P. carinii*. The Gomori methenamine–silver nitrate (Fig. 4 *A*) and toluidine blue O (Fig. 4 *B*) stains are most useful for localizing organisms in specimens. These stains clearly outline the cyst forms but not the trophozoites. The Gomori stain is more complex and requires some four hours to complete, whereas the toluidine blue O method requires only 10 to 20 minutes. These methods also stain fungi and nonbudding yeasts, which may resemble *P. carinii* cysts. The Giemsa, polychrome methylene blue (Fig. 4*C* and *D*), Wright and Gram-Wei-

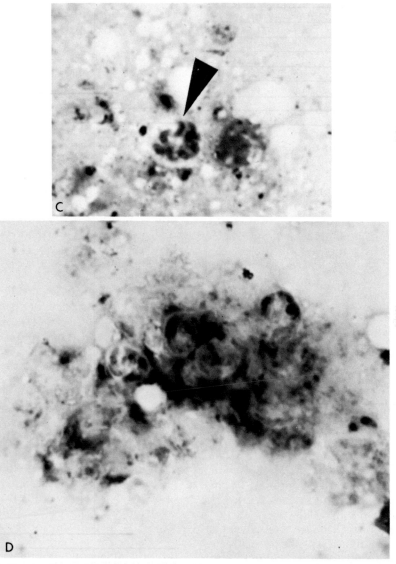

Figure 4 *(Continued).* *C.* Polychrome methylene blue stain showing cysts with crescent-shaped sporozoites. The cyst wall does not stain, resulting in a clear zone or "halo" around the intracystic sporozoites *(arrow).* The cytoplasm of the sporozoites stains light blue with a dark-staining nucleus. As many as eight sporozoites may be seen in one cyst. (Original magnification × 1440.) *D,* Polychrome methylene blue stain showing a massive cluster of cysts and trophozoites. The trophozoites are 2 to 4 microns in diameter with light blue cytoplasm and small punctate, sometimes eccentrically located, nuclei. They are pleomorphic, with a marked affinity for clustering in masses. The trophozoite is not sufficiently unique for identification as *P. carinii,* since platelet and cell remnants may mimic this stage of the organism. (Original magnification × 1440.)

gert stains are most useful for detailed study of the organisms, since the cyst with sporozoites as well as trophozoites is identifiable. The cyst wall does not stain with these reagents. Fluorescein-labeled antibody methods have been applied to clinical specimens but offer no significant advantages over the other staining procedures.

SEROLOGY. In the epidemic-infantile type, antibodies to *P. carinii* may be detected by the complement-fixation test in 75 to 95 per cent of the cases. Seroconversion usually occurs during the second week of the illness; however, this test has not been sufficiently sensitive for diagnostic purposes in the immunodeficient child and adult with the infection.

An immunofluorescence method developed at the Center for Disease Control detected antibody in the sera of 35 per cent of suspected or confirmed cases of *P. carinii* pneumonitis of the child-adult type and was more sensitive than the complement-fixation test. Unfortunately, antibody was detected in patients without *P. carinii* infection, thus limiting its use in the diagnosis of active infection.

Treatment

SPECIFIC DRUGS. Three drugs have been evaluated in the treatment of *P. carinii* pneumonitis.

Pentamidine isethionate, a diamidine with antifungal and antiprotozoan activity, was the first drug used successfully. With the infantile interstitial plasma cell pneumonitis, the mortality rate was reduced from 50 to about 3 per cent with pentamidine therapy. This drug became available in the United States in 1967 solely through the Center for Disease Control in Atlanta. The mortality rate in untreated cases of *P. carinii* pneumonitis in this country is about 100 per cent. Data from the CDC have shown that 43 per cent of 163 pentamidine-treated cases recovered (Walzer and coworkers, 1974). More favorable results have come from specific medical centers with recovery rates up to 75 per cent. Pentamidine is administered as a single daily dose of 4.0 mg. per kilogram intramuscularly for 10 to 14 days. The total dose should not exceed 56 mg. per kilogram. Unfortunately, an inordinate number of toxic and adverse side effects are associated with pentamidine therapy. Adverse effects can be expected in one-half the patients, and these include impaired renal or liver function, hypoglycemia, injection site reactions, anemia, thrombocytopenia, neutropenia, hypotension, skin rashes and hypocalcemia.

Recently, the drug combination trimethoprim-sulfamethoxazole has been evaluated for the treatment of this infection. In animal studies, this drug was effective in both treatment and prevention of *P. carinii* pneumonitis (Hughes and coworkers, 1974). The dosage of 20 mg. trimethoprim–100 mg. sulfamethoxazole per kilogram per day, orally, in four divided doses for two weeks has been shown to be the preferred one for human cases (Hughes and coworkers, 1975a: Lau and Young, 1976).

A recent study has compared the therapeutic efficacies of pentamidine isethionate and trimethoprim-sulfamethoxazole (Hughes and coworkers, 1976). To date we have studied 42 children with *P. carinii* pneumonitis randomized in a controlled investigation. Of the 21 treated with pentamidine, 16 (76 per cent) recovered, and 17 (81 per cent) of the 21 treated with trimethoprim-sulfamethoxazole recovered. No significant adverse effects occurred in the drug combination group; on the other hand, the high incidence of reactions as found in other studies occurred with the pentamidine group. Thus, trimethoprim-sulfamethoxazole is as effective as pentamidine but has the advantage of less adverse side-effects. The Federal Drug Administration has approved trimethoprim-sulfamethoxazole for use in this infection.

The drug combination pyrimethamine and sulfonamide has proved effective in the treatment of this infection in animals (Frenkel and coworkers, 1966). However, clinical studies in man have been limited and results are equivocal.

SUPPORTIVE MEASURES. Oxygen should be administered as required to keep the arterial oxygen tension (Pa_{O_2}) above 70 mm. Hg. The fraction of inspired oxygen ($F_{I_{O_2}}$) should be kept below 50 volumes per cent, if possible, to prevent oxygen intoxication. Assisted or controlled ventilation is indicated when the Pa_{O_2} is less than 60 mm. Hg at $F_{I_{O_2}}$ of 50 volumes per cent or greater. The use of a continuous negative pressure system (Sanyal and coworkers, 1975) has been useful in the management of patients requiring assisted ventilation.

Since the mode of transmission of *P. carinii* is not known, and since some instances of possible man-to-man transmission have been reported, it is probably wise to admit patients to contagious isolation rooms.

Our policy has been to withhold immunosuppressive drugs during the acute phase of the infection if the status of the primary disease permits.

Atypical Cases

The majority of cases of *P. carinii* pneumonitis follow a characteristic pattern from onset to demise or recovery. However, in a small number of patients, unexpected features of the infection have occurred. In some cases the pulmonary infiltrate presents as a lobar pneumonitis resembling that of bacterial origin, a solitary nodular lesion suggestive of malignancy, or pneumonitis in areas of previous therapeutic irridiation suggestive of radiation pneumonitis.

Rare cases of disseminated *P. carinii* infection involving hematopoietic tissues of liver, spleen, thymus, lymph nodes and bone marrow have been reported. A few descriptions of *P. carinii* pneumonitis in neonates have strongly suggested the possibility of intrauterine infection.

Recurrent infection or reinfection has occurred several months to a year after recovery from an initial episode of *P. carinii* pneumonitis. The clinical manifestations and response to treatment are similar to the primary infection.

REFERENCES

Dutz, W., Post, C., Kohout, E., and Aghamohammadi, A.: Cellular reaction to *Pneumocystis carinii*. Z. Kinderheilkd., *114*:1, 1973.

Frenkel, J. K., Good, J. T., and Schultz, J. A.: Latent pneumocystis infection of rats, relapse and chemotherapy. Lab Invest., *15*:1449, 1966.

Gajdusek, D. C.: *Pneumocystis carinii* — etiologic agent of interstitial plasma cell pneumonia of premature and young infants. Pediatrics, *19*:543, 1957.

Hughes, W. T.: Current status of laboratory diagnosis of *Pneumocystis carinii* pneumonitis. C. R. C. Crit. Rev. Clin. Lab. Sci., *6*:145, 1975.

Hughes, W. T., Feldman, S., and Sanyal, S. K.: Treatment of *Pneumocystis carinii* pneumonitis with trimethoprim-sulfamethoxazole. Can. Med. J., *112* (Suppl.): 47, 1975a.

Hughes, W. T., Feldman, S., Aur, R. J. A., Verzosa, M. S., Hustu, H. O., and Simone, J. V.: Intensity of immunosuppressive therapy and incidence of *Pneumocystis carinii* pneumonitis. Cancer, *36*:2004, 1975b.

Hughes, W. T., Feldman, S., Chaudhary, S., Ossi, M. J., and Sanyal, S. I.: Comparison of trimethoprim-sulfamethoxazole and pentamidine in the treatment of *Pneumocystis carinii* pneumonitis. Pediatr. Res. (abstract), *10*:399, 1976.

Hughes, W., McNabb, P. C., Makres, T. D., and Feldman, S.: Efficacy of trimethoprim and sulfamethoxazole in the prevention and treatment of *Pneumocystis carinii* pneumonitis. Antimicrob. Agents Chemother., *5*:289, 1974.

Lau, W. K., and Young, L. S.: Co-trimoxazole treatment of *Pneumocystis carinii* pneumonia in adults. N. Engl. J. Med., *295*:716, 1976.

Pifer, L., and Hughes, W. T.: Cultivation of *Pneumocystis carinii* in vitro. Pediatr. Res. (abstract), *9*:344, 1975.

Price, R., and Hughes, W.: Histopathology of *Pneumocystis carinii* infestation and infection of malignant disease of childhood. Hum. Pathol., *5*:737, 1974.

Sanyal, S. K., Mitchell, C., Hughes, W. T., Feldman, S., and Caces, J.: Continuous negative chest wall pressure as therapy for severe respiratory distress in older children. Chest, *68*: 143, 1975.

Walzer, P. D., Perl, D. P., Krogstad, D. J., Rawson, P. G., and Schultz, M. G.: *Pneumocystis carinii* pneumonia in the United States. Ann. Intern. Med., *80*:83, 1974.

CHAPTER TWENTY-ONE

VIRAL ETIOLOGY OF RESPIRATORY ILLNESS

Vincent V. Hamparian, Ph.D., and Henry G. Cramblett, M.D.

The application of modern cell culture methodology to the study of viruses launched the field of virology into an era of intense activity with the consequent rapid accumulation of an overwhelming body of new knowledge. In the decade 1953 to 1963 alone, approximately 150 new viruses were recovered from human patients, an average of 15 viruses per year. Most of these agents are either proved or probable causes of respiratory tract illness. This chapter will endeavor to acquaint the physician with exemplary methods for

TABLE 1. VIRUSES AFFECTING THE RESPIRATORY TRACT OF MAN

Virus Designation*	Number of Known Serotypes
RNA Viruses	
A) Picornaviruses	
⇥Enteroviruses	
Polioviruses	3
Coxsackieviruses	24 group A, 6 group B
ECHO viruses	34
⇥Rhinoviruses	at least 100 types
B) Orthomyxoviruses	
Influenza A	at least 4 subtypes
Influenza B	at least 2 subtypes
Influenza C	1
C) Paramyxoviruses	
Parainfluenza	4
Respiratory syncytial	1
Rubeola	1
D) Coronaviruses	at least 2
E) Togaviruses (e.g., rubella)	1
F) Diplornaviruses (e.g., reovirus)	3
G) Arenaviruses (e.g., lymphocytic choriomeningitis)	1
DNA Viruses	
A) Adenoviruses	31
B) Poxviruses (e.g., variola)	1
C) Herpesviruses	
Varicella	1
Cytomegalovirus	1
Herpes simplex	2
Epstein-Barr	1

*Because of structural differences between influenza C and other influenza viruses, influenza C virus may be reclassified and removed from the orthomyxovirus group. For similar reasons, it has been suggested that respiratory syncytial virus be placed into a third myxovirus group for which the name metamyxovirus has been proposed.

the laboratory diagnosis of viral respiratory disease and to summarize the salient aspects of the clinical picture produced by viruses infecting the respiratory tract of man. The mycoplasma, rickettsiae and chlamydiae are not viruses and are considered elsewhere in this volume. Table 1 shows the viruses or groups of viruses known to be associated with respiratory tract illness in man. Table 2 presents an overall interpretive estimate of the relative importance of viral respiratory disease agents in pediatric populations according to clinical syndrome. The data in this table are derived primarily from studies dependent upon isolation of virus from clinical specimens. Undoubtedly, many known viruses were missed because of poor sampling and the known insensitivity of viral isolation procedures. Hence the figures given in Table 2 are very conservative. Approximately 40 per cent of the viral etiologic agents of acute respiratory diseases in infants and children have been delineated.

Laboratory Diagnosis: General Considerations

For viral diagnostic procedures, it is axiomatic that acute-phase serum samples and materials for virus recovery attempts be obtained as early in the course of the illness as possible. Convalescent-phase serum specimens should be taken three to four weeks after the onset of illness. In general, serologic procedures alone are not practical for diagnostic purposes. The great number of known respiratory viruses, the difficulties and expense of preparing potent, specific antigens, and in many cases the undependable specificity of the antibody response all serve to preclude the routine use of serologic procedures for laboratory diagnosis. Serologic examination is most useful after the recovery of a virus from a patient. The presence of a fourfold or greater increase in neutralizing antibody titer with paired patient's sera for a particular virus provides added assurance that the virus caused an infection in the patient and is not a laboratory contaminant. In addition, serologic procedures are often of particular value for obtaining seroepidemiologic data on individual viruses or on a single group of viruses.

For laboratory diagnosis, viral isolation procedures are preferable because they yield specific, meaningful answers and are suitable for routine application on a large scale. Ideally, clinical specimens such as throat washings should be collected in a menstruum rich in protein and should arrive in the laboratory

TABLE 2. ESTIMATE OF RELATIVE IMPORTANCE OF VIRUSES IN ACUTE RESPIRATORY TRACT ILLNESSES OF CHILDREN. SUMMARY OF SELECTED EXEMPLARY REPORTS*

Etiologic Agent	Percentage Contribution to Clinical Syndrome				
	Uri	Croup	Bronchitis	Pneumonia	Bronchiolitis
Respiratory syncytial virus	8–15	2–10	9	10–20	10–30
Parainfluenza virus	4	30–40	15	5–10	15
Adenovirus	10	4	6	4–7	6
Rhinovirus	5–15	unknown	unknown	unknown	unknown
Influenza virus	3	5	1	3–9	1
Coronavirus	5	unknown	unknown	unknown	unknown

*The nature of the reports precludes separation of hospitalized patients from outpatients. However, respiratory syncytial, parainfluenza and influenza viruses are more often associated with illnesses requiring hospitalization.

with minimal delay. Specimens should be kept in wet ice during transportation over short distances or frozen in dry ice if time in transit is longer than 24 hours. Information such as the kind of specimen, the clinical diagnosis and the date of the onset of the illness should be forwarded with the specimen.

Although the recovery and identification of most viruses are relatively slow procedures (compared with the overnight isolation of *Streptococcus pyogenes*) and specific therapeutic drugs are not available for most viral diseases, the diagnostic laboratory performs a vital function by keeping under constant surveillance the prevalence of viruses within a given population. Such surveillance can alert public health officials to the need for instituting measures to prevent or interrupt epidemic disease. The laboratory can help the physician to reduce the unnecessary use of antibacterial drugs and can increase accurate diagnosis and prognosis. In addition, it can provide the necessary epidemiologic data to help determine which viruses are worthy candidates for inclusion in vaccines or for attempts at other methods of control.

PICORNAVIRUSES

General Properties

The picornaviruses (*pico* — very small; *rna* — ribonucleic acid) are one of the largest groups of viruses known. They contain a ribonucleic acid core and range in size from 15 to 30 millimicrons in diameter. The few types adequately studied by electron microscopy have cubic, icosahedral symmetry. The viruses do not have an outer envelope and are not susceptible to lipid solvents. As can be seen in Table 1, the picornaviruses are divided into two major subgroups — the enteroviruses and the rhinoviruses.

Biologically, these subgroups differ in that the enteroviruses primarily inhabit the gastrointestinal tract and are most commonly isolated from the feces and throat of the infected person. The enteroviruses are capable of causing a spectrum of illness ranging from common colds to aseptic meningitis. They do not appear to be associated with lower respiratory tract illness. Rhinoviruses, on the other hand, are rarely if ever found in the feces and have been found associated only with respiratory tract illness. In the laboratory these two subgroups can be differentiated easily on the basis of stability at pH 3.0. Rhinoviruses are extremely labile under these conditions, while the enteroviruses are unaffected. The lability of rhinoviruses at acid pH might explain their absence from the gastrointestinal tract.

ENTEROVIRUSES

Clinical Aspects

The enteroviruses cause a wide spectrum of illnesses in which the respiratory tract is not involved or is involved only to a minor degree. These include aseptic meningitis with or without paralysis, pleurodynia, exanthems, gastroenteritis, myocarditis and pericarditis. Only diseases with major involvement of the respiratory tract will be discussed in this section.

As with most viruses, the enteroviruses rarely cause clinically distinguishable respiratory disease. Rhinitis, tonsillitis, pharyngitis and croup due to various enteroviruses have been reported. These syndromes, however, do not differ sufficiently from those due to other viruses to permit the clinician to make an etiologic diagnosis on clinical grounds alone.

Herpangina is most often caused by group A coxsackieviruses types 2, 4, 5, 6, 7, 8, 9, 10, 16 and 22 but may also be caused less often by group B coxsackieviruses and ECHO viruses. It is a disease in which the clinical diagnosis can be made with some certainty. The disease occurs most commonly in children between the ages of one and four years. There is usually fever, irritability and occasionally vomiting and diarrhea associated with abdominal pain. The lesions characteristic of the disease begin as papules that progress to fragile vesicles which are easily broken, leaving behind small ulcers surrounded by inflammatory areolae. The lesions are characteristically located on the soft palate, uvula and tonsillar fauces. This is in contradistinction to the lesions caused by herpes simplex virus, which are located in the anterior portion of the oral cavity. There is no specific therapy. Since immunity is type-specific, an individual child may have recurrent episodes of herpangina due to different serotypes of enteroviruses.

Other clinically distinguishable illnesses due to group A coxsackieviruses include hand, foot and mouth disease and lymphonodular pharyngitis. The former is most often due to coxsackievirus A–16, and the latter to coxsackievirus A–10.

Laboratory Diagnosis

On a routine basis, enteroviruses are best isolated by the inoculation of clinical specimens, such as washings from rectal swabs and throat swabs, into rhesus monkey renal cell cultures. All known enteroviruses with the exception of some of the coxsackie A group and ECHO virus type 21 can be recovered in such cell cultures. Some coxsackie A viruses do not propagate in cell cultures, but can be isolated by inoculation of newborn mice. The isolation, standardization and identification of coxsackie A viruses using mice is so time-consuming and laborious that few laboratories use this procedure. Usually, coxsackie A viruses can be presumptively identified by the type of pathologic changes produced in infant mice. These agents primarily involve the skeletal muscles, causing a flaccid type of paralysis. Since herpangina is the usual clinical finding in humans infected with coxsackie A viruses, and since few

other viruses have been associated with this syndrome, the cause can be determined with reasonable certainty on a clinical basis.

To the experienced person, the type of cytopathologic changes produced by a virus in cell culture and the insensitivity of some cell types to certain viruses provide important clues to the identity of the agent. The cytopathic effects produced by picornaviruses are typical, and if the agent recovered is stable at pH 3.0, this is good presumptive evidence that it is an enterovirus. For specific identification, the virus can be tested against immune serum pools utilizing the "intersecting serum scheme" or combinatorial serum pools[*] in which each type-specific serum is present in one or more pools. The unknown virus is presumptively identified when it is neutralized by the appropriate pool or pools sharing identical antisera. An additional aid in simplifying the identification of an unknown enterovirus is the ability of a large number of such viruses to agglutinate type O human erythrocytes. If demonstrable, this property can provide a clue to the identity of the virus, thus reducing the amount of serologic testing necessary. Hemagglutinating enteroviruses include ECHO virus types 3, 6, 7, 11–13, 19–21, 24, 25, 29, 30, 33 and coxsackievirus types B_1, B_3, B_5, B_6, A_7, A_{20}, A_{21} and A_{24}.

RHINOVIRUSES

Clinical Aspects

More data are available concerning clinical illnesses resulting from rhinovirus infections in adults than in children. These viruses have been shown to be responsible for approximately 30 per cent of the upper respiratory tract illnesses in adults. For the most part,

*Combinatorial serum pools for typing enteroviruses can be obtained from the Reference Reagents Branch (RRB) of the National Institute of Allergy and Infectious Diseases (NIAID).

the predominant signs and symptoms have included rhinorrhea, coryza, and minimal soreness or "scratchiness" of the throat, usually without fever. In children, rhinovirus infections are associated with lower almost as commonly as with upper respiratory tract illnesses. Further, upper respiratory tract illness in children is frequently accompanied by fever. Croup, bronchitis, pneumonia and bronchiolitis have been observed in children from whom rhinoviruses have been recovered. However, attempts to determine the exact role of rhinoviruses in lower respiratory tract illnesses of children are complicated by the presence of other known viral pathogens in this age group. Data are not available to determine the relative importance of the various serotypes as causes of respiratory disease in children. Present data indicate that rhinoviruses are associated with up to 15 per cent of the respiratory diseases in infants and children.

Laboratory Aspects

The initial virus in this group to be isolated and described in detail was the 2060 strain, formerly known as ECHO 28 virus. Although the 2060 virus was isolated in monkey kidney cell cultures, success in the isolation of a number of agents from common colds in adults was accomplished by using cell cultures derived from human tissues. The early laboratory methods necessary to propagate these agents were different from those routinely used for other viruses. A unique property of these agents is the necessity to roll inoculated cell cultures at 33° C. during the viral isolation procedure. The cell culture system consisted of primary human fetal kidney cultures maintained on a relatively low pH medium. Human fetal tissues are not routinely available and do not have the desirable quality of uniformity of susceptibility to viruses.

The first significant technologic advance for simplifying work with these agents was provided by the development of diploid cell strains from human fetal tissue. Such cells can be made available in quantity, maintain a normal karyotype throughout their useful life span and do not have the properties of "malignant" cells. Human diploid cell strains are highly sensitive to rhinoviruses, which produce distinct and easily recognizable cytopathologic changes in these cells. Although other picornaviruses produce a similar cytopathic effect, the rhinoviruses are easily distinguished by their lability at pH 3.0.

At present, specific identification of rhinoviruses is not feasible for the ordinary virus laboratory. It seems likely that a multiplicity of serotypes are present in the population at any one time. The great diversity and the rapid turnover of serotypes in a given geographic area suggest that the total number of antigenic types may be very large. In the relatively short time period in which these agents have been recognized as a distinct group, 89 serotypes have been described. Typing sera for routine use are not yet available from commercial or federal sources, and isolates must be stored for identification at some future date unless the individual laboratory is willing to expend the time, labor and expense in preparing suitable antisera. Small amounts of reagent-grade antisera for the 89 numbered serotypes are available for reference purposes only from the RRB of the NIAID.

ADENOVIRUSES

General Properties

The adenoviruses are composed of a DNA core enclosed in a protein shell about 70 millimicrons in diameter. No outer envelope is present. These agents are not affected by lipid solvents or by exposure to pH 3.0. All human adenoviruses share a common complement-fixing antigen. With the exception of types 12 and 18, all human types agglutinate rat or monkey erythrocytes. These agents propagate and mature within the nucleus of the infected cell, producing type B intranuclear inclusions and a characteristic cytopathic effect. A property of certain members of this group is the ability to induce the formation of malignant tumors when inoculated into newborn hamsters. This is the first recognized example of tumor induction in animals by viruses of human origin.

Clinical Aspects

The adenoviruses are responsible for approximately 5 per cent of all respiratory tract disease in infants and children. They may infect any portion of the respiratory tract and hence cause a wide spectrum of disease ranging from rhinitis to bronchiolitis. Adenovirus types 3, 4 and 7 are the most frequent serotypes causing respiratory tract disease. Types 1, 2 and 5 are less common causes of disease and apparently cause illness only in infants and younger children.

Pharyngoconjunctival fever is the only clinically distinguishable syndrome caused by the adenoviruses. Most patients with this disease are infected with either adenovirus type 3 or 7, with occasional cases due to types 4 and 14. The signs and symptoms of pharyngoconjunctival fever include erythema and injection of the palpebral and bulbar conjunctivae (unilateral or bilateral) and erythema of the tonsils and pharynx, occasionally accompanied by exudate and coryza and fever. As the child recovers, there may be enlargement and tenderness of the posterior cervical and preauricular lymph nodes. Pharyngoconjunctival fever is clinically similar to prodromal measles prior to the appearance of Koplik spots and exanthem.

Other respiratory tract diseases due to adenoviruses are not clinically distinguishable. Nevertheless, the presence of conjunctivitis associated with respiratory disease is suggestive of adenovirus infection.

Adenovirus types 1, 2, 3 and 7 have been recovered by postmortem examination of lung tissue of children with primary viral pneumonia. Adenovirus pneumonia, however, is not clinically different from pneumonia due to other viruses.

Laboratory Aspects

Most laboratories utilize stable cell lines such as HeLa, KB and Hep-2 for the isolation of adenoviruses from throat or rectal specimens. For optimum recovery of adenoviruses, cell cultures of primary fetal kidney tissue also should be used. Such cultures can be maintained for long periods of time and are particularly useful for certain slow-growing adenoviruses. Identification of an isolate as an adenovirus is relatively easy. These agents produce a characteristic cytopathic effect in cell cultures. In addition, all human adenoviruses possess a group-specific complement-fixing antigen that is best demonstrated by use of a specific, standardized antiserum prepared in animals. When utilizing the complement-fixation reaction for the identification of viruses, a negative test should be interpreted with caution, since it may be due to inadequate complement-fixing antigen content in the preparation used.

Specific identification of adenoviruses can be accomplished by use of type-specific antisera in neutralization or hemagglutination-inhibition tests. The hemagglutination-inhibition test is particularly helpful, since the type of red cell agglutinated and the pattern of agglutination obtained place the virus in a subgroup, substantially reducing the number of antisera needed for final identification. Knowledge of adenovirus types most likely to be encountered in a given clinical situation is also helpful in the rapid identification of isolates.

ORTHOMYXOVIRUSES

General Properties

The orthomyxoviruses contain a ribonucleoprotein core enclosed in an outer envelope and range in particle size from 80 to 120 millimicrons. These agents contain essential lipid and are inactivated by lipid solvents. Orthomyxoviruses are also inactivated at pH 3.0. Orthomyxoviruses combine with host cells and agglutinate erythrocytes by attachment to mucoprotein receptor sites on cell membranes. Similar receptor substances are present in serum, urine, tissue extracts and secretions of the respiratory tract. These viruses possess an enzyme (neuraminidase) which splits off N-acetylneuraminic acid residues from mucoprotein receptors. Once the enzyme substrate is destroyed, the virus particle elutes and can attach to fresh receptor material to repeat the process. Orthomyxoviruses cause hemadsorption, a phenomenon in which erythrocytes adsorb to cells in infected cultures and which is used extensively for demonstrating the presence of virus.

The three subtypes of influenza virus (A, B and C) can be differentiated from each other by complement-fixation tests. All strains of the same subtype share a common internal ribonucleoprotein antigen distinct from that of strains of other subtypes. Viruses within a subtype can be distinguished from each other by either complement-fixing or hemagglutinating antigens found on the surface of the virion. The influenza viruses, particularly type A, are notorious for instability of antigenic composition. For example, since 1933, when the first human influenza virus was isolated, about four major and many minor changes have occurred in the influenza A virus, while only two demonstrable antigenic changes have occurred in influenza B virus since its original isolation in 1940. No changes have occurred in the antigenic structure of influenza C virus. The antigenic instability of influenza viruses contributes to our inability to control the disease effectively with vaccines.

Clinical Aspects

Illnesses due to influenza types A, B and C are similar. Most pandemics and epidemics of influenza are due to strains of type A virus, while type B virus is usually endemic or epidemic. Type C influenza virus causes only sporadic cases of disease.

In children the most common symptoms of influenza are headache, cough, sore throat and nasal discharge or obstruction. Other symptoms include substernal pain or pressure lacrimation, vomiting, abdominal pain and weakness or dizziness. On physical examination, fever is usually present with an impressive absence of physical findings. There may be mild to moderate erythema of the pharynx and erythema of the conjunctivae, and coarse rhonchi may be present.

Laboratory Aspects

The classic technique for the isolation of influenza viruses has been the inoculation of throat specimens into the amniotic cavity of the ten-day-old embryonated chicken egg. The presence of the virus in amniotic fluid is detected by hemagglutination, and the exact identity can be established by the use of specific, inhibitor-free antiserum in hemagglutination-inhibition tests. Primary rhesus monkey kidney cell cultures also appear to be useful for the recovery of influenza viruses from clinical materials. Viruses recovered in cell culture can be identified in neutralization tests with specific antisera which usually can be obtained from commercial sources.

During recognized epidemics, hemagglutination-inhibition and complement-fixation tests can be used to great advantage for diagnostic purposes. Antigens can be prepared in the laboratory or obtained commercially. When sera collected from patients during the acute and convalescent phases of illness are available, antibody increases can be demonstrated with a minimum of labor and cost. An advantage of the complement-fixation technique is that nonspecific inhibitors of hemagglutination present in most sera do not affect the outcome of the test.

PARAMYXOVIRUSES

General Properties

Although the parainfluenza and orthomyxoviruses share many common properties, they have certain distinguishing characteristics. The parainfluenza viruses are larger, ranging between 100 and 300 millimicrons in diameter. Many paramyxoviruses not only can cause hemagglutination but can also lyse certain kinds of erythrocytes. In addition, polykaryocytosis is commonly produced in infected cell cultures. Although they share common antigens, there is no single antigen common to all parainfluenza viruses.

In contrast to influenza A and B viruses, there is no evidence that any important antigenic changes have occurred in members of the paramyxovirus group.

Clinical Aspects

The parainfluenza viruses have been recovered from children with syndromes varying from mild rhinitis to severe bronchiolitis. In general, infections with types 1 and 3 viruses are more common than those with type 2. The significance of type 4 virus in the causation of respiratory illness is uncertain at present. Collectively, parainfluenza viruses types 1, 2 and 3 are the most important agents etiologically associated with croup. In contrast to types 1 and 3 viruses, which cause a diverse number of respiratory illnesses, type 2 virus is usually associated only with croup.

Laboratory Aspects

Serologic procedures such as the complement-fixation and hemagglutination-inhibition tests are useful, but suffer from lack of specificity of the antibody response. Heterotypic antibody responses following parainfluenza virus infections in humans are not uncommon, and in the absence of virus isolation studies, serologic results are difficult to interpret precisely; however, they can be utilized to delegate causation to the parainfluenza virus group.

The development of the hemadsorption technique has simplified the virus isolation and identification methodology for the parainfluenza viruses. Primary rhesus monkey renal cell cultures appear to be the most sensitive system for the recovery of these agents from clinical materials. The cytopathic effects produced by these agents on initial inoculation into such cultures are subtle at best, making the hemadsorption phenomenon basic to the early and certain recognition of these agents in cell cultures. The specific identification of a hemadsorbing agent is carried out by use of type-specific antisera in neutralization tests. Antisera for this purpose are available from commercial sources. The number of known hemadsorbing viruses recoverable from human sources in monkey renal cell culture is at present relatively small, and antisera are needed for only seven or eight viruses. It is worthy of note that some lots of monkey kidney cell cultures harbor endogenous simian viruses capable of causing cytopathic effects or the hemadsorption phenomenon. The isolation of "new" viruses in such cell cultures or even in nonsimian cell culture systems must be interpreted with caution, especially if monkey cell cultures are used routinely in the laboratory.

RESPIRATORY SYNCYTIAL VIRUS

General Properties

With a few exceptions, the presently recognized biological and physical properties of the respiratory syncytial virus are similar to those of other paramyxoviruses. It is of medium size and contains an RNA core. It is inactivated by lipid solvents and is extremely labile at pH 3.0. In contrast to parainfluenza viruses, it lacks the ability to agglutinate erythrocytes or to cause hemadsorption. In addition, respiratory syncytial virus has some structural characteristics that are not shared by other paramyxoviruses.

Clinical Aspects

The respiratory syncytial virus is the most important single virus causing respiratory tract disease in infants and children. It is estimated that as many as 15 per cent of the cases of respiratory disease seen in outpatients and a minimum of 25 per cent of the cases of respiratory disease in hospitalized infants and young children are due to the respiratory syncytial virus.

Bronchiolitis is the most severe illness caused by this virus. The virus is responsible for over 50 per cent of the cases of this syndrome. It may also cause pneumonia, bronchitis, croup and rhinitis. The less severe upper respiratory tract illnesses are often the clinical expression of reinfections with the virus.

Laboratory Aspects

This agent is particularly susceptible to inactivation, a factor that emphasizes the importance of the careful collection and handling of clinical specimens. Stable cell line cultures such as HeLa, KB and Hep-2 are highly sensitive to respiratory syncytial virus, although some reports indicate that certain strains propagate best in monkey kidney cell cultures. In addition, human diploid cell strains such as WI–38 also appear to be very sensitive for primary isolation of this agent. The cytopathologic features are characteristically lytic in nature with the formation of syncytia, cell rounding and swelling. Absence of hemadsorption concomitant with this kind of cytopathic effect suggests the presence of respiratory syncytial virus. Specific identity can be established by the neutralization technique using specific hyperimmune serum which is available from commercial sources. Since the virus produces a potent complement-fixing antigen, some laboratories prefer to use the complement-fixation test for identification of isolates.

CORONAVIRUSES

The coronaviruses are a recently recognized group of agents consisting of a number of human and animal viruses (infectious bronchitis virus of chickens, mouse hepatitis virus) with similar physicochemical and morphologic properties. The human coronaviruses include some strains that propagate in cell culture and others that grow only in human embryonic tracheal and nasal organ cultures. These viruses are 80 to 160 millimicrons in diameter, are sensitive to lipid solvents and low pH and contain a ribonucleic acid core. They possess a characteristic surface structure — petal-shaped (coronalike) projections distributed uniformly around the surface of the virion. The human and mouse strains appear to be antigenically related. Based on serologic studies, there appear to be at least two antigenically distinct human coronaviruses.

Clinical Aspects

The coronaviruses are apparently important causes of the common cold. Volunteers infected with these viruses develop severe manifestations of rhinitis and many have complaints of sore throat and cough. Study of naturally occurring cases of coronavirus infection in adults reveals that coryza is frequently present with nasal congestion, sneezing and sore throat. Less common complaints include headache, cough, muscular and general aches, chills and "feverishness." Epidemiologic observations suggest that the coronaviruses may be the etiologic agents of a portion of the respiratory tract illnesses that occur in adults during the winter season when prevalence of rhinoviruses and other known respiratory virus pathogens is often low. The role of coronaviruses in the causation of respiratory disease in infants and children is unknown, but it has been suggested that they are responsible for up to 5 per cent of upper respiratory tract infections in children.

Laboratory Diagnosis

Present methodology for isolation and identification of coronaviruses is too difficult for routine application by the ordinary diagnostic laboratory. Although some strains can be isolated in cell cultures and produce cytopathic effects, specific antisera are not routinely available for identification. This necessitates use of the electron microscope to identify an isolate as a coronavirus. In organ cultures, examination with the electron microscope also is necessary to detect the presence of these agents with any degree of certainty. Thus, the diagnosis of illness caused by coronaviruses is still a research procedure.

COMMENT

Although a number of viruses, including rubeola, rubella, varicella, variola, cytomegalovirus and lymphocytic choriomeningitis, are capable of causing symptoms of acute respiratory disease, their primary manifestations are not usually in the respiratory tract, and for this reason they will not be discussed here. (See chapters on Measles Pneumonia, Varicella Pneumonia and Cytomegalic Inclusion Disease.) The reoviruses also are omitted from discussion, since there is no definite proof that they play a significant role in the causation of human respiratory disease. Moreover, the existing evidence is merely suggestive, and final judgment

must await the results of future investigations.

It must be emphasized that the methodology for laboratory diagnosis of virus infections varies considerably from laboratory to laboratory. The techniques utilized are often governed by the special interests, experience and background of the laboratory personnel. These differences are not vital as long as the laboratory adequately performs the task for which it exists.

It is hoped that the techniques described in this chapter will be improved in the future and replaced by more rapid, more accurate and less costly means for laboratory diagnosis of viral infections. Methods presently being explored in a number of laboratories with varying degrees of success include the use of fluorescent antibody techniques, radioimmune assays for antigen and antibody, immune electron microscopy, direct application of electron microscopy to clinical materials, and miniaturized cell cultures and microtiter equipment.

REFERENCES

Beem, M. O.: Acute respiratory illness in nursery school children: a longitudinal study of the occurrence of illness and respiratory viruses. *Am. J. Epidemiol., 90*:30, 1968.

Bradburne, A. F.: Antigenic relationships amongst coronaviruses. *Arch. Gesamte. Virusforsch., 31*:352, 1970.

Chanock, R. M., Mufson, M. A., and Johnson, K. M.: Comparative biology and ecology of human virus and Mycoplasma respiratory pathogens. *Prog. Med. Virol., 7*:208, 1965.

Conference on newer respiratory disease viruses. *Am. Rev. Resp. Dis., 88*:part 2 of two parts, September 1963.

D'Alessio, D., Williams, S., and Dick, E. C.: Rapid detection and identification of respiratory viruses by direct immunofluorescence. *Appl. Microbiol., 20*:233, 1970.

Estola, T.: Coronaviruses. A new group of animal RNA viruses. *Avian Diseases, 14*:No. 2, 1970.

Gwaltney, J. M., Jr., and Jordan, W. S., Jr.: The present status of respiratory viruses. *Med. Clin. North Am., 47*:1155, 1963.

Hamparian, V. V., Hilleman, M. R., and Ketler, A.: Contributions to characterization and classification of animal viruses. *Proc. Soc. Exp. Biol. Med., 112*:1040, 1963.

Hendley, J. O., Gwaltney, J. M., Jr., and Jordan, W. S., Jr.: Rhinovirus infections in an industrial population. IV. Infections within families of employees during two fall peaks of respiratory illness. *Am. J. Epidemiol., 89*:184, 1968.

Herrmann, E. C., Jr.: The tragedy of viral diagnosis, *Postgrad. Med. J., 46*:545, 1970.

Herrmann, E. C., Jr.: New concepts and developments in applied diagnostic virology. *Prog. Med. Virol., 17*:221, 1974.

Hilleman, M. R., Hamparian, V. V., Ketler, A., Reilly, C. M., McClelland, L., Cornfeld, D., and Stokes, J., Jr.: Acute respiratory illnesses among children and adults. Field study of contemporary importance of several viruses and appraisal of the literature. *J.A.M.A., 180*:445, 1962.

Hsiung, G. D. (Ed.): *Diagnostic Virology: An Illustrated Handbook.* 1st Ed. (Revised.) New Haven, University Press, 1973.

Hsiung, G. D., Pinheiro, F., and Gabrielson, M. O.: The virus diagnostic laboratory: functions and problems based on three years' experience. *Yale J. Biol. Med., 36*:104, 1963.

Kapikian, A. Z., Kim, H. W., Wyatt, R. G., Rodriguez, W. J., Cline, W. L., Parrott, R. H., and Chanock, R. M.: Reovirus agent in stools: association with infantile diarrhea and development of serologic tests. *Science, 185*:1049, 1974.

Kaye, H. S., and Dowdle, W. R.: Seroepidemiologic survey of coronavirus (strain 229E). Infections in a population of children. *Am. J. Epidemiol., 101*:238, 1975.

Lennette, E. H., and Schmidt, N. J. (Eds.): *Diagnostic Procedures for Viral and Rickettsial Infections.* 4th Ed. New York, American Public Health Association, 1969.

Loda, F. A., Clyde, W. A., Jr., Glezen, W. P., Senior, R. J., Sheaffer, C. I., and Denny, F. W., Jr.: Studies on the role of viruses, bacteria, and *M. pneumoniae* as causes of lower respiratory tract infections in children. *J. Pediatr., 72*:161, 1968.

McIntosh, K., Kapikian, A. Z., Turner, H. C., Hartley, J. W., Parrott, R. H., and Chanock, R.

M.: Seroepidemiologic studies of coronavirus infection in adults and children. *Am. J. Epidemiol., 91*:585, 1970.

McQuillin, J., Gardner, P. S., and McGuckin, R.: Rapid diagnosis of influenza by immunofluorescent techniques. *Lancet, 2*:690, 1970.

McQuillin, J., Gardner, P. S., and Sturdy, P. M.: The use of cough/nasal swabs in the rapid diagnosis of respiratory syncytial virus infection by the fluorescent antibody technique. *J. Hyg. (Camb.), 68*:283, 1970.

Melnick, J. L.: Classification and nomenclature of animal viruses. *Progr. Med. Virol., 13*:462, 1971.

Mufson, M. A., Krause, H. E., Mocega, H. E., and Dawson, F. W.: Viruses, *Mycoplasma pneumoniae* and bacteria associated with lower respiratory tract disease among infants. *Am. J. Epidemiol., 91*:192, 1970.

Nagahama, H., Eller, J. J., Fulginiti, V. A., and Marks, M. I.: Direct immunofluorescent studies of infection with respiratory syncytial virus. *J. Infect. Dis., 122*:260, 1970.

Rosenbaum, M. J., Kory, R. C., Siegesmund, K. A., Pedersen, H. J., Sullivan, E. J., and Peckinpaugh, R. O.: Electron microscope methods for identification of adenoviruses isolated in micro tissue cultures. *Appl. Microbiol., 23*:141, 1972.

Schmidt, N. J.: Trends in the laboratory diagnosis of viral infections. *Postgrad Med., 35*:488, 1964.

Sullivan, E. J., and Rosenbaum, M. J.: Isolation and identification of adenoviruses in microplates. *Appl. Microbiol., 22*:802, 1971.

Valters, W. A., Boehm, L. G., Edwards, E. A., and Rosenbaum, M. J.: Detection of adenovirus in patient specimens by indirect immune electron microscopy. *J. Clin. Microbiol., 1*:472, 1975.

Vassall, J. H., II, and Ray, C. G.: Serotyping of adenovirus using immune electron microscopy. *Appl. Microbiol., 28*:623, 1974.

Wulff, H., Kidd, P., and Wenner, H. A.: Etiology of respiratory infections. Further studies during infancy and childhood. *Pediatrics, 33*:30, 1964.

CHAPTER TWENTY-TWO

VIRAL PNEUMONIA

Floyd W. Denny, M. D.

Respiratory infections are the major cause of morbidity due to acute illnesses in the United States; many of these infections will involve the lower respiratory tract, particularly in infancy. Mortality resulting from acute lower respiratory tract disease is a serious problem in children under five years of age. A large proportion of these illnesses, possibly most, are due to specific respiratory viruses and *Mycoplasma pneumoniae.* Despite this information and the great scientific and technical advances made in the understanding and control of many diseases, surprisingly little progress has been made in our knowledge regarding the diagnosis and management of viral infections of the lower respiratory tract.

The term "pneumonia" is usually used to designate involvement of terminal airways and alveoli of the lung, but many infections of the lung are not restricted to such a narrow anatomic site. It is now accepted that many children with bronchiolitis, tracheobronchitis, croup and possibly at times even upper respiratory tract infections will also have pneumonia. The biggest problem facing the clinician caring for the child with pneumonia, with or without involvement of other sites, is the differentiation of viral infections, for which no specific treatment is available, from bacterial and mycoplasmal infections, which respond to particular antimicrobial agents. In the child with pneumonia, there are few clinical characteristics or readily available, rapid and accurate laboratory diagnostic tests that allow this differentiation. Fortunately, however, several of the respiratory viruses produce characteristic clinical syndromes in addition to pneumonia that suggest their involvement; furthermore, they occur in epidemiologic patterns that are predictable from year to year. It is imperative, therefore, that the pediatric clinician have a thorough understanding of the epidemiology of lower respiratory tract infections.

Incidence

The true incidence of viral pneumonia is unknown, owing at least in part to the lack of an accurate way of differentiating viral pneumonia from that due to other agents. There have been many studies on the hospital occurrence of pneumonia, but the lack of knowledge regarding the population from which the cases came has made these data difficult to interpret.

The incidence of pneumonia varies with age. A study by Foy and coworkers (1973) from Seattle, Washington, showed the highest attack rate for pneumonia due to respiratory viruses and *M. pneumoniae* to be in children less than five years old, in whom the incidence was 40 episodes per 1000 children per year. The majority of these episodes occurred in children under three years of age. These data are comparable to studies by Glezen and Denny (1973) in Chapel Hill, North Carolina, which have shown the incidence of *total* lower respiratory tract disease in a private pediatric practice to be 134 per 1000 children per year. The rate ranged from 240 per 1000 children per year in infants under one year of age to only 34 illnesses per 1000 in late adolescence. Even though

TABLE 1.   VIRUSES CAUSING PNEUMONIA

Common Causes	Less Common Causes	In Neonates or Compromised Hosts
Respiratory syncytial virus	Rhinoviruses	Cytomegalovirus
Parainfluenza viruses 1, 2 and 3	Enteroviruses	Herpesvirus hominis
Adenoviruses	Coronaviruses	Rubella virus
Influenza viruses A and B	Rubeola virus	
	Varicella virus	

precise rates for pneumonia are unknown, it is clear that this entity is predominantly a disease of young children and its occurrence decreases rather sharply with age.

Etiology

Table 1 shows the viruses that are the most frequent causes of pneumonia in children. Those agents listed as less common causes are associated with generalized diseases — measles and chickenpox — or are encountered infrequently as causes of pneumonia. Pneumonia due to these uncommon agents, that seen in neonates and compromised hosts, and that due to influenza viruses A and B, which are discussed in another chapter, will not be considered further. Respiratory syncytial virus (RSV), parainfluenza viruses 1, 2 and 3 (Para 1, 2 and 3) and several types of adenoviruses (Adenos) are common causes of pneumonia and will be considered in greater detail.

Epidemiology

The clinical manifestations of pneumonia, with the possible exception of pneumococcal lobar pneumonia in the older child, are such that it is usually impossible to implicate a specific etiologic agent on clinical grounds alone. There are other reasons why the etiologic diagnosis of pneumonia is difficult to make: ① pulmonary infections can be caused by organisms of all classes, including bacteria, fungi, viruses, rickettsia, chlamydia and M. pneumoniae; ② diagnostic tests, including isolation and identification of agents and serologic confirmation of infections, are frequently difficult and time-consuming to perform or are not readily available; and ③ pulmonary secretions for culture are difficult to obtain without contamination with normal upper respiratory tract flora, which often include bacteria with the potential for pulmonary pathogenicity. All of the pathogens listed above must be considered in one clinical-epidemiologic setting or another; however, the most frequent diagnostic dilemma for physicians managing community-acquired pneumonia in previously healthy children is differentiating those patients with viral pneumonia from those who have disease due to bacteria and M. pneumoniae. It has been found that infections due to RSV and to Para 1, 2 and 3 occur in epidemiologic patterns that are sufficiently characteristic for the clinician to make an etiologic diagnosis in many instances. The information to be collected includes the age and sex of the patient, season of the year, associated anatomic sites of involvement within the respiratory tract (bronchiolitis, tracheobronchitis and croup) and characteristics of illness occurring simultaneously in the community, the family or other epidemiologic niches of which the patient is a member (day care center or school). This type of information can assume major diagnostic importance in the differentiation of nonbacterial from bacterial pneumonias, which rarely occur in epidemic patterns.

RESPIRATORY SYNCYTIAL VIRUS. RSV is the most common cause of

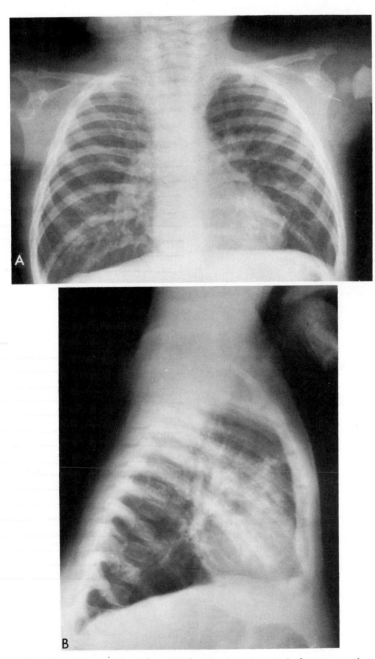

Figures 1 to 4.   Chest roentgenograms from children having pneumonia due to several common respiratory viruses. Diagnosis established by culture techniques. Note wide diversity of types of pulmonary involvement.

Figure 1.   Bronchiolitis and diffuse pulmonary infiltrates in an infant with respiratory syncytial virus infection. (From Collier, A. M.: Presented at the Bronchiolitis Workshop held at the National Institutes of Health. *Pediatr. Res., 11*:209, 1977.)

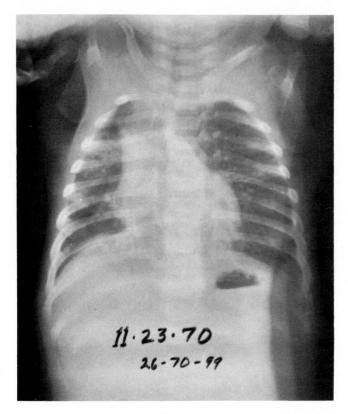

Figure 2. Fatal pneumonia due to parainfluenza virus type 1 in a small child.

Figure 3. Diffuse pneumonitis and atelectasis of the right upper lobe due to parainfluenza virus type 3. Virus grown from lung aspirate.

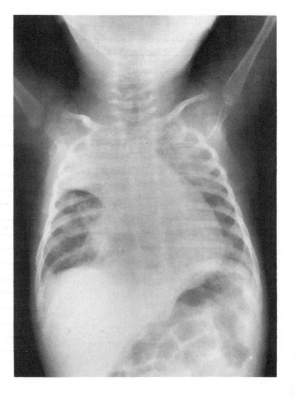

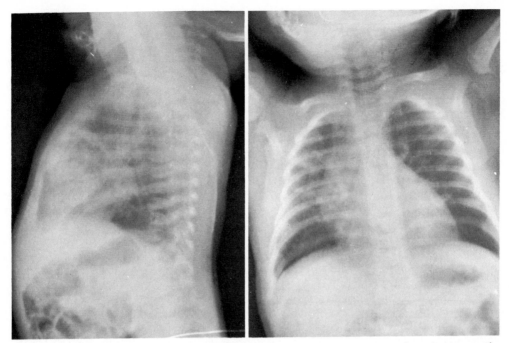

Figure 4. Diffuse pneumonitis in an infant. Parainfluenza virus type 3 was grown from the throat and a pneumococcus from the blood. This is an example of the problem facing the pediatrician in making an etiologic diagnosis in patients with pneumonia.

bronchiolitis and pneumonia in infancy and early childhood. Infections occur any time after birth, with little evidence of protection by maternal antibody, which is found in varying amounts in all newborns. The majority of pneumonia due to RSV occurs in the first three years of life, with occasional cases up to age five to seven years. During the first six months of life, bronchiolar obstruction and interstitial pneumonia may cause severe respiratory compromise with an occasional fatal outcome. Bronchiolitis and pneumonia due to RSV are more common in boys than in girls.

RSV disease occurs in yearly epidemics of six to eight weeks of duration almost exclusively in the winter and spring. When RSV infections occur in families, older children and adults will manifest mild upper respiratory tract symptoms if they become ill. When RSV is prevalent in the community, there will be an increase in bronchiolitis and pneumonia visits to health care facilities and increased pneumonia hospitalizations in infants and young children. There will be little or no associated increase in pneumonia in school age children and normal adults. Adults with chronic obstructive lung disease may have exacerbations of lower respiratory tract difficulty associated with RSV infections.

PARAINFLUENZA VIRUSES. Para 1, 2 and 3 are responsible for the majority of human parainfluenza respiratory illnesses. Illnesses due to types 1 and 2 are clinically and epidemiologically distinct from type 3 disease, especially in children.

The primary significance of Para 1 and 2 infections in children is their etiologic association with croup. During periods of prevalence of parainfluenza virus croup, occasional infants and young children with pneumonia due to these agents will be seen. When this occurs, the clinical illness is indistinguishable from RSV or Para 3 pneumonia. Para 1 and 2 infections occur in both endemic and epidemic patterns. The relationship of community population size to these patterns is unclear.

When Para 1 and 2 appear in epidemic fashion, they demonstrate a predilection for the fall season.

Para 3 is second only to RSV as a cause of bronchiolitis and pneumonia in infants and children. As with RSV, there is little evidence of protection afforded by transplacentally acquired antibody. Pneumonia is most frequently a manifestation of infection during the first three years of life. Infants less than six months of age are at risk for severe respiratory compromise secondary to bronchiolar obstruction and interstitial pneumonia.

Although there is no basis for clinical distinction of RSV and Para 3 disease, the two agents have different epidemiologic patterns of occurrence. Para 3 infections are endemic and occur throughout the year. There may be short periods of minor increased prevalence of this virus, but it is usually not associated with community-wide epidemics and consequently is not associated frequently with periods of increased pneumonia incidence in infants and young children.

Parainfluenza infections in families usually result in mild upper respiratory tract illness in older children and adults; however, there is a low incidence of parainfluenza virus–associated pneumonia in normal adults.

ADENOVIRUSES. Adenoviruses types 1, 2 and 5 are endemic in the population, and while they are most commonly associated with febrile upper respiratory tract infections, there is a low incidence of bronchiolitis and pneumonia in infants and young children accompanying infections by these serotypes. Adenovirus types 3, 7, 14 and 21 infections occur less frequently in infancy and early childhood, yet they account for many of the severe episodes of bronchiolitis and pneumonia occurring in children less than two years of age. Severe lower respiratory tract infections with these types have occurred both sporadically and in epidemic patterns. Epidemics have been both institutional and community-wide, but have been few in number. All adenovirus infections increase in frequency in winter months.

Pathology and Pathogenesis

Knowledge of the pathology and pathogenesis of viral pneumonias is meager because of the limited number of fatal cases, the lack of application of specific diagnostic tests and the difficulty in establishing animal models. Data from human cases are frequently hard to interpret because of the severity of the fatal lesion, superinfection with bacteria or fungi which occurs frequently in severely ill, hospitalized patients, and the inevitable damage wrought by assisted ventilation in these patients. This section will summarize data from human cases and animal models, when available, infected with respiratory syncytial virus, the parainfluenza viruses and the adenoviruses.

RESPIRATORY SYNCYTIAL VIRUS. Examination of fatal cases has shown extensive bronchopneumonia with patchy atelectasis and areas of overaeration. There may be signs of acute necrotizing bronchiolitis with sloughing of the bronchiolar epithelium and exudate into the lumen, sometimes leading to complete occlusion. In other areas there may be proliferative changes of bronchiolar epithelium. Eosinophilic cytoplasmic inclusions may be found. Peribronchiolar monocytic infiltration, including lymphocytes, plasma cells and macrophages, is widespread, and there may be hemorrhage and edema of the bronchiolar walls. Exudate may be seen in alveoli adjacent to bronchioles, and there is infiltration of cells in interstitial tissues. There is usually wide variation in the severity of lesions in different parts of the lungs.

The pathologic changes in nonfatal cases are unknown, and a suitable animal model for RSV infections has not been developed. Thus, knowledge regarding milder pathologic changes and their temporal sequence is speculative at this time and awaits further study.

It has been suggested that immune mechanisms may play a role in the pathogenesis of serious diseases due to RSV occurring in infants who possess maternal antibody. There are two hypotheses about the possible mechanism. Chanock and coworkers (1970) have advanced the theory that the maternal antibody may complex with viral antigen to produce a destructive process, while Gardner and coworkers (1970) have suggested that an anaphylactoid reaction may occur with the second exposure to the virus after a mild, sensitizing infection under the cover of maternal antibody. There is little direct evidence to support either theory, but it is of obvious importance to determine if any immune mechanisms are operative in the pathogenesis of RSV infections, particularly in reference to vaccine development.

PARAINFLUENZA VIRUSES. Descriptions of fatal pneumonia cases in humans are meager and incomplete. Para 3 infections in the Syrian hamster cause reproducible pathologic changes, however, and are the basis of most of our knowledge in this area. In this model, focal, necrotic lesions are noted in the bronchial epithelium 24 hours after infection. By 48 to 72 hours, there are further degenerative changes in the bronchial epithelium with the appearance of giant cells; there are also intraluminal exudates and the accumulation of polymorphonuclear and mononuclear cells in the peribronchial and perivascular spaces. In three to five days, there is involvement of terminal bronchioles, and if there is alveolar involvement, it appears to be an extension of the bronchiolar lesion. By five to seven days, the peribronchial and perivascular exudate is made up mostly of mononuclear cells; thereafter complete clearing occurs.

Data on the pathology and pathogenesis of Para 1 and 2 infections are not available.

ADENOVIRUSES. Fatal cases have been due almost invariably to types 3, 4, 7 and 21. In these cases there are multiple areas of consolidation along with thick mucopurulent tracheobronchial secretions. The lung between involved areas frequently is hyperaerated. Large hilar lymph nodes are also described. Microscopic examination shows severe bronchiolitis with infiltration into the lamina propria of lymphocytes, plasma cells, macrophages and a few polymorphonuclear leukocytes. There is interstitial and alveolar involvement, including infiltration with round cells. Typical adenovirus intranuclear inclusions are found in epithelial cells and histiocytes. In severely involved lungs, there is marked necrosis of bronchioles and alveoli.

An animal model has not been developed for this group of viruses, so further details regarding pathology are not available.

Clinical Manifestations

In the individual patient there are no readily available means to differentiate between pneumonia caused by a virus and that due to bacteria or *M. pneumoniae*, the other frequent causes of childhood pneumonia. Commonly, upper respiratory tract symptoms of several days' duration, including fever, coryza, hoarseness and cough, precede the pulmonary illness. Virus pneumonias are frequently associated with clinical findings of pathologic involvement throughout the lower respiratory tract. Cough and coarse rhonchi characteristic of tracheobronchitis are common, as is wheezing indicative of bronchiolitis. Headache, malaise and myalgia may be present in older children. High fever occurs frequently in viral pneumonia, and some children have severe respiratory compromise; since these findings are common to viral and bacterial pneumonias, they are not good differentiating clinical features in including or excluding an etiologic bacterial agent. Most patients recover in seven to ten days, but illnesses lasting longer are not unusual.

Roentgenographic Appearance

The classic radiographic appearance of viral pneumonia is that of a patchy bronchopneumonia; however, lobar consolidation indistinguishable from pneumococcal lobar pneumonia occurs in many childhood viral pneumonias. The presence of pleural fluid, pneumatoceles, abscesses, circular pneumonia and lobar consolidation with evidence of volume expansion of the involved lobe should be considered inconsistent with viral disease, although small amounts of pleural fluid may be seen in occasional children with viral pneumonia.

Laboratory Findings

Peripheral white blood cell counts are usually within the normal range or slightly elevated and have not generally been useful in differentiating viral pneumonia from that due to bacteria. Children with bacteremic pneumococcal pneumonia frequently have markedly elevated white blood cell counts. Therefore, a peripheral white blood cell count that is normal or slightly elevated is not helpful, whereas a markedly elevated count increases the likelihood of a bacterial cause.

Bacterial cultures of sputum and of the upper respiratory tract have limited usefulness in differentiating viral pneumonias from that due to bacteria. Many normal children have pneumococci or *Hemophilus influenzae* in their upper respiratory tracts, so their presence in cultures is difficult to interpret. Cultures of blood, pleural fluid and material obtained directly from an involved lobe will be bacteriologically sterile in viral pneumonia cases; such cultures can be very useful in establishing a specific etiologic factor in bacterial pneumonia and should be obtained in severely ill patients.

Specific diagnosis of a viral infection depends on isolation of the agent from the respiratory tract or detection of an antibody rise. Acute phase serum should be obtained on the day of diagnosis, and convalescent phase serum ten days to three weeks later.

Rapid virus diagnosis may be available in some centers by fluorescence antibody staining of exfoliated respiratory epithelial cells. Detection of respiratory viral antigens in body fluids — pleural fluid, serum and urine — by techniques such as counter-current immunoelectrophoresis or radioimmunoassay has not been reported.

Diagnosis

Since pneumonia due to bacteria and *M. pneumoniae* responds to appropriate antimicrobial treatment and pneumonia due to viruses does not, it is important to make a specific etiologic diagnosis when possible. As noted previously, there are few clinical and laboratory findings that will allow this differentiation. In contrast, viral infections of the lung follow certain clinical and epidemiologic patterns, and these are useful in determining proper management of the patient with pneumonia. The clinician caring for children is urged, therefore, to familiarize himself or herself with these patterns and manage these patients accordingly.

Complications

It is becoming clear that otitis media is found commonly in children with infections due to respiratory viruses, especially RSV. Present data suggest that these cases of otitis media are initiated by the infecting virus; whether or not there is superimposed bacterial infection is not clear at this time. Other acute complications of viral pneumonia are unusual, including secondary bacterial invasion of the lung.

Long-term complications of viral pneumonia are unknown; adequate studies to answer this important question have not been done. It is clear, however, that some children have very severe chronic lung disease following adenovirus pneumonia.

Management

The course of viral pneumonia is not altered by the administration of antibiotics, and bacterial superinfections are so rare that the routine use of antimicrobials is not warranted. Symptomatic therapy, including bed rest, analgesics and antipyretics, maintenance of fluid intake and increased humidity is indicated.

Severely ill patients should be hospitalized; in-patient management should include maintenance of an adequate airway, postural drainage to ensure clearance of secretions, oxygen as necessary and adequate hydration.

Prevention

Vaccines for the prevention of viral pneumonia are not available. Hall and coworkers (1975) have demonstrated that RSV infections are highly contagious in hospitals, so special precautions should be taken to isolate children with pneumonia that could be due to RSV. Although it has not been demonstrated that lower respiratory tract infections due to other agents are similarly contagious, it would seem prudent to isolate all children with viral pneumonia while in hospital.

Prognosis

The prognosis of the individual child with viral pneumonia would seem to be excellent. In spite of this, pneumonia, presumably viral in most instances, continues to be a leading cause of death in small children. When this is coupled with the possible association of lower respiratory tract infections in childhood with chronic lung disease in adults, one should be cautious in considering viral pneumonia a benign disease. Obviously, much work is required to answer the many problems associated with this clinical entity.

REFERENCES

Acute respiratory illnesses reported to the U. S. National Health Survey during 1957–1962. *Am. Rev. Res. Dis., 88*:14, part 2, 1963.

Aherne, W., Bird, T., Court, S. D. M., Gardner, P. S., and McQuillin, J.: Pathologic changes in virus infections of the lower respiratory tract in children. *J. Clin. Pathol., 23*:7, 1970.

Becroft, D. M. O.: Histopathology of fatal adenovirus infection of the respiratory tract in young children. *J. Clin. Pathol., 20*:561, 1967.

Brandt, C. D., Kim, H. W., Arrobio, J. O., Jeffries, B. C., Wood, S. C., Chanock, R. M., and Parrott, R. H.: Epidemiology of respiratory syncytial virus infection in Washington, D. C. III. Composite analysis of eleven consecutive yearly epidemics. *Am. J. Epidemiol., 98*:355, 1973.

Brown, R. S., Nogrady, M. B., Spence, L., and Wiglesworth, F. W.: An outbreak of adenovirus type 7 infection in children in Montreal. *Can. Med. Assoc. J., 108*:434, 1973.

Buthala, D. A., and Soret, M. G.: Parainfluenza type 3 virus infections in hamsters: virologic, serologic, and pathologic studies. *J. Infect. Dis., 114*:226, 1964.

Chanock, R. M., and Parrott, R. H.: Acute respiratory disease in infancy and childhood: present understanding and prospects for prevention. *Pediatrics, 36*:21, 1965.

Chanock, R. M., Kapikian, A. Z., Mills, J., Kim, H. W., and Parrott, R. H.: Influence of immunological factors in respiratory syncytial virus diseases of the lower respiratory tract. *Arch. Environ. Health, 21*:347, 1970.

Chany, C., Lepine, P., Lelong, M., Le-Tan-Vinh, Satge, P., and Virat, J.: Severe and fatal pneumonia in infants and young children associated with adenovirus infections. *Am. J. Hyg., 67*:367, 1958.

Child health in the European region. *W.H.O. Chron., 25*:319, 1971.

Dingle, J. H., Badger, G. F., and Jordon, W. S., Jr.: *Illness in the Home: A Study of 25,000 Illnesses in a Group of Cleveland Families.* Cleveland, Press of Case Western Reserve University, 1964.

Foy, H. M., Cooney, M. K., McMahan, R., and Grayston, J. T.: Viral and mycoplasmal pneumonia in a prepaid medical care group during an eight-year period. *Am. J. Epidemiol., 97*:93, 1973.

Gardner, P. S., McQuillin, J., and Court, S. D. M.: Speculation on pathogenesis in death from respiratory syncytial virus infection. *Br. Med. J., 1*:327, 1970.

Glezen, W. P., and Denny, F. W.: Epidemiology of acute lower respiratory disease in children. *N. Engl. J. Med., 288*:498, 1973.

Glezen, W. P., and Fernald, G. W.: Effect of passive antibody on parainfluenza virus type 3 pneumonia in hamsters. *Infect. Immunol., 14*:212, 1976.

Glezen, W. P., Loda, F. A., Clyde, W. A., Jr., Senior, R. J., Sheaffer, C. I., Conley, W. G., and Denny, F. W.: Epidemiologic patterns of acute lower respiratory disease of children in a pediatric group practice. *J. Pediatr.*, 78:397, 1971.

Hall, C. B., Douglas, R. G., Jr., Geiman, J. M., and Messner, M. K.: Nosocomial respiratory syncytial virus infections. *N. Engl. J. Med.*, 293:1343, 1975.

Hope-Simpson, R. E., and Higgins, P. G.: A respiratory virus study in Great Britain: review and evaluation. *Prog. Med. Virol.*, 11:354, 1969.

Kim, H. W., Arrobio, J. O., Brandt, C. D., Jeffries, B. C., Pyles, G., Reid, J. L., Chanock, R. M., and Parrott, R. H.: Epidemiology of respiratory syncytial virus infection in Washington, D. C. I. Importance of the virus in different respiratory tract disease syndromes and temporal distribution of infection. *Am. J. Epidemiol.*, 98:216, 1973.

Lang, W. R., Howden, C. W., Laws, J., and Burton, J. F.: Bronchopneumonia with serious sequelae in children with evidence of adenovirus type 21 infection. *Br. Med. J.*, 1:73, 1969.

Loda, F. A., Glezen, W. P., and Clyde, W. A., Jr.: Respiratory disease in group day care. *Pediatrics*, 49:428, 1972.

McIntosh, K., Ellis, E. F., Hoffman, L. S., Lybass, T. G., Eller, J. J., and Fulginiti, V. A.: The association of viral and bacterial respiratory infections with exacerbations of wheezing in young asthmatic children. *J. Pediatr.*, 82:578, 1973.

Parrott, R. H., Kim, H. W., Arrobio, J. O., Hodes, D. S., Murphy, B. R., Brandt, C. D., Camargo, E., and Chanock, R. M.: Epidemiology of respiratory syncytial virus infection in Washington, D. C. II. Infection and disease with respect to age, immunologic status, race and sex. *Am. J. Epidemiol.*, 98:289, 1973.

Rice, R. P., and Loda, F. A.: A roentgenographic analysis of respiratory syncytial virus pneumonia in infants. *Radiology*, 87:1021, 1966.

Rooney, J. C., and Williams, H. E.: The relationship between proved viral bronchiolitis and subsequent wheezing. *J. Pediatr.*, 79:744, 1971.

World Health Statistics Report, 24:258, 1971.

Wright, H. T., Jr., Beckwith, J. B., and Gwinn, J. L.: A fatal case of inclusion body pneumonia in an infant infected with adenovirus type 3. *J. Pediatr.*, 64:528, 1964.

Zweiman, B., Schoenwetter, W. F., Pappano, J. E., Jr., Tempest, B., and Hildreth, E.: Patterns of allergic respiratory disease in children with a past history of bronchiolitis. *J. Allergy Clin. Immunol.*, 48:283, 1971.

CHAPTER TWENTY-THREE

INFECTIONS OF THE RESPIRATORY TRACT DUE TO MYCOPLASMA PNEUMONIAE

FLOYD W. DENNY, M.D.

Mycoplasmas, formerly called pleuropneumonia-like organisms (PPLO), have been known for many years to be important causes of veterinary diseases, but *Mycoplasma pneumoniae* is the only member of this group of agents proved to be pathogenic for humans. *M. pneumoniae* was first isolated in the 1940s by Eaton and his coworkers from a case of primary atypical pneumonia; it was considered a virus until the early 1960s, when it was shown to be a mycoplasma. Subsequently, this mycoplasma has been demonstrated to be a major cause of respiratory infections, especially pneumonia, in school-aged children and young adults.

Incidence

The incidence of *M. pneumoniae* pneumonia varies greatly with the age of the patient and the epidemicity of the organism. Clinical illnesses are unusual before the age of four or five years; the peak incidence is between 10 and 15 years. In school-aged children, college students and military personnel during epidemic periods, *M. pneumoniae* causes 40 to 60 per cent of pneumonia cases. The incidence of infections of other parts of the respiratory tract is unknown.

The Organism

M. pneumoniae is a small (approximately 0.150 μm wide) filamentous structure, without a cell wall, which is variable in length and has a specialized tip that measures 0.100 × 0.300 μm. This tip consists of a dense central core surrounded by a lucent space that is enveloped by an extension of the triple-layered unit membrane of the organism. A very dense central filament can be seen within the central core of the organism. This tip is the site of the attachment of *M. pneumoniae* to host cells, which will be described in a later section.

M. pneumoniae grows well in a special medium containing yeast extract and serum; it is thus the smallest known free-living organism in nature. Colonies appear after five to ten days of incubation as spherical, granular structures half submerged in the agar, measuring 30 to 100 microns in diameter; they rarely reveal the "fried-egg" morphology typical of many mycoplasmas. *M. pneumoniae* can be identified tentatively by its ability to hemolyze red blood cells and to reduce glucose. Specific identification is made by inhibition of growth in the presence of homotypic antibody.

Epidemiology

M. pneumoniae infections have been found worldwide, wherever an adequate search has been made. They are endemic in large communities. On this background of activity, prolonged, smoldering epidemics occur at irregular intervals. These periods of increased prevalence usually begin in the fall and last one or two years. In small communities, the endemic pattern of infection may be less apparent, and clinical illnesses are recognized only during epidemic periods.

The occurrence of *M. pneumoniae* illnesses is dictated at least in part by the age and specific antibody status of the patient. Children under five years of age apparently have frequent infections but usually are not ill; the implications of this in the pathogenesis of *M. pneumoniae* disease are discussed in the following section. It has been demonstrated in adults that there is an inverse relationship between levels of antibody and susceptibility. In the absence of antibody, the infection rate is high; in individuals with elevated titers there are few infections.

It would appear that *M. pneumoniae* is not highly communicable, since it may take several weeks to spread among members of a family. In spite of this, a very high percentage of susceptible contacts may become infected eventually. The prolonged carriage of *M. pneumoniae* in the infected host may be an important factor in the indolent epidemics caused by this organism.

Pathology, Immunology and Pathogenesis

PATHOLOGY. Little information is available on the histopathologic features of *M. pneumoniae* disease in humans because the disease is rarely fatal. In the few cases that have been reported, the essential features are interstitial pneumonia and acute bronchiolitis. Thickening of bronchiolar walls with edema, vascular congestion, and infiltrates of mononuclear and plasma cells are described. Polymorphonuclear leukocytes, when present, are usually confined to the bronchiolar lumen, where they are admixed with sloughed epithelial cells and debris.

Further insight into the pathologic changes of human disease is limited by the fact that material from these cases represents terminal disease upon which other complications may be superimposed. Several experimental models have been developed to study the pathophysiologic process of the disease; the most prominent of these are the Syrian hamster and the tracheal organ culture.

In the hamster model, animals are inoculated intranasally; infection is established by the end of the second week, and positive cultures persist for two to three months. Pneumonia appears shortly after infection; the characteristic lesion is peribronchial in location. The lung parenchyma is usually spared, although at times areas of interstitial edema and congestion or atelectatic changes secondary to bronchiolar obstruction may occur. The peribronchial infiltration involves the connective tissue, blood vessels, muscularis, lamina propria and basement membrane. Intraluminal exudation is usually present, ranging from small crescents of cells to enough material to produce obstruction of the airway. The chief intraluminal cell types are sloughed epithelial cells, polymorphonuclear leukocytes and macrophages; the submucosal cells are mainly lymphocytes and plasma cells.

Collier and Clyde (1974) have used hamster tracheal organ cultures to study host-cell injury by *M. pneumoniae*. In this model, ciliostasis occurs 48 to 72 hours after inoculation and appears specific for *M. pneumoniae*; other human mycoplasma species do not produce ciliostasis. Injury to epithelial cells is seen as early as 24 hours after inoculation and consists of cytoplasmic vacuolization, nuclear swelling with marginated cromatin and loss of cilia from some cells. Mycoplasma colonies appear on the epithelial surfaces by 48 hours; subsequently, the epithelial cells lose polarity and organization, and through cytoplasmic and nuclear disruption the surface layer is destroyed.

Immunofluorescent methods have identified the surface colonies as *M. pneumoniae;* in addition, specific antigen is seen extending into the epithelial layer. Applications of electron microscopy to comparable specimens has revealed the attachment of *M. pneumoniae* by the specialized terminal structure to cilia and to the epithelial cell surface. Organisms have been found in the intercellular spaces between and beneath the epithelium, but no structures resembling mycoplasmas have been found within infected cells. Similar changes have been observed in human tracheal organ cultures.

The electron microscopic techniques developed to study attached *M. pneumoniae* in tracheal organ cultures have been extended to the intact hamster model and to exfoliated cells from cases of human *M. pneumoniae* pneumonia. All studies have confirmed the attachment of the organism by the specialized tip to ciliated epithelial surfaces. Attachment involves specific neuraminidase-sensitive receptors on the respiratory epithelium. Studies have demonstrated that only living *M. pneumoniae* attach to cell surfaces and that following attachment there is alteration in host-cell macromolecular synthesis and carbohydrate metabolism, which precedes cytopathologic tissue change.

IMMUNOLOGY. A variety of serologic responses occurs following *M. pneumoniae* infections. Cold hemagglutinins are usually the first antibodies detected and the first to disappear; it has been demonstrated that the frequency and height of the cold hemagglutinin response are related directly to the severity of the pneumonic involvement. It should be recognized that cold hemagglutinins are nonspecific and can develop in patients with other diseases, including pneumonia due to other agents. Specific immunologic responses

persist for long periods after infection and can be demonstrated by several techniques, including complement-fixation, growth inhibition and radioimmunoprecipitation. Complement-fixing antibody tests, in which commercially available antigen is used, are satisfactory for usual diagnostic purposes. Characterization of the specific immunoglobulin composition of convalescent human sera has shown that IgM, IgA and IgG appear successively; IgM appears early and is followed by IgA and IgG, which persists the longest.

Studies have shown that humans who possess antibody to *M. pneumoniae* following natural disease are protected from subsequent infections and that this protection may be correlated with the height of circulating antibody. Experiments in hamsters infected by the natural route have shown similar protection. Animals inoculated by a route other than the respiratory tract showed less protection to a challenge infection, although the level of circulating antibody was equal to or greater than that found in animals infected by the natural route. These studies suggest that local immunity formed in the lung following infection, either humoral or cellular, is primarily responsible for protection. IgA-specific antibody has been found in tracheobronchial secretions by Brunner and coworkers (1973), but the amount detected is less than that found usually following viral respiratory tract infections. Furthermore, its biologic activity has not been determined. Whether this IgA has antiattachment qualities has not been demonstrated, but this could be an important protective mechanism in *M. pneumoniae* infections.

Studies using the hamster model have shown that the peribronchial round cells contain immunoglobulins. IgM appears early and is followed by IgG during the period of maximum pneumonia at two weeks. IgA-containing cells increase but are the least affected. Nonimmunoglobulin stainable lymphocytes tending to surround small blood vessels have been noticed to increase in number during the period of infection; this has suggested that cell-mediated immune mechanisms might be a factor in *M. pneumoniae* lung infections.

The role of cell-mediated immunity has been clarified further by the work of Fernald and coworkers (1976), who demonstrated that *M. pneumoniae*–reactive lymphocytes appear in peripheral blood following natural and experimental infections in humans. It was subsequently shown that ablation of thymus function by antithymocyte serum in the hamster prevented the typical pathologic changes of round cell accumulation in the peribronchial and perivascular spaces following *M. pneumoniae* infection. Since the formation of nonimmunoglobulin as well as immunoglobulin cells was inhibited, it was suggested that T cells had a direct and a helper function in this model.

PATHOGENESIS. The role of immunity in the pathogenesis of *M. pneumoniae* infections has been clarified further by observations of human infections. Several studies have shown that small children are infected commonly with *M. pneumoniae* but infrequently become ill. Observations in a day care center in Chapel Hill confirmed this observation and also demonstrated that reinfections occur commonly. Further studies in these children showed that those under five years of age developed circulating antibodies, but circulating lymphocytes could not be stimulated by *M. pneumoniae* antigen. In contrast, children over five years of age, in addition to the development of circulating antibodies, developed lymphocytes that responded to specific antigen.

All of the studies outlined have suggested that the pneumonic lesion following *M. pneumoniae* infection is an immunologic reaction that can be characterized best as "anamnestic pneumonia." Thus, the immunologic response of the host is responsible for the disease itself or for protection against it, depending on the qualitative and quanti-

tative balance of humoral and cellular immunity. Since this is inherently and inevitably linked to the aging process, it possibly answers some of the questions about the clinical and epidemiologic characteristics of *M. pneumoniae* disease.

Clinical Manifestations

Respiratory and nonrespiratory sites are involved in *M. pneumoniae* infections. The lung is the primary site of infection. The incubation period of pneumonia is somewhat variable, but is probably between two and three weeks. The onset of illness is gradual. No symptoms or signs are diagnostic of infection, but headache and malaise, fever, and cough are the predominant findings; sore throat occurs frequently. Usually the severity of symptoms is greater than the physical signs that occur later in the disease. Rales are the most prominent sign, but dullness to percussion and sputum production occur frequently. It is common for *M. pneumoniae* to be isolated from the sputum or the upper respiratory tract for several weeks to months after recovery.

The association of *M. pneumoniae* infections with illness in parts of the respiratory tract other than the lung has been reported in several population groups. As with *M. pneumoniae* pneumonia, there are no clinical characteristics of nonpneumonic infections that allow their easy identification, but undifferentiated upper respiratory infections, pharyngitis, croup, tracheobronchitis and bronchiolitis have been described. In addition, otitis media, otitis externa and bullous myringitis have all been described in association with *M. pneumoniae* infection.

Nonrespiratory sites of involvement include the skin, central nervous system, blood, heart and joints. In contrast to the proved and constant relationship between *M. pneumoniae* and respiratory tract infections, the relationship between *M. pneumoniae* and other organ systems is either tenuous or at best uncommon. The skin lesions include maculopapular rashes, erythema nodosum and the Stevens-Johnson syndrome. Some patients with infections due to *M. pneumoniae* have had meningoencephalitis, and patients with the Guillain-Barré syndrome have been described. Hemolytic anemia is the most common hematologic disorder encountered, but thrombocytopenia and coagulation defects have been reported. The heart has been involved infrequently, but myocarditis and pericarditis have been described, as has a rheumatic fever-like syndrome.

The spectrum of illnesses associated with *M. pneumoniae* infections may vary from severe, and on occasion fatal, pneumonia to asymptomatic infection. Severity may be determined in part by epidemiologic setting, age and antibody status.

Complications following infections due to *M. pneumoniae* have not been described frequently; specifically, bacterial superinfection has not been a common observation. It should be made clear, however, that follow-up studies of *M. pneumoniae* illnesses are insufficient for any definite conclusions to be made regarding long-term complications. With the recognition that *M. pneumoniae* reinfections occur and that these can lead to disease, the possibility exists that this organism could play a role in the development of chronic lung problems.

Roentgenographic Appearance

As with the other aspects of clinical infection, there is nothing diagnostic about roentgenogram findings. The pneumonia is usually described as interstitial or bronchopneumonic, and involvement is usually in one of the lower lobes. Pleural fluid is unusual, and its presence would suggest another diagnosis in most instances.

Laboratory Findings

The peripheral leukocyte count is normal most of the time, as is the differential white blood cell count. Swabs of the throat or sputum cultured on special mycoplasma medium may demonstrate *M. pneumoniae;* as mentioned previously, these patients remain colonized for long periods of time.

Acute phase serum should be obtained at the time of diagnosis and a cold hemagglutinin titer determined. Convalescent phase serum should be obtained in ten days to three weeks; a specific antibody rise during this time indicates the presence of an *M. pneumoniae* infection.

Rapid diagnosis by a study of exfoliated cells with fluorescent antibody or electron microscopic techniques is possible, but these tests are too cumbersome and expensive at this time for routine use.

Diagnosis

As outlined previously, there are no specific clinical, epidemiologic or laboratory tests that will allow a definite diagnosis of *M. pneumoniae* illnesses early in their course. Certain observations are suggestive of the presence of infection due to this organism, however, and can be helpful to the practicing physician. The occurrence of pneumonia in school-aged children and young adults, especially if cough is a prominent symptom, is always suggestive of *M. pneumoniae* pneumonia. The presence of cold hemagglutinins in a titer equal to or greater than 1:64 supports the diagnosis. The diagnosis can be confirmed by the isolation of the organism and the demonstration of the development of specific antibodies. If the presence of *M. pneumoniae* in a community can be confirmed in a few patients by isolation of the organism or by serologic techniques, the probability of other patients with characteristic clinical manifestations having *M. pneumoniae* illnesses is greatly increased.

Management

M. pneumoniae shows exquisite in vitro sensitivity to erythromycin and to most of the tetracyclines. The agent has

Figures 1 to 6. Chest-roentgenograms from patients having *Mycoplasma pneumoniae* pneumonia established by culture and serologic techniques. Note diversity of types of pulmonary involvement. (From Clyde, W. A., Jr., in Gallagher, Heald and Garrell (Eds.): *Medical Care of the Adolescent.* New York, Appleton-Century-Crofts.)

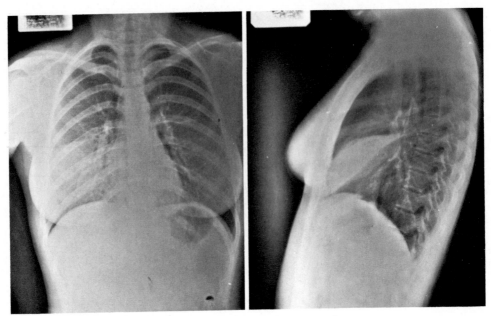

Figure 1. Right middle lobe pneumonia.

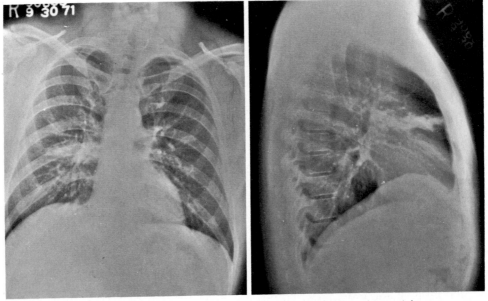

Figure 2. Pneumonitis involving segments of the right middle and lower lobes.

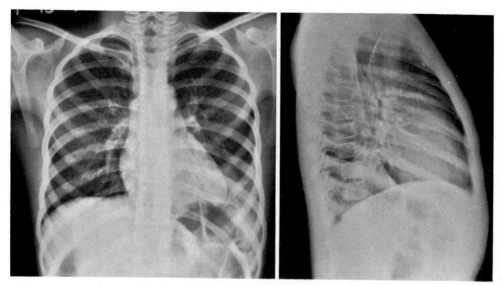

Figure 3.   Left lower lobe pneumonia.

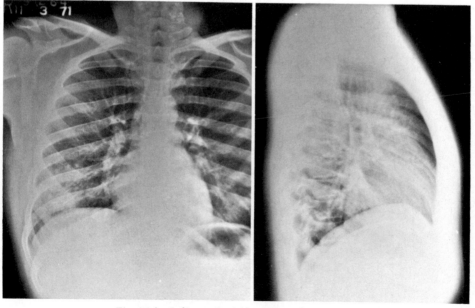

Figure 4.   Infiltrates in right middle and lower lobes.

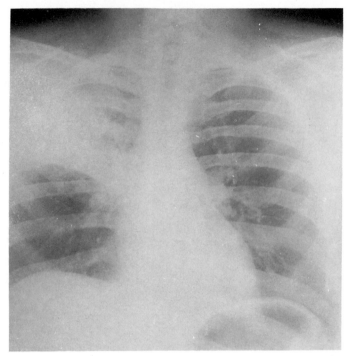

Figure 5. Consolidation of the anterior segment of the right upper lobe.

variable sensitivity to some of the other commonly used antibiotics; as anticipated, because of the absence of a cell wall in mycoplasmas, it is quite resistant to the penicillins. The effectiveness of erythromycin and the tetracyclines in shortening the course of *M. pneumoniae* pneumonia has been demonstrated in several population groups. Erythromycin is the drug of choice in children

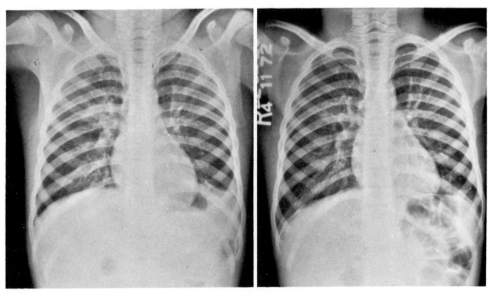

Figure 6. *Left,* Pleural effusion, left costophrenic angle. *Right,* Clearing two days later.

because of the untoward effects of the tetracyclines in this group; it should be exhibited in full therapeutic doses for several days after defervescence, usually a total of seven to ten days. In spite of the efficacy of those antibiotics in ameliorating the course of *M. pneumoniae* illnesses, the organism is not eradicated.

Symptomatic therapy, including bed rest, analgesics and antipyretics, maintenance of fluid intake and increased humidity, is indicated.

Prevention

Efforts have been made to produce an effective vaccine against *M. pneumoniae* infections; inactivated and live attenuated vaccines have been developed and evaluated. Inactivated vaccines have been most extensively evaluated in military personnel; in one study, Mogabgab (1973) reported 87 per cent reduction in bronchitis and 66 per cent reduction in pneumonia due to *M. pneumoniae*. Other studies have demonstrated that inactivated vaccines are rather poorly antigenic and protective. This, plus the suggestion in one study that vaccinated individuals who did not develop an immune response had more severe disease following challenge with virulent *M. pneumoniae* than did similarly inoculated controls, has led to attempts to develop live attenuated vaccines. At the present time, neither type of vaccine has been licensed for commercial use. In view of the data suggesting that *M. pneumoniae* pneumonia is an immunologically mediated disease, the use of any vaccine in children would seem unwise at this time.

Prognosis

The prognosis in the individual patient with an *M. pneumoniae* infection would seem to be excellent, but fatalities have been reported. This, and the role this organism could possibly play in the development of chronic lung disease, should be a constant reminder that *M. pneumoniae* illnesses are not always completely benign.

REFERENCES

Brunner, H., Greenberg, H. B., James, W. D., Horswood, R. L., Couch, R. B., and Chanock, R. M.: Antibody to *Mycoplasma pneumoniae* in nasal secretions and sputa of experimentally infected human volunteers. *Infect. Immunol.*, 8:612, 1973.

Clyde, W. A., Jr.: Models of *Mycoplasma pneumoniae* infection. *J. Infect. Dis.*, 127:S69, 1973.

Collier, A. M., and Clyde, W. A., Jr.: Appearance of *Mycoplasma pneumoniae* in lungs of experimentally infected hamsters and sputum from patients with natural disease. *Am. Rev. Resp. Dis.*, 110:765, 1974.

Denny, F. W., Clyde, W. A., Jr., and Glezen, W. P.: *Mycoplasma pneumoniae* disease: clinical spectrum, pathophysiology, epidemiology, and control. *J. Infect. Dis.*, 123:74, 1971.

Fernald, G. W.: Role of host response in *Mycoplasma pneumoniae* disease. *J. Infect. Dis.*, 127:S55, 1973.

Fernald, G. W., and Clyde, W. A., Jr.: Pulmonary immune mechanisms in *Mycoplasma pneumoniae* disease. In Kirkpatrick, C. H., and Reynolds, H. Y. (Eds.): *Immunologic and Infectious Reactions in the Lung.* New York, Marcel Dekker, Inc., 1976, pp. 101–130.

Fernald, G. W., Collier, A. M., and Clyde, W. A., Jr.: Respiratory infections due to *Mycoplasma pneumoniae* in infants and children. *Pediatrics*, 55:327, 1975.

Foy, H. M., Grayston, J. T., and Kenny, G. E.: Epidemiology of *Mycoplasma pneumoniae* infection in families. *J.A.M.A.*, 197:859, 1966.

Mogabgab, W. J.: Protective efficacy of killed *Mycoplasma pneumoniae* vaccine measured in large-scale studies in a military population. *Am. Rev. Resp. Dis.*, 108:899, 1973.

Steinberg, P., White, R. J., Fuld, S. L., Gutekunst, R. R., Chanock, R. M., and Senterfit, L. B.: Ecology of *Mycoplasma penumoniae* infections in Marine recruits at Parris Island, South Carolina. *Am. J. Epidemiol.*, 89:62, 1969.

Taylor, G., Taylor-Robinson, D., and Fernald, G. W.: Reduction in the severity of *Mycoplasma pneumoniae*–induced pneumonia in hamsters by immunosuppressive treatment with antithymocyte sera. *J. Med. Microbiol.*, 7:343, 1973.

Wilson, M. H., and Collier, A. M.: Ultrastructural study of *Mycoplasma pneumoniae* in organ culture. *J. Bacteriol.*, 125:332, 1976.

CHAPTER TWENTY-FOUR

INFLUENZA

ROBERT H. PARROTT, M.D.

The Virus

Influenza illness has been defined epidemiologically for centuries; influenza viruses were the first viral agents proved to be respiratory tract pathogens. Nonetheless, the terms "influenza" and "flu" are among the most overused diagnoses for nondescript infectious diseases in both lay and medical circles. Perhaps this is because the spectrum of clinical response to influenza infection is broad and the most practical clue to the probable diagnosis of influenza is epidemiologic—the knowledge that influenza infection is prevalent in the community.

Influenza viruses are members of the myxovirus group. They are essentially spherical virions, 80 to 100 nm. in diameter, and they contain a ribonucleic acid nucleoprotein central helix surrounded by an envelope of lipoprotein. The envelope has periodic projections or spikes that house the hemagglutinin (HA) and neuraminidase (NA) antigens, which are the basis for the newer W.H.O. nomenclature for influenza.

There are three antigenically distinct influenza viruses in regard to their ribonucleoprotein: A, B and C. Within the A and B serotypes, variation in antigenic composition occurs from time to time. The changes may be major, such as a complete shift in either HA or NA or both HA and NA at once. Minor mutations or "antigenic drift" may take place within a single type of HA or NA. Kilbourne (1973) believes that pandemic or epidemic severity "reflects principally the extent of antigenic change from pre-existing virus;" Table 1 both displays the W.H.O. nomenclature for influenza A viruses and shows the basis for Kilbourne's belief. This antigenic shifting largely accounts for the ability of influenza to produce epidemics even in populations of persons who have previously experienced influenza infection or immunization and has serious implications for the preparation and availability of effective vaccines.

Epidemiology and Immunity

Influenza infection often occurs in epidemics that may sweep through a community in a matter of one or two months. Morbidity in a susceptible population may be high and is particularly severe in infants and those over 65 years of age. The incidence of infection

TABLE 1. ANTIGENIC VARIATIONS IN HEMAGGLUTININ (HA) AND NEURAMINIDASE (NA) OF THE VIRUS AND PANDEMIC SEVERITY OF INFLUENZA

Year	Virus		Change in	Extent of Change	Result
1918	H-sw	N1	?	?	Pandemic (severe)
192?	H0	N1	HA	++	No pandemic
			NA	+	
1947	H1	N1	HA	++	Pandemic (mild)
			NA	+	
1957	H2	N2	HA	+++	Pandemic (severe)
			NA	+++	
1968	H3	N2	HA	+++	Pandemic (moderate)

From Kilbourne, E. D.: The molecular epidemiology of influenza. *J. Infect. Dis.*, 127:478, 1973. University of Chicago Press, Publisher.

and illness is highest, however, in children of school age. Type- and subtype-specific immunity after natural infection exists, based on anti-HA and anti-NA antibodies, but is not of high order; children may become infected several times within a matter of years by the same or related strains. Detectable type-specific serum antibodies, however, do occur and persist. There is evidence that antibody developed against earlier strains may rise during a subsequent infection with a related strain of influenza virus. Perhaps this is the reason that the incidence of influenza infection and clinical illness is lower in older persons than in school-age children.

Influenza A virus activity was demonstrated in infants and young children from metropolitan Washington, D.C., during each of 17 successive August-July respiratory disease years; during 15 of these years, at least 2 per cent of hospitalized respiratory disease patients yielded an influenza A or B virus or showed an influenza A or B (CF) serum complement-fixing antibody response. Overall, 14 per cent of 812 croup patients and 5 per cent of 5313 hospitalized patients with respiratory infection showed evidence of influenza A or B virus infection. Infection with influenza A virus was about four times more common than infection with influenza B virus, though the mean period of hospitalization with either virus was the same, 7.9 days. Both influenza viruses were recovered more than twice as frequently from respiratory disease outpatients than from respiratory disease inpatients. Influenza A infections were particularly common during the period 1968-1974, after the appearance of the H3N2 virus subtype. Patients with serious influenza A virus infections were especially likely to have croup, to be seen during December through February, and to be infant Negro males. During the peak month of a composite of 11 consecutive influenza A virus outbreaks, influenza A virus infection was demonstrated in 70 per cent of croup patients and in 36 per cent of all hospitalized respiratory patients. During the peak month of a composite of 6 consecutive influenza B virus outbreaks, influenza B virus infection was demonstrated in 27 per cent of croup patients and in 10 per cent of all hospitalized respiratory disease patients.

Laboratory Diagnosis

Laboratory demonstration of influenza virus infection may include either recovery of the virus from throat washings and swabbings or evidence of a significant rise in serum antibody during convalescence from illness. Chick embryo has been the traditional laboratory host for isolation of influenza viruses. The clinical specimen is preferably inoculated into the amniotic sac of 10- or 11-day-old chick embryos. The amniotic fluid is harvested in two or three days and tested for hemagglutinins with chicken or guinea pig red blood cells. The inoculation of monkey kidney cell cultures, however, and the subsequent development of hemadsorption, which occurs with myxovirus-infected tissue culture, seems to be a simpler and more sensitive method, although certain influenza A strains do grow best in chick embryo. Type-specific animal sera are used to identify the virus recovered in egg or tissue culture. Sera obtained from patients early and about three weeks after the onset of illness are tested for antibodies to influenza virus by complement-fixation, hemagglutination inhibition or tissue culture neutralization methods.

Pathogenesis

One of the predominant pathogenic characteristics of influenza viruses in susceptible hosts, such as chick embryos, ferrets or humans, is a peculiar affinity for epithelial cells of the respiratory tract mucosa. Typically, influenza virus infection destroys ciliated epithelium, and there is metaplastic hyperplasia of the tracheal and bronchial epithelium with associated edema. The alveoli may become distended with a hyaline-like material.

Clinical Features

Infection in humans may be subclinical or may be accompanied by mild, moderate or severe clinical manifestations. In most cases of overt illness, the throat and nasal mucous membranes are dry and there is a dry cough with a tendency toward hoarseness. There is fever of sudden onset accompanied by flushed facies, photophobia with retrobulbar pain, myalgia, hyperesthesia and sometimes prostration. In uncomplicated cases, these symptoms last for four or five days. Usually, a child wiith influenza infection has a more sudden onset of these "toxic" signs than do children with parainfluenza, respiratory syncytial virus or adenovirus infection.

Croup is a common manifestation, especially in infants. Complications of influenza infection include severe viral pneumonia, often hemorrhagic, and encephalitis or encephalopathy. Influenza infection, particularly that due to type B, has been found in significant numbers of children with Reye's syndrome. Influenza virus infection has also been associated with sudden infant death syndrome. Bacterial infection due to *H. influenzae,* beta hemolytic streptococci, or especially *Staphylococcus aureus* may complicate influenza infection, apparently with a higher frequency than in other viral illnesses. Pneumonia is the principal clinical manifestation of bacterial invasion.

Treatment

There is no specific therapy for influenza virus infection; thus, antibiotics should not be used in uncomplicated influenza. Experimentally, the drug amantadine has been shown to have some effect in preventing and possibly ameliorating influenza virus infection due to certain strains of virus. However, the drug has not been widely studied in children, and the ratio of therapeutic to toxic dose is narrow. Also, it must be used prior to infection, and specific viral diagnosis in anticipation of exposure is impractical.

Multivalent inactivated type A and B influenza virus vaccines are available for immunization. To be effective, such vaccines must contain antigens similar to those that will be encountered in nature within a few months to a year following vaccine administration. Because influenza viruses show progressive antigenic variation, suitable vaccine strains are likely to be those recovered in the recent past. Worldwide surveillance is maintained with the hope of identifying major antigenic shifts so that new strains can be included in vaccines.

There is increasing recognition that influenza infections produce more illness in infants and children than was previously believed. Also, children are a major link in the spread of influenza infection throughout the community. Broad use of an effective vaccine in children, particularly those of school age, might well reduce the spread of virus and lessen the total impact of influenza in a community.

However, except in the face of a pandemic, routine immunization with killed vaccine has not been recommended for infants and children. Children, and particularly infants, have a greater rate of febrile reactions to killed vaccine, probably related to viral protein itself.

Studies to determine optimal dosage of killed vaccine for children in the recent national "swine flu" immunization program showed ① doses of "whole virus" vaccine that regularly produced antibody also produced an undesirable level of local and febrile reactions, and ② children responded with fewer reactions and reasonable antibody levels after two doses of "split product" vaccines given four weeks apart.

In these studies, certain guidelines were reached for pediatric dosage of inactivated vaccine containing a new antigen, such as the Nsw1 N1 virus found in military personnel and others in early 1976, and designated Asw/NJ/76. Essentially, it was determined that children 3 to 17 years of age who had no prior exposure to the influenza strain in the vaccine could tolerate a split virus vaccine dosage of 200 CCA units without significant reactions, but this dosage failed to produce satisfactory antibody responses. However, a second dose of 200 CCA units about 4 weeks after the first did provide significant antibody levels in most. The addition of 200 CCA units per dose of another influenza A antigen in a "bivalent" preparation did not add untoward reactions. Half this dosage (100 CCA units) was also acceptable and immunogenic in a limited study of children six months to three years of age. These guidelines should be helpful in determining dosage of such vaccines in the future.

Several research groups are developing potential attenuated influenza vaccines with inhibitor-resistant or temperature-sensitive strains. Prototypes of such vaccines have been shown to be attenuated for adults and older children. However, mild residual pathogenicity has been demonstrated in infants who had no prior experience with any influenza virus. Further attenuated prototypes are under study.

Routine influenza immunization is recommended for patients in disease categories that result in the highest mortality rates following influenza infection. Primary influenza immunization and annual renewal doses are indicated for infants and children with (1) rheumatic heart disease, especially those with mitral stenosis; (2) other cardiovascular disorders, such as congenital or hypertensive heart disease, especially those with evidence of frank or incipient cardiac insufficiency; (3) chronic bronchopulmonary disease, such as cystic fibrosis, chronic asthma, chronic bronchitis, bronchiectasis and pulmonary tuberculosis, and patients with weak or paralyzed respiratory muscles; (4) chronic metabolic disease; (5) chronic glomerulonephritis or nephrosis; and (6) chronic neurologic disorders. Consideration should also be given to the immunization of children in institutions, particularly during years of expected high incidence.

Since formulations and content of vaccines are likely to change, the physician is advised to consult the most recent statements from the Public Health Service Advisory Committee on Immunization Practices or the American Academy of Pediatrics Committee on Infectious Diseases.

REFERENCES

Kilbourne, E. D.: The molecular epidemiology of influenza. *J. Infect. Dis., 127*:478, 1973.
Jackson, G. G., and Muldoon, R. L.: Viruses causing common respiratory infections in man. V. Influenza A (Asian). *J. Infect. Dis., 131*:308, 1975.

CHAPTER TWENTY–FIVE

BRONCHIECTASIS

Rosa Lee Nemir, M.D.

Bronchiectasis, meaning dilatation of bronchi, was first described by Laennec in 1819 in his *Traité de l'Auscultation Médiate*. Since this first report, extensive literature has accumulated giving the natural history of the disease based on both clinical and experimental observations. Currently, reports are appearing on effective surgical procedures, as well as follow-up studies comparing similar groups treated either surgically or entirely by medical means.

Incidence

The true incidence of bronchiectasis is not reflected by any statistical report, and an accurate statement of its frequency is difficult. Bronchography, the most reliable diagnostic test, is not used often enough in those asymptomatic patients whose history suggests the possibility of bronchial damage; nor is it applied to many of those recovering from such infections as measles, recurrent pneumonia or respiratory tract illness in which continuing symptoms and persistent roentgenographic findings suggest an underlying pulmonary pathologic change.

Clark (1963), reviewing the experience in Great Britain, suggested an annual incidence in 1951 of 1.06 per 10,000 children. In the United States, Ruberman and coworkers (1957) reviewed 1711 patients with pneumonia and studied by bronchography 69 children whose chest roentgenograms showed residual findings. Bronchiectasis was present in 29, or 1.7 per cent. In Copenhagen, in a follow-up study of 151 patients who had pneumonia or pertussis possibly complicated by pneu-

monia, Biering (1956) found only one child with bronchiectasis. Between 1966 and 1971, 0.3 per cent of all patients admitted to New Delhi hospitals were found to have bronchiectasis (Malhotra and coworkers, 1973).

Certainly children with the classic symptoms of bronchiectasis have not been seen with frequency in recent years. The decreased incidence results from several factors: the impressive decline in the childhood infections pertussis and measles, both formerly common precursors of bronchiectasis; the effective use of antibacterial agents in preventing and curing common lower respiratory tract infections; the decreased incidence of primary pulmonary tuberculosis in infancy and early childhood; and the better management of atelectasis and damaged lung by bronchial drainage and physiotherapy.

Factors Associated with the Development of Bronchiectasis

A. CONGENITAL BRONCHIECTASIS. This category is now accepted as being responsible for a small percentage of cases of bronchiectasis. It is thought to be the result of developmental arrest. In postnatal developmental arrest, the involved areas may result in the formation of cysts which retain fluid or air and which may become infected, resulting in saccular bronchiectasis. The signs of disease usually appear early, but are contingent on the frequency of the predisposing respiratory infections.

A defect in the development of bronchial cartilage in young infants, first described by Williams and Campbell in 1960, has also gained attention as a cause of congenital bronchiectasis. There are 18 such patients in the literature. Characteristically, these patients have mild respiratory illness associated with wheezing, cough and a predilection to recurrent episodes of respiratory infections. Autopsy reports from two patients by Mitchell and Bury (1975) describe obliterative bronchiolitis, as well as deficiency of cartilage in the fourth division of segmental bronchi. One pathologist maintains that infection rather than a congenital factor is responsible, but the very young age of the patients argues against this theory. Moreover, Wayne and Taussig's recent report (1976) of cartilage defect (Williams-Campbell syndrome) in siblings suggests, etiologically, a congenital factor. This is the first description of a familial incidence in the literature.

Tracheobronchomegaly, first described by Mounier-Kuhn (1932), is associated with the development of bronchiectasis and attributed to a congenital developmental failure of elastic and muscular tissues of the trachea and main bronchi. The original cases were in adults, but later an eight-year-old child and recently an 18-month-old infant were described. Such instances are quite rare, the disease being described chiefly in adults; but the symptoms of chronic respiratory disease and of bronchiectasis often date to early childhood. The markedly dilated trachea, almost the size of the vertebral body, is apparent on chest films.

ACQUIRED BRONCHIECTASIS. Most of the patients belong in this group. Many clinical studies involving large numbers of children have established that the three most frequent antecedent infections are pertussis, measles and pneumonia. Accumulating evidence points to the respiratory virus infections, especially the adenovirus, as a predisposing factor in the development of bronchiectasis. Other factors are those associated with bronchial obstruction: foreign body aspiration, enlarged bronchopulmonary nodes of primary tuberculosis or other causes, mediastinal masses and tumors, and anatomic pulmonary anomalies.

In 1933 Kartagener described a syndrome consisting of the triad of bronchiectasis, sinusitis and situs inversus. The greater frequency of bronchiectasis in such instances has been documented by reports of over 400 patients from many countries. According to Adams and Churchill (1937) and Olsen (1943), who also described an accompanying nasal polyposis in many of his cases, the frequency of bronchiectasis in congenital dextrocardia is from 15 to 20 per cent. The rarity of this triad among all patients with bronchiectasis is apparent in Perry and King's report (1940) of 400 patients, only six of whom were found to have the Kartagener syndrome. The incidence of situs inversus in Japan following a mass roentgenographic chest survey by Katsuhara and coworkers (1972) is 1 in 4100, twice the rate in Caucasians. A genetic recessive factor was postulated, and its greater frequency was explained on the basis of the higher incidence of consanguineous marriages in Japan. Bronchiectasis occurred in 0.25 per cent of these patients, again a higher incidence. With a different approach to the study of the frequency of Kartagener's syndrome, Miller and Divertie (1972) in the United States, using clinical, radiographic and electrographic diagnostic observations, reviewed 106 patients with complete or partial situs inversus seen at the Mayo Clinic during a 27-year period. Kartagener's syndrome was found in 19 of these, but most significant was the longevity of one patient, a 72-year-old woman.

The familial nature of bronchiectasis is indicated by a report of two children in one family, and the genetic factor, postulated by Cockayne (1938) and developed by Torgersen (1947), is supported by its presence in identical twins, and further suggested by the Japanese studies.

The cause of the high incidence of bronchiectasis among the Maoris in New Zealand has not been determined, but among the 65 described by Hinds (1958), none had dextrocardia or cystic fibrosis. Similarly, the greater

frequency of bronchiectasis reported by
Fleshman and coworkers (1968) among
Alaskan native children 16 years of age
or under (88 of the 100 patients were
Eskimos) is not understood, although it
appears to be associated with the
greater frequency of lower respiratory
tract disease in this same segment of
Alaskan population. Maxwell (1972)
found a high incidence of bronchiectasis among the Australian Aboriginal
children suffering from chronic chest
disease in an area where measles, pertussis and tuberculosis have virtually
been eradicated. The 83 children with
bronchiectasis and the 35 with chronic
bronchitis responded to good medical
care but reverted to illness when returned to their homes, where poor social factors and malnutrition appeared
to influence the recrudescence. In this
study and in all the above, there were
no patients with agammaglobulinemia,
cystic fibrosis or situs inversus.

It is understandable that the diffuse,
frequent respiratory infections in patients with cystic fibrosis of the pancreas may produce extensive bronchial
damage resulting ultimately in pulmonary complications such as bronchiectasis. The pathologic features and pathogenesis of the pulmonary lesions have
been well described. The frequency of
cystic fibrosis was surprisingly high in
one study from Australia, with 57 cases
among 241 patients studied (1959).

Similarly, patients with agammaglobulinemia have acquired bronchiectasis.
Collins and Dudley (1955) reported the
pathologic findings in two such cases
and Visconti in another. Among 187
patients with bronchiectasis reported by
Glauser and coworkers (1966), congenital hypogammaglobulinemia occurred
in four boys, and acquired hypogammaglobulinemia in one girl. Nevertheless, gamma globulin deficiency does
not appear to be commonly associated
with bronchiectasis. Pittman (1960), for
example, studied the gamma globulin
concentrations in 52 patients with long-
standing bronchiectasis. She failed to
find any with agammaglobulinemia, but
found one patient with hypogamma-

globulinemia whom she treated over a
four-year period.

Asthma and chronic sinusitis are frequently present in patients with bronchiectasis, but whether they occur as
antecedent or complication is not yet
clear. Today, with the liberal use of antibiotics, sinusitis is less common, and
when it occurs, is usually amenable to
medical therapy. The causal or sequential relationship is not clear.

REVERSIBLE AND IRREVERSIBLE BRON-
CHIECTASIS. The type of pneumonia
preceding bronchiectasis is more often
interstitial or bronchopneumonic. Such
infection is associated with bronchial
disease because of peribronchial infiltration and endobronchial edema, mucosal swelling and obstruction by muco-
secretions. Serial bronchograms in
patients with prolonged atypical pneumonia have demonstrated that bronchial dilatation may clear within two to
three months in many instances.

The term *reversible bronchiectasis* is
generally applied to this pathologic
state, and Blades and Dugan (1944)
called these cases *pseudobronchiectasis*. It
has become clear that bronchial dilatation described as cylindrical may be reversible, but saccular bronchiectasis is irreversible. Lees (1950) has shown that
cylindrical bronchiectasis is relatively
common after pertussis in which viscid
secretions are abundant. This concept
of reversible bronchiectasis, entailing
the disappearance of the compensatory
bronchial dilatation following the expansion of a previously collapsed portion of the lung, is important to the clinician, pointing up the need for a
follow-up bronchogram before pulmonary resection is recommended. Nelson
and Christoforidis (1958), for example,
reported four patients who were
thought to have cylindrical bronchiectasis shortly after pneumonia, but were
spared operation by a second bronchogram, interpreted as normal. In reporting a similar experience with two children, Crausaz (1970) discussed the
factors influencing the reversibility of
bronchial dilatation, such as the time
interval following the damaging agent,

the etiologic relation to infection or foreign body, the age of the patient, and the success of the immediate treatment. Drapanas and coworkers (1966) described a patient who sustained a poststenotic injury to the left main bronchus following a car accident. Extensive cylindrical and saccular bronchiectasis in the left lung, demonstrated by cinebronchography, was reversed shortly after surgical repair was performed one month after the accident.

Pathogenesis

A number of experimental studies and extensive publications have clarified our understanding of the pathogenesis of bronchiectasis. It is now generally agreed that infection and obstruction of the bronchi are the two important etiologic factors in the production of acquired bronchiectasis. It is also clear that mechanical stress and obstruction alone may not result in permanent damage to the bronchi. It is still not certain in which order these two underlying causes need to occur. Certainly they complement each other in the development of damaged bronchi.

In atelectatic areas produced by the obstruction of major bronchi or peripheral bronchi where the dilatation compensates for the decreased parenchymal lung volume, the retained bronchial secretions favor anaerobic growth, which results in damage to bronchial walls. The pressure of tuberculous bronchopulmonary nodes damages the bronchi early, often eroding the bronchus and injuring its elastic tissue and muscular wall. Stenosis alone may occur, or bronchiectasis may develop later.

In patients with pneumonia, severe bronchial infection may produce abnormal physiology associated with decreased ciliary action and necrosis of the bronchial walls. These factors, together with retained bronchial secretions, may lead to weakening of the walls of the bronchi and resultant dilatation.

Clinically and experimentally, atelectasis over a period of time may occur without subsequent ectasia of the bronchi. Lees (1950), in a report of 150 children with pertussis, found atelectasis in 65, or 43 per cent, and yet found only four cases of bronchiectasis, three reversible and one showing possible permanent damage on follow-up. On the other hand, similar observations by others in children with bronchiectasis have stressed atelectasis as an antecedent factor.

Anspach (1934) described the triangular shadow adjacent to the heart as atelectasis of the lower lobe of the lung and pointed out the direct relation of the long duration of such obstruction to the development of bronchiectasis. Indeed, necropsies in infants dying early in the course of such lower lobe collapse failed to show bronchial dilatation even though thick exudate filled the smaller bronchi.

The well known experimental work in rabbits done by Tannenberg and Pinner (1942) showed that ligation of the bronchi alone did not lead to bronchiectasis. They concluded that the mechanical forces operating when air is absorbed after bronchial occlusion tend to constrict, not dilate, bronchi and that uncomplicated pulmonary atelectasis would not cause bronchiectasis unless accompanied by infection. Such an infection may produce, within three to four weeks, an extensive saccular bronchiectasis in an atelectatic lung.

Experimental work on dogs by Croxatto and Lanari (1954) also demonstrated the effect of bronchial ligation on dilatation of the bronchi by retained secretions. Within two months the bronchial dilatation became stabilized. "Infection superimposed to the dilatation produced by retained secretions led to the production of bronchiectasis and...in some cases, even though the dilating material was extracted, the bronchus remained dilated." Clearly, in some instances, the bronchial dilatation was reversible.

A controlled experimental study was done by Cheng (1954), who subjected rats to both sham and actual bronchial ligation, using antibiotic therapy in some. From his investigation, Cheng suggested that bronchitis and stagnation of the accompanying secretions and exudate are two essential factors in the development of bronchiectasis. He concluded that bronchiectasis is apparently due to the pressure of accumulated stagnant secretions on bronchial walls weakened by inflammation.

Parenchymal collapse of varying extent occurs early in bronchiectasis on the basis of bronchial obstruction alone, extrinsic or intrinsic, and late in the disease on the basis of resultant bronchial wall pathologic changes. The normal flexibility of the bronchi is lost when the elastic and muscular tissues are destroyed and replaced by fibrous tissues.

Pathology

Until several decades ago the pathology of bronchiectasis was based on postmortem specimens of advanced disease. Large ectatic bronchi filled with purulent material were grossly characteristic of the disease, and the adjacent parenchyma was usually infected, showing diffuse pneumonia or abscesses and sometimes emphysema. Such pathologic features are seen less frequently today because antibiotic therapy has prevented many advanced inflammatory lesions, and immunologic protection (with vaccines) from rubeola and pertussis have dramatically decreased the former predominant antecedent causes of bronchiectasis. Surgical resection, in suitable cases, has cured many patients. Surgery has also made available for pathologic study ample material which reflects the stages in the development of bronchiectasis, so that mild, moderate and severe instances may be analyzed. Macroscopically, in acquired bronchiectasis, there are dilated bronchi, whether fusiform, cylindrical or saccular; often parenchymal collapse of the involved lobe; and usually pleural thickening with strong adhesions. If the disease is early, cylin-

drical or fusiform bronchi are found; if late, the saccular variety occurs, often filled with mucopurulent material. Occasionally an accompanying bronchopneumonia or fibrosis and patchy emphysema in the area distal to the diseased bronchi may be found.

Under microscopic examination, the chief lesion is found in the bronchi; the duration and nature of infection determine the tissue reaction. There is relatively severe bronchial destruction with inflammatory changes. The progression of bronchial wall damage is, first, destruction of elastic tissue; next, damage to the muscular coat; and finally, damage to the cartilage of the bronchi. Hayward and Reid (1952) described the extent of damage to the bronchial cartilage and demonstrated that the greatest pathologic change is found in saccular bronchiectasis, in which cartilage is always absent in the walls of saccular dilatation, whereas the cartilages are normal in cylindrical bronchiectasis. Calcifications have also been described in the cartilage. These sequential changes have been especially well analyzed by Whitwell (1952), who used 200 consecutive specimens from the bronchial epithelial lining. The columnar cells are replaced by cuboidal and then by squamous cells, which are sometimes heaped into layers. Notably, long-standing bronchiectasis is associated with epithelial cells that show absence of or scanty cilia. The bronchial lining may be ulcerated, fibrosed or denuded, sometimes immediately overlying distended blood vessels. Such areas may lead to hemoptysis. Ogilvie (1941) described these and other lesions and emphasized, as did Whitwell, the pronounced increase in size of the bronchial glands, lymphoid hyperplasia, and hypertrophy of mucous glands that may obstruct the bronchi. Important changes in the vascular structure of both bronchial and pulmonary arteries may occur in the diseased lung. In human beings there may be enlarged aneurysmal structures often associated with a history of hemoptysis. The walls of the bronchial arteries may be thickened, and there may be hyperplasia of the intima.

Other pathologic findings at autopsy may reveal the systemic disease partially responsible for the bronchiectasis, such as tuberculous hilar lymph nodes, tumors in adults though rarely in children, cystic fibrosis of the pancreas, evidence of asthma, situs inversus, or other vascular congenital anomalies.

SITE OF BRONCHIECTASIS. The left lower lobe is most frequently affected, with both lower lobes more often involved than the upper lobes. The right middle lobe is the common site of foreign body aspiration and of collapse from the pressure of tuberculous bronchial lymph nodes. When bronchiectasis is bilateral, it is usually patchy; the most common pattern is a combination of left lower lobe and lingula and right middle and lower lobes. Perry and King (1940) reported a 54 per cent incidence of left lower lobe bronchiectasis (usually including the lingula as well) in 400 patients of all ages. In children, Strang (1960) and later Clark (1963) also reported that bronchiectasis occurred more often in the left lower lobe. Swierenga (1957), in a critical analysis of 221 children under 16 years of age with bronchiectasis, related the site of the disease to the history and found that the right side predominated when tuberculosis or aspiration of a foreign body was responsible.

The predisposition of the left lower lobe to atelectasis and bronchiectasis may be due to the fact that the left main bronchus is two-thirds the size of the right main bronchus and, second, that the left main bronchus crosses the mediastinum at an acute angle behind the aorta, by which it can be readily compressed. Whitwell (1952), who also found the left lower lobe involved three times more frequently than the right in 200 consecutive resection specimens, explained the bilateral lesions as follows: "Clinical evidence is against the view that bronchiectasis spreads from one lobe to another; a more likely explanation is that at the onset of disease

the bronchi are subjected to varying degrees of injury."

The unique findings by Fleshman and coworkers (1968) of the preponderance of right upper lobe bronchiectasis in Alaskan native children under 18 months of age, especially in the nontuberculous group, may well be associated with the greater frequency of right upper lobe pneumonia previously described. In our own experience at New York University–Bellevue Medical Center, the right upper lobe is the area most frequently affected by pneumonia in the patient under two years of age.

Clinical Features

Bronchiectasis may present a broad spectrum of clinical features from the full-blown classic picture of the chronically ill patient to the healthy-appearing, fully active child whose only evidence of pulmonary disease is found in the bronchogram. The former group is rare today. The majority present minimal symptoms and physical findings.

ONSET. The onset may be acute, immediately following an infection such as pneumonia, pertussis or measles, in which continued bronchial obstruction producing collapse suggests the possibility of bronchiectasis in a child who fails to recover or whose chest roentgenograms fail to clear. Another group of patients are those with recurring and chronic pulmonary disease such as asthma, bronchitis and pneumonia in whom increasing or persistent symptoms of illness suggest the need for complete investigation, often including a bronchogram.

It is commonly recognized that tuberculous hilar adenopathy often leads to long-standing parenchymal atelectasis and subsequent bronchial dilatation, but these dilatations usually remain free from disturbing secondary bacterial infection. Consequently they are usually asymptomatic, detectable only on bronchographic study.

In earlier studies, the average age of the patient at onset was in childhood, before the age of five years. In these reports, percentages varied from 66 to 80 per cent; in more recent reports they are much lower. In Clark's (1963) study of 116 children, 35 gave a history of symptoms for five years and only 25 had symptoms for less than one year.

The nature of the initial illness varies according to authors, the composition of the population (such as the peculiar susceptibility to bronchiectasis seen among the Maoris), and the geographic areas by countries. In Scotland, Clark observed 116 children between 1946 and 1955 and ascribed the illness in more than half to pneumonia, pertussis and measles.

The findings of Williams and O'Reilly (1959) in Melbourne included two unusual features: the frequency of cystic fibrosis of the pancreas, and the greater number of patients whose bronchiectasis dated from bronchiolitis or interstitial pneumonia in early childhood. Indeed, those authors grouped their patients clinically into two categories, which also differed in response to surgery—the first favorably, the second less successfully. The first group included those patients with subacute pyogenic collapse occurring at all ages, usually beginning as an acute illness associated with pathogenic organisms, and terminating in a unilateral bronchiectasis. In these the genetic history for chronic respiratory disease was negative. The second group consisted of those with nonspecific infectious bronchiolitis, or interstitial pneumonia, occurring under three years of age, unassociated with culturable pathogens, and terminating in diffuse disease and positive bronchographic findings. There appeared to be a strong genetic factor in this latter group; the family history revealed definite bronchiectasis in 14 per cent and chronic sinusitis, bronchitis and probable bronchiectasis in an additional 38 per cent. It must be remembered that this series was heavily weighted by patients with cystic fibrosis, in which the genetic factor is known to exist.

In New Zealand, Lang and coworkers (1969) described an unusual causal relationship between an acute bronchopneumonia due to adenovirus type 21 and the development of bronchiectasis. Severe pneumonitis in 25 infants (all except two were Polynesians), aged three to 18 months, was followed by a high incidence of permanent lung damage in the 21 survivors. Bronchiectasis was shown by contrast medium in five and seen at autopsy in another.

In Finland, two of 29 young children severely ill with adenovirus type 7 pneumonia developed bronchiectasis, and two developed fibrosis of the lung (Similä and coworkers, 1971).

Similarly, a viral cause was postulated by Macpherson and coworkers (1969) for the six patients reported from Canada with *unilateral hyperlucent lung syndrome*. A significant rise in viral antibody titers for adenovirus in four patients and for respiratory syncytial virus in one was found. Bronchiectasis developed in four of these six patients. The bronchograms showed cylindrical dilatation with abrupt cut-off of peripheral bronchi described as the "pruned tree" appearance.

The importance of pneumonia as an antecedent to bronchiectasis is well recognized. In the United States, 28 per cent of the 400 patients reported by Perry and King (1940) had a history of pneumonia, and approximately two-thirds of the children in an earlier study by Raia (1938) had pneumonia, with or without pertussis, and measles. One-third of the series of patients seen by Avery and coworkers (1961) between 1940 and 1960 gave a history of pneumonia at onset, but rubeola held a less conspicuous position than in earlier studies.

The growing significance of viral pneumonia as an etiologic agent is being substantiated by long-term follow-up in various reports. Swierenga (1973) observed ten such in serologically-virologically diagnosed viral pneumonia. This infection may produce bronchiolitis obliterans, which in turn may predispose to bronchiectasis.

SIGNS AND SYMPTOMS. The most frequent symptom of bronchiectasis is a cough that may be dry or productive of sputum varying in amount, but greatest in the early morning. Foul-smelling sputum has seldom been encountered in children during the last two decades. Franklin (1958), in his six-year-long observations of 171 children in the Meath School of Recovery for bronchiectatic children, noted that there was no relation between the degree of health and the amount of sputum and cough. Patients with saccular bronchiectasis produce more sputum. Hemoptysis resulting from erosion of the bronchi, particularly in the well advanced saccular variety, is not common (Field), even though bronchiectasis is the most frequent cause of hemoptysis. Irregular episodes of fever may indicate infection in the diseased lung and may be associated with bronchitis or pneumonia. Disturbances of nutrition are seen occasionally in the severe cases. In general, the patients appear well. Dyspnea on exertion and fatigability are found in those with severe chronic disease.

In the early reports, clubbing of the fingers varied in frequency from 25 to 50 per cent. This finding is relatively uncommon in more recent reports with less severely ill patients. In a series of long-term studies, including 160 patients, Field reported a change in the incidence of clubbing from 43.7 per cent in 1949 to 6.5 per cent in her 1969 follow-up. Most observers believe that the occurrence of clubbing is correlated with the activity of disease, but Whitwell (1952) found no correlation between the presence of clubbing of the fingers and the extent or severity of pulmonary lesions; nor was there correlation with the nature of the patient's sputum. Long-term observations have demonstrated that clubbing of the extremities is reversible in both medically and surgically treated patients. Laurenzi (1970) related digital clubbing to the longevity of symptoms and history of recurrent infection rather than to the extent or type of disease.

Occasional medium moist rales over the ectatic lung, which vary in relation to the bronchial drainage of retained secretions and to the extent of such secretions, may be present. When the bronchi are filled, there may be only some diminution of breath sounds and impairment of resonance. After complete clearing for a period of time, there may be no abnormal physical findings. Patients with asthma complicated by bronchiectasis are more apt to have abnormal lung findings, and also have more diffuse pathologic changes with bilateral signs. Such patients are more difficult to treat successfully. Atelectatic areas are often undiagnosed by physical findings, and the collapsed segments of the lung are diagnosed only by chest roentgenograms.

As the child approaches adolescence, he shows improvement. Even patients with known extensive disease may become asymptomatic for a period, sometimes indefinitely; they may have no more respiratory infections than the average adult. But others show greater susceptibility to colds, influenza, sinusitis and chronic bronchitis. Frequent cough, lingering on after the acute episode, is the distinguishing feature of bronchiectasis.

Diagnosis

Three particular categories should lead to further investigation of the bronchial tree: a history of chronic cough, the persistence of atelectasis from whatever cause, and the failure of the chest roentgenogram to clear after respiratory infections or, particularly, after pertussis, measles, bronchiolitis and interstitial pneumonia. Bronchoscopy may be especially indicated for patients with prolonged or recurrent atelectasis, or with abnormal localized lung findings. Occasionally an unsuspected foreign body, such as timothy grass in summer, may be aspirated, or the cause of obstruction may be intrabronchial mucous plugs or the pressure of surrounding tissue such as lymph nodes.

DIAGNOSTIC AIDS. Since the introduction of radiopaque contrast media for the visualization of the bronchial tree by Sicard and Forestier in 1922, a definitive diagnostic tool has been available. Bronchography, as done by the trained physician, is safe, provided a test is given for the rare case of sensitivity to the dye used, and provided the procedure is instituted only after the acute infection has subsided and after a period of proper postural drainage of the bronchial tree. Bronchograms made shortly after acute inflammation show some cylindrical dilatation, probably owing to the loss of muscle tone secondary to the infection. The lung should be free of secretions and relatively clear from treatable bacterial infections when a bronchogram is performed. Therefore, a period of appropriate antimicrobial therapy may be indicated prior to bronchography. If these methods fail to clear the tracheobronchial tree, preliminary bronchoscopy may be desirable before bronchography is attempted. Some authorities recommend that bronchoscopy precede a bronchogram. Fiberoptic bronchoscopy has facilitated this procedure, and is tolerated by older children. Bilateral bronchograms may be obtained at one time, except when there is definite impairment of respiratory function; in this case, the lung with the greater pulmonary disease should be observed first. Differences in the size of the bronchioles during the inspiratory and expiratory phases in the bronchograms of patients with bronchiectasis as compared with normal subjects have been noted by Isley and others (1962). The patient with bronchiectasis shows a decrease in size during forced expiration.

The ordinary roentgenogram of the chest is helpful in suggesting bronchiectasis in some cases, although the four tenets described by Andrus (1937) are not always found in bronchiectasis: namely, 1) an increase in pulmonary markings, 2) chronic pneumonia, 3) ring shadows, and 4) displacement of heart and mediastinum. The last, of course, applies only when there is accompanying atelectasis. Lateral and oblique views are needed to clarify and often to diagnose pulmonary collapse. Negative chest roentgenograms may be found in some patients with bronchiectasis.

The honeycombed lung is characterized by areas of circular or polygonal translucencies surrounded by dense fibrous bands. This characteristic finding of advanced disease is correlated in pathologic specimens with pronounced peribronchial fibrosis and emphysema.

In most cases, flat plates of the chest and bronchograms are adequate for diagnosis. In some cases in which better understanding of parenchymal shadows at the periphery of bronchi is desired, tomobronchography may be helpful. This procedure is infrequently indicated in children. Pulmonary function studies are helpful in the management of the patient and in deciding on the suitability of surgical therapy.

The microbial flora in the patient with bronchiectasis is varied and in many instances has no causal relation to the disease symptoms or even to the exacerbations. A mixed flora of bacteria, pneumococci, streptococci and staphylococci, fusiform bacilli, and spirochetes has been described. *Hemophilus influenzae* has repeatedly been isolated by many workers, recently by Allibone and coworkers (1956). The search for infectious agents in 137 Naval recruits with cylindrical bronchiectasis by Rytel and coworkers (1964) included cultures for mycoplasma and bacteria grown from material obtained by bronchoscopy from the diseased lung. Viral tissue culture studies and complement-fixation tests for adenovirus infections also were made. This study resulted in an unusually small percentage of *Hemophilus influenzae* (5.5 per cent); the finding of a high incidence of antibody titer to adenovirus of 1:64 or greater (present in 46 per cent of those with bronchiectasis as compared with 27 per cent with bronchopneumonia), although a virus (influenza B) was isolated in only two patients; and finally, the failure to isolate mycoplasma from a single case.

In adults, a preliminary study of the

value of transtracheal aspiration for cultures in 34 symptomatic patients with bronchiectasis and bronchitis was compared with the results from sputum samples (Bjerkestrand and coworkers, 1975). Organisms from the latter were often the same as those found in tracheal aspirates. The frequency of anaerobic organisms (from five of 18 bronchiectatic patients) emphasizes the need to request such anaerobic cultures. Transtracheal aspiration is not indicated in children, who are usually asymptomatic. When pneumonia occurs, a well obtained sputum sample will be as helpful as transtracheal aspirate for bacterial analysis.

Contraindications to the procedure are hypoxia, acidosis, severe cardiac disease and bleeding disorders. Complications are mild hemoptysis and moderate subcutaneous emphysema.

Of course, appropriate skin testing for tuberculosis should always be made, keeping in mind the likelihood of diminished tuberculin reactions following measles and certain viral infections and vaccines. If the tuberculin reaction is positive, the interrelationship between the tuberculous infection and bronchiectasis should be carefully studied. (See section on Tuberculosis, p. 456.) If mediastinal gland enlargement is found or if disease is suspected, search for the explanation by suitable tests, such as angiography, is required. Because of the role alpha₁-antitrypsin plays in the pathogenesis of lung disease, patients with bronchiectasis should be tested for this deficiency. One such patient, a 34-year-old woman, was recently reported (Longstreth and coworkers, 1975).

Disease States Associated with Bronchiectasis

SINUSITIS. The frequent association of sinusitis with bronchiectasis has been noted by clinicians, especially in the earlier studies. More recent observers find that sinusitis is much less frequent and troublesome.

The interrelation of sinusitis and lower respiratory tract infection associated with chronic productive sputum is apparent. The determination of the identity of the original offender required study. Ormerod contributed evidence that iodized poppy seed oil (Lipiodol) could be found in the nasal passages shortly after use of the oil in bronchography. Previously, McLaurin (1943) had demonstrated Lipiodol in the bronchial tree 24 to 48 hours after injection into the sinuses.

The continuity of the epithelial lining of the upper and lower respiratory tract facilitates the spread of infection from one area to another. The antibiotic era is associated with the decreased incidence of persistent infection in sinuses. Since the organisms most commonly cultured from the sinuses (*Staphylococcus aureus*, coagulase-positive, or Streptococcus) are usually susceptible to antimicrobial therapy, effective clearing of infected sinuses may be accomplished, even though Hogg (1951) and Brock (1951) have suggested that severe bronchiectasis will continue to reinfect the sinuses.

There is a cycle of infection between upper and lower tract infection until the bronchiectasis is cleared. In many instances the edematous sinuses reflect an allergic state that underlies the bronchiectasis.

ASTHMA. The frequency of asthma in patients with bronchiectasis has varied in different groups. Wheezing, a common finding in bronchiectatic patients, does not always denote allergic asthma. In Field's group, a high proportion of children were found to have asthma, and she emphasized the poorer prognosis in this group. Protracted and poorly controlled asthma may be associated with bronchiectasis and should lead to investigation. The seriousness of asthma as a diffuse disease underlying bronchiectasis when the two coexist is illustrated by the pulmonary function studies made by Strang (1960), who found that abnormal pulmonary function tests associated with obstruction to airflow persisted between attacks of overt wheezing, suggesting an association with either bronchial obstruction or pulmonary fibrosis or a combination of both.

③ TUBERCULOSIS. The association of childhood tuberculosis with bronchiectasis has been indicated repeatedly and is related to the bronchial obstruction by the hilar and mediastinal lymph nodes. The greater frequency of right lung disease has also been noted.

Respiratory infections occur more often in children with *serum protein deficiency, dysgammaglobulinemia* and *agammaglobulinemia*. The bronchial damage and resultant bronchiectasis will depend on the sequence and the type of infection.

④ CYSTIC FIBROSIS. Similarly, the diffuse pathologic changes of the bronchial epithelium of the uncontrolled patient with fibrocystic disease of the pancreas make these patients fertile ground for the development of bronchiectasis. Diarrheal episodes in patients with bronchiectasis, especially early in life, should lead to an investigation of the chlorides by sweat tests and other suitable methods (see Cystic Fibrosis, Chapter 45).

⑤ SYSTEMIC DISEASES. An increasing volume of literature indicates the association between bronchiectasis and such systemic diseases as xanthomatosis, tuberous sclerosis, scleroderma, and cystic lung disease with fibrotic changes. Bronchiectasis in two patients with systemic lupus erythematosus has been reported; one case was verified by surgical and necropsy material. The bronchiectasis in all these diseases is not distinctive, and pathologic specimens of the lungs do not suggest these underlying disease states.

⑥ HEROIN ADDICTION. Two mechanisms play a role in predisposing heroin addicts to the development of bronchiectasis, usually connected with overdosage, pulmonary edema and vomiting. Pulmonary edema is associated with a propensity to pulmonary infections, and in one reported case, diffuse bronchiectasis occurred within eight months. Vomiting results in atelectasis and may be followed by local infection and thereby lead to localized bronchiectasis.

Medical Treatment

Once the diagnosis of bronchiectasis is established, it should be determined whether or not the damage is irreversible, remembering the tendency of the bronchial tree to dilate after certain pneumonias and to produce cylindrical reversible or "pseudo" bronchiectasis. Drainage of the retained secretions is essential and is usually accomplished by postural drainage, but sometimes requires bronchoscopy. Postural drainage exercises, occasional use of positive pressure breathing, bronchodilators, and warm, moist inhalations are helpful in promoting drainage.

Relief of atelectasis, which entails investigation of its cause, is essential for the ultimate success of bronchiectasis therapy. Bronchoscopy is indicated for the persistent segmental or lobar atelectasis that fails to respond to postural drainage. Fiberoptic bronchoscopy is more easily tolerated than rigid bronchoscopy and is equally successful in achieving drainage. (See section on Diagnostic Aids, p. 453.)

The possibility of sinusitis coexisting with bronchiectasis should always be remembered. Attention should be given to the general health of the patient, and tests should be made for the study of any underlying predisposing disease as described in the preceding section. Antibiotics and chemotherapy may be used for the acute episodes, as indicated by bacterial cultures and antibiotic resistance determinations.

The introduction of penicillin marked the beginning of a new era in the medical treatment of bronchiectasis. In 1945, Kay and Meade reported the value of penicillin in preoperative treatment, and its effectiveness in reducing sputum in some patients after parenteral therapy.

After many studies, chiefly in adults, long-term administration of antibiotics, whether continuous or interrupted, is not recommended. In 1969, Laterjet, Galy and Préault emphasized this principle in their medical treatment of a large group of children and adolescents. They used antibiotics sparingly and only as specifically indicated for verified acute infections. Relatively short courses of appropriate antibiotic therapy of a few days to several weeks are desirable for acute infections, and decisions should be based on the results obtained from sputum cultures and sensitivity studies. Many infections, especially in young children, are of viral origin and are not responsive to such therapy. The possibility of side-effects from the long-standing use of such medication, as well as interference with microbial balance and the possible subsequent invasion by mycotic infections, is also an important consideration.

Surgical Treatment

Before surgical treatment is considered for any patient, a period of observation while on medical treatment is essential to determine the degree of possible improvement, to make certain that the bronchiectasis is not reversible (if cylindrical type), and to clear the airways of as much secretion as possible. Pulmonary resection is seldom an emergency measure. The indications for surgery in bronchiectasis are extensive or repeated hemoptysis, a history suggesting foreign body aspiration, and a well localized saccular or advanced fusiform bronchiectasis with associated recurrent pneumonia or bronchitis. A patient without symptoms need not be subjected to resection even though bronchiectasis is apparent in the bronchogram. A child should be at least eight years of age, and preferably ten to 15 years of age, before such an elective operative procedure is carried out.

Sanderson and coworkers (1974), in their review of 393 patients with bronchiectasis, concur with others on the relatively safe age period between puberty and late teens for surgical therapy.

Patients with upper lobe lesions where the site of the lesion favors drainage rarely fail to respond to adequate medical therapy. Patients with extensive bilateral disease offer a problem, in part because of limited pulmonary reserve, and should be carefully evaluated. Bilateral resection in two stages has been successfully achieved, taking full cognizance of the pulmonary function prior to surgery. The more severely damaged area is removed first. Sometimes improvement is so great that the second operation may be unnecessary. When bilateral bronchiectasis is part of a general systemic disease, conservative treatment is usually preferable. Bronchiectasis in patients with tuberculosis usually responds well to medical treatment. The current literature continues to furnish evidence of the success of surgical treatment. Relapses may occur when some portion of diseased lung remains; this is usually the result of poor preoperative visualization in the bronchogram or, frequently, the sparing of the apical or superior segment in lower lobe resection. Surgeons agree on the wisdom of removing this segment when lower lung resection is performed.

To summarize, *medical treatment* is preferred for patients whose disease is minimal and asymptomatic, for patients with far advanced disease who may not tolerate surgery well because of other associated diseases or much diminished pulmonary function, and for patients whose bronchiectasis has been diagnosed too recently to determine the degree to which it can be cleared by adequate medical treatment.

Surgical resection is preferred when the lesion is localized to one segment or lobe and the patient is symptomatic, as when there is persistent or recurring bronchial obstruction; when there is failure to control localized infection by antimicrobial therapy; when there is repeated hemorrhage; when, despite medical treatment over a period of time, the patient fails to do well; or when there is a known or suspected foreign body irretrievable by bronchoscopy. Of 233 patients with bronchiectasis treated surgically by Stolf and coworkers (1974), 15 (or 6.4 per cent) had bronchiectasis due to foreign body aspiration. There are always patients who do not fall into clear-cut categories and whose treatment requires painstaking evaluation. Carefully accumulated facts and knowledge of the individual case over a fairly long observation period are essential in making a wise choice between surgical resection and medical treatment.

Complications

In patients with extensive disease, the medical complications that were more common before the use of antibiotics are abscess of the brain or lung, empyema, bronchopleural fistula, emphysema, and severe, sometimes fatal pneumonia. In addition, there is always the possibility of hemoptysis, and in those with advanced chronic disease, cor pulmonale with fatal outcome, and amyloidosis.

For the past two decades, atelectasis has been the most frequent postoperative complication. Other complications, such as empyema, fistula with empyema, or fistula with pneumothorax, are uncommon. Stolf and associates (1974), reporting the results of surgery on 233 patients, 77 of whom were 20 years of age or under, noted a 4.6 per cent incidence of these complications. Sanderson and coworkers (1974) also found these complications (none with pneumothorax) occurring with the same frequency in 272 operations. A mild postoperative bronchitis may develop. All these patients recovered within a short time. Before 1960, the incidence of complications was approximately 16 per cent. The changed picture with its excellent surgical results is due in large measure to improved surgical techniques and to better control of infection.

Chest deformity is minimal in children because of the compensatory growth of the remaining pulmonary tissues. Modern physiotherapy has also added to the improved results following surgery in childhood.

Prognosis

The outlook for patients with bronchiectasis has greatly improved in the past few decades, owing in large measure to a decrease in the predisposing childhood infections (especially measles and pertussis) and to the control of bacterial infections of the respiratory tract made possible by antimicrobial therapy. In addition, associated diseases such as cystic fibrosis and tuberculosis are better controlled. The management of the asthmatic patient still remains a challenge, and patients with asthma and bronchiectasis have the poorest prognosis.

As compared with earlier reports from the preantibiotic period, recent studies have shown that the general health of the patients has been improved and that response to medical treatment has been rewarding. Such observations in children correspond to long-term studies chiefly in adults, in whom asymptomatic bronchiectasis has been found not uncommonly in those 50 years of age and over and even in older age groups (70 to 80 years). The need for eradicating segments of the lung or a lung in which the bronchial tree is damaged or ectatic is no longer urgent or even necessary to maintain health. This is borne out by Field's experience, reported in 1969, covering 16 to 25 years of observation and follow-up of both medically and surgically treated young patients in England.

Although the only real cure for bronchiectasis is eradication of the diseased lung by surgical resection, the patient may remain asymptomatic for very long periods of time. It has been repeatedly shown that bronchiectasis is not progressive, but remains localized. Its apparent spread to adjacent areas postoperatively is thought to be in reality residua of a previously infected area reactivated after surgery. Evidence for this statement may be found in long-term studies of children and adults.

The postoperative fatality rate is low and has declined from 1.3 to 1.7 per cent for the year between 1950 and 1960 (Davis and coworkers, 1962; Peräsalo and coworkers, 1960) to less than 1 per cent (Sanderson and colleagues, 1974; Stolf and associates, 1974; Swierenga, 1973).

In children, the prognosis is particularly good. For example, in 1969, Glauser and others reported no deaths in children since 1945. In New Zealand, Borrie and Lichter (1965) reported no deaths in their 45 patients under 19 years of age during the decade 1952–1962.

More recently, Ripe (1971) reviewed the surgical treatment of bronchiectasis between 1958 and 1965 in 66 adult patients (26 to 64 years of age). There were eight deaths. The factors associated with a good prognosis were absence of rhinosinusitis, unilateral bronchiectasis, lower lobe lesions, age of patient (younger patients fared better), and absence of signs of obstructive lung disease as determined by pulmonary function studies. As might be predicted, the underlying cause of the bronchiectasis influenced the prognosis. Thus, surgical treatment of foreign body aspiration and of congenital cyst in three patients resulted in a cure, whereas those with asthmatic symptoms were much less benefited by surgical treatment and sometimes remained unimproved.

Pulmonary function studies from the Children's Service at Bellevue Hospital made by Filler (1964) on 15 adolescents who had surgical resections showed that these patients made good physiologic and functional adjustments after operation. When the lung resections were small (bisegmentectomies or right middle lobectomies), there was no reduction in lung volume or in respiratory capacity. In those with more extensive surgery (removal of one-fourth to one-third of the lung) the decrease in vital capacity was less than anticipated, perhaps because of the overdistention of the remaining lung tissue. No reduction in maximal breathing capacity was observed. Follow-up observation of most of these patients in the Chest Clinic of New York University Medical Center has revealed normal-functioning youths who exercise and pursue an unmodified school program.

Pulmonary function studies are essential to measure the extent of underlying pathologic conditions not only postsurgically but also for continuing observation of medically treated patients.

Prevention

Control of the childhood diseases underlying the development of bronchiectasis is the essence of prevention. Pertussis and measles vaccines have had a great impact on the reduction of these diseases in both frequency and severity. Early prophylactic isoniazid therapy of tuberculosis has greatly reduced the incidence of bronchial lymph node complications. Interstitial or viral pneumonias, unlike bacterial pneumonias, still offer a therapeutic challenge, particularly since parenchymal atelectasis occurs frequently. Attention to segmental collapse, especially if persistent or recurrent, using proper therapeutic measures, is essential in the prevention of bronchiectasis. Because of the urgency for prompt therapy by bronchoscopy, foreign body apiration must always be remembered. Patients with recurrent lung infections and especially those with bronchiectasis, even though asymptomatic, must be cautioned against the harm of cigarette smoking to their lungs.

Case Reports

CASE 1. Tuberculosis was diagnosed in a two-year-old Negro boy one year before admission to the Children's Chest Service, Bellevue Hospital. A right upper lobe infiltrate was found, and isoniazid therapy was begun. He was admitted to the Hospital in August 1962 because of recent weight loss, a persistent pulmonary shadow and a history of irregular isoniazid medication.

Physical examination was not remarkable except for undernutrition and an enlarged liver, an infected pharynx and cervical adenopathy. All gastric cultures and culture

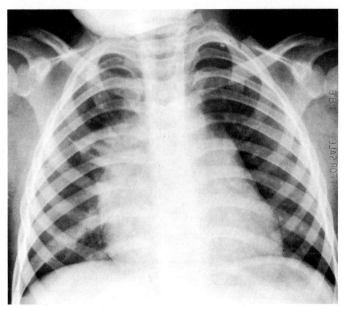

Figure 1. Case 1. Irregular triangular density extending out from the hilus and above the fissure line to the right upper lobe, which is displaced upward.

from bronchoscopic aspiration were negative for acid-fast bacilli.

Bronchoscopy one month after admission showed a nipple of granulation tissue inside the right upper lobe bronchus at the carina between the segmental orifices. Figure 1 shows the chest roentgenogram one day previously. A bronchogram two weeks later (Fig. 2) showed a saccular bronchiectasis of the anterior and posterior segments of the right upper lobe.

Shortly afterward the child was discharged home and was followed up regularly in the Bellevue Hospital Children's Chest Clinic. He has received isoniazid and PAS therapy for 18 months. One episode of persistent low-grade fever required inpatient study in the winter of 1965. All cultures for acid-fast bacilli were negative. Bronchoscopy of the right upper lobe revealed a patent and normal bronchus, but the mucosa was red and swollen at the seg-

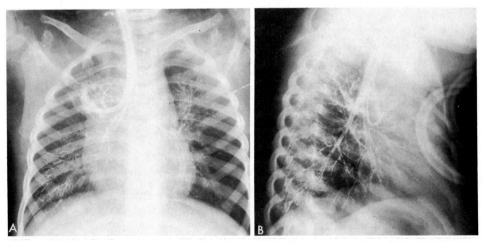

Figure 2. Case 1. *A,* In the right upper lobe there are crowding of the bronchi and irregular dilatations. *B,* Irregularly enlarged and tortuous bronchi of the posterior segment of the right upper lobe are demonstrated in the lateral view.

mental spurs. The lungs were clear, and there was no cough and no weight loss. This patient, observed in regular clinic visits since 1965, was still doing well when last seen in April 1976.

CASE 2. Repeated attacks of pneumonia throughout childhood resulted in saccular bronchiectasis of the right upper lobe in a nine-year-old girl. A successful lobectomy was followed by improved pulmonary function, loss of clubbing of fingers, and improved health. Follow-up for seven years

shows no recurrence of bronchiectasis. (See Fig. 3.)

CASE 3. A 5 1/2-year-old girl was seen at Bellevue Hospital Children's Chest Out-Patient Department approximately five months before her death in the Hospital on January 29, 1960. A premature baby whose first year of life was marked by failure to thrive, she was the subject of many attacks of pulmonary disease throughout her short life, beginning at two years of age with her first attack of asthma. She had four bouts of

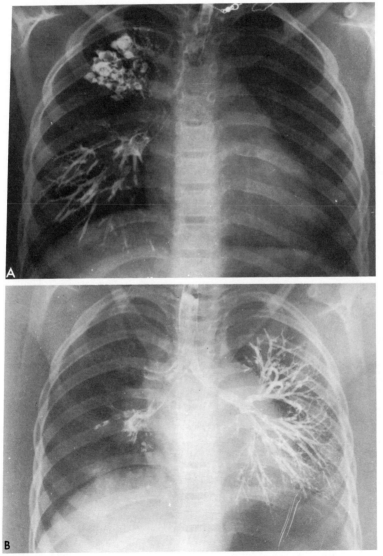

Figure 3. Case 2. *A,* Bronchogram taken two months before operation shows a saccular bronchiectasis in a shrunken right upper lobe. *B,* Normal left lung demonstrated shortly after operation.

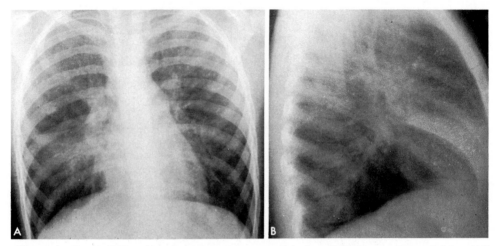

Figure 4. Case 3. Diffuse bronchopneumonia one month before death. Note collapse of right middle lobe, especially well visualized in the lateral view (*B*).

pneumonia, including the terminal one. She was considered to be an asthmatic child, although no allergen was found to which she was sensitive. (See Figs. 4 to 9.)

Gamma globulin studies and sweat tests gave essentially normal results. During her first admission to the Children's Service for respiratory distress, she was found to have bronchopneumonia and bronchiectasis of the right middle lobe with impaired pulmonary function. There was decreased oxygen saturation and some carbon dioxide retention. The fingers showed clubbing. After two months she recovered sufficiently to re-

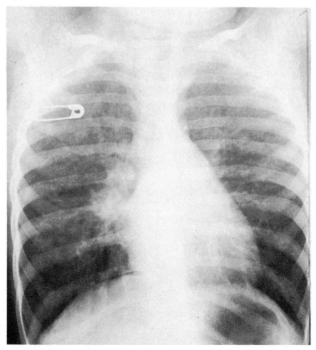

Figure 5. Case 3. Four days before death there is distention of the lungs and diffuse increase in bronchial markings with bilateral mottling in the upper third and hyperaeration at the bases. The large right root in the right middle lobe appears to have expanded.

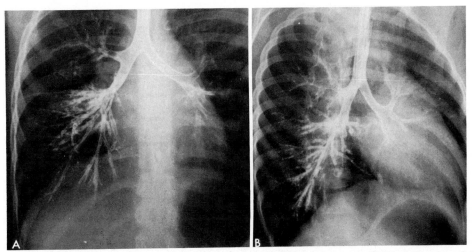

Figure 6. Case 3. *A*, Bronchogram taken three months before death shows cylindrical dilatation of the right middle and adjacent right lower lobe bronchi with some crowding of these bronchi. A fine horizontal pleural line is visible on the right. *B*, The lateral view shows the sudden stublike termination of some of these bronchi.

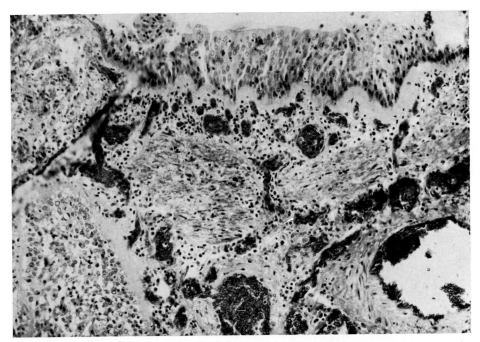

Figure 7. Case 3. A microscopic section of the bronchus (× 500) shows a thick basement membrane beneath the epithelial lining. There is extensive inflammation involving the muscular tissue as well, where there is also some destruction of muscle.

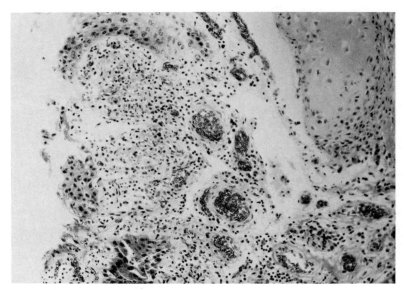

Figure 8.   Case 3. Squamous cell metaplasia of the lining epithelium of the bronchus. There is also destruction of smooth muscle and beginning alteration of the cartilage. (× 500.)

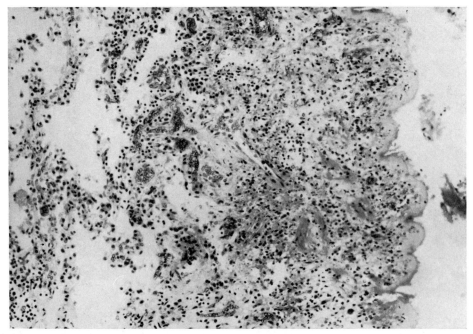

Figure 9.   Case 3. A microscopic section of a bronchiole (× 500) shows the destruction of the wall. There is loss of mucosa and a thickened basement membrane.

turn home and receive ambulatory care. The terminal diffuse pneumonia occurred two months later.

Autopsy revealed bilateral interstitial pneumonia and cylindrical bronchiectasis of the right middle lobe and a portion of the right lower lobe.

REFERENCES

Adams, R., and Churchill, E. D.: Situs inversus, sinusitis and bronchiectasis. Report of 5 cases, including frequency statistics. *J. Thorac. Surg., 7*:206, 1937.

Allibone, E. C., Allison, P. R., and Zinnemann, K.: Significance of *H. influenzae* in bronchiectasis of children. *Br. Med. J., 1*:1457, 1956.

Andrus, P. M.: Bronchiectasis, an analysis of its causes. *Am. Rev. Tuberc., 36*:46, 1937.

Andrus, P. M.: Chronic nonspecific pulmonary disease. *Am. Rev. Tuberc., 41*:87, 1940.

Anspach, W. E.: Atelectasis and bronchiectasis in children. Study of 50 cases presenting triangular shadow at base of lung. *Am. J. Dis. Child., 47*:1011, 1934.

Avery, M. E., Riley, M. C., and Weiss, A.: The course of bronchiectasis in childhood. *Bull. Johns Hopkins Hosp., 109*:20, 1961.

Bachman, A. L., Hewitt, W. R., and Beekley, H. C.: Bronchiectasis—a bronchographic study of 60 cases of pneumonia. *Arch. Intern. Med., 91*:78, 1953.

Banner, A. S., Muthuswany, P., Shah, R. S., Rodriguez, J., Saksena, F. S., and Addington, W. W.: Bronchiectasis following heroin-induced pulmonary edema. *Chest, 69*:552, 1976.

Bartlett, J. G., Rosenblatt, J. E., and Finegold, S. M.: Percutaneous transtracheal aspiration in the diagnosis of anaerobic pulmonary infection. *Ann. Inter. Med., 79*:535, 1973.

Becroft, D. M. O.: Bronchiolitis obliterans, bronchiectasis, and other sequelae of adenovirus type 21 infection in young children. *J. Clin. Pathol., 24*:72, 1971.

Berg, G., and Nordenskjöld, A.: Pulmonary alterations in tuberous sclerosis. *Acta Med. Scand., 125*:428, 1946.

Bergstrom, W. H., Cook, C. D., Scannell, J., and Berenberg, W.: Situs inversus, bronchiectasis and sinusitis; report of a family with two cases of Kartagener's triad and two additional cases of bronchiectasis among six siblings. *Pediatrics, 6*:573, 1950.

Biering, A.: Childhood pneumonia, including pertussis, pneumonia, and bronchiectasis. A follow-up study of 151 patients. *Acta Paediatr., 45*:348, 1956.

Bjerkestrand, G. A., Digranes, A., and Schreiner, A.: Bacteriological findings in transtracheal aspirates from patients with chronic bronchitis and bronchiectasis. *Scand. J. Resp. Dis., 56*:201, 1975.

Blades, B., and Dugan, D. J.: Pseudo bronchiectasis in atypical pneumonia. *J. Thorac. Surg., 13*:40, 1944.

Blasi, A., and Marsico, S. A.: Congenital bronchiectasis (bronchiectasis due to prenatal malformative factors). *Bronches, 25*:343, 1975.

Borrie, J., and Lichter, I.: Surgical treatment of bronchiectasis: ten-year survery. *Br. Med. J., 2*:908, 1965.

Bradshaw, H. H., Myers, R. T., and Cordell, A. R.: Bronchiectasis; a fourteen-year appraisal. *Ann. Surg., 145*:644, 1957.

Brock, R. C.: Problem of sinusitis in bronchiectasis. *J. Laryngol. Otol., 65*:449, 1951.

Brody, J. A., and McAlister, R.: Depression of tuberculin sensitivity following measles vaccination. *Am. Rev. Resp. Dis., 90*:607, 1964.

Brody, J. A., Overfield, T., and Hammas, L. M.: Depression of the tuberculin reaction by viral vaccines. *N. Engl. J. Med., 271*:1295, 1964.

Campbell, P. E.: Congenital lobar emphysema: etiological studies. *Aust. Paediatr. J., 5*:226, 1969.

Carter, M. G., and Welch, K. J.: Bronchiectasis following aspiration of timothy grass. *N. Engl. J. Med., 238*:832, 1948.

Cheng, K-K.: The experimental production of bronchiectasis in rats. *J. Pathol. Bacteriol., 67*:89, 1954.

Cherniack, M. S., Vosti, K. L., Dowling, H. F., Lepper, M. H., and Jackson, G. G.: Long-term treatment of bronchiectasis and chronic bronchitis. *Arch. Intern. Med., 103*:345, 1959.

Clark, N. S.: Bronchiectasis in childhood. *Br. Med. J., 1*:80, 1963.

Clause, H., Sanger, P. W., Taylor, F. H., and Robicsek, F.: Systemic lupus erythematosus associated with bronchiectasis: report of two cases. *Dis. Chest, 45*:219, 1964.

Cockayne, E. A.: The genetics of transposition of the viscera. *Q. J. Med., 7*:479, 1938.

Collins, H. D., and Dudley, H. R.: Agammaglobulinemia and bronchiectasis. A report of two cases in adults, with autopsy findings. *N. Engl. J. Med., 252*:255, 1955.

Corpe, R. F., and Hwa, E. C.: A correlated bronchographic and histopathologic study of bronchial disease in 216 TBC patients. *Am. Rev. Tuberc., 73*:681, 1956.

Crausaz, P. H.: Pulmonary artery circulatory defect and etiology of bronchiectasis. *Rev. Med. Suisse Rom., 90*:55, 1970.

Crausaz, P. H.: Reversible bronchiectasis or temporary dilatation during an acute pneumopathy. *Rev. Med. Suisse Rom., 90*:45, 1970.

Crausaz, P. H., and Raball, J. A.: Bronchectasies réversibles. *J. Fr. Otorhinolaryngol, 23*:337, 1974.

Croxatto, O. C., and Lanari, A.: Pathogenesis of bronchiectasis. Experimental study and anatomical findings. *J. Thorac. Surg., 27*:514, 1954.

Culiner, M. M.: Intralobar bronchial cystic disease, the "sequestration complex" and cystic bronchiectasis. *Dis. Chest, 53*:462, 1968.

Davis, M. B., Jr., Hopkins, W. A., and Wansker, W. C.: The present status of the treatment of bronchiectasis. *Am. Rev. Resp. Dis., 85*:816, 1962.

Denney, M. K., Berkus, E. M., Snider, T. H., and Nedwicki, E. G.: Foreign body bronchiectasis. *Dis. Chest. 53*:613, 1968.

Dickey, L. B.: Pulmonary diseases associated with cystic fibrosis of the pancreas. *Dis. Chest, 17*:153, 1950.

Drapanas, T., Siewers, R., and Feist, J. H.: Reversible poststenotic bronchiectasis. *N. Engl. J. Med., 275*:917, 1966.

Dutau, G., and Fardou, M. M.: Bronchography in children. *Poumon Coeur, 31*:119, 1975.

Dyggve, H., and Gudbjerg, C. E.: Bronchiectasis in children. *Acta Paediat., 47*:193, 1958.

Edward, F. R.: The long-term results of the surgical treatment of bronchiectasis. *Acta Chir. Belg., 46*:668, 1954.

Field, C. E.: Bronchiectasis in childhood. I. Clinical survey of 160 cases. *Pediatrics, 4*:21, 1949.

Field, C. E.: Bronchiectasis in childhood. II. Aetiology and pathogenesis, including a survey of 272 cases of doubtful irreversible bronchiectasis. *Pediatrics, 4*:231, 1949.

Field, C. E.: Bronchiectasis in childhood. III. Prophylaxis, treatment and prognosis. *Pediatrics, 4*:335, 1949.

Field, C. E.: Bronchiectasis, third report on a follow-up study of medical and surgical cases from childhood. *Dis. Child., 44*:551, 1969.

Filler, J.: Effects upon pulmonary function of lobectomy performed during childhood. *Am. Rev. Resp. Dis., 89*:801, 1964.

Fine, A., and Baum, G. L.: Long-term follow-up of bronchiectasis. *Lancet, 86*:505, 1966.

Finke, W.: The reversibility of early bronchiectasis. Its implication for therapy and prevention. *N. Y. J. Med., 5*:1163, 1951.

Fleischner, F.: Reversible bronchiectasis. *Am. J. Roentgenol., 46*:166, 1941.

Fleshman, J. K., Wilson, J. F., and Cohen, J. J.: Bronchiectasis in Alaska native children. *Arch. Environ. Health, 17*:517, 1968.

Foster, J. H., Jacobs, J. K., and Daniel, R. A.: Pulmonary resection in infancy and childhood. *Ann. Surg., 163*:658, 1961.

Franklin, S. W.: The prognosis of bronchiectasis in childhood. *Arch. Dis. Child., 33*:19, 1958.

Galy, P.: Anatomical evolution of "Bronchitis" of the childhood bronchiectasis, correlations with the therapeutic resection. *Respiration, 27*(Suppl.):224, 1970.

Galy, P., and Dorsit, O.: Facteurs congénitaux dans la genèse de la bronchite chronique et les bronchectasies y compris les syndromes de Kartagener et de Mounier-Kuhn. *Poumon Coeur, 27*:133, 1971.

Gandevia, B.: Combined tomography and bronchography (tomobronchography) in the investigation of pulmonary disease. *Med. J. Aust., 2*:813, 1957.

Ginsberg, R. L., Cooley, J. C., Olsen, A. M., Kirklin, J. W., and Clagget, O. T.: Prognosis of bronchiectasis after resection. *Surg. Gynecol. Obstet., 101*:99, 1955.

Glauser, E. M., Cook, C. D., and Harris, G. B. C.: Bronchiectasis: a review of 187 cases in children with follow-up pulmonary function studies in 58. *Acta Paediatr. Scand., 165*(Suppl.):1, 1966.

Goodman, D. H.: Bronchiectasis, eosinophilia, asthma pneumonitis (Beap syndrome). *Ann. Allergy, 33*:289, 1974.

Gottlieb, O., and Storm, O.: The results of surgical resection for bronchiectasis. *Acta Chir. Scand., 3*:228, 1956.

Gratecos, L., Oddo, G., Louchet, E., Coinget, J., and Orsini, A.: Aspect évolutif des bronchiectasies traitées et surveillées dans un centre pédiatrique sur une période de dix ans. *Ann. Pediatr., 16*:1443, 1969.

Gudbjerg, C. E.: Roentgenologic diagnosis of bronchiectasis. *Acta Radiol., 43*:209, 1955.

Gudbjerg, C. E.: Bronchiectasis. Radiologic diagnosis and prognosis after operative treatment. *Acta Radiol., 143*:11, 1957.

Hartline, J. V., and Zelkowitz, P. S.: Kartagener's syndrome. *Am. J. Dis. Child., 121*:349, 1971.

Hayward, J., and Reid, L. McA.: The Cartilage of the intrapulmonary bronchi in normal lungs, in bronchiectasis, and in massive collapse. *Thorax, 7*:98, 1952.

Helm, W. H., and Thompson, V. C.: The long-term results of resection for bronchiectasis. *Q. J. Med., 27*:353, 1958.

Hentel, W., Longfield, A. N., and Gordon, J.: A re-evaluation of bronchiectasis using fume fixation. I. The broncho-alveolar structures: a preliminary study. *Dis. Chest., 41*:44, 1962.

Heusfeldt, E.: Bronchiectasis: etiology, surgical treatment and prevention. *Acta Chir. Scand., 245*(Suppl.):76, 1959.

Hinds, J. R.: Bronchiectasis in the Maori. *N. Z. Med. J., 57*:328, 1958.

Hogg, J. C.: Discussion on the role of sinusitis in bronchiectasis. *J. Laryngol. Otol., 65*:442, 1951.

Hunter, T. B., Kuhns, L. R., Roloff, M. A., and Holt, J. F.: Tracheobronchomegaly in an 18 month old child. *Am. J. Roetgenol. Radium Ther. Nucl. Med., 123*:687, 1965.

Hutchinson, J. H.: The pathogenesis of epituberculosis in children, with a note on obstructive emphysema. *Glasgow Med. J., 30*:271, 1949.

Isley, J. K., Jr., Bacos, J., Hickam, J. B., and Baylin, G. J.: Bronchiolar behavior in pulmonary emphysema and in bronchiectasis. *Am. J. Roentgenol., 87*:853, 1962.

Jennings, G. H.: Re-expansion of the atelectatic lower lobe and disappearance of bronchiectasis. *Br. Med. J., 2*:963, 1937.

Johansson, L., and Silander, T.: Surgery for bronchiectasis. Primary results in 61 cases. *Acta Chir. Scand., 124*:419, 1962.

Jones, E. M., Peck, W. M., Woodruff, C. E., and Willis, H. S.: Relationship between tuberculosis and bronchiectasis. A study of clinical and of post-mortem material. *Am. Rev. Tuberc., 61*:387, 1950.

Jones, O. R., and Cournand, A.: The shrunken pulmonary lobe with chronic bronchiectasis. *Am. Rev. Tuberc., 28*:293, 1933.

Kartagener, M.: Zur Pathogenese der Bronchiektasien: Bronchiektasien bei Situs Viscerum Inversus. *Beitr. z. Klin. d. Tuberk., 83*:489, 1933.

Kartagener, M., and Horlacher, A.: Zur Pathogenese der Bronchiektasien; Situs Viscerum inversus und Polyposis nas: in einem Falle Familiärer Bronchiektasien. *Beitr. Klin. Tuberk., 87*:331, 1935.

Kartagener, M., and Stucki, P.: Bronchiectasis with situs inversus. *Arch. Pediatr., 79*:193, 1962.

Katsuhara, K., Kawamoto, S., Wakabayashi, T., and Belsky, J. L.: Situs inversus totalis and Kartaganer's syndrome in a Japanese population. *Chest, 61*:56, 1972.

Kay, E. B.: Bronchiectasis following atypical pneumonia. *Arch. Intern. Med., 75*:89, 1945.

Kay, E. B., and Meade, R. H., Jr.: Penicillin in the treatment of chronic infections of the lungs and bronchi. *J.A.M.A., 129*:200, 1945.

Kergin, F. G.: The surgical treatment of bilateral bronchiectasis. *J. Thorac. Surg., 19*:257, 1950.

Klimanskii, V. A., Klimanskaya, E. V., and Grudovsky, L. M.: Evaluation of the results of lung resection in children with chronic nonspecific pneumonia. *Khirugiia* (Mosk.), *45*:22, 1969.

Konietzko, N. F. J., Carton, R. W., and Leroy, E. P.: Causes of death in patients with bronchiectasis. *Am. Rev. Resp. Dis., 100*:852, 1969.

Kürklü, E. U., Williams, M. A., and le Roux, B. T.: Bronchiectasis consequent upon foreign body retention. *Thorax, 28*:601, 1973.

Laennec, R. T. H.: De l'Auscultation Médiate, un Traite du Diagnostie des Maladies des Poumons et de Coeur, Fondé Principalement sur ce Nouveau Moyen D'Exploration. Paris, Brosson et Chaude, 1819.

Lander, F. P. L.: Bronchiectasis and atelectasis; temporary and permanent changes. *Thorax, 1*:198, 1946.

Lang, W. R., Howden, C. W., Laws, J., and Burton, J. F.: Bronchopneumonia with serious sequelae in children with evidence of adenovirus type 21 infection. *Br. Med. J., 1*:73, 1969.

Latarjet, M., Galy, P., and Préault, M.: Le traitement médicale de la maladie bronchiectasique de l'enfance et de l'adolescence. *Ann. Pediatr. 16*:349, 1969.

Laurenzi, G. A.: A critical reappraisal of bronchiectasis. *Med. Times, 98*:89, 1970.

Lees, A. W.: Atelectasis and bronchiectasis in pertussis. *Br. Med. J., 2*:1138, 1950.

Lévêque, B., Jean, R., Benoit, Mme., Cloup, Mme., Mischler, Mlle., and Marie, J.: Pronostic évolution à long terme et retentissement social de la dilatation des bronches de l'enfant. *Ann. Pediatr., 16*:314, 1969.

Liebow, A. A., Hales, M. R., and Lindskog, G. E.: Bronchiectasis and abnormal changes in pulmonary bronchial vessels, *Am. J. Pathol., 25*:211, 1949.

Lindskog, G. E., and Hubbell, D. S.: An analysis of 215 cases of bronchiectasis. *Surg. Gynecol. Obstet., 100*:643, 1955.

Logan, W. D., Jr., Abbott, O. A., and Hatcher, C. R., Jr.: Kartagener's triad. *Dis Chest, 48*:613, 1965.

Longstreth, G. F., Weitzman, S. A., Browning, R.

J., and Lieberman, J.: Bronchiectasis and homozygous alpha₁-antitrypsin deficiency. *Chest, 67*:233, 1975.

McKim, A.: Bronchiectasis as seen in an ambulant clinic service. A follow-up study of 49 cases over a minimum period of nine years. *Am. Rev. Tuberc., 66*:457, 1952.

McLaurin, J. G.: Review of interrelationship of paranasal sinus disease and certain chest conditions, with especial consideration of bronchiectasis and asthma. *Ann. Otol. Rhinol. Laryngol., 44*:344, 1935.

McLaurin, J. G.: Interrelationship of upper and lower respiratory infections emphasizing routes of infection. *Ann. Otol. Rhinol. Laryngol., 52*:589, 1943.

Macpherson, R. I., Cumming, G., and Chernick, V.: Unilateral hyperlucent lung in childhood: a complication of viral pneumonia. *J. Can. Assoc. Radiol., 20*:225, 1969.

Malhotra, O. P., Pande, J. N., and Guleria, J. S.: Clinical profile in bronchiectasis. *J. Assoc. Physicians India, 21*:414, 1973.

Maxwell, G. M.: Chronic chest disease in Australian aboriginal children. *Arch. Dis. Child., 47*:897, 1972.

Mayer, E., and Rappaport, I.: Developmental origin of cystic, bronchiectatic and emphysematous changes in the lungs. *Dis. Chest, 21*:146, 1952.

Miller, R. D., and Divertie, M. B.: Kartagener's syndrome. *Chest, 62*:130, 1972.

Mitchell, R. E., and Bury, R.: Congenital bronchiectasis due to deficiency of bronchial cartilage (Williams-Campbell syndrome): A case report. *J. Pediatr., 87*:230, 1975.

Montorsi, W.: Bronchiectasis. *Minerva Med., 64*:546, 1973.

Morlock, H. V., and Pinchin, A. J. S.: Congenital bronchiectasis. *Br. Med. J., 2*:780, 1933.

Mounier-Kuhn, P.: Dilation de la trachée constatations radiographiques et bronchoscopiques, *Lyon Med., 150*:106, 1932.

Nelson, S. W., and Christoforidis, A.: Reversible bronchiectasis. *Radiology, 71*:375, 1958.

Niculescu, N., Gavrilita, N., and Ionescu, G.: Our experience in the surgical treatment of bronchiectasis in children. (From *Pediatria* [Bucur.], *18*:179, 1969.) English translation: *Paediatrics, 13*:41, 1969.

Ochsner, A., DeBakey, M., and De Camp, P. T.: Bronchiectasis: its curative treatment by pulmonary resection. An analysis of 96 cases. *Surgery, 25*:518, 1949.

Ogilvie, A. C.: The natural history of bronchiectasis: a clinical, roentgenologic and pathologic study. *Arch. Intern. Med., 68*:395, 1941.

Olsen, A. M.: Bronchiectasis and dextrocardia. Observations on the aetiology of bronchiectasis. *Am. Rev. Tuberc., 47*:435, 1943.

Pastore, P. N., and Olsen, A. M.: Absence of frontal sinuses and bronchiectasis in identical twins. *Proc. Staff Meet. Mayo Clin., 16*:593, 1941.

Peräsalo, O., Scheinin, T. M., and Pantzar, P.: On the surgical treatment of bronchiectasis. *Acta Chir. Scand., 119*:198, 1960.

Perry, K. M. A., and King, D. S.: Bronchiectasis: a study on prognosis based on a follow-up of 400 patients. *Am. Rev. Tuberc., 41*:531, 1940.

Pittman, H. S.: Gamma globulin concentrations in ambulatory patients with bronchiectasis. *Am. Rev. Resp. Dis., 81*:251, 1960.

Prolonged antibiotic treatment of severe bronchiectasis. A report by a Subcommittee of the Antibiotics Clinical Trials (Non-Tuberculous) Committee of the Medical Research Council. *Br. Med. J., 2*:255, 1957.

Raia, A.: Bronchiectasis in children with special reference to prevention and early diagnosis. *Am. J. Dis. Child., 56*:582, 1938.

Ripe, E.: Bronchiectasis. I. A. follow-up study after surgical treatment. *Scand. J. Resp. Dis., 52*:96, 1971.

Ripe, E., Selander, H., and Wolodarski, J.: Bronchiectasis. II. A model for prognosticating the results of surgery. *Scand. J. Resp. Dis., 52*:113, 1971.

Rivera, G. E.: Bronchoscopy in thoracic pathology. Analysis of 1000 Cases. *J. Fr. Otorhinolaryngol., 23*:710, 1974.

Rosenzweig, D. W., and Stead, W. W.: The role of tuberculosis and other forms of bronchopulmonary necrosis in the pathogenesis of bronchiectasis. *Am. Rev. Resp. Dis., 93*:769, 1966.

Ruberman, W., Shauffer, I., and Biondo, T.: Bronchiectasis and acute pneumonia. *Am. Rev. Tuberc., 76*:761, 1957.

Rytel, M. W., Conner, G. H., Welch, C. C., Kraybill, W. H., and Edwards, E. H.: Infectious agents associated with cylindrical bronchiectasis. *Dis. Chest, 46*:23, 1964.

Sanderson, J. M., Kennedy, M. C. S., Johnson, M. F., and Manley, D. C. E.: Bronchiectasis: results of surgical and conservative management. A review of 393 cases. *Thorax, 29*:407, 1974.

Sant' Agnese, P. A. di: The pulmonary manifestation of fibrocystic disease of the pancreas. *Dis. Chest, 27*:654, 1955.

Schachter, E. N., and Basta, W.: Bronchiectasis following heroin overdose: a report of two cases. *Chest, 63*:363, 1973.

Shafir, R., Jaffe, R., and Kalter, Y.: Bronchiectasis: a cause of infantile lobar emphysema. *J. Pediatr. Surg., 11*:107, 1976.

Shahwan, M. M.: Right sided abscess in the region of the diaphragm associated with bronchiectasis. *Proc. R. Soc. Med., 66*:356, 1973.

Sicard, J. A., and Forestier, J.: Iodized oil as contrast medium in radioscopy. *Bull. Mém. Soc. Med. Hop. Paris, 46*:463, 1922.

Similä, S. Ylikorkala, O., and Wasz-Höckert, O.: Type of adenovirus pneumonia. *J. Pediatr., 79*:605, 1971.

Smith, K. R., and Morris, J. F.: Reversible bronchial dilatation. Report of a case. *Dis. Child, 42*:652, 1962.

Soloman, M. H., Winn, K. J., White, R. D., Bulkley, B. H., Kelly, D. T., Gott, V. L., and Hutchins, G. M.: Selected reports: Kartagener's syndrome with corrected transposition. *Chest, 69*:678, 1976.

Spain, D., and Thomas, A. G.: The pulmonary manifestations of scleroderma. *Ann. Intern. Med., 32*:152, 1949.

Spain, D. W., and Lester, C. W.: Time demand in the development of irreversible bronchiectasis. *J. Pediatr., 32*:415, 1948.

Starr, S., and Berkovich, S.: Effect of measles, gamma-globulin-modified measles and vaccine measles on tuberculin test. *N. Engl. J. Med., 270*:386, 1964.

Stiles, Q. R., Meyer, B. W., Lindesmith, G. G., and Jones, J. C.: The effects of pneumonectomy in children. *J. Thorac. Cardiovasc. Surg., 58*:394, 1969.

Stolf, N. A. G., Lemos, P. A. P., Curi, N., de Arrude, R. M., and Zerbini, E. J.: Tratamento cirúrgico de 233 pacientes portadores de bronquectasia. *Rev. Hosp. Clin. Fac. Med. São Paulo, 29*:80, 1974.

Strang, C.: The fate of children with bronchiectasis. *Ann. Intern. Med., 44*:630, 1956.

Strang, L. B.: Abnormalities of ventilatory capacity in children with asthma and bronchiectasis. *Arch. Dis. Child., 35*:224, 1960.

Swierenga, J.: Childhood bronchiectasis. *Dis. Chest, 32*:154, 1957.

Swierenga, J.: So-called idiopathic bronchiectasis (special review about therapy and results). *Bronches, 23*:84, 1973.

Szpunar, J., and Okrasinka, B.: Sinusitis in children with bronchiectasis. The influence of allergy on its development. *Arch. Otolaryngol., 76*:352, 1962.

Tannenberg, J., and Pinner, M.: Atelectasis and bronchiectasis. An experimental study concerning their relationship. *J. Thorac. Surg., 11*:571, 1942.

Temple, A. D., Smoling, L., and Aubert, E.: Long-term antibiotic therapy in chronic chest disease. *Med. Serv. J. Can., 19*:473, 1963.

Torgersen, J.: Transposition of viscera—bronchiectasis and nasal polyps. Genetical analysis and contributions to problem of constitution. *Acta Radiol., 28*:17, 1947.

Van Creveld, S., and Ter Poorten, F. H.: Reticuloendotheliosis chiefly localized in the lungs, bone marrow and thymus. *Arch. Dis. Child., 10*:57, 1935.

Visconti, R. J.: Agammaglobulinemia with bronchopulmonary manifestations. *Dis. Chest, 48*:530, 1965.

Wanderer, A. A., Elliot, F. E., Gultz, R. W., and Cotton, E. K.: Tracheobronchiomegaly and acquired cutis laxa in a child: Physiologic and immunologic studies. *Pediatrics, 44*:709, 1969.

Warnock, M. L., Ghahremani, G. G., Rattenborg, C., Ginsberg, M., and Valenzuela, J.: Pulmonary complications of heroin intoxication: aspiration pneumonia and diffuse bronchiectasis. *J.A.M.A., 219*:1051, 1972.

Wayne, K. S., and Taussig, L. M.: Probable familial congenital bronchiectasis due to cartilage deficiency (Williams-Campbell syndrome). *Am. Rev. Resp. Dis., 114*:15, 1976.

Whitwell, F.: A study of the pathology and pathogenesis of bronchiectasis. *Thorax*, 7:213, 1952.

Williams, H., and Anderson, C.: Bronchiectasis and bronchostenosis following primary tuberculosis in infancy and childhood. *Q. J. Med.*, 22:295, 1953.

Williams, H., and Campbell, P.: Generalized bronchiectasis associated with deficiency of cartilage in the bronchial tree. *Arch. Dis. Child.*, 35:182, 1960.

Williams, H., and O'Reilly, R. N.: Bronchiectasis in children: its multiple clinical and pathological aspects. *Arch. Dis. Child.*, 34:192, 1959.

Williams, H. F., Landau, L. I., and Phelan, P. D.: Generalized bronchiectasis due to extensive deficiency of bronchial cartilage. *Arch. Dis. Child.*, 47:423, 1972.

Wissler, H.: Zur Landzeit-Prognose der Bronchiektasen im Kindesalter. *Respiration, 27* (Suppl.):183, 1970.

Wolfe, R. R.: Kartagener's syndrome: a pediatric responsibility. *Chest, 69*:573, 1976.

Wurnig, P.: Die Rolle der antibiotischen Inhalationstherapie bei Bronchiecktasien (Rückbildungsfähigkeit und Operabilität). *Respiration, 27*(Suppl.):216, 1970.

Wynn-Williams, N.: Bronchiectasis: a study centered in Bedford and its environs. *Br. Med. J., 1*:1194, 1953.

Wynn-Williams, N.: Observations on the treatment of bronchiectasis and its relation to prognosis. *Tubercle (London), 38*:133, 1957.

Zuckerman, H. S., and Wurtzebach, L. R.: Kartagener's triad. Review of the literature and report of a case. *Dis. Chest, 19*:92, 1951.

Zuelzer, W. W., and Newton, W. A.: The pathogenesis of fibrocystic disease of the pancreas. *Pediatrics, 4*:53, 1949.

CHAPTER TWENTY-SIX

PULMONARY ABSCESS

Robert H. High, M.D.

Pulmonary abscess develops when a portion of the pulmonary parenchyma is infected and subsequently becomes suppurative and necrotic. Occlusion of the bronchial segments leading to the involved area often occurs. The frequency with which lung abscess is noted has decreased in children, owing in part to the more prompt and effective treatment of pneumonia and to the more widespread use of endotracheal intubation during anesthesia, especially for surgical procedures in the oropharynx.

Pulmonary abscess may be multiple or single. In the former instance, septicemia, especially staphylococcal, is commonly the cause. Septicemia occurring in children who have had shunts of cerebrospinal fluid, in particular those using the ventriculojugular route with a valve in the drainage system, is likely to produce multiple pulmonary abscesses. Multiple abscesses may also complicate extensive pneumonia, especially that caused by staphylococci or Friedländer's bacillus. Multiple abscesses often develop in the presence of chronic suppurative bronchopulmonary disease associated with cystic fibrosis of the pancreas, extensive bronchiectasis, or congenital hypogammaglobulinemia and other immune deficiencies. In the latter group, pulmonary abscesses often develop during the terminal phase of the disease.

Single lung abscesses (Fig. 1) often follow the aspiration of infected material or a foreign body, and they may also be produced by infected emboli. Many times solitary lung abscesses develop during the course of acute pneumonia, especially that caused by staphylococci. Occasionally, anomalous cysts or sequestered lobes become infected with the subsequent development of pulmonary abscess (Fig. 2).

Abscesses that follow the aspiration of secretions or a foreign body are often caused by a variety of bacteria, chiefly those of the oral cavity, including fusospirochetal organisms, Bacteroides species and streptococci that are not of the group A type. Such abscesses are often called anaerobic or putrid abscesses.

Pulmonary abscesses complicating the course of pulmonary tuberculosis and that of the pulmonary mycotic infections are considered elsewhere.

In response to the infecting material, the pulmonary parenchyma undergoes intense acute inflammatory changes, thrombosis of the vascular supply and edema, with resulting obstruction of the bronchi draining the area (Fig. 3). Necrosis and central liquefaction of the involved area occur. After about ten days the abscess is likely to rupture into a bronchus, and the contents may be evacuated by coughing; sometimes the material is aspirated, producing a widespread bronchopneumonia. After evacuation of an abscess, the granulation tissue lining the walls may bleed. In the older child such hemorrhage may be manifested by hemoptysis, but this is not likely in the younger patient. After evacuation of a pulmonary abscess, fibrosis often occurs; many abscesses heal spontaneously, often with no sequelae.

Pulmonary abscesses located near the

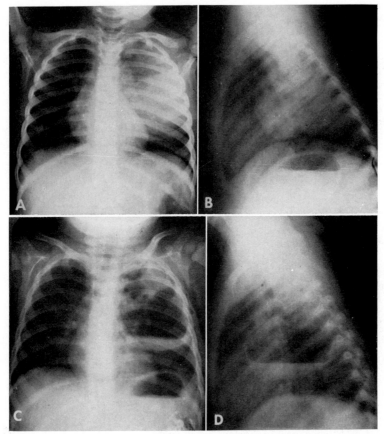

Figure 1. Solitary pneumococcal abscess. *A* and *B*, Preaspiration films. *C* and *D*, Postaspiration films (same day). The outcome was complete recovery.

periphery of the lung are likely to cause inflammation of the overlying pleura with a resultant plastic pleuritis. Sometimes such peripheral abscesses rupture into the pleural cavity, and a bronchopleural fistula associated with a pyopneumothorax develops (Fig. 4). These latter circumstances are serious

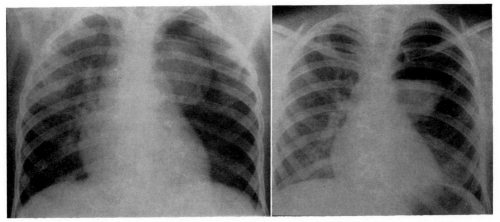

Figure 2. Infected congenital cyst. Note the fluid levels.

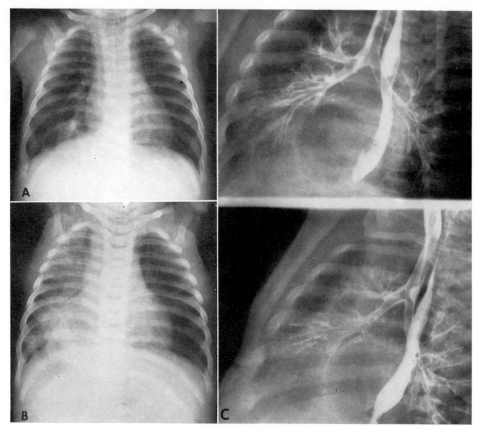

Figure 3. *A*, Recurrent pulmonary abscess, right lower lobe (7/26/65). *B*, Extension of abscess (9/17/65). *C*, Demonstration of lack of filling by bronchography (9/23/65). Subsequent thoractomy revealed sequestered lobe. Removal was followed by cure.

consequences of a pulmonary abscess, particularly if the abscess is produced by anaerobic organisms.

Aerobic (nonputrid) pulmonary abscesses secondary to septicemia, pneumonia, cystic fibrosis of the pancreas, and the like may be difficult to recognize because of the manifestations of the primary disease. Physical examination may suggest the presence of pulmonary consolidation. Roentgenographic examination shows segmental areas of pneumonia which resolve slowly. When the abscess communicates with the bronchial tree, air will displace some or all of the purulent material, and a cavity with or without a fluid level will be apparent. An area of inflammatory reaction will be noted surrounding the abscess. If the abscess ruptures into the pleural space, the physical and roentgenographic findings will be those of pyopneumothorax.

In *putrid (anaerobic) pulmonary abscesses* there is often a history of aspiration of secretions or of a foreign body, recent tonsillectomy, general anesthesia, or the like, but such is not always the case. After aspiration, a latent period of a few days may be noted before symptoms and signs of pulmonary infection develop. Occasionally the onset is insidious, but more commonly it is sudden with the appearance of fever, cough, chest pain, dyspnea, tachypnea, occasionally hemoptysis in the older child, as well as general manifestations of infection such as malaise and anorexia. Leukocytosis is often marked. The cough is usually dry and nonproductive in the early stages of the disease. After the abscess has liquefied and communicates with the bronchial tree, a large amount of purulent material may be raised by coughing.

Physical examination of the chest may suggest the presence of consolidation of the lung. Occasionally a pleural friction rub may be heard. Sometimes, especially if the diseased area is surrounded by normally aerated lung tissue, localized changes cannot be detected by physical examination. Under such circumstances, the diagnosis of pulmonary disease is suggested by the presence of such findings as cough, chest pain and dyspnea.

Symptoms and abnormal physical findings tend to subside after the contents of the abscess have been evacuated. If the abscess persists for several weeks, clubbing of the fingers may develop.

Roentgenographic examinations show changes similar to those described above (aerobic pulmonary abscess).

Antimicrobial treatment of the basic disease, when such is present, is imperative. In the presence of acute pneumonia or septicemia, such therapy may be all that is required. Most of the bacteria causing pulmonary abscess are the common pathogens of the respiratory tract. Infections with Friedländer's bacilli are fortunately uncommon in children. Accordingly, penicillin G should be administered in large doses initially by parenteral routes and later by the oral route. Whenever staphylococci are suspected of causing the abscess, initial

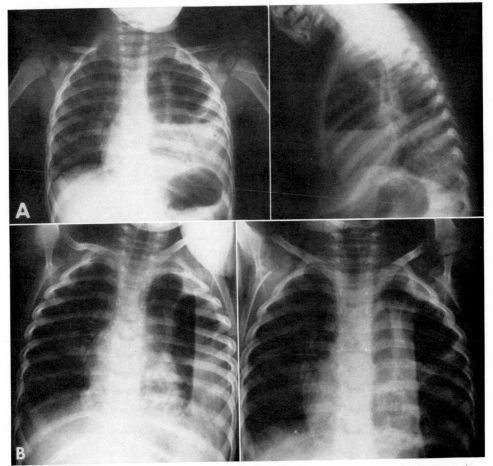

Figure 4. A two-year-old male child with staphylococcal pulmonary abscesses and pyopneumothorax. Note the fluid levels and shift of fluid with change in position. The outcome was complete recovery.

therapy should include the administration of one of the semisynthetic penicillin preparations, which are resistant to degradation by staphylococcal penicillinase. (See Staphylococcal Pneumonia, p. 388.) Kanamycin, colistin, methacillin, oxacillin, cloxacillin, dicloxacillin or nafcillin may be given in addition to penicillin until the results of cultures and sensitivity tests are available. Sulfonamide drugs are not recommended when purulent collections are present.

When an abscess has formed, bronchoscopic examination should be performed to aspirate as much of the purulent material as possible, to remove a foreign body or to exclude its presence and, of much importance, to secure material for culture and sensitivity tests. Cultures should be made for pyogenic bacteria, fungi and mycobacteria. Subsequent therapy may be guided by the results of such cultures. Bronchoscopic aspirations should be repeated until the amount of purulent material is minimal. Some recommend the instillation of proteolytic enzymes or antimicrobial agents, or both, during the bronchoscopic examination. The efficacy of such topical applications is difficult to evaluate, but theoretical considerations favor their use.

Postural drainage, aided by appropriate physical therapy to the chest (see p. 109), should also be used.

The aerosol administration of antibiotics and agents that help to liquefy mucus, such as N-acetylcystine, has been recommended, but their efficacy remains to be established. Systemic absorption of antibiotic agents is minimal after aerosol administration, and systemic toxic reactions are infrequent. Aerosol therapy is an addition to, but not a substitute or alternative for, intensive systemic therapy.

In those instances in which the foregoing measures fail to provide adequate and prompt drainage of a pulmonary abscess, direct aspiration under biplane fluoroscopic guidance is recommended. After aspiration of as much purulent material as possible, instillation of antibiotics and proteolytic enzymes may be made directly into the abscess cavity. Repeated aspirations and instillations may be made in those instances in which resolution is slow.

In most instances, a pulmonary abscess will resolve when treated as outlined above. In general, those caused by staphylococci or pneumococci respond well. In those patients in whom abscess closure does not occur after a trial of conservative treatment of perhaps a month's duration, surgical removal of the involved lobe or portion of a lobe is indicated.

Children who have healed pulmonary abscesses should be observed for the possible development of bronchiectasis in the involved area.

REFERENCES

Bernard, W. F., Malcolm, J. A., and Wylie, R. H.: Lung abscess: a study of 148 cases due to aspiration. *Dis. Chest, 43*:620, 1963.

Burnett, W. E., Rosemond, G. P., Caswell, H. T., Hall, J. H., and Bucher, R. M.: The topical treatment of lung abscess. *Pa. Med. J., 52*:719, 1949.

Cook, C. D.: Pulmonary abscess. In Gellis, S. S., and Kagan, B. M. (Eds.): *Current Pediatric Therapy 4.* Philadelphia, W. B. Saunders Company, 1970, pp. 198–199.

Eichenwald, H. F., and McCracken, G. H., Jr.: Pulmonary abscess. In Nelson, W. E. (Ed.): *Textbook of Pediatrics.* 9th Ed. Philadelphia, W. B. Saunders Company, 1969, pp. 938–939.

High, R. H.: Pulmonary abscesses. In Shirkey, H. C. (Ed.): *Pediatric Therapy* 1975. 5th Ed. St. Louis, C. V. Mosby Company, 1975, p. 692.

Thomas, D. M.: Management of postoperative pulmonary complications. *J. Ky. Med. Assoc., 61*:869, 1963.

CHAPTER TWENTY-SEVEN

PLEURISY AND EMPYEMA

Reynaldo D. Pagtakhan, M.D.,
and Victor Chernick, M.D.

Pleural inflammation is associated with minimal or considerable accumulation of liquid in the pleural cavity and remains an important cause of pulmonary disability and death in pediatric patients. In Chapter 40 we review the anatomic features of the pleura and the physiology of liquid movement across it in health and disease, present a classification of pleural effusions based on pathophysiology and chemistry of their contents and discuss the management of noninflammatory, hemorrhagic and chylous effusions. This chapter considers the etiologic spectrum, pathogenesis, functional pathology, diagnosis, management and prognosis of inflammatory pleural disorders.

Etiology and Pathogenesis

Inflammation of the pleural membranes (pleurisy; pleuritis) usually is a consequence of diseases elsewhere in the body and, rarely, of disturbances primarily residing in the pleura. The inciting process may be infection, neoplasm, trauma, pulmonary vascular obstruction, systemic granulomatous disease or some generalized inflammatory disorder affecting serous membranes. Infection from adjacent pulmonary and subdiaphragmatic foci reaches the visceral pleura by contiguous spread. Occasionally, bacteria reach the pleural cavity via a bronchopleural fistula or by way of the circulation from distant sites of suppuration. Neoplastic involvement of the pleura may be primary or metastatic. Metastases may occur through parenchymal lung involvement or directly into the pleura. Neoplasms may also obstruct lymphatic channels and interfere with pleural drainage, particularly clearance of proteins from the pleural cavity. Trauma following certain diagnostic and therapeutic cardiothoracic procedures irritates the pleura, which may become secondarily infected. Pulmonary embolism results in focal parenchymal necrosis that spreads to involve a pleural surface, causing pleurisy with or without effusion.

Irrespective of the origin and inflammatory nature of the inciting process, the initial exudative stage of pleural inflammation is characterized by accumulation of a small amount of thin fibrin along with a few polymorphonuclear cells. Liquid exudation into the pleural cavity is minimal or not detectable (dry or plastic pleurisy). The liquid remains uninfected for some time, even in those cases where the inciting underlying disorders are infectious in nature. Subsequently, permeability of the pleural capillaries is greatly enhanced, resulting in considerable accumulation of fibrin exudates (pleurisy with effusion). Since exudates have high protein concentration, the pleural liquid oncotic pressure is increased, thereby favoring further transport of liquid into the pleural cavity. These changes ultimately exceed lymphatic drainage, and significant pleural effusion ensues. When the underlying disturbance is an infection, the stage of pleurisy with effusion is followed by a so-called fibrinopurulent phase characterized by further increased accumulation of fibrin and polymorphonuclear leukocytes and by bacterial invasion of the pleural cavity. Effusions tend to loculate during this stage. Thick, purulent exudate resulting from pleural bacterial infection is termed empyema. It may be associated with a penetrating putrid odor characteristic of anaerobic infection. The bacterial agent, however, may not be identified if antimicrobial therapy had been given prior to evacuation of empyema. If the fibrinopurulent effusion is not drained in time, fibroblasts grow from both pleural surfaces and form an inelastic membrane. Thus, the nature of the underlying clinical disorder, stage of pleurisy, specific type of infecting agent and onset of antimicrobial therapy determine the degree and final character of the pleural exudate.

Table 1 classifies the clinical disorders that may cause pleurisy and empyema according to the original site and nature of the inciting inflammatory process. Primary neoplasms of the pleura include benign and malignant mesothelioma. They are rare causes of exudative pleural effusions in children. Pleural irritation may follow certain diagnostic (e.g., needle aspiration of the lung and percutaneous pleural biopsy) and therapeutic (e.g., radiation therapy to mediastinal malignancy; cardiothoracic operations) procedures performed on the chest. Fortunately, occurrence of secondary purulent pleurisy due to medical intervention has remained low in contrast to the valuable yield and salutary results these procedures offer the physician and his patient.

Thoracoabdominal infections constitute the major origin of pleurisy with effusion. Up to 20 per cent of children with viral and mycoplasma pneumonia develop effusions, which are usually transient and of minor importance. On occasion, however, the effusions can be massive and cause respiratory distress, necessitating prompt drainage, or may be recalcitrant and cause prolonged morbidity in infants with concurrent malnutrition. Nonetheless, the effusions usually remain thin. Pulmonary tuberculosis usually causes dry pleurisy until the caseous materials containing the tuberculous antigen leak into the pleura. Considerable effusion then occurs as a result of the specific allergic reaction of the pleural membranes.

TABLE 1. ETIOLOGIC SPECTRUM OF PLEURISY AND EMPYEMA

Origin and Nature of Inflammation	Illustrative Clinical Disorders
Primary in Pleura	
Neoplasm	Primary pleural mesothelioma
Trauma	Following cardiothoracic surgery, lung aspiration and percutaneous pleural biopsies, thoracic irradiation therapy
Contiguous Structures	
Lung infection	Pneumonia (aerobic and anaerobic bacterial, tuberculous, fungal, viral, mycoplasma, echinococcal), bronchopleural fistula
Chest wall and subdiaphragmatic infection	Chest wall contusion and abscess, intra-abdominal abscess (subphrenic and hepatic), acute hemorrhagic pancreatitis, pancreaticopleural fistula
Mediastinal infection and neoplasm	Acute mediastinitis (secondary to esophageal rupture); mediastinal tumors
Systemic Diseases	
Septicemia	Distant sites of suppuration
Malignancy	Lymphoma, leukemia, neuroblastoma, hepatoma, multiple myeloma
Vascular obstruction	Pulmonary infarction
Connective tissue or collagen disorders	Systemic lupus erythematosus, polyarteritis, Wegener's granulomatosis, rheumatoid arthritis, scleroderma, rheumatic fever
Granulomatous disease	Sarcoidosis

The cellular character of the exudate is lymphocytic. Effusion is usually on the side of the primary parenchymal focus. Bilateral effusions indicate hematogenous dissemination from some remote focus. Frank tuberculous empyema is rare, occurring in only about 2 per cent of tuberculous pleurisy, particularly when bronchopleural fistula complicates the disease.

Nontuberculous bacterial pneumonias constitute the most frequent origin of inflammatory pleural effusions, also referred to as parapneumonic effusions. The effusion may loculate owing to pleural adhesions or may be purulent. Table 2 lists in order of descending prevalence the predominant aerobic and anaerobic isolates of empyema. In any given patient, either or both types may be isolated, but the actual occurrence rate is difficult to ascertain. The opportunity to establish a specific etiologic agent may depend on the patient's age, nature of the underlying disease, standard of laboratory culture methods and onset of antimicrobial therapy.

The advent of the antimicrobial era has brought about not only a significant drop in the overall incidence of bacterial infection but also a shift in bacteriologic predominance. Thus, staphylococcus has emerged as the single most

TABLE 2. BACTERIOLOGY OF NONTUBERCULOUS EMPYEMA

Aerobic Bacteria
  Staphylococcus aureus
  Hemophilus influenzae
  Streptococcus pyogenes
  Diplococcus pneumoniae
  Escherichia coli
  Klebsiella species
  Pseudomonas aeruginosa

Anaerobic Bacteria
  Microaerophilic streptococcus
  Fusobacterium nucleatum
  Bacteroids melaninogenicus
  Bacteroids fragilis
  Peptococcus
  Peptostreptococcus
  Catalase-negative, non–spore-forming, gram-positive bacilli

common aerobic pathogen of empyema. Infants and children are prone to develop septicemia from staphylococcal pneumonia, perhaps related to their appreciably low serum titer of coagulase-reacting factor. Clinical settings that favor consideration of staphylococcal empyema include the presence of superficial skin lesions, osteomyelitis, lung abscess, bronchopleural fistula and cystic fibrosis. Another common aerobic isolate is *Hemophilus influenzae*, associated with otitis media and pneumonia in older children. Paracolon bacteria and pneumococcus are common in infants. Pseudomonas is seen with increased frequency in debilitated patients requiring prolonged respirator therapy.

Anaerobic pleuropulmonary infections have their distinctive clinical settings. More than 90 per cent of the patients manifest periodontal infections and have altered consciousness and dysphagia. Thus, aspiration of a large volume of oropharyngeal secretions occurs in the presence of disturbed clearing mechanisms. It is therefore not surprising that the three predominant pleural anaerobic isolates, namely microaerophilic streptococcus, *Fusobacterium nucleatum* and *Bacteroides melaninogenicus* (Table 2), compose the normal flora of the upper respiratory tract and that localization of the primary pulmonary disease (e.g., lung abscess and necrotizing pneumonia) is usually in gravity-dependent lung segments. The clinical course is generally insidious and indolent. Mediastinal and subdiaphragmatic foci of infections are also common sites of origin for anaerobic empyema.

Except for septicemia from contiguous or distant sites of suppuration, systemic origins of pleurisy generally produce nonpurulent effusion. Effusion secondary to pulmonary embolism of venous thrombi, fat or gas is rare in childhood, although it may be a serious consequence of malignancy. Pleurisy may be associated with connective tissue disorders, such as lupus erythematosus and rheumatoid arthritis, and is part of the more widespread inflammatory process.

In summary, a variety of clinical disorders of protean inflammatory origins can induce pleurisy and empyema. Certain clinical settings are distinctive for specific bacterial isolates.

Functional Pathology

Pulmonary disability is a function of duration, rapidity of onset and extent of pleural involvement and is modified by concurrent complication and status of cardiopulmonary reserve. Early in the phase of pleurisy, chest pain on inspiration diminishes thoracic excursion, induces rapid shallow breathing and increases dead space:tidal volume ratio. As a result of hypoventilation, hypoxemia and hypercapnia ensue. Later, significant effusion displaces the mediastinum. This reduces lung volume and impedes venous return. With concurrent complication, such as pneumatocele seen in staphylococcal infection, ventilation-perfusion imbalance is further compromised and work of breathing is aggravated. Reflex bronchospasm may occur. Thus, severe pleural disease may produce striking abnormalities in lung volume, airflow and pulmonary blood flow with ensuing disturbances of gas exchange.

Diagnosis

History and Physical Examination. The physician is first alerted to a diagnosis of pleurisy as he listens to a narration of symptoms produced by pleural inflammation per se and those due to the underlying clinical disorder. Symptoms of direct pleural involvement include chest pain, chest tightness and dyspnea. The older child may complain of sharp pleuritic pain on inspiration due to stretching of the parietal pleura. The pain is accentuated by breathing and coughing because of greater motion of the visceral surface over the parietal surface. The locus of pleurisy determines the site of pain,

which may be felt in the chest overlying the site of inflammation, or referred to the shoulder if the central diaphragm is involved or to the abdomen if the peripheral diaphragm is involved. Severe chest pain inhibits respiratory movement and causes dyspnea. As effusion increases and separates the pleural membranes, pleuritic pain becomes a dull ache and may disappear. However, increased pleural liquid accumulation aggravates dyspnea. Infants and younger children may present with dyspnea and cough that vary with changes in body position.

The patient may present with manifestations related to the underlying inciting process. High fever, chills, vomiting, anorexia, lethargy and severe prostration suggest an infectious etiologic agent and increasing toxicity (e.g., staphylococcal empyema). Abdominal distention may be present owing to partial paralytic ileus. A symptomless interval may intervene between the onset of the pleural complication and apparent cure of underlying pneumonia. Relentless pneumonia in the presence of pancreatitis suggests pancreaticopleural fistula. A history of rapid reaccumulation of effusion associated with weight loss should suggest a malignancy. Pleurisy with effusion is one of the hallmarks of systemic lupus erythematosus and may occur in other connective tissue disorders. Thus, systemic manifestations of pleurisy vary with the nature of the underlying disorders and their protean clinical picture. Moreover, steroid therapy may mask the common constitutional symptoms.

Attention to the chest finding on physical examination is important, particularly if only a small amount of pleural exudate is present. Pleural rub due to roughened pleural surfaces may be the only finding early in the disease and may be heard during inspiration or expiration. Diminished thoracic wall excursion, dull or flat percussion, decreased tactile and vocal fremitus, diminished whispering pectoriloquy, fullness of the intercostal spaces and decreased breath sounds are easily demonstrated over the site involved in the older child with moderate effusion. Breath sounds in the neonate can come through loud and clear because of his small chest volume. The trachea and the cardiac apex are displaced toward the contralateral side.

History-taking and physical examination do not stop after admission of the patient to the hospital. Events in the clinical course during hospitalization may suggest emergence of certain complications of empyema. Expectoration of an increasing quantity of purulent sputum with or without hemoptysis may herald the onset of bronchopleural fistula and ensuing pyopneumothorax. Bronchopleural fistula may be due to rupture of neglected empyema into the lung or rupture of pulmonary suppuration into the pleura. Findings of chest wall abscess and costal chondritis may suggest extension (empyema necessitans) of tuberculous or fungal em-

pyema. Muffling of the heart tones and pericardial rub indicate extension into the pericardium. Another complication is acute mediastinitis, which with its clinical picture of increasing toxicity is as serious as pericarditis.

CHEST ROENTGENOGRAM. A chest roentgenogram is most useful in substantiating the physical findings of pleural effusion, irrespective of its nature and underlying cause (see also Chapter 40, Liquid in the Pleural Space). Obliteration of the costophrenic sinus (Fig. 1, *arrow*) may be the earliest radiologic sign of minimal liquid accumulation, best demonstrated in the decubitus position. Moderate effusion causes layering of liquid density along the lateral chest wall. In the absence of pleural adhesions, the liquid density shifts with change in body position from upright to decubitus views. Failure of the liquid to shift indicates loculation, as commonly seen in staphylococcal empyema. Massive effusion may

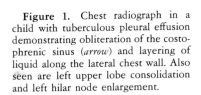

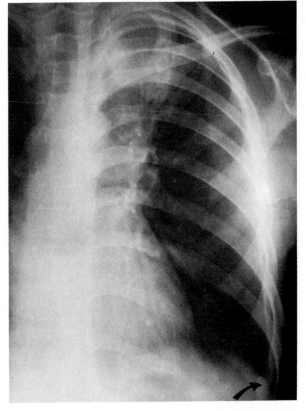

Figure 1. Chest radiograph in a child with tuberculous pleural effusion demonstrating obliteration of the costophrenic sinus (*arrow*) and layering of liquid along the lateral chest wall. Also seen are left upper lobe consolidation and left hilar node enlargement.

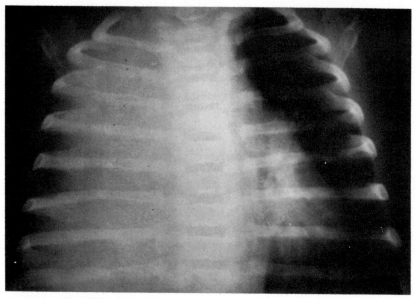

Figure 2. Chest radiograph in a child with staphylococcal empyema demonstrating complete opacification of the right hemithorax with displacement of the heart and mediastinum to the left.

occupy one hemithorax, which demonstrates a uniform water density and displacement of the mediastinum toward the contralateral side (Fig. 2).

A chest roentgenogram is also important in documenting the presence of pyopneumothorax, which appears in the upright view as an air-liquid level extending to the lateral portion of the hemithorax. This picture can be differentiated from a huge lung abscess by obtaining a decubitus view. Further radiologic assessment of bronchopleural fistula may be obtained by a variety of methods. One approach is by sinography. Radiopaque contrast material is injected into the affected pleura through a needle or existing chest tube (Fig. 3). As the patient coughs, the contrast material opacifies the fistula and spreads throughout the bronchial tree. This is the procedure of choice for peripherally situated small fistulas. Selective bronchography is employed to delineate multiple, centrally located fistulas.

EXAMINATION OF THE PLEURAL LIQUID. The pleural liquid may provide the only evidence on which to make a specific etiologic diagnosis or exclude others (also see Chapter 40). Thus, thoracentesis is mandatory. It must be performed by experienced personnel after careful planning. The procedure is explained to patients old enough to comprehend. Local anesthetic is used. Size and length of the needle are determined by chest wall thickness and anticipated character of the fluid. Interposing a three way stopcock between needle and syringe allows a large quantity of liquid to be removed without danger of air entry. In addition to being guided by the chest roentgenogram, the point of maximum dullness must be ascertained to localize the site of needle entry. The seventh posterolateral intercostal space is sufficient for most cases of nonloculated effusions. Once inserted, the needle is clamped at skin level to prevent inadvertent shifting. Vigorous cough is dangerous, and the needle should be withdrawn quickly. A post-thoracentesis chest film is obtained to look for any complication and underlying parenchymal disease.

The gross appearance of the liquid is noted and a Gram stain made. The remainder of the specimen is sent for cytologic examination, biochemical studies, pH and P_{CO_2} determinations and microbiologic cultures. Thin and clear pleural effusions suggest noninfectious inflammatory exudates, which must be differentiated from transudates (see Chapter 40, Table 2). Nontraumatic sanguineous exudates may be due to underlying malignancy, pulmonary infarction, pancreaticopleural fistula, connective tissue disorder or tuberculosis. Thick, purulent effusion is diagnostic of empyema. If it is putrid, anaerobic infection is incriminated. Thin, clear effusions, however, do not rule out an infectious basis. Gram stain is particularly useful if the patient had prior antimicrobial therapy. Cytologic findings of malignant cells are diagnostic. In addition to biochemical studies for protein and lactic dehydrogenase, which separate exudate from transudate, determination of amylase helps establish a diagnosis of underlying pancreatitis (amylase concentration is elevated). A new immunoprecipitin method—countercurrent immunoelectrophoresis (CIE)—has recently proved useful for the diagnosis of certain bacterial antigens (e.g., staphylococcal) in the body fluids, including pleural liquid. CIE may provide a presumptive etiologic diagnosis for certain infectious pleural effusions in the event Gram stain and culture return negative. A definitive etiologic diagnosis rests on the result of microbiologic cultures.

Infectious pleural effusions developing during the course of bacterial pneumonias may be categorized as ① empyema, that is, purulent with positive Gram stain and/or culture, and ② nonempyema. Nonempyemic effusions either remain free or loculate, depending on the stage of pleurisy. Table 3 compares empyema, loculated exudates and nonloculated effusions according to gross appearance, bacteriologic confirmation, biochemical characteristics, and P_{CO_2} and pH determinations. The specimen for pH and P_{CO_2} determinations is collected anaerobically and placed in ice during its transport to the blood gas laboratory. Arterial pH is determined simultaneously, since it influences pleural liquid pH. It appears that pleural liquid pH can discriminate free-moving, nonloculated effusions (pH>7.30) from locu-

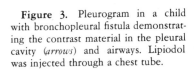
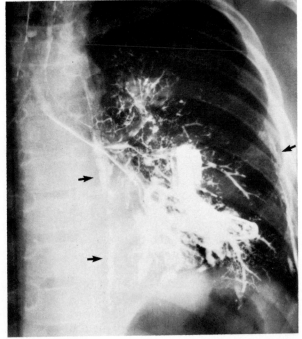

Figure 3. Pleurogram in a child with bronchopleural fistula demonstrating the contrast material in the pleural cavity (*arrows*) and airways. Lipiodol was injected through a chest tube.

TABLE 3. PHYSICAL AND CHEMICAL CHARACTERISTICS OF
PARAPNEUMONIC PLEURAL EFFUSIONS*

Characteristics	Empyema	Loculated Exudates	Nonloculated Effusions
Appearance	Purulent and predominantly turbid	Nonpurulent and predominantly less turbid	Nonpurulent and predominantly less turbid
Gram stain and/or Culture	Positive	Negative	Negative
Glucose (mg./dl)	Majority <50 (mean = 36)	Majority <50 (mean = 36)	Majority >100 (mean = 134)
Protein (gm./dl)	Invariably >3.0 (mean = 4.7)	Invariably >3 (mean = 6.0)	Majority <3 (mean = 2.7)
P$_{CO_2}$ (mm. Hg)	Majority >60 (mean = 100)	Majority >60 (mean = 71)	Majority <40 (mean = 45)
pH (units)	Invariably <7.30 (mean = 6.93)	Invariably <7.30 (mean = 6.94)	Invariably >7.30 (mean = 7.38)

*Modified from Potts, D. E., Levin, D. C., and Sahn, S. A.: *Chest, 70*:328, 1976.

lated exudates and frank empyema (pH<7.30). Thus, low pleural liquid pH may have therapeutic and prognostic importance. It is imperative to emphasize, however, that the use of pleural liquid pH below and above 7.30 is valid only with effusions due to nontuberculous bacterial pneumonias. Tuberculous and other noninfectious inflammatory exudates may also have a low pleural liquid pH, and their differentiation must be based on clinical information and results of other laboratory tests. Moreover, the usefulness of pleural liquid pH as a criterion for the initiation of thoracotomy drainage needs prospective evaluation in children with varying types of empyema, particularly those due to anaerobic bacteria.

PLEURAL BIOPSY. Parietal pleural biopsy is indicated in patients with unexplained inflammatory pleural effusion. The procedure may be performed either percutaneously at the bedside, using a specially designed needle, or by open thoracotomy under general anesthesia. A variety of special cutting needles have been used, namely, Cope, Abrams, Ballestero, Vim-Silverman and Harefield. The Harefield needle allows aspiration of liquid at the time of pleural biopsy. The tissue specimen includes portions of intercostal muscles and adjoining parietal pleura approximately 4 mm. in diameter and is sent for histologic and culture studies. The liquid in the pleural space prevents the needle from puncturing the lung. Thus, the biopsy is most easily accomplished at the time of initial thoracentesis when there is the least chance of lacerating the underlying lung. The greatest value of percutaneous parietal biopsy is in clinical disorders that cause widespread involvement of the pleural surface (e.g., tuberculosis, tumors).

The technique of percutaneous pleural biopsy is as follows: The patient is seated and adequately supported. The appropriate site for needle entry is infiltrated to the parietal pleura with local anesthesia. A small incision is made on the skin to facilitate introduction of the trocar. The Harefield needle, with the notch closed, is carefully advanced into the pleural space. The pleural effusion is aspirated. Thereafter, the needle with the notch open is withdrawn slowly while lateral pressure is applied in the direction of the notch, which is indicated by the small rounded knob on the hub of the needle. A catch is felt as the notch becomes engaged on the parietal pleura. The inner cutting core is advanced, obtaining the specimen, and the needle is then withdrawn. Careful technique is associated with a minimal occurrence of complications such as pneumothorax or hemothorax. Since morbidity from the procedure is low and repetition of the biopsy increases the diagnostic yield, a repeat biopsy becomes indicated when an etiologic diagnosis has not been established.

OTHER LABORATORY INVESTIGATIONS. Additional appropriate tests are carried out to elucidate a suspected underlying disease state. For example, a positive Mantoux reaction, particularly a recent conversion, strongly suggests tuberculosis; a negative skin test does not rule it out. Examination of bronchopulmonary secretions obtained by sputum induction, by gastric fluid aspiration and during bronchoscopy may be indicated. Certain immunologic tests (e.g., anti-DNA) are indicated to clarify the causative role of some connective tissue or collagen disorders. Blood culture is performed when sepsis is suspected. A negative sweat test rules out cystic fibrosis. Roentgenograms of other organs are ordered when underlying malignancy is a consideration. As well, repeat physical examination may reveal findings that lead to a specific diagnosis.

Management

Treatment of inflammatory pleural disorders is aimed at specific management of the underlying cause and relief of functional disturbances caused by the inciting clinical disorder, pleural involvement and concurrent complication. Therapy is medical and surgical. A prompt and specific etiologic diagnosis is optimal for management.

General supportive measures include bedrest for the acutely ill child and chloral hydrate for restlessness and irritability. It is imperative to recognize that irritability may be due to pain, high fever, distressing cough or hypoxia. Relief of sharp pain occurring with every phase of respiration—characteristic of dry pleurisy—demands immediate attention. Mild cases promptly respond to such simple measures as local heat and acetylsalicylic acid. Aspirin is also indicated for very high fever to minimize discomfort to the child and avert febrile convulsion, particularly among young infants. Severe pleuritic pain may require the use of oral codeine sulfate, which will also suppress dry cough due to irritation of the airways. Alternative analgesic measures include topical ethyl chloride spray and intravenous calcium gluconate. Response of some patients to the latter drugs indicates that muscle spasm may play a role in the genesis of pain. Lying on the affected side may provide temporary relief by splinting the involved thorax. Excruciating pain, as may be seen in pleuritis due to neoplasm, requires an exceptional approach. Repeated subcutaneous morphine injection may be indicated in terminal cases. Moreover, intercostal nerve block using 1 to 2 ml. of 1 per cent lidocaine solution has been tried. It is injected via a 23-gauge, 2-inch long needle into the area near the nerves involved.

Humidified oxygen is given to relieve hypoxemia; an inspired oxygen concentration is used to keep arterial P_{O_2} between 50 and 100 mm. Hg. Oxygen therapy may help hasten absorption of excess gastrointestinal gas. More direct measures for relief of abdominal distention, which can hinder respiration, include the use of gastric suction, insertion of rectal tubes and administration of Prostigmin methyl sulfate. Fluid and electrolytes are provided to replace water and sodium lost via the skin and the lungs by evaporation, a process aggravated by fever. Parenteral alimentation may be indicated when underlying malnutrition is present.

The stage of effusion following dry pleurisy usually provides a permanent relief from pain. However, accumulation of an excessive amount of pleural liquid necessitates a thoracentesis to relieve dyspnea. Repeat thoracentesis and, eventually, <u>continuous chest tube drainage are indicated if rapid reaccumulation of effusion induces dyspnea and dominates the clinical picture as is commonly seen in neoplasm.</u> Although most effusions due to a noninfectious inflammatory process require only drainage to relieve dyspnea, additional specific measures may be indicated in the presence of certain underlying systemic disease. Systemic and intrapleural instillation of chemotherapeutic agents and mediastinal irradiation of the involved nodes or primary tumor sites control pleural effusion in lymphoma. Prednisone ameliorates dyspnea as well as cough, anorexia and weight loss in sarcoidosis. Steroid will increase the rate with which tuberculous effusion resolves and fever returns to normal, but definitive proof of its value on eventual ventilatory function has not been shown. Tuberculous effusions usually clear within six months on isoniazid and para-aminosalicylic acid or ethambutol therapy alone. Indeed, asymptomatic noninfectious pleural exudates need only management of the

TABLE 4. A GUIDE TO ANTIMICROBIAL THERAPY OF BACTERIAL PLEURISY AND EMPYEMA

Infecting Agent	Drug and Dosage (per kg. per day) Route and Duration*	Target Organs for Side-Effects
A. Aerobic bacteria	✓ Oxacillin	
1. Staphylococcus	1.a. Methicillin, 200–400 mg. divided in 3–4 doses IV initially; for 3–4 weeks	Kidney, bone marrow, allergy
	b. Cloxacillin, 100–200 mg. divided in 3–6 doses IV initially; for 3–4 weeks	Same as A.1.a
2. *Hemophilus influenzae*	2.a. Ampicillin, 50–200 mg. divided in 2–4 doses IV initially; for 7–10 days	Skin, gastro-intestinal, bone marrow, CNS
	✓ b. Chloramphenicol, 25–100 mg. divided in 4 doses IV initially; for 7–10 days	Bone marrow, skin, gastro-intestinal, cardiocirculatory, optic nerve
3. Pneumococcus and streptococcus	3. Penicillin G, 50,000–300,000 units divided in 3–4 doses IV or IM; for 7–10 days	Allergy, CNS
4. *E. coli* and Klebsiella	✓ 4. Gentamicin, 5–7 mg. divided in 2–3 doses IV, for 14 days or longer	Kidney, auditory nerve
5. Pseudomonas	5.a. Carbenicillin, 100–600 mg. divided in 4 doses IV, for 10 days or longer	Skin, gastro-intestinal, bone marrow, CNS
	b. Tobramycin, 5–7 mg. divided in 2 doses	Same as A.4
B. Anaerobic bacteria		
1. *Bacteroides fragilis*	1. Chloramphenicol, same as A.2.b	Same as A.2.b
2. All except *Bacteroides fragilis*	2.a. Penicillin G, same as A.3	Same as A.3
	b. Ampicillin, same as A.2.a	Same as A.2.b

IV = intravenously; IM = intramuscularly; CNS = central nervous system; kg. = kilogram body weight.
*Note:

1. The lower dose in the dosage range and less frequent intervals of administration are recommended for newborn infants.

2. Duration of therapy for anaerobic pneumonitis requires an adjustment if the lung lesions go on to cavitate. Often, 6 to 12 weeks are required before the lung lesions clear or only a small stable residual disease is left.

underlying disorder. Improvement in the underlying systemic disease is paralleled by resolution of the accompanying pleural exudation.

Pleural effusions due to infection require specific antimicrobial treatment and certain surgical considerations. Antimicrobial therapy should be initiated on the strength of a positive Gram stain or grossly purulent liquid. Initial choice of antimicrobial agents is based on a consideration of the clinical data, the bacterial epidemiology in the community, and known pharmacologic properties of the drugs. Dosage must be adequate, and administration initally should be via the intravenous route. Since infection may be polymicrobial, more than one antimicrobial drug has to be given initially. Subsequent changes in antimicrobial coverage are guided by the results of culture and sensitivity tests. A guide to antimicrobial therapy of nontuberculous bacterial pleurisy and empyema is presented in Table 4. Duration of drug treatment must be long enough to prevent relapse. The physician must always be aware of the potential side-effects of the drugs on various target organs and must be prepared to use alternative drugs at the appropriate time.

With appropriate antimicrobial therapy, the patient should recover completely from an episode of aerobic bacterial pleurisy and empyema. Pleural drainage initiated to relieve symptoms can often be stopped after 24 hours. Pleural drainage is not necessary if the patient remains asymptomatic, despite the slow resolution of the roentgenographic changes.

In contrast, anaerobic pneumonitis and pleural sepsis more often produce thick, loculated empyema which is difficult to evacuate by multiple thoracenteses. Moreover, these patients tend to remain febrile for an average of three weeks after the first drainage procedure, and most fatalities (10.6 per cent) have been ascribed to delay or failure to obtain optimal surgical drainage. Thus, anaerobic empyema may often require longer antimicrobial therapy and open thoracotomy drainage.

Table 5 lists current surgical considerations in the management of bacterial pleurisy and empyema. A rational choice of a surgical drainage procedure requires knowledge of the specific etio-

TABLE 5. SURGICAL MANAGEMENT OF BACTERIAL PLEURISY AND EMPYEMA

Procedure	Rationale and Comments
1) Thoracentesis (needle aspiration)	For prompt relief of dyspnea and initial step for diagnostic study of the liquid. May be repeated two or three times and most of effusion removed during tap.
2) Intercostal tube drainage (closed thoracotomy)	For massive, relatively thin effusion in the presence of overwhelming toxicity (e.g., secondary to lung abscess).
3) Tube thoracotomy with rib resection (open thoracotomy)	For symptomatic thick, encapsulated empyema not controlled by antibiotics and early obliteration of empyema cavity is expected (e.g., postlobectomy empyema).
4) Open flap drainage	For larger symptomatic empyema (e.g., postpneumonectomy empyema). Easy to care for technique for septic and debilitated patients.
5) Pleural decortication	For removal of restrictive fibrous tissue layer on surface of lungs. Indicated for symptomatic chronic empyema with lung entrapment.
6) Extrapleural thoracoplasty	To obliterate pleural cavity and lessen space into which lung has to expand. May be a deforming procedure and now very rarely indicated.

logic diagnosis and clinical course of the disease. With the availability of current antimicrobial agents and prompt medical therapy, open flap drainage, pleural decortication and thoracoplasty now almost never need be done. Perhaps the only remaining indication for these surgical procedures is concurrent bronchopleural fistula, which may require, if recalcitrant, grafting with pedicled muscle. On occasion, surgical drainage may be indicated for a large, symptomatic pneumatocele. Usually, however, the pneumatocele subsides spontaneously with resolution of the underlying inflammation. Concurrent extrapulmonary complications (e.g., pericarditis) are managed appropriately.

Prognosis

The outlook of inflammatory pleural disorders basically depends upon the ① nature of the underlying clinical problem, ② nature and extent of pleural disease, ③ age of the patient, ④ onset of therapy and ⑤ occurrence of complications. Malignant pleurisy carries an extremely grave prognosis, whereas viral and mycoplasma pleural diseases generally resolve spontaneously with time. Empyemic versus nonempyemic, free-moving pleural liquid is associated with a more prolonged and complicated hospital course and may require longer follow-up at home. Empyema carries a far higher mortality in infants under two years of age if treatment is delayed. Prompt and adequate therapy during the acute phase should result in complete recovery. Complications such as bronchopleural fistula and tension pneumatocele are rare but may delay onset of full recovery.

Noninfectious pleurisy and effusions resolve with the resolution of the underlying systemic clinical problems. The outcome of bacterial pleurisy and empyema has remarkably improved in recent years. Only 25 years ago, the mortality from empyema was approximating 100 per cent; now, virtually no death should occur with prompt therapy. Fibrothorax is extremely rare. In contrast to adults, infants and children have a remarkable ability to resolve a thickened pleura with no effect on subsequent lung growth and function.

REFERENCES

Bartlett, J. G., and Finegold, S. M.: Anaerobic infections of the lung and pleural space. Am. Rev. Resp. Dis., 110:56, 1974.

Bechamps, G. J., Lynn, H. B., and Wenzl, J. E.: Empyema in children: review of Mayo Clinic experience. Mayo Clin. Proc., 45:43, 1970.

Berger, H. W., and Mejia, E.: Tuberculous pleurisy. Chest, 63:88, 1973.

Cho, C., Hiatt, W. D., and Behbehan, A. M.: Pneumonia and massive pleural effusion associated with adenovirus type 7. Am. J. Dis. Child., 126:92, 1973.

Dorman, J. P., Campbell, D., Grover, F., and Trinkle, J. K.: Open thoracostomy drainage of postpneumonic empyema with bronchopleural fistula. J. Thorac. Cardiovasc. Surg., 66:979, 1973.

Eichenwald, H. F.: Antimicrobial therapy in children. Curr. Probl. Pediatr., 4:3, 1974.

Fine, N. L., Smith, L. R., and Sheedy, P. F.: Frequency of pleural effusions in mycoplasma and viral pneumonias. N. Engl. J. Med., 288:790, 1970.

Grix, A., and Giammona, S. T.: Pneumonitis with pleural effusion in children due to mycoplasma pneumoniae. Am. Rev. Resp. Dis., 109:665, 1974.

Hsu, J. T., Bennett, G. M., and Wolff, E.: Radiologic assessment of bronchopleural fistula with empyema. Diag. Radiol., 103:41, 1972.

Kissane, J. M.: Pathology of Infancy and Childhood. 2nd Ed. St. Louis, The C. V. Mosby Company, 1975.

Krugman, S., and Ward, R.: Infectious Diseases of Children and Adults. 5th Ed. St. Louis, The C. V. Mosby Company, 1973.

Lampe, R. M., Chottipitayasunondh, T., and Sunakorn, P.: Detection of bacterial antigen in pleural fluid by counter-immunoelectrophoresis. J. Pediatr., 88:557, 1976.

Light, R. W.: Management of parapneumonic effusions. Chest, 70:325, 1976.

Lincoln, E. M., Davies, P. A., and Bovornkitti, S.: Tuberculous pleurisy with effusion in children. Am. Rev. Tuberc., 77:271, 1958.

Potts, D. E., Levin, D. C., and Sahn, S. A.: Pleural fluid pH in parapneumonia effusions. Chest, 70:328, 1976.

Sahn, S. A., Lakshminarayan, S., and Char, D. C.: "Silent" empyema in a patient receiving corticosteroids. Am. Rev. Resp. Dis., 107:873, 1973.

Shackelford, P. G., Campbell, J., and Feigin, R.

D.: Countercurrent immunoelectrophoresis in the evaluation of childhood infections. *J. Pediatr.,* 85:478, 1974.

Stead, W. W., and Sproul, J. M.: Pleural effusion. *D. M.,* July 1964.

Stiles, Q. R., Lindesmith, G. G., Tucker, B. L., Meyer, B. W., and Jones, J. C.: Pleural empyema in children. *Ann. Thorac. Surg.,* 10:37, 1970.

Thornton, G. F.: The role of corticosteroids in the management of tuberculous infections. In Johnson III, J. E. (Ed.): *Rational Therapy and* *Control of Tuberculosis.* Gainsville, University of Florida Press, 1970, pp. 113–125.

Weick, J. K., Killy, J. M., Harrison, E. G., Carr, D. T., and Scanlon, P.: Pleural effusion in lymphoma. *Cancer, 31*:848, 1973.

Wise, M. B., Beaudry, P. H., and Bates, D. V.: Long term follow-up of staphylococcal pneumonia. *Pediatrics, 38*:398, 1966.

Wolfe, W. G., Spick, A., and Bradford, W. D.: Pleural fluids in infants and children. *Am. Rev. Resp. Dis., 98*:1027, 1968.

SECTION V

NONINFECTIOUS
DISORDERS
OF THE RESPIRATORY
TRACT

CHAPTER TWENTY-EIGHT

LUNG INJURY FROM HYDROCARBON ASPIRATION AND SMOKE INHALATION

ROBERT B. MELLINS, M.D.

LUNG INJURY FROM HYDROCARBON ASPIRATION

Hydrocarbon toxicity resulting from the ingestion of petroleum solvents: dry cleaning fluids, lighter fluids, kerosene, gasoline and liquid polishes and waxes (mineral seal oil) has continued to be a common occurrence in the small child over the past 20 years (Mellins and coworkers, 1956; Eade and coworkers, 1974). The decrease in the frequency of kerosene poisoning during this period may reflect the concomitant decrease in the use of kerosene space heaters. On the other hand, the availability of an increasing number of cleaning fluids, furniture polishes and liquid floor waxes within the home and all too frequently within the easy reach of the toddler accounts for the persistence of hydrocarbon poisoning.

Although central nervous system abnormalities (including weakness, confusion and coma), gastrointestinal irritation, myocardiopathy and renal toxicity all occur, the most frequent as well as the most serious complication is pneumonitis. Deaths from hydrocarbon poisoning are almost always from pneumonitis rather than from central nervous system toxicity.

Supported in part by NIH grant HL 06012.

Pathology

Pathologic changes in the lung of fatal cases have included necrosis of bronchial, bronchiolar and alveolar tissue, atelectasis, interstitial inflammation, hemorrhagic pulmonary edema, vascular thromboses, necrotizing bronchopneumonia and hyaline membrane formation. Injury to the myocardium has also been reported (James and coworkers, 1971). At the experimental level, hydrocarbon pneumonitis in rats is characterized by an acute alveolitis that is most severe at three days, subsides at ten days, and is followed by a chronic proliferation phase that may take weeks to resolve (Gross and associates, 1963). These experimental studies, when taken in conjunction with the observation in the human that the chest roentgenographic abnormalities are present for some time after the physical findings have cleared, suggest that the pulmonary lesions may also persist for some time in the human.

Pathophysiology

Low surface tension facilitates the spread of hydrocarbons along mucus membranes, and when coupled with choking and gagging probably accounts for the aspiration of hydrocarbon liquids into the lungs. Low viscosity and high volatility may facilitate deep penetration into the lungs.

There is experimental evidence to suggest that hydrocarbons increase the minimum surface tension, presumably by altering surfactant, thus predisposing to alveolar instability, small airway closure and atelectasis (Giammona, 1967). These alterations in the lung would account for the combination of hyperinflation and atelectasis seen on the chest roentgenogram as well as the hypoxemia. Because they are liquid solvents, it is possible that hydrocarbons injure cells by disrupting cell membranes. The observation that there is a decrease in the ability to clear bacteria following experimental kerosene poisoning suggests that hydrocarbon aspiration also impairs pulmonary defense mechanisms.

Initially, considerable controversy centered around how much of the toxicity resulted from aspiration as against gastrointestinal absorption with subsequent transport to the lungs and other organs by the blood. The bulk of evidence now suggests that the pulmonary lesions are caused by aspiration and not by gastrointestinal absorption (Richardson and Pratt-Thomas, 1951; Gerarde, 1959; Huxtable and coworkers, 1964; Giammona, 1967; Wolfe and coworkers, 1970; Wolsdorf and Kundig, 1972). Experimental evidence suggests that the hydrocarbons are removed by the first capillary bed they encounter (Bratton and Haddow, 1975; Wolsdorf, 1976), again reinforcing the notion that pulmonary damage occurs from aspiration, not from pulmonary excretion following gastrointestinal absorption. Indeed, the liver and the lung filter out sufficient amounts of kerosene to protect the brain from damage (Bratton and Haddow, 1975).

Although drowsiness, tremor and occasionally convulsions have been presumed to result from direct injury of the central nervous system, it seems more reasonable to attribute the central nervous system involvement to hypoxia from lung damage (Bratton and Haddow, 1975). Fatalities are rarely attributed to central nervous system involvement per se. The available experimental evidence indicates that small amounts of hydrocarbons, when aspirated, may produce more serious disease than larger amounts retained in the stomach.

Clinical Findings

Intercostal retractions, grunting, cough and fever may appear within 30 minutes of aspiration or may be delayed for a few hours. Initially, auscultation of the chest may reveal only coarse or decreased sounds. When severe injury occurs, hemoptysis and pulmonary edema develop rapidly, cyanosis becomes more severe and death may occur within 24 hours of aspiration. Roentgenographic signs of chemical pneumonitis are present usually within 24 hours or sooner. The findings vary from punctate, mottled densities to pneumonitis or atelectasis or both, and tend to be more prominent in dependent portions of lung. Air trapping with overdistention of the lungs, pneumatoceles and pleural effusions may also develop. The radiographic abnormalities reach their maximum by 72 hours, and then usually clear within a few additional days. Occasionally, the roentgenographic findings are said to persist for several weeks. There is a very poor correlation between clinical symptoms, physical findings and radiographic abnormalities. In general, the radiographic changes are more prominent than the findings on physical examination, and tend to persist for a longer period of time.

Blood gas studies reveal hypoxemia without hypercapnia, suggesting that ventilation-perfusion abnormalities, rather than alveolar hypoventilation, are the primary physiologic defect. Destruction of the epithelium of the airways together with bronchospasm caused by surface irritation accounts for the ventilation-perfusion abnormalities.

Long-term follow-up studies of the pulmonary function in patients who have had hydrocarbon pneumonitis to determine whether irreversible changes occur are not available, but would seem to be highly desirable.

Management

Since large volumes of hydrocarbon appear to do less damage when ingested into the gastrointestinal tract than when aspirated into the lungs, it seems reasonable to avoid emetics or gastric lavage. Studies in animals and humans have failed to demonstrate either a therapeutic or prophylactic role for adrenocorticosteroids in this condition (Hardman and coworkers, 1960; Albert and Inkley, 1968; Steele and coworkers, 1972; Marks and coworkers, 1972; Wolsdorf and Kundig, 1973).

Although superimposition of bacterial infection is always of concern, there is no good evidence to suggest that this occurs often. Since leukocytosis and pyrexia are common findings following hydrocarbon aspiration, it is extremely difficult, perhaps impossible, to tell whether bacterial superinfection has occurred. One thoughtful review (Eade and coworkers, 1974) concludes that bacterial complications do not occur in the majority of patients. Until there is further evidence on this subject, we believe that antimicrobial therapy should be reserved for the patient who is severely compromised by undernutrition, debilitation or underlying disease, or in whom the pneumonia is especially severe. Nor do we believe that focusing on the possibility of infection should obscure or delay initiation of other forms of therapy when pulmonary disease is severe. Since airway closure and collapse may be a significant part of the disease, the use of some form of continuous distending airway pressure of the lung would seem to be desirable, especially since this may make it possible to reduce the concentration of inspired oxygen necessary to maintain a reasonable Pa_{O_2}. The use of bronchodilators would also seem to be reasonable in order to relieve bronchospasm.

Prevention of the accidental ingestion of products containing hydrocarbons should be a high priority. Education of parents to keep potentially toxic materials out of the reach of young children would seem to be self-evident.

RESPIRATORY COMPLICATIONS OF SMOKE INHALATION

A great deal of the morbidity and mortality of victims of fires is now recognized to result from pulmonary injuries due to smoke inhalation. The severity of the lung injury depends on (1) the nature of the material involved in the conflagration and the products of incomplete combustion that are generated, and (2) whether the victim has been confined in a closed space. Although we will focus in this section on the serious consequences of smoke inhalation from fires, it is worth pointing out that some of the same compounds that are generated in fires are now considered part of the industrial pollution of the environment. Thus, the lung injury that occurs in victims of smoke inhalation may represent an extreme form of a challenge to which we are all exposed in smaller doses.

Pathogenesis

In a general way, the pathogenesis of lung injury from smoke inhalation includes thermal and chemical factors. Because the upper air passage is such an effective heat exchanger, it is likely that most of the heat from inhaled smoke is dissipated by the time the inhaled material reaches the carina. On theoretical grounds, it is conceivable that continuous oxidation of incompletely combusted material as it descends into the lung may result in thermal injury of the small and more peripheral lung units.

Depending upon the material involved in fires, a wide variety of noxious gases may be generated. These include the oxides of sulfur and nitrogen, acetaldehydes, hydrocyanic acid and carbon monoxide. Irritant gases such as NO_2 or CO_2 may combine with water in the lung to form corrosive acids. Aldehydes that form from the combustion of furniture and cotton materials induce denaturation of protein, cellular damage and pulmonary edema. The combustion of wood is also likely to generate considerable quantities of carbon monoxide (CO). Plastics, if heated to sufficiently high temperatures, may be the source of very toxic vapors. Thus, chlorine and hydrochloric acid may be generated from polyvinylchloride, and hydrocarbons, aldehydes, ketones and acids from polyethylene. Although the particulate matter carried in the smoke (soot) probably does not of itself produce injury, toxic gases may be absorbed on the surface of the particles and carried into the lungs; the soot particles may also be responsible for inducing reflex bronchoconstriction.

CARBON MONOXIDE POISONING. Carbon monoxide poisoning is an especially serious complication of smoke inhalation and is likely to occur soon after exposure. The mechanism of toxicity results from the reversible combination of CO with hemoglobin to form HbCO. Carbon monoxide not only has a high affinity for hemoglobin, but it also shifts the oxyhemoglobin dissociation curve to the left, making it necessary for the oxygen tension in the tissues to decrease to very low levels before appreciable amounts of oxygen are released in the hemoglobin. For this reason, the toxicity of CO poisoning is greater at high altitude and in the presence of anemia. It is important to emphasize that while the oxygen content of the arterial blood is low in CO poisoning, the oxygen tension (Pa_{O_2}) is not reduced. Since the carotid body is believed to respond to the Pa_{O_2}, ventilation may not be stimulated until serious acidosis has resulted. This, together with the fact that HbCO is bright red, makes the clinical diagnosis very difficult. The reduction in hemoglobin

available to oxygen in carbon monoxide poisoning is much more serious than an equivalent reduction in anemia because there is a leftward shift as well as a change in the shape of the O_2 dissociation curve, which therefore requires a considerably lower oxygen tension at the tissue level before oxygen is unloaded.

Pathology

A variety of different pathologic lesions have been described in patients following smoke inhalation. Part of the variation in pathologic lesions described may be attributed to differences in the toxic products generated in fires. However, many of the changes seen may not result simply from the direct chemical injury to the respiratory tract. Rather, they may reflect secondary circulatory, metabolic or infectious complications of surface burns, or may be induced by tracheostomy tubes, the administration of oxygen, the use of mechanical ventilators, and the administration of intravenous fluids in volumes in excess of maintenance needs.

The use of animal models to study the pathologic process has been of limited value because steam rather than the toxic products present in smoke have usually been used, and the modifying effects of the upper air passages have been eliminated by the use of tracheal cannulas. The lesions following smoke inhalation are likely to resemble those seen following the inhalation of toxic gases, such as phosgene or chlorine. The inhalation of small amounts of these gases results in alveolar and bronchiolar epithelial damage leading to an obliterative bronchiolitis. Severe exposure also produces damage to the alveolar capillaries, with hemorrhage, edema and the formation of hyaline membranes.

In a group of infants carefully studied following exposure to smoke in a newborn nursery, there was necrosis of bronchial and bronchiolar epithelium with vascular engorgement and edema, and with the formation of dense membranes or casts that partially obstructed the large and small airways. Bronchiolitis and bronchopneumonia were present in some, as well as interstitial and alveolar edema. There was carbonaceous material in the alveoli with alveolar hemorrhage.

Patients who die following severe surface burns have had necrotizing bronchitis and bronchiolitis with intra-alveolar hemorrhage and hyaline membrane formation and massive pulmonary edema. In these patients, it is difficult to know how much to attribute to direct pulmonary injury from smoke as against the complex metabolic, infectious and circulatory derangements that complicate surface burns.

Pathophysiology

Severe damage to the upper air passages leads to stridor, with increases in both inspiratory and expiratory resistance. Bronchiolitis and alveolitis are likely to lead to impaired gas exchange, exaggerating the hypoxemia. Depending on the severity and the distribution of the airway obstruction, there may be atelectasis or air trapping with hyperinflation. The latter is especially likely to occur because of premature closure of small airways.

Although reflex bronchoconstriction is likely to contribute to the increase in airway resistance, it is difficult to assess the magnitude of this because airway resistance is already high as the result of bronchial and bronchiolar edema and inflammation.

Clinical Findings

The initial assessment of a victim of a fire should focus on central nervous system damage as the result of hypoxemia. Hypoxemia, whether the result of asphyxia or CO poisoning, may produce irritability or depression. If there is any change in the state of the sensorium, oxygen should be administered while awaiting the results of blood gas studies, including the level of carbon monoxide.

The clinical manifestations of carbon monoxide poisoning vary with the level of CO hemoglobin. Mild varieties of intoxication lead to headache, diminution in visual acuity, irritability and nausea. More severe intoxication produces confusion, hallucination, ataxia and coma. Carbon monoxide may increase cerebral blood flow, increase the permeability of cerebral capillaries, and increase the pressure in the cerebrospinal fluid. There is also reason to believe that carbon monoxide may have some long term effects on the central nervous system.

Carbon monoxide levels may be reduced in half in less than an hour when breathing pure oxygen. If severe carbon monoxide poisoning is suspected, it may be necessary to administer oxygen by mask with nonbreathing valves in order to achieve concentrations close to 100 per cent. Furthermore, if clinical or arterial blood gas studies suggest alveolar hypoventilation, mechanical control of ventilation will also be necessary.

Although there may be some delay in the clinical evidence of respiratory tract injury resulting from smoke inhalation, manifestations of respiratory distress (including tachypnea, cough, hoarseness and stridor) and auscultatory evidence of respiratory tract damage (including decreased breath sounds, wheezes, rhonchi and rales) are usually present by 12 to 24 hours, and perhaps sooner. Roentgenographic evidence of pulmonary disease is usually not very helpful in the early diagnosis, since positive findings may lag several hours or more after auscultatory evidence of damage is present.

Respiratory insufficiency may occur early in the course of smoke inhalation not only as the result of asphyxia and CO poisoning, but also as the result of airway obstruction. This may result from edema anywhere along the laryngotracheobronchial tree. Since it may be difficult to localize the level of obstruction, whenever there is clinical evidence of severe obstruction, the upper airways should be assessed by direct or indirect laryngoscopy before swelling of the head, neck or oropharynx and trismus make this examination difficult.

Intubation of the trachea may be necessary when there are (1) severe burns of the nose, face or mouth, because of the likelihood that nasopharyngeal edema and obstruction will develop; (2) edema of the vocal cords with laryngeal obstruction; (3) difficulty in handling secretions; and (4) progressive respiratory insufficiency requiring mechanical assistance to ventilation. Although there is considerable disagreement as to when to perform tracheostomy, in general it makes more sense to perform tracheostomy when the obstruction is proximal to the larynx, and to reserve nasotracheal intubation for when lower portions of the respiratory tract are involved.

Treatment

As already indicated, the initial treatment should focus on reversing CO poisoning, if present, by administration of humidified oxygen. Subsequently, the administration of oxygen may be important because of the hypoxemia resulting from bronchiolitis and alveolitis with premature closure of small airways. Constant distending airway pressure, whether administered positively at the mouth or negatively around the body, may also be necessary to maintain reasonable levels of Pa_{O_2} without using excessively high concentrations of inspired oxygen.

In addition to the increase in airway resistance resulting from edema in and around the walls of the airways, it is likely that some reflex bronchoconstriction occurs from irritation of airway receptors. For this reason, it seems reasonable to administer bronchodilators such as isoproterenol or theophylline, or some of the newer, relatively selective bronchodilators, such as terbutaline.

As in many other conditions, the role of chest physiotherapy is yet to be clearly defined. Nevertheless, the encouragement of deep breathing and cough or gentle endotracheal suction in the presence of endotracheal intubation coupled with postural drainage would seem to be reasonable.

Although the use of corticosteroids is frequently advocated in the hope of suppressing inflammation and edema, most control studies evaluating their use in other conditions, such as pneumonitis resulting from aspiration of gastric contents or hydrocarbons, have failed to demonstrate a significant effect. Thus, it is difficult to marshal strong support for the use of corticosteroids based on the experience with other forms of chemical injury to the lung. Furthermore, the long-term use of steroid therapy in victims of fire is likely to be deleterious because it increases the susceptibility to infection. Until further evidence is available, it may not be unreasonable to give one large dose of corticosteroids early in the course of smoke inhalation and then to focus on other therapeutic modalities, including the use of bronchodilators, constant distending airway pressures and mechanical support of ventilation.

The available evidence indicates that the use of antimicrobial agents does not prevent the subsequent development of infection and may only predispose to the emergence of resistant organisms. Since fever, white blood cell count and erythrocyte sedimentation rate may all be elevated as a result of smoke inhalation, and since the chest roentgenogram may show nonspecific opacities that represent either atelectasis or edema, it may be extremely difficult to establish the presence of an infection in the absence of positive blood cultures. Under these circumstances, it would seem preferable at the present time to reserve the use of antimicrobial therapy for those patients in whom there is clinical deterioration in spite of supportive therapy. Since the prevention of infection is clearly an important part of the therapy in victims of fires, aseptic care of the trachea and humidifying equipment is essential.

The Relation of Pulmonary Injury from Smoke Inhalation to the Pulmonary Complications of Surface Burns

It is our present view that pulmonary damage from smoke inhalation declares itself during the first 24 hours. Individuals with widespread surface burns may develop pulmonary complications after several days, but it is our current notion that these complications are not the result of direct chemical or thermal injuries to the respiratory tract from smoke inhalation. We think it more than likely that the pulmonary injury is attributable to complex metabolic, infectious or circulatory derangements complicating the surface burns. Because of the present tendency to administer fluids aggressively to patients who are victims of fires, especially when there are surface burns with loss of serum proteins, it seems likely that some of the increase in pulmonary opacities seen in chest roentgenograms after two or three days may represent pulmonary edema that is in part, at least, the result of aggressive fluid therapy.

REFERENCES

Lung Injury from Hydrocarbon Aspiration

Albert, W. C., and Inkley, S. R.: The efficacy of steroid therapy in the treatment of experimental kerosene pneumonitis. *Am. Rev. Resp. Dis.*, 98:888, 1968.

Bratton, L., and Haddow, J. E.: Ingestion of charcoal lighter fluid. *J. Pediatr.*, 87:633, 1975.

Eade, N. R., Taussig, L. M., and Marks, M. I.: Hydrocarbon pneumonitis. *Pediatrics*, 54:351, 1974.

Gerarde, H. W.: Toxicological studies on hydrocarbons. V. Kerosene. *Toxicol. Appl. Pharmacol.*, 1:462, 1959.

Giammona, S. T.: Effects of furniture polish on pulmonary surfactant. *Am. J. Dis. Child.*, 113:658, 1967.

Gross, P., McNerney, J. M., and Babyak, M. A.: Kerosene pneumonitis: an experimental study with small doses. *Am. Rev. Resp. Dis.*, 88:656, 1963.

Hardman, G., Tolson, R., and Baghdassarian, O.: Prednisone in the management of kerosene pneumonia. *Indian Practitioner*, 13:615, 1960.

Huxtable, K. A., Bolande, R. P., and Klaus, M.: Experimental furniture polish pneumonia in rats. *Pediatrics*, 34:228, 1964.

James, J. W., Kaplan, S., and Benzing, G.: Cardiac complications following hydrocarbon ingestion. *Am. J. Dis. Child.*, 121:431, 1971.

Marks, M., Chicoine, L., Legere, G., and Hillman, E.: Adrenocorticosteroid treatment of hydrocarbon pneumonia in children—a cooperative study. *J. Pediatr.*, 81:366, 1972.

Mellins, R. B., Christian, J. R., and Bundesen, H. N.: The natural history of poisoning in childhood. *Pediatrics*, 17:314, 1956.

Richardson, J. A., and Pratt-Thomas, H. R.: Toxic effects of varying doses of kerosene administered by different routes. *Am. J. Med. Sci.*, 221:531, 1951.

Steele, R. W., Conklin, R. H., and Mark, H. M.: Corticosteroids and antibiotics for the treatment of fulminant hydrocarbon aspiration. *J.A.M.A.*, 219:1434, 1972.

Wolfe, B. M., Brodeur, A. E., and Shields, J. B.: The role of gastrointestinal absorption of kerosene in producing pneumonitis in dogs. *J. Pediatr.*, 76:867, 1970.

Wolsdorf, J.: Kerosene intoxication: an experimental approach to the etiology of the CNS manifestation in primates. *J. Pediatr.*, 88:1037, 1976.

Wolsdorf, J., and Kundig, H.: Kerosene poisoning in primates. *S. Afr. Med. J.*, 46:617, 1972.

Wolsdorf, J., and Kundig, H.: Dexamethasone in the management of kerosene pneumonia. *Pediatr. Res.*, 7:432, 1973.

Respiratory Complications of Smoke Inhalation

Cox, M. E., Heslop, B. F., Kempton, J. J., and Ratcliff, R. A.: The Dellwood fire. *Br. Med. J.*, 1:942, 1955.

Grunnet, M. L.: Long-term nervous system effects resulting from carbon monoxide exposure. In *Physiological and Toxicological Aspects of Combustion Products.* International Symposium, Washington, D.C., National Academy of Sciences, 1976, p. 119.

Lloyd, E. L., and MacRae, W. R.: Respiratory tract damage in burns. *Br. J. Anaesth.*, 43:365, 1971.

Mellins, R. B., and Park, S.: Respiratory complications of smoke inhalation in victims of fires. *J. Pediatr.*, 87:1, 1975.

Root, W. S.: Carbon monoxide. In Fenn, W. O., and Rahn, H. (Eds.): *Handbook of Physiology, Section 3.* Respiration. Volume II. Washington, D.C., American Physiological Society, 1965, p. 1087.

CHAPTER TWENTY-NINE

DROWNING AND NEAR-DROWNING

Jerome H. Modell, M.D.

Drowning is one of the three leading causes of accidental death in the United States. During the past 25 years, over 135,000 persons have died of drowning (Zugzda, 1969, 1973). Over the last two decades, the death rate, approximately three in 100,000 persons, has remained fairly constant (Zugzda, 1969, 1973), even though the explosive growth of the aquatic industry and the increased popularity of water sports would seem to indicate an increasing rate of drowning. This suggests that resuscitation and treatment of the victim of submersion is improving. Unfortunately, there are no national statistics to reflect the large group of persons who "near-drown" and then either recover uneventfully or suffer permanent neurologic damage. A recent report demonstrated an 89 per cent survival rate among patients admitted to three hospitals from 1963 to 1974 with a diagnosis of near-drowning (Modell and coworkers, 1976). If these figures are extrapolated to the national population using the previously mentioned mortality rate, as many as 1,226,000 patients may have been treated for near-drowning during the past 25 years. In addition, many persons are resuscitated at the scene of the accident and are never admitted to a hospital. Therefore, this figure of over one million victims is probably an underestimation.

The highest incidence of death from drowning occurs in the second decade of life (Press and coworkers, 1968). Most of these individuals are healthy and have a normal life expectancy be-fore their acute catastrophe. Unlike the patient who is treated for a progressive, incapacitating illness, successful therapy for the near-drowning victim usually is followed by several decades of health and productivity.

Approximately 65 per cent of those who die from drowning are unable to swim (Webster, 1967). Over half of those who drown in swimming pools in the United States are children under the age of ten (Webster, 1967). These statistics emphasize the importance of early swimming instruction. Approximately one-third of the drowning victims are known to be adequate swimmers who overexerted themselves by attempting to swim distances beyond their capability, either by swimming long distances under water after hyperventilating, or by disregarding boating and fishing safety rules, e.g., failing to use life preservers (Press and coworkers, 1968). Thus, it is important not only to offer proper swimming instruction early in life, but also to emphasize continually the potential hazards of inadequate safety measures for water sports. Unfortunately, in spite of intensified educational and instructional efforts, loss of life from aquatic accidents continues. It is necessary, therefore, to understand in depth the pathophysiologic changes that occur during near-drowning to ensure an orderly approach to resuscitation.

Ten per cent of drowning victims do not actually aspirate water (Cot, 1931), but die from acute asphyxia while submerged, perhaps because of reflex

498

laryngospasm or breath-holding. Furthermore, no two near-drowning victims aspirate exactly the same quantity of water. In addition, humans can aspirate fresh water, seawater, or brackish water. One also must realize that no two near-drowning victims are exactly alike physiologically. The state of health of each individual immediately before the accident may have differed considerably. Varying quantities of water may have been aspirated. Some patients may have submerged after maximum inhalation, and others after maximum exhalation. Thus, the length of time before irreversible hypoxia occurs may vary. The circumstances of the accident also influence pathophysiologic effects. One patient may succumb in the water from physical exhaustion. Another may fall into the water, hit his head, and suffer a concussion. The victim may have become severely ill or may have died of some disease, and then subsequently have fallen into the water. For example, an elderly patient may suffer a myocardial infarction during swimming, lose consciousness, and then aspirate fluid as a terminal event. All these factors must be considered when describing an individual patient (Davis, 1971). Therefore, review of the pathophysiologic studies reported after drowning and near-drowning should serve as valuable background for understanding the problems that arise in treating the individual patient.

PATHOPHYSIOLOGY

Changes in Blood Gas, Acid-Base, and Pulmonary Status

The single most important consequence of near-drowning is hypoxemia (Modell and coworkers, 1966). The degree and duration of hypoxemia depend on the length of submersion and on whether or not the patient aspirates fluid. Initially, hypoxemia is accompanied by hypercarbia and acidosis (Modell

and coworkers, 1966). A mammal responds to total immersion in liquid by holding his breath or closing his vocal cords, or both (Coryllos, 1938; Lougheed and coworkers, 1939). Approximately 10 per cent of human drowning victims die without actually aspirating fluid (Cot, 1931). Experiments using anesthetized intubated dogs demonstrate that when laryngospasm is simulated by occluding the endotracheal tube, the carbon dioxide tension increases only 3 to 6 torr per minute, and the pH decreases approximately 0.05 unit per minute. However, arterial oxygen tension (Pa_{O_2}) drops precipitously from the normal control values that existed immediately before tracheal obstruction to approximately 40 torr after one minute of obstruction, to 10 torr after three minutes, and to 4 torr after five minutes (Modell and coworkers, 1972). In other studies, Kristoffersen and coworkers (1967) reported that a decrease in Pa_{O_2} to 10 to 15 torr was uniformly fatal in dogs. However, Modell and colleagues (1972) have shown that 80 per cent of dogs anesthetized with barbiturates could be resuscitated by ventilating their lungs with air five minutes after the onset of tracheal obstruction, even though their mean Pa_{O_2} was 4 torr. Whether the barbiturate anesthetic protected these animals is speculative. However, it is known that barbiturates can protect the hypoxic brain (Michenfelder and Theye, 1973).

In two studies in 1961, Craig demonstrated the importance of hypoxia. In studying the breaking point of breath-holding in human volunteers during simulated underwater swimming, he found that point to be 87 seconds at rest, at which time the carbon dioxide tension of alveolar air ($P_{A_{CO_2}}$) was 51 torr and the oxygen tension ($P_{A_{O_2}}$) was 73 torr. After hyperventilation, breath-holding could be maintained for 146 seconds. In this instance, the $P_{A_{CO_2}}$ rose to only 46 torr, but the $P_{A_{O_2}}$ dropped to 58 torr. When exercise followed hyperventilation, the breath-holding point dropped to 85 seconds and the $P_{A_{CO_2}}$ remained fairly constant at 49 torr. However, the $P_{A_{O_2}}$ dropped further to 43 torr. Craig postulated that if the swimmer hyperventilated before swimming underwater, the Pa_{CO_2} would remain low. The swimmer, therefore, could consciously repress the urge to breathe. He then would develop cerebral hypoxia, lose consciousness, and begin to breathe while submerged (Craig, 1961a).

In treating 91 human victims of near-drowning, this author and his colleagues have seen 10 patients (12 per cent) who probably suffered near-drowning without aspiration (Modell and coworkers, 1976). This diagnosis was made based on the patients' histories and on the fact that their Pa_{O_2} levels were over 80 torr while the patients spontaneously breathed room air immediately upon admission to the hospital. In these cases, mouth-to-mouth resuscitation was given promptly at the scene of the accident, and spontaneous ventilation returned rapidly. If victims of near-drowning without aspiration are ventilated artificially before circulation ceases or before irreversible damage to the central nervous system occurs, recovery will be dramatic and complete. If spontaneous ventilation begins while the patient is still under water, however, aspiration will occur and treatment will be more complicated.

If aspiration occurs in the near-drowning victim, even though the initial hypercarbia may be reversed rapidly by increasing the patient's minute alveolar ventilation, and even though respiratory acidosis may disappear, the patient frequently is left with persistent arterial hypoxemia and metabolic acidosis (Modell and coworkers, 1968a). A Pa_{O_2} as low as 21 torr and a pH as low as 6.77 have been reported (Modell and coworkers, 1976). The metabolic acidosis frequently requires administration of sodium bicarbonate. In 76 patients who had bicarbonate levels calculated after a near-drowning episode, 55 had levels of 20 mEq. per liter or less. In 10 of the patients, the levels

were as low as 6 to 10 mEq. per liter (Modell and coworkers, 1976). The arterial hypoxemia that occurs can be profound and will persist as long as significant intrapulmonary pathologic conditions continue.

Although hypoxia occurs after aspiration of either fresh water or seawater, the factors contributing to the hypoxia may be different with the two fluid media. In either case, pulmonary compliance decreases (Colebatch and Halmagyi, 1961, 1962, 1963; Halmagyi and Colebatch, 1961). However, after aspiration of seawater, the primary problem is fluid-filled but perfused alveoli (Modell and coworkers, 1967). They respond as they would in atelectasis and produce a large intrapulmonary shunt. Since seawater is hypertonic, fluid is drawn from the plasma into the alveolus. For example, in animals that aspirate 22 ml. per kilogram of seawater, an average of 33 ml. per kilogram can be drained from the lungs after five minutes (Modell and coworkers, 1973). On the other hand, when experimental animals aspirate fresh water, significant amounts of fluid cannot be drained from their lungs; the fluid is absorbed into the circulation (Modell and Moya, 1966). When fresh water is aspirated, the surface tension properties of pulmonary surfactant are altered (Giammona and Modell, 1967). As a result, the alveolus becomes unstable and atelectasis occurs, producing an intrapulmonary shunt and hypoxemia (Modell and coworkers, 1968b). Other factors that might contribute to pulmonary edema and alteration of ventilation-to-perfusion ratio in these patients are pulmonary hypertension and cerebral hypoxia (Moss and coworkers, 1972).

A variety of microscopic findings have been reported after fluid aspiration. Using electron microscopy, no changes were seen in rats that had aspirated small quantities of fresh water (Halmagyi, 1961). On the other hand, when lungs of rats were perfused through the trachea with large quantities of fresh water, the alveolar septae widened, the capillaries collapsed, the number of red blood cells decreased, the endothelial and septal cell nuclei became engorged, the mitochondria became swollen, and the cell outlines were obliterated (Reidbord and Spitz, 1966). After aspiration of small quantities of seawater, the lung weight increased and intra-alveolar hemorrhages were seen (Halmagyi, 1961). After aspiration of large volumes of seawater, however, the changes were less marked than those observed after the aspiration of large quantities of fresh water (Reidbord and Spitz, 1966). Thus, the microscopic changes that occur differ when very small or very large quantities of water are aspirated. This may account for some of the differences reported during autopsies of human drowning victims.

Another frequent finding at autopsy soon after death by drowning is hyperexpansion of the lungs with areas that resemble those occurring in acute emphysema (Davis, 1971). This could result from rupture of the alveoli when the airway pressure that is generated widely fluctuates during violent ventilatory efforts against a closed glottis, or from obstruction by a column of water in the airway during submersion. If the patient survives for at least 12 hours after near-drowning only to die later, the lungs frequently show evidence of bronchopneumonia, multiple abscesses, mechanical injury, and deposition of hyaline material in the alveoli (Fuller, 1963a, 1963b; Modell and coworkers, 1968a).

Recent studies report the effect that various ventilatory patterns have on improving Pa_{O_2} after near-drowning with seawater (Modell and coworkers, 1974). The evidence indicates that placing positive end-expiratory pressure (PEEP) on the airway will increase markedly the Pa_{O_2} in animals that either breathe spontaneously or are ventilated mechanically. These studies suggest that the use of PEEP increases functional residual capacity, thereby minimizing intrapulmonary shunting and ventilation-to-perfusion abnormalities and promoting better oxygenation.

Similar studies conducted on fresh water aspiration demonstrated an improvement in Pa_{O_2} when mechanical ventilation was combined with PEEP. However, no improvement in Pa_{O_2} was seen when 10 cm. H_2O PEEP was applied in spontaneously breathing animals (Ruiz and coworkers, 1973). The difference in results of these two studies may be that in order to overcome the surfactant changes that occur after aspiration of fresh water, the alveoli must be inflated mechanically before PEEP can effectively maintain the alveolus in an inflated state. On the other hand, since pulmonary surfactant is normal after seawater aspiration, the spontaneous respiratory movement of the animal might be sufficient to inflate the alveoli, and the PEEP might help to maintain them in a state of partial inflation.

It should be emphasized that in the above two studies, PEEP was set at 10 cm. H_2O in all animals. Clinically, it is our practice to titrate PEEP in order to produce the minimum degree of pulmonary venous admixture or intrapulmonary shunt without affecting cardiac output (Kirby and coworkers, 1975). Had such an approach been taken in these animal studies, it is entirely possible that animals subjected to aspiration of fresh water also would have benefited from PEEP, even without receiving controlled mechanical ventilation. It has been demonstrated in human victims of near-drowning that titration of PEEP does improve ventilation-to-perfusion ratios and arterial oxygenation, not only when the patient's ventilation is controlled, but also when he breathes spontaneously and receives intermittent mandatory breaths from a ventilator, as needed, to clear carbon dioxide (Modell and Downs, 1976).

Blood Volume and Serum Electrolytes

In addition to the acute pulmonary effects and changes in blood gas tensions and acid-base balance that occur, aspiration of hypo- or hypertonic fluid can result in a number of changes in other systems. The extent and direction of these changes will depend upon the quantity and nature of the fluid aspirated.

In general, the greater the volume of water that is aspirated, the greater are the changes. If 11 ml. per kilogram or less of fluid is aspirated, it is unlikely that persistent changes other than those caused by fluid in the lungs will occur in any system (Modell, 1968). However, if quantities of water greater than 11 ml. per kilogram are aspirated, the blood volume increases after aspiration of hypotonic fluid in direct proportion to the quantity of fluid aspirated (Modell, 1968). Conversely, blood volume decreases linearly as the quantity of seawater aspirated increases (Modell and coworkers, 1967). In instances of total immersion, blood volume may increase as much as 160 per cent after fresh water aspiration (Modell and Moya, 1966) and may decrease to approximately 65 per cent of the normal value after seawater aspiration (Modell and coworkers, 1967).

It is important to stress that most patients do not aspirate enough fluid to produce changes in blood volume great enough to threaten life. Thus, while it is important to note the effective circulating blood volume by recording the patient's central venous pressure and pulmonary capillary wedge pressure as appropriate, blood volume changes requiring urgent treatment usually are not seen. When a significant decrease in effective circulating blood volume is evident, it usually results from the loss of fluid from the vascular space into the lung. In victims of severe near-drowning, significant amounts of fluid can be lost into the lung as pulmonary edema and will require replacement.

Changes that occur in serum electrolyte concentrations after drowning and near-drowning also depend upon both the type and volume of water aspirated and are inversely proportionate to changes in blood volume. Experiments have shown that if dogs aspirate 22 ml. per kilogram or less of fresh water, significant persistent changes in extracellular serum electrolytes do not occur (Modell and Moya, 1966). Another study demonstrated that less than 15 per cent of human drowning victims who died in the water had serum electrolyte concentrations indicating aspiration of more than 22 ml. per kilogram of water (Modell and Davis, 1969). This might explain why significant changes in serum electrolyte concentrations have not been reported in human victims of near-drowning.

This author and his colleagues studied electrolyte concentrations in 83 patients who near-drowned in either fresh water, seawater or brackish water (Modell and coworkers, 1976). In the fresh water victims, mean concentrations were as follows: serum sodium, 138 mEq. per liter; serum chloride, 97 mEq. per liter; and serum potassium, 3.9 mEq. per liter. Victims of seawater near-drowning had these mean concentrations: serum sodium, 146 mEq. per liter; serum chloride, 103 mEq. per liter; and serum potassium, 3.9 mEq. per liter. The ranges of values in the total group, regardless of type of water aspirated, were as follows: serum sodium, 126 to 160 mEq. per liter; serum chloride, 86 to 126 mEq. per liter; and serum potassium, 2.4 to 6.3 mEq. per liter. Although the seawater near-drowning victims showed a slight increase in the concentration of extracellular serum electrolytes, this could not be considered life-threatening. This suggests that the importance of immediate therapy for electrolyte changes after near-drowning has been overestimated, and that each patient's electrolyte status should be evaluated before corrective therapy is initiated.

Hemoglobin and Hematocrit Values

In instances of seawater aspiration, one might predict an increase in the hemoglobin and hematocrit values of whole blood because of hemoconcentration, and after fresh water aspiration, a decrease resulting from hemodilution. However, when the hemoglobin and hematocrit values of 83 near-drowning victims were analyzed, the mean value for hemoglobin in the fresh water drowning victims was 13.2 gm. per 100 ml. The value was 13.4 gm. per 100 ml. for those near-drowned in seawater (Modell and coworkers, 1976). Likewise, there was no difference in mean hematocrit concentration between the two groups of patients. Marked changes in hemoglobin and hematocrit values rarely are reported, further substantiating the hypothesis that human victims of near-drowning do not aspirate huge quantities of fluid.

When large volumes of fresh water are absorbed, hemolysis of red cells can occur, causing plasma hemoglobin to increase. This hemolysis is not due solely to hypotonicity but is strongly related to the Pa_{O_2}. In animals that had 44 ml. per kilogram of distilled water injected rapidly into their superior vena cava and were permitted to breathe spontaneously so that Pa_{O_2} remained within reasonable limits, the plasma hemoglobin levels were not significantly elevated. On the other hand, when tracheal obstruction was combined with the infusion of the same quantity of water, plasma hemoglobin concentrations in excess of 1000 mg. per 100 ml. were seen (Modell and coworkers, 1972). This further emphasizes the importance of establishing adequate arterial oxygenation in the near-drowning victim.

Cardiovascular System

Most human near-drowning victims show remarkable stability of the cardiovascular system. Experimental evidence suggests that changes in cardiovascular function during near-drowning are caused predominantly by changes in Pa_{O_2} and acid-base balance (Noble and Sharpe, 1963; Modell and Moya, 1966; Modell and coworkers, 1967, 1968a, 1968b, 1976). Obviously, variations in blood volume and serum electrolyte concentrations also can contribute to cardiovascular changes. However, less than 15 per cent of drowning victims aspirate sufficient water to cause such changes (Modell and Davis, 1969).

A wide variety of electrocardiographic changes have been reported in experimental studies of drowning in both fresh water and seawater. The early literature emphasizes that ventricular fibrillation occurs secondary to fresh water drowning (Swann and coworkers, 1947; Swann and Brucer, 1949). It has been shown, however, that death from ventricular fibrillation does not occur in dogs that aspirate 22 ml. per kilogram or less of fresh water (Modell and Moya, 1966). On the other hand, when at least 44 ml. per kilogram was aspirated, ventricular fibrillation occurred in as many as 80 per cent of the animals studied (Modell and Moya, 1966). Only two cases of ventricular fibrillation after near-drowning have been documented in humans (Middleton, 1962; Redding, 1965).

Arterial blood pressure after near-drowning has been reported to be normal, elevated or low (Rath, 1953; Dumitru and Hamilton, 1963; Fainer, 1963; Modell, 1963; Munroe, 1964). These changes seem to be secondary to the state of oxygenation, acid-base balance, cardiac function, and the level of circulating catecholamines. Measurements of central venous pressure and pulmonary capillary wedge pressure usually reflect the effective circulating blood volume. Low values in near-drowning victims usually indicate the acute decrease in blood volume that occurs when plasma is lost in the lungs.

Neurologic and Renal Functions

Frequently the question is asked, How long can a patient remain submerged and still be resuscitated? There are reports of patients being resuscitated after submersion in fresh water for 10 (Ohlsson and Beckman, 1964), 20 (Ohlsson and Beckman, 1964), 22 (Kvittingen and Naess, 1963), and 40 (Siebke and coworkers, 1975) minutes, and in seawater for 17 minutes (King and Webster, 1964). All of these patients were hypothermic, and three of them developed prolonged neurologic deficits. However, approximately one year later, they all functioned normally.

The fear of resuscitating a near-drowning victim who may have a prolonged neurologic deficit is always present. However, the cases just cited indicate the tremendous variation that exists in the individual's ability to tolerate submersion and subsequent hypoxemia, and should encourage physicians and rescuers to maintain resuscitative efforts as long as possible. In a series of 81 survivors from a total of 91 near-drowning victims, the author and his colleagues have seen only two patients who had residual neurologic damage. In both instances, the patient was still in a state of cardiac arrest when brought to the emergency room. Although cases of resuscitation with permanent neurologic damage are reported in the literature, during the past decade the measuring of arterial blood gas tensions and pH has become commonplace in most hospitals, and the incidence of persons having residual brain damage after near-drowning seems to be decreasing.

Adequate renal function remains intact in most patients who are resuscitated after near-drowning, although albuminuria, hemoglobinuria, oliguria or anuria can occur (Rath, 1953; Fuller, 1963b; Kvittingen and Naess, 1963; King and Webster, 1964; Munroe, 1964; Redding and Pearson, 1964; Gambino, 1969). Renal damage also may progress to acute tubular necrosis (Fuller, 1963b). It is not known whether this is secondary to severe lactic acidosis or hypoxemia, or both, or to the biochemical effects of the aspirated water. In any event, such severe changes are rare.

THERAPY

The prime objective of emergency therapy for the near-drowning victim is to restore arterial blood gas and acid-base levels to normal as rapidly as possible. Thus, immediate rescue and initial management of the near-drowning victim are crucial in determining the outcome. Although, theoretically, the use of appliances would facilitate water rescue, such items are rarely available at the scene of the accident. Since the degree of hypoxia increases rapidly with each second of apnea, it is imperative that emergency measures be taken immediately to initiate ventilation. Some rescuers can deliver mouth-to-mouth or mouth-to-nose respiration while the victim is still in the water. Others find this impossible because it limits their swimming ability. Artificial respiration should be given to the apneic near-drowning victim as soon as possible. Many external chest methods have been reported over the years as means of administering artificial ventilation. Yet, there is little question that the most effective methods available today are still mouth-to-mouth and mouth-to-nose ventilation (Safar and coworkers, 1958). To ensure adequate ventilation in these methods, the rescuer must obtain an adequate airway by inspecting the patient's mouth for foreign objects, and by supporting the airway by elevating the jaw and soft tissues. Placing an appliance, such as a nasopharyngeal, oropharyngeal or endotracheal airway, is necessary occasionally. However, in most patients an adequate airway can be achieved without using such devices. Furthermore, inserting an appliance in a partially reactive patient may precipitate laryngospasm, vomiting or aspiration of stomach contents.

If the victim has not aspirated water and if effective ventilation is established before permanent circulatory or neurologic changes occur, the prognosis is excellent. If water has been aspirated, as discussed earlier in this chapter, persistent alterations of pulmonary function probably will occur. In general, time should not be wasted trying to drain water from the lungs of a victim of near-drowning in fresh water (Ruben and Ruben, 1962). On the other hand, because seawater is hypertonic, fluid is drawn from the circulation into the lungs (Modell and coworkers, 1967, 1974). It has been shown that the survival rate of animals that have aspirated large quantities of seawater can be increased if their lungs are drained by gravity (Modell and colleagues, 1974). Since human drowning victims rarely aspirate large quantities of water, it is more important to initiate artificial ventilation than to drain the fluid. However, if the victim of a seawater accident can be placed in a head-down position to promote drainage by gravity without compromising artificial ventilation, this is, of course, preferable.

Victims of drowning and near-drowning frequently swallow large quantities of water before losing consciousness. Thus, it is even more important to ensure a free airway, so that the stomach is not overdistended during resuscitation. If gastric distention occurs, the patient may regurgitate and may aspirate acid gastric contents, thereby causing aspiration pneumonitis (Wynne, in press). And although time should not be wasted draining the stomach during the initial phase of resuscitation, extreme care should be taken to avoid causing aspiration of gastric contents.

If near-drowning victims remain hypoxic after initial resuscitative attempts, supplemental oxygen must be given as soon as possible. When the proper equipment for mechanical ventilation is available, it should replace mouth-to-mouth resuscitation. A method of intermittent positive pressure ventilation should be used that also can supply a high inspired oxygen concentration. Hand-operated units frequently are preferable to pressure-cycled units in the emergency situation, since most automatic devices are pressure-limited, and in a patient who has a very low pulmonary compliance, the apparatus can be shut off before adequate volumes of inspiratory gases are delivered. This is particularly true if the patient requires

simultaneous closed-chest cardiac massage. The pressure generated on chest compression frequently will cycle the ventilator before an adequate tidal volume is delivered. In selecting a device to replace mouth-to-mouth ventilation, consider whether the appliance or mechanical ventilator is capable of producing PEEP. Most emergency resuscitators cannot be adapted to produce PEEP. However, as was stated earlier, the use of PEEP significantly increases Pa_{O_2} in victims of near-drowning.

If the patient does not have an effective heart beat, closed chest cardiac massage should be instituted immediately. In this situation, the presence or absence of ventricular fibrillation should be confirmed to determine whether electrical defibrillation is indicated.

Even when the patient breathes spontaneously after rescue or begins to breathe after initial resuscitative efforts, the rescuer should not be lulled into a false sense of security. A patient who is able to converse with the rescuer still may have an extremely low Pa_{O_2}. Supplemental oxygen therapy should be continued until actual measurement of Pa_{O_2} confirms it to be unnecessary. Since the pulmonary lesion may not be readily reversible if the patient has aspirated water, and since the rescuer cannot always determine at the scene of the accident whether or not water has been aspirated, it is imperative that all near-drowning victims be taken to a hospital for further evaluation and therapy. During transport to the hospital, supplemental oxygen should be given, regardless of the patient's apparent clinical condition. Ventilatory and circulatory assistance should be provided as indicated.

Initial hospital therapy should emphasize pulmonary care, which may range from simply increasing the fractional concentration of inspired oxygen ($F_{I_{O_2}}$) in a spontaneously breathing patient to providing continuous ventilatory support by establishing a patent airway with an endotracheal tube that is connected to a mechanical ventilator. Although strict guidelines that establish when endotracheal intubation is necessary are not available, it has been shown that in a series of 20 near-drowning victims, all of whom had normal chest roentgenograms on admission to the hospital, only one required endotracheal intubation, even though some patients had oxygen tensions as low as 50 torr (Modell and coworkers, 1976). In retrospect, perhaps this one patient could have been treated more conservatively as well. Even when the chest roentgenogram is normal, patients must be followed with serial analyses of arterial blood gases, since the findings on chest roentgenogram frequently lag behind the actual intrapulmonary status (Modell and coworkers, 1976).

Based on this author's experience, approximately 70 per cent of near-drowning victims have a significant degree of metabolic acidosis accompanying their hypoxia (Modell and coworkers, 1976). Therefore, we recommend that if the patient is unresponsive and if arterial blood gas results are not immediately available, sodium bicarbonate (1.0 mEq. per kilogram of body weight) should be given empirically to the near-drowning victim. Of course, samples of arterial blood must be taken as soon as possible to evaluate oxygen and carbon dioxide tensions, pH and bicarbonate level. These values will determine the extent of ventilatory support, the appropriate $F_{I_{O_2}}$, the amount of additional bicarbonate to be administered, and the pattern of mechanical ventilatory support necessary to produce normal carbon dioxide elimination, adequate oxygenation and acid-base balance.

Recently, it has been shown that adding PEEP, both with and without concomitant mechanical ventilation, can increase Pa_{O_2} significantly in both animals and humans after aspiration of seawater (Modell and coworkers, 1974). Similarly, PEEP combined with mechanical ventilation has been shown to increase Pa_{O_2} significantly in fresh water near-drowning victims (Ruiz and coworkers, 1973; Rutledge and Flor, 1973). The exact amount of PEEP that is supplied to any patient should be determined on an individual basis. If the patient requires PEEP to maintain an acceptable Pa_{O_2}, the level of PEEP should be increased gradually. The effect on oxygen tension and on cardiovascular function is then assessed. An optimum level will be reached when PEEP is producing the lowest intrapulmonary shunt or intrapulmonary venous admixture, and when the adverse effects on circulation are minimal. If this level of PEEP is exceeded, Pa_{O_2} may decrease rather than increase. The use of PEEP frequently permits the physician to maintain adequate arterial oxygenation with a lower $F_{I_{O_2}}$, thus minimizing the possibility of oxygen toxicity.

Many clinicians fear that an increase in PEEP always decreases cardiac output. This can occur in the presence of hypovolemia. However, if a normal effective circulating blood volume is maintained, cardiac output actually may increase as PEEP increases and as Pa_{O_2} improves (Downs and coworkers, 1973).

If bronchospasm is present because of aspiration of fluid, it can be treated by administering an aerosol of bronchodilating agent, such as racemic epinephrine. Pulmonary edema frequently is seen after near-drowning with aspiration. If frothy pulmonary edema fluid is felt to be present in the airway, administering nebulized 20 to 30 per cent ethyl alcohol has been advocated to change the surface tension of the bubbles, thereby causing them to lose their stability and to rupture. This would reduce the mechanical blockage to ventilation. Applying PEEP appears to be excellent therapy for pulmonary edema, and once PEEP is titrated to an optimum level, aerosols of ethyl alcohol are rarely necessary.

Until recently, many physicians advocated the use of steroids and prophylactic broad-spectrum antibiotics to treat near-drowning victims (Modell and coworkers, 1968a; Sladen and Zauder, 1971). Evidence now suggests that steroid therapy may not improve arterial oxygenation or survival rate in animals that have aspirated hydrochloric acid (Chapman and coworkers, 1974a, 1974b; Downs and coworkers, 1974). Similar studies in our laboratory with a model of fresh water drowning also failed to demonstrate any significant improvement in either arterial oxygenation or survival rate with the use of steroids (Calderwood and coworkers, 1975). Retrospective analysis of a large series of consecutive human near-drowning victims also failed to demonstrate any superiority of therapy using steroids and prophylactic antibiotics (Modell and coworkers, 1976). Therefore, we now give steroids only to those patients who fail to respond appropriately to other active measures taken to improve pulmonary function and arterial oxygenation. Also flora normally found in the lungs may be disrupted by the routine use of broad-spectrum antibiotics, thereby encouraging secondary infection with organisms such as Pseudomonas. Perhaps it is better to culture secretions from the trachea on a daily basis and to treat infection with specific antibiotics when it occurs, rather than to administer antibiotics prophylactically.

Many near-drowning victims vomit during the accident or emergency resuscitative efforts and may aspirate solid debris or particles of undigested food. Serial physical examinations and chest roentgenograms will prove helpful in diagnosing regional or lobar atelectasis caused by aspiration of particulate matter. If regional atelectasis occurs, bronchoscopic examination is indicated. By using the fiberoptic bronchoscope, the presence of foreign material in the airway can be confirmed without disconnecting the patient from mechanical ventilatory devices. This minimizes the period of hypoxia that otherwise might occur during bronchoscopic examination.

The patient's hematocrit should be determined early in the therapy. Unless this value is markedly abnormal or unless obvious hemolysis is present in the plasma fraction after fresh water aspiration, the problems in treating the patient will be limited almost exclusively to ventilation, oxygenation and acid-base balance, and significant fluid and electrolyte disturbances are unlikely to occur.

All near-drowning victims should be monitored closely. At the minimum, every patient should have vital signs monitored, i.e., pulse, respiration, blood pressure and temperature. It is imperative that all near-drowning victims also have serial determinations made of arterial blood gas tensions and pH. Electrocardiographic monitoring and urine output should be observed closely in patients who require any type of prolonged support. Arterial catheters facilitate blood sampling for reliable determination of blood gas tensions. In addition, if the patient shows any degree of circulatory instability, venous pressure should be monitored. However, central venous pressure is only an approximate guide in the complete assessment of cardiac function and blood volume balance, since it reflects only what may be happening proximal to the right atrium. It frequently is necessary to separate the effects of hypovolemia from those of cardiac failure when a low cardiac output and hypotension are present. These conditions suggest placing a Swan-Ganz pulmonary arterial catheter so that pulmonary artery and pulmonary capillary wedge pressures can be obtained (Swan and coworkers, 1970). The latter value is a better indicator of the function of the left side of the heart and is, therefore, a more useful guide in determining whether the patient requires additional fluid or supplemental cardiac support. The presence of a catheter in the pulmonary artery also permits analysis of mixed venous blood so that the arterial-venous oxygen content difference can be monitored. When oxygen consumption is reasonably constant, this value will give an indirect indication of whether the cardiac output is increasing, decreasing or remaining stable (Colgan and Mahoney, 1969; Gustafson and Nordström, 1970). Pulmonary venous admixture then can be measured, and if a pulmonary catheter with a thermodilution tip is used, serial determinations of direct cardiac output can be obtained.

In addition to monitoring the patient with serial determinations of Pa_{O_2}, Pa_{CO_2}, pH and bicarbonate level, laboratory evaluation should consist of hemoglobin, hematocrit and serum electrolyte determinations; urinalysis; culture of tracheal secretions; and chest roentgenograms. These evaluations should be made routinely, and other tests should be added as appropriate.

If serum electrolyte concentrations are abnormal, administering the appropriate physiologic salt solution is indicated. Since most of these patients do not have marked abnormalities of serum electrolyte levels, recommending a "routine" approach to fluid administration is not advised. In general, intravenous fluid therapy should begin with administering lactated Ringer's solution and should then change to use the specific fluid required. If clinical signs and monitoring indicate the presence of hypovolemia, giving blood or volume expanders, or both, should be considered. After near-drowning in seawater, administering blood is rarely necessary, because usually there is no loss of red blood cells. On the other hand, volume expanders may have to be given to replace the plasma lost into the lung. After aspiration of large quantities of fresh water, hemolysis of red blood cells can occur. This is most marked during severe hypoxemia. Hemoglobin and hematocrit concentrations of whole blood may not reflect the extent of hemolysis immediately upon admission to the hospital. Serial determinations sometimes will show a gradual decrease in these values (Modell and coworkers, 1968a). Since pulmonary edema almost always accompanies near-drowning, the physician may be faced with the necessity of having to replace blood volume in the face of pulmonary edema. This requires constant, simultaneous attention to both blood volume and pulmonary status. It may be necessary to infuse fluid on the one hand while applying PEEP (or occasionally use potent diuretics to mobilize and remove interstitial pulmonary water) on the other.

The two most important drugs in treating near-drowning victims are oxygen and bicarbonate solution. If proper attention is paid to balancing the effective circulating blood volume with fluid replacement based on urine output, CVP, and pulmonary capillary wedge pressure measurements, vasopressor therapy rarely will have to be considered for these patients. Occasionally, it may be advisable to employ drugs that primarily stimulate the beta receptors to increase temporarily the cardiac output until blood volume can be stabilized. For similar reasons, digitalis has been used to improve cardiac function during this very critical period. Prolonged use of any type of vasopressor is not suggested. At best, it should be considered a "crutch" rather than a specific mode of therapy. In addition, diuretics may be helpful in promoting renal output, particularly in patients having high concentrations of plasma hemoglobin. Potent diuretics also have been recommended to help mobilize intrapulmonary water in an attempt to shorten the course of pulmonary insufficiency (Sladen and coworkers, 1968).

Deliberately induced hypothermia (Ohlsson and Beckman, 1964) and exchange transfusions (Kvittingen and Naess, 1963) have been advocated on occasion in the treatment of the drowning victim. The rationale for inducing hypothermia is that it will decrease cerebral oxygen consumption. However, to be effective, hypothermia should be induced before hypoxia occurs. Obviously, this is not possible in the near-drowning patient. As a result, the rationale for using induced hypothermia is questionable.

Some physicians have recommended exchange transfusions for fresh water near-drowning victims because of a potentially high plasma hemoglobin level that might affect the kidneys adversely (Kvittingen and Naess, 1963). Since patients with plasma hemoglobin levels in excess of 500 mg. per 100 ml. have not been reported (Modell and coworkers, 1968a), exchange transfusion is probably not necessary and only further delays the institution of proper therapy.

In summary, the near-drowning victim must be treated immediately for ventilatory insufficiency, hypoxia, and the resulting acidosis. The cause and pathophysiologic changes of pulmonary insufficiency vary, depending upon the type and volume of fluid aspirated. Success or failure of the overall resuscitative effort frequently will depend upon the adequacy of prompt emergency resuscitation and on effective intensive pulmonary care. Each patient should be evaluated and treated individually, since abnormalities of multiple organ systems can occur, their degree and form varying considerably from patient to patient.

REFERENCES

Calderwood, H. W., Modell, J. H., and Ruiz, B. C.: The ineffectiveness of steroid therapy for treatment of fresh-water near-drowning. *Anesthesiology, 43*:642, 1975.

Chapman, R. L., Jr., Downs, J. B., Modell, J. H., and Hood, C. I.: The ineffectiveness of steroid therapy in treating aspiration of hydrochloric acid. *Arch. Surg., 108*:858, 1974a.

Chapman, R. L., Jr., Modell, J. H., Ruiz, B. C., Calderwood, H. W., Hood, C. I., and Graves, S. A.: Effect of continuous positive-pressure ventilation and steroids on aspiration of hydrochloric acid (pH 1.8) in dogs. *Anesth. Analg., 53*:556, 1974b.

Colebatch, H. J. H., and Halmagyi, D. F. J.: Lung mechanics and resuscitation after fluid aspiration. *J. Appl. Physiol., 16*:684, 1961.

Colebatch, H. J. H., and Halmagyi, D. F. J.: Reflex airway reaction to fluid aspiration. *J. Appl. Physiol., 17*:787, 1962.

Colebatch, H. J. H., and Halmagyi, D. F. J.: Reflex pulmonary hypertension of fresh-water aspiration. *J. Appl. Physiol., 18*:179, 1963.

Colgan, F. J., and Mahoney, P. D.: The effects of major surgery on cardiac output and shunting. *Anesthesiology, 31*:213, 1969.

Coryllos, P. N.: Mechanical resuscitation in advanced forms of asphyxia. A clinical and experimental study in the different methods of resuscitation. *Surg. Gynecol. Obstet., 66*:698, 1938.

Cot, C.: Les Asphyxies Accidentelles (submersion, electrocution, intoxication oxycarbonique). Étude clinique, thérapeutique et préventive. Paris, Éditions Médicales N. Malaine, 1931.

Craig, A. B., Jr.: Causes of loss of consciousness during underwater swimming. *J. Appl. Physiol., 16*:583, 1961a.

Craig, A. B., Jr.: Underwater swimming and loss of consciousness. *J.A.M.A., 176*:255, 1961b.

Davis, J. H.: Autopsy findings in victims of drowning. In Modell, J. H.: *The Pathophysiology and Treatment of Drowning and Near-drowning.* Springfield, Illinois, Charles C Thomas, 1971.

Downs, J. B., Chapman, R. L., Jr., Modell, J. H., and Hood, C. I.: An evaluation of steroid therapy in aspiration pneumonitis. *Anesthesiology, 40*:129, 1974.

Downs, J. B., Klein, E. F., Jr., and Modell, J. H.: The effect of incremental PEEP on PaO$_2$ in patients with respiratory failure. *Anesth. Analg., 52*:210, 1973.

Dumitru, A. P., and Hamilton, F. G.: A mechanism of drowning. *Anesth. Analg., 42*:170, 1963.

Fainer, D. C.: Near drowning in sea water and fresh water. *Ann. Intern. Med., 59*:537, 1963.

Fuller, R. H.: The clinical pathology of human near-drowning. *Proc. R. Soc. Med., 56*:33, 1963a.

Fuller, R. H.: The 1962 Wellcome prize essay. Drowning and the post-immersion syndrome. A clinicopathologic study. *Milit. Med., 128*:22, 1963b.

Gambino, S. P.: Personal communication. January 13, 1969.

Giammona, S. T., and Modell, J. H.: Drowning by total immersion. Effects on pulmonary surfactant of distilled water, isotonic saline, and sea water. *Am. J. Dis. Child., 114*:612, 1967.

Gustafson, I., and Nordström, L.: Central venous PO$_2$ and open-heart surgery. *Acta Anaesthesiol. Scand., 37*(Suppl.):112, 1970.

Halmagyi, D. F. J.: Lung changes and incidence of respiratory arrest in rats after aspiration of sea and fresh water. *J. Appl. Physiol., 16*:41, 1961.

Halmagyi, D. F. J., and Colebatch, J. H. J.: The drowned lung. A physiological approach to its mechanism and management. *Aust. Ann. Med., 10*:68, 1961.

King, R. B., and Webster, I. W.: A case of recovery from drowning and prolonged anoxia. *Med. J. Aust., 1*:919, 1964.

Kirby, R. R., Downs, J. B., Civetta, J. M., Modell, J. H., Dannemiller, F. J., Klein, E. F., and Hodges, M.: High level positive end expiratory pressure (PEEP) in acute respiratory insufficiency. *Chest, 67*:156, 1975.

Kristoffersen, M. B., Rattenborg, C. C., and Holaday, D. A.: Asphyxial death: the roles of acute anoxia, hypercarbia and acidosis. *Anesthesiology, 28*:488, 1967.

Kvittingen, T. D., and Naess, A.: Recovery from drowning in fresh water. *Br. Med. J., 5341*:1315, 1963.

Lougheed, D. W., Janes, J. M., and Hall, G. E.: Physiological studies in experimental asphyxia and drowning. *Can. Med. Assoc. J., 40*:423, 1939.

Michenfelder, J. D., and Theye, R. A.: Cerebral protection by thiopental during hypoxia. *Anesthesiology, 39*:510, 1973.

Middleton, K. R.: Cardiac arrest induced by drowning: Attempted resuscitation by external and internal cardiac massage. *Can. Med. Assoc. J., 86*:374, 1962.

Modell, J. H.: Resuscitation after aspiration of chlorinated fresh water. *J.A.M.A., 185*:651, 1963.

Modell, J.: Die physiologischen Grundlagen für die Behandlung von Ertrunkenen. *Therapie Woche, 43*:1928, 1968.

Modell, J. H., and Davis, J. H.: Electrolyte changes in human drowning victims. *Anesthesiology, 30*:414, 1969.

Modell, J. H., and Downs, J. B.: Patterns of respiratory support aimed at pathophysiology. *1976 ASA Refresher Course Lectures*, 1976, pp. 223–1 to 223–9.

Modell, J. H., and Moya, F.: Effects of volume of aspirated fluid during chlorinated fresh water drowning. *Anesthesiology, 27*:662, 1966.

Modell, J. H., Calderwood, H. W., Ruiz, B. C., Downs, J. B., and Chapman, R., Jr.: Effects of ventilatory patterns on arterial oxygenation after near-drowning in sea water. *Anesthesiology, 40*:376, 1974.

Modell, J. H., Davis, J. H., Giammona, S. T., Moya, F., and Mann, J. B.: Blood gas and electrolyte changes in human near-drowning victims. *J.A.M.A., 203*:337, 1968a.

Modell, J. H., Gaub, M., Moya, F., Vestal, B., and Swarz, H.: Physiologic effects of near drowning with chlorinated fresh water, distilled water and isotonic saline. *Anesthesiology, 27*:33, 1966.

Modell, J. H., Graves, S. A., and Ketover, A.: Clinical course of 91 consecutive near-drowning victims. *Chest, 70*:231, 1976.

Modell, J. H., Kuck, E. J., Ruiz, B. C., and Heinitsch, H.: Effect of intravenous vs. aspirated distilled water on serum electrolytes and blood gas tensions. *J. Appl. Physiol., 32*:579, 1972.

Modell, J. H., Moya, F., Newby, E. J., Ruiz, B. C., and Showers, A. V.: The effects of fluid volume in seawater drowning. *Ann. Intern. Med., 67*:68, 1967.

Modell, J. H., Moya, F., Williams, H. D., and Weibley, T. C.: Changes in blood gases and A-aDO$_2$ during near-drowning. *Anesthesiology, 29*:456, 1968b.

Moss, G., Staunton, C., and Stein, A. A.: Cerebral etiology of the "shock lung syndrome." *J. Trauma, 12*:885, 1972.

Munroe, W. D.: Hemoglobinuria from near-drowning. *J. Pediatr., 64*:57, 1964.

Noble, C. S., and Sharpe, N.: Drowning: its mechanism and treatment. *Can. Med. Assoc. J., 89*:402, 1963.

Ohlsson, K., and Beckman, M.: Drowning—reflections based on two cases. *Acta Chir. Scand., 128*:327, 1964.

Press, E., Walker, J., and Crawford, I.: An interstate drowning study. *Am. J. Public Health, 58*:2275, 1968.

Rath, C. E.: Drowning hemoglobinuria. *Blood, 8*:1099, 1953.

Redding, J. S.: Treatment of near drowning. *Int. Anesthesiol. Clin., 3*:355, 1965.

Redding, J. S., and Pearson, J. W.: Management of drowning victims. *G. P., 29*:100, 1964.

Reidbord, H. E., and Spitz, W. U.: Ultrastructural alterations in rat lungs. Changes after intratracheal perfusion with freshwater and seawater. *Arch. Pathol., 81*:103, 1966.

Ruben, A., and Ruben, H.: Artificial respiration. Flow of water from the lung and the stomach. *Lancet, 1*:780, 1962.

Ruiz, B. C., Calderwood, H. W., Modell, J. H., and Brogdon, J. E.: Effect of ventilatory patterns on arterial oxygenation after near-drowning with fresh water: a comparative study in dogs. *Anesth. Analg., 52*:570, 1973.

Rutledge, R. R., and Flor, R. J.: The use of mechanical ventilation with positive end-expiratory pressure in the treatment of near-drowning. *Anesthesiology, 38*:194, 1973.

Safar, P., Escarraga, L. A., and Elam, J. O.: A comparison of the mouth-to-mouth and mouth-to-airway methods of artificial respiration with chest-pressure arm-lift methods. *N. Engl. J. Med., 258*:671, 1958.

Siebke, H., Breivik, H., Rød, T., and Lind, B.: Survival after 40 minutes' submersion without sequelae. *Lancet, 1*:1275, 1975.

Sladen, A., and Zauder, H. L.: Methylprednisolone therapy for pulmonary edema following near drowning. *J.A.M.A., 215*:1793, 1971.

Sladen, A., Laver, M. B., and Pontoppidan, H.: Pulmonary complications and water retention in prolonged mechanical ventilation. *N. Engl. J. Med., 279*:448, 1968.

Swan, H. J. C., Ganz, W., Forrester, J., Marcus, H., Diamond, G., and Chonette, D.: Catheterization of the heart in man with use of a flow-directed balloon-tipped catheter. *N. Engl. J. Med., 283*:447, 1970.

Swann, H. G., and Brucer, M.: The cardiorespiratory and biochemical events during rapid anoxic death. VI. Fresh water and sea water drowning. *Tex. Rep. Biol. Med., 7*:604, 1949.

Swann, H. G., Brucer, M., Moore, C., and Vezien, B. L.: Fresh water and sea water drowning: a study of the terminal cardiac and biochemical events. *Tex. Rep. Biol. Med., 5*:423, 1947.

Webster, D. P.: Pool drownings and their prevention. *Public Health Rep., 82*:587, 1967.

Wynne, J. W., and Modell, J. H.: Aspiration of stomach contents. A review. *Ann. Intern. Med.* (in press).

Zugzda, M. J.: Personal communications, July 25, 1969, and November 2, 1973.

CHAPTER THIRTY

HYPOSTATIC PNEUMONIA

William Curtis Adams, M.D.

Hypostatic pneumonia is a complication of those conditions predisposing to prolonged maintenance of a supine position. In this position, the diaphragm is at a relatively high level and there is a tendency for small airways in the basal lung lobes to collapse. Inability to take a deep breath may lead to atelectasis, and an ineffective cough may be associated with pooling of pulmonary secretions in the dependent parts of the lung. Subsequent bacterial infection causes a pneumonia, initially localized to the dependent portions of the lung, which may become more widespread. The use of antibiotics has decreased the risk of bacterial infection in this situation. Severe scleroderma, dermatomyositis, tetanus, and poliomyelitis are examples of debilitating conditions that may be complicated by hypostatic pneumonia.

Trauma may also play a very important role. Trauma peripheral to the chest area may be involved as readily as trauma to the chest. The constant supine position of the patient in leg, pelvic, or cervical (head) traction sets the scene. Any patient with multiple system trauma is likely to be kept supine for long periods. Chest trauma causing spontaneous splinting of rib action because of pain quite naturally leads to hypostatic pneumonia, as does a flail chest. Central nervous system trauma affecting the respiratory control center, causing improper lung function, may lead directly to hypostatic pneumonia. Abdominal trauma may cause significant reduction in diaphragmatic excursions, thus leading to abnormal respiratory function.

The early classic symptoms of pneumonia are characteristically absent, and the physical signs of dullness and rales must be carefully looked for in the dependent lung fields. Roentgenographic evidence of consolidation in the dependent areas will confirm the diagnosis in questionable cases.

Prevention by frequent change of position and maintenance of good pulmonary function is the primary therapeutic approach. The development of arterial blood gas determinations has added a singularly important diagnostic tool to our armamentarium. Careful monitoring of the arterial blood gases permits early detection of the problem and may be an excellent guide to therapeutic needs. Postural drainage and respiratory physiotherapy are cornerstones of both prophylactic and active treatment. However, the conditions present will often prevent postural drainage techniques, thus placing dependence upon respiratory physiotherapeutic mechanisms.

The tracheobronchial tree secretions have a pH of 6.5 to 8.5 in health and disease. The most effective inhalant medications should have a pH within that range. The medication should enhance the escalator action of the ciliary mucous membrane, and promote thin, watery secretions by the serous gland. A 20 per cent alcohol in water mixture provides a pH of 6.8 to 7.0 and does not change the surface tension. The addition of racemic epinephrine (a normal body catecholamine that is automatically destroyed and eliminated) stimulates both the escalator activity of the ciliary mucous membrane and the production of thin, watery secretions by the serous glands. This mixture also promotes vasoconstriction, thus counteracting peribronchial edema and aiding in the elimination of secretions. If the patient is unable to breathe deeply, the mixture is delivered by intermittent positive pressure respiratory support. The underlying condition will dictate the degree of respiratory gas support required. Generally, compressed air will be preferable to O_2 as the vehicle, but the arterial blood gases will aid in the proper selection.

If bacterial infection of the lung is present, appropriate antibiotic therapy must be instituted.

CHAPTER THIRTY-ONE

FOREIGN BODIES IN THE AIR PASSAGES

James W. Brooks, M.D., and Arnold M. Salzberg, M.D.

Foreign bodies aspirated into and retained in the tracheobronchial tree in infancy and childhood may threaten life or produce severe lung damage.

In a review of 55 respiratory foreign bodies in 54 pediatric patients during the past 15 years, the most frequent offender was a peanut in the right main stem bronchus (Tables 1, 2 and 3).

Diagnosis

Foreign body aspiration is often accompanied by sudden, violent coughing, gagging, wheezing, vomiting, cyanosis and brief episodes of apnea. If the foreign body is small and not obstructive, these findings may be minimal. After the initial dramatic symptoms, an annoying cough and wheezing persist without respiratory distress, unless the trachea is involved.

Physical examination can be helpful in diagnosis and localization. Observation may demonstrate unilateral thoracic overexpansion from obstructive emphysema or underexpansion from atelectasis. Wheezing can be heard with and without the stethoscope, and decreased breath sounds over the affected side are constant.

Fluoroscopy and chest roentgenogram in various projections are indispensable. A radiopaque foreign body offers no problem in identification (Fig. 1). The usual radiologic findings associated with nonopaque foreign bodies are atelectasis or obstructive em-

TABLE 2. FOREIGN BODIES IN AIR PASSAGE, 1960–1975

Object	Number
Peanut	26
Plastic bullet	6
Safety pin	1
Screw	2
Sewing needle	1
	36

TABLE 1. FOREIGN BODIES IN AIR PASSAGE, 1960–1975

Portion of Bronchial Tree	Number
Trachea	10
Right main stem bronchus	16
Right upper lobe	0
Right intermediate bronchus	6
Right lower lobe	5
Left main stem bronchus	12
Left upper lobe	2
Left lower lobe	4
	55

TABLE 3. FOREIGN BODIES IN AIR PASSAGE

Objects found in air passages of pediatric patients: (19) picture hook, bone, pinto bean, ball pen top, chestnut, crayon, tacks; (2) soy bean, corn kernel, egg shell, tooth, marble, hat pin, bean, rubber balloon; (2) watermelon seed, sunflower seed.

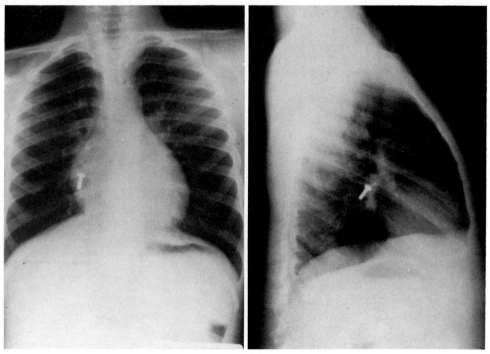

Figure 1. Posteroanterior and lateral roentgenograms of screw aspirated into the right lower lobe of the lung.

physema, except for those occasions when a lateral chest roentgenogram may demonstrate the object in a well outlined air tracheogram (Fig. 2). Fluoroscopy and lateral decubitus chest roentgenograms may document the dynamics of air trapping and localize the obstructive emphysema (Fig. 3). After the first 24 hours, the roentgenographic findings may progress from those of partial to complete atelectasis; the situation may be complicated by pneumonitis (Fig. 4).

Occasionally, the initial symptoms and physical findings may be minimal or overlooked and the presenting problem is persistent, localized, recurrent pneumonia that does not completely clear

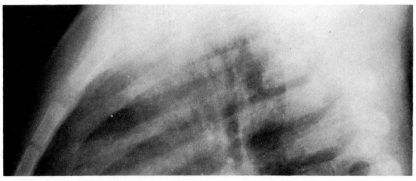

Figure 2. Lateral chest roentgenogram showing aspirated peanut in thoracic trachea just proximal to carina.

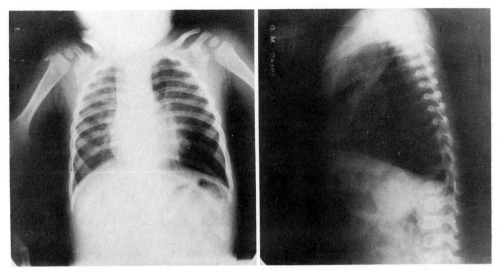

Figure 3. "Air trapping" of left lower lobe of lung due to aspirated peanut.

with adequate therapy. Bronchoscopy should be done if the possibility of foreign body exists, especially if hemoptysis is concurrent.

Respiratory distress may accompany obstructing foreign bodies of the high esophagus and pharyngoesophageal junction and this area should be scrutinized endoscopically if roentgenograms are suggestive and dysphagia occurs.

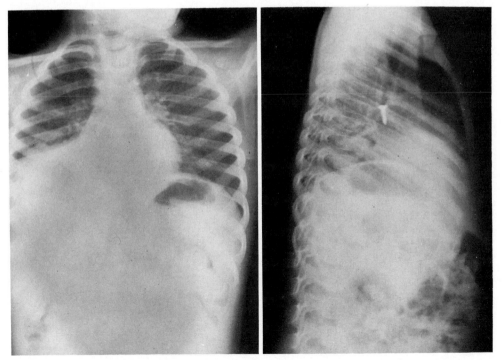

Figure 4. Atelectasis and pneumonia of right lower lobe of lung due to aspirated screw in right lower lobe of lung approximately 96 hours previously.

Treatment

Foreign bodies in the tracheobronchial tree should be removed promptly by bronchoscopy under general anesthesia. Early extraction will reduce local damage and distal parenchymal complications.

The ventilating bronchoscope surrounding the Storz-Hopkins telescope provides a closed, safe, efficient route for general anesthesia and mechanical ventilation. A separate channel in the bronchoscope sheath permits the insertion of foreign body forceps without obstruction of vision, and manipulation can be done under magnification. Even under these superior circumstances, extraction is often difficult and tedious, especially with those foreign objects that tend to crumble, such as peanuts.

Following removal of a foreign body from the lower airway, edema of the glottis from manipulation or of the bronchus from contact or chemical bronchitis can be annoying. Corticosteroid therapy for 24 to 48 hours and a course of antibiotic therapy should be helpful. Postoperative chest films may demonstrate a pneumothorax, which on rare occasions follows overenthusiastic anesthesia or excessive coughing. Chest tube drainage becomes necessary under these circumstances.

In less than 5 per cent of our patients, endoscopic extraction was not possible in spite of repeated attempts, and thoracotomy with bronchotomy became necessary. No unusual morbidity followed these procedures (Fig. 5). Failure of bronchoscopy on two occasions would seem to be an indication for open operation, since nonoperative resolution is highly unlikely and delay is associated with pulmonary morbidity.

Small respiratory foreign bodies have

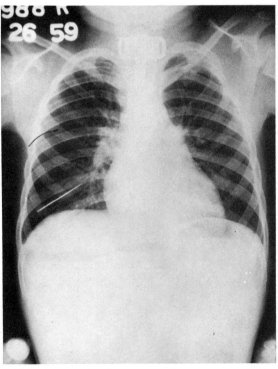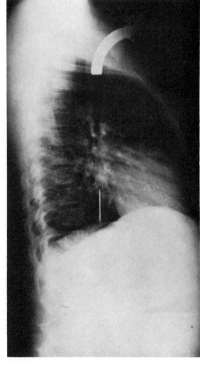

Figure 5. Aspirated sewing needle that could not be located with the bronchoscope, thus requiring thoracotomy for successful removal.

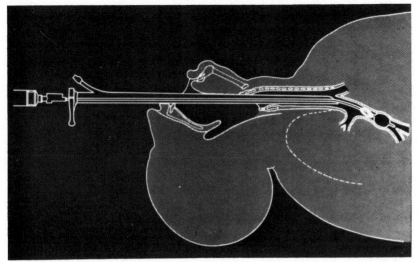

Figure 6. Technique of use of Fogarty catheter to extract small bronchial foreign body from distal bronchus.

been removed by a Fogarty catheter (Fig. 6) and by inhalation of bronchodilators with postural drainage.

Results

Bronchoscopic removal of foreign bodies was successful in 51 patients, while in four others thoracotomy and bronchotomy were required. One unfortunate child with a rubber balloon in the trachea expired while en route to the emergency room.

Cardiac arrest occurred in two instances of foreign body in the trachea; however, immediate resuscitation and bronchoscopic removal of the foreign body were successfully carried out.

It is apparent that foreign bodies in the tracheobronchial tree are particularly life-threatening in the pediatric population. Parents should be made aware of the hazards, and exclude small objects from the environment and peanuts and fruit seeds from the diet.

REFERENCES

Brown, B. S. J., et al.: Foreign bodies in the tracheobronchial tree in childhood. *J. Can. Assoc. Radiol., 14*:158, 1963.

Bunker, P. G.: Unrecognized foreign bodies in the air and food passages. *G. P., 29*:78, 1964.

Camarata, S. J., and Salyer, J. M.: Management of foreign bodies in air passages and esophagus under general anesthesia. *Am. Surg., 31*:725, 1965.

Carter, R.: Bronchotomy: the safe solution for an infarcted foreign body. *Ann. Surg., 10*:93, 1970.

Clery, A. P., Ellis, F. H., and Schmidt, H. W.: Problems associated with aspiration of grass heads (Inflorescences). *J.A.M.A., 171*:1478, 1959.

Jackson, C.: Grasses as foreign bodies in bronchus and lung. *Laryngoscope, 62*:897, 1952.

Kassay, D.: Observations on 100 cases of bronchial foreign bodies. *Arch. Otolaryngol., 71*:42, 1960.

Kassay, D.: Management of bronchial foreign bodies. *Eye Ear Nose Throat Mon., 42*:54, 1963.

Laurance, B.: Hemoptysis, bronchiectasis and foreign body in lung. *Br. Med. J., 1*:125, 1954.

Law, D., and Kosloske, A. M.: Management of tracheo-bronchial foreign body in children. *Pediatrics, 58*:362, 1976.

Linton, J. S. A.: Long-standing intrabronchial foreign bodies. *Thorax, 12*:164, 1957.

CHAPTER THIRTY-TWO

CRYPTOGENIC OR IDIOPATHIC FIBROSING ALVEOLITIS
(Usual Interstitial Pneumonia)

WILLIAM M. THURLBECK, M.B., CH.B.

A wide variety of terms has been used to describe interstitial inflammatory disease of the lung associated with interstitial fibrosis. Included are such terms as organizing interstitial pneumonia, idiopathic pulmonary fibrosis, chronic interstitial pneumonitis, idiopathic diffuse interstitial fibrosis of the lung, bronchiolar emphysema, muscular cirrhosis of the lung, chronic diffuse sclerosing alveolitis, and the Hamman-Rich syndrome. "Cryptogenic" or "idiopathic fibrosing alveolitis" or just "fibrosing alveolitis" are the most commonly used terms at present, although, as Liebow (1975) has pointed out, these are not completely satisfactory terms in that they stress only one possible end result of lung injury, and he thus prefers the term "usual" chronic interstitial pneumonia (UIP). It is now apparent that a useful purpose can be served by classifying the interstitial pneumonias into several categories. This chapter will deal with the "usual" form of interstitial pneumonia, and the subsequent chapter will deal with described variants.

Definition and Pathology

Fibrosing alveolitis is characterized by interstitial inflammation of the lung accompanied by gross disorganization of the lung so that the periphery of the lung consists of small cystic spaces lined by bronchiolar cells and type I and II alveolar epithelial cells. The spaces are separated from each other by dense connective tissue (Figs. 1 and 2). The exact mode of development of the lesion is uncertain, but it is postulated that there is an initial injury to the alveolar wall that results in destruction of the alveolar basement membrane and in the formation of an exudate in the alveolar spaces. Organization of the exudate results in extensive loss of distal air spaces (alveolar ducts and sacs) and dilatation of the proximal part of the acinus (respiratory bronchioles), which becomes largely lined by continuous bronchiolar epithelium. This leads to the microcystic appearance of the lung, but in reality the majority of the "cysts" connect with airways and are dilated distal airways. Since bronchiolar secretions accumulate in many of the proximal spaces, the airway connections are imperfect or absent in many instances. Most of these spaces are less than 2 mm. in diameter. The process is usually most prominent, and the cysts largest, in the basal parts of the lung. There is extensive fibrosis with varying degrees of proliferation of smooth muscle be-

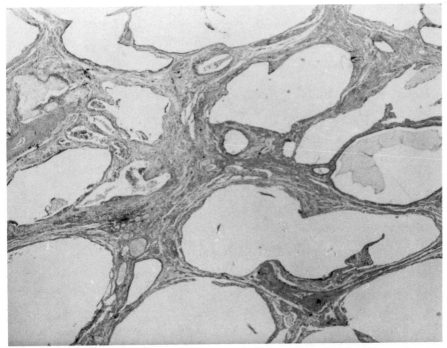

Figure 1.   The normal lung architecture is grossly disorganized and replaced by cystic spaces 0.5 to 2 mm. in diameter and separated from each other by dense fibrous tissue (× 30).

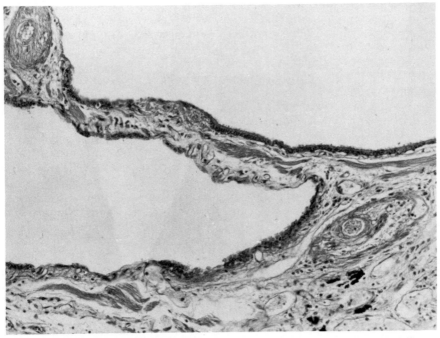

Figure 2.   The air spaces are lined by bronchiolar epithelium and there is dense interstitial fibrosis. Note the presence of smooth muscle and the scattering of inflammatory cells (× 150).

tween the spaces. An infiltrate of mononuclear cells of varying severity is present in the interstitium.

Etiology

By definition, the condition must be of unknown cause, but identical lesions may be found in the lungs of patients with systemic sclerosis, rheumatoid arthritis, dermatomyositis and systemic lupus erythematosus. This has led to the concept that fibrosing alveolitis is a "collagen" disease, with a probable underlying immunologic mechanism. Further credence is given to this notion by the occurrence of abnormal immunoglobulins in up to two-thirds of patients with fibrosing alveolitis, and autoantibodies and antinuclear antibodies may be present in up to 40 per cent of cases (Turner-Warwick and Haslam, 1971).

Identical pulmonary findings may occur in patients with neurofibromatosis, celiac disease and renal acidosis. Fibrosing alveolitis may also occur as a familial, autosomal dominant condition (Swaye and coworkers, 1969). It was originally thought that up to 25 per cent of examples of fibrosing alveolitis might be familial (Donohue and coworkers, 1959); it now appears that the true incidence of the familial disorder is closer to 3 per cent (Solliday and associates, 1973). Finally, known agents may produce similar or identical pulmonary lesions, and these include asbestos, drugs that may be cytotoxic (busulfan, bleomycin, methotrexate, cyclophosphamide, hexamethonium, mecamylamine, melphalan, hydralazine and hydantoin), drugs that act through hypersensitivity (nitrofurantoin), and viral infections. A similar lesion may result from chronic eosinophilic pneumonia or, most important, hypersensitivity pneumonitis (extrinsic allergic alveolitis). The list of agents that may produce the latter syndrome grows each year, and the chronic form may be nonspecific and may closely mimic idiopathic fibrosing alveolitis (Lopez and Salvaggio, 1976). It is thus important in any given case of fibrosing alveolitis to make a detailed questioning of the patient to try to determine possible etiologic agents.

Clinical Manifestations

The condition is relatively uncommon in children, but in one series, 3 of 13 patients with fibrosing alveolitis were less than 14 years of age; in another, 5 of 87 patients were below the age of 10 years, and 3 others were between 10 and 19 years of age (Donohue and coworkers, 1959). Fibrosing alveolitis has been reported in a 4-month-old child. The familial form of the disease manifests in childhood in about the same proportion of children to adults as the nonfamilial cases do. In adults, the condition is more common in males than in females, but the sex incidence is about equal in children. In the familial variant, females are more commonly affected.

The onset is insidious; dyspnea is usually the earliest symptom, first appearing on exertion but later present at rest. Cough, either productive or nonproductive, is the presenting complaint in less than 15 per cent of patients. Chest pain is not uncommon and is sometimes pleuritic in nature. Hemoptysis is an occasional presenting complaint and complication of the condition. Fever is very unusual; when it occurs, it may be a manifestation of superimposed infection, which can represent a serious clinical problem. Anorexia, weight loss, fatigue and weakness are usual features as the disease progresses. Clubbing is a characteristic feature. Obvious cyanosis appears late in the disease process, but hypoxemia or mild cyanosis is quite common. Examination of the chest may disclose few abnormalities, but the classic abnormalities consist of showers of fine, late inspiratory crepitations. Spontaneous pneumothorax occurs in about 3 per cent of cases (Gaensler and coworkers, 1972). The appearance of peripheral edema, hepatomegaly, accentuation of the second pulmonic sound and an elevated venous pressure indicates the presence of right ventricular failure, which is common in the terminal stages of the disease.

The chest radiograph is sometimes entirely normal even when there are both physiologic abnormalities and clinical symptoms. The characteristic roentgenographic features are of a diffuse reticulonodular pattern, more striking in the lower zones of the lung (Fig. 3), and of diminished lung volumes. The latter feature may be present even when the pulmonary parenchymal changes appear relatively slight or absent on the roentgenogram. Pleural involvement, as manifested by blunting of one or both costophrenic angles, has been described in 8 of 11 patients in one series (Dill and coworkers, 1975). Right ventricular hypertrophy and dilatation appear as a terminal event.

There are no pathognomonic laboratory features, but as noted previously, hypergammaglobulinemia is frequent, and antinuclear factor and rheumatoid factor are present in 25 to 40 per cent of cases.

Diagnosis

Patients with diffuse interstitial fibrosis have restrictive lung disease with a reduction in the diffusing capacity. Characteristically, all lung volumes and lung capacities are reduced, and lung compliance is diminished, sometimes up to 50 per cent of predicted. Tests of expiratory flow may also show reduced values, but when this is found, it is usually due to diminished lung volumes. When correction is made for the reduced lung volumes, the expiratory flow rates are often supernormal, reflecting the increased elastic recoil of the lung. At rest, arterial P_{O_2} may be nearly normal, but there is a reduction during exercise. Arterial P_{CO_2} is usually low normal or low, reflecting the increase in minute ventilation that occurs in these patients. The reason for this increase beyond that required to restore normal blood gases remains unexplained. Hypoxemia is thought to be due more to abnormalities of ventilation to perfusion matching than to the diminished diffusing capacity. Pulmo-

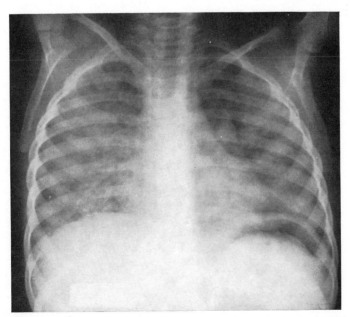

Figure 3.   There are diffuse reticulonodular densities in the middle and lower zones of the lungs ($\times 150$). (Courtesy of W. W. Waring, M.D., Tulane School of Medicine, New Orleans.)

nary function studies are thus an excellent means of identifying a patient with restrictive lung disease due to pulmonary fibrosis, and these tests may be abnormal in patients whose chest roentgenographs are normal. However, the definitive delineation of the type of fibrosis and exclusion of other causes of restrictive lung disease can be made only by lung biopsy, which is the definitive diagnostic procedure.

Differential diagnosis should include the collagen diseases, sarcoidosis, and other granulomatous diseases as well as a multitude of conditions that may produce diffuse pulmonary infiltration. Every effort should be made to determine possible exogenous causes for the condition.

Course and Complications

The clinical signs and symptoms depend on the extent of lung involvement and the degree to which lung function has been altered. The disease is usually inexorably progressive and appears to be due to involvement of increasing amounts of lung tissue. Complete and permanent arrest of the condition is unusual. A superimposed acute inflammatory process produces exacerbation of the symptoms and may precipitate cardiac failure or respiratory insufficiency. The latter conditions are the usual causes of death.

Treatment

Treatment is generally symptomatic and supportive, with emphasis on the prevention and treatment of respiratory infections. Corticosteroids have generally been used, occasionally with apparent symptomatic relief. However, there is seldom evidence of improvement of lung function, and there remains some doubt as to the suitability of this treatment, particularly in growing children. However, in view of the subjective improvement in a number of subjects and the fact that it is the only effective drug, a trial dose of corticosteroids is generally recommended. Prednisone is the drug of choice, and the dosage used must be high, maintained for long periods, and tapered slowly.

REFERENCES

Dill, J., Ghose, T., Landrigan, P., MacKeen, A. D., and MacNeil, A. R.: Cryptogenic fibrosing alveolitis. *Chest, 67*:411, 1975.

Donohue, W. L., Laski, B., Uchida, I., and Mann, J. D.: Familial fibrocystic pulmonary dysplasia and its relation to the Hamman-Rich syndrome. *Pediatrics, 24*:786, 1959.

Gaensler, E. A., Carrington, C. B., and Coutu, R. E.: Chronic interstitial pneumonias. *Clin. Notes Resp. Dis., 10*:3, 1972.

Liebow, A. A.: Definition and classification of interstitial pneumonias in human pathology. *Hum. Pathol. Prog. Resp. Res., 8*:1, 1975.

Lopez, M., and Salvaggio, J.: Hypersensitivity pneumonitis: current concepts of etiology and pathogenesis. *Ann. Rev. Med., 27*:453, 1976.

Solliday, N. H., Williams, J. A., Gaensler, E. A., Coutu, R. E., and Carrington, C. B.: Familial chronic interstitial pneumonia. *Am. Rev. Resp. Dis., 108*:193, 1973.

Swaye, P., Van Ordstrand, H. S., McCormack, L. J., et al.: Familial Hamman-Rich syndrome. Report of eight cases. *Chest, 55*:7, 1969.

Turner-Warwick, M., and Haslam, P.: Antibodies in some chronic fibrosing lung diseases. I. Nonspecific autoantibodies. *Clin. Allergy, 1*:83, 1971.

Turner-Warwick, M., and Parkes, W. R.: Circulating rheumatoid and antinuclear factors in asbestos workers. *Br. Med. J., 3*:492, 1970.

CHAPTER THIRTY-THREE

DESQUAMATIVE INTERSTITIAL PNEUMONIA AND OTHER VARIANTS OF INTERSTITIAL PNEUMONIA

WILLIAM M. THURLBECK, M.B., CH.B.

There are several morphologically distinct variants of interstitial pneumonia, and it is important to recognize these variants. This is particularly true for desquamative interstitial pneumonia, the most common variant, since its prognostic implications are very different from fibrosing alveolitis discussed in the preceding chapter. It is also true that in the past, distinctions have not been made among the various types of interstitial pneumonia, and they have been grouped together as "fibrosing alveolitis" or "Hamman-Rich" disease. Thus, some of the reports in the literature concerning fibrosing alveolitis are hard to interpret because they likely include several separate histologic and, perhaps, clinical entities.

DESQUAMATIVE INTERSTITIAL PNEUMONIA (DIP)

Like fibrosing alveolitis, DIP is much commoner in adults than in children, but at least 18 cases have been reported in children, and the youngest child had

symptoms dating from $2\frac{1}{2}$ weeks of age (Howatt and coworkers, 1973). In adults, idiopathic fibrosing alveolitis is about four times as common as DIP is (Gaensler and coworkers, 1972), and the same may be true in children. DIP is defined and diagnosed on histologic criteria. The two characteristic features of DIP are (1) the proliferation of cells lining the alveolar spaces, and (2) the presence of cells lying free and packing the alveolar spaces (Fig. 1 E and F). The cells lining the air spaces are type II alveolar cells, and the cells lying free in the spaces are macrophages containing brown granules that stain positively with periodic acid—Schiff stain. Occasionally, the macrophages may fuse to form multinucleated cells. Less conspicuous are the interstitial changes, which consist of a reduction in the number of blood-filled capillaries, and an interstitial infiltrate, which consists of lymphocytes, plasma cells and eosinophils. Generally, lymphocytes predominate and eosinophils are scanty. Nodular accumulations of lymphocytes occur, often near bronchioles but also near the pleura within parenchyma. Eosinophilic intranuclear inclusions have been described in 5 to 80 per cent of cases

523

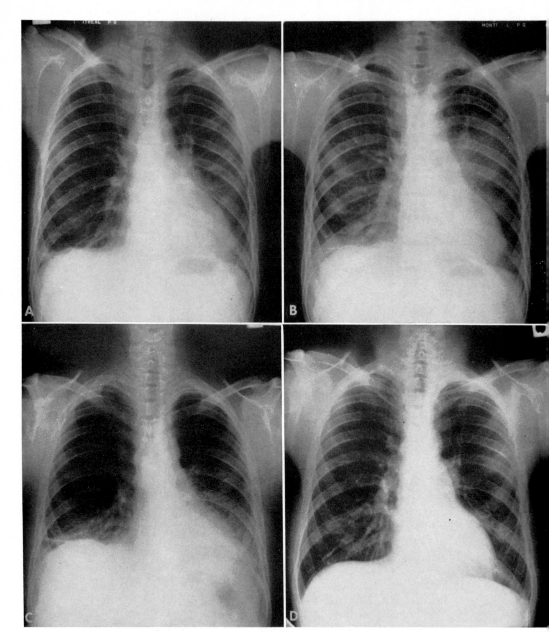

Figure 1. Radiographs and histologic sections of an 11-year-old boy with desquamative interstitial pneumonia. The symptoms dated from an onset of influenza and responded to steroids. An initial biopsy was done on presentation and a second biopsy was performed three years subsequently, and the patient remained reasonably well until killed in an automobile accident five years later. Physiologically, the patient showed mild restrictive lung disease. (From Bates, D. V., Macklem, P. T., and Christie, R. V.: *Respiratory Function in Disease.* 2nd Ed. Philadelphia, W. B. Saunders Company, 1971. Reproduced courtesy of Dr. David Bates.)

Radiologic examination (A to D). At the time of initial presentation in 1959, the chest roentgenogram (*A*) shows loss of volume of both lower lobes and there is a similar change in the lingular segment. The pulmonary infiltrations become more obvious in the radiograph taken in January 1960 (*B*). Some improvement is noted by October 1960 (*C*), and there is almost complete resolution in November 1962 (*D*).

Histopathologic examination (E) shows the initial biopsy and illustrates the relative preservation of the architecture of the lung. The alveolar spaces can still be recognized as such, but are lined by columnar (Type II) epithelial cells. The air spaces contain many of the characteristic desquamated cells, which are macrophages. The second lung biopsy (*F*) done three years later shows extensive resolution of the cellular proliferation of the cells lining the air spaces and absence of cells within the air spaces. There is modest interstitial pulmonary fibrosis, but the lung architecture is essentially intact.

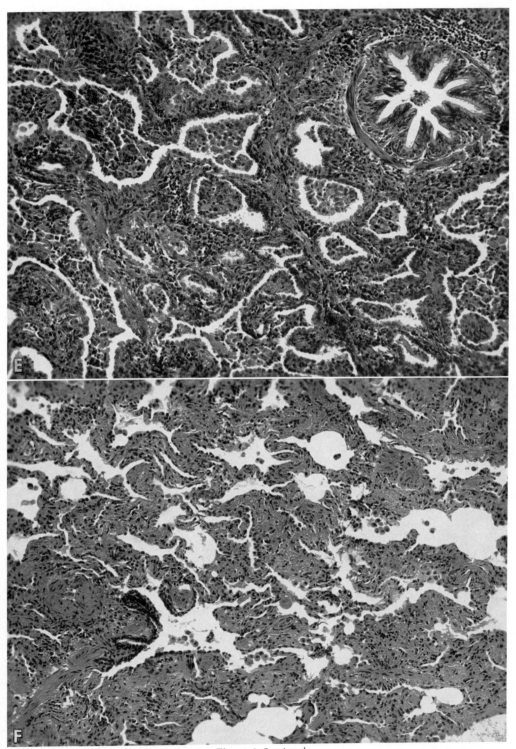

Figure 1 *Continued.*

(Liebow and coworkers, 1965; Patchefsky and coworkers, 1971). They occur in both the alveolar lining cells and the desquamated cells. They have been described as "virus-like," but electron microscopic studies have shown that these inclusions correspond to degenerative changes and consist of myelin figures (McNary and Gaensler, 1971) and that there is clumping of the chromatin at the nuclear membrane. In classic cases, the alveolar framework is preserved (Fig. 1 E) and there is none of the alveolar collapse and gross distortion of the lung architecture as is seen in fibrosing alveolitis. Fibrosis may be minimal. There is clearly a transition between DIP and fibrosing alveolitis, and cases have been recorded showing the development of fibrosing alveolitis some years after lung biopsy had shown classic DIP (McCann and Brewer, 1974). Nonetheless, the great differences in prognosis make it important to differentiate the two conditions.

Etiology

The cause is unknown, but because of the overlap in some cases between DIP and fibrosing alveolitis, an immunologic mechanism is often invoked. However, the presence of rheumatoid factor and antinuclear factor is much less frequent than in fibrosing alveolitis, and DIP is not encountered in the collagen diseases with the same frequency as is fibrosing alveolitis. Histologic findings identical with DIP have been found in asbestosis, but this likely represents a response to diffuse alveolar damage rather than implies that asbestos is often a specific etiologic agent.

Clinical Features

The condition is about equally frequent in males and females. In general, the clinical features are similar to fibrosing alveolitis. The onset in most cases is insidious, but in two reported cases the onset appeared to be related to influenza in the family. All members of the family were involved, but the two patients were left with dyspnea. Dyspnea is the most striking feature, and in young children, tachypnea and tachycardia are prominent findings. Fatigability, anorexia and weight loss also occur. Cyanosis is usual, as is clubbing. Fever, usually not exceeding 38°C., may be present. Physical examination of the chest may be entirely normal despite the presence of functional abnormalities. The most classic findings are those of fine rales at both bases.

Radiologic Findings

In about two-thirds of the cases, an almost unique roentgenographic picture is seen (Gaensler and coworkers, 1972). This consists of a faint triangular haziness radiating out from the hila, along the heart borders to both bases, sparing the costophrenic angles. The opacities have been described as having a "ground-glass" appearance. In children, however, the shadows are likely to be more irregularly distributed (Fig. 1 A to D), although the ground-glass characteristic is usually present. Thus, in the 16-year-old boy reported in the original series of cases (Liebow and coworkers, 1965), lesions were first seen in the left upper lobe and superior segment of the left lower lobe with no involvement of the diaphragmatic region. The process then evolved in the more characteristic adult way. The radiologic changes clear more slowly than do the symptoms when the patients are treated with steroids. The radiologic lesions may recur, together with clinical symptoms, when steroids are interrupted.

Laboratory Data

Leukocytosis, usually not exceeding 15,000 white blood cells per mm.^{3}, is sometimes found. A few patients, including a child, have been reported to have eosinophilia. Originally, it was thought that serum protein abnormalities were absent in DIP, but occasional patients had positive LE preparations, rheumatoid factor or ANF, or abnormal immunoglobulin levels (Patchefsky and coworkers, 1973).

The pulmonary function abnormalities in DIP are similar to those of fibrosing alveolitis (see Chapter 32), consisting mainly of a restrictive pulmonary defect and diminished diffusing capacity. These changes tend to be less severe than in fibrosing alveolitis, and in some instances lung volumes may be normal or nearly so. Blood gases follow a similar pattern to that described in fibrosing alveolitis.

Treatment and Course in DIP

The majority of cases in children have had a gratifying response to corticosteroid therapy even when there has been extremely severe respiratory distress. One eight-year-old child appeared in extremis, yet three weeks after commencement of treatment with prednisone, she was breathing normally without oxygen, and ten years later was free of pulmonary symptoms (Bhagwat and coworkers, 1970). Discontinuation of cortiscosteroids may result in relapse, but in these instances, reinstitution of steroids in high dosages is usually followed by improvement. In the patient described in this chapter, this was the case. A good response to corticosteroids has not been uniform; poorly responsive cases have been reported, including a patient who did not respond and died after a short illness. The presence of pulmonary fibrosis in lung biopsies is a poor prognostic sign, and the pathologist should always indicate the extent and severity of the fibrosis as seen in the specimen. In adults, an excellent response is found in 80 per cent of patients; the same is likely true of children.

LYMPHOID INTERSTITIAL PNEUMONIA (LIP)

This condition is less common than DIP, and only three cases have been reported in children (Halprin and co-workers, 1972; Liebow and Carrington 1973). It is likewise defined morphologically, and it is characterized by an exquisitely interstitial infiltrate of lymphocytes and plasma cells. Lymphocytes are present in all cases and they are usually the dominant cells, although occasionally plasma cells may be prominent. In about 20 per cent of cases, there is an infiltrate of large mononuclear and reticuloendothelial cells, and some of these patients appear to overlap with malignant lymphoma of the lung. Touton-type giant cells sometimes occur.

Clinical Features

Since the number of cases in children is so few, the precise features of LIP are uncertain, and the following remarks refer to LIP in both adults and children. Serum protein abnormalities are usually found in LIP (Liebow and Carrington, 1973). In about two-thirds of the cases that have abnormal proteins, there is hypergammaglobulinemia and usually an increase in IgG; in the remaining one-third of cases there is hypogammaglobulinemia. Two-thirds of the cases have been female, and nearly all the cases with hypogammaglobulinemia or IgM hypergammaglobulinemia have been seen in women. About one-fourth of the cases with abnormal proteins have had Sjögren's syndrome, and the hypothesis has been suggested that LIP may be a variant of this disease, and that those cases that do not have overt Sjögren's disease represent Sjögren's disease limited to involvement of the lung.

The onset of the condition is insidious and its course is slowly progressive. Dyspnea and cough are the usual presenting complaints, but in the occasional patient, a definite episode of pneumonia has marked the onset of the symptoms. Fever occurs in about 40 per cent of patients, and all the signs and symptoms of Sjögren's disease are present in those with this condition. Physical signs are usually minimal, despite obvious radiologic and functional abnormalities. Pulmonary function data are available on only three cases: one had normal tests of pulmonary function; one had a restrictive defect; and one had a mild obstructive pattern (Halprin and coworkers, 1972).

Radiologic Changes

About half of patients have had a fine reticulonodular pattern and the remainder have had a coarsely reticulonodular or nodular pattern on their chest roentgenograms. The reticular pattern is characteristically linear or slightly curved, more obvious at the bases where it often has a fernlike or feathery appearance. The nodular densities are sharply defined and round. Pleural effusions have been seen in about one-sixth of cases.

Treatment and Prognosis

Very little information is available, and such data that do exist relate to steroid treatment, which has produced radiologic improvement in about half the cases; the majority of these patients have had Sjögren's syndrome. The course appears to be a protracted one.

GIANT CELL INTERSTITIAL PNEUMONIA (GIP)

This variant of interstitial pneumonia is characterized by the presence of many large, rather bizarre multinucleated cells in the alveolar spaces (Liebow, 1975). These cells are "cannibalistic," i.e., they engulf other cells. In addition, discrete desquamated macrophages fill the alveolar spaces, and alveoli are lined by type II cells; there is also an interstitial infiltrate of monocytes, predominantly lymphocytes.

Only seven cases have been reported in detail, and none of them has been in children (Reddy and coworkers, 1970; Sokolowski and coworkers, 1972). The clinical presentation has been similar to fibrosing alveolitis or DIP—progressive dyspnea, cough, chest pain, fatigue and weight loss, with clubbing and fine basal rales being present on physical examination. The chest roentgenogram usually shows bilaterally patchy nodular infiltrates involving the midlung fields or upper zones of the lung, and the apices and costophrenic angles have generally been spared. In other cases, flame-shaped opacities have been described; in yet others, the roentgenogram has resembled that seen in DIP. The majority of patients have benefited from steroid treatment, but this has not been a uniform result. It seems likely that this rare condition may be a variant of DIP.

BRONCHIOLITIS OBLITERANS (Bronchiolitis obliterans with interstitial pneumonia—BIP)

Only one report has dealt specifically with this condition (Gosink and coworkers, 1973). This term clearly includes several different conditions, and there is some question whether any real relationship between BIP and other forms of interstitial pneumonia and fibrosing alveolitis exists. However, some examples of BIP show a prominent interstitial mononuclear infiltrate and interstitial fibrosis with honeycombing, and microcyst formation has been found in about 10 per cent of cases. The most characteristic feature of BIP is the presence of an exudate within the lumen of respiratory bronchioles that undergoes varying states of organization. The intrabronchiolar lesions vary in appearance. In what is presumably an earlier stage, the lesions are cellular with an infiltrate predominantly of lymphocytes but including an admixture of polymorphonuclear leukocytes. Subsequently, organization leads to fibrous polyps, sometimes lined by bronchiolar epithelium. In some instances, the lesions lie predominantly around bronchioles and lead to marked constriction and even obliteration. The distal alveolar parenchyma is variably involved. Most commonly, lipid-laden macrophages, characteristic of obstructive pneumonitis, fill many of the distal alveolar spaces. In other instances, organizing exudate, similar to that seen in the bronchioles, may be seen in the alveolar spaces. Interstitial inflammation and fibrosis are usually not prominent, but in some cases they may be the predominant lesion.

It is clear that several conditions may present with this histologic lesion. In about a third of patients, the lesions have appeared following a pneumonic episode, and in a further fifth, the patients have had chronic respiratory disease, suggesting an infectious etiologic agent for these two groups of cases. A further 10 per cent of patients with GIP have been associated with inhalation of toxic substances. In the remainder, about one-third, no etiologic agent could be implicated. The roentgenographic pattern has been quite variable. The majority of patients have had alveolar opacities of varying size and distribution, two patients had pulmonary overinflation, and the remainder had nodular and reticulonodular opacities.

Seven of the 52 reported patients were under the age of 20 years. The clinical presentation has been variable. Cough, dyspnea and malaise are almost always present, and 78 per cent of patients have produced sputum. Fever and a leukocytosis of more than 10,000 cells per mm.^{3} have been present in about two-thirds of cases, and rales have been heard in about 80 per cent of cases. While the onset of the condition has generally been insidious, the course has been rather more rapid and has been measured in terms of weeks rather than months or years, as is the case of interstitial pneumonias. In general, the presentation is therefore different from the forms of interstitial pneumonias described previously. Some of the patients in whom the disease had an apparently infectious origin were submitted to lung resection for localized disease, with apparent cure. In the remainder of the infectious group, in the post-toxic inhalation group and in the idiopathic group, patients have been treated with steroids or antibiotics or both. About two-thirds of patients have shown a significant improvement, and the idiopathic group of BIP showed the highest proportion with improvement.

REFERENCES

Bhagwat, A. G., Wentworth, P., and Conen, P. E.: Observations on the relationship of desquamative interstitial pneumonia and pulmonary alveolar proteinosis in childhood: a pathologic and experimental study. *Chest*, 58:326, 1970.

Gaensler, E. A., Carrington, C. B., and Coutu, R. E.: Chronic interstitial pneumonias. *Clin. Notes Resp. Dis.*, 10:3, 1972.

Gosink, B. B., Friedman, P. J., and Liebow, A. A.: Bronchiolitis obliterans: roentgenologic-pathologic correlations. *Am. J. Roentgenol. Radium Ther. Nucl. Med.*, 117:816, 1973.

Halprin, G. M., Famirez-R., J., and Pratt, P. C.: Lymphoid interstitial pneumonia. *Chest*, 62:418, 1972.

Howatt, W. F., Heidelberger, K. P., LeGlovan, D. P., and Schnitzer, B.: Desquamative interstitial pneumonia: case report of an infant unresponsive to treatment. *Am. J. Dis. Child.*, 126:346, 1973.

Liebow, A. A.: Definition and classification of interstitial pneumonias in human pathology. Alveolar Interstitium of the Lung. International Symposium, Paris, 1974. *Prog. Resp. Res.*, 8:1, 1975.

Liebow, A. A., and Carrington, C. B.: Diffuse pulmonary lymphoreticular infiltrations associated with dysproteinemia. *Med. Clin. North Am.*, 57:809, 1973.

Liebow, A. A., Steer, A., and Billingsley, J. G.: Desquamative interstitial pneumonia. *Am. J. Med.*, 39:369, 1965.

McCann, B. G., and Brewer, D. B.: A case of desquamative interstitial pneumonia progressing to "honeycomb lung." *J. Pathol.*, 112:199, 1974.

McNary, W. F., and Gaensler, E. A.: Intranuclear inclusion bodies in desquamative interstitial pneumonia. Electron microscopic observations. *Ann. Intern. Med.*, 74:404, 1971.

Patchefsky, A. S., Banner, M., and Freundlich, L. M.: Desquamative interstitial penumonia: significance of intranuclear viral-like inclusion bodies. *Ann. Intern. Med.*, 74:322, 1971.

Patchefsky, A. S., Fraimow, W., and Hoch, W. S.: Desquamative interstitial pneumonia: pathological findings and follow-up in 13 patients. *Arch. Intern. Med.*, 132:222, 1973.

Reddy, P. A., Gorelick, D. F., and Christianson, C. S.: Giant cell interstitial pneumonia. *Chest*, 58:319, 1970.

Sokolowski, J. W., Cordray, D. R., Cantow, E. F., Elliot, R. C., and Seal, R. B.: Giant cell interstitial pneumonia: report of a case. *Am. Rev. Resp. Dis.*, 105:417, 1972.

CHAPTER THIRTY-FOUR

PULMONARY ALVEOLAR PROTEINOSIS

Harris D. Riley, Jr., M.D.

Pulmonary alveolar proteinosis is a syndrome of unknown cause that is characterized by progressive dyspnea and cough. It was first described in 1958 by Rosen, Castleman and Liebow, who reported 27 instances of the disorder, and was considered a new disease. However, retrospective studies suggest that the condition may have existed as far back as 1941. In 1969, Davidson and Macleod reviewed the literature and stated that 139 cases had been reported up to that time, 100 from the United States and 39 from other parts of the world, especially Great Britain and France. There were four children and seven teenagers, but 85 of the patients were between the ages of 30 and 50 years. Since that time, sporadic cases, usually in adults, have been described, and by 1972, 224 case reports had appeared in the world literature. Of the patients initially described by Rosen and colleagues, two were children, 2 years 4 months and 15 years of age, respectively. However, the number of cases occurring in infants and children among the total cases described is small. Danigelis and Markarian reported in December 1969 that only 10 cases in the pediatric age group had been described, but subsequently Sunderland and coworkers (1972) stated that 34 cases in children 15 years of age or less had been reported in the world literature.

Pathology

The gross pathologic appearance of the lung is characteristic, although the extent and distribution of the disease may vary. Multiple firm gray or yellow nodules of varying size are often located subpleurally throughout the lung and the weight of the lungs is increased. The bronchial tree appears normal, and there is usually evidence of alveolar wall damage. Although hyperplasia of the alveolar epithelium is usually present, inflammation and fibrous thickening of the interalveolar septa are conspicuously absent, and, in the absence of infection, fibrous tissue organization to the stage of honeycombing has never been reported. The most striking feature is the microscopic appearance, which is characterized by interalveolar deposition of granular, eosinophilic, PAS-positive proteinaceous material (Fig. 1). Special stains have shown the presence of carbohydrates, protein and increased amounts of phospholipids in the alveolar debris. The material in the alveoli, which has been identified as a lipoprotein with many chemical similarities to pulmonary surfactant but with different physical properties, is thought to be derived from granular pneumocytes.

These pathologic findings are believed by some investigators to result from the transformation of alveolar

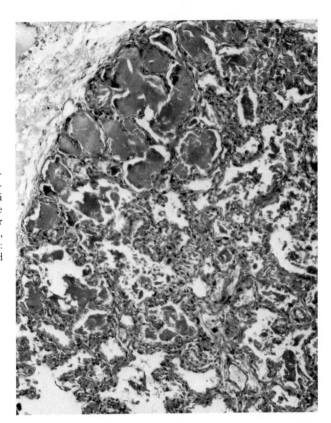

Figure 1. Photomicrograph of a typical section of the lung in a three-month-old infant with pulmonary alveolar proteinosis. Peripheral alveoli are filled with dense, PAS-positive homogeneous material with acicular spaces. (From Wilkinson, R. H., Blanc, W. A., and Hagstrom, J. W. C.: *Pediatrics, 41*:510, 1968. Reproduced with permission.)

pneumocytes, which increase in both size and number and project into the alveolar lumen. Subsequently, these cells slough and degenerate, and the alveolar accumulation leads to an alveolar-capillary block type of diffusion defect and an increase in pulmonary venous shunt. Other workers have postulated that the alveolar deposits could represent a response to an infectious agent or to a toxic substance in the environment, such as quartz crystsls. Pulmonary changes similar to the disease in humans have been produced in pathogen-free rats exposed to quartz inhalation. The disease has also been considered to be due to an abnormal generation of a surface-active substance normally present in small amounts in the lung, to a plasma infiltrate secondary to inherent defects in the pulmonary alveolar capillaries, or to deficient pulmonary cellular clearance, a concept that has received some support from the studies of Ramirez and Harlan

(1968). All attempts to isolate a bacterial or parasitic agent have been unsuccessful, and the alveolar accumulation does not impair migration of macrophages. There are certain pathologic similarities in the lung to changes produced by infection with *Pneumocystis carinii.* Plenck and coworkers (1960) reported the presence of complement-fixing antibodies to *Pneumocystis carinii* in four of nine patients, but the organism was not recovered in any instance; patients with pulmonary alveolar proteinosis are liable to secondary infection with this parasite.

Pathogenesis

In 1965, Liebow and coworkers first described desquamative interstitial pneumonia, a disease also of unknown cause, characterized by proliferation of alveolar lining cells with desquamation of alveolar cells into the distal air spaces. These workers believed it to be a separate entity from pulmonary alveolar proteinosis, but pointed out that the two diseases had striking similarities. Recently, Bhagwat, Wentworth and Conen (1970) reported the case of a nine-month-old infant with necropsy findings that resembled both desquamative interstitial pneumonia and pulmonary alveolar proteinosis. They also experimentally produced similar histopathologic changes of both disorders in the same rabbit lung. These investigators have suggested that pulmonary alveolar proteinosis and desquamative interstitial pneumonia may have a common pathogenesis or that they may represent different stages or components of a single disease, previous sensitization to an unknown agent being an important factor in determining which components of the disease process will predominate.

There is no definitive correlation of pulmonary alveolar proteinosis with exposure to a variety of inhalants, occupation, race, nationality or geographic location. It has been postulated that pulmonary alveolar proteinosis may be another manifestation, perhaps earlier or to a less evocative insult, of the same spectrum of reactions that includes desquamative interstitial pneumonia and diffuse interstitial fibrosis. A patient has been described in whom lung biopsy showed typical pulmonary alveolar proteinosis without thickening or inflammatory infiltration of the alveolar septa and who died 12 years later of pulmonary insufficiency secondary to lung fibrosis.

Kunstling, Goodwin and DesPrez (1976) have detailed the pathologic and pathogenetic findings and relationships of diseases that are characterized by proliferation of granular pneumocystis along the alveolar surface and, in some instances, shedding into the alveolar spaces.

Clinical Manifestations

The clinical manifestations of pulmonary alveolar proteinosis are extremely varied. The usual clinical picture is characterized by progressive dyspnea and cough, which, in older children, may be productive of yellow sputum; there is also cyanosis, fatigue and weight loss. In cases in the pediatric age range, which often present before one year of age, vomiting and diarrhea may be the earliest manifestations. The onset may be abrupt or insidious and not infrequently is ushered in by a febrile illness. Hemoptysis occasionally occurs. Physical findings are relatively few and usually consist of only a few scattered rales and, rarely, clubbing of the fingers and toes. The disease, in some instances, may assume a comparatively chronic course; in such instances, growth failure is common.

The vital capacity is reduced to a variable degree. The maximum breathing capacity is normal or slightly reduced. The oxygen saturation of the hemoglobin of the arterial blood may be normal or reduced.

Immunologic examination of some children with the disease has revealed various types of immunologic deficiency states, including thymic alymphoplasia. Not surprisingly, therefore, complicating infections occur frequently. Fungal infection is common, Nocardia being the most frequent offending organism.

The disease may be suspected from changes noted on the chest roentgenogram. Typically, there is a fine, diffuse, feathery perihilar increase in lung density radiating in a butterfly pattern similar to that seen in pulmonary edema, but without cardiac enlargement (Fig. 2). Occasionally, the infiltration assumes a slightly nodular pattern, but is more homogeneous than that usually seen in idiopathic pulmonary hemosiderosis. The roentgenographic changes are due to the presence of the alveolar fluid.

If sputum specimens can be obtained, PAS-positive material may be demonstrated by cytologic examination. Elevation of the serum lactic acid dehydrogenase (LDH) in the absence of hepatic disease is reported to occur

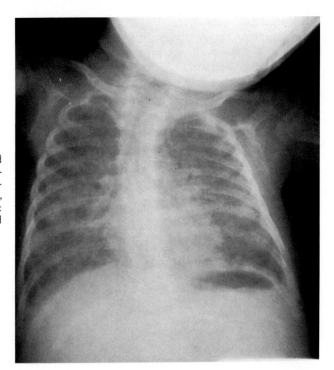

Figure 2. Posteroanterior chest roentgenogram in a three-month-old infant with pulmonary alveolar proteinosis showing diffuse, feathery infiltration. (From Wilkinson, R. H., Blanc, W. A., and Hagstrom, J. W. C.: *Pediatrics, 41*:510, 1968. Reproduced with permission.)

commonly; the LDH returns to normal levels in patients who recover. Lung biopsy is the more frequently used method of making the diagnosis antemortem.

Pulmonary alveolar proteinosis must be differentiated from diseases of the heart with associated pulmonary edema and from the pulmonary disorders characterized by fibrosis, sarcoidosis and fungal infections of the lung. *Pneumocystis carinii* infection can present a similar clinical picture. Lung biopsy is necessary to clarify the diagnosis in most instances.

Prognosis

The prognosis is generally unfavorable. In adults, the disease may remain stable for considerable periods of time and spontaneous improvement may occur; however, death eventually occurs in about one-half of the patients from progressive filling of alveoli or from secondary infection. However, in children, the mortality to date is more than 75 per cent, with the illness ranging from a few days up to several months. Secondary bacterial and mycotic infections are particularly common in infants and children and are frequently the cause of death.

Treatment

Various methods of treatment have been attempted. Some degree of reversibility in certain patients is suggested by the clearing of pulmonary roentgenographic changes and improvement in gaseous exchange following aerosol therapy with proteolytic enzymes or pulmonary lavage with saline, heparinized saline or *N*-acetylcysteine, alone or in combination. Of these, lavage appears to be the most promising. Only one lung is irrigated at a time, and several liters of solution and several separate irrigators may be necessary. Irrigation should yield large quantities of surfactant and alveolar macrophages. When there is progression of symptoms, functional impairment and roentgenographic evidence of alveolar filling, pulmonary lavage is indicated. Antibiotics appear to be indicated only in the presence of secondary bacterial infection. In contrast to the results in desquamative interstitial pneumonia, adrenocorticosteroids seem to have no demonstrable benefit.

REFERENCES

Bhagwat, A. G., Wentworth, P., and Conen, P. E.: Observations on the relationship of desquamative interstitial pneumonia and pulmonary alveolar proteinosis in childhood: a pathologic and experimental study. *Dis. Chest, 58*:326, 1970.

Colon, A. R., Lawrence, R. D., Mills, S. D., and O'Connell, E. J.: Childhood pulmonary alveolar proteinosis. *Am. J. Dis. Child., 121*:481, 1971.

Cugell, D. W.: Pulmonary alveolar proteinosis. *J.A.M.A., 234*:80, 1975.

Dangelis, J. A., and Markarian, B.: Pulmonary alveolar proteinosis including pulmonary electron microscopy. *Am. J. Dis. Child., 118*:871, 1969.

Davidson, J. M., and Macleod, W. M.: Pulmonary alveolar proteinosis. *Br. J. Dis. Chest, 63*:13, 1969.

Heppleston, A. G., and Young, A. E.: Alveolar lipo-proteinosis: an ultrastructural comparison of the experimental and human forms. *J. Pathol., 107*:107, 1972.

Hudson, A. R., Halprin, G. M., Miller, J. A., and Kilburn, K. H.: Pulmonary insterstitial fibrosis following alveolar proteinosis. *Chest, 65*:700, 1974.

Kunstling, R. R., Goodwin, R. W., Jr., and DesPrez, R. M.: Diffuse interstitial pulmonary fibrosis (cryptogenic fibrosing alveolitis). *South. Med. J., 69*:479, 1976.

Liebow, A. A., Steer, A., and Billingsley, J. C.: Desquamative interstitial pneumonia. *Am. J. Med., 39*:369, 1965.

Plenck, H. P., et al.: Pulmonary alveolar proteinosis—a new disease? *Radiology, 74*:928, 1960.

Ramirez, R. J.: Pulmonary alveolar proteinosis, treatment by massive bronchopulmonary lavage. *Arch. Intern. Med., 119*:147, 1967.

Ramirez, R. J., and Harlan, W. R., Jr.: Pulmonary alveolar proteinosis. Nature and origin of the alveolar lipid. *Am. J. Med., 45*:502, 1968.

Rosen, S. H., Castleman, B., and Liebow, A. A.: Pulmonary alveolar proteinosis. *N. Engl. J. Med., 258*:1123, 1958.

Spitler, L., Keuppers, F., and Fundenberg, H. H.: Normal macrophage function in pulmonary alveolar proteinosis. *Am. Rev. Resp. Dis., 102*:975, 1970.

Sunderland, W. A., Campbell, R. A., and Edwards, M. J.: Pulmonary alveolar proteinosis and pulmonary cryptococcosis in an adolescent boy. *J. Pediatr., 80*:450, 1972.

Wilkinson, R. H., Blanc, W. A., and Hagshom, J. W. C.: Pulmonary alveolar proteinosis in three infants. *Pediatrics, 41*:510, 1968.

CHAPTER THIRTY-FIVE

IDIOPATHIC PULMONARY ALVEOLAR MICROLITHIASIS

Robert H. High, M.D.

Idiopathic pulmonary alveolar microlithiasis is a rare disease and is uncommonly noted in children. In most instances the abnormality is noted in chest roentgenograms taken because of unrelated suspected or definite bronchopulmonary or cardiac disease. Occasionally the disease is identified in routine "survey" films. To date, somewhat under 200 cases have been reported in the English literature. Most have been reported in adults, although some adolescent patients have been diagnosed and even fewer children and infants have been identified as having this disturbance.

The disease has been reported from many areas of the world. Most patients have been Caucasian or Oriental, although at least one has been reported in a Black. The patients have not had any consistent history of unusual environmental exposure to toxic substances or air-borne agents. No recognized geographic clustering of patients has been detected. No recognized infectious agent has been identified.

Roughly two-thirds of the cases have been in family members. In these instances, females outnumber males in a ratio of approximately two to one. This observation is questioned by some. In nonfamilial cases, the sex prevalence is roughly equal.

The disease is characterized by the intra-alveolar deposition of calcific granules of less than 0.1 to approximately 0.3 mm. in diameter. The deposits initially are most prominent in the lung bases, and gradually, as the disease progresses, involve more and more of the alveoli. The individual deposits are laminated, "onionskin" granules consisting almost exclusively of various calcium and phosphate complexes. Other substances are present in variously small amounts. Occasionally pleural abnormalities are noted.

The mechanism by which the intra-alveolar microliths are produced is, as yet, undefined. There are hypotheses that there are some alveolar or intra-alveolar enzyme abnormalities. Calcium, phosphorus and other metabolic abnormalities have been searched for, but none has been found. Parathyroid function studies have been normal, as have been pathologic studies of the parathyroid tissues. Roentgenographic studies of the bones have been normal. The only extrapulmonary changes in specimens obtained at autopsy are those consistent with anoxemia and cor pulmonale. Other observed abnormalities have been regarded as coincidental.

There have not been enough pulmonary function studies reported in pediatric patients to determine any consistent pattern. In adults, reduction in residual pulmonary volume is definite, with a relentlessly progressive reduction in various pulmonary functions until death ensues from pulmonary insufficiency or cor pulmonale, or both, with right-sided heart failure. The disease is usually fatal by mid-adult life, although occasional patients with this disease have survived into their sixties.

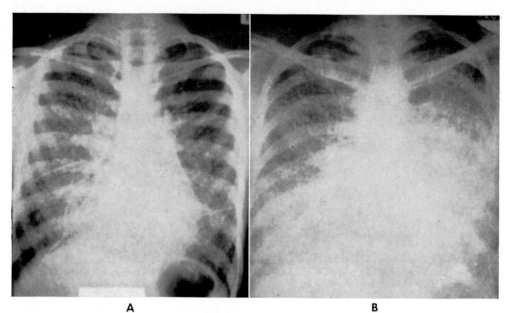

Figure 1. *A,* Roentgenogram taken in February 1954, showing minute miliary dissemination except at the apex and peripheral parts of both lungs. Hairline densities were seen from the hilus to peripheral parts. *B,* Roentgenogram taken in April 1964. Minute miliary dissemination became confluent at the hilus and striated at the peripheral parts of both lungs. (From Oka, S., et al.: *Am. Rev. Resp. Dis.,* 93:612, 1966.)

In children, the disease is usually unassociated with any symptoms, although occasional patients have had chronic cough. As far as can be determined, hemoptysis and the occasional expectoration of an identifiable microlith have not been reported in children. Physical examination is usually nonspecific or normal until the degree of pulmonary insufficiency is great enough to cause clubbing of the fingers, cyanosis and the like.

The diagnosis is generally made roentgenographically and is based on the characteristic "sandstorm" appearance of the lungs (Fig. 1). The changes usually are greatest in the lung bases and gradually involve more of the lungs in adult life until almost all of the alveoli are involved. Occasionally, in adults with long-standing disease, emphysematous blebs may be observed. In this country, one of the most common diseases from which idiopathic pulmonary alveolar microlithiasis is to be differentiated is healed disseminated histoplasmosis. This can readily be done roentgenographically and with other appropriate tests.

The diagnosis can be confirmed with a biopsy of the lungs. Percutaneous needle biopsy is not likely to be successful because the thick fibrous changes in the lung commonly prevent obtaining an adequate specimen of pulmonary tissue. Open biopsy of the lung is therefore recommended. Open biopsy of the lung may be regarded as unnecessary because the roentgenographic changes and the clinical course of the disease are quite characteristic. Open biopsy of the lung is recommended, however, if additional studies can be obtained that add to our knowledge of this rare disease of obscure causation. Roentgenograms of other members of the family should obviously be obtained.

There is no known specific treatment of this disease; until such is found, the disease will pursue a relentlessly progressive course ending in death, usually in early adult life. Supportive and symptomatic treatment is indicated when necessary. Fortunately, most children are asymptomatic and do not require such treatment. Appropriate counseling and sympathetic support are obviously part of the overall management.

REFERENCES

Clark, R. B., and Johnson, F. C.: Idiopathic pulmonary alveolar microlithiasis. *Pediatrics*, 28:650, 1961.

Fuleihan, F. J. D., Abboud, R. T., Balikian, J. P., and Nucho, C. K. N.: Pulmonary alveolar microlithiasis: Lung Function in five cases. *Thorax*, 24:84, 1969.

Hossein, E.: Pulmonary alveolar microlithiasis. *Mich Med.*, 72:691, 1973.

Oka, S., et al.: Pulmonary alveolar microlithiasis. *Am. Rev. Resp. Dis.*, 93:612, 1966.

O'Neill, R. P., Cohn, J. E., and Pellegrino, E. D.: Pulmonary alveolar microlithiasis—a family study. *Ann. Intern. Med.*, 67:957, 1967.

Sosman, M. C., Dodd, G. D., Jones, W. D., and Pillmore, G. U.: Familial occurrence of pulmonary microlithiasis. *Am. J. Roentgenol.*, 77:947, 1957.

Thurairajasingam, S., Dharmasena, B. D., and Kasthuriratna, T.: Pulmonary alveolar microlithiasis. *Australas. Radiol.*, 19:175, 1975.

CHAPTER THIRTY-SIX

PULMONARY HEMOSIDEROSIS

Douglas C. Heiner, M.D.

The term "pulmonary hemosiderosis" indicates an abnormal accumulation of iron as hemosiderin in the lungs. It results from bleeding into the lungs and is much more likely to follow diffuse alveolar hemorrhage than bleeding from large arteries or arterioles. It may be primary in the lungs or secondary to cardiac or systemic disease. In most instances in which it is primary, the cause is unknown, but a significant proportion of cases occurring in infants and a small percentage in older children appear to be related to the ingestion of cow milk. Pulmonary hemosiderosis in adults is commonly secondary to cardiac disease involving left ventricular failure or pulmonary venous hypertension such as occurs in mitral stenosis. This elevation of venous pressure may result in recurrent or chronic capillary oozing of blood into the alveoli with resultant hemosiderosis (brown induration) of the lungs. In children, on the other hand, primary pulmonary hemosiderosis is more frequent than the secondary varieties. The majority of all primary cases occur during childhood.

Although the first description of the pathologic features of brown induration of the lungs was by Virchow in 1864, the clinical picture of idiopathic pulmonary hemosiderosis was not reported until Ceelen's description in 1931. The first antemortem diagnosis was recorded by Waldenström in 1940, and knowledge of the disease has since been amplified by many authors. In Europe, the idiopathic form is frequently referred to as "Ceelen's disease" or "Ceelen-Gellerstedt's disease."

It seems likely that several disease processes may lead to primary as well as to secondary pulmonary hemosiderosis, and as time progresses, the diagnosis of idiopathic pulmonary hemosiderosis should apply to a smaller and smaller proportion of patients. At present, it is convenient to classify and describe pulmonary hemosiderosis as follows:

Primary pulmonary hemosiderosis
1. Isolated
2. With cardiac or pancreatic involvement
3. With glomerulonephritis (Goodpasture's syndrome)
4. With sensitivity to cow milk

Secondary pulmonary hemosiderosis
1. With primary cardiac disease
2. With primary collagen vascular or purpuric disease

ISOLATED PRIMARY PULMONARY HEMOSIDEROSIS

This diagnosis refers to those instances in which no cause and no significant associated disease are apparent. It may occur at any age, but occurs chiefly in children and young adults. It is commonly referred to as idiopathic pulmonary hemosiderosis.

Symptoms and Physical Findings

The most helpful clinical signs are iron deficiency anemia, recurrent or chronic pulmonary symptoms including cough, hemoptysis, dyspnea, wheezing and often cyanosis, and characteristic abnormalities on chest roentgenograms. Hemoptysis in children is an especially helpful clue to the diagnosis, although one must be aware that sometimes it is difficult to determine the origin of blood when there are both coughing and vomiting. In some infants, swallowed blood from the lungs is vomited without coughing, so that the possibility of a pulmonary source of bleeding should be kept in mind in children with unexplained hematemesis, particularly when there are roentgenographic abnormalities in the lungs. Any of the features noted above may be the first manifestation of the disease. For example, subjects have been recorded in whom there was apparently an asymptomatic iron deficiency anemia as an initial single abnormal finding. Others have had hemoptysis, persistent cough or another pulmonary symptom before anemia was apparent. Pulmonary symptoms may occur with or without detectable roentgenographic abnormalities, or there may be striking roentgenographic changes before pulmonary symptoms or other features are clearly manifest. The clinical picture is usually characterized by recurrent episodes of pulmonary bleeding during which there is fever, tachycardia, tachypnea, leukocytosis, an elevated sedimentation rate, abdominal pain and often other findings suggesting a bacterial pneumonia. Occasionally, pneumonia appears to be confirmed by positive sputum or throat cultures, and only long-term follow-up combined with an awareness of the possibility of pulmonary hemosiderosis leads to the correct diagnosis. Poor weight gain and easy fatigue are common in subjects with moderate to severe disease. Physical findings vary, depending on the status of the patient at the time of examination. There may be pallor, dyspnea, bronchial or suppressed breath sounds, rales, rhonchi, wheezing and an emphysematous chest. Liver or spleen enlargement is sometimes found and may be transient.

Laboratory and Roentgenologic Findings

The anemia is typically microcytic and hypochromic, and the serum iron concentration is low in spite of an excessive accumulation of iron in the lungs. Trace labeling of red blood cells with radioisotopes has shown that large volumes of blood may exude into the lungs, the iron subsequently becoming largely sequestered in macrophages where it is unavailable for use in the formation of new red blood cells. Animal experiments suggest, however, that there may be slow utilization of hemosiderin iron from the lungs for hematopoiesis, and it is possible that in human pulmonary hemosiderosis the rate of deposition of iron in the lungs in most instances merely exceeds the rate of utilization. The fact that symptoms, chest roentgenograms and anemia sometimes clear completely indicates that in remission there may be significant net removal of iron from the lungs.

There is a variable hematologic response to oral or intramuscular iron. Some patients have a good reticulocyte and hemoglobin response, but others appear to have defective hematopoiesis while the disease process is active. Many have reticulocytosis during periods of active pulmonary bleeding whether or not iron therapy is administered, and this, along with mild jaundice and an elevated urobilinogen excretion, may lead to an erroneous diagnosis of hemolytic anemia. This diagnosis seems even more credible in the few subjects who have a positive direct Coombs test result, suggesting that anti-red blood cell antibodies are adherent to the erythrocyte surfaces. Circulating cold agglutinins may also be found, and like a positive Coombs test result, suggest the presence of an unusual immune response.

Eosinophilia has been present in one-fifth to one-eighth of the reported cases, but experience suggests that eosinophil counts fluctuate markedly in this disease and that the likelihood of finding eosinophilia is proportional to the number of times it is looked for in a given case. If frequent differential leukocyte or absolute eosinophil counts are obtained, more than this proportion of subjects will be found to have eosinophilia.

Stool guaiac test results are frequently positive, and the presumption is that this is due to swallowed blood from the tracheobronchial tree. Reasonable evidence for this presumption comes from the fact that most patients with pulmonary hemosiderosis produce bloody sputum, some of which is obviously swallowed. In addition, the gastric juice usually contains iron-laden macrophages (siderophages) from the lungs even when there is no obvious hemoptysis.

The finding of siderophages in the stomach in the presence of otherwise unexplained pulmonary disease is good presumptive evidence of pulmonary hemosiderosis (Fig. 1). It is the simplest reliable diagnostic laboratory test in in-

fants and young children. The Prussian blue reaction with potassium ferrocyanide and hydrochloric acid provides a good stain, the hemosiderin granules within macrophages acquiring an easily recognized deep blue color. Siderophages may also be found in the sputum or in washings of the tracheobronchial tree, or within the alveoli of biopsy specimens obtained by needle aspiration or open operation. Most workers accept siderophages in gastric or bronchial secretions as diagnostic if typical clinical features are present and are not accompanied by evidence of extrapulmonary disease.

A biopsy diagnosis is considered necessary by some workers. The pathologic findings by light microscopy of lung tissue have been summarized in detail by Soergel and Sommers (1962). They include alveolar epithelial hyperplasia and degeneration with excessive shedding of cells, large numbers of siderocytes, varying amounts of interstitial fibrosis and mast cell accumulation,

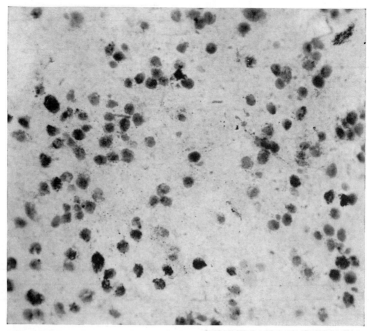

Figure 1.   Siderophages in gastric washings of a 15-year-old boy with chronic pulmonary disease, recurrent hemoptysis and iron deficiency anemia. Bronchial washings showed similar iron-laden macrophages. There was no evidence of cardiovascular, renal, collagen or purpuric disease, but multiple precipitins to cow milk were present in high titer. Chronic cough and hemoptysis ceased coincidentally with removal of milk from the diet. Prussian blue stain × 150.

elastic fiber degeneration, and sclerotic vascular changes. Most of these features were present in the specimen shown in Figure 2. Vasculitis is usually absent, but, if found, suggests that the disorder may not be primary, but rather secondary to a systemic collagen vascular disease.

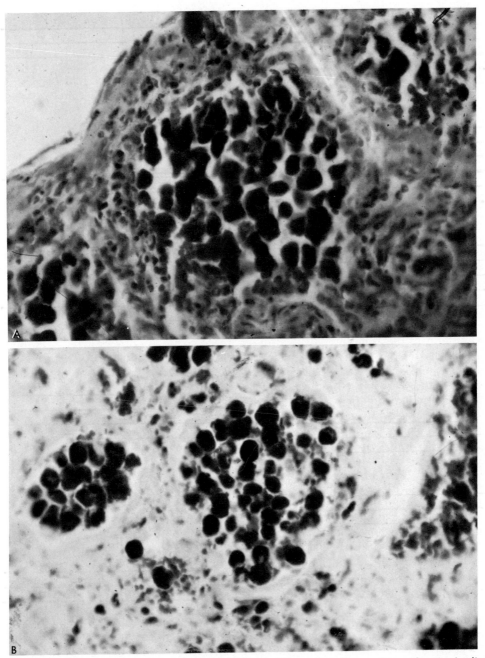

Figure 2. Microscopic sections of lung from three-year-old boy with pulmonary hemosiderosis who died several hours after a diagnostic needle biopsy of the lung. *A,* Hematoxylin and eosin stain showing iron-containing macrophages filling an alveolus, marked alveolar epithelial proliferation, fibrosis and fresh intra-alveolar bleeding. *B,* Prussian blue stain showing hyperplastic alveolar walls and alveoli containing red cells and many deeply stained iron-laden macrophages ($\times$ 500).

Immunofluorescent studies reveal fibrinogen or fibrin in the alveolar spaces, but immunoglobulin deposits and complement are usually not demonstrable. Electron microscopy has revealed focal ruptures of the capillary basement membranes with collagen deposition and hydropic changes in the pneumocytes, but normal endothelial cells. These findings are thought to distinguish the histologic features of primary or idiopathic pulmonary hemosiderosis from those of Goodpasture's syndrome, in which linear immunoglobulin and complement deposition along the basement membrane has been shown by immunofluorescence, and vascular damage with wide endothelial gaps and a diffusely fragmented basement membrane with a thin electron dense margin have been shown by electron microscopy. However, some subjects with Goodpastrure's syndrome do not have demonstrable immunoglobulin deposits in the lung, and some patients with "idiopathic pulmonary hemosiderosis" have immunofluorescent evidence of linear immunoglobulin deposition in the renal glomeruli without clinical evidence of renal disease. Hence, there may be some overlapping between these two diseases, especially in the young adult patient.

Lung biopsy is justified in infants or young children in whom clinical findings are atypical, or if the diagnosis is still in doubt after all simpler procedures have been done, including a careful search for siderophages in several specimens of gastric juice, sputum or bronchial washings. Needle aspiration biopsy may be as risky as open biopsy under anesthesia, or more risky. The author observed one subject in whom the clinical picture suggested primary pulmonary hemosiderosis with active pulmonary lesions and in whom needle biopsy was performed under local anesthesia. The procedure was considered benign when it was done, but seemed to be the turning point to deterioration with a rapidly progressive downhill course, massive pulmonary hemorrhage and a fatal termination several hours later. Postmortem examination confirmed the clinical diagnosis. Other authors have suggested that needle biopsy is not without danger in this disease.

A search should be made for serum precipitins to cow milk and for circulating antiglomerular basement antibody in every case, since these constitute noninvasive studies that may be helpful in arriving at the more specific diagnoses of pulmonary hemosiderosis with sensitivity to cow milk or Goodpasture's syndrome, respectively.

Roentgenographic abnormalities vary from minimal transient infiltrates to massive parenchymal involvement with secondary atelectasis, emphysema and hilar lymphadenopathy. The findings are somewhat variable from patient to patient and may change in a given subject with each new bleeding or with clinical remission. Diffuse, soft perihilar infiltrates are common. In some subjects, the appearance is similar to that of pulmonary edema. In others it is more like bronchial or lobar pneumonia, and in still others it may resemble the findings in miliary tuberculosis, Gaucher's disease or Wegener's granulomatosis. Thus, there frequently is thickening of interlobar septa with horizontal lines and fine nodulations suggesting interstitial fibrosis. The resulting reticular or reticulonodular pattern may be widespread, but is often present chiefly in the lower lobes and is likely to persist for months or years after acute infiltrative lesions have cleared in those who survive. Illustrative roentgenograms are shown in Figures 3 and 4.

Pulmonary function tests have demonstrated impaired diffusion, decreased compliance (stiff lungs) and airway obstruction. The findings are most marked during and immediately after active intrapulmonary bleeding. One may find reductions in vital capacity, total lung capacity, one-second forced expiratory volume, maximal breathing capacity, arterial oxygen tension, arte-

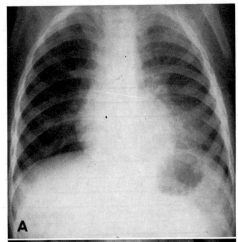

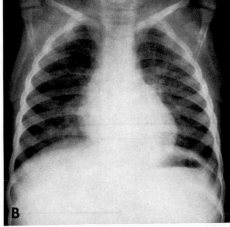

Figure 3. *A*, Roentgenogram of a boy with primary pulmonary hemosiderosis of two years' duration during an exacerbation at 27 months of age. Note soft perihilar infiltrates, most evident along the left cardiac border. *B*, Same subject four months later when asymptomatic. Note decrease in soft infiltrates, but prominent bilateral reticulonodular pattern suggesting interstitial fibrosis.

rial carbon dioxide tension and arterial oxygen saturation in individual subjects.

Cardiac catheterization has revealed variable findings, some patients showing no abnormalities, others having pulmonary arterial hypertension and even right ventricular failure as a result of cor pulmonale. Significant abnormalities in pulmonary function and demonstrated pulmonary hypertension indicate a more guarded prognosis than if these physiologic parameters

are normal, although most deaths are due to active bleeding rather than to pulmonary or cardiac insufficiency.

Complications

The potential danger of needle biopsy in idiopathic pulmonary hemosiderosis has been mentioned. From the use of radioiodinated serum albumin for pulmonary scanning, severe reactions have been recorded that were perhaps due to iodine sensitivity associated with the use of oral Lugol's solu-

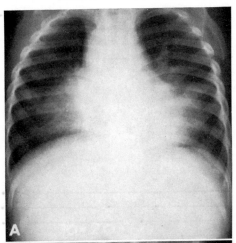

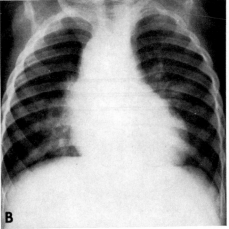

Figure 4. *A*, Roentgenogram of a boy with primary pulmonary hemosiderosis at two years of age, showing diffuse, soft perihilar infiltrates, somewhat suggestive of pulmonary edema. *B*, Same subject six months later, showing less pronounced infiltrates in right middle lobe and left hilar regions, and some horizontal septal lines suggesting fibrosis.

tion to block thyroidal uptake of radioiodine. One subject has been reported who had an exacerbation of pulmonary symptoms when given aerosolized Isuprel for wheezing; he improved markedly when the inhalations were ceased. One must be on guard against requesting unnecessary studies and should be alert to untoward reactions from drugs. Occasionally there is sudden unexpected death, and in some subjects this can occur during the first apparent episode of pulmonary bleeding. In such cases there may be minimal or no frank hemoptysis, the diagnosis being first suspected at postmortem examination. The usual cause of death is respiratory failure or shock associated with massive intrapulmonary hemorrhages.

Treatment

When possible, treatment should be preceded by vigorous attempts to rule out known factors that might be important in the causation of or that might aggravate idiopathic hemosiderosis. These include appropriate studies to detect heart disease, diffuse collagen vascular disease and thrombocytopenic purpura, and attempts to uncover sensitivity to drugs, inhaled substances and foods. Acute crises should be treated with oxygen. Severely dyspneic patients may benefit from its administration by intermittent positive pressure, and persistent bleeding occasionally may be reversed by more prolonged periods of positive end-expiratory pressure (PEEP) breathing. Blood transfusions are indicated to correct severe anemia or shock. The blood should be obtained from a healthy nonallergic donor and carefully cross-matched. It should be given under close supervision, since several acutely ill patients have been thought to do less well during and immediately after transfusions. ACTH, 10 to 25 units daily, or hydrocortisone, 4 mg. per kilogram of body weight per day, by intravenous infusion is recommended. Critically ill subjects are prob-

ably best kept on intravenous fluid therapy with nothing by mouth for 24 to 48 hours. After this, foods may be introduced, and prednisone, 2 mg. per kilogram, may be given orally instead of ACTH or hydrocortisone. After a clinical remission has been well established, the corticosteroid level can be gradually decreased until the drug is discontinued or until pulmonary symptoms recur. If maintenance corticosteroid therapy is necessary, an attempt should be made to establish the minimum dose that will suppress symptoms, but not produce undesirable side-effects. The drug should be continued at this dose for three months before again trying to discontinue it. Growth retardation and other steroid side-effects may be minimized in some patients by administering the corticosteroid on three consecutive days of each week, or by giving the amount calculated for two days as a single dose every second day at breakfast. If pulmonary disease recurs at any time, corticosteroids should be reinstituted, or the dosage temporarily increased, in an attempt to suppress the process. Control of the disease should be judged by symptoms, hematologic studies and roentgenographic findings. Many subjects with idiopathic pulmonary hemosiderosis are in constant danger of relapse and even death; hence, careful long-term medical supervision is indicated.

Three additional approaches to therapy are worth consideration. The first is a concerted effort to provide a hypoallergenic diet. There is evidence that milk restrictions may be of significant benefit in certain infants who are ingesting large amounts of milk (see section on Pulmonary Hemosiderosis with Sensitivity to Cow Milk). In older children and adults, milk restriction usually has proved to be of little or no obvious benefit. If "idiopathic" pulmonary hemosiderosis is in fact usually an allergic or "immunoallergic" disorder, the situation may be analogous to gastrointestinal and food allergies in which milk sensitivity is common in infancy but is much less important in older subjects. A two- or three-month trial period on a milk-free diet is innocuous and should always be considered, particularly if there was chronic rhinitis, recurrent or persistent otitis media, atopic dermatitis, wheezing or frequent respiratory symptoms early in life while the child was ingesting relatively large amounts of milk. Subjects who have the onset of symptoms only later in life when milk intake has been reduced are unlikely to respond to a milk-free diet; nevertheless, it is the author's belief that meticulous efforts to identify allergens, including the judicious use of diets from which likely allergens have been eliminated, may be fruitful. Recording of the food and beverages ingested for the 24 hours before the onset of each exacerbation may give a clue to an allergenic food. Efforts to quantitate reaginic and precipitating antibodies to food proteins and to demonstrate a decrease in total serum IgE on elimination of a dietary item followed by an increased IgE when the food is again ingested may prove helpful in individual cases.

The second measure to consider is the use of additional immunosuppressant drugs, such as azathioprine, cyclophosphamide or chlorambucil. Azathioprine (Imuran) has been administered most frequently with apparent success. The dose ranged from 1.2 to 5 mg. per kg. per day. Two or 3 mg. per kg. per day is the usually recommended initial dose. Under most circumstances, this would be given in combination with prednisone in doses of 5 to 20 mg. every six hours during episodes of acute bleeding. The steroids are then gradually shifted as the clinical course permits to single doses of 10 to 40 mg. administered every second morning. Each immunosuppressive drug may be expected to have the effect of lowering the required dose of the other, thereby minimizing undesirable side-effects. Each may be increased at times of exacerbation or decreased in the presence of side-effects. An attempt should probably be made to stop all drugs after a year has elapsed in which there are no symptoms, anemia or roentgen evidences of disease activity. There should be little hesitation, however, in reinstituting single or double drug immunotherapy should the disease again become active. Splenectomy has been suggested as an additional method of attaining nonspecific suppression of the immune response, but its value remains uncertain.

A final measure that may be worthy of trial in subjects who respond poorly to other measures or who have chronic pulmonary symptoms or persistent roentgenologic findings is the use of the iron-chelating drug deferoxamine (desferrioxamine). This agent has been found to be useful in removing excessive accumulations of tissue iron from subjects with transfusion hemosiderosis, acute iron toxicity, idiopathic hemochromatosis in whom repeated phlebotomies are not feasible, and other conditions. Although experience to date suggests that hemosiderin sequestered in pulmonary macrophages is quite resistant to deferoxamine chelation, Cavalieri (1963) was encouraged by the use of the drug. Present evidence indicates that urinary iron excretion in subjects with excessive iron accumulation is proportional to the number of grams of deferoxamine administered up to 1.6 gm. daily or about 25 mg. per kilogram per day. The drug seems to be most effective when given intramuscularly in divided doses eight hours apart. Levels of 24-hour urinary iron excretion should be studied for several days before and after institution of chelate therapy. If the daily urinary iron excretion is increased by more than 3 or 4 mg. per gram of administered deferoxamine or by 8 to 10 mg. per 24 hours, there is evidence of the removal of excessively accumulated iron. An increase in serum iron levels should also occur, and if iron deficiency anemia is present, it may improve. Periodic checks of 24-hour urinary iron excretion should be made with any long-term chelate therapy in order to indicate its continued value.

PRIMARY PULMONARY HEMOSIDEROSIS WITH CARDIAC OR PANCREATIC INVOLVEMENT

Some subjects with idiopathic pulmonary hemosiderosis have been found at postmortem examination to have inflammatory infiltrates in the myocardium. These have varied from minimal scattered lesions to extensive myocardial disease. If significant myocardial disease is present when the pulmonary disease is discovered, it may be difficult or impossible to decide whether the pulmonary hemosiderosis is a primary or secondary phenomenon. There may be distinctive alterations demonstrable on lung biopsy that may help in the differential diagnosis. From a clinical point of view, when myocarditis is the primary disorder, the heart should be large and other evidences of congestive failure should be present early in the course of the disease; whereas if the heart is normal in size at the time pulmonary hemosiderosis is recognized and then enlarges, one can assume that the lung disease is primary rather than secondary to myocarditis.

The treatment of idiopathic pulmonary hemosiderosis is the same whether or not myocarditis is present, with one exception. If congestive failure is detected, it should be treated appropriately with digitalis, diuretics and other measures of recognized value.

One subject has been reported who developed both exocrine pancreatic deficiency and diabetes mellitus, his clinical course suggesting elements of hemachromatosis as well as idiopathic pulmonary hemosiderosis. A second subject with idiopathic pulmonary hemosiderosis developed diabetes, bilateral penetrating corneal ulcerations

and myocarditis. In such cases, it may be extremely difficult to decide whether the pulmonary disease is most appropriately classified as the primary disorder or whether it is simply a major secondary manifestation of a more generalized connective tissue or "immunoallergic" disease. At present, pulmonary hemosiderosis may be classified as primary or idiopathic if it is the major manifestation and if the associated findings do not fit into any well recognized syndrome such as polyarteritis nodosa.

PRIMARY PULMONARY HEMOSIDEROSIS WITH GLOMERULONEPHRITIS (GOODPASTURE'S SYNDROME)

In 1918, Goodpasture described a patient with pulmonary bleeding and glomerulonephritis. Although it is not certain that his patient had primary pulmonary hemosiderosis, the eponym "Goodpasture's syndrome" has been applied to the association of primary pulmonary hemosiderosis and proliferative or membranous glomerulonephritis. There is some debate as to whether Goodpasture's syndrome is different from or related to isolated pulmonary hemosiderosis. Several authors have pointed out possible differences in the clinical picture and in pathologic findings in the lung to support the contention that they are distinct entities. Thus, it is known that Goodpasture's syndrome usually occurs in young adult males and is rare or nonexistent in infants. It is more likely to be fatal than is isolated pulmonary hemosiderosis, although neither disease has a generally good prognosis. Examination of lung tissue in Goodpasture's syndrome has been reported to show necrotizing alveolitis with degenerative changes of the alveolar capillary basement membranes, occasional arteritis, and relatively little alveolar epithelial proliferation or hemosiderosis, all of which are somewhat in contrast with the findings in isolated pulmonary disease. The finding by immunofluorescence of immunoglobulin and complement deposits along the alveolar septal walls has been thought to be more characteristic of Goodpasture's syndrome, as has ultrastructural evidence of diffuse vascular disease with wide endothelial gaps and fragmented capillary basement membranes having electron-dense margins. Linear immunofluorescence of renal glomeruli has generally been considered characteristic of Goodpasture's syndrome, but even this finding is not present in all patients with "idiopathic" pulmonary hemosiderosis associated with glomerulonephritis. In any event, the clinical disease usually is characterized by initial pulmonary involvement with hemoptysis, iron deficiency anemia and typical siderophages. Thus, in the early stages before evidences of renal disease appear, the disease may be clinically indistinguishable from isolated pulmonary hemosiderosis. Death may result either from the renal disease or from pulmonary hemorrhage. In a few subjects, renal disease becomes apparent before, or concomitantly with, the pulmonary disease.

Treatment is the same as that described for isolated pulmonary hemosiderosis, corticosteroids being the most helpful single therapeutic agent. Results of therapy are much better when kidney lesions have not progressed to the point of renal insufficiency. If a remission occurs, careful follow-up is mandatory, and attempts should be made to suppress recurrent pulmonary or renal disease as soon as either appears. There have been reports of cessation of pulmonary hemorrhaging in subjects with Goodpasture's syndrome following bilateral nephrectomy. Whether this will prove to be a generally applicable procedure remains to be determined. It may be an approach worth considering when renal disease is severe or pulmonary disease is otherwise uncontrollable.

PRIMARY PULMONARY HEMOSIDEROSIS WITH SENSITIVITY TO COW MILK

In 1962, four patients were described who fulfilled the criteria for primary pulmonary hemosiderosis in that each had recurrent pulmonary disease, hemoptysis, iron deficiency anemia, and iron-laden macrophages in gastric or bronchial washings or at lung biopsy. Additional distinctive features included unusually high titers of serum precipitins to multiple constituents of cow milk, positive intradermal skin tests to various cow milk proteins, chronic rhinitis, recurrent otitis media, and growth retardation. The symptoms of each patient improved when cow milk was removed from the diet, and returned with reintroduction of milk. Since this report, the author has attended several subjects with proved pulmonary hemosiderosis and multiple precipitins to cow milk in high titer who improved after removal of milk from the diet. Serums from other patients with an established diagnosis have been sent to the author, and about half of these have been found to have multiple precipitins to cow milk. Each of those with precipitins was felt by his physician to have much less hemoptysis or none at all and to show general improvement when cow milk was removed from his diet. An almost immediate clearing of chronic rhinitis and cough in several subjects who were placed on a milk-free diet seems to have provided an early clue that a lasting improvement would result in the pulmonary status. Most of the subjects having an important element of sensitivity to cow milk were small infants, although one was 15 years of age.

A few subjects with this disorder have mild to moderate enlargement of the liver or spleen. Others have hypertrophy of the tonsils and adenoids, sometimes of sufficient degree to cause respiratory obstruction with secondary pulmonary hypertension and cor pulmonale. In addition, there often is an increase in the levels of serum immunoglobulins, particularly IgA and IgE. These findings in conjunction with high levels of precipitating antibodies to food proteins suggest a general stimulation of the immunologic apparatus. This is further substantiated by the fact that these findings usually return to normal upon institution of a milk-free diet.

It should be emphasized that not all subjects with primary pulmonary hemosiderosis have unusual precipitins to cow milk, and some without this finding do not change dramatically when on a milk-free diet. Nevertheless, two subjects with proved diagnoses, but without multiple precipitins, have been felt by competent pediatricians to clearly improve on a milk-free diet, and the one who was challenged with milk reintroduction had an immediate recurrence of symptoms. This suggests that in at least some subjects with pulmonary hemosiderosis and clinical sensitivity to milk, demonstrable precipitins may not be an essential part of the disease. One must conclude either that antibodies in subprecipitating quantities can be etiologic factors or that antibodies per se may simply indicate a vigorous immune response and may be unrelated to the pathogenesis of the hypersensitive state. The point is unsettled. A few subjects continue to have active pulmonary disease with bleeding and succumb while on a milk-free diet. This suggests either multiple etiologies or diverse exacerbating factors. In some instances, it may be impossible to sort out etiologic and aggravating factors, but every effort should be made to relate these to relapses, and their avoidance to remissions. The characteristic remitting nature of all forms of primary pulmonary hemosiderosis makes this a particularly challenging task.

There are several similarities between subjects having pulmonary hemosiderosis with sensitivity to cow milk and infants who have milk-induced gastrointestinal bleeding and iron deficiency anemia. Both are likely to have multiple precipitins to cow milk in high titer, and both are usually recognized between the ages of six months and two years. Symptoms and abnormal bleeding can be repeatedly induced in each by the ingestion of cow milk, and symptom-free intervals without bleeding occur on a milk-free diet. There seems to be a direct relation between the amount of milk ingested and the severity of symptoms and bleeding in both groups. Some in each category become less sensitive to cow milk as they grow older. One observable difference is that most patients with milk-induced gastrointestinal bleeding and iron deficiency anemia seldom have positive intradermal skin test results to milk proteins, whereas those with milk-related pulmonary hemosiderosis do. However, neither group commonly has reaginic antibodies to milk demonstrable by Prausnitz-Küstner reactions or by the radioallergosorbent test (RAST).

The treatment of subjects with milk-related pulmonary hemosiderosis is identical with that described previously under Idiopathic Pulmonary Hemosiderosis. Cow milk and milk products should be removed from the diet until a complete remission has been attained. Subsequent challenge with cow milk in moderate amounts (16 to 32 ounces daily) for several weeks is probably justified in a patient who is not critically ill in an effort to confirm a relation of milk ingestion to symptoms. If respiratory tract symptoms of any kind recur when milk is reintroduced and clear when it is again eliminated, a milk-free diet should be maintained indefinitely. The same may be said if a drop in total serum IgE follows elimination of cow milk from the diet and a subsequent rise follows milk reintroduction. An aliquot of each serum should be frozen and retested at one time under identical conditions in order to confirm the validity of any observed variations in IgE levels. Some subjects are able to tolerate milk with minimal symptoms after a milk-free diet for six months to a year. Nevertheless, persistent and recurrent pulmonary infiltrates have been found in several such subjects, suggesting that a milk-free diet should have been continued.

The possibility that foods other than cow milk may play a role in occasional instances of pulmonary hemosiderosis should be considered, and if a food comes under suspicion as a result of history, skin tests or immunologic studies, temporary elimination of and a careful diagnostic challenge with the food is warranted. A suggested technique to help identify other offending dietary constituents is that of placing the subject on a protein-free synthetic diet such as Vivonex* for three weeks. If symptoms become quiescent, well cooked meats, vegetables and fruits are added one at a time at intervals of four days. They are given twice daily in generous proportions. If it is possible to demonstrate a relation between the ingestion of a specific food and the occurrence of respiratory tract symptoms on two separate occasions with amelioration when the food is carefully avoided, that food is completely withheld from the diet for a year, and thereafter is permitted only infrequently and in minimal quantities. Cereals, eggs, fish and other foods can also be added in this manner after a satisfactory basic diet has been achieved.

PULMONARY HEMOSIDEROSIS SECONDARY TO HEART DISEASE

Any form of heart disease that results in a chronic increase in pulmonary venous and capillary pressure may theoretically lead to diapedesis of red cells into the alveoli and secondary pulmonary hemosiderosis. The most common defect causing this sequence of events is mitral stenosis, but it has occurred in chronic left ventricular failure of several varieties. If significant heart disease is present, therefore, one must

*Eaton Laboratories.

consider this in the interpretation of iron-laden macrophages in gastric and bronchial washings, in sputum and even in lung biopsies. In these instances, the burden of proof is on the person who suggests an origin other than cardiac. According to some authors, even the pathologic findings in biopsy sections may look enough like those of idiopathic pulmonary hemosiderosis to be difficult to distinguish. Others, however, report distinctive features in hemosiderosis secondary to heart disease, and list concentric hypertrophy of pulmonary arterioles, thickened alveolar capillary basement membranes, and an interstitial diapedesis of red blood cells as findings that are not seen in the primary pulmonary forms of the disease.

If mitral stenosis, cor triatriatum or infradiaphragmatic drainage of the pulmonary veins is present in association with pulmonary hemosiderosis, a vigorous program of medical therapy followed by surgical repair of the obstructive lesion is mandatory, since reversal of the disease process is otherwise unlikely. Special diagnostic procedures, including cardiac catheterization with measurement of the gradient across the mitral valve or other sites of obstruction, and selective angiocardiograms to define precisely the pathologic anatomy, may be necessary to establish an accurate diagnosis.

If chronic myocardial disease or another cause of left ventricular failure is primarily at fault, every effort must be made to determine the cause of the disorder and to provide appropriate medical and surgical therapy.

PULMONARY HEMOSIDEROSIS AS A MANIFESTATION OF DIFFUSE COLLAGEN-VASCULAR OR PURPURIC DISEASE

A number of instances have been recorded in which the lesions of polyarteritis nodosa have been limited to a few organs, including pulmonary involvement with hemosiderosis. In such instances, it may initially be impossible to distinguish this disease from primary pulmonary hemosiderosis except by biopsy. Nevertheless, with or without therapy, the passage of time may result in involvement of other organs, and this may lead to a suspicion of polyarteritis and also provide more accessible material for biopsy. Sometimes pulmonary hemosiderosis occurs as part of Wegener's granuloma, which is considered by some to be a variant of polyarteritis nodosa involving chiefly the nasal septum, lungs, spleen, liver and kidney. Other connective tissue diseases, including lupus erythematosus, rheumatic fever and rheumatoid arthritis, have occasionally occurred in association with pulmonary hemosiderosis, often with a diffuse vasculitis. Treatment of diffuse collagen-vascular disease with pulmonary hemosiderosis is much the same as that outlined for idiopathic pulmonary hemosiderosis. It should also include any measures or precautions indicated for the management of the connective tissue disease itself.

Several subjects have been reported to have pulmonary hemosiderosis in association with anaphylactoid purpura, and others in association with thrombocytopenic purpura. When either occurs, treatment must be directed at the basic disease as well as at the pulmonary complication. Splenectomy is likely to be particularly helpful in thrombocytopenic purpura with pulmonary hemosiderosis if an early and lasting remission does not occur with steroid therapy alone.

REFERENCES

Anspach, W. E.: Pulmonary hemosiderosis. *Am. J. Roentgenol., 41*:592, 1939.

Apt, L., Pollycove, M., and Ross, J. F.: Idiopathic pulmonary hemosiderosis: a study of the anemia and iron distribution using radioiron and radiochromium. *J. Clin. Invest., 36*:1150, 1957.

Azen, E. A., and Clatanoff, D. V.: Prolonged sur-

vival in Goodpasture's syndrome. *Arch. Intern. Med., 114*:453, 1964.

Boat, T. F., Polmar, S. H., Whitman, V., Kleinerman, J. I., Stern, R. C., and Doershuk, C. F.: Hyperreactivity to cow milk in young children with pulmonary hemosiderosis and cor pulmonale secondary to nasopharyngeal obstruction. *J. Pediatr., 87*:23, 1975.

Beirne, G. J., and Brennan, J. T.: Glomerulonephritis associated with hydrocarbon solvents: mediated by anti-glomerular basement membrane antibody. *Arch. Environ. Health, 25*:365, 1972.

Bronson, S. M.: Idiopathic pulmonary hemosiderosis in adults: report of a case and review of the literature. *Am. J. Roentgenol., 83*:269, 1960.

Browning, J. R., and Houghton, J. D.: Idiopathic pulmonary hemosiderosis. *Am. J. Med., 20*:374, 1956.

Byrd, R. B., and Gracey, D. R.: Immunosuppressive treatment of idiopathic pulmonary hemosiderosis. *J.A.M.A., 226*:458, 1973.

Campbell, S.: Pulmonary haemosiderosis and myocarditis. *Arch. Dis. Child., 34*:218, 1959.

Canfield, C. J., Davis, T. E., and Herman, R. H.: Hemorrhagic pulmonary-renal syndrome. *N. Engl. J. Med., 268*:230, 1963.

Case Records of the Massachusetts General Hospital (Case 17–1976). *N. Engl. J. Med., 294*:944, 1976.

Cavalieri, S.: Desferrioxamine with corticosteroids in a case of idiopathic pulmonary hemosiderosis. *Fracastoro, 56*:389, 1963.

Cavalieri, S., and others: Study of two cases of idiopathic pulmonary hemosiderosis. *Minerva Pediatr., 15*:683, 1963.

Ceelen, W.: Die Kreislaufstörungen der Lungen. In Henke, F., and Lubarsch, O. (Eds.): *Handbuch der speziellen pathologischen Anatomie und Histologie.* Vol. 3. Berlin, J. Springer, 1931, pp. 1–163.

Cook, C. D., and Hart, M. C.: Cited by Hill, L. W.: Some advances in pediatric allergy in the last ten years. *Pediatr. Clin. North Am., 11*:17, 1964.

Cooper, A. S.: Idiopathic pulmonary hemosiderosis: report of a case in an adult treated with triamcinolone. *N. Engl. J. Med., 263*:1100, 1960.

DeGowin, R. L., Oda, Y., and Evans, R. H.: Nephritis and lung hemorrhage. Goodpasture's syndrome. *Arch. Intern. Med., 111*:16, 1963.

DeGowin, R. L., Sorensen, L. B., Charleston, D. B., Gottschalk, A., and Greenwald, J. H.: Retention of radio iron in the lungs of a woman with idiopathic pulmonary hemosiderosis. *Ann. Intern. Med., 69*:1213, 1968.

DiMaio, D. J., Zeichner, M. B., and DiMaio, V. J.: Sudden death in a woman with unsuspected idiopathic pulmonary hemosiderosis. *J.A.M.A., 206*:2520, 1968.

Dolan, C. J., Jr., Srodes, C. H., and Duffy, F. D.: Idiopathic pulmonary hemosiderosis. Electron microscopic, immunofluorescent, and iron kinetic studies. *Chest, 68*:577, 1975.

Donald, K. J., Edwards, R. L., and McEvoy, J. D.:

Alveolar capillary basement membrane lesions in Goodpasture's syndrome and idiopathic pulmonary hemosiderosis. *Am. J. Med., 59*:642, 1975.

Editorial: Idiopathic pulmonary haemosiderosis. *Lancet, 1*:979, 1963.

Elgenmark, O., and Kjellberg, S. R.: Hemosiderosis of the lungs—typical roentgenological findings. *Acta Radiol., 29*:32, 1948.

Everett, E. D., Newcomer, K. L., Anderson, J., Bergen, J., and Overholt, E. L.: Goodpasture's syndrome. Response to mercaptopurine and prednisone. *J.A.M.A., 213*:1849, 1970.

Fuleihan, F. J., Abboud, R. T., and Hubaztar, F.: Idiopathic pulmonary hemosiderosis. Case report with pulmonary function studies and review of the literature. *Am. Rev. Resp. Dis., 98*:93, 1968.

Gellerstedt, N.: Über die essentielle anamisierende Form der braunen Lungeninduration. *Acta Pathol. Microbiol. Scand., 16*:386, 1939.

Gilman, P. A., and Zinkham, W. H.: Severe idiopathic pulmonary hemosiderosis in the absence of clinical or radiologic evidence of pulmonary disease. *J. Pediatr., 75*:118, 1969.

Goodpasture, E. W.: Significance of certain pulmonary lesions in relation to the etiology of influenza. *Am. J. Med. Sci., 158*:863, 1919.

Gurewich, V., and Thomas, M. A.: Idiopathic pulmonary hemorrhage in pregnancy. Report of a case suggesting early pulmonary hemosiderosis with clinical recovery after steroid therapy. *N. Engl. J. Med., 261*:1154, 1959.

Halvorsen, S.: Cortisone treatment of idiopathic pulmonary hemosiderosis. *Acta Paediatr., 45*:139, 1956.

Harkavy, J.: Vascular allergy and its systemic manifestations. Washington, D. C., Butterworths, 1963.

Heiner, D. C.: Pulmonary hemosiderosis. In Gellis, S., and Kagan, B. M. (Eds.): *Current Pediatric Therapy, 1966–1967.* Philadelphia, W. B. Saunders Company, 1966, pp. 147–148.

Heiner, D. C., and Rose, B.: Elevated levels of γE (IgE) in conditions other than classical allergy. *J. Allergy, 45*:30, 1970.

Heiner, D. C., Sears, J. W., and Kniker, W. T.: Multiple precipitins to cow's milk in chronic respiratory disease. A syndrome including poor growth, gastrointestinal symptoms, evidence of allergy, iron deficiency anemia, and pulmonary hemosiderosis. *Am. J. Dis. Child., 103*:634, 1962.

Holland, H. H., Hong, R., Davis, N. C., and West, C. D.: Significance of precipitating antibodies to milk proteins in the serum of infants and children. *J. Pediatr., 61*:181, 1962.

Holzel, A.: Primary hemosiderosis followed by exocrine and endocrine pancreatic deficiencies. *Proc. R. Soc. Med., 61*:302, 1968.

Hukill, P. B.: Experimental pulmonary hemosiderosis. The liability of pulmonary iron deposits. *Lab. Invest., 12*:577, 1963.

Hwang, Y-F., and Brown, E. B.: Evaluation of deferoxamine in iron overload. *Arch. Intern. Med., 114*:741, 1964.

Irvin, J. M., and Snowden, P. W.: Idiopathic pulmonary hemosiderosis: report of case with apparent remission from cortisone. *J. Dis. Child., 93*:182, 1957.

Irwin, R. S., Cottrell, T. S., Hsu, K. C., Griswold, W. R., and Thomas, H. M.: Idiopathic pulmonary hemosiderosis. An electron microscopic and immunofluorescent study. *Chest, 65*:41, 1974.

Jaklovszky, A., Balla, A., and Petres-Brassay, I.: Essential pulmonary hemosiderosis as a differential diagnostic problem in anemic states in children. *Rev. Pediatr. Obstet. Gynecol., 24*:61, 1975.

Johnson, J. R., and McGovern, V. J.: Goodpasture's syndrome and Wegener's granulomatosis. *Australas. Ann. Med., 11*:250, 1962.

Kennedy, W. P.: Idiopathic pulmonary hemosiderosis. *Am. Rev. Resp. Dis., 99*:967, 1969.

Kilman, J. W., Clatworthy, H. W., Hering, J., Reiner, C. B., and Klassen, K. P.: Open pulmonary biopsy compared with needle biopsy in infants and children. *J. Pediatr. Surg., 9*:347, 1974.

Launay, C., and others: Idiopathic pulmonary hemosiderosis. *Ann. Pediatr. (Paris), 10*:379, 1963.

Lewis, E. J., Schur, P. H., Busch, G. J., et al.: Immunopathologic features of a patient with glomerulonephritis and pulmonary hemorrhage. *Am. J. Med., 54*:507, 1973.

Lexow, P., and Sigstad, H.: Glomerulonephritis with initial lung purpura. *Acta Med. Scand., 168*:405, 1960.

Livingstone, C. S., and Boczarow, B.: Idiopathic pulmonary hemosiderosis in a newborn. *Arch. Dis. Child., 42*:543, 1967.

Lockwood, C. M., Boulton-Jones, J. M., and Wilson, C. B.: Plasmapheresis: the role of this new technique in the recovery of a patient with Goodpasture's syndrome and severe renal failure. Presented at the Sixth International Congress of Nephrology, Florence, Italy, June 8–12, Poligrafici Luigi Parma, Bologna, Italy, 1975, p. 818.

Loftus, L. R., Rooney, P. A., and Webster, C. M.: Idiopathic pulmonary hemosiderosis and glomerulonephritis. Report of a case. *Dis. Chest, 45*:93, 1964.

McCanghey, W. T., and Thomas, B. J.: Pulmonary hemorrhage and glomerulonephritis. The relation of pulmonary hemorrhage to certain types of glomerular lesions. *Am. J. Clin. Pathol., 38*:577, 1962.

McDonald, R.: Chelating agents in chronic iron overload. *Clin. Pediatr., 5*:457, 1966.

MacGregor, C. S., Johnson, R. S., and Turk, K. A. D.: Fatal nephritis complicating idiopathic pulmonary haemosiderosis in young adults. *Thorax, 15*:198, 1960.

MacMahon, H. E., Derow, H. A., and Patterson, J. F.: Clinicopathologic conference. *Bull. N. Engl. Med. Center, 15*:161, 1953.

Maddock, R. K., Jr., Stevens, L. E., Reemtsma, K., and Bloomer, H. A.: Goodpasture's syndrome. Cessation of pulmonary hemorrhage after bilateral nephrectomy. *Ann. Intern. Med., 67*:1258, 1967.

Mathew, T. H., Hobbs, J. B., Kalowski, S., et al.: Goodpasture's syndrome: normal renal diagnostic findings. *Ann. Intern. Med.*, 82:215, 1975.

Mathews, T. S., and Soothill, J. F.: Complement activation after milk feeding in children with cow's milk allergy. *Lancet*, 2:893, 1970.

Matsaniotis, N., Karpouzas, J., Apostolopoulou, E., and Messaritakis, J.: Idiopathic hemosiderosis in children. *Arch. Dis. Child.*, 43:307, 1968.

Montaldo, G.: Sopra un caso di anemia emolitica con emosiderosi pulmonare. *Hematologica*, 19:353, 1938.

Negoita, C., and others: Idiopathic pulmonary hemosiderosis. An immuno-allergic disease. *Med. Intern. (Bucur)*, 15:1085, 1963.

Nickerson, H. J.: Idiopathic pulmonary hemosiderosis in a 5-month-old infant. *Clin. Pediatr.*, 7:416, 1968.

Nitschke, A.: Das klinische Bild der Eisenlunge. *Klin. Wochenschr.*, 23:348, 1944.

O'Donohue, W. J., Jr.: Idiopathic pulmonary hemosiderosis with manifestations of multiple connective tissue immune disorders: treatment with cyclophosphamide. *Am. Rev. Resp. Dis.*, 109:473, 1974.

Ognibene, A. J.: Rheumatoid disease with unusual pulmonary manifestations. Pulmonary hemosiderosis, fibrosis and concretions. *Arch. Intern. Med.*, 116:567, 1965.

Parish, W. E.: Short-term anaphylactic IgG antibodies in huma sera. *Lancet*, 2:591, 1970.

Ploem, J. E., DeWail, J., Verloop, N. A. C., and Punt, K.: Sideruria following a single dose of desferrioxamine. *Br. J. Haematol.*, 12:396, 1966.

Repetto, G., Lisboa, C., Emparaza, E., Ferretti, R., Neiru, M., Etchart, M., and Meneghello, J.: Idiopathic pulmonary hemosiderosis. Clinical, radiological and respiratory function studies. *Pediatrics*, 40:24, 1967.

Rose, G. A., and Spencer, H.: Polyarteritis nodosa. *Q. J. Med.*, 26:43, 1957.

Saltzman, P. W., West, M., and Chomet, B.: Pulmonary hemosiderosis and glomerulonephritis. *Ann. Intern. Med.*, 56:409, 1962.

Schaar, F. E., and Rigler, L. G.: Idiopathic pulmonary hemosiderosis: essential brown induration of the lungs; report of a case and review of literature. *Lancet*, 76:126, 1956.

Schuler, D.: Essential pulmonary hemosiderosis. *Ann. Paediatr.*, 192:107, 1959.

Soergel, K. H., and Sommers, S. C.: Idiopathic pulmonary hemosiderosis and related syndromes. *Am. J. Med.*, 32:499, 1962a.

Soergel, K. H., and Sommers, S. C.: The alveolar epithelial lesions of idiopathic pulmonary hemosiderosis. *Am. Rev. Resp. Dis.*, 85:540, 1962b.

Sprecace, G. A.: Idiopathic pulmonary hemosiderosis. Personal experience with six adults treated within a ten-month period, and a review of the literature. *Am. Rev. Resp. Dis.*, 88:830, 1963.

Steiner, B.: Essential pulmonary hemosiderosis as an immunohematological problem. *Arch. Dis. Child.*, 29:391, 1954.

Steiner, B.: Immunoallergic lung purpura treated with azathioprine, and with splenectomy. *Helv. Acta Paediatr.*, 24:413, 1969.

Sutherland, J. C., Markham, R. V., Jr., and Mardiney, M. R., Jr.: Subclinical immune complexes in the glomeruli of kidneys postmortem. *Am. J. Med.*, 57:536, 1974.

Thomas, A. M.: A case of Wegener's granulomatosis. *J. Clin. Pathol.*, 11:146, 1958.

Thomas, H. M., and Irwin, R. S.: Classification of diffuse intrapulmonary hemorrhage. *Chest*, 68:483, 1975.

Turner-Warwick, M.: Autoantibodies in allergic respiratory disease. In *Progress in Immunology II*. Vol. 4: Clinical Aspects 1. Amsterdam, North-Holland Publishing Company, 1974.

Valassi-Adam, H., Rouska, A., Karpouzas, J., and Matsaniotis, N.: Raised IgA in idiopathic pulmonary hemosiderosis. *Arch Dis. Child.*, 50:320, 1975.

Waldenström, J.: Anemia and iron deficiency. Blodbust och jarubrist. *Nord. Med.*, 6:940, 1940.

Walsh, J. R., Mass, R. E., Smith, F. W., and Lange, V.: Desferrioxamine effect on iron excretion in hemochromatosis. *Arch. Intern. Med.*, 113:435, 1964.

Wilson, C. B., and Dixon, F. J.: Anti-glomerular basement membrane antibody-induced glomerulonephritis. *Kidney Int.*, 3:74, 1973.

Wilson, C. B., Marquardt, H., and Dixon, F. J.: Radioimmunoassay (RIA) for circulating antiglomerular basement membrane (GBM) antibodies. *Kidney Int.*, 6:114A, 1974.

Wilson, J. F., Heiner, D. C., and Lahey, M. E.: Studies on iron metabolism. IV. Milk-induced gastrointestinal bleeding in infants with hypochromic microcytic anemia. *J.A.M.A.*, 189:568, 1964.

Wyllie, W. G., Sheldon, W., Bodian, M., and Barlow, A.: Idiopathic pulmonary hemosiderosis, essential brown induration of the lungs. *Q. J. Med.*, 17:25, 1948.

Ziai, M.: Anemia, shortness of breath and asthma in an infant. *Clin. Pediatr.*, 14:976, 1975.

CHAPTER THIRTY–SEVEN

ATELECTASIS

ROSA LEE NEMIR, M.D.

The term "atelectasis," although meaning imperfect expansion, is used to refer to the nonaerated lung, a clinical concept known for more than a century. It was described in 1819 by Laennec from necropsy findings, and was produced experimentally in 1845 by Traube. This chapter deals with *acquired* atelectasis and refers to postnatal collapse of a segment, lobe or lobes of the lung.

Causes

Acquired atelectasis may arise under a variety of circumstances: ① *bronchial obstruction* due to causes in the bronchial lumen, such as mucous plugs or foreign bodies; due to causes in the wall of the bronchus, such as mucosal edema and inflammation; from tumors or smooth muscle spasm; or from peribronchial factors such as pressure from tumors, from cysts or from lymph nodes enlarged by infections or lymphomas; ② *abnormal alveolar surface tension* following alteration of the alveolar lining layer; ③ direct local *pressure on parenchymal tissue* from contiguous masses, from enlargement of heart or adjacent vascular structures or from misplaced viscera, such as diaphragmatic hernia or eventration of the diaphragm; ④ *increased intrapleural pressure*, resulting from exudate, blood, pus or air in the pleural space; ⑤ *neuromuscular disease*, such as paralysis of the diaphragm in poliomyelitis and diphtheria and in congenital anomalies, such as amyotonia congenita. Contraction of the "myoelastic fibers" in the terminal pulmonary alveolar passages

under the control of the autonomic nervous system has also been implicated as a cause of atelectasis, especially massive collapse.

Pathophysiology

When a bronchus becomes occluded, air is trapped in the part of the parenchyma ventilated by the affected bronchus, and the trapped gases are absorbed into the blood perfusing that part of the lung. The rate at which absorption occurs depends on the solubility of the constituent gases: atmospheric air, nitrogen and helium are absorbed in two to three hours; oxygen is absorbed in a few minutes, leading to rapid collapse. Rahn (1959–1960), in a study of a dog breathing oxygen, has reported experimental collapse of a lung within six minutes. This observation has serious implications when applied to operative procedures utilizing oxygen.

The rate and extent of collapse are further modified by collateral ventilation through interalveolar pores and through bronchiole-alveolar communications. The presence of interalveolar pores described by Kohn (1893) has been confirmed in several studies. The experimental work of Van Allen and Lindskog (1931) in dogs and human specimens first called attention to this collateral ventilation.

More recently, a different and even more significant collateral ventilating mechanism has been described by Lambert (1955), who found short epithelium-lined communications, approximately 30 microns in diameter,

553

between the distal bronchioles and neighboring alveoli. These tubules are about three times the diameter of most interalveolar pores, and can aerate hundreds of alveoli adjacent to a peripheral bronchiole.

After the collapse of a segment or lobe, ventilation of the affected parenchyma becomes minimal, while perfusion of the area may be only slightly decreased, resulting in abnormality of ventilation-perfusion relations in the involved area of the lung. Yet shunting of blood from the collapsed portion of the lung to normally ventilated areas results in a circulatory adjustment. If the obstructed area is large enough, cyanosis may result.

Another important change that occurs after obstruction of a bronchus is the accumulation and stasis of secretions; these furnish a favorable site for the growth of microorganisms. As the secretions accumulate, they may distend a collapsed segment to more than its normal size ("drowned lung"). Later, with the absorption of fluids, the affected portion contracts. In terms of the hemodynamics, experimental studies on dogs demonstrated that arterial tortuosity occurs in the atelectatic lobe, as shown by angiograms (Hobbs and colleagues, 1972).

The internal surface of mammalian lungs is lined by a film containing a surface-acting factor that reduces alveolar tension. Von Neergaard (1929) first called attention to the importance of this factor in maintaining alveolar patency. This lining layer, surfactant (dipalmitoyl lecithin), has the unusual property of varying surface tension with changes in area, thereby preventing collapse and the emptying of the smaller alveoli into the larger lung units. By histochemical techniques this film has been identified as a lipoprotein with a high phospholipid content. The unusual property of variable surface tension is probably attributable to the phospholipid component. The lining layer appears to be synthesized in the mitochondria of the epithelial cells. The normal lining layer may be dam-

aged or inactivated under a variety of pathologic conditions, promoting collapse of the affected alveoli. Extracts of abnormal lungs have been found to have high surface tensions in a variety of conditions—immature newborns, respiratory distress syndrome, following pulmonary artery ligation and pulmonary edema—and in adults with pneumonia and collapse. The high surface tensions found in these conditions imply that increased retractive forces are operating on the involved alveoli, promoting collapse of the smaller units.

The mechanical effect of the decreased volume of the collapsed segment is to distend the adjacent parenchyma. This compensatory effect may be so great that small collapsed areas, sometimes called focal atelectasis, are not noticed clinically or on roentgenogram. This is especially true for those areas or segments adjacent to the heart where the small triangular paracardiac shadow may go unnoticed. The heart and the mediastinum may also take part in the adjustment of intrathoracic pressures, and may be displaced toward the atelectatic lung to fill the space previously occupied by expanded lung. The diaphragm on the affected side is often elevated.

Nonobstructive pulmonary collapse has provoked extensive study and analysis. In addition to the surface tension factor (surfactant) and the neurogenic factor, such as paralysis of the diaphragm and intercostal muscles, another concept for nonobstructive atelectasis is based on the altered normal pulmonary physiology affecting the neuromuscular structure of the terminal air passage. Much evidence has accumulated to support the belief that the lung contains smooth muscle fibers which in the most distally located portion of the air passages, including the alveolar sacs, are interwoven with elastic fibers. This "myoelastic" element is responsible for maintaining a state of contraction of pulmonary tissue similar to the continuous tonus provided by smooth muscle elsewhere—such as the stomach, intestines, bladder, arteries and veins. The precipitating factor may be severe pain, as in broken ribs, thoracic surgery, abdominal surgery, or the stimulation of bronchi as in bronchography. Corssen (1964) described photomicrographs of diseased and apparently normal lung tissue obtained from 26 patients during various surgical procedures. Muscular tissue was found extending beyond the terminal bronchioles.

Similarly, abnormal alterations in the depth of breathing have been suggested as a basis for atelectasis. In an experimental study conducted on the influence of morphine on dogs, Egbert and Bendixen (1964) showed a decrease in the depth of breathing; they suggested a causal relation of this drug effect to atelectasis.

Segmental atelectasis is commonly seen in young infants with respiratory infections and less frequently in older children. The larger bronchial lumen and the stiffer cartilaginous structure of bronchi in the older child make atelectasis less likely than in the infant. In addition, the more rigid thoracic walls favor the clearing of obstructed bronchi in the older child.

Incidence

The incidence of postnatal or acquired atelectasis in childhood depends on several factors: the age of the patient, the kind of population sampled, the awareness and interest of the physician in the discovery of atelectasis, and the utilization of different views in chest roentgenograms.

A report by an anesthesiologist may feature postoperative atelectasis, although improved anesthesiology has rendered this complication infrequent; in a report by a physician who sees many children with infectious diseases, pneumonia, bronchiolitis, measles and pertussis (the latter two diseases now infrequently encountered in communities with adequate health services) may predominate; a bronchoscopist may emphasize aspiration of a foreign body, or vomitus, or obstruction by mucous plugs during infections and, less commonly, bronchial obstruction by extrinsic masses from lymph nodes in the hilar or mediastinal areas. The neonatologist will be concerned with atelectasis related to many factors at birth and those resulting from the use of mechanical respirators and intubation. (See Chapter 10.)

In a retrospective study of 165 bronchograms performed between 1938 and 1969, radiologists Robinson and colleagues (1971) found some evidence of transient segmental collapse in 45 per cent of the patients whose ages ranged from 4 days to 16 years. There was greater frequency among asthmatic patients and those with other allergic manifestations. Atelectasis has become an uncommon complication of bronchography during the recent past years owing to changes in anesthesia and in contrast material, and because of improved technique in performing bronchograms.

In an effort to avoid the error of bias from a study of selected material, James and coworkers (1956) analyzed every known case (845 patients) of pulmonary collapse seen on x-ray study in a London hospital during the period 1945 to 1952. Pertussis was the leading cause of "pulmonary collapse," occurring in 18.9 per cent; upper and lower respiratory tract infections, sinobronchitis and pneumonia accounted for 58.2 per cent, all four in approximately equal proportion. The remainder of the group was associated with asthma, tuberculosis (6 per cent each), measles, and miscellaneous and postoperative causes, 2.3 to 3.6 per cent. Since 1954, the time of termination for this study, several changes have occurred. Pertussis and measles pneumonia are rarely seen now because of the wide use of prophylactic vaccines in infancy. In the United States, sinusitis, although still present and often overlooked, is becoming uncommon; this is probably due in large measure to the successful use of appropriate antimicrobial therapy for respiratory infection, especially against such microorganisms as the streptococcus and the pneumococcus. Meanwhile, asthma continues to be a pediatric problem at all ages.

On the pediatric service of New York University — Bellevue Medical Center, the most common causes of atelectasis in the first two years of life are respiratory infections, especially bronchiolitis, bronchopneumonia, tuberculosis and asthmatic bronchitis. In the school-age child, pneumonia and asthma are more frequent and tuberculosis is less common. Similar experience has been reported from the Mayo Clinic by Logan and Leonardo (1970) for the period 1940 to 1965. They analyzed the causes of atelectasis in 81 selected children under 16 years of age, excluding trauma, neoplasm, foreign body aspiration, surgery and the respiratory distress syndrome as factors. Pneumonia alone was responsible for 20 per cent of the cases; pneumonia with other associated conditions for 15 per cent; and asthma for 17 per cent (only 4 of 14 patients had uncomplicated asthma). Segmental atelectasis was found in 7.4 per cent in a survey of 530 acutely ill asthmatic children in Philadelphia (Lecks and coworkers, 1967).

Aspiration of vomitus is an uncommon but often serious cause of atelectasis, especially in the young, debilitated or physically handicapped infant. Organized diverse efforts to prevent foreign body aspiration are constantly being made by many medical and lay groups, including the American Academy of Pediatrics, local and national health organizations, voluntary agencies, the toy and drug industries, and insurance companies. Much educational material is available and distributed widely to parents and other groups, with special emphasis on the preschool ages, one through four years.

Atelectasis Due to Bronchial Obstruction

The most common cause of extrabronchial obstruction leading to atelectasis is compression of the adjacent bronchi by hilar and mediastinal lymph nodes. Such nodal enlargement may be due to infection of the lungs and pleura or, rarely, may result from descending drainage into the bronchi from an infection in the upper respiratory tract. The most common agents are tubercle bacilli, respiratory viruses (rarely measles), and bronchiolitis in infants. Other causes are lymphomas, Hodg-

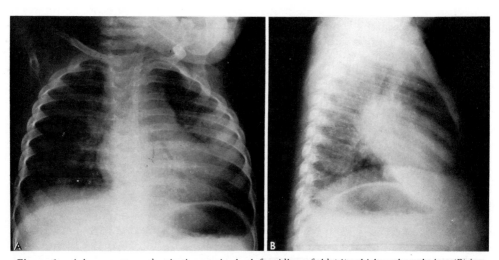

Figure 1. A homogeneous density is seen in the left midlung field *(A)*, which on lateral view *(B)* is apparently segmental, involving the entire lingula. This corresponds to the bronchoscopic findings as reported. These roentgenographic findings remained unchanged for many months. Tuberculous cause was clearly established.

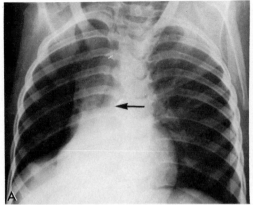
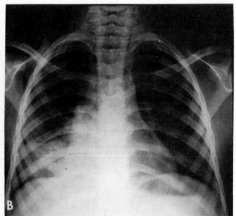
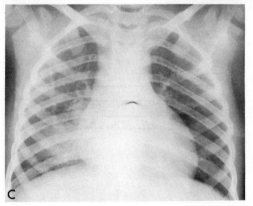

Figure 2. *A,* There is a homogeneous dense shadow above the right diaphragm extending from the periphery to the heart border, bounded superiorly by a straight edge at the level of the fifth rib anteriorly, consistent with atelectasis. There is hypoaeration in the right lung above this area. There is also displacement of the heart and mediastinum to the right (even discounting the effect of some torsion to the right). The bronchi to the right middle and lower lobes were obstructed as determined by bronchoscopy. *B,* Four days later, after bronchoscopy and suction of caseous material from the right middle and lower lobes, there is partial expansion of the atelectatic segment. The costophrenic angle is clear. The shadow is less dense in the right base, but there is still displacement of the heart and mediastinum. Note the large dense shadow in the right hilar area. *C,* One month later, after a second bronchoscopy and suction of large amounts of cloudy fluid material, there is almost complete clearing of the atelectasis and return of the mediastinal structures to normal position. Tuberculous endobronchial disease associated with tuberculosis of hip.

kins' disease, leukemias, and metastasis from malignancy in other organs, such as Wilms' tumor, adrenal neuroblastoma, retinoblastoma, osteogenic sarcoma and teratoma of the testes. Tuberculous lymph node bronchial compression resulting in obstruction is described elsewhere (see Chapter 46). Two patients are shown in Figures 1 and 2, one illustrating atelectasis due to tuberculous nodal compression of the bronchus, and the second demonstrating atelectasis due to caseous material filling the bronchus after rupture of the infected gland into the bronchus. Compression of a lung by a markedly enlarged heart may produce atelectasis. In infants and young children with acyanotic congenital heart disease, the distended pulmonary arteries and an enlarged left atrium result in airway obstruction. The most common sites thus affected are the left upper bronchus, left main bronchus and middle bronchus.

Primary malignant tumors of the lung are rare in childhood. Dargeon (1960), in his wide experience at Memorial Hospital, New York, has reported only one case, a leiomyosarcoma in a four-year-old boy in whom atelectasis of the right middle and lower lobes was demonstrated on x-ray film. Total collapse of the left lower lobe may give a rounded appearance on roentgenogram and simulate a paraspinal tumor, as illustrated by Melamed and colleagues (1975) with case reports.

Congenital anomalies of the diaphragm (eventration, hiatus hernia)

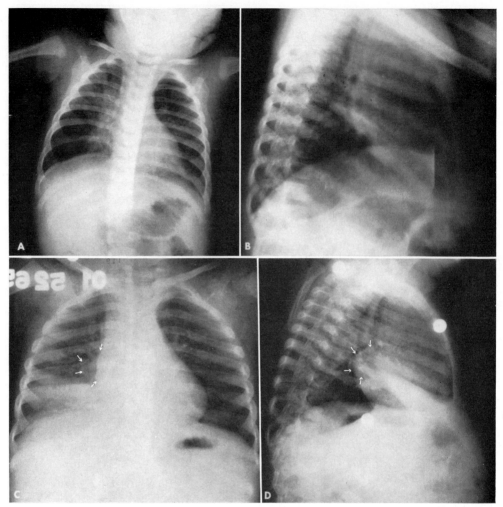

Figure 3. *A,* There is an increase in the bronchovascular markings extending from the right root, and some patchy infiltration is seen in the hilar area along the heart border and extending upward into the right upper lobe. *B,* In the lateral view there is a mottled density in the medial aspect of the lung extending from the bronchial bifurcation and overlying the heart shadow, but this is not definitely segmental in distribution. *C,* There is some displacement of trachea, heart and mediastinum to the right. A rounded, fairly dense area in the right hilar area suggests nodal enlargement. There is a homogeneous shadow above the diaphragm extending as a wedge-shaped shadow to the periphery. The costophrenic angle is clear. *D,* A shrunken right middle density may be seen, suggesting atelectasis of the entire right middle lobe with questionable hilar density surrounding the apex of the lobe. These films were taken during two months of recurrent pneumonia that failed to respond to antibiotics. Bronchoscopy was negative. Atelectasis may be due to disturbed respiration from disease of the central nervous system in this hydrocephalic infant.

may permit sufficient pressure on the bronchi by *displaced viscera* to produce atelectasis of the parenchyma supplied by the bronchus (Fig. 3). Certainly this is a rare cause of pulmonary collapse in our experience. Presenting symptoms of the atelectasis are minimal or absent;

those of the hernia may be unnoticed for years and consist of fleeting pain and discomfort. Occasionally bleeding or intestinal obstruction may lead to the diagnosis. Sweet (1953), in an analysis of 130 patients with hiatus hernia, found only ten instances of pulmonary complications: six of these had transitory atelectasis, and four had pulmonary emboli from which they recovered.

The cause of *intrabronchial obstruction* may be endogenous or exogenous; an example of the latter is aspiration of a foreign body; the former may originate within the bronchus as a part of disease or infection, such as granulomatous tissues, chiefly tuberculous in origin, or mucous material frequently secondary to cystic fibrosis or asthma (Fig. 4).

The course and duration of such atelectasis in children depend on many factors, most important of which is the physiologic state of the obstructed bronchus. In asthmatic patients, the smooth muscle spasm promotes narrowing of the lumen and facilitates obstruction. Other factors, such as increased viscosity of mucus and reduction in pulmonary surfactant, also play a part. Effective medication with bronchodilators, fluid therapy, and mu-

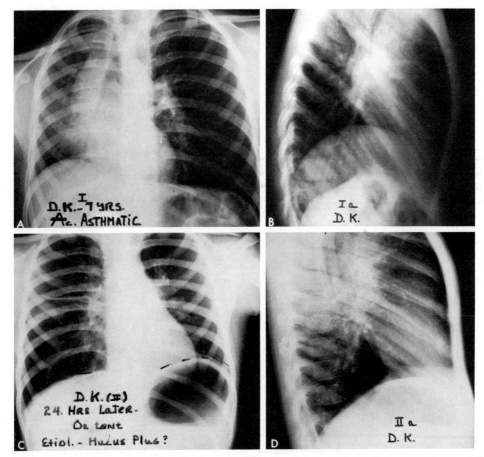

Figure 4. This seven-year-old boy has been known as an allergic child for four years and treated for asthmatic attacks from time to time. *A* and *B*, Roentgenograms taken a few hours after an acute, severe asthmatic attack. There is obvious massive displacement of mediastinal structure to the right with elevation of the right diaphragm. Extensive distention of the left hemithorax, widening of the interspaces and flattening of the diaphragm. In the lateral film *(B)* the increased anteroposterior diameter of the chest, the elevated diaphragm, and the hyperaeration anteriorly and posteriorly are apparent. *C* and *D*, Roentgenograms taken the following day after the patient has spent the night in an oxygen tent. Return of structures to relatively normal position may be seen. Horizontal fissures on the right are visualized, and widened intercostal spaces are present bilaterally.

This patient is shown to illustrate sudden massive (partial) obstruction of the right main bronchus that clears spontaneously within 24 hours. The cause of the obstruction is not definitely known. It is plausible to suggest a mucous plug as the etiologic factor.

colytic agents may quickly restore the bronchial lumen to relatively normal diameter. On the other hand, in bronchopneumonia, bronchiolitis and cystic fibrosis, the inherent disease of the bronchi manifested by both edema and swelling within the bronchi, the peribronchial exudate, and the mucoid material filling the bronchus favors obstruction at various areas, which, even when relieved in one area, may appear in another as long as the infection thrives.

The special qualities of the material producing obstruction affect the outcome and also influence the kind of therapy. (For foreign body aspiration, see below.) The viscid quality of the mucus in cystic fibrosis (mucoviscidosis) favors atelectasis and makes ordinary medication ineffective; mucolytic agents are frequently required.

The chronicity of the infection, which results in damage to bronchi, and the sort of material obstructing the lumen of the bronchus also determine the outcome of the atelectasis. Frequently these intrabronchial plugs cannot be removed by bronchoscopy. Shaw (1951) described mucus plugs in ten asthmatic patients, eight of whom required surgical resection. These plugs were greenish gray, and had a thick, tenacious consistency; on cut section there was lamination, and they varied in size from 2.5 to 3.5 cm. in length and from 0.9 to 2.3 cm. in diameter. In patients with cystic fibrosis, mucoid impaction of the bronchi, described by Waring and colleagues (1967), accounts for the airway obstruction, focal or segmental, in this disease.

Foreign bodies aspirated into the lung usually enter a noninfected lung with healthy bronchi. The sequence of events in this circumstance will depend on the patient, his age, state of consciousness and health, the nature of aspirated material, the promptness of correct diagnosis, and the speed and success of appropriate therapy. The younger the patient, the more rapidly atelectasis occurs when the bronchi are occluded. In the young infant it can de-

velop within a few hours, while in the older child a longer period is usually required. Metallic aspirants may produce obstruction because of their size, and injury because of their shape, but vegetal aspirants have a particularly irritating quality, resulting in prompt mucosal swelling and obstruction (Fig. 5). Some of these, such as peanuts, beans, maize, peas and watermelon seed, swell to many times their size and consistute a most serious problem; diagnosis is often obscure, too, because nonopaque aspirant is not visible on roentgenogram and the history is incomplete. The right lung is involved more often than the left, probably because of the sharper angulation of the left main bronchus.

Signs and Symptoms of Bronchial Obstruction

Obviously these vary, depending on the cause of the pulmonary collapse. In general, atelectasis that occurs during the course of tuberculosis, lymphoma, neoplasm, asthma or infections such as bronchiolitis, bronchitis, bronchopneumonia and sinobronchitis produces no change in the clinical picture unless the obstructed area is a main bronchus. This is rare in the course of these pulmonary infections. The patients are already sick, with considerable cough and some fever. Because of the diminished aeration of lung associated with obstruction, the symptoms of tachypnea, dyspnea, cough and stridor, when present, may be increased.

Occasionally a localized constant wheeze, diminished breath sounds and impaired resonance may suggest atelectasis; diagnosis is confirmed by chest roentgenogram. Careful observation may reveal a difference in respiratory expansion; there may be diminished expansion and contraction of the ribs over the atelectatic area and fullness and widened intercostal spaces over the adjacent, compensating, overdistended portion of the lung. Displacement of the heart and the mediastinum and elevation of the diaphragm are detecta-

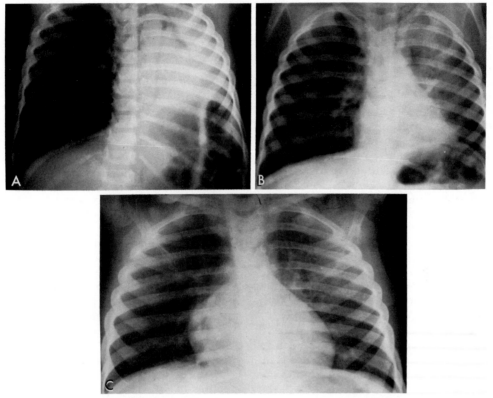

Figure 5. *A,* Complete shift of heart and mediastinal structures into the left hemithorax, where there is a homogeneous density filling the chest. Signs are suggestive of massive atelectasis of the left lung. A peanut was removed from the left main stem bronchus by bronchoscopy, immediately clearing the obstruction *(B).* Within a few days the patient completely recovered *(C).*

ble only if the atelectasis involves a large area.

In young infants, the mobility of the mediastinum makes evaluation of the tracheal position important; examination should be carried out for epigastric pulsations.

When a previously well child has aspirated a foreign body, there is usually a definite history of respiratory disturbance. The signs may go unnoticed until secondary signs of infection and obstruction become prominent. Coughing, choking and gagging occur at the time of aspiration. If a large bronchus is involved, cyanosis or asphyxia may occur. A wheeze is heard, sometimes without the use of a stethoscope. If the obstruction is at the site of the main bronchus, bilateral wheezing will be evident; otherwise the wheeze is localized to the area obstructed. In many instances, and especially if the obstructed area is limited to a segment or a subsegment, the incident of choking may be followed by a symptomless period of many days; then infection in the area of atelectasis results in fever, cough and malaise. If the infection has involved other parts of the lung, there may be an increased respiratory rate. At this point the clinical picture is that of pneumonitis with atelectasis; the severity of the pneumonitis is related to the virulence of the infecting organism and the nature of the aspirated foreign body.

Diagnosis

When there is lobar atelectasis, the differential diagnosis includes pneumonia and, in the case of the swollen, wet, atelectatic lung, pleural effusion. Embolism is a rare complication in childhood. In differential diagnosis, the position of the heart, mediastinum and diaphragm and the nature of both tactile and vocal fremitus are most helpful. Egophony or nasal voice sounds suggest the presence of fluid. Rales are usually present in patients with pneumonia, especially in bronchopneumonia when crackling rales are often heard. Rales are usually absent in the atelectatic lung, especially after clearing of the "wet" stage. The etiologic agent of the pleural fluid may be the determining factor in the production of rales. In an effusion caused by the staphylococcus, rales are often heard over the lung. They are usually absent when there is a pneumococcus effusion, and in tuberculosis. With effusion the heart and the mediastinum are displaced toward the normal side, unless there is an underlying collapse of lung; there is no displacement in patients with pneumonia, and the displacement is toward the affected side in atelectasis. The position of the diaphragm is best established on x-ray film, but occasionally physical examination may be helpful in determining free movement of the diaphragm. Lateral views of the chest are essential in clarifying the diagnosis of atelectasis and differentiating it from pneumonia. Other clinical features commonly associated with pneumonia are fever, cough, tachypnea or dyspnea, and evidence of infection. When atelectasis is present in patients with tracheal intubation who are receiving mechanical ventilation, infection may be present and related to bacterial colonization of the tracheobronchial tree rather than to an infection of the pulmonary tissue, at least in the beginning.

Laboratory aids in determining the presence of infection, such as blood cell counts, sedimentation rates, and cultures from the nose and throat, the blood and other sources, are valuable guides both in understanding the clinical picture and in treating the patient. The tuberculin skin test, as well as other skin tests when indicated, may be necessary to establish the diagnosis.

The most valuable diagnostic tool is the roentgenogram of the chest. The earliest roentgenographic evidence of atelectasis may be a swollen lung with fissure lines extending beyond its normal areas, thus indicating a swollen or larger segment or lobe; there are often convex curves instead of the usual straight pleural line. Shortly afterward, as the lung becomes truly atelectatic or airless, the fissure lines become concave and the segment of lobe contracts to a much smaller size. This progression of change is best exemplified in atelectasis of the right middle lobe, especially if the atelectasis has been present over a period of time; the lobe may become so small that on x-ray film it is seen as a dense band suggesting pleural thickening rather than a completely atelectatic lobe.

Understanding of these roentgenographic findings can best be obtained by a review of Spain's (1954) experimental production of "acute nonaeration of the lung" in dogs. The earliest pathologic change consisted of congestion and edema. Within 36 hours, however, there was some reduction in the size of the lung, and inflammatory cells appeared. The correlation with serial roentgenograms in patients with obstructed bronchi is obvious.

Robbins and Hale (1945) have pointed out that there is x-ray evidence of elevation of the hilus on the atelectatic side, but in such interpretation it must be remembered that the left hilus is normally higher than the right. The position of the septa and the hilus should therefore be recorded in the study of the chest roentgenograms. Elevation of the diaphragm and an elevated position of the hilus on the affected side reflect the smaller volume of the lung containing an atelectatic area or areas. The position of the diaphragm may be of diagnostic aid; it is usually unaffected in lobar pneumonia, and is displaced downward and often flattened on the side of pleural effusion; it sometimes cannot be visualized if fluid overlies it. For proper interpretation and diagnosis of atelectasis, roentgenograms should be obtained in both lateral and posteroanterior views. Films taken during inspiratory and expiratory phases of respiration are also helpful, especially when aspiration of a nonopaque foreign body is the cause of atelectasis. Tomography can be most helpful, especially in the interpretation of rounded lesions. (See Chapter 5.)

Atelectasis may occur in any lobe or segment of the lung. The least frequently affected is the left upper lobe, except in congenital heart disease when the left upper lobe is most often involved. When all causes for obstruction of the airway are considered, the right lower and left lower lobes are most frequently collapsed. The age of the patient and the cause of the atelectasis determine the frequency of lobe obstruction. In lower respiratory tract infections, the left lower and right middle lobes are most frequently involved. The right middle lobe is most vulnerable when there is enlargement of the hilar lymph nodes; it is also the most commonly affected lobe in asthmatic patients. Some writers have referred to this frequency as the "right middle lobe syndrome" (Dees and Spock, 1966). In childhood tuberculosis, the right upper and middle lobes are more frequently obstructed than any other lobes. Aspirated material in young infants more often produces right upper lobe obstruction; this probably results because of the recumbent position of the baby and because of the sharp angulation of the right upper lobe bronchus, which tends to trap aspirated material rather than permit expulsion into the main bronchus.

Treatment

Atelectasis associated with acute infections of the lower respiratory tract is usually short-lived and clears with or before the acute infection. This is especially true in acute bronchitis, bronchiolitis and pneumonia in infants. In such instances, therefore, it is pointless to treat the atelectasis; therapy should be directed toward the respiratory infection. Change in the position of the patient, maintenance of moisture in the air, and sometimes bronchodilators are indicated. Bronchoscopy is not advisable during the early stages of an acute infection.

When atelectasis occurs in a patient who has had chronic or recurrent pulmonary disease, the bronchi may be damaged, and the secretions in such areas may be retained or expelled more slowly. These children require careful investigation of the underlying cause of recurrent or chronic infection, including special studies if they are asthmatic or have cystic fibrosis. Tests should be made for immunologic deficiencies, such as gamma globulin and alpha$_1$-antitrypsin enzymes. Cultures for the etiologic agent should be carried out; postural drainage with chest percussion should be used, and the administration of a bronchodilator is often helpful. In those with recurrent episodes of pulmonary obstruction, positive pressure breathing exercises may be of value. Adequate medical treatment, including attention to hydration, especially important for patients with asthma and cystic fibrosis, must always be given proper trial before bronchoscopy is done.

On the other hand, if there is a history of aspiration, or a serious coughing or choking spell followed by a wheeze, or an unexplained *unilateral* wheeze, bronchoscopy should immediately be considered. Only about 2 to 4 per cent (Jackson and Jackson, 1959) spontaneously cough up the aspirated material. Delay in removal of the foreign body seriously alters the prognosis. The foreign body not only becomes embedded, injures the bronchus and generates infection, but may also descend deeper into the smaller bronchi, thereby making removal by bronchoscopy more difficult.

In general, the object of therapy in obstructive atelectasis is to locate the cause of bronchial obstruction, to remove it as soon as possible by appropriate methods, and to maintain good pulmonary ventilation at all times. Infection, when the cause of obstruction, should be suitably treated. If it is not, secondary infection usually develops. Removal of secretions or similar intrabronchial material, the use of antispasmodics and bronchodilators in an effort to increase the lumen of the obstructed bronchi, the liquefaction of secretions (aerosols), and the use of postural drainage should be utilized as needed. If these measures are ineffectual, mechanical suction or bronchoscopy is indicated. Proper administration of oxygen to maintain healthy pulmonary ventilation may be necessary.

When atelectasis persists for many months, damage to the lung is likely (fibrosis) and renders this portion of the lung parenchyma functionless. If medical treatment and bronchoscopy have been ineffectual in reaerating the lung, surgical removal of the lobe or segment should be considered. Bronchograms and pulmonary function studies are necessary to arrive at such a decision. James and coworkers (1956) suggest a waiting period of two years before final decision because they observed 15 patients whose lungs re-expanded between one and two years. Many factors will influence the ultimate choice of surgical removal of the diseased portion of the lung: the age of the patient, the location of the diseased lobe or segments, the extent of damage to the lung, the result of pulmonary functional studies, the underlying cause of the atelectasis, the presence of infection, and the general health of the child. (See Chapter 25, Bronchiectasis.) Successful medical management of respiratory infections with antibiotics, greater ease in the therapeutic use of the bronchoscope, and skillful and effective thoracic surgery offer an optimistic outlook in either choice for many children. Fortunately, persistent collapse is uncommon.

Preventive therapy, especially in obstructive atelectasis, should succeed in decreasing the incidence of this pulmonary complication. Attention has been directed toward the efforts to educate all those responsible for small children as to the common causes of aspiration of foreign bodies and their prevention. Antibiotics, mucolytic agents, detergents as inhalants, postural drainage and other physiotherapeutic measures on a prophylactic basis may greatly reduce the incidence of pulmonary collapse associated with bronchial obstruction by secretions. Occasionally, liquefaction of secretions by expectorants is also indicated.

Complications

Permanent damage to the proximal bronchi occluded often follows prolonged atelectasis. Fibrosis and bronchiectasis frequently follow atelectasis. (See pages 446 and 518 for a discussion of these conditions.)

Overdistended or hyperaerated areas may exist simultaneously with atelectatic areas and result from the same etiologic factors. In the former instance the occlusion is partial; in the latter the occlusion may be complete, resulting in an airless lung. Prolonged overdistention also causes damage to the lung. In children this is a rare complication.

Prognosis

Many factors are involved in the prognosis of the patient with atelectasis; among these are the cause of the collapse, the duration of the atelectasis, the extent of the concomitant infection, the age of the patient, and the effectiveness of therapy in preventing superimposed infection and in clearing the airways. The two aspects for consideration are prognosis for recovery or fatality, and prognosis in terms of permanent damage to the lung as a result of the airlessness of the lung parenchyma.

A fatal outcome is likely only (1) when the underlying cause for the atelectasis is life-threatening, or (2) when extensive loss of the ventilating function follows a massive lung area involvement that is unresponsive to treatment. Foreign body aspiration unrecognized or untreated may fall in the first category, because of acute secondary pneumonia. Hence, diagnostic acumen in such cases is vital, and suspicion should be aroused when pneumonia follows collapse, when the disease progresses despite apparently proper therapy, when constant, localized wheezing is heard, or when the clinical picture is atypical. Bronchoscopy in such cases may be a lifesaving measure. To illustrate further, in patients who have atelectasis during the course of cystic fibrosis or extensive heart disease, the ultimate prognosis is not favorable, not because of the pulmonary collapse, but because of the advanced pathologic stage of the two disease processes.

Permanent damage to the lung following atelectasis is not uncommon, the damage being to the architecture of the bronchial tree. Two decades ago, pertussis, measles and bronchopneumonia were among the most common offenders in producing bronchiectasis. Today these diseases are increasingly rare as forerunners of severe pulmonary complications. Long-standing bronchial obstruction in childhood tuberculosis is associated with a high incidence of bronchopulmonary damage. This complication of childhood tuberculosis (endobronchial) is still seen despite early and adequate antimicrobial tuberculosis therapy, but with decreasing frequency. (See Chapter 25, Bronchiectasis.)

In general, pulmonary collapse during the course of acute infections has a good immediate and long-range prognosis.

Careful medical follow-up care to ensure proper pulmonary hygiene is valuable and essential to continued good health.

NONOBSTRUCTIVE ATELECTASIS

There is evidence that this etiologic category for the airless lung is more common than was previously suspected. The surface tension factor (surfactant), sometimes called the "antiatelectasis" factor, seems most important during infancy, especially as related to hyaline membrane disease (Avery and Mead, 1959). Changes in the pulmonary surfactants may occur at any age. The lungs of two children dying in status asthmaticus showed atelectasis and diminished antiatelectasis surfactant factor attributed to pulmonary arterial vasoconstriction (Lecks and associates, 1966). Conversely, there is experimental evidence in animals that transient reduction of surface activity may also result from lung collapse; this quickly returns to normal, however. Burbank and coworkers (1961) have suggested that the lung is an actively contractile organ and that, under the stimulus of unusual pain, a reflex mechanism is responsible for the terminal alveolar muscular spasm that, together with the resultant changes in surface tension and intraluminal air pressure, results in collapse. This may occur in pneumonia and nonobstructive atelectasis, with fracture of ribs, after abdominal or thoracic surgery, and during the course of bronchography.

The importance of the neurogenic factor affecting the muscles of respiration was described by Pasteur. Churchill (1953) has also called attention to this factor in the nonobstructive cause of atelectasis as a weakened force in respiratory muscle action.

Patients undergoing thoracotomy or abdominal surgery are especially likely to develop atelectasis. Swartz (1974), in his textbook on surgery, states that atelectasis is responsible for 90 per cent of all postoperative pulmonary complications. Hypoventilation associated with shallow breathing and diminished cough due to pain is an important etiologic factor.

Atelectatic episodes have been described also during extensive poliomyelitis, during diphtheria, and in patients with neuromuscular anomalies, such as amyotonia congenita or injuries to the spinal cord. Berry and Sanislow (1963) have described "acute respiratory insufficiency" which they called atelectasis and defined as characterized by an "un-obstructive, nontransudative alveolar collapse and intense interstitial pulmonary capillary congestion" following intensive parenteral fluid therapy. Atelectasis, although occurring in only 2 to 3 per cent of 380 burned patients at Brooke Army Medical Center, was the commonest cause of the "infrequent" pulmonary complications and was most frequently seen in the early postburn period.

The *clinical features* and *diagnostic aspects of nonobstructive atelectasis* are dependent on the underlying cause and on the extent of the atelectasis. Some patients are acutely ill with respiratory symptoms resulting from disturbed pulmonary physiologic functions; others are symptomless or show little difference in the symptoms already existing with the illness.

A silent, apparently symptomless atelectasis in 14 heroin addicts (now a tragic responsibility of pediatricians also) was described by Gelfand and associates (1967). Atelectasis was found in these patients, admitted to the hospital for detoxification, by chest roentgenograms. Two possible explanations suggested for the pulmonary collapse were pulmonary emboli and the heroin effect in depressing respiration or decreasing sighing. Pulmonary complications, such as edema and bronchial obstruction from vomitus, continue to be reported in addict patients with heroin overdose. Rapid development of pneumonia and bronchiectasis may occur. (See Chapter 25, Bronchiectasis.)

The roentgenograms for both nonobstructive and obstructive atelectasis are similar. Absence of opaque foreign bodies and of mediastinal or hilar masses is a differential feature between obstructive and nonobstructive atelectasis.

Treatment

Analysis of the underlying cause of the atelectasis and evaluation of the presenting symptoms are essential to intelligent therapy.

When the etiologic agent appears to be related to surfactant, attempt may be made to repair the defective alveolar lining layer by inhalations of aerosols of substances with similar physical properties. In contrast to the natural surfactant, most synthetic surface-active agents have fixed surface tensions that are not altered with changes in the alveolar area. Such agents are the detergents, the Tweens (hydrophilic nonionic surfactants) and the Spans (lipophilic surfactants); if administered in an aerosol, these tend to replace the normal lining by a film of fixed surface tension, increasing the retractive forces in the lung. Experimental study of excised lung lined with synthetic surfactant demonstrates the beneficial effect on inflation and deflation pressure-volume curves. Radigan and King (1960) have demonstrated the value of detergents in preventing postoperative atelectasis. The object of this therapy is to stimulate involuntary and forceful coughing. In pediatrics, a similar objective may be achieved by inhalation in nonsurgical patients when coughing is desired.

An ingenious therapeutic device for massive atelectasis of the right lung due to amyotonia congenita in a three-year-old child was used by Townsend and Squire (1956). A jacket encircling the chest attached to a 3-pound weight designed to concentrate traction along the midaxillary line was successful in relieving the collapse within a few days. The patient remained clear for months and, in subsequent bouts of atelectasis, responded to similar treatment without the use of bronchoscopy.

In other respects the treatment of obstructive and nonobstructive atelectasis does not differ. Massive postoperative atelectasis may also be nonobstructive; the additional aspect of treatment for these postoperative patients is given in the succeeding section.

MASSIVE PULMONARY COLLAPSE

Acute massive pulmonary collapse may occur under a variety of circumstances, but most commonly follows upper abdominal or thoracic surgery or bronchial obstruction, resulting from foreign body aspiration or more frequently from mucoid material or the aspiration of vomitus. It is also seen after chest trauma. In the last instance the collapse is usually on the injured side, but may occur on the opposite side, possibly owing to aspiration of blood. Although diaphragmatic paralysis or paresis is also associated with massive atelectasis, it is rarely seen now, because the two most frequent offenders, diphtheria and poliomyelitis, are rapidly disappearing. This section will be devoted to a discussion of massive postoperative collapse.

Incidence

From our own experience at Bellevue Hospital and from the recent literature, it is clear that this massive atelectasis in children is uncommon, especially as a postoperative complication. A comprehensive study by two large city hospitals for the period 1931 to 1941 reported only 21 cases. A later study in a Philadelphia hospital, covering 1941 to 1945, analyzed 1240 patients with upper abdominal surgery and reported massive atelectasis in 22 children.

Pathogenesis

Massive postoperative atelectasis of the lung may be due to obstructive or nonobstructive factors, although it is thought that the latter, such as hypoventilation or ineffectual respirations, are much more frequent. The same etiologic mechanisms described under both obstructive and nonobstructive atelectasis apply here. In addition, there are other factors directly related to the surgical procedures. These are preoperative and postoperative medications, increased bronchial secretions associated with the operation, excessive pain (especially in thoracic and abdominal surgery), effects on respiration of injury to abdominal muscles, direct effects of anesthetics on the respiratory tract, absence of cough reflex, and inactivity of the patient from both positioning and surgical bandages.

The importance of deep breathing and occasional sighing in normal respirations has been demonstrated. Severe abdominal pain affects the kind and depth of respiration, and morphine has been shown to affect the breathing pattern by causing respiratory depression and eliminating the occasional normal spontaneous deep breaths.

The experimental work of de Takats and associates (1942) has led them to conclude that the essential basis for postoperative atelectasis is a combination of increased bronchial secretion associated with reflex bronchoconstriction and bronchial obstruction. Bronchial secretions may be increased in intra-abdominal manipulation during operation, by blunt injury to the chest wall or by pulmonary embolism. Lindskog (1941) has postulated the release of a histamine-like substance from the sites of operation; theoretically, this provokes the secretions and bronchiolar constriction. This is found less frequently in newborn and very young infants.

Anesthesia resulting in hypoxia may also be a mechanism leading to atelectasis. The early experimental work of Briscoe (1919–1920) pointed out the importance of position of the patient with regard to the development of atelectasis. Long periods in a supine position with constricting abdominal bandages affect the diaphragmatic movements, leading to inadequate ventilation and collapse.

Clinical Features

Symptoms of massive collapse usually appear on the first postoperative day. They consist of fever, respiratory distress, dyspnea, cyanosis and anxiety. The diagnosis is easily made by physical examination and roentgenograms. The heart and the mediastinum are displaced toward the affected side, and there is dullness and markedly diminished to absent breath sounds, and tactile and vocal fremitus; tachypnea and tachycardia are present. There may be a lag in respiration and narrowing of the interspaces on the affected side. By roentgenogram, the diaphragm is elevated.

The diagnosis may be verified by various tests to determine the perfusion of the nonventilated parenchyma, such as arterial blood desaturation, a useful and relatively accurate test using the technique of earpiece oximetry. Pulmonary function studies are more tedious, but more accurate. These tests may be valuable in determining postoperative pulmonary complications.

The differential diagnosis includes pneumonia, pulmonary embolism, pleural effusion and pneumothorax. The last two may be distinguished by the shift of the heart and mediastinal structures to the opposite side. Pneumonia may coexist with or follow atelectasis; the degree of fever, presence of rales, and other clinical signs and laboratory tests such as bacterial cultures are diagnostic aids. Pulmonary embolism occurs rarely in childhood. It is accompanied by symptoms of shock and often hemoptysis.

Prognosis

The prognosis in this alarming picture is good unless there is an underlying complication such as pneumonia or embolism. Most patients recover spontaneously with the use of simple mechanical measures such as coughing and positioning.

Treatment

Active treatment consists in the removal of the obstruction to airways by coughing (often accompanied by forceful blows to the thorax or supplemented by tracheal suction), by oxygen inhalation, by medications directed toward liquefying secretions, by mucolytic solutions, and by the inhalation of bronchodilators. If voluntary coughing cannot be relied on, positive pressure breathing may be used after careful evaluation of the airway obstruction and estimation of the probable pres-

sure in the pleural spaces. The use of appropriate antibiotics and the application of the preventive measures, with special attention to the exclusion of medications that depress cough and respiration, are indicated. It is important to remember that atelectasis may clear spontaneously and that good general care of the patient and encouragement of deep inspiration are desirable for a short time before extensive therapeutic measures are used.

Bronchoscopy for postoperative atelectasis has long been recognized as a lifesaving measure, and the techniques and methods are fully described. The experienced, well equipped endoscopist has no difficulty with children, even the very young.

The best results with intermittent positive pressure breathing are obtained when the treatment is begun on the first postoperative day and used three or four times daily for 15 minutes each time; 40 per cent oxygen and 60 per cent helium or air under 10 to 12 cm. of water pressure, at a rate of eight to ten respirations per minute, are utilized. Medication consisting of bronchodilators, antibiotics, expectorants or detergents may be added as indicated.

Preventive Therapy

Cooperative efforts by the team of physicians, nurses and paramedical persons involved in the care of the surgical patient are most important in the prevention of atelectasis. The absence of respiratory infection preoperatively, the choice of the site for abdominal surgical incision to minimize muscular injury, economy of time during the operation, care in the choice of the anesthetic, depth of anesthesia, together with postoperative supervision encouraging cough, changes of position, and elimination of secretions or vomitus, or blood, are all essential elements of good prophylactic care. Some patients can be encouraged to use intermittent positive pressure breathing the day before operation. Collart and Brenneman (1971) give valuable, detailed suggestions for the care of surgical patients to prevent the development of atelectasis.

The science of anesthesiology and the growth of this specialty by excellent teaching have made massive atelectasis of the lung a rare occurrence. The many research contributions by physiologists, surgeons, internists, pediatricians and other physicians continue to be helpful in understanding the causes and in developing effective preventive measures.

REFERENCES

Auspach, W. E.: Atelectasis and bronchiectasis in children. *Am. J. Dis. Child., 47*:1011, 1934.

Avery, M. E.: The alveolar lining layer. A review of studies on its role in pulmonary mechanics and in the pathogenesis of atelectasis. *Pediatrics, 30*:324, 1962.

Avery, M. E., and Mead, G.: Surface properties in relation to atelectasis and hyaline membrane disease. *Am. J. Dis. Child., 97*:517, 1959.

Barino, C.: Brief clinical consideration of the pathogenesis of "functional" atelectasis. *Riv. Ital. Radiol. Clin., 6*:41, 1956.

Becker, A., Barak, S., Braun, E., and Meyers, M. P.: The treatment of postoperative and pulmonary atelectasis with intermittent positive pressure breathing. *Surg. Gynecol. Obstet., 111*:517, 1960.

Bendixen, H. H., Smith, G. M., and Mead, J.: Pattern of ventilation in young adults. *J. Appl. Physiol., 19*:195, 1964.

Berry, R. E. L., and Sanislow, C. A.: Clinical manifestations and treatment of congestive atelectasis. *Arch. Surg., 87*:153, 1963.

Bowen, T. E., Fishback, M. F., and Green, D. C.: Treatment of refractory atelectasis. *Ann. Thorac. Surg., 18*:584, 1974.

Brashear, R. E., Meyer, S. C., and Manion, M. W.: Unilateral atelectasis in asthma. *Chest, 63*:847, 1973.

Briscoe, J. C.: The mechanism of postoperative massive collapse of the lungs. *Q. J. Med., 13*:293, 1919–1920.

Briscoe, J. C.: The muscular mechanism of respiration and its disorders. *Lancet, 1*:637; 749; 859, 1927.

Brock, R. C.: *The Anatomy of the Bronchial Tree.* London, Oxford Medical Publications, 1954.

Brown, E. S., Johnson, R. P., and Clements, J. A.: Pulmonary surface tension. *J. Appl. Physiol., 14*:717, 1959.

Bryant, L. R., Trinkle, J. K., Mobin-Uddin, K., Baker, J., and Griffen, W. O., Jr.: Bacterial colonization profile with tracheal intubation and mechanical ventilation. *Arch. Surg., 104*:647, 1972.

Bryant, L. R., Mobin-Uddin, K., Dillon, M. L., and Griffen, W. O., Jr.: Misdiagnosis of pneu-

monia in patients needing mechanical respiration. *Arch. Surg., 106*:286, 1973.

Burbank, B., Cutler, S. S., and Sbar, S.: Nonobstructive atelectasis: its occurrence with pneumonitis. *J. Thorac. Cardiovasc. Surg., 41*:701, 1961.

Bush, G. H.: Intermittent pressure breathing in children. In Evans, F. T., and Gray, T. C. (Eds.): *Modern Trends in Anesthesia.* New York, Appleton-Century-Crofts, 1967, p. 217.

Churchill, E. D.: Pulmonary atelectasis, with special reference to massive collapse of the lung. *Arch. Surg., 11*:489, 1925.

Churchill, E. D.: The segmental lobular physiology and pathology of the lung. *J. Thor. Surg., 18*:279, 1949.

Churchill, E. D.: The architectural basis of pulmonary ventilation. *Ann. Surg., 137*:1, 1953.

Clements, J. A.: Surface active materials in the lung. In Liebow, A. A. (Ed.): *The Lung.* Baltimore, Williams & Wilkins Company, 1968, p. 31.

Clinical Anesthesia Conference: Massive atelectasis incident to anesthesia. *N.Y. State J. Med., 73*:1317, 1973.

Colgan, F. J., Mahoney, P. D., and Fanning, G. L.: Resistance breathing (blow bottles) and sustained hyperinflations in the treatment of atelectasis. *Anesthesiology, 32*:543, 1970.

Collart, M. E., and Brenneman, J. K.: Preventing postoperative atelectasis. *Am. J. Nursing, 71*:1982, 1971.

Collins, C. D., Darke, C. S., and Knowelden, J.: Chest complications after upper abdominal surgery: their anticipation and prevention. *Br. Med. J., 1*:401, 1968.

Corbett, D. P., and Washington, J. E.: Respiratory obstruction in the newborn and excess pulmonary fluid. *Am. J. Roentgenol. Radium Ther. Nucl. Med., 112*:18, 1971.

Corssen, G.: Changing concepts of the mechanism of pulmonary atelectasis, a study of smooth muscle elements in the human lung. *J.A.M.A., 188*:485, 1964.

Coryllos, P. N., and Birnbaum, G. L.: The circulation in the compressed atelectatic, and pneumonic lung. *Arch. Surg., 19*:1346, 1929.

Crocker, D., Horne, J. A., Ahlgren, E. W., and Kirby, R. R.: Treatment of post-thoracotomy atelectasis in infants. *Anesth. Analg. (Cleve.), 53*:113, 1974.

Culiner, M. M., Reich, S. B., and Abouav, J.: Nonobstructive consolidation-atelectasis following thoracotomy. *J. Thor. Surg., 37*:371, 1959.

Dargeon, H. W.: *Tumors of Childhood.* New York, Paul B. Hoeber, Inc., 1960.

Dawson, J.: Valvular bronchial obstruction. A report of three cases. *Br. J. Radiol., 25*:557, 1952.

Dees, S. C., and Spock, A.: Right middle lobe syndrome in children. *J.A.M.A., 197*:8, 1966.

Della Porta, G., and De Ritis, L.: Pulmonary atelectasis in bronchial asthma. *Minerva Pediatr., 25*:765, 1973.

DeTakats, G., Beck, W. C., and Fenn, G. K.: Pulmonary embolism. *Surgery, 6*:339, 1939.

DeTakats, G., Fenn, G. K., and Jenkinson, E. L.:

Reflex pulmonary atelectasis. *J.A.M.A., 120*:686, 1942.

Dripps, R. D., and Deming, van M.: Postoperative atelectasis and pneumonia. *Am. Surg., 124*:94, 1946.

Egbert, L. D., and Bendixen, H. H.: Effect of morphine on breathing pattern. A possible factor in atelectasis. *J.A.M.A., 188*:485, 1964.

Ehrlick, R., and Arnon, R. G.: The intermittent endotracheal intubation technique for the treatment of recurrent atelectasis. *Pediatrics, 50*:144, 1972.

Ferris, B. J., Jr., and Pollard, D. S.: Effect of deep and quiet breathing on pulmonary compliance in man. *J. Clin. Invest., 39*:143, 1960.

Fletcher, B. D., and Avery, M. E.: The effects of airway occlusion after oxygen breathing on the lungs of newborn infants. *Radiology, 109*:655, 1973.

Foley, F. D., Moncrief, J. A., and Mason, A. D., Jr.: Pathology of the lung in fatally burned patients. *Ann. Surg., 167*:251, 1968.

Fung, Y. C.: Stress, deformation and atelectasis of the lung. *Circ. Res., 37*:481, 1975.

Galvis, A. G., White J. J., and Oh, K. S.: A bedside washout technique in infants. *Am. J. Dis. Child., 127*:824, 1974.

Gelfand, M. L., Hammer, H., and Hevizy, T.: Asymptomatic pulmonary atelectasis in drug addicts. *Dis. Chest, 52*:782, 1967.

Gerami, S., Richardson, R., Harrington, B., and Pate, J. W.: Obstructive emphysema due to mediastinal bronchogenic cysts in infancy. *J. Thorac. Cardiovasc. Surg., 58*:432, 1969.

Goodwin, T. C.: Lipoid cell pneumonia. *Am. J. Dis. Child., 48*:309, 1934.

Gordon, R. A.: Bronchoscopy in the treatment of pulmonary atelectasis. *Can. Med. Assoc. J., 54*:6, 1946.

Griffiths, M. I.: Pulmonary atelectasis in young children. *Arch. Dis. Child., 28*:170, 1953.

Hamilton, W. K.: Atelectasis, pneumothorax and aspiration as postoperative complications. *Anesthesiology, 22*:708, 1961.

Hamilton, W. K., McDonald, J. S., Fischer, H. W., and Bethards, R.: Postoperative respiratory complications: a comparison of arterial gas tensions, radiographs and physical examination. *Anesthesiology, 25*:607, 1964.

Harboyan, G., and Nassif, R.: Tracheobronchial foreign bodies — a reivew of 14 years' experience. *J. Laryngol., 84*:403, 1970.

Hayward, J., and Reid, L. McA.: The cartilage of the intrapulmonary bronchi in normal lungs, in bronchiectasis, and in massive atelectasis. *Thorax, 7*:98, 1952.

Herfarth, C.: Errors of indication in pulmonary atelectasis of newborns and infants. *Langenbecks Arch. Chir., 327*:593, 1970.

Hobbs, B. B., Hinchcliffe, W. A., and Greenspan, R. H.: Effects of acute lobar atelectasis on pulmonary hemodynamics. *Invest. Radiol., 7*:1, 1972.

Hoffstaedt, E. G. W.: Modern concept of pulmonary collapse: study in functional pathology. *Tubercle, 34*:234, 1953.

Hogg, J. C., Williams, J., Richardson, J. B., Mach-

lem, P. T., and Thurlbeck, W. M.: Age as a factor in the distribution of lower-airway conductance and in the pathologic anatomy of obstructive lung disease. *N. Engl. J. Med., 282*:1283, 1970.

Hughes, W. F., and Reisman, R. E.: Migratory atelectasis in an asthmatic child following steroid withdrawal. *J. Allergy, 43*:301, 1969.

Huppler, E. G., Clagett, O. T., and Grindlay, J. H.: Elimination and transport of mucus in the lung. *J. Thorac. Surg., 32*:661, 1956.

Ikard, R. W.: Bronchogenic cyst causing repeated left lung atelectasis in an adult. *Ann. Thorac. Surg., 14*:434, 1972.

Inselman, L. S., Mellins, R. B., and Brasel, J. A.: Effect of atelectasis on compensatory lung growth. *Am. Rev. Resp. Dis., 113*(Suppl.):41, 1976.

Jackson, C., and Jackson, C. L.: *Diseases of the Nose, Throat and Ear.* Philadelphia, W. B. Saunders Company, 1959, pp. 842–55.

Jacobaeus, H. C.: A study of acute massive atelectatic collapse of the lung. *Br. J. Radiol., 3*:50, 1930.

Jacobaeus, H. C.: Spontaneous collapse of the lung. *Med. Klin., 38*:673, 1932.

James, U., Brumblecombe, F. S. W., and Wells, J. W.: The natural history of pulmonary collapse in childhood. *Q. J. Med., 25*:121, 1956.

Johanssen, L., and William-Olsson, G.: Foreign bodies in the bronchi. *Acta Chir. Scand., 283*(Suppl.):153, 1961.

Kersten, T. E., and Humphrey, E. W.: Pulmonary shunt mechanism in atelectasis. *Surg. Forum, 26*:211, 1975.

Klaus, M., Reiss, O. K., Tolley, W. N., Piel, C., and Clements, J. A.: Alveolar epithelial cell mitrochondria as source of the surface-active lung lining. *Science, 137*:750, 1962.

Kohn, H. H.: Zur Histologie des indurirenden fibrinosen Pneumonie. *Munch. Med. Wochenschr., 40*:42, 1893.

Kuhns, L. R., and Poznanski, A. K.: Endotracheal tube position in the infant. *J. Pediatr., 78*:991, 1971.

Krahl, V. E.: Microscopic anatomy of the lungs. *Am. Rev. Resp. Dis., 80*(Suppl.):24, 1959.

Laennec, R. T. H.: *Diseases of the Chest* (1819). 4th Ed. Translated by John Forbes in 1834. London.

Lambert, M. W.: Accessory bronchiole-alveolar communications. *J. Pathol. Bacteriol., 70*:311, 1955.

Lambert, M. W.: Accessory bronchiolo-alveolar channels. *Anat. Rec., 127*:472, 1957.

Lance, J. S., and Latta, H.: Hypoxia, atelectasis and pulmonary edema. *Arch. Pathol., 75*:373, 1963.

Lecks, H. I., Whitney, T., Wood, D., and Kravis, L. P.: Newer concepts in occurrence of segmental atelectasis in acute bronchial asthma and status asthmaticus in children. *J. Asthma Res., 4*:65, 1966.

Lecks, H. L., Wood, D. W., Kravis, L. P., and Sutnick, A. I.: Pulmonary surfactants, segmental atelectasis and bronchial asthma. *Clin. Pediatr. (Phila.), 6*:270, 1967.

Liebow, A. A.: The genesis and functional implications of collateral circulation of the lungs. *Yale J. Biol. Med., 22*:637, 1950.

Lindskog, G. E.: Studies on the etiology of postoperative pulmonary complications. *J. Thorac. Surg., 10*:635, 1941.

Logan, G. B., and Leonardo, E.: The obstructive lobe syndrome. *J. Asthma Res., 7*:119, 1970.

McAsian, T. C., Matjasko-Chiu, J., Turney, S. Z., and Crowley, R. A.: Influence of inhalation of 100 per cent oxygen on intrapulmonary shunt in severely traumatized patients. *J. Trauma, 13*:811, 1973.

Macklem, P. T.: Airway obstruction and collateral ventilation. *Physiol. Rev., 51*:368, 1971.

Macklin, C. C.: The musculature of the bronchi and lungs. *Physiol. Rev., 9*:1, 1929.

Mead, J., Wittenberger, J. L., and Radford, E. P., Jr.: Surface tension as a factor in pulmonary volume pressure hysteresis. *J. Appl. Physiol., 10*:191, 1957.

Melamed, M., Langston, H. T., Reynes, C., and Barker, W. L.: Simulated paraspinal tumor or abscess by rounded atelectasis of the lower lobe. *Chest, 67*:497, 1975.

Messer, J. W., Peters, G. A., and Bennett, W. A.: Causes of death and pathologic findings in 304 cases of bronchial asthma. *Chest, 38*:616, 1960.

Michael, P.: *Tumors of Infancy and Childhood.* Philadelphia, J. B. Lippincott Company, 1964, p. 251.

Moersch, H. J.: Bronchoscopy in treatment of postoperative atelectasis. *Surg. Gynecol. Obstet., 77*:435, 1943.

Molonoy, C. J.: Postoperative pulmonary collapse in childhood. *Am. J. Dis. Child., 66*:280, 1943.

Munt, P. M.: Middle lobe atelectasis in sarcoidosis. Report of a case with prompt resolution. *Am. Rev. Resp. Dis., 108*:357, 1973.

Nathan, M. A., and Reis, D. J.: Hypoxemia, atelectasis and the elevation of arterial pressure and heart rate in paralyzed artifically ventilated rat. *Life Sci., 16*:1103, 1975.

Newell, J. C., Levitzky, M. G., and Lowers, S. R., Jr.: Influence of methylprednisolone on perfusion of acutely atelectatic lung. *Surg. Forum, 26*:106, 1975.

O'Connor, M. J.: Comparison of two methods of postoperative pulmonary care. *Surg. Gynecol. Obstet., 140*:615, 1975.

Ngai, S. H.: The pharmacological aspects of the control of respiration. In Evans, F. T., and Gray, T. C. (Eds.): *Modern Trends in Anesthesia.* Vol. 3. New York, Appleton-Century-Crofts, 1967, p. 171.

O'Brien, E.: Vegetal bronchitis. A summation of thoughts on its etiology. Presentation of 23 Cases. *Laryngoscope, 58*:1013, 1948.

O'Driscoll, M.: Postoperative pulmonary atelectasis and collapse, and its prophylaxis with intravenous bicarbonate. *Br. Med. J., 4*:26, 1970.

Oh, K. S., Stitik, F. P., Galvis, A. G., Bearman, S. B., Heller, R. M., and Dorst, J. P.: Radiologic manifestations in patients on continuous positive pressure breathing. *Radiology, 110*:627, 1974.

Ophsahl, T., and Berman, E. J.: Bronchogenic mediastinal cysts in infants. *Pediatrics, 30*:372, 1962.

Palamarchuk, V. P.: Atelectasis of the lungs in the burned. *Vestn. Rentgenol. Radiol., 43*:3, 1968.

Palley, A.: Factors leading to production of bronchiectasis in childhood and its prevention. *S. Afr. Med. J., 22*:169, 1948.

Pasteur, W.: Respiratory paralysis after diphtheria as a cause of pulmonary complications, with suggestions as to treatment. *Am. J. Med. Sci., 100*:242, 1890.

Pasteur, W.: Massive collapse of the lung. *Lancet, 2*:1351, 1908.

Pasteur, W.: Active lobar collapse of the lung after abdominal operations. *Lancet, 2*:1080, 1910.

Pattle, R. E.: Properties, function and origin of the alveolar lining layer. *Proc. R. Soc. Lond., (Biol.) Series, B, 148*:217, 1958.

Pattle, R. E., and Thomas, L. C.: Lipoprotein composition of the film lining the lung. *Nature, 189*:844, 1961.

Perna, A. M., Brawley, R. K., Bender, H. W., and Gott, V. L.: Fatal respiratory distress syndrome after prolonged mechanical ventilation: its pathogenesis and prevention. *J. Surg. Res., 11*:584, 1971.

Pinck, R. L., Burbank, R., Cutler, S. S., Sbar, S., and Mangieri, M.: Nonobstructive atelectasis. *Am. Rev. Resp. Dis., 91*:909, 1965.

Pruitt, B. A., Jr., DiVincenti, F. C., Mason, A. D., Jr., Foley, F. D., and Flemma, R. J.: The occurrence and significance of pneumonia and other pulmonary complications in burned patients: comparison of conventional and topical treatments. *J. Trauma, 10*:519, 1970.

Radford, E. P., Jr.: Method for estimating respiratory surface area of mammalian lungs from their physical characteristics. *Proc. Soc. Exp. Biol. Med., 87*:58, 1954.

Radford, E. P., Jr.: Recent studies of mechanical properties of mammalian lungs. In Remington, J. W., (Ed.): *Tissue Elasticity.* Washington, D. C., American Physiological Society, 1957, pp. 177–190.

Radigan, L. R., and King, R. D.: A technique for the prevention of postoperative atelectasis. *Surgery, 47*:184, 1960.

Rahn, H.: The role of N_2 gas in various biological processes, with particular reference to the lung. *Harvey Lectures.* Series 55, 1959–1960, p. 173.

Reilly, B. J.: Neonatal radiology. Regional distribution of atelectasis and fluid in the neonate with respiratory distress. *Radiol. Clin. North Am., 13*:225, 1975.

Reinhardt, K.: Total left pulmonary atelectasis following bronchography. *J. Radiol. Electrol. Med. Nucl., 32*:470, 1951.

Robbins, L. L., and Hale, C. H.: Roentgen appearance of lobar and segmental collapse of lung. Technic of examination. *Radiology, 44*:107, 1945.

Robinson, A. E., Hall, K. D., Yokoyama, K. N., and Capp, M. P.: Pediatric bronchography: the problems of segmental pulmonary loss of volume. I. A retrospective study of 165 pediatric bronchograms. *Invest. Radiol., 6*:89, 1971.

Rose, M., and Lindsberg, D. A. B.: Effect of pulmonary pathogens on surfactant. *Dis. Chest, 53*:541, 1968.

Ross Conference on Pediatric Research #37: Normal and abnormal respiration in children. 1960, pp. 36–45.

Rudy, N. E., and Crepeau, J.: Role of intermittent positive pressure breathing postoperatively. *J.A.M.A., 167*:1093, 1958.

Sachdeva, S. P.: Treatment of postoperative pulmonary atelectasis by active inflation of the atelectatic lobe(s) through an endobronchial tube. *Acta Anaesthesiol. Scand., 18*:65, 1974.

Safar, P., Grenvik, A., and Smith, J.: Progressive pulmonary consolidation: a review of cases and pathogenesis. *J. Trauma, 12*:955, 1972.

Scarpelli, E. M.: Pulmonary surfactants and their role in lung disease. *Adv. Pediat., 16*:177, 1969.

Schwartz, M. L., Northrup, W. F., Nicoloff, D. M., and Humphrey, E. W.: The effect of steroids on adaptation to atelectatic shunting. *J. Thorac., 68*:822, 1974.

Shaw, R. R.: Mucoid impaction of the bronchi. *J. Thorac. Surg., 22*:149, 1951.

Siebecker, K. L., Sadler, P. E., and Mendenhall, J. T.: Postoperative ear oximeter studies in patients who have undergone pulmonary resection. *J. Thorac. Surg., 36*:88, 1958.

Singer, J. J., and Graham, E. A.: Roentgen-ray study of bronchiectasis. *Am. J. Roentgenol., 15*:54, 1926.

Skatrud, J., Gilbert, R., Auchincloss, J. H., Jr., and Rana, S.: Blood clot cast following hemoptysis and resulting in atelectasis. *Chest, 69*:131, 1976.

Sladen, A., Laver, M. B., and Pontoppidan, H.: Pulmonary complications and water retention in prolonged mechanical ventilation. *N. Engl. J. Med., 279*:448, 1968.

Smith, T. C., and Siebecker, K. L.: Postoperative ear oximeter studies in thoracotomy patients. II. Variations with operative procedures and with the stir-up regime. *J. Thorac. Cardiovasc. Surg., 39*:478, 1960.

Smith, T. C., Cook, F. D., De Kornfield, T. J., and Siebecker, K. L.: Pulmonary function in the immediate postoperative period. *J. Thorac. Cardiovasc. Surg., 39*:788, 1960.

Spain, D. M.: Acute nonaeration of lung: pulmonary edema versus atelectasis. *Dis. Chest, 25*:550, 1954.

Stein, M., Koota, G. M., Simon, M., and Frank, H. A.: Pulmonary evaluation of surgical patients. *J.A.M.A., 181*:765, 1962.

Stranger, P., Lucas, R. V., Jr., and Edwards, J. E.: Anatomical factors causing respiratory distress in a cyanotic congenital cardiac disease. *Pediatrics, 43*:760, 1969.

Strum, A.: Der Lungenkrampf: Kontraktionatektase durch pulmonalen Spasmus. *Dtsch. Med. Wochenschr., 71*:201, 1946.

Strum, A.: Ist die Lunge Kontraktil? *Schweiz. Med. Wochenschr., 81*:859, 1951.

Sutnick, A. O., and Soloff, L. A.: Pulmonary surfactant and atelectasis. *Anesthesiology, 25*:676, 1964.

Swartz, S. T.: Complications. In Swartz, S. T., et al. (Eds.): *Principles of Surgery.* 2nd Ed. New York, McGraw-Hill Book Company, Inc., 1974, pp. 467–469.

Sweet, R. H.: Analysis of 130 cases of hiatus hernia treated surgically. *J.A.M.A., 151*:367, 1953.

Tannenberg, O., and Pinner, M.: Atelectasis and bronchiectasis. *J. Thorac. Surg., 11*:571, 1942.

Thomas, P. A.: A comparative study of lung compliance and pulmonary surfactant activity in human subjects. *Ann. Thorac. Surg., 11*:133, 1971.

Tichy, S., Skerik, P., Pitha, J., and Vanousova, E.: Treatment by bronchoscopic aspiration in cases of pulmonary atelectasis following thoracic and abdominal operations. *Rozhl. Chir., 49*:70, 1970.

Tooley, W., Gardner, R., Thung, N., and Finley, T.: Factors affecting the surface tension of lung extracts. *Fed. Proc., 20*:428, 1961.

Townsend, E. H., Jr., and Squire, L.: Treatment of atelectasis by thoracic traction. *Pediatrics, 17*:250, 1956.

Traube, L.: Die Ursachen und die Beschaffenheit der jenigen Veranderungen, Welche das Lungenparenchym nach Durchschneidung der Nn. Vagi erleidet. Kritisch-experimenteller Beitrag zur Lehre von der Pneumonie und Atelektase. *Beitr. Exp. Pathol. Physiol., 1*:65, 1846.

Van Allen, C. M., and Lindskog, G. E.: Collateral respiration in the lung. *Surg. Gynecol. Obstet., 53*:16, 1931.

Von Neergaard, K.: Neue Auffassungen ober einen Grundbegriff der Atemmechanik. Die Retraktions Kraft der Lunge, abhangig von der Oberflachenspannung in den Alveolen. *Ztachr. Ges. Exp. Med., 66*:373, 1929.

Voss, T. J. V.: Ways of reducing atelectasis and improving oxygen uptake from the lungs. *S. Afr. Med. J., 47*:761, 1973.

Wahrenbrock, E. A., Carrico, C. J., Amundsen, D. A., Trummer, M. J., and Severinghaus, J. W.: Increased atelectatic pulmonary shunt during hemorrhagic shock in dogs. *J. Appl. Physiol., 29*:615, 1970.

Waldbott, G. L.: Complications of bronchial asthma. *South. Med. J., 56*:407, 1963.

Wanner, A., Landa, J. F., Nieman, R. E., Jr., Vevaina, J., and Delgado, I.: Bedside bronchofiberscopy for atelectasis and lung abscess. *J.A.M.A., 224*:1281, 1973.

Waring, W. W., Brunt, C. H., and Hillman, B. C.: Mucoid impaction of the bronchi in cystic fibrosis. *Pediatrics, 39*:166, 1967.

Wesenberg, R. L., and Struble, R. A.: Selective bronchial catheterization and lavage in the newborn. A new therapeutic procedure for diagnostic radiology. *Radiology, 105*:397, 1972.

Wittig, H. J., and Chang, C. H. (Joseph): Right middle lobe atelectasis in childhood asthma. *J. Asthma, 39*:245, 1967.

Xalabarder, C.: What is atelectasis? *Tubercle, 30*:266, 1949.

Yeh, T. J., Manning, H., Ellison, L. T. and Ellison, R. G.: Alveolar surfactant in chronic experimental atelectasis. *Am. Rev. Resp. Dis., 93*:953, 1966.

CHAPTER THIRTY-EIGHT

PULMONARY EDEMA

ROBERT B. MELLINS, M.D., and S. ALEX STALCUP, M.D.

One by-product of the availability of potent diuretics and the modern trend toward intensive care and monitoring of patients with serious illnesses has been a greater appreciation of the significance of fluid movement into the lung as a complication of a variety of conditions. This, coupled with an improved understanding of the pathogenesis of pulmonary edema, summarized in several recent reviews (Fishman, 1972; Robin and coworkers, 1973; Staub, 1974; Guyton and coworkers, 1975; Levine and Mellins, 1975), has enhanced our ability to treat a variety of illnesses in which pulmonary edema develops.

Anatomic Considerations

Certain structural features of the lung are worth pointing out because they have a bearing on gas exchange during pulmonary edema. The capillaries are placed eccentrically within the alveolar septum (Fig. 1 *A*). In some areas, the basement membrane of the capillary endothelium and the alveolar epithelium are fused with no additional space between them, even during edema formation. This would seem to be an ideal situation for preserving gas exchange, at least until such time as the alveoli themselves are filled with liquid. In other areas, there is an interstitial space between the endothelial and epithelial basement membrane that

contains a ground substance and connective tissue elements. In addition to supplying support to the capillary network, this widened portion of the alveolar-capillary membrane provides a channel for water and protein en route to the lymphatics and larger interstitial fluid spaces (Fig. 1 *B*). As long as water can be confined to these channels, gas exchange can be preserved.

Pulmonary capillaries, like muscle capillaries, have a continuous endothelium with relatively tight intercellular junctions. The bronchial microvasculature, much like visceral capillaries, is discontinuous, with intercellular fenestrations or gaps. Whether this accounts for increased fluid movement across the bronchial but not the pulmonary capillaries (for example, in response to bradykinin as shown by Pietra and coworkers, 1971) remains to be determined. It may be that the role of the bronchial circulation in the genesis of pulmonary edema has been underestimated.

At the ultrastructural level, the available evidence from tracer studies indicates that the alveolar epithelial membrane contains tighter cellular junctions than does the capillary endothelial membrane. Thus, edema in diseases that alter pulmonary vascular permeability is likely to be confined initially to the interstitial and lymphatic spaces; alveolar edema results only when the volume that can be handled by these is overwhelmed.

Although the alveoli are generally conceived as spherical in shape, there is increasing evidence that a polyhedral

Supported in part by NIH grants HL 06012 and HL 14218 (SCOR), with additional support from the New York Lung Association.

573

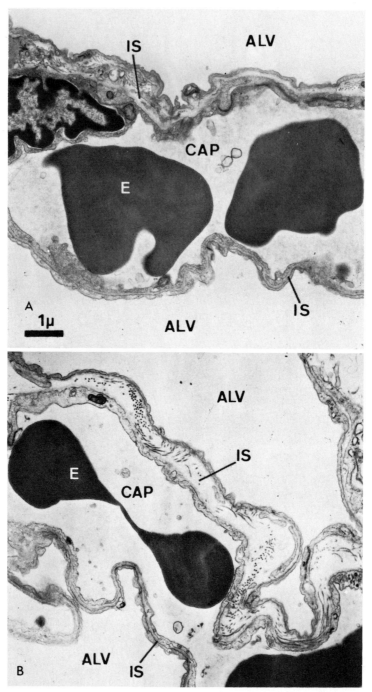

Figure 1. *A,* The normal alveolar septum in which the epithelial and endothelial basement membranes are fused in some areas and separated by an interstitial space of connective tissue in others. *B,* The alveolar septum in pulmonary edema. The areas where the basement membranes are fused remain thin; only the areas with a connective tissue interstitial space widen. ALV, alveolar lumen; CAP, capillary; E, erythrocyte; IS, interstitial space. (From Mellins, R. B., Levine, O. R., and Fishman, A. P.: *Circ. Res., 24*:197, 1969.)

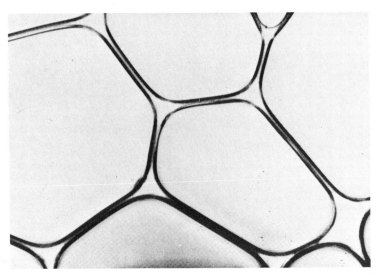

Figure 2. Surfactant foam obtained from the lung by bronchial rinsing assumes a polyhedral shape. (From Reifenrath, R.: *Resp. Physiol., 24*:115, 1975.)

model is closer to reality. Figure 2 shows that this is indeed the shape that is assumed by surfactant removed from the lung. From the point of view of fluid movement in the lung, the importance of this shape is that the walls of the alveolar septa are flat, except at the corners where the septa meet. Thus, it is only at the corners where the alveolar air-liquid interface is curved that the force exerted by surface tension can lower alveolar fluid and interstitial fluid pressures as predicted by the Laplace relationship (Fig. 3).

Pulmonary blood vessels have been defined anatomically and physiologically. Anatomically, the vessels have been traditionally classified by their morphologic characteristics as either arteries, arterioles, capillaries, veins or venules. Functionally, these divisions are included under two broad classifications based upon their behavior relative to the hydrostatic pressures of the interstitium surrounding the vessels, the interstitial fluid pressure. These are the alveolar vessels and the extra-alveolar vessels. The alveolar vessels are in the alveolar walls or septae and behave as if they were exposed to alveolar pressure. These vessels may collapse if airway pressures exceed vascular pressures (zone I conditions of West). Extra-alveolar vessels lie in the larger interstitial spaces and behave as if surrounded by a pressure that is as negative or more negative than pleural pressure, and that tends to vary with pleural pressure. In addition, there are vessels lying in the intersections of alveolar septal walls (corner vessels) that are exposed to more negative pressures than the alveolar vessels, at least in part because of the acute radius of curvature found at the alveolar corners as described previously (Fig. 3). The functional classification is important because it predicts the pressures surrounding the vessels participating in fluid exchange, and it will be used in subsequent analyses of fluid movement and edema. Unfortunately, there is no clear-cut correlation between the functional and the anatomical classifications.

Although fluid exchange is generally considered to occur at the capillary level, it is now clear that a large amount of fluid movement also occurs at the level of the arterioles and venules, and that under certain circumstances more

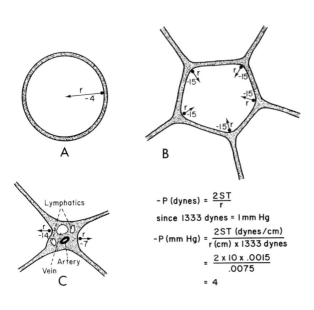

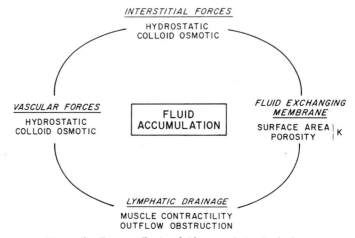

Figure 3. Effect of surface tension on the alveolar fluid and interstitial fluid pressure. *A*, Assuming a spherical model of the alveolus with a radius of 75 microns and a surface tension of 10 dynes/cm., we calculate that the fluid lining the alveolus would be pulled away with a pressure of minus 4 mm. Hg. *B*, Assuming a polyhedral model, with the radius of curvature at the corners of 20 microns, the negative pressure in the corners would be minus 15 mm. Hg. The pressure at the angles (not shown) where the alveolar air-liquid interface is cylindrical and where $-P = \dfrac{ST}{r}$ would be minus 7.5 mm. Hg. *C*, Dynamics at alveolar angles adjacent to interstitial spaces surrounding larger blood vessels and lymphatics; pressures of minus 7 to minus 14 mm. Hg can be calculated, depending on the radius of curvature at the angles. (Modified from Guyton, A. C., et al.: In *Lung Liquids.* Ciba Symposium 38. Amsterdam, North Holland, American Elsevier Publishing Company, 1976.)

than 50 per cent of pulmonary edema fluid originates from extra-alveolar vessels (Iliff, 1971).

Forces Responsible for Fluid Movement

The factors responsible for fluid accumulation are shown in Figure 4. These include intravascular and interstitial hydrostatic and colloid osmotic pressures, the permeability character-istics of the fluid-exchanging membrane, and lymphatic drainage.

The equilibrium of fluid across fluid-exchanging membranes is generally expressed as follows:

$$Q_f = K_f \, (Pmv - Ppmv) - \sigma(\pi mv - \pi pmv)$$

wherein

Q_f = the net transvascular flow;

K_f = the filtration coefficient of the

Figure 4. Factors affecting fluid accumulation in the lung.

fluid-exchanging vessels and includes both the contribution of the permeability of the vessels and the surface area across which fluid exchange occurs;

Pmv = microvascular hydrostatic pressure;

Ppmv = perimicrovascular (interstitial fluid) hydrostatic pressure;

πmv = colloid osmotic pressure in the microvasculature;

πpmv = colloid osmotic pressure in the perimicrovasculature, the interstitial fluid colloid osmotic pressure;

σ = the reflection coefficient and describes the transvascular protein osmotic pressure difference; it is a measure of the resistance of the membrane to the flow of protein.

The term "microvasculature" is used because, as previously indicated, fluid exchange is not limited to the capillaries alone. In the following discussion, each of the above factors and the pathophysiologic influences on them will be described in detail.

VASCULAR FORCES. The pressure in the pulmonary microvasculature, Pmv (generally but not precisely referred to as pulmonary capillary pressure), is believed to be above left atrial pressure by 40 per cent of the difference between left atrial (LA) and pulmonary arterial (PA) pressure. Hence, an increase in either PA or LA pressure will tend to increase the hydrostatic pressure, favoring movement out of the fluid-exchanging vessels. For example, Pmv may be increased by the elevation in LA pressures in left-sided heart failure, or by increases in PA pressure as seen in large left-to-right shunts. Because of the large capacity of the pulmonary vascular bed, considerable elevation in blood flow can occur (as in exercise, or shunts) without raising PA pressures appreciably. At the experimental level, ligation of one pulmonary artery, directing all flow through the contralateral lung, results in only a slight elevation of PA pressure at rest. A clinical illustration of the capacity of the pulmonary vascular bed to handle an increase in blood flow was provided by a five-month-old infant we studied with congenital absence of the left lung and total anomalous pulmonary venous connection t the right atrium. Surgical correction of pulmonary venous obstruction reduced PA pressures to normal, despite the continued diversion of the total cardiac output to the right lung.

Because the pulmonary vascular membrane is only very slightly permeable to proteins, the plasma proteins normally are responsible for osmotic pressure (πmv) well in excess of the pulmonary microvascular hydrostatic pressure. The plasma colloid osmotic pressure may be markedly reduced in clinical conditions in which the plasma proteins are low, e.g., malnutrition, nephrosis and massive burns.

It should also be emphasized that the rapid infusion of non-colloid-containing fluids not only raises vascular hydrostatic pressures, but also lowers the colloid osmotic pressure because of hemodilution. On the other hand, the infusion of colloid-containing fluids may raise microvascular hydrostatic pressure because of the absorption of fluid throughout the body, thus limiting its usefulness as a therapeutic agent in edema.

INTERSTITIAL FORCES AND MECHANICAL INTERDEPENDENCE. Although still a matter of controversy, we believe that the weight of evidence provided by Guyton, Taylor, and Granger (1975) favors the conclusion that the interstitial hydrostatic pressure throughout the lung is normally negative. The degree of negativity that one calculates using the classic Starling formulation depends upon the values one uses for the perimicrovascular or interstitial colloid osmotic pressure. Because the concentration of protein in the lymph from the lung is relatively high as compared with lymph from an extremity, some have assumed that the protein in the perimicrovascular space is also high. On the other hand, considering the delicate nature of the lymphatic walls and the fact that lymphatics can generate considerable pressures, it seems likely that concentration of the protein occurs in the lung lymphatics and that the protein concentration in the pulmonary interstitial spaces is considerably lower than in the lung lymph. This concentrating ability of the lymphatics together with its strong pumping action would seem to be necessary for the maintenance of a negative interstitial fluid pressure and a dry lung.

Some recent studies on the manner in which pleural pressures are transmitted to the interstitium of the lung have special relevance to the development of pulmonary edema, especially in diseases that affect the lung nonuniformly. As previously indicated, the pressure surrounding the corner and extra-alveolar vessels is believed to be less than pleural pressure, and can become considerably more negative at high lung volumes (Permutt, 1973). In disease, these negative pressures may be amplified many fold because of "mechanical interdependence" of lung units (Mead and coworkers, 1970; Macklem and Murphy, 1974). When the expansion of some units of the lung lags behind surrounding lung units because of disease, the force (pleural pressure) per unit area distending the lagging unit is increased. Amplification of transpulmonary (distending) pressures by mechanical interdependence is seen in situations of increased respiratory resistance, decreased lung compliance, or expansion of the lung from the airless state. Mechanical interdependence can act on diseased areas of the lung to produce distending pressures that are exceedingly large. When transmitted to the interstitial space around blood vessels, these pressures can enhance edema formation and may cause the rupture of vessels. Indeed, this may be a central mechanism in the formation of hyaline membranes. These considerations become especially important when various forms of constant distending pressures are used therapeutically. Although only 5 to 10 cm. H_2O may be applied, if the pressure does not distend some areas of the lung as quickly as others, the pressure surrounding lagging units may be consid-

erably greater because of amplification of pressures. Another approach that has led to much the same conclusions has been provided by Reifenrath (1975), who suggests that it is mechanical interdependence that is primarily responsible for lung stability.

MICROVASCULAR FILTRATION COEFFICIENT. Several groups of workers have attempted to characterize the ease with which water crosses the pulmonary fluid-exchanging vessels by calculating K_f, the filtration coefficient. K_f includes both the surface area of the membrane and its porosity. There are at least two kinds of questions to be addressed. First, is the pulmonary capillary more or less leaky than fluid-exchanging vessels in other tissues? Second, is the lung of the young animal more or less leaky than the lung of the adult?

Some studies have suggested that the K_f of the pulmonary capillaries is about one-tenth of the muscle capillaries (Levine and coworkers, 1967). On the other hand, other studies (Perl and associates, 1975) provide evidence that the filtration coefficient of the pulmonary vessels is approximately the same as that of the skeletal muscle capillaries.

Some of the apparent differences in K_f obtained by different workers (Staub, 1974) may be explained by Guyton's observations that normally there is a great deal of resistance to the flow of fluid in the narrow interstitial spaces of the alveolar septal wall, resulting in a very low "effective" pulmonary capillary filtration coefficient. As fluid accumulates and the septum widens, the resistance falls and the "effective" filtration coefficient is higher.

There is experimental evidence to suggest that the microvascular permeability to protein is greater in the young as compared with the adult dog (Taylor and associates, 1967; Boyd and coworkers 1969), and that the filtration coefficient of the puppy lung is greater than that of the adult dog (Levine and coworkers, 1973). However, uncertainties about the difference in magnitude of the interstitial forces, the lymphatic drainage and the surface area of the alveolar capillary membrane in the immature and mature lung make it impossible to calculate K_f with any precision.

Our understanding of the factors that alter microvascular membrane permeability are primitive. Contrary to much that is written, there is evidence that hypoxia alone does not alter permeability (Goodale and colleagues, 1970). Histamine, which appears to increase the permeability of systemic vascular beds (including the bronchial vessels), has been considered to have little effect on the pulmonary microvasculature. However, Brigham and Owen (1975) have shown an increase in lymph flow in response to histamine infusions, but it is not clear whether this response can be attributed to a change in vascular permeability or to changes in the balance of hydrostatic pressures. The role of potent vasoactive chemical mediators with known permeability effects, such as bradykinin and the prostaglandins, is just beginning to be studied.

LYMPHATIC CLEARANCE. Whether there is fluid accumulation in the lung depends upon the balance between fluid filtration into the lung and lymphatic clearance. Early in the onset of interstitial edema, lymphatic drainage of fluid is an important protective mechanism preventing alveolar flooding. Although the lymphatics may not be able to handle large amounts of fluid acutely, there is experimental evidence to indicate that under conditions of chronic edema the ability of the lymphatics to clear fluid may increase several fold.

Since the lymphatics ultimately drain into the great veins, elevation of systemic venous pressure might be expected to increase fluid accumulation not only by raising pressure in the fluid-exchanging vessels but also by impairing lymphatic drainage. While impairment of clearance by this mechanism may occur under conditions of chronic right-sided heart failure, especially if lymphatic valve incompetence

occurs, a variety of acute experiments indicate that the lymphatics can actively generate pressures in excess of 25 mm. Hg (Hall and coworkers, 1965; Pang and Mellins, 1975). Although earlier work had indicated that increased motion or ventilation of the lung increased lymphatic fluid drainage, suggesting a passive milking action, it now appears that the contribution of active contractions of the smooth muscle of the lymphatics is also significant. To what extent drugs that affect smooth muscle also affect lymphatic pumping is unknown, but could be appreciable.

Active contraction of the lymphatics, together with the presence of lymphatic valves, helps to explain how fluid moves "uphill" from the negative pressures in the pulmonary interstitium (minus 9 mm. Hg) to the great veins at a pressure of zero or above.

SURFACE TENSION. Surface tension on the inner surface of the alveolus tends to pull fluid away from the alveolar epithelium with a force of at least minus 4 mm. Hg (Fig. 3 A). This figure is based upon the assumption that the alveolar surface is spherical and that the surface tension is 10 dynes per cm., which is low presumably because of the presence of the surfactant. However, because the alveoli are polyhedral in shape, there are many angles where two alveoli come together and corners where more than two alveoli abut. Although the shape of the alveolar air-liquid interface is spherical in the corners as well as in crypts in the alveolar walls, it is cylindrical at the angles, and therefore $-P = \frac{ST}{r}$ would be the appropriate formula to use at the angles. Because the radii of curvature at the angles and corners of the alveoli are much smaller, the pressures will therefore be much more negative (Fig. 3 B). Surface tension at the alveolar air-liquid interface would be expected to expand the perivascular space and to lower perimicrovascular pressure, thus promoting the formation of interstitial edema. The effect of the change in radius of curvature of the alveolar air-liquid interface on surface forces is further illustrated in Figure 5. Initially, as fluid collects in the corners, the radius of curvature becomes greater and the pressure becomes less negative (Fig. 5 *B*). Once the fluid layer becomes spherical throughout the inner surface of the alveoli, additional fluid will decrease the radius, and the pressure will become more negative (Fig. 5 *C*). This explains why the filling of an alveolus with fluid is self-accelerating once there is a critical amount of fluid in the alveolus.

From the above reasoning, Guyton, Taylor and Granger (1975) have concluded that for alveoli of normal size, the interstitial fluid pressure around alveoli (and around alveolar vessels) would have to be at least minus 2 mm. Hg to prevent alveolar flooding; for smaller alveoli, the interstitial pressure would have to be still more negative.

Surface tension at the alveolar air-liquid interface opposes the transmission of alveolar pressure to the fluid-exchanging vessels (Mellins and co-workers, 1969). Therefore, the beneficial effects of positive pressure breathing in the treatment of pulmonary edema probably do not relate to an increase in the pressure surrounding the fluid-exchanging vessels, but rather to (1) an increase in intrathoracic pressures, impeding venous return to the thorax, thus lowering the hydrostatic pressures within the pulmonary vascular bed, and (2) the prevention of airway collapse, thus enhancing blood gas exchange.

Safety Factors Against Edema

A variety of clinical observations have indicated that vascular hydrostatic pressures must be raised 15 to 20 mm. Hg, or plasma colloid osmotic pressures reduced an equivalent amount, before edema develops. Several factors contribute to this safety factor against edema. The interstitial fluid pressure, which we believe to be about minus 9 mm. Hg, is not a fixed value, but will rise to approximately zero with minimal amounts of fluid filtration into the lung. At the same time, the filtered

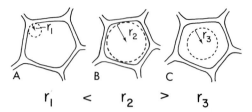

Figure 5. Effect of fluid accumulation on the radius of curvature at the alveolar air-liquid interface. See text for description.

fluid will dilute the interstitial plasma protein, thus lowering the interstitial colloid osmotic pressure. Lymphatic drainage of fluid and protein also contributes to this margin of safety. The ability of the lymphatics to concentrate protein by filtration of fluid through the walls of the lymphatics, although still an area of controversy, probably also contributes by keeping the interstitial osmotic pressure low.

Pathophysiologic Consequences

The effect of pulmonary edema on the function of the lung is complex. Increased pulmonary blood volumes result in a fall in lung compliance, i.e., increased lung recoil, at normal or high lung volumes (Levine and coworkers, 1965); however, there is a decrease in lung recoil at low lung volumes, which leads to premature airway closure, and an increase in the resistance of the peripheral airways (Macklem, 1976). Increase in interstitial edema does not further reduce the compliance at high lung volumes until the extravascular fluid volumes increase at least threefold (Hauge and coworkers, 1975). Peribronchiolar cuffs of fluid would be expected to lead to an increase in airway closure and an increase in airway resistance. Studies in adult animals (Levine and coworkers, 1965) have shown some increase in total airway resistance. If the small airways contribute a relatively greater proportion of the total airway resistance in infants than in adults, one might expect pulmonary edema to lead to a greater increase in airway resistance in the infant. Indeed, airway obstruction has been a presenting sign of a group of infants with ventricular septal defects and left-to-right shunts (Hordof and coworkers, 1977), presumably, at least in part, because of interstitial pulmonary edema. In addition, some children with interstitial edema as a result of left atrial obstruction, e.g., cor triatriatum, have also presented with a picture of recurrent asthmatic attacks. To minimize the markedly increased work of moving their stiff lungs, a pattern of rapid, shallow breathing is used. It is also believed that stimulation of vagal juxtaalveolar or J-receptors within the interstitium by edema contributes to the hyperventilation as well as the tachypnea and dyspnea so characteristic of early pulmonary edema. It is not clear whether increased ventilation enhances or impedes fluid accumulation. Increased ventilation is known to promote the removal of excess water by the lymphatics. However, if there are inhomogeneities of disease within the lung, we have already indicated that mechanical amplification of pressures could lead to enhanced edema formation.

Initially, edema fluid collects around the larger blood vessels and airways. The tethering action of the lung on airways is thus reduced, and the airways are narrowed and more likely to close at higher than normal lung volumes. Airway resistance is thus increased, and alveolar gas exchange is impaired. As edema worsens and alveolar flooding occurs, there is further hypoxemia as the blood shunts past nonventilating alveoli. Respiratory acidosis may supervene if the patient is depressed by the use of sedation or if exhaustion develops. The extent to which bronchial mucosal edema intensifies the increase in airway resistance when pulmonary edema is accompanied by elevated systemic venous pressure is not known.

The rightward shift of the oxygen dissociation curve produced by the increased red cell 2, 3-diphosphoglyceric acid seen with chronic hypoxemia may not occur with acute pulmonary edema, thus limiting the unloading of oxygen at the tissue level. Respiratory alkalosis, more commonly seen in older children and adults with pulmonary edema, may shift the oxygen dissociation curve to the left, which also impairs oxygen unloading.

Pulmonary edema has been shown to impair intrapulmonary antibacterial activity in vivo, and the antibacterial activity of alveolar macrophages harvested from edematous lungs has also been shown to be impaired (La Force and coworkers, 1973).

Although the dynamics of pleural fluid formation are discussed in Chapter 40, it is worth pointing out here that there is no simple correlation between the accumulation of pulmonary and pleural fluid. Thus, in an experimental preparation in which the effects on fluid accumulation in the thorax of systemic and pulmonary venous hypertension were compared, there was a greater accumulation of pleural fluid in systemic venous hypertension, while there was more pulmonary edema with pulmonary venous hypertension (Mellins and coworkers, 1970).

Etiologic Considerations

INCREASED HYDROSTATIC PRESSURE IN THE PULMONARY MICROVASCULATURE. A variety of clinical conditions are associated with increased hydrostatic pressures in the pulmonary vascular bed, either as the result of elevation of vascular pressures distal to the lung or as the result of increased blood flow and pulmonary arterial hypertension. Those resulting from elevation of pressures distal to the lung include left-sided heart failure, congenital hypoplastic left heart syndrome, cor triatriatum, mitral stenosis, congenital obstruction of pulmonary venous drainage, and pulmonary veno-occlusive disease.

Pulmonary edema as a result of left-sided heart failure is seen in severe aortic stenosis, in coarctation of the aorta (usually accompanied by a left ventricular overload in infants), in intrinsic myocardial disease (cardiac glycogen storage diseases, endocardial fibroelastosis, anomalous left coronary artery, viral and rheumatic myocarditis), and in large congenital arteriovenous fistulas. Pulmonary edema is a frequent complication of acute renal disease when systemic hypertension is accompanied by expansion of the extracellular fluid in excess of urine output.

A variety of congenital heart lesions, including ventricular septal defects and patent ductus arteriosus, are associated with increased blood flow and pressure in the pulmonary vascular bed, leading to vascular engorgement and edema. When the burden on the left ventricle becomes too great as a result of the large left-to-right shunt and left-sided heart failure supervenes, pulmonary vascular pressures are increased by both high flow and increased left atrial pressures.

Pulmonary edema is sometimes seen as a complication of surgically performed systemic-to-pulmonary artery shunts for congenital lesions with insufficient pulmonary blood flow, such as Fallot's tetrad. This is more likely to occur following a Waterston type shunt than with a Blalock procedure, because the margin of safety between an insufficient shunt and one that is too great is very narrow in the former.

Overzealous administration of fluids may also intensify the development of pulmonary edema by raising hydrostatic pressures and by diluting plasma proteins. To what extent the inappropriate secretion of antidiuretic hormone complicates and intensifies the development of pulmonary edema in diseases is not known. This has been reported to occur with severe pneumonia (Mor and coworkers, 1975) and asthma (Baker and coworkers, 1976), and could accompany other diseases.

DECREASED PLASMA COLLOID OSMOTIC PRESSURE. For any given level of vascular pressure, pulmonary edema is more likely to develop when the plasma proteins are low. This is seen with severe malnutrition, massive burns, protein-losing enteropathies and nephrosis.

It can also be seen in patients with a variety of other conditions when withdrawal of multiple blood samples for diagnostic purposes is coupled with the administration of large amounts of non-colloid-containing fluids.

DECREASED INTERSTITIAL HYDROSTATIC PRESSURE. We have already emphasized that because of mechanical interdependence of adjacent lung units, when inflation of some units lags behind others, large negative interstitial pressures can be generated around and within the lagging units. We believe that these negative pressures can be transmitted to the fluid-exchanging vessels, enhancing edema formation, especially in obstructive lung disease like asthma and bronchiolitis as well as in the repiratory distress syndrome. Although one might argue that all pressures, including the vascular pressures, would fall a similar amount, at least three factors keep vascular pressures high relative to interstitial pressures:

1. The decrease in intrathoracic pressures will enhance venous return, increasing cardiac output.

2. As pulmonary microvascular pressures decrease below alveolar pressure, alveolar vessels will be compressed and perfusion obstructed; this, in turn, will increase afterload on the right ventricle, producing an increase in cardiac output, and maintaining forward flow by raising intravascular hydrostatic pressures.

3. Exposure of the surfaces of the left ventricle to large negative pleural pressures is analogous to imposing an afterload. As a consequence of this, theory would predict that there will be increased end-diastolic filling pressures, which will be reflected in elevated left atrial and pulmonary microvascular pressures. It should also be recalled that when airway resistance is high, e.g., during croup, large negative alveolar pressures may be generated during inspiration (Newth and coworkers, 1972), and these too would be expected to be transmitted to the fluid-exchanging vessels.

We believe these considerations have

special relevance to a variety of clinical conditions in which there is a lag in the expansion of the lung in spite of the development of very negative intrathoracic pressures (Stalcup and Mellins, 1977). One such example is seen in children with heart failure complicating hypertrophied tonsils and adenoids (Luke and coworkers, 1966; Bland and associates, 1969; Cayler and coworkers, 1969). Although many have assumed that cor pulmonale with right-sided heart failure is the principal complication, we, like others (Levin and coworkers, 1975), have been struck by the clinical and radiographic findings of pulmonary edema in several children with this condition. At the bedside, one cannot but be impressed with the severe intercostal retractions during inspiration. Indeed, this inspiratory pattern comes very close to simulating a Müller maneuver, i.e., a strong inspiration against a closed glottis or obstructed upper airway. The negative pressures surrounding and restraining the left ventricle are analogous to an afterload, and would be expected to raise the pressures on the left side of the heart relative to pleural pressures. Thus, we believe that the large negative intrathoracic pressures are at least in part responsible for cardiomegaly, pulmonary vascular engorgement and edema.

A dramatic example of the change in heart size following removal of the tonsils and adenoids is shown in Figure 6. Figure 6 *A* shows the chest roentgenogram of a three-year-old boy with chronic hypertrophied tonsils and adenoids at the time of presentation with clinical evidence of left- and right-sided heart failure. Figure 6 *B* shows the improvement following removal of the tonsils and adenoids. While the obstruction in this condition has been attributed solely to the size of the tonsils and the adenoids, the observation that the obstruction is considerably less during wakefulness than during sleep indicates that oropharyngeal muscle control is also a contributing factor. Indeed, it may be that it is variations in the latter, especially during sleep, rather than simply the size of the tonsils and adenoids that explains why some children get into cardiopulmonary difficulty while others with apparently just as much hypertrophy of the tonsils and adenoids do not.

Sudden marked lowering of the interstitial fluid pressure may be the mechanism responsible for edema in at least nine patients, mostly young adults, who have been reported with the sudden development of pulmonary edema following re-expansion of pneumothorax (Childress and coworkers, 1971; Wagaruddin and Bernstein, 1975). In some, this has occurred after conventional closed underwater drainage, while in others this has occurred after application of very negative pressures by suction. Although the mechanism has not been established, it seems likely that very negative interstitial pressures as the result of the simultaneous occurrence of bronchial occlusion or some factor restraining lung expansion and very negative pleural pressures is the cause (Childress and coworkers, 1971). In most of the reported patients, lung collapse had been present for some time prior to re-expansion. Whether this factor alone restrains rapid expansion, as, for example, by a decrease in surfactant in the collapsed area, remains unclear.

INCREASED VASCULAR PERMEABILITY IN FLUID-EXCHANGING VESSELS. There are at least two ways that the permeability of a membrane can be increased. The total number of pores may increase or the diameter of the pores may increase. The distinction between pulmonary edema induced by increases in hydrostatic pressure and that induced by increases in permeability, while clinically useful, is sometimes blurred by the observation that as intravascular pressures rise the pores may be stretched, thus altering permeability. It is our impression that relatively large pressures, i.e., pressures in excess of 30 mm. Hg, are necessary to produce the stretched-pore phenomenon. It may be, however, that the sensitivity of the methods available to detect small increments in the rate of fluid movement is not sufficient to demonstrate the phenomenon at lower pressures.

A variety of clinical conditions are believed to alter the permeability of the alveolar capillary membrane, presumably by damage to epithelial or endothelial cells. In addition, there is now in-creasing evidence that the release of potent chemical mediators may be involved in the genesis of pulmonary edema in these conditions. For example, histamine, prostaglandins and bradykinin, all of which may be released during acute asthma, are capable of increasing vascular permeability under some circumstances. These agents may be responsible for pulmo-

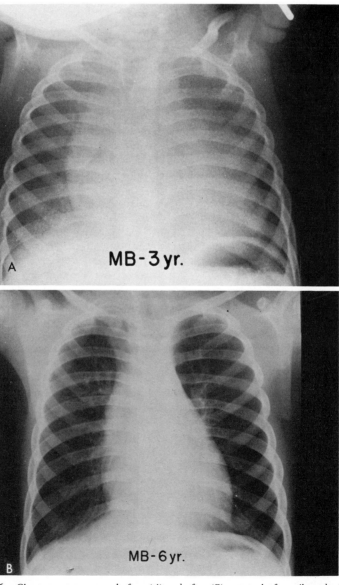

Figure 6. Chest roentgenogram before (*A*) and after (*B*) removal of tonsils and adenoids.

nary edema when released by autoimmune mechanisms in hypersensitivity pneumonitis or alveolitis, as well as in Goodpasture's disease and systemic lupus erythematosus. Whether idiopathic pulmonary hemosiderosis falls into this group remains unknown.

The inhalation of a variety of noxious gases, many of which may be generated during fires, produce denaturation of proteins, cellular damage and pulmonary edema. These include the oxides of sulfur and nitrogen, hydrocyanic acid and several aldehydes. More recently, the inhalation of herbicides, such as paraquat, has been associated with the development of pulmonary edema, presumably on the basis of a change in permeability. Even before morphologic evidence of alveolar injury is apparent, there is an increase in surface tension, presumably as the result of inactivation or impaired synthesis of pulmonary surfactant (Robertson, 1973).

The auscultatory evidence of pulmonary edema resulting from inhalation of smoke with damage to the alveolar capillary membrane is always manifest within 24 hours and usually precedes roentgenographic changes (Mellins and Park, 1975). The diffuse haziness on chest roentgenograms that first appears several days following massive burns probably results from the loss of plasma proteins coupled with the administration of large amounts of intravenous fluids, or from other circulatory complications.

A variety of circulating toxins, for example, snake venom, produce pulmonary edema by altering the alveolar capillary membrane. Experimental evidence has been presented indicating that gram-negative bacteremia can produce a sustained increase in lung vascular permeability as well as a transient elevation of pulmonary vascular pressures (Brigham and coworkers, 1974). Although the lymphatics have been shown to have the ability to clear large volumes of filtered fluid and protein in this condition, eventually this mechanism can also be overwhelmed. There-

fore, fluid therapy should be adjusted to keep vascular pressures low when permeability is increased.

OTHER CAUSES. There are a number of other conditions in which the mechanisms responsible for pulmonary edema are not clear. In some of these, one suspects that alterations in vascular pressures in conjunction with increases in permeability may be responsible.

The improvement seen in ventilation following administration of diuretics suggests that some patients with cor pulmonale may also have pulmonary edema. We believe this does occur, but it is difficult to prove. Whether the mechanism is increased systemic venous hypertension, and therefore bronchial microvascular hypertension, or more negative interstitial pressures as the result of obstructive airway breathing is not clear.

Pulmonary edema is seen following large doses of radiation and in uremia. While vascular hydrostatic pressures may be elevated and colloid osmotic pressures lower, there is reason to think that permeability is altered as well.

The mechanism responsible for the pulmonary edema following lesions of the brain is not fully understood. In most cases, a neurally mediated increase in peripheral systemic vascular resistance initiated by the release of catecholamines (Nathan and Reis, 1975) results in a shift of blood from the systemic to the pulmonary circulation. Increased pulmonary blood volume, perhaps accompanied by left-sided heart failure, leads to an increase in pulmonary vascular pressures. Pulmonary hypertension and hypervolemia result in increased fluid transudation, which apparently persists even after the systemic and pulmonary vascular hypertension subside (Theodore and Robin, 1976).

A variety of conditions referred to as shock lung or adult respiratory distress syndrome result in edema by mechanisms that are not entirely clear. One can speculate that the release of a variety of vasoactive substances alters pulmonary capillary permeability. Although hypoxia, especially when accompanied by acidosis, is believed to enhance pulmonary edema, one recent and thoughtful review (Staub, 1974) comes to the conclusion that there is no good experimental evidence that hypoxia per se alters pulmonary capillary permeability. On the other hand, high concentrations of oxygen are known to produce lung damage and edema.

The pathogenesis of high altitude edema remains unclear. It affects some highlanders who return home after a brief stay at sea level. It also occurs in some sea level dwellers soon after arriving at high altitude. In addition to a constitutional predisposition to pulmonary hypertension with hypoxia (Hultgren and coworkers, 1971), some have assumed that nonuniform increases in precapillary resistance are responsible for the very high pressures seen at least in some pulmonary capillaries (Viswanathan and coworkers, 1969).

Heroin and other narcotics have also been associated with pulmonary edema. Pulmonary capillary wedge pressure has been elevated in some patients (Paranthaman and Khan, 1976), but has been normal in others. The protein concentration in pulmonary edema fluid from the trachea has been very close to serum levels, suggesting alterations in pulmonary capillary permeability (Katz and coworkers, 1972). Whether hypoxia and acidosis or neurogenic pulmonary edema as the result of cerebral edema play a role is not known. Clinical and roentgenographic evidence of pulmonary edema have occurred following the intravenous administration of paraldehyde (Sinal and Crowe, 1976). Although a direct toxic action on the pulmonary vascular bed has been proposed, the cause remains obscure.

Pulmonary edema has been seen as a late complication of severe salicylate poisoning. The mechanism remains unknown. Since prostaglandins may play a role in maintaining normal pulmonary vascular pressures, it is intriguing to speculate that inhibition of prostaglandin synthesis by salicylates may result in pulmonary edema.

Pulmonary Edema in Asthma, Bronchiolitis and Neonatal Respiratory Distress Syndrome

There are three important clinical conditions discussed in greater detail in Chapters 41, 17 and 10 in which pulmonary edema may be an important part of the pathogenesis, namely, asthma, bronchiolitis and neonatal respiratory distress syndrome (RDS).

There are at least five factors that are important in the genesis of pulmonary edema in *asthma*:

1. The release of a number of vasoactive substances, including histamines, prostaglandins and bradykinin, in part, at least, as the result of IgE interaction at the surface of the mast cell, causes edema of the airways. Presumably, increased vascular permeability plays a role.

2. The thick edematous walls together with bronchospasm narrows the airway lumen, with a tendency to early closure except at the highest lung volumes. To prevent airway closure and allow adequate ventilation, the patient must maintain a high inspiratory position, i.e., a high lung volume, which is accomplished by maintaining very negative pleural pressures. This has been demonstrated to occur in adults with asthma (Permutt, 1973). We have found the *average* pleural pressure throughout the entire ventilating cycle to be minus 16 cm. H_2O in a group of children with acute asthma of widely varying severity (Stalcup and Mellins, 1977).

3. Because of increased airway resistance, the negative swing in pleural pressure during inspiration is increased. In all probability, there is also very negative alveolar pressure during inspiration.

4. The negative pleural and alveolar pressures would be expected to lower both interstitial (perimicrovascular) and vascular pressures. However, as alveolar pressure exceeds microvascular

pressure, there is increased resistance to right ventricular emptying. Under these circumstances, the Frank-Starling mechanism would be expected to raise right ventricular and pulmonary arterial blood pressures. This would be facilitated by the increased venous return to the thorax as a result of the very negative pleural pressures. Thus, the gradient favoring filtration of fluid is increased because vascular hydrostatic pressures are elevated while perimicrovascular pressures are decreased.

Although the effect of acute asthma on left heart dynamics has not been studied, the markedly negative pleural pressures would be expected to dilate the left ventricle and could conceivably lead to elevation of left ventricular end-diastolic pressure, left atrial pressure and pulmonary microvascular pressures.

5. In a disease like asthma in which the extent of airway obstruction is uneven, we have already shown not only that the interstitial pressures in units that lag during inflation are negative, but also that the magnitude of negativity is amplified by mechanical interdependence.

In summary, elevated vascular pressures, more negative perimicrovascular pressures and increased vascular permeability all promote the development of edema of the lung. In addition, vigorous administration of fluids dilutes plasma proteins, lowers colloid osmotic pressures and raises vascular hydrostatic pressures. Thus, the aggressive administration of fluids so commonly advocated in asthma is likely to intensify the development of edema.

Because the small airways are the principal site of airway obstruction in *bronchiolitis*, there is also a tendency to early airway closure in this condition. To oppose this and to ventilate these lungs, markedly negative pleural pressures are also generated, indicated by severe intercostal and substernal retractions on inspiration. It is our hypothesis that many of the same mechanical factors leading to pulmonary edema in asthma also occur in bronchiolitis.

It is unlikely that appreciable edema will be present early in the course of the disease, except perhaps for that resulting from inflammation, since fluid intake is initially low and the children are often dehydrated. However, with hospitalization, at least two therapeutic procedures may alter this. The administration of humidified oxygen will reduce fluid losses from the respiratory tract. The liberal administration of intravenous fluids traditionally advocated will reduce the plasma colloid osmotic pressure, and together with the mechanisms discussed previously will raise pulmonary vascular hydrostatic pressures. This, together with the very negative interstitial pressures, will lead to interstitial edema. A vicious cycle then occurs in which peribronchial cuffs of fluid intensify the small airway obstruction, necessitating the development of still more negative pleural pressures to ventilate the lungs. We have seen a dramatic decrease in the severity of bronchiolitis with reversal of hypercapnia following the use of diuretics under these circumstances. However, early in the course we would not expect diuretics to be helpful, and in fact, if dehydration is present, they may be contraindicated.

In *neonatal RDS*, pleural pressures can be inferred to be very negative, at least during part of the inspiratory cycle, from the bedside observations of pronounced inspiratory retractions. The lungs, which are stiff, at least in part because of surfactant deficiency, have an increased tendency to collapse. The patient must develop very negative pleural pressures in order to ventilate these stiff lungs. However, the highly compliant chest wall of the newborn infant may limit the magnitude of negative pressures that the infant can generate spontaneously. Insofar as negative pleural pressures are generated, interstitial or perimicrovascular pressures will become more negative, enhancing edema. On the other hand, in the absence of surfactant, surface forces will become extremely large at low lung volumes. At the alveolar level, this will tend to lower the interstitial pressure surrounding at least some of the fluid-exchanging vessels. Areas of microatelectasis will be subjected to increased distending pressures from adjacent inflated lung. Because the forces are operating over a smaller area in the collapsed lung, they will be amplified by mechanical interdependence. However, the very negative interstitial pressures generated in the perimicrovascular space will favor edema formation.

There are at least two possible explanations for the development of hyaline membranes in neonatal RDS: (1) if amplified pressures are applied to the surface of units of lung with complete airway closure and if there is diminished or absent collateral ventilation, as probably occurs in small infants, the absorption of gas will result in sufficiently low alveolar pressures to induce transudation of fluid and hemorrhagic atelectasis (Pang and Mellins, 1975), and (2) release or altered metabolism of vasoactive substances associated with the events of birth may increase vascular permeability.

Diagnosis

In a general way, small increases in lung water are too subtle to detect by currently available clinical methods, i.e., auscultation and chest radiology, until the interstitial and extravascular water has doubled or tripled. The presence of rales indicates that peripheral lung units (alveoli and alveolar ducts) are opening. Whether the quality of sounds is different when the fluid is confined to the interstitial spaces as contrasted to its presence in the alveolar lumen is not known. When the fluid moves up to larger airways, rhonchi and wheezes are to be expected. The contribution of bronchial wall edema and bronchospasm to rhonchi and wheezes is not known.

Acute changes in fluid accumulation may not be detectable by chest roentgenogram unless massive. Under conditions of chronic edema formation, lymphatics and interstitial accumulations of fluid may be visible as Kerley lines (see under Radiographic Findings). Because peribronchiolar collection of fluids can narrow airways, airway closure is more likely to occur at high lung volumes, producing air trapping. Thus, low diaphragms may be a useful sign of interstitial edema, provided there are no other reasons for airway obstruction. Other signs that are useful in following the severity of pulmonary engorgement and edema include the rapidity and shallowness of breathing, the magnitude of inspiratory intercostal retractions, and changes in body weight. Grunting is a common accompaniment of pulmonary edema and represents a useful maneuver to prevent lung collapse (Pang and Mellins, 1975).

Once the magnitude of pulmonary edema is sufficiently severe to lead to persistent airway closure or alveolar flooding, it is very difficult to separate edema, atelectasis and inflammation on chest roentgenograms.

Radiographic Findings

Although most of the radiographic signs of pulmonary edema are nonspecific, improved radiographic techniques, when taken in conjunction with improved understanding of the pathophysiology of pulmonary edema, have enhanced the usefulness of the chest roentgenogram in the diagnosis of pulmonary edema (Hublitz and Shapiro, 1974).

The A and B lines of Kerley represent interlobular sheets of abnormally thickened or widened connective tissue that are tangential to the x-ray beam; the A lines are in the depths of the lung near the hilum, and the B lines are at the periphery or surface of the lung (Fig. 7). These are more properly referred to as septal lines. While thickening may occur from a variety of processes, including fibrosis, pigment deposition and pulmonary hemosiderosis, when they are transient they are usually caused by edema. These septal lines of edema are more clearly visible

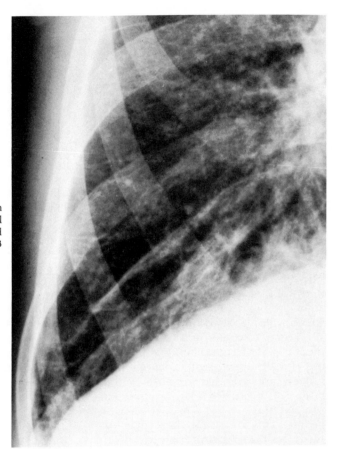

Figure 7. Chest roentgenogram of 18-year-old with congenital mitral stenosis demonstrating horizontal septal lines of edema (Kerley B lines) at the periphery of the lung.

in older children and adults with chronic edema (Fig. 7) than in infants, presumably because they are wider.

Perivascular and peribronchial cuffing are other radiographic signs of interstitial edema fluid. Another radiographic sign of early pulmonary edema is prominent upper lobe vessels, which appear in conjunction with basal interstitial edema. For hydrostatic reasons, perivascular edema is greatest at the bases, and the normal tethering action of the lung is therefore less in this region. With increased resistance to the lower lobe vessels, there is redistribution to the upper lobes. This sign is, of course, of limited value in infants because they are most likely to be in the supine position. The recognition of interstitial pulmonary edema depends on the highest quality radiographic techniques, including short exposure times.

More severe forms of pulmonary edema commonly produce a perihilar haze, presumably because the large perivascular and peribronchial collections of fluid are in this location. A reticular or lattice-like pattern may also be present and is more common at the base in the upright individual.

Therapy

Reversing hypoxemia remains the essential first step. When this cannot be done by simply increasing the O_2 concentration of the inspired mixture, mechanical ventilation may be necessary. Mechanical aid not only reduces the oxygen consumption by reducing the work of breathing, but when coupled with positive end-expiratory pressure improves oxygenation by preventing collapse of lung units. The positive intrathoracic pressure generated by positive pressures at the mouth may reduce fluid filtration in the lung by impeding venous return and therefore decreasing pulmonary vascular volume and pressure. The experimental evidence reviewed previously suggests that when vascular volume and pressures are maintained, positive pressure ventilation may actually enhance fluid accumulation in the lung. The improved oxygenation suggests that the fluid must be sequestered in interstitial spaces that do not impair gas exchange.

When the pulmonary edema results from heart failure, with elevation of pulmonary microvascular pressures, several therapeutic approaches are helpful. These include (1) measures that improve cardiac contractility and allow the heart to achieve an increased stroke volume at a lower filling pressure, e.g., oxygen and digitalis; (2) measures that reduce preload, including the sitting position, rotating tourniquets and positive pressure ventilation; (3) measures that reduce both preload and afterload primarily by relieving anxiety, e.g., morphine; (4) measures that improve contractility and afterload and also produce bronchodilation, e.g., aminophylline; and (5) measures that decrease plasma volumes and left atrial pressure and increase plasma colloid osmotic pressures, e.g., diuretics.

When it is possible to anticipate alterations in one or another of the factors responsible for fluid accumulation in the lung, the best overall plan for fluid management would seem to be to replace fluid deficits while correcting acid-base abnormalities and then to administer maintenance needs, carefully calculated to take into consideration decreased or increased losses.

When a decreased plasma colloid osmotic pressure is a complicating factor of pulmonary edema, intravenous administration of albumin may be helpful. However, since this will initially promote the absorption of fluid from the entire body, vascular pressures may rise transiently, thus minimizing the gain. For this reason, colloid administration must be done slowly and cautiously, and probably in conjunction with the administration of diuretics. It should also be borne in mind that while too large a vascular volume may promote edema formation by elevating vascular hydrostatic pressure, too small a vascular volume may lead to poor perfusion of vital organs. This may occur during periods when venous return is impaired by the positive intrathoracic pressures that accompany mechanical ventilation.

Previous approaches to therapy of asthma have included the administration of generous amounts of fluid (well in excess of maintenance requirements), presumably to loosen secretions. If, as we have shown, the transvascular gradient favoring filtration and the vascular permeability are already increased in asthma, once deficits are corrected, the administration of fluids in excess of maintenance needs would be expected to aggravate the disease by fostering edema formation.

As we have already indicated, dehydration may be present early in the course of bronchiolitis, and diuretics may be contraindicated. Later in the hospital course, especially after liberal amounts of fluid have been given, pulmonary edema may be present and may be a cause for increased airway obstruction, in which case diuretics may be very helpful.

In addition to the general therapeutic measures already discussed, treatment of neurogenic pulmonary edema should focus on the reduction in intracranial pressure, when this is possible, and by the pharmacologic reduction in systemic arterial blood pressure.

The treatment of pulmonary edema resulting from altered pulmonary permeability is on less secure grounds. Thus, some have advocated large doses of corticosteroids in patients with gram-negative infection. When pulmonary edema is a complication of severe shock with disseminated intravascular coagulation, low molecular weight dextran and heparin have been used.

Whenever increased capillary permeability is responsible for pulmonary edema, the rate and volume of intravenous fluids should be adjusted to keep vascular pressures low.

A recurrent theme throughout this chapter has been the potential role of vasoactive substances in the genesis of pulmonary edema by altering vascular pressures and permeability. Although the information about them is still very limited, we have chosen to emphasize their importance because we believe that a more fundamental understanding of their role in the genesis of pulmonary edema is likely to lead to more specific forms of therapy.

REFERENCES

Baker, J. W., Yerger, S., and Segar, W. E.: Elevated plasma antidiuretic hormone levels in status asthmaticus. *Mayo Clin. Proc., 51*:31, 1976.

Bland, J. W., Edwards, F. K., and Brinsfield, W.: Pulmonary hypertension and congestive heart failure with chronic upper airway obstruction. *Am. J. Cardiol., 23*:830, 1969.

Boyd, R. D. H., Hill, J. R., Humphreys, R. W., Normand, I. C. S., Reynolds, E. O. R., and Strang, L. B.: Permeability of lung capillary to macromolecules in fetal and newborn lambs and sheep. *J. Physiol. (Lond.), 201*:567, 1969.

Brigham, K. L., and Owen, P. J.: Increased sheep lung vascular permeability caused by histamine. *Circ. Res., 37*:647, 1975.

Brigham, K. L., Woolverton, W. C., Blake, L. H., and Staub, N.: Increased sheep lung vascular permeability caused by pseudomonas bacteremia. *J. Clin. Invest., 54*:792, 1974.

Cayler, G. G., Johnson, E. E., Lewis, B. E., Kortzeborn, J. W., Jordan, J., and Fricker, G. A.: Heart failure due to enlarged tonsils and adenoids. *Am. J. Dis. Child., 118*:708, 1969.

Childress, M. E., Moy, G., and Mottram, M.: Unilateral pulmonary edema resulting from treatment of spontaneous pneumothorax. *Am. Rev. Resp. Dis., 104*:119, 1971.

Fishman, A. P.: Pulmonary edema. The water-exchanging function of the lung. *Circulation, 46*:390, 1972.

Goodale, R. L., Goetzman, B., and Visscher, M. B.: Hypoxia and iodoacetic acid and alveolocapillary barrier permeability to albumin. *Am. J. Physiol., 219*:1226, 1970.

Guyton, A. C., Taylor, A. E., and Granger, H. J.: *Circulatory Physiology II: Dynamics and Control of the Body Fluids.* Philadelphia, W. B. Saunders Company, 1975.

Guyton, A. C., Taylor, A. E., Drake, R. E., and Parker, J. C.: Dynamics of subatmospheric pressure in the pulmonary interstitial fluid. In *Lung Liquids*, Ciba Symposium 38. North-Holland, Amsterdam, American Elsevier Publishing Company, 1976, p. 77.

Hall, J. G., Morris, B., and Wooley, G.: Intrinsic rhythmic propulsion of lymph in the unanesthetized sheep. *J. Physiol. (Lond.), 180*:336, 1965.

Hauge, A., Gunnar, B., and Waaler, B. A.: Interrelations between pulmonary liquid volumes and lung compliance. *J. Appl. Physiol., 38*:608, 1975.

Hordof, A. J., Mellins, R. B., Gersony, W. M., and Steeg, C. N.: Reversibility of chronic obstructive lung disease in infants following repair of ventricular septal defects. *J. Pediatr., 90*:187, 1977.

Hublitz, U. F., and Shapiro, J. H.: The radiology of pulmonary edema. *CRC Crit. Rev. Clin. Radiol. Nucl. Med., 5*:389, 1974.

Hultgren, H. N., Grover, R. F., and Hartley, L. H.: Abnormal circulatory responses to high altitude in subjects with a history of high-altitude pulmonary edema. *Circulation, 44*:759, 1971.

Iliff, L.: Extra-alveolar vessels and edema development in excised dog lungs. *Circ. Res., 28*:524, 1971.

Katz, S., Aberman, A., Frand, U. I., Stern, I. M., and Fulop, M.: Heroin pulmonary edema. *Am. Rev. Resp. Dis., 106*:472, 1972.

La Force, F. M., Mullane, J. F., Boehme, R. F., Kelly, W. J., and Huber, G. L.: The effect of pulmonary edema on antibacterial defenses of the lung. *J. Lab. Clin. Med., 82*:634, 1973.

Levin, D. L., Muster, A. J., Pachman, L. M., Wessel, H. U., Paul, M. H., and Koshaba, J.: Cor pulmonale secondary to upper airway obstruction. *Chest, 68*:166, 1975.

Levine, O. R., and Mellins, R. B.: Liquid balance in the lung and pulmonary edema. In Scarpelli, E., and Auld, P. A. (Eds.): *Pulmonary Physiology of the Fetus, Newborn and Child.* Philadelphia, Lea and Febiger, 1975, p. 239.

Levine, O. R., Mellins, R. B., and Fishman, A. P.: Quantitative assessment of pulmonary edema. *Circ. Res., 27*:414, 1965.

Levine, O. R., Mellins, R. B., Senior, R. M., and Fishman, A. P.: The application of Starling's law of capillary exchange to the lungs. *J. Clin. Invest., 46*:934, 1967.

Levine, O. R., Rodriguez-Martinez, F., and Mellins, R. B.: Fluid filtration in the lung of the intact puppy. *J. Apply. Physiol., 34*:683, 1973.

Luke, M. J., Mehrizi, A., Folger, G. M., Jr., and Rowe, R. D.: Chronic nasopharyngeal obstruction as a cause of cardiomegaly, cor pulmonale and pulmonary edema. *Pediatrics, 37*:762, 1966.

Macklem, P. T.: Influence of left atrial pressure on lung mechanics. *International Congress on Cardiac Lung.* Sponsored by European Society of Cardiology and European Society for Clinical Respiratory Physiology. Florence, December 1976.

Macklem, P. T., and Murphy, B.: The forces applied to the lung in health and disease. *Am. J. Med., 57*:371, 1974.

Mead, J., Takishima, T., and Leith, D.: Stress distribution in lungs: a model of pulmonary elasticity. *J. Appl. Physiol., 28*:596, 1970.

Mellins, R., and Park, S.: Respiratory complications of smoke inhalation in victims of fires. *J. Pediatr., 87*:1, 1975.

Mellins, R. B., Levine, O. R., Skalak, R., and Fishman, A. P.: Interstitial pressure of the lung. *Circ. Res., 24*:197, 1969.

Mellins, R. B., Levine, O. R., and Fishman, A. P.: Effect of systemic and pulmonary venous hypertension on pleural and pericardial fluid accumulation. *J. Appl. Physiol., 29*:564, 1970.

Mor, J., Ben Galim, E., and Abrahamov, A.: Inappropriate antidiuretic hormone secretion in an infant with severe pneumonia. *Am. J. Dis. Child., 129*:133, 1975.

Nathan, M. A., and Reis, D. J.: Fulminating arterial hypertension with pulmonary edema from release of adrenomedullary catecholamines after lesions of the anterior hypothalamus in the rat. *Circ. Res., 37*:226, 1975.

Newth, C. J. L., Levison, H., and Bryan, A. C.: The respiratory status of children with croup. *J. Pediatr., 81*:1068, 1972.

Pang, L. M., and Mellins, R. B.: Neonatal cardiorespiratory physiology. *Anesthesiology, 43*:171, 1975.

Paranthaman, S., and Khan, F.: Acute cardiomyopathy with recurrent pulmonary edema and hypotension following heroin overdosage. *Chest, 69*:117, 1976.

Perl, W., Chowdhury, P., and Chinard, F. P.: Reflection coefficients of dog lung endothelium to small hydrophilic solutes. *Am. J. Physiol., 228*:797, 1975.

Permutt, S.: Physiologic changes in the acute asthmatic attack. In Austen, K. F., and Lichtenstein, L. M. (Eds.): *Asthma: Physiology, Immunopharmacology and Treatment.* New York, Academic Press, 1973, p. 15.

Pietra, G. G., Szidon, J. P., Leventhal, M. M., and Fishman, A. P.: Histamine and interstitial pulmonary edema in the dog. *Circ. Res., 29*:323, 1971.

Reifenrath, R.: The significance of alveolar geometry and surface tension in the respiratory mechanics of the lung. *Resp. Physiol., 24*:115, 1975.

Robertson, B.: Paraquat poisoning as an experimental model of the idiopathic respiratory distress syndrome. *Bull. Physiopathol. Resp., 9*:1433, 1973.

Robin, E. D., Cross, C. E., and Zelis, R.: Pulmonary edema. *N. Engl. J. Med., 288*:239, 292, 1973.

Sinal, S. H., and Crowe, J. E.: Cyanosis, cough and hypotension following intravenous administration of paraldehyde. *Pediatrics, 57*:158, 1976.

Stalcup, S. A., and Mellins, R. B.: Mechanical forces producing pulmonary edema in acute asthma. N. Engl. J. Med. (in press).

Staub, N. C.: Pulmonary edema. *Physiol. Rev., 54*:678, 1974.

Taylor, P. M., Boonyaprakob, U., Waterman, V., Watson, D., and Lopata, E.: Clearance of plasma proteins from pulmonary vascular beds of adult dogs and pups. *Am. J. Physiol., 213*:441, 1967.

Theodore, J., and Robin, E. D.: Speculations on neurogenic pulmonary edema (NPE). *Am. Rev. Resp. Dis., 113*:405, 1976.

Viswanathan, R., Jain, S. K., and Subramanian, S.: Pulmonary edema of high altitude. III. Pathogenesis. *Am. Rev. Resp. Dis., 100*:342, 1969.

Waqaruddin, M., and Bernstein, A.: Reexpansion pulmonary oedema. *Thorax, 30*:54, 1975.

CHAPTER THIRTY-NINE

EMPHYSEMA AND ALPHA₁-ANTITRYPSIN DEFICIENCY

RICHARD C. TALAMO, M.D.

The term "emphysema" has been applied to a wide variety of pulmonary conditions. When defined as "overaeration of lung," it has been used in association with congenital lobar emphysema, hyperinflation resulting from extrinsic or intrinsic airway obstruction, cystic fibrosis, asthma, bronchiolitis, compensatory hyperinflation and the localized hyperlucency of lung that may occur in early infantile respiratory distress syndrome or in bronchopulmonary dysplasia. Most of these conditions are discussed in detail in other sections of this book.

More recently, a strict pathologic definition of emphysema has evolved: dilatation of distal air spaces, accompanied by disruption of alveolar walls. This definition clearly fits the emphysema seen in adult lungs as a result of elastic tissue destruction. Pulmonary pathologists can generally agree that there are two major types of emphysema among adults: the more common centrilobular variety, which is associated with a preceding history of chronic bronchitis in cigarette-smoking middle-aged adult males; and panlobular (or panacinar) emphysema, which is much less common, involves diffuse damage of elastic tissue in alveolar septae, is not necessarily associated with chronic bronchitis or cigarette smoking, but which is highly characteristic of severe alpha₁-antitrypsin deficiency.

It is now clear that true panacinar emphysema can occur in childhood in association with severe alpha₁-antitrypsin deficiency. While only a small number of infants and children with this disease have been well described thus far in the world literature, the common occurrence of the genes associated with alpha₁-antitrypsin deficiency in many populations suggests that this clinical condition may be more common than is currently appreciated.

Severe serum alpha₁-antitrypsin deficiency in association with chronic obstructive pulmonary disease with onset in young adult life was first described in Sweden in 1963 (Laurell and Eriksson, 1963). The familial nature of this deficiency was well described in 1965 (Eriksson, 1965). The first report of the deficiency in association with emphysema in a child was in 1971 (Talamo and coworkers, 1971).

Severe alpha₁-antitrypsin deficiency has also been described in infants with onset of liver disease in the early months of life, often progressing to cirrhosis (Sharp and coworkers, 1969). In a few instances, young children have been described with a combination of cirrhosis and chronic, progressive, obstructive pulmonary disease (Glasgow and associates, 1973; Kaiser and colleagues, 1975).

This chapter will present current knowledge with regard to the alpha₁-antitrypsin as a serum protein, its measurement, its genetics, the pathogenesis and clinical features of the pulmonary disease associated with alpha₁-antitrypsin deficiency, as well as the differential diagnosis, treatment and prognosis of this disease.

Alpha₁-antitrypsin Biology

Alpha₁-antitrypsin is the major alpha₁ globulin in human serum, and is a glycoprotein of 54,000 molecular weight. It is one of the six well characterized protease inhibitors in human serum; in terms of concentration and function, alpha₁-antitrypsin is the major serum protease inhibitor. While this protein is able to inhibit a wide spectrum of enzymes in vitro, its major protective function in humans is thought to be the inhibition of tissue enzymes, particularly one or more elastases released under normal circumstances from polymorphonuclear leukocytes. Thus, the alpha₁-antitrypsin, which is small enough to diffuse readily into the interstitial space and a variety of body fluids, is able to inhibit elastase and possibly other proteases, preventing the damage of tissue, particularly elastin. Alpha₁-antitrypsin may function as a "shuttle protein," bringing enzymes released in tissue back into the circulation for transfer to other serum protease inhibitors and disposal in the reticuloendothelial system.

Alpha₁-antitrypsin is synthesized in the liver cell and secreted into serum, where its half-life is four to six days. In addition to being a major serum protein and appearing in body fluids and tissues, the alpha₁-antitrypsin is known to occur in the cytoplasm of pulmonary alveolar macrophages, on the cell surface of polymorphonuclear leukocytes, along the normal adult human airway at the level of the terminal bronchiole, and in platelet granules.

Serum alpha₁-antitrypsin is an acute phase reactant; its level may double or triple as a result of a variety of nonspecific acute inflammatory processes, during pregnancy, immediately following the stress of surgery, and in individuals being treated with estrogens.

Alpha₁-antitrypsin Measurement

Alpha₁-antitrypsin is responsible for over 90 per cent of the trypsin inhibitory capacity of normal human serum; functional assays are readily available for measurement of its ability to inhibit trypsin in vitro. A variety of quantitative immunochemical methods can be used for specific measurement of the alpha₁-antitrypsin, including radial immunodiffusion and electroimmunoassay. Commercial materials are currently widely available for simple immunochemical quantitation. In all known clinical circumstances, alpha₁-antitrypsin function and immunochemical quantitative measurements have correlated very highly; a nonfunctioning inhibitor protein has not yet been identified.

Genetics and Incidence of Deficiency

It was first demonstrated that serum alpha₁-antitrypsin is inherited via a series of codominant alleles, which determine both the serum concentration of the protein and its electrophoretic mobility (Fagerhol and Laurell, 1967). It was discovered that the alpha₁-antitrypsin migrates toward the anode as a series of multiple bands on starch gel electrophoresis at acid pH. To the present time, more than 25 different alleles and more than 48 combinations of them have been described in the world's literature. This system of alpha₁-antitrypsin alleles has been named the Pi (protease inhibitor) system. Pi^M, the major allele in most populations, has an intermediate electrophoretic mobility, while a variety of faster alleles are named by the earlier letters of the alphabet; slower alleles are named by the later letters. Normal individuals are of Pi MM phenotype, and those with severe alpha₁-antitrypsin deficiency are of the phenotype Pi ZZ. (By agreement, these homozygous types are named Pi M and Pi Z, unless complete family typing has been done.) Serum levels of alpha₁-antitrypsin in Pi ZZ individuals are 10 to 15 per cent of those in the Pi M normals. Pi MZ heterozygotes have intermediate levels. A Pi^{null} (or Pi$^-$) allele has been recently described, which is associated with no detectable alpha₁-antitrypsin (Talamo, 1975).

In Caucasian populations, Pi M individuals compose approximately 90 per cent of the total population, Pi MZ 2 or 3 per cent, and Pi MS 3 to 5 per cent; miscellaneous other types make up the remainder. In several large population studies, the incidence of Pi Z individuals is approximately one per 3000 to one per 6000 live births, somewhat lower than the incidence of cystic fibrosis (one per 1500 live births).

Molecular Abnormality

Pi Z alpha₁-antitrypsin deficiency is accompanied by abnormal storage in the hepatocyte cytoplasm of a material that cross reacts immunologically with serum alpha₁-antitrypsin; this storage appears to be in the granules of rough endoplasmic reticulum. This abnormal form of the protein lacks the complete biochemical structure necessary for normal release into serum, resulting in the very low serum levels characteristic of Pi Z alpha₁-antitrypsin deficiency. Purified preparations of Pi M and Pi Z alpha₁-antitrypsin have been compared structurally and have been found to differ by a single amino acid substitution in one peptide. The major substitution appears to be a lysine residue in the Z protein in place of a glutamic acid residue in the M protein (Jeppsson, 1976; Yoshida and coworkers, 1976). This substitution is consistent with the slower electrophoretic mobility of the Z protein. Pi S alpha₁-antitrypsin has been reported to have a valine in place of a glutamic acid in the M protein.

Pathogenesis of Pulmonary Disease

Several lines of evidence have suggested the course of events that leads to elastin destruction and results in panacinar emphysema in this disease: (1) aging circulating granulocytes

normally marginate along the capillary endothelium in the pulmonary circulation, dying and releasing their enzymatic contents into pulmonary tissue. While a variety of enzymes is released, the most significant appear to be one or more elastases, which can degrade the elastin present in alveolar septae. Other granulocyte enzymes, such as collagenase, have been found to be much less effective in experimental models of emphysema than elastase is. In fact, purified granulocyte elastase has been shown to localize in alveolar septae after tracheal installation.

In the lung of a normal Pi M individual, significant amounts of alpha₁-antitrypsin are found in pulmonary tissue and secretions, probably in a sufficient amount to inhibit the digestion of elastic tissue. In deficient Pi Z individuals, alpha₁-antitrypsin levels are markedly decreased, allowing elastic tissue destruction to occur. It is thought that any infectious or toxic injury to the lung that might increase the numbers of granulocytes or alveolar macrophages in pulmonary tissue could enhance the release of elastase and hasten the progression of elastin destruction in deficient individuals.

Clinical Course

In most individuals with familial emphysema and alpha₁-antitrypsin deficiency, there is a subtle increase in dyspnea, usually beginning near the end of the third decade of life. Dyspnea is generally progressive and not often associated with cough or sputum production. Chest radiographs demonstrate increasing hyperaeration of the lung fields, beginning especially at the lung bases, while pulmonary function studies document the progression of irreversible chronic obstructive pulmonary disease. Intravenous administration of radio-labeled materials demonstrates diminished perfusion at the lung bases in the upright position, a concomitant of many chronic pulmonary conditions. As the disease progresses, recurrent infections with bronchitis and severe bronchiectasis may become superimposed upon the diffuse, underlying emphysematous process. The progression of this disease can clearly be hastened by smoking or recurrent pulmonary infections. The vast majority of individuals with familial emphysema and alpha$_1$-antitrypsin deficiency are of the phenotype Pi Z. A few have been described with Pi types SZ, S or PZ. Quantitative analysis of alpha$_1$-antitrypsin function or concentration will almost always make the diagnosis of severe deficiency of these types, while definitive genetic analysis of the alpha$_1$-antitrypsin, as described above, will assure it.

The pathologic change of the lung in patients with severe alpha$_1$-antitrypsin deficiency is quite characteristic. Its hallmark is diffuse panacinar emphysema, demonstrated well in many autopsied cases, using appropriate morphometric techniques involving whole lung slices. This process appears to begin at the lung bases, advancing progressively toward the apices. In a few instances, striking widespread bronchiectasis has been found superim-

posed upon the underlying emphysema. A variety of other pathologic processes have been described in association with the Pi Z phenotype in adults. These include certain types of liver disease (cirrhosis, hepatic carcinoma); renal disease with glomerular deposits of alpha$_1$-antitrypsin, immunoglobulin and complement; recurrent pancreatitis; peptic ulcer; and severe panniculitis. Among these various clinical manifestations, the lung and liver disease are most closely correlated with severe alpha$_1$-antitrypsin deficiency, while the other findings have been observed in only a few cases.

Only a small number of cases has been reported in the pediatric age range with severe alpha$_1$-antitrypsin deficiency and chronic, progressive pulmonary disease definitely attributable to the deficiency (Table 1). In only three instances has pathologic confirmation been available. One of these children has been definitely typed as Pi ZZ, while in the other two, strong presumptive evidence of the Pi ZZ phenotype was presented. Patient 4 is a Pi ZZ sibling of patient 3, who had patholog-

TABLE 1.

Patient	Age	Sex	Age at Onset	Pi Type	Pulmonary Function	Pulmonary Pathology	X-ray
Talamo et al. (1971)	13 yrs.	F	18 mos.	ZZ*	Severe obstructive lung disease	Consistent with panacinar emphysema	Marked hyperinflation
Houstek et al. (1973)	13 yrs.	M	2 yrs.	†	Severe obstructive lung disease	Panacinar emphysema	Hyperinflation; "bullous emphysema"
Glasgow et al. (1973)	Died at 11½ yrs.	F	6 yrs.	‡	ND	Panacinar emphysema, diffuse bronchiectasis	Hyperinflation with bullae
Glasgow et al. (1973)	12½ yrs.	M	§	ZZ	Moderate airway obstruction	ND	Mild hyperinflation
Dunand et al. (1976)	14 yrs.	F	3½ yrs.	SZ	Severe obstructive lung disease	ND	Marked hyperinflation

*Typing confirmed after original case report.

†No typing reported, but levels of alpha$_1$-antitrypsin function and concentration in the range of Pi ZZ patients. Levels in mother and brother consistent with Pi MZ.

‡Alpha$_1$ globulin band missing on serum electrophoresis (consistent with Pi ZZ).

§Mild chest symptoms, including intermittent wheezing and unproductive nocturnal cough, one episode of pneumonia, but no exact age of onset noted.

ically proved emphysema. Patient 4 was early in the course of his disease at the time of the report. Patients 3 and 4 had a 12½-year-old male sibling of Pi ZZ phenotype who was reported to have normal pulmonary function. Patients 3 and 4 also had the characteristic clinical picture of infantile liver disease, progressing to cirrhosis, associated with severe alpha₁-antitrypsin deficiency. Another Pi ZZ child with cirrhosis and clinical and roentgenographic evidence of emphysema has recently been described. No information concerning lung function or pulmonary disease was included (Kaiser and coworkers, 1975).

Patient 5 has strong clinical evidence for panacinar emphysema at the age of 14 years, following onset of symptoms at age 3½ years. An asymptomatic brother of patient 5, also of Pi SZ phenotype, has laboratory evidence of mild airway obstruction.

In this group of well documented patients, the most prominent symptoms have been chronic cough, progressive dyspnea and wheezing, either continuous or intermittent. Digital clubbing is described in the severely affected patients. As noted in Table 1, the age of onset ranged from 18 months to 3½ years. Of significance is the fact that other causes of chronic pulmonary disease in infancy and childhood were ruled out in each case. These included cystic fibrosis, immunodeficiency and allergic disease. Four of these individuals had either definite or strongly suggestive evidence of the Pi ZZ phenotype. Other children with less convincing evidence of true emphysema have been reported to have chronic pulmonary disease in association with Pi phenotypes ZZ, MZ and S.

Very little is known about the natural clinical history of individuals born with the Pi Z phenotype. While a certain number will develop serious liver disease in infancy or early childhood, most will undoubtedly be well until young adult life, when there is a rather high likelihood of development of clinical emphysema. In fact, there are several reported individuals in the fifth decade (or older) of Pi type Z who have been said to be totally asymptomatic. When some of these individuals have been examined closely in the pulmonary function laboratory, a variety of physiologic abnormalities, including mildly impaired air flow rates, hypoxemia, increased alveolar-arterial oxygen gradients and decreased carbon monoxide diffusing capacity have been found. Altered distribution of pulmonary perfusion with loss of the normally occurring perfusion gradient from base to apex (in the upright position) is often present in such older individuals. On the other hand, a few children of Pi type ZZ have been studied and found to be physiologically normal. In one 14-year-old girl of Pi type ZZ, an alteration in the distribution of pulmonary blood flow was found, although all other parameters of lung function were normal. Thus, there is some evidence that the earliest physiologic manifestation of severe alpha₁-antitrypsin deficiency in the lung is an alteration in the distribution of pulmonary blood flow. It is conceivable that this abnormality could result from destruction of elastin in the early stages of emphysema.

A recent screening program in Sweden involved the quantitative determination of alpha₁-antitrypsin levels in 200,000 neonates over a two-year period (Sveger, 1976); 120 infants of Pi type Z were discovered. Among these, there were 9 with prolonged obstructive jaundice with severe clinical symptoms. In addition, there were five Pi Z infants with prolonged jaundice and no clinical symptoms. At follow-up at the age of two to three years, only a few of these infants had definite clinical evidence of liver disease. Of the remaining Pi Z infants, about one-half had abnormal tests of hepatocellular function at three, six and 12 months of age, without any clinical evidence of liver disease. On the other hand, the number of alpha₁-antitrypsin deficient children with severe respiratory disease during the first three years of life was not impressive. Seven Pi Z infants and one Pi SZ infant had bronchitis with wheezing more than twice a year. Two Pi Z children with coexisting cirrhosis had persistent cough for more than six months, and three Pi Z infants had recurrent croup. One Pi Z infant had severe pneumonia with cyst formation. No control group was available.

Abundant evidence from epidemiologic studies is now available concerning the clinical health and pulmonary physiology in Pi MZ individuals. The incidence of respiratory signs, symptoms and illnesses is no different from a control population during the childhood years. There appears to be no significant abnormality in pulmonary function tests in the Pi MZ children studied. Further, there is no increased incidence of the Pi MZ phenotype in large groups of children with asthma or cystic fibrosis. When adults of the Pi MZ phenotype are examined, there is a clearly demonstrable deterioration of lung function with age, which is abnormal in comparison with a control group of Pi MM individuals. Smoking appears to worsen this deficit. There is still some disagreement about whether the prevalence of overt chronic pulmonary disease is higher among groups of Pi MZ adults.

Diagnosis

The diagnosis of emphysema with severe alpha$_1$-antitrypsin deficiency involves the demonstration of an obstructive pulmonary defect by lung function analysis, by the presence of bilateral, diffuse hyperinflation of the lungs on chest roentgenogram, and by the confirmation of the serum protein abnormality by biochemical and immunochemical techniques.

The physiologic abnormalities include an increase in total lung capacity, a decrease in vital capacity, an increase in residual volume and functional residual capacity, an increase in airways resistance accompanied by an abnormal diffusing capacity, blood gas derangements consistent with obstructive pulmonary disease, and alterations in pulmonary ventilation and perfusion as demonstrated by radioisotope techniques. The obstructive pulmonary defect should be irreversible or only slightly reversible with bronchodilators, unless there is also a coexisting second pulmonary disease, such as asthma.

Routine chest films demonstrate hyperinflation (Fig. 1), sometimes accompanied by bulla formation, often at the lung bases. Evidence of superimposed

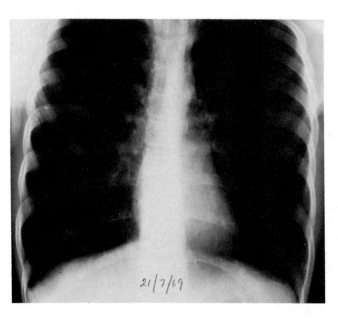

Figure 1. Anteroposterior chest roentgenogram of a 13-year-old female with Pi Z alpha$_1$-antitrypsin deficiency and biopsy evidence of panacinar emphysema. A striking degree of radiolucency is present.

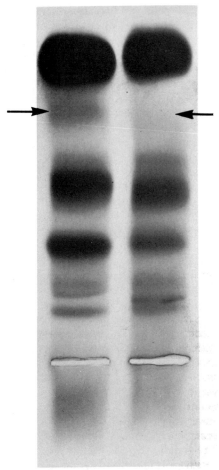

Figure 2. Agarose serum protein electrophoresis of samples from a normal Pi M individual (*left*) and a deficient Pi Z patient (*right*). The alpha₁-antitrypsin region is indicated by the arrow in each pattern. The anode is at the top.

pulmonary infection or bronchiectasis may be present. Chest fluoroscopy reveals poor movement of the diaphragms with respiration bilaterally. Bronchography may be necessary to delineate the presence of bronchiectasis whenever it is suspected.

Routine serum protein electrophoresis should reveal a missing alpha₁ globulin band (Fig. 2); this is presumptive evidence of the existence of Pi Z, Pi SZ or Pi — alpha₁-antitrypsin deficiency. These electrophoretic findings should be confirmed by quantitative measurement of alpha₁-antitrypsin function, using biochemical techniques, and of concentration, using specific immunochemical techniques. When alpha₁-antitrypsin quantitation is in the range of severe alpha₁-antitrypsin deficiency, the genetic typing procedures, using acid starch gel and antigen-antibody crossed electrophoresis or isofocusing electrophoresis (currently an experimental method), should be used. These procedures are available in an increasing number of medical centers.

Differential Diagnosis

The disease states that could easily be confused with emphysema and alpha₁-antitrypsin deficiency are also characterized by chronic obstructive pulmonary defects. These include (1) cystic fibrosis, which can be diagnosed by an abnormal sweat test, the coexistence of pancreatic insufficiency and the presence of similar disease in siblings; (2) asthma, which can be diagnosed by reversibility with bronchodilators and evidence of the atopic state, including blood eosinophilia, positive skin tests to inhalant allergens and, often, elevated IgE levels; (3) bronchiectasis, which may be associated with an earlier history of severe pulmonary infection, the production of copious amounts of sputum, chronic bacterial infection and characteristic bronchographic changes; and (4) immunodeficiency diseases, such as agammaglobulinemia, thymic aplasia or combined immunodeficiency disease, which are associated with persistent, recurrent or unusual pulmonary infections and laboratory evidence of abnormalities in the T cell or B cell system, or in both. While each of these clinical syndromes is usually distinctive enough to lead one to the correct diagnosis, it should be remembered that any of them might co-exist with emphysema and severe alpha₁-antitrypsin deficiency. In fact, both cystic fibrosis and asthma have been described in association with alpha₁-antitrypsin deficiency. Presumably, these are chance associations.

There are several situations in which the diagnosis of severe alpha$_1$-antitrypsin deficiency should be strongly considered. Any infant or child with chronic cough, wheezing or dyspnea, especially when the exact diagnosis is not clear, should have serum alpha$_1$-antitrypsin analyses performed. When there is a family history of siblings or first cousins with chronic respiratory symptoms, analysis should also be performed. The clinical setting of severe pneumonia that does not resolve might also be accompanied by alpha$_1$-antitrypsin deficiency. Finally, when chronic pulmonary symptoms occur in an infant or child with clinical liver disease, the diagnosis of severe alpha$_1$-antitrypsin deficiency should be considered.

Treatment

While no specific treatment is currently available for this pulmonary disease, much benefit can be derived from a variety of measures. Since there is definite evidence that the emphysema associated with alpha$_1$-antitrypsin deficiency can progress more rapidly in the presence of noxious inhalants, it is imperative to emphasize the elimination of environmental smoke and fumes. The patient and his family should be urged to eliminate all tobacco smoking. In addition, since the occurrence of pulmonary infection would enhance the number of inflammatory cells (granulocytes and alveolar macrophages) in the lung, appropriate antibiotics should be provided early in its course. There is no evidence for the usefulness of prophylactic antibiotics in this situation.

Pulmonary physical therapy and breathing exercises would become of definite benefit when recurrent infection and bronchiectasis are features of this disease.

While there is no evidence that bronchodilators can reverse the course of emphysema in this disease, or provide symptomatic relief, they should be used when their benefit can be demonstrated, such as in the presence of superimposed infection. There is no evidence whatsoever of a beneficial effect of corticosteroids. They should be used only if indicated for coexistent asthma.

In the advanced stages of the disease, intermittent or continuous oxygen therapy may be necessary. Rarely, dramatic improvement has resulted from the surgical removal of one or more of the large areas of bullous emphysema that can occur, especially in the lower lobes.

Possibilities exist for the treatment of the underlying alpha$_1$-antitrypsin deficiency in the future. These might include the long-term use of synthetic inhibitors of granulocyte elastase and the possible stimulation of release of stored alpha$_1$-antitrypsin from the liver. There is no evidence of the potential benefits of infusing large amounts of serum alpha$_1$-antitrypsin over an extended period of time. This approach would be somewhat impractical, in view of the short survival time of this protein in the circulation.

Prognosis

Since the number of infants and children described with this disease has been small up to the present time, there is no good information on the prognosis. In all of the documented cases, there has not been any reversal of lung damage, and one would expect a downhill progression in most cases. However, observations in large numbers of adults with this disease suggest that the rate of progression of pulmonary disease can be quite variable.

REFERENCES

Dunand, P., Cropp, G. J. A., and Middleton, E.: Severe obstructive lung disease in a 14-year-old girl with alpha$_1$-antitrypsin deficiency. *J. Allergy Clin. Immunol.*, 57:615, 1976.

Eriksson, S.: Studies in alpha$_1$-antitrypsin deficiency. *Acta Med. Scand.*, 177:432, 1965.

Fagerhol, M. K., and Laurell, C. B.: The polymorphism of "prealbumins" and alpha$_1$-antitrypsin in human sera. *Clin. Chim Acta*, 16:199, 1967.

Glasgow, J. F. T., Lynch, M. J., Hercz, A., Levison, H., and Sass-kortsak, A.: Alpha$_1$-antitrypsin deficiency in association with both cirrhosis and chronic obstructive lung disease in two sibs. *Am. J. Med.*, 54:181, 1973.

Houštek, J., Copová, M., Zapletal, A., Tomášova, H., and Samánek, M.: Alpha₁-antitrypsin deficiency in a child with chronic lung disease. *Chest*, 64:773, 1973.

Jeppsson, J.: Amino acid substitution Glu→Lys in alpha₁-antitrypsin Pi Z. *FEBS Letters*, 65:195, 1976.

Kaiser, D., Rennert, O. M., Joller-Jemelka, H., Gotze, H., Sollberger, H., and Kehrli, P.: Alpha₁-antitrypsin-Mangel: Kombination von Lungenemphysem und Lebercirrhose im fruhen Kindesalter. *Klin. Wochenschr.*, 53:117, 1975.

Laurell, C. B., and Eriksson, S.: The electrophoretic alpha₁-globulin pattern of serum in alpha₁-antitrypsin deficiency. *Scand. J. Clin. Lab. Invest.*, 15:132, 1963.

Sharp, H., Bridges, R. A., Krivit, W., and Freier, E. F.: Cirrhosis associated with alpha₁-antitrypsin deficiency: a previously unrecognized inherited disorder. *J. Lab. Clin. Med.*, 73:934, 1969.

Sveger, T.: Liver disease in alpha₁-antitrypsin deficiency detected by screening of 200,000 infants. *N. Engl. J. Med.*, 294:1316, 1976.

Talamo, R. C.: Basic and clinical aspects of the alpha₁-antitrypsin. *Pediatrics*, 56:91, 1975.

Talamo, R. C., Levison, H., Lynch, M. J., Hercz, A., Hyslop, N. E., and Bain, H. W.: Symptomatic pulmonary emphysema in childhood associated with hereditary alpha-1-antitrypsin and elastase inhibitor deficiency. *J. Pediatr.*, 79:20, 1971.

Yoshida, A., Lieberman, J., Gaidulis, L., and Ewing, C.: Molecular abnormality of human alpha₁-antitrypsin variant (Pi ZZ) associated with plasma activity deficiency. *Proc. Natl. Acad. Sci.*, 73:1324, 1976.

CHAPTER FORTY

LIQUID AND AIR IN THE PLEURAL SPACE

Reynaldo D. Pagtakhan, M.D.
and Victor Chernick, M.D.

Disorders of the pleura constitute an important cause of morbidity and mortality in infants and children. Their prompt recognition and appropriate management can avert the occurrence of a more serious cardiorespiratory catastrophe. In this chapter we shall discuss the anatomic features of the pleural "space," the physiology of liquid transport in the potential space and the various noninflammatory disorders of liquid accumulation and their management. (Inflammatory disorders of the pleura are discussed in Chapter 27.) Finally, the process and treatment of gas accumulation in the pleural space because of leakage of air from the alveoli will be considered.

LIQUID IN THE PLEURAL SPACE

ANATOMIC FEATURES

The pleural membranes, which cover the outer surface of the lungs (visceral pleura) and the inner surface of the thoracic wall (parietal pleura), are in intimate contact, which leaves a gas-free space with only a thin film of liquid covering its surface. The membranes are lined with a single layer of ciliated, flat mesothelial cells, 6 to 7 microns thick, along with a connective tissue layer, 30 to 40 microns thick, of collagen and elastic fiber. Between the connective tissue layer and the limiting membrane of the lung lies a region, 20 to 50 microns thick, of blood vessels and lymphatics. Branches of the pulmonary artery supply the visceral pleura, while the parietal pleura is supplied by branches of the intercostal arteries. Lymphatic vessels are located in the subepithelial layer of the parietal pleura. The parietal pleura drains into the internal mammary system ventrally, the intercostal lymph node dorsally and the mediastinal lymph nodes inferiorly. The entire visceral pleura drains into the mediastinal nodes. The thoracic and right lymphatic ducts then drain into the systemic venous circulation.

PHYSIOLOGY OF LIQUID IN THE PLEURAL SPACE

The pleural membranes are permeable to liquid. In contrast to a normally totally gas-free pleural space, complete emptying of the pleural liquid does not occur, and a small but measurable amount (approximately 1.0 milliliter) of liquid remains. A rational understanding of pleural liquid accumulation in various disease states requires a thorough knowledge of normal liquid transport into and out of the pleural cavity. Normally, close to 90 per cent of the original amount of pleural liquid filtered out of the arterial end of the capillaries is reabsorbed at the venous end. The remainder (10 per cent) of

602

the filtrate is returned via the lymphatics. The imbalance between filtration and reabsorption forces determines the direction of liquid movement. Starling described a classic approach to convective (bulk) liquid movement between vascular and extravascular compartments, which can be expressed as

$$\dot{Q}_v = K_f [(P_c - P_{is}) - (\pi_{pl} - \pi_{is})]$$

$$30 \sim 11 \sim$$

where $\dot{Q}_v$ = rate of net liquid movement per unit surface area of capillary; K_f = capillary filtration coefficient; P_c = capillary hydrostatic pressure; P_{is} = hydrostatic pressure in interstitial space (equivalent to intrapleural pressure); π_{pl} = plasma oncotic pressure; and π_{is} = interstitial space oncotic pressure (equivalent to oncotic pressure of pleural liquid).

Liquid movement across the pleural capillaries generally obeys the foregoing law of transcapillary liquid exchange. The filtration coefficient (K_f) is an index of capillary wall permeability that depends on the structural integrity of the intercellular junctions of the endothelial lining. The oncotic pressure (π) is a function of the molal concentration of protein, mainly albumin. Normal plasma with a protein concentration of 7.0 gm./100 ml. has an oncotic pressure of 32 to 35 cm. H_2O, whereas pleural liquid with a protein concentration of 1.77 gm./100 ml. has an estimated oncotic pressure of about 5.8 cm. H_2O. The mean hydrostatic pressures (P_c) in the parietal and visceral pleural capillaries are 30 and 11 cm. H_2O, respectively. Since the intrapleural pressure (equivalent to P_{is}) at resting lung volume is about 5 cm. H_2O subatmospheric, there is a net pressure of 9 cm. H_2O (filtration pressure) at the parietal pleural capillary level tending to drive liquid into the pleural space. In contrast, a net driving pressure of minus 10 cm. H_2O (absorption pressure) is acting on the visceral pleural capillaries, driving liquid from the pleural space into the capillaries (Table 1). Net liquid absorption from the pleural space occurs because there is more extensive vascularity in the visceral than in the parietal pleura. As the pleural liquid volume is reduced, a more intimate contact between the lungs and chest wall occurs. Increased negative pressure develops in the liquid between the contact points of visceral and parietal pleura owing to deformation at the sites of increased local stretching. Ultimately, the negative pleural liquid pressure equilibrates with the absorption pressure. Thus, the pleural space is kept only nearly liquid-free, a state that represents an equilibrium between filtration and absorption.

The pleural liquid is sterile and contains an average of nearly 2.0 gm./100 ml. proteins. Particulate matter from the pleural liquid is returned to the systemic circulation via the lymphatics or directly into the pleural capillaries. Large molecular weight particles, such as proteins and erythrocytes, are cleared solely via the lymphatic channels in the parietal pleura through preformed stomas formed by direct continuity of the endothelial cells of

TABLE 1. STARLING RELATIONSHIP IN PARIETAL AND VISCERAL PLEURA

	Parietal Pleura	Visceral Pleura
Force Moving Liquid Into Pleural Space (cm. H_2O)		
Capillary hydrostatic pressure	30	11
Interstitial hydrostatic pressure (pleural pressure)	5	5
Oncotic pressure of pleural liquid	6	6
Total (cm. H_2O)	41	22
Force Moving Liquid Into Pleural Capillaries (cm. H_2O)		
Plasma oncotic pressure	32	32
NET Force (cm. H_2O)	9 (out)	9 (in)

lymphatic vessels with pleural mesothelial cells. Clearance of proteins occurs independently of net liquid movement. A major propelling force in the transport of pleural content into the circulation is respiratory movement, since hypoventilation is known to decrease absorption of particulate matter from the pleural space. Smaller ions, such as sodium, and low molecular weight dyes, such as methylene blue, are rapidly absorbed directly into the visceral pleural circulation. Pleural absorption of both liquid and particles is hastened by augmenting intercostal and diaphragmatic activity, e.g., deep breathing exercises, which result in increased vascular and lymphatic uptake owing to dehiscences formed between mesothelial cells of the visceral pleura.

Normally, the pleural liquid is alkaline. The pH of the liquid is determined by several factors, namely ① pH, P_{CO_2} and bicarbonate of arterial blood, ② P_{CO_2} of the local pleural tissue, ③ metabolism of cells in the pleural liquid and ④ transfer of H^+, CO_2 and bicarbonate between the pleural cavity and the surrounding blood and tissue.

ACCUMULATION OF EXCESS PLEURAL LIQUID

Etiology and Pathogenesis

The normal state of a nearly liquid-free pleural cavity represents an equilibrium between pleural liquid formation (filtration) and removal (absorption). Fundamentally, excess liquid accumulates in the pleural cavity (effusion) whenever filtration exceeds removal mechanisms as a result of either: ① increased filtration associated with normal or impaired absorption or ② normal filtration associated with inadequate removal. Thus, disequilibrium may be due to disturbances in Starling forces that govern filtration and absorption or to alterations in lymphatic drainage, or both.

A variety of clinical disorders can alter vascular filtration and absorption

in the pleural capillaries as well as lymphatic flow (Table 2). The capillary filtration coefficient (K_f) may be increased owing to damage in the basement membrane as a result of inflammation (e.g., pleural infection, rheumatoid arthritis, systemic lupus erythematosus, pulmonary infarction) or direct toxic damage on the endothelium. Local blood flow may increase, resulting in an increase in capillary hydrostatic pressure (P_c). Moreover, protein is lost from the capillaries and accumulates in the pleural cavity, thereby increasing pleural fluid oncotic pressure (π_{is}). The net consequence of these changes is increased liquid and protein transudation into the pleural cavity that exceeds the normal capacity of lymphatic drainage. Hydrostatic pressure (P_c) may also be increased because of systemic venous hypertension (e.g., pericarditis, right-sided heart failure from overinfusion of blood or fluid, superior vena cava syndrome) or because of pulmonary venous hypertension (e.g., congestive heart failure). The resulting increased pleural liquid accumulation (hydrothorax) is due not only to increased driving pressure in the systemic capillaries but also to a higher filtration coefficient. The creation of a markedly subatmospheric pleural pressure (e.g., following thoracentesis), even in the presence of a normal hydrostatic pressure in the pleural capillaries, may also result in increased fluid filtration from the pleural capillaries. This mechanism explains cases of recurrent effusion following repeated thoracenteses or increasing effusion in tuberculosis with visceral pleural thickening and fibrosis and permanently atelectatic lungs.

Oncotic pressure (π) determines how effectively fluid is reabsorbed. Net absorption by the visceral pleura is reduced to zero by an increase in pleural liquid protein higher than 4 gm./100 ml. (e.g., infection) in the presence of normal plasma protein concentration. When plasma oncotic pressure is significantly reduced (e.g., hypoalbuminemia; nephrosis), parietal pleural filtration is increased and visceral pleural

TABLE 2. PATHOPHYSIOLOGY OF PLEURAL LIQUID ACCUMULATION

Primary Mechanism	Clinical Disorders	Pleural Effusion
Altered Starling Forces		
Increased capillary permeability (K_f)	Pleuropulmonary infection; circulating toxins; systemic lupus erythematosus; rheumatoid arthritis; sarcoidosis; tumor; pulmonary infarction; viral hepatitis	Exudate
Increased capillary hydrostatic pressure (P_c)	Overhydration; congestive heart failure; venous hypertension; pericarditis	Transudate
Decreased hydrostatic pressure of the interstitial space (P_{is})	Trapped lung with chronic pleural space; post-thoracentesis	Transudate
Decreased plasma oncotic pressure (π_{pl})	Hypoalbuminemia; nephrosis; hepatic cirrhosis	Transudate
Increased oncotic pressure of interstitial space (π_{is})	Pulmonary infarction	Exudate
Inappropriate Lymphatic Flow		
Inadequate outflow	Hypoalbuminemia; nephrosis	Transudate
Excessive inflow	Hepatic cirrhosis with ascites; peritoneal dialysis	Transudate
Impaired flow (Mediastinal lymphadenopathy and fibrosis; thickening of parietal pleura; obstruction of thoracic duct; developmental hypoplasia or defect)	Mediastinal radiation, superior vena caval syndrome, pericarditis; tuberculosis; lymphoma, mediastinal hygroma; hereditary lymphedema, congenital chylothorax	Exudate or Transudate or Chyle
Disruption of diaphragmatic lymphatics	Pancreatitis; subphrenic abscess	Exudate
Vascular Leak	Trauma, spontaneous rupture, vascular erosion by neoplasm, hemorrhagic disease	Blood

absorption is reduced even with normal concentration of pleural protein. If lymphatic channels are unable to provide adequately for drainage, pleural effusion ensues. Lymphatic drainage, however, may be impeded as a result of ① systemic venous hypertension, ② mediastinal lymphadenopathy (e.g., lymphoma or fibrosis), ③ thickening of parietal pleura (e.g., tuberculosis), ④ obstruction of thoracic duct (e.g., chylothorax) and ⑤ developmental hypoplasia of lymphatic channels (e.g., hereditary lymphedema). On occasion, the lymphatic system is overloaded by absorption of peritoneal fluid (e.g., liver cirrhosis with ascites; peritoneal dialysis) via the diaphragmatic lymphatics. The result is escape of excess lymphatic fluid under increased pressure into the pleural cavity where pressure is normally subatmospheric.

From the foregoing discussion, it is evident that a single clinical disorder may cause a pleural effusion as a result of one or several mechanisms. Moreover, it is possible that clinical disorders may coexist. This may explain the varying character of pleural effusion seen clinically.

Classically, pleural effusions have been classified into transudate and exudate. This classification can be of great value, since certain disease states produce transudates almost exclusively (e.g., congestive heart failure) and others produce exudates (e.g., pleural infections). A transudate usually occurs when the mechanical forces of hydrostatic and oncotic pressures are so altered as to favor liquid filtration. The pleural surfaces are not involved by the underlying disorder. In contrast, exudates result either from inflammatory

TABLE 3.   CHEMICAL SEPARATION OF TRANSUDATES AND EXUDATES

Type of Effusion	Pleural Liquid Concentration		Pleural/Serum Concentration Ratio	
	PROTEIN	LDH	PROTEIN	LDH
Transudate	<3 gm./100 ml.	<200 I.U.	<0.5	<0.6
Exudate	≥3 gm./100 ml.	≥200 I.U.	≥0.5	≥0.6

LDH = lactic dehydrogenase.

diseases that affect the pleural surfaces, causing increased capillary permeability, or from disorders that impede lymphatic drainage. A pleural liquid protein concentration of 3.0 gm./100 ml. separates transudates (<3 gm./100 ml.) from exudates (>3 gm./100 ml.). Another approach classifies exudates as having any one of the following features: a pleural liquid-to-serum protein ratio greater than 0.5; a pleural liquid lactic dehydrogenase (LDH) greater than 200 I.U.; and a pleural liquid-to-serum LDH greater than 0.6 (Table 3).

Pleural effusion may also be classified as chylous (Table 4), chyliform or hemorrhagic. Chylothorax refers to an accumulation of chyle in the pleural cavity and results from obstruction of either the thoracic duct or left subclavian vein (e.g., neoplastic, parasitic and inflammatory conditions), from congenital lymph fistula of undetermined cause or from traumatic rupture of lymphatic channels (e.g., following extracardiac vascular operations or diaphragmatic hernia repair). Chylothorax is the most common type of pleural effusion in the newborn period.

When the type of pleural liquid only assumes the appearance of chyle (milky white and opalescent) but does not demonstrate fat globules (pseudochyle), the effusion is called chyliform. The milky appearance represents the fatty degeneration of pus and endothelial cells. It may be seen in long-standing cases of purulent effusion.

Frank blood in the pleural cavity is referred to as hemothorax. It may be caused by trauma to the chest wall, vascular erosion by neoplasm (e.g., pleural mesothelioma), spontaneous rupture of subpleural bleb or great vessels (patent ductus arteriosus, coarctation of aorta) and strangulated diaphragmatic hernia.

Functional Pathology

The degree of dysfunction is determined by the severity and rapidity of development of pleural effusion as well as by the nature of the underlying disorder and the status of cardiopulmonary function. Moderate to large pleural effusions increase elastic resistance to distention, thereby reducing lung volume on the ipsilateral side. Thus, the vital capacity is reduced. Airflow remains normal, since the nonelastic resistance is usually unaffected. The corresponding hemidiaphragm is depressed, and contralateral lung func-

TABLE 4.   CERTAIN PHYSICAL AND CHEMICAL CHARACTERISTICS OF CHYLE

Sterile
Ingested lipophilic dyes stain the effusion
Cells predominantly lymphocytes
Sudan stain: fat globules
Total fat content = exceeds that of plasma (e.g., up to 660 mg./100 ml.)
Protein content = ½ or same as that of plasma (usually ≥ 3.0 gm./100 ml.)
Electrolytes = same as plasma
BUN = same as plasma
Glucose = same as plasma

tion and vascular flow may be compromised by mediastinal displacement. Thus, alveolar gas exchange may be seriously impaired and cardiac function disturbed. Malnutrition secondary to loss of chyle (rich in proteins, lipids and fat-soluble vitamins) and shock due to blood loss are additional hazards.

Diagnosis

HISTORY AND PHYSICAL EXAMINATION. Pleural effusion is usually secondary to an underlying disorder. The basic disease determines most of the systemic symptoms. Until accumulation of pleural liquid increases enough to cause cardiorespiratory difficulties (e.g., dyspnea, orthopnea), a pleural effusion may be asymptomatic. Thus, attention to the chest findings on physical examination is important, particularly if only a small amount of liquid is present. Pleural rub may be the only finding during the early phase. Diminished thoracic wall excursion, dull or flat percussion, decreased tactile and vocal fremitus, diminished whispering pecto-riloquy, fullness of the intercostal spaces and decreased breath sounds are easily demonstrated over the site involved in the older child with moderate effusion. Breath sounds in the neonate can come through loud and clear because of his small chest volume. The trachea and the cardiac apex are displaced toward the contralateral side. Careful physical examination, even in the neonate, will enable the physician to suspect a pleural effusion.

CHEST ROENTGENOGRAM. In general, a minimum of approximately 400 milliliters of pleural liquid are required for roentgenographic visualization in upright views of the chest. A small quantity of pleural liquid is seen best at end-expiration as a straight radiodense line. It should be differentiated from the undulating outline of soft tissues unaffected by the respiratory phase. Lateral decubitus films taken with the patient lying on the affected side can detect as little as 50 milliliters of liquid. Recent experimental evidence indicates that as little as 5 milliliters of pleural liquid can be visible on properly ex-

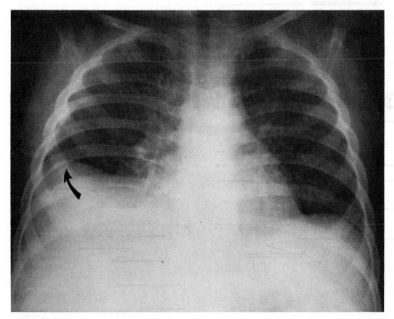

Figure 1. Upright chest radiograph in a child with nephrotic syndrome demonstrating right infrapulmonary pleural effusion. The right hemidiaphragm shows peak elevation laterally (*arrow*) with relative lucency of the costophrenic sinus, signs which are indicative of an infrapulmonary location of the liquid.

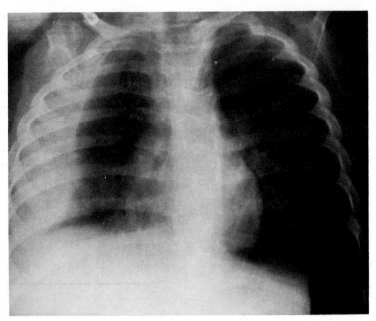

Figure 2. Decubitus chest radiograph with right side dependent in same patient as in Figure 1, confirming the presence of free-flowing right pleural effusion.

posed radiographs. It is demonstrable as a layering of liquid density in the dependent portion of the thoracic cavity. Decubitus films may also demonstrate an infrapulmonary pleural effusion (Figs. 1 and 2). When effusion is moderate, chest radiographs demonstrate uniform water-density and widened interspaces on the affected side with displacement of the mediastinum to the contralateral hemithorax. A roentgenogram taken after thoracentesis may demonstrate the underlying parenchymal involvement obscured by the effusion.

EXAMINATION OF THE PLEURAL LIQUID. Evacuation of liquid by thoracentesis confirms the clinical and radiologic diagnosis of effusion. The specimen may provide the only evidence on which to make the diagnosis of certain specific disease states or to exclude others.

The gross appearance of the liquid may be a clue to the cause of the effusion. Thus, a pale yellow liquid suggests serous effusion. Aspiration of chylous liquid suggests injury to the

lymphatic channels (e.g., postsurgical; neoplasm, tuberculosis) or spontaneous anatomic leakage of chyle (e.g., congenital chylothorax). The characteristic milky appearance in congenital chylothorax is seen only after oral feeding has begun a few days earlier. A bloody fluid implies vascular erosion from malignant tumor or damage to intercostal or chest wall vessels from blunt thoracic trauma. Brisk and massive bleeding is apt to be seen when the systemic circulation is involved, since systemic pressure is sixfold higher than the pulmonary pressure. A purulent specimen indicates bacterial infection of the pleura (see Chapter 27).

Total counts of red and white blood cells are of negligible value and need not be done routinely unless chest trauma is suspected, in which case eosinophilia may be present. Differential cell counting can identify tumor cells and is done if a neoplasm is suspected. Parts of the liquid are sent for cytologic studies for malignant cells, for biochemical determinations (fat content; protein and lactic dehydrogenase along with their serum determinations) and for microbiologic studies (cultures and Gram stain) to rule out infection.

In summary, physical and chemical characterizations of pleural liquid differentiate inflammatory pleural effusion from transudate, chyle or frank blood (Tables 3 and 4) caused by a variety of clinical disorders (Table 2). In the group of conditions associated with noninflammatory pleural effusion, the pleural membranes remain basically healthy. The underlying primary mechanisms are fundamentally a result of physical imbalance between increased liquid formation and inappropriate lymphatic flow. Pleural transudation occurs as a consequence of any of the following alterations in Starling forces: ① increased pulmonary capillary hydrostatic pressure, ② decreased plasma oncotic pressure and ③ markedly subatmospheric pleural pressure. These changes favor increased liquid filtration at the parietal pleural surface. Liquid accumulates in the pleural cavity because lymphatic drainage is inadequate to cope with the increased liquid load. A transudate may also occur as a result of excessive lymphatic inflow and pressure at the level of the diaphragmatic lymphatic channels. Impaired lymphatic flow may produce either a transudate or an exudate, depending on the dominant underlying or concurrent pathologic process. Thoracic duct obstruction can produce pure chylous effusion. Chylothorax in later childhood may also be traumatic. In contrast, overt trauma and underlying pathologic states are usually not recognizable in neonatal chylothorax. Frank bloody pleural liquid is almost invariably (except for vascular erosion by neoplasm that is associated with inflammation) a result of noninflammatory vascular leak.

Management

Treatment of noninflammatory, hemorrhagic and chylous pleural effusions is directed at supportive therapy of the functional disturbances and at specific management of the underlying disorder. Evacuation of noninflammatory liquid following the initial diagnostic thoracentesis is indicated only for relief of dyspnea and other cardiorespiratory disturbances caused by mediastinal displacement. Intercostal tube drainage is provided when repeated thoracenteses are necessary, since repeated needle drainage may be traumatic to a child. Diuretics administered to some patients may slow reaccumulation of transudate and thereby decrease or eliminate the need for frequent thoracentesis. Specific treatment of the underlying disorder emphasizes the need for thorough history taking and meticulous physical examination to arrive promptly at an accurate clinical diagnosis. Cardiovascular and renal causes (e.g., congestive heart failure; nephrosis) as well as lymphatic disorders causing inappropriate lymphatic flow are managed accordingly. Fluid overload (e.g., from intravenous infusion or peritoneal dialysis) as a cause of pleural transudation may require only a diuresis or spontaneous resolution with time.

The treatment of hemothorax when associated with shock requires immediate expansion of vascular volume and direct surgical repair of bleeders. Smaller bleeds should be evacuated, since healing is often associated with pleural adhesions. Fibrinolytic enzymes instilled into the pleural cavity may help when clots have formed. Chest pain is relieved by analgesics.

Chylothorax poses unique problems in management. Immediate and repeat thoracentesis is required for life-threatening cardiorespiratory embarrassment. In the absence of a life-threatening situation, initial treatment modalities for neonatal and most cases of surgical traumatic chylothorax involve ① single thoracentesis with complete drainage of chyle, ② use of medium-chain triglycerides (MCT) as the major source of dietary fat and ③ replacement of nutrient losses. Some cases of traumatic chylothorax would immediately require direct surgical intervention. The use of an MCT diet and avoidance of fatty meals containing long-chain fatty acids significantly reduce lymph flow up to tenfold because MCT are absorbed directly into the portal venous blood and contribute little to chylomicron formation. Cessation of chylous effusion largely occurs toward the end of the second week of treatment. In an occasional patient to whom chyle reaccumulates rapidly, a subsequent trial of fasting and parenteral hyperalimentation (via a vein other than the left subclavian) becomes indicated. The nonoperative treatment program is continued for a total duration of four to five weeks to allow sufficient time for closure of lymphatic channel fistulae. Concurrently, intravenous protein and electrolyte-containing solutions are infused to replace protein loss and prevent hypovolemia. Vitamin supplements are added to avoid deficiency states. With the foregoing therapeutic program, most patients respond favorably with progressive weight gain and cessation of chylothorax; only a few should be recalcitrant and require thoracotomy.

AIR IN THE PLEURAL SPACE

In this section we will consider the physiology of gas in the pleural space, and the process, clinical spectrum, diagnosis and treatment of gas accumulation in the pleural cavity and adjacent tissues because of leakage of air from the alveoli.

BASIC CONSIDERATIONS

Under physiologic conditions, the pleural membranes are permeable to gas. In view of the nature of dissociation curves for oxygen and carbon dioxide, the partial pressure (torr) of gases in the venous blood at sea level are: $P_{O_2} = 40$, $P_{CO_2} = 46$, $P_{N_2} = 573$ and $P_{H_2O} = 47$. They add up to 706 torr, that is, 54 torr (73 cm. H_2O) less than atmospheric pressure (at sea level). Since the total gas pressure in the venous blood is about 73 cm. H_2O subatmospheric, and the intrapleural pressure at resting lung volume is ap-

proximately 5 cm. H_2O subatmospheric, there exists a pressure gradient of about 68 cm. H_2O favoring continuing absorption of gas from the pleural space into the circulation. Thus, any gas volume within the pleural space diffuses out of it until all the gas phase disappears, and normally the pleural space is kept totally gas-free.

This process of absorption can be hastened considerably (approximately sevenfold) if the gas is loculated (and there is no further air leak) by breathing 100 per cent oxygen. Oxygen breathing will wash out nitrogen from the body without significantly increasing venous P_{O_2}. Because under ordinary circumstances arterial blood is nearly completely saturated with oxygen during air breathing, oxygen breathing changes arterial oxygen content by increasing only that amount of oxygen dissolved in plasma. The increase in dissolved oxygen from air to oxygen breathing is approximately 1.5 volumes per cent. Since arteriovenous oxygen content difference remains on average 5 volumes per cent, and the steep part of the oxyhemoglobin dissociation curve is in effect, breathing 100 per cent oxygen will raise venous P_{O_2} only from 40 to, say, 50 torr. This is accomplished while P_{N_2} goes to nearly zero, and therefore the total venous gas pressure is approximately 143 mm. Hg or some 617 torr (800 cm. H_2O) less than atmospheric pressure. Thus, 100 per cent oxygen breathing will hasten the absorption of loculated gas, independent of its location.

CLINICAL CONSIDERATIONS

Etiology and Pathogenesis

Intrapleural accumulation of air (pneumothorax) ensues whenever the pleural space develops a free communication with the atmosphere, either from a chest wall defect through the parietal pleura or from alveolar rupture, or both. A chest wall defect can result from surgical procedures and penetrating injury from missiles and projectiles. Thoracic trauma, including compressive blunt injury from vehicular accidents, falls and external cardiac massage, can rupture the lung. Infants and children are prone to internal injury from blunt trauma because of the greater compressibility of their chest wall. Thus, laceration or transection of major airways has been reported accompanying chest trauma even without fractured rib fragments or obvious external injury.

Fundamentally, three factors determine the extent of alveolar distention, namely (1) degree of transpulmonary pressure exerted, (2) duration of pressure applied and (3) ratio of inexpansible to expansible portion of the lung. Alterations of these factors with concomitant lung rupture can occur during the patient's own respiratory efforts, but more commonly during resuscitation and artificial ventilation and in the presence of incomplete airways obstruction and parenchymal consolidation seen in a variety of lower respiratory tract diseases. Positive intra-alveolar inflation pressure increases air volume but decreases blood volume in the adjacent vessels. Given this disproportionate change in blood volume and air volume, the tissue that tethers the perivascular sheath to the alveolar wall tends to attenuate. Since the mechanical forces in the alveolar wall and the tethering elements are angular to each other, rupture of the base of the alveoli occurs when the critical shear or traction force is exceeded and allows gas to escape into the perivascular space. The escaping air dissects itself along perivascular planes centrifugally to the hilum, where it ruptures into the mediastinum (pneumomediastinum) and then ruptures through the visceral pleura into the pleural space. Alternatively, when under tension in the interstitial space, air may rupture directly through the visceral pleura into the pleural space. When the air leak is confined to the interstitium of the lung, the condition is known as pulmonary interstitial emphysema (Fig. 3). Chest roentgenograms demonstrating pneumothorax and pneumomediastinum are illustrated in Figures 4 and 5, respectively. When under sufficient pressure, air may dissect out of the thorax

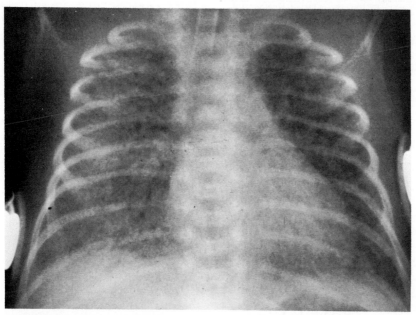

Figure 3. Chest radiograph in a newborn infant with hyaline membrane disease demonstrating interstitial emphysema of the right lung.

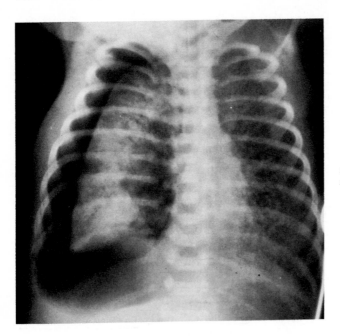

Figure 4. Chest radiograph in a neonate demonstrating right pneumothorax.

along subcutaneous tissue planes (subcutaneous emphysema) (Fig. 5) or into the peritoneal cavity (pneumoperitoneum) (Fig. 5). Air may become loculated in lobar fissures to produce pulmonary pseudocysts. Elevated intraalveolar tension less commonly allows subsequent dissection of air into the pericardial space (pneumopericardium); the exact mechanism remains unknown. Table 5 summarizes the clinical spectrum of air leak phenomena secondary to lung rupture. In the neonatal period, lung rupture can result from prolongation of the high transpulmonary pressure required during the first few breaths to open an airless lung, which opens sequentially. Prolonged application of high transpulmonary pressure across the normally aerated portions of the lung occurs because some of the airways may be occluded by aspirated blood, mucus, meconium or squamous epithelium. The incidence of spontaneous pneumothorax in the newborn period is about 1 per cent. The newborn is particularly susceptible to uneven alveolar distention owing to the underdeveloped pores of Kohn, which normally allow interalveolar air distribution.

Hyaline membrane disease (HMD)

with multiple areas of atelectasis can also lead to rupture of alveoli. Spontaneous air leak occurs in about 5 to 8 per cent of patients with HMD. There is conflicting evidence on whether a continuous distending pressure during spontaneous ventilation increases the incidence of lung rupture in HMD. Continuous negative pressure is not associated with an increase in the incidence of air leak in HMD above the spontaneous incidence, while nasal CPAP (continuous positive airway pressure) has been associated with an increased incidence in some studies. The introduction of PEEP (positive end-expiratory pressure) during artificial ventilation has doubled the incidence of air leak.

TABLE 5. CLINICAL SPECTRUM OF AIR LEAK PHENOMENA SECONDARY TO RUPTURE OF ALVEOLI

Interstitial emphysema
Pneumomediastinum
Pneumothorax
Subcutaneous emphysema
Pneumoperitoneum
Pneumopericardium
Pulmonary pseudocyst
Pulmonary venous gas embolism

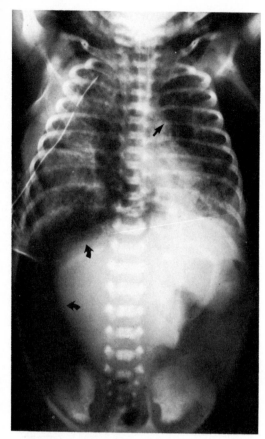

Figure 5. Chest radiograph in a newborn infant with hyaline membrane disease demonstrating pneumomediastinum (*small arrow*), massive subcutaneous emphysema, and pneumoperitoneum pushing the liver down (*two large arrows*).

The pathogenesis of pneumothorax in the older child can be disease-specific. In cavitary or progressive tuberculosis, subpleural caseous infiltrates undergo liquefaction, resulting in pleural necrosis and rupture. Although an inflammatory response is elicited that attempts to seal off the rupture, bronchopleural fistula often persists. Pneumothoraces sometimes seen in miliary pulmonary tuberculosis are unexplained. Pulmonary metastases of a sarcoma have been postulated to grow very rapidly, outgrow their blood supply and become necrotic, thereby rupturing the bronchus and pleural space, creating a bronchopleural fistula. Alternatively, tumor emboli cause lung infarction and necrosis and eventually air

leak. Primary or metastatic pulmonary tumor may also cause lung rupture by ball-valve obstruction of an airway. In cystic fibrosis, pneumothorax results from rupture of subpleural blebs and large bullae—a result of chronic air trapping in patients with long-standing, more advanced obstructive lung disease. Rupture of blebs and bullae usually occurs during exacerbation of pulmonary infection. In asthma, it is postulated that the visceral pleura is thinner and thus has increased susceptibility to rupture at transpulmonary pressures that would not allow rupture under normal circumstances. Moreover, mucoid impaction may be associated with expiratory obstruction, leading to overdistention and rupture of alveoli.

Functional Pathology

Irrespective of the age of the patient and the underlying cause of pneumothorax, massive or continued air leak elevates the intrapleural pressure to above atmospheric, so-called tension pneumothorax. The ipsilateral lung collapses because its elastic recoil can no longer be counteracted by the outward pull of a previously subatmospheric pleural pressure. The contralateral lung is overexpanded during inspiration and develops a greater retractive force, thereby pulling the mediastinum toward it during expiration, impeding venous return to the heart. Hypoxemia and hypercapnia result. Since ventilation is impaired, greater inspiratory efforts develop in an attempt to generate sufficient negative pleural pressure to ventilate the normal lung, thereby aggravating the tension pneumothorax, shifting the mediastinum further and severely impeding systemic venous return to the heart. Compensatory tachycardia occurs and further decreases diastolic filling and ventricular output, with cardiac standstill imminent unless pulmonary tamponade is decompressed. Lung collapse per se does not contribute in a major way to poor gas exchange because there is a redistribution of pulmonary blood flow to the normal lung with lower vascular resistance.

In addition to the intrapleural pressure developed and the inherent elastic recoil of the lung, the degree of lung collapse also varies with the cause of pneumothorax and the presence of visceroparietal adhesions. Chronic lung disease that decreases lung elastic recoil as well as concomitant pleural adhesions will restrain total collapse that ordinarily will occur with atmospheric pressure in the pleural space in the presence of otherwise normal lung and pleura.

Diagnosis

Symptoms of pneumothorax vary according to the extent of lung collapse, degree of intrapleural pressure, rapidity of onset, age and respiratory reserve of the patient. A patient can present suddenly in cardiorespiratory collapse without any clinical warning or antecedent roentgenographic change, or may be asymptomatic with the diagnosis initially made on chest roentgenogram. Early recognition of lung rupture requires keen awareness of its possibility, particularly when dealing with diseases and clinical situations known to be associated with this complication (Table 6).

In an otherwise normal neonate, symptoms of spontaneous pneumothorax are often subtle and physical findings misleading, since no obvious abnormal physical findings may be discernible. Certain clinical features, however, have been observed on close observation: tachypnea above 60 per minute is invariably seen, chest bulging is usually noticeable, especially if unilateral pneumothorax is present, and the infant is unusually irritable. A shift of the cardiac impulse away from the site of the pneumothorax is useful but often not confidently detected. As well, it is difficult to appreciate diminished air entry on the ipsilateral side because of the small size of the newborn chest. Grunting, retraction and cyanosis are

TABLE 6. CONDITIONS ASSOCIATED WITH ALVEOLAR RUPTURE

First breath

Diagnostic and therapeutic maneuvers
  Thoracentesis
  Aspiration lung biopsy
  Percutaneous pleural biopsy
  Cardiothoracic surgery
  Resuscitation
  Respirator therapy, especially with PEEP

Lower respiratory tract diseases

  Hyaline membrane disease
  Aspiration syndrome
  Asthma
  Cystic fibrosis
  Tuberculosis (cavitary; miliary)
  Pneumonia and bronchiolitis
  Malignancy (primary or metastatic)

Blunt thoracic trauma

Spontaneous

noted late in the progression of the complication.

In a newborn with underlying lung disease requiring some form of mechanical respiratory assistance, certain observations are useful to note. Rapid increase in inspiratory pressure reading on the respirator accompanied by sudden deterioration should immediately suggest a diagnosis of tension pneumothorax, which necessitates prompt needle decompression. Changes in vital signs include decreases in heart rate, blood pressure and respiratory rate and narrowing of pulse pressure. An ominous clinical presentation is cardiorespiratory arrest. Even when deterioration is gradual, auscultation is often unreliable, since breath sounds from the remaining expansible lungs are clearly transmitted across the small newborn chest during mechanical ventilation. It is obvious that serial chest roentgenograms every 12 to 24 hours are essential during the early phase of ventilatory treatment of the newborn even in the absence of clinical signs of pneumothorax, since the latter can occur without forewarning. Moreover, in the presence of interstitial emphysema, pneumomediastinum or hyperlucency of any lung zone, particularly when the infant is on continuous distending pressure, the clinician must be alert to the increased threat of impending serious air leak and pneumothorax.

Although certain limitations of physical examination of the chest have been alluded to previously, periodic physical reappraisal remains important and must be done whenever clinical worsening or deterioration in arterial gas tensions, or both, are observed. Additional nonroentgenographic tools for monitoring infants for the presence of pneumothorax in high-risk situations, e.g., hyaline membrane disease, meconium aspiration and during mechanical ventilation, should be utilized and include continuous electrocardiographic display on the oscilloscope or intermittent recording. A sudden decrease (40 per cent or more) or variability in the QRS voltage seen in the left precordial and standards leads I, II and III should alert one to the occurrence of a pneumothorax. Care must be taken to avoid misdiagnosis from electronic artifacts such as a change in standardization. Recently, chest transillumination utilizing a powerful fiberoptic light probe has been effectively applied to diagnose pneumothorax at the bedside and has distinct advantage on that basis. Wider application of these techniques can indicate the necessity for an early radiologic examination.

Roentgenographic confirmation is essential when the physical findings are minimal and cardiorespiratory function is only modestly altered. An anteroposterior chest film supplemented by a horizontal-beam cross-table lateral view with the patient supine or in decubitus position can detect even relatively small amounts of intrapleural or mediastinal air. Pneumothorax has to be differentiated from lung cyst and lobar emphysema, in which the lower border of the radiolucency is crescentic; in addition, attenuated lung markings are seen in lobar emphysema. A skin fold is seen as a radiodense line extending beyond the skeletal chest wall boundary into the surrounding soft tissues, and lung markings may appear lateral to this line. A congenital diaphragmatic hernia can be readily distinguished if a nasogastric tube with radiopaque tip that is used to decompress is left, and may be seen in the thoracic cavity on the roentgenogram.

In an older child, certain disease conditions, e.g., bronchiolitis, asthma, cystic fibrosis, pertussis syndrome, hydatid cyst, progressive primary pulmonary tuberculosis, metastatic sarcoma, staphylococcal pneumonia, and blunt thoracic injury, alert the clinician to the relative risk of pneumothorax, particularly when a patient suddenly develops severe cardiorespiratory collapse or, less seriously, sudden chest or referred shoulder pain associated with dyspnea, cyanosis and rapid shallow breathing. Contributory factors to the foregoing clinical setting include frequent paroxysms of cough, severity of the underlying lung disease and respirator therapy. Moreover, occurrence of this complication is not as difficult to detect in this age group as it is in the newborn infant, since it is easier to ascertain abnormal physical findings in the older child. Nonetheless, it must be realized that in children with diffuse obstructive lung disorders the physical signs of the underlying disease may be similar to those of the pneumothorax and may be quite unchanged by the addition of this complication, except for the shift of the trachea and the apex beat. Even the latter may be difficult to locate in light of the overinflation. A positive scratch sign—loud and harsh sound heard over the midsternum when the affected side is stroked with a dull instrument or finger—may be elicited.

Radiologic confirmation during full expiration is helpful. Bullae, massive lung cyst or partial obstruction with secondary overinflation may be mistaken for a chronic pneumothorax. Careful attention to details of history and assessment of the lung edge on chest film usually clarify the diagnosis. Another consideration is traumatic diaphragmatic hernia, which usually occurs on the left because of the shielding effect of the liver on the right and possible inherent weakness of the left leaf of the diaphragm. Attention should be directed to the convex shadow cast by the upper border of the stomach and to the linear opacities representing bowel wall. Definitive diagnosis is made with a chest roentgenogram taken following a barium swallow. Avoidance of error in diagnosis is important to avoid trauma to the stomach, spleen or other abdominal organs located in the chest cavity and to prevent the development of a tension pneumothorax during attempts to needle an intrapulmonary air space.

Arterial gas tensions and pH may be initially normal, with P_{CO_2} even below normal at times. In the presence of unrelieved tension, however, acidosis, hypoxemia and hypercapnia are invariably present.

Management

The functional consequences of a tension pneumothorax or of even a small pneumothorax in patients with respiratory insufficiency pose an immediate threat to life unless the intrapleural air is immediately evacuated. Effective management requires early clinical recognition and prompt radiologic investigation. Frequent utilization of electrocardiographic monitoring and chest transillumination hasten confirmation of the diagnosis and increase the chances of successful treatment.

A rational approach to therapeutic management of air leak complications should take into account clinical severity, presence and nature of the underlying lung disease, gestational and postnatal age, precipitating event and history of recurrence. Attention must be equally directed to the treatment of the underlying disease process. In small, nonprogressive asymptomatic or mildly symptomatic pneumothorax not associated with any underlying disease and occurring in the term newborn infant, expectant care is frequently satisfactory, since the pleura has the physiologic capacity to remain totally gas-free. Conservative measures include frequent small feedings, mild sedation to minimize crying and oxygen-enriched air. Spontaneous resolution is achieved in an average period of 48 hours (range one to three days). Approximately 1.25 per cent of lung volume reexpands each day in room air. Absorption of the loculated pneumothorax is hastened sevenfold by oxygen inhalation, which increases the pressure gradient of gases between the pleura and the venous blood. Prolonged oxygen administration is dangerous to premature infants for fear of retinal toxicity, and to any patient for fear of direct toxicity to the lungs. Thus, this approach should not be relied upon in the presence of continued air leak. Moreover, in the absence of a definitive roentgenographic picture that excludes the usual differential diagnosis, it is best to defer needle aspiration unless clinical worsening indicates a contrary approach. Needle perforation of a tension pulmonary cyst, congenital lobar emphysema, or a traumatic tear of the lung can add or lead to tension pneumothorax and result in a more precarious clinical situation.

In the presence of underlying disease, such as meconium aspiration or hyaline membrane disease in a premature infant, direct mechanical evacuation of intrapleural air should be performed unless the size of pneumothorax is very small, the underlying disorder is mild, and the clinical status is stable. However, close clinical and blood gas monitoring are integral parts of management. Appropriate measures must be taken as soon as clinical or biochemical deterioration is detected.

Mechanical evacuation of air from the pleural cavity is achieved either via a catheter attached to a one-way flutter valve (Heimlich valve) requiring no underwater seal or suction, or via an underwater seal tube drainage with suction applied. The choice depends upon the clinical circumstances. Direct needle aspiration into the second or third intercostal space along the midclavicular line should precede either of the foregoing for prompt decompression that is warranted in tension pneumothorax requiring emergency evacuation.

For a neonate with minimal underlying disease and small to moderately sized pneumothorax, an Argyle thoracic semirigid catheter size French 12 is used. The catheter is mounted on a trocar to facilitate its introduction, and has terminal and side holes for better air evacuation and a radiopaque sentinel line for radiographic visualization. With strict asepsis and under local anesthesia, the catheter is inserted through a small skin incision over the anterior second or third intercostal space just lateral to the midclavicular line and introduced deeply enough to ensure the side holes are within the pleural cavity; otherwise, surgical emphysema may develop if the side holes lie immediately underneath the skin. The catheter is then secured to the skin, using a pursestring suture technique. After the initial evacuation of intrapleural air with a syringe, a one-way flutter drain valve (e.g., Heimlich valve) is fitted directly onto the external end of the catheter, requiring no adaptor. The valve allows air to escape but prevents its reflux and functions equally well in the presence of fluid that may drain. Since fluid can cause sticking of the one-way rubber valve, it should be cleaned at least once every 12 hours or whenever any significant fluid drainage occurs. The connection between the catheter and the valve is sealed off with adhesive tape, and the area around the tube insertion is similarly sealed. The entire setup is then attached to the anterior chest wall, ensuring that the distal end is unimpeded.

An underwater seal system, however, has to be used when there is large or continued air leak that exceeds the outflow capacity of the Heimlich valve, when the patient is on intermittent positive pressure ventilation, particularly with concomitant application of a continuous distending pressure at end-expiration, or when associated fluid drainage interferes with the free exit of air. Care is taken to ensure the drainage tube is not deeper than 2 cm. under water, lest air will not drain until a higher pressure builds up in the pleural space. Suction is applied at a pressure of minus 5 to minus 15 cm. H_2O.

Shortly after the procedure, a chest film should be taken to assess expansion of the lungs. The drainage tube is left in site for an average period of three days. The time to extubate is crucial, and once the decision has been made, extubation must be a sequential process. First, suction is discontinued after continued air leak has ceased. Cessation of air leak is recognized by cessation of air bubbling in the drainage tube under the water seal during the respiratory cycle. Patency of the tube is assured by observing the swing of the water meniscus, which normally oscillates during respiration. After cessation of air leak is established and complete lung expansion is confirmed by roentgenography, the tube is deliberately clamped overnight prior to its final withdrawal. A chest tube still decompressing an air leak must never be clamped lest a tension pneumothorax develop.

Pneumomediastinum per se seldom causes severe cardiorespiratory difficulty. However, if the gas does not decompress by extension to the pleural or subcutaneous spaces, high pressures may result. Direct decompression of the mediastinum may be achieved by placing a needle behind the sternum from below (xiphoid approach) or by a small incision at the sternal notch.

Pulmonary interstitial emphysema may be treated by increasing inspired O_2 concentration or reducing ventilator pressures. Occasionally, interstitial emphysema of the lung may persist as loculated gas spaces and require surgical removal, particularly in small premature infants requiring ventilator therapy for hyaline membrane disease.

Pneumopericardium may be managed conservatively by lowering ventilatory flow rates and end-expiratory pressure. Should the cardiac size be markedly reduced or there is rapid onset of hypotension associated with muffled heart tones, bradycardia and cyanosis, cardiac tamponade is imminent. In this situation, immediate pericardiocentesis is indicated.

Pneumoperitoneum from alveolar rupture must be differentiated from that due to a perforated viscus, which requires immediate surgical intervention. When the pneumoperitoneum is associated with extensive pulmonary air leak in an infant who is otherwise in relatively good condition, conservative medical therapy utilizing high inspired oxygen and adjustment of ventilator pressures may suffice. Paracentesis is done when increased abdominal pressure adds to dyspnea.

The foregoing therapeutic approach of management outlined for the neonate applies to any pediatric patient. Drainage by a one-way flutter valve usually suffices for the older child with mild or moderately symptomatic spontaneous pneumothorax. Special considerations, however, are taken in the management of older children in whom the predisposing or underlying clinical conditions may be asthma, tuberculosis, metastatic sarcoma or cystic fibrosis. Immediate closed thoracotomy with insertion of a waterseal intercostal tube is the treatment of choice for pneumothorax complicating acute asthma or progressive pulmonary tuberculosis, since any added reduction in pulmonary function should be avoided. In tuberculosis, too much suction is avoided, since it can sometimes keep the fistula patent. In those with a large fistula, subsequent decortication may be necessary.

Management of the complication in patients with cystic fibrosis involves several considerations. In the first attack of a small asymptomatic unilateral pneumothorax, expectant care in the hospital and treatment of acute pulmonary infection are usually followed by resolution. In the case of bilateral occurrence, one may initally elect to decompress only the side associated with greater lung collapse and anticipate spontaneous resolution of the other, less severely involved side. If spontaneous resolution in either situation does not occur or if the initial episode is a large pneumothorax, mechanical drainage is done. Whenever feasible, use of a portable device (e.g., Heimlich valve) is recommended, since it permits early mobilization, which is particularly important in this group of children. Otherwise, the underwater seal system under suction is used. The latter is indicated whenever the complication reduces lung volume by 50 per cent or more, is increasing in size and causes dyspnea in patients with tenuous respiratory reserve. After most of the intrapleural air has been evacuated, pleurodesis is recommended for those patients with persistent or recurrent pneumothorax, since major pulmonary surgery is a great risk for them. The sclerosing agent favored by most is quinacrine hydrochloride, which is instilled into the pleura at an initial dose of 100 mg. in 15 ml. of saline, and the patient is positioned hourly for gravitational distribution of the drug. Three additional doses, 100 mg. each, are repeated during the next three consecutive days. If this approach fails, open thoracotomy with segmental resection and pleurectomy are undertaken, except in patients with far advanced respiratory insufficiency and cor pulmonale. A similar surgical procedure is indicated in any child with chronic (longer than three months) pneumothorax, irrespective of cause.

Prognosis

Prognosis is a function of the severity (i.e., with or without tension) and type of pneumothorax (i.e., spontaneous, traumatic or associated with parenchymal disease), the nature of the underlying lung disorder and the promptness of diagnosis and evacuation of the intrapleural air. Preparedness is the key factor to an excellent outcome. Thus, in hospital areas where high-risk patients are cared for, that is, in intensive care units for the newborn, infants and older children and in emergency departments, an equipment tray containing a 50-ml. syringe, a three-way stopcock, an 18-gauge needle, a kidney basin and a bottle of sterile saline should always be at hand. Medical and nursing personnel should have an ongoing program of preparedness and should be able to intervene promptly and appropriately when the emergent occasion arises.

REFERENCES

Liquid in the Pleural Space

Badrinas, F., Rodriguez-Roisin, R., Rives, A., and Picada, C.: Multiple myeloma with pleural involvement. *Am. Rev. Resp. Dis., 110*:82, 1974.

Black, L. F.: The pleural space and the pleural fluid. *Mayo Clin. Proc., 47*:493, 1972.

Chernick, V., and Reed, M. H.: Pneumothorax and chylothorax in the neonatal period. *J. Pediatr., 76*:624, 1970.

Dines, D., Pierre, R. V., and Franzen, S.: The value of cells in the pleural fluid in the differential diagnosis. *Mayo Clin. Proc., 50*:571, 1975.

Dippel, W. F., Doty, D. B., and Ehrenhaft, J. L.: Tension hemothorax due to patent ductus arteriosus. *N. Engl. J. Med., 288*:353, 1973.

Hyde, R., Hall, C., and Hall, W. J.: New pulmonary diagnostic procedures. *Am. J. Dis. Child., 126*:292, 1973.

Kosloske, A. M., Martin, L. W., and Schubert, W. K.: Management of chylothorax in children by thoracentesis and medium-chain triglyceride feedings. *J. Pediatr. Surg., 9*:365, 1974.

Light, R. W., and Luchsinger, P. C.: Metabolic activity of pleural liquid. *J. Appl. Physiol., 34*:97, 1973.

Light, R. W., Macgregor, M. I., Luchsinger, P. C., and Ball, W. C.: Pleural effusions: diagnostic separation of transudates and exudates. *Ann. Intern. Med., 77*:507, 1972.

Mellins, R. B., Levine, D. R., and Fishman, A. P.: Effect of systemic and pulmonary venous hypertension on pleural and pericardial fluid accumulation. *J. Appl. Physiol., 29*:564, 1970.

Moskowitz, H., Platt, R. T., Schachar, R., and Mellins, R.: Roentgen visualization of minute pleural effusion. *Radiology, 109*:33, 1973.

Murchison, W. G., Harper, W. K., and Putnam, J. S.: Traumatic diaphragmatic hernia: late presentation as bloody pleural effusion. *Chest, 66*:734, 1974.

Nelson, D. G., and Loudon, R. G.: Sarcoidosis with pleural involvement. *Am. Rev. Resp. Dis., 108*:647, 1973.

Staub, N. C.: Pathogenesis of pulmonary edema. *Am. Rev. Resp. Dis., 109*:358, 1974.

Wang, N.: The preformed stomas connecting the pleural cavity and the lymphatics in the parietal pleura. *Am. Rev. Resp. Dis., 111*:12, 1975.

Air in the Pleural Space

Aranda, J. V., Stern, L., and Dunbar, J. S.: Pneumothorax with pneumoperitoneum in a newborn infant. *Am. J. Dis. Child., 123*:163, 1972.

Dines, D. E., Cortese, D., Brennan, M.D., Hahn, R., and Payne, W. S.: Malignant pulmonary neoplasms predisposing to spontaneous pneumothorax. *Mayo Clin. Proc., 48*:541, 1973.

Glauser, F. L., and Bartlett, R. H.: Pneumoperitoneum in association with pneumothorax. *Chest, 66*:536, 1974.

Heimlich, H. J.: Valve drainage of the pleural cavity. *Dis. Chest, 53*:282, 1968.

Kattwinkel, J., Taussig, L. M., McIntosh, C. L., di Sant'Agnese, P. A., Boat, T. F., and Wood, R. E.: Intrapleural instillation of quinacrine for recurrent pneumothorax. *J.A.M.A., 226*:557, 1973.

Katz, S., and Horres, A. D.: Medullary respiratory neuron response to pulmonary emboli and pneumothorax. *J. Appl. Physiol., 33*:390, 1972.

Kirkpatrick, B. V., Felman, A. H., and Eitzman, D. V.: Complications of ventilator therapy in respiratory distress syndrome. *Am. J. Dis. Child., 128*:496, 1974.

Kuhns, L. R., Bednarck, F. J., Wyman, M. L., Roloff, D. W., and Borer, R. C.: Diagnosis of pneumothorax or pneumomediastinum in the neonate by transillumination. *Pediatrics, 56*:355, 1975.

Kuritzky, P., and Goldfarb, A. L.: Unusual electrocardiographic changes in spontaneous pneumothorax. *Chest, 70*:535, 1976.

Lackey, D. A., Ukrainski, C. T., and Taber, P.: The management of tension pneumothorax in the neonate using the Heimlich flutter valve. *J. Pediatr., 84*:438, 1974.

Macklin, C. C.: Transport of air along sheaths of pulmonic blood vessels from alveoli to mediastinum. *Arch. Intern. Med., 64*:913, 1939.

Malan, A. F., and de V. Helse, H: Spontaneous pneumothorax in the newborn. *Acta Pediatr. Scand., 55*:224, 1966.

Merenstein, G. B., Dougherty, K., and Lewis, A.: Early detection of pneumothorax by oscilloscope monitor in the newborn infant. *J. Pediatr., 80*:98, 1972.

Ogata, E. S., Gregory, G. A., Kitterman, J. A., Phibbs, R. H., and Tooley, W. H.: Pneumothorax in the respiratory distress syndrome: incidence and effect on vital signs, blood gases, and pH. *Pediatrics, 58*:177, 1976.

Pomerance, J. J., Weller, M. H., Richardson, C. J., Soule, J. A., and Cato, A.: Pneumopericardium complicating respiratory distress syndrome: role of conservative management. *J. Pediatr., 84*:883, 1974.

Summers, R. S.: The electrocardiogram as a diagnostic aid in pneumothorax. *Chest, 63*:127, 1973.

Wilson, J. L.: Factors involved in the production of alveolar rupture with mechanical aids to respiration. *Pediatrics, 13*:146, 1954.

Liquid and Air in the Pleural Space

Agostoni, E.: Mechanics of the pleural space. *Physiol. Rev., 52*:57, 1972.

Grosfeld, J. L., and Ballantine, T. V. N.: Surgical respiratory distress in infancy and childhood. *Curr. Probl. Pediatr., 6*:1, 1976.

Murray, J. F.: *The Normal Lung: The Basis for Diagnosis and Treatment of Pulmonary Disease.* Philadelphia, W. B. Saunders Company, 1976.

CHAPTER FORTY-ONE

ASTHMA

Susan C. Dees, M.D.

Bronchial asthma, a reversible obstructive airway disease, is a common, capricious disorder of respiration affecting persons of all ages with repeated attacks of difficulty in breathing; this may develop into continuous respiratory embarrassment. Its characteristic features are wheezing, labored breathing, an irritative tight cough and tenacious sputum. The symptoms range from the mildest cough and wheeze to the most severe respiratory distress, which may result in prostration and fatal asphyxia. A combination of edema of the bronchial mucosa and bronchospasm decreases the caliber of bronchioles and bronchi and produces bilateral obstructive hyperinflation.

The usual cause for this sequence of events in children is an allergic reaction in the bronchi. In some instances no allergic or immunologic process can be recognized, however, and the assumption is then made that some degree of bronchial obstruction is produced by factors other than those resulting from antigen-antibody union. This has led to the classification of asthma into *allergic* (reaginic) and *nonallergic* (nonreaginic) types. Although most asthma in children is of the allergic type, there may be nonallergic causes for wheezing, such as compression of the bronchi by external pressure, by foreign body in the airway, by a diffuse endobronchial inflammatory reaction, or by bronchoconstriction following exercise. Rackemann (1940) suggested separating asthma into *extrinsic asthma*, caused by allergens or external factors, and *intrinsic asthma*, caused by nonallergic factors. Intrinsic asthma

has been used to designate asthma due to bacterial infection, which in the strict sense is not of intrinsic origin. This term has also been applied to asthma attacks provoked by emotional stimuli, and to a different type of asthma, usually seen in elderly patients, which is associated with pulmonary fibrosis. Asthma is further described as *spasmodic*, if isolated attacks occur with long symptom-free intervals; as *continuous*, when some daily wheezing is present; as *intractable*, when symptoms are constant and unrelieved by bronchodilators; and as *status asthmaticus*, when little or no response is obtained with bronchodilators such as epinephrine, and the patient's respiratory metabolism is greatly unbalanced. Kraepelien and coworkers (1958) developed a helpful classification for asthma according to severity: grade I, consisting of less than five attacks per year; grade II, of five to ten attacks per year; and grade III, of ten or more attacks per year or the presence of continuous symptoms.

Incidence

Familiarity with asthma as a common condition in children and adults has tended to blind both the public and the medical profession to its true significance as a health hazard. Mild forms are confused with trivial respiratory tract infections that people are resigned to endure periodically, and the severe forms are often mistaken for pneumonia or bronchitis. The serious lung damage which can result from asthma

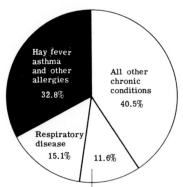

Figure 1. Incidence of asthma among chronic diseases of children under 17 years of age. Based on United States National Health Survey data as reported in interviews during period July 1959–June 1961. (From Schiffer, C. G., and Hunt, E. P.: *Illness Among Children.* Children's Bureau Publ. No. 405, Washington, D.C., United States Department of Health, Education, and Welfare, 1963, p. 14.)

is obscured by the comforting but misleading belief that all children "outgrow" asthma.

It came as a surprise to many to learn from the United States National Health Survey (1959–1961) that asthma, hay fever and other allergies accounted for one-third of *all* chronic conditions occurring annually in children under 17 years of age (Schiffer and Hunt, 1963) (Fig. 1). The rate of prevalence of asthma, hay fever and other allergies was 74.3 per 1000 children, divided equally among asthma (25.8), hay fever without asthma (24.5) and other allergies (24.0). This information is summarized for allergies and other chronic diseases in Table 1, which shows the average annual number of conditions,

the percentage distribution and the rate per 1000 children. Since one child in five, or nearly 14 million children, had some kind of chronic condition, this means that at least 4 to 6 million children had some chronic allergic condition, and more than 1.5 million had asthma. The distribution of chronic conditions by age is shown in Fig. 2, in which it will be seen that allergies comprise one-quarter of the chronic medical problems even at 15 and 16 years of age.

Other surveys with slightly different design, but still based on household interview technique, made in Connecticut and metropolitan New York, found that one in five children of school age suffered from allergy (Rapaport, Appel and Szanton, 1960). A study of allergic diseases in adolescents, done in Denver, Colorado, showed asthma to be present in 28 per 1000, the same prevalence given in the National Health Survey (Freeman and coworkers, 1964). In 1965 a survey of a rural Iowa population of 1760 families yielded an allergic population of 611 persons; 199 of these were children with asthma or hay fever, and of these 95 had asthma (Smith, 1968).

In a summary of various reported studies of the incidence of asthma in school-age children, Smith (1974) called attention to the variation in different countries. While some variations can be attributed to differences in sampling techniques and definitions, there may be some real differences in geographic and demographic factors. The

TABLE 1. CHRONIC CONDITIONS IN CHILDREN UNDER 17 YEARS OF AGE

Condition	Number (in 1000s)	% Distribution	Rate/1000 Children
All chronic conditions	13,996	100	226.1
Infective parasitic*	154	1.1	2.5
Hay fever	1,518	10.8	24.5
Asthma	1,595	11.4	25.8
Other allergies	1,485	10.6	24.0
Total allergy	4,598		73.3

(handwritten: 74.3/1000)

Condensed from *Illness Among Children.* Children's Bureau Publication No. 405, United States Department of Health, Education, and Welfare, Washington, D.C., 1963, p. 72.
*Excludes tuberculosis.

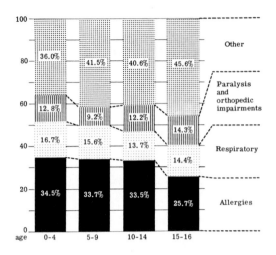

Figure 2. Distribution of chronic conditions by age. (From Schiffer, C. G., and Hunt, E. P.: *Illness Among Children.* Children's Bureau Publ. No. 405, Washington, D.C., United States Department of Health, Education, and Welfare, 1963.)

lowest rates are in Finland (0.5 per cent) and Scandinavia (1.6 per cent); the highest rates are in the British Isles in Aberdeen (4.8 per cent), in Birmingham (4.0 per cent), in Australia (3.7 per cent), and in New Zealand (9.2 per cent in boys and 4.9 per cent in girls).

The surveys cited for the United States include that of Nathanson and Rhyne for Maryland elementary school children with an incidence of wheezing of 6.9 per cent, and that of Broder and coworkers (1974) for Tecumseh, Michigan, for children aged six to eight years with an incidence of 4.7 per cent. A second follow-up survey of this city four years later showed rates for asthma of 5.3 per cent for boys and 3.0 per cent for girls aged five to nine years.

A recent study of the frequency of asthma in 10,971 English school children from rural and urban Kent between the ages of five and 14 years was reported to be 3.8 per cent by parent questionnaires (Hamman, Halil and Holland, 1975). These asthmatic children had lower peak flow expiratory rates than their nonasthmatic peers. The study also confirmed the early age of onset of asthma, as one-third of the children had the first attack of asthma before two years of age. Asthma was more common in boys than in girls and in the more affluent social classes.

There was no evidence that bronchitis predisposed to asthma, or vice versa.

Morbidity

The United States National Health Survey of 1959–61 reports that "the single chronic condition causing the highest percentage of days lost from school was asthma; 22.9 per cent of all days lost from school because of chronic conditions was due to asthma." Allergic diseases that were the chief cause of restricted activity, along with respiratory disease, caused 55.2 per cent of days lost from school (Fig. 3). The survey found that nearly 33 mil-

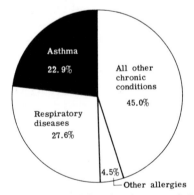

Figure 3. School days lost because of chronic conditions. (From Schiffer, C. G., and Hunt, E. P.: *Illness Among Children.* Children's Bureau Publ. No. 405, Washington, D.C., United States Department of Health, Education, and Welfare, 1963.)

TABLE 2. DAYS OF ILLNESS DUE TO CHRONIC CONDITIONS

	Activity Restricted (Age 0–16 yrs.)	Bed Days (Expressed in 1000s)	School Days Lost (Age 6–16 yrs.)
All chronic conditions	136,660	54,633	32,927
Hay fever without asthma	2,517	725	566
Asthma with or without hay fever	24,163	11,656	7,524
Other allergies	7,095	822	967
Heart disease	3,507	1,200	859
Paralysis	2,587	1,681	743
Impairment of extremities:			
Upper extremities	1,009	234	76
Lower extremities and hip	6,482	818	303

Condensed from *Illness Among Children.* Children's Bureau Publication No. 405, United States Department of Health, Education and Welfare, Washington, D.C., 1963, p. 80.

lion school days were lost because of chronic conditions, or three days for each child with at least one chronic condition. When one analyzes these days of illness by condition, the large part asthma contributed to the overall averages of disability can be seen more clearly. Table 2, which outlines the days of illness caused by chronic conditions, shows 24,163,000 restricted activity days, 11,656,000 bed days, and 7,524,000 school days lost because of asthma. This is more than twice the combined total restricted activity days for heart disease, paralysis and orthopedic impairment; it is three times the bed days, and nearly four times the lost school days for these other, more obviously disabling conditions.

Mortality

Fortunately, the high frequency of asthma in childhood is largely offset by a low death rate, the mortality rate being much lower than in the later years of life. Yet because of the large number of asthmatics, asthma still ranks among the 60 leading causes of death in the United States (Vital Statistics of the United States, 1972). To evaluate properly the meaning of the mortality from asthma, it must be considered against the background of the rates for some conditions that have special importance in childhood, either as preventable, hereditary or major

causes of illness. For several decades the death rate for asthma was stationary but from 1954 to 1967 the total rate for asthma declined from the level of 3.8 to 2.1, and by 1972 to 1.1 per 100,000 (rates for specific diseases are given per 100,000 population). During this same time, death rates from other diseases fell much more impressively: rates for tuberculosis, for example, fell from 10.2 to 1.7; rheumatic fever and chronic rheumatic heart disease went from 12.1 to 6.8; the total death rate for acute poliomyelitis, diphtheria, pertussis, measles, dysentery and meningococcal infections is 0.0 per 100,000.

The conditions that are compared with asthma as a cause of childhood deaths are listed in Table 3.

TABLE 3. NUMBER OF DEATHS IN CHILDREN UNDER 15 YEARS OF AGE, UNITED STATES, 1967, 1972, DUE TO SELECTED CONDITIONS

Conditions	1967	1972
Asthma	159	96
Rheumatic fever with heart disease	123	66
Tuberculosis	78	34
Measles	73	22
Cystic fibrosis	506	400
Poliomyelitis, acute	5	—
Diphtheria	26	4

From U.S. Department of Health, Education and Welfare: *Vital Statistics of the United States,* Vol. IIA, pp. 1–100 to 1–133, 1967, and Vol. IIA, pp. 1–186 to 1–228, 1972.

Death from asthma occurs so rarely in the experience of any one physician that it is always a shocking and unexpected outcome. Nevertheless, an ominous and impressive series of reports appeared in the 1960s that point specifically to a significant, upward trend in sudden unexpected asthma deaths in both children and adults (Alexander, 1963; Richards and Patrick, 1965; Stolley, 1972). In this period in England, Wales and Australia there was a 45 per cent increase overall in the death rate, primarily in the age group four to 15 years. Similar trends have been noted in Scandinavian countries, and in all there has been a progressive decline since then to the levels comparable to those in the 1950s (Macdonald and coworkers, 1976; Graff-Lonnevig and Kraepelien, 1976).

Speizer (1969) reported an eightfold increase in asthma deaths in England and Wales in the period between 1960–1966 from less than 1 per cent to 7 per cent in the ages of ten to 14 years. In a six-month period in 1966, there were 184 deaths in asthmatics five to 34 years old, and of these 80 per cent were sudden and unexpected; 84 per cent were using some form of pressurized aerosol bronchodilator. While two-thirds or more of the patients had been using steroids, Speizer and coworkers (1968) called attention to the fact that steroids had been in widespread general use for ten years before the rapid increase in the death rate occurred. They suggested that the rise in mortality is or may be related to the use of pressurized aerosol bronchodilators. The increased over-the-counter sales of a very much more concentrated isoproterenol pressurized aerosol than had been used in bulb-type nebulizers coincided with this rise in death rates, and later, a restriction in its sale coincided with the fall in death rates and sudden death from asthma in England and Australia. These observations along with the stable asthma death rates in countries such as the United States and Canada in which the high-concentration aerosols were not sold led to the conclusion that the toxic effect of isoproterenol was highly suspect as a cause for this upward trend.

Studies by Patterson and coworkers (1968) and Reisman (1970) have shown that inhalation of large doses of isoproterenol (isoprenaline) is associated with resistance to the usual cardiac stimulation effect of the drug. Part of it is converted into 3-methoxyisoprenaline, which is a weak beta adrenergic receptor antagonist which may contribute to the arrhythmias, bradycardia and cardiac arrest that are noted in these fatal cases. Even more recently, Taylor and Harris (1970) have described a cardiac toxic effect from Freon (Fluoroalkane) gases on mice, rat and dog hearts. In the presence of asphyxia this gas causes sinus bradycardia, AV block and T-wave depressions that are rapid, long-lasting and lethal. They suggest that Freon is not an inert gas, and its toxic effects may be the mechanism of sudden death in youths who sniff Freon aerosols and in asthmatics who overuse pressurized aerosols.

These observations on asthma deaths are being made at the same time that we are more alert to the toxic effects of aminophylline and oversedation and are more vigorous in treating acidosis, thus decreasing these contributive lethal factors in asthma. It is imperative that we reassess asthma mortality in terms of these reports to determine whether the aerosols or some other yet unrecognized agent is responsible for these changes in sudden mortality from asthma.

Pathogenesis

Allergic asthma is the most important from of spontaneously occurring human hypersensitivity. Asthma, hay fever, infantile eczema, urticaria and angioedema are the diseases for which the term "atopy' (strange disease) was coined by Coca and Cooke in 1923. They are characterized by a hereditable tendency (Cooke and Vander Veer, 1916; Spain and Cooke, 1924) and by the presence of a unique sort of circulating antibody. Initially, it was believed that this sort of sensitivity occurred only in human beings, but in recent years atopic conditions have been found in dogs, horses, walruses and other animals. Furthermore, patients with these disorders have been found in whom neither the circulating antibodies nor the hereditary features are present. The converse has also been demonstrated by the detection of naturally occurring or induced reagin in some normal nonatopic persons.

Prior to 1966, when the Ishizakas identified a new and different immunoglobulin which was designated IgE, the reaginic antibody was recognized only by certain unique properties. These were heat lability at 56° C. for two hours, sensitization of skin and other tissues in allergic subjects, and the ability to sensitize passively the skin of a normal subject (Prausnitz-Küstner reaction).

The Ishizakas (1976) have summarized the current knowledge of the immunochemical characteristics of IgE based on their studies and those of others (Johansson, 1967). IgE is an immunoglobulin with a sedimentation coefficient of 8S and a molecular weight of 200,000. Structural studies have shown that it is composed of two heavy (ϵ) and two light polypeptide chains, with the antigenic determinants present in the F_C portion of the heavy chains. It is a very minor component of the serum protein, with a turnover rate of two to three days.

In normal sera, the average concentration is 100 ng. (55 IU; International Unit = 2.2 to 2.4 ng.) per milliliter. In atopic persons the level may rise to several thousand nanograms per milliliter. IgE is present on mast cells and human basophils but not on the other granulocytes or small lymphocytes.

The minimum dose of IgE antibody necessary to elicit a positive P–K reaction in human beings is 10^{-6} to 10^{-5} ng. N – much less than is necessary to produce guinea pig PCA reaction with other immunoglobulins. The antibody has been shown to be multivalent, and

as two adjacent molecules appear to be required to produce a skin-reactive complex or histamine release, this indicates that a hypersensitivity reaction is produced by the bridging of two cell-fixed IgE molecules.

Ishizaka has determined that human basophils possess 10,000 to 40,000 IgE molecules per cell and that the total number of receptor sites for IgE is 40,000 to 90,000 per cell. The minimum concentration of anti-ragweed IgE antibody required to sensitize human skin is 0.25 ng./ml. Human skin, leukocytes and primate lung tissue can be passively sensitized with IgE with subsequent release of histamine on incubation with allergen. Sensitized lung fragments also release histamine, SRS–A (slow-reacting substance of anaphylaxis) and eosinotactic factor on exposure to allergens. Since these are the chemical mediators incriminated in allergic reactions, the importance of IgE is apparent. The high affinity of basophils and mast cells for IgE and the small amount required to produce a reaction explain the small amount of antigen needed to cause a reaction in highly sensitive cells and the persistence of the sensitization. Since the nature of the antibodies involved in allergy is the subject of much active investigation and concepts are constantly being modified as new data are presented, the reader should consult current reviews on the subjects of allergy and immunology for up-to-date information.

The atopic antibodies appear after sensitization to environmental substances, which are often poor but complete antigens or are haptens which combine with serum protein to form a sensitizing antigen. Pollen, dust, animal dander, foods, fungi, bacteria, insect stings and certain drugs (such as penicillin and iodides) that are not noxious agents are examples of allergens which sensitize and are incriminated in asthma. Injections of animal serums may produce both atopic and precipitating antibodies.

In spite of the many large gaps in the

knowledge of the nature and properties of atopic antibody, the earliest investigators made a practical application of their observations on skin and mucous membrane sensitization, passive transfer and heat lability in developing the clinical diagnostic tests for specific sensitization in allergic patients. These observations form the basis on which modern clinical allergy rests; current immunologic investigation should ultimately produce additional aids that will elucidate the basic pathophysiology of the allergic diseases.

Pathology

Extreme overinflation of the lungs in fatal asthma is a remarkably constant autopsy finding, irrespective of the patient's age. The lungs seem to "pop" out of the chest cage as it is opened, and it is difficult to compress the lung or to force any air out of it. On the pleural surface, emphysematous blebs are seen, tending to be small in children and to increase in size with age. The lungs still retain an elastic but somewhat stiff and rubbery consistency.

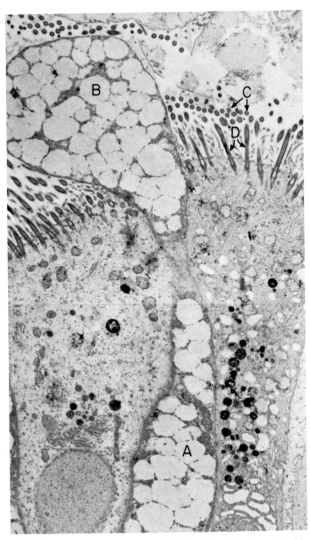

Figure 4. Normal human bronchus, showing epithelial cells. (× 23,000.) *A,* Mucus in a goblet cell. *B,* Mucous droplet being extruded from cell. *C* and *D,* Cilia in cross section and longitudinal section.

From the cut surface, gelatinous sticky mucus protrudes from the bronchioles and bronchi; only with gross infections do these mucous plugs become purulent. Varying degrees of atelectasis may be encountered, ranging from partial atelectasis of a small area of one lobe to collapse of an entire lobe or, more rarely, an entire lung.

The characteristic microscopic findings are increased thickness and hyalinization of the basement membrane of the bronchi and hypertrophy of the mucous and goblet cell glands of the bronchial and bronchiolar mucosa. Droplets of mucus are extruded into the bronchial lumen and coalesce to form mucus plugs, which often occlude the lumen. Bronchiolectasis of the respiratory bronchioles may result in panlobular emphysema with airway obstruction without any alveolar destruction (Sanerkin, 1970). When it occurs in lesser degree, this is a normal process, as shown in sections of normal bronchus (Fig. 4). In the mucus from

an asthmatic patient, desquamated bronchial epithelial cells and eosinophils are seen. Eosinophils also may be seen infiltrating the mucosa and bronchial wall. There may be a loss of cilia in patches or apparently in large areas. The mucosa may become redundant, with strong infoldings that may become almost polypoid. In some patients, especially very young children, the lymph nodes are greatly enlarged, and clumps of lymphocytes are present along the bronchial wall. Hypertrophy of smooth muscle of the bronchial wall has been confirmed by Dunnill and coworkers (1969), who found that muscle accounts for approximately 11.9 per cent of the volume of the wall of the segmental bronchi in status asthmaticus, in contrast to approximately 4.6 per cent in normal subjects. Spasm of the smooth muscle is impossible to detect in pathologic sections, and for this reason some investigators have questioned whether muscle spasm is actually a feature of asthma. Their objection is

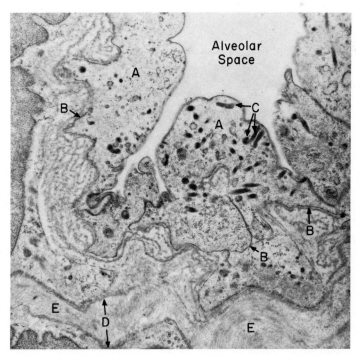

Figure 5.   Alveolar wall from young asthmatic, showing *(A)* alveolar epithelial cells, *(B)* basal membrane, *(C)* lysosomes, *(D)* septal membrane, *(E)* collagen fibrils in septal membrane. The capillary endothelium is at lower margin of section. (× 23,000.)

at variance, however, with the well known relief from asthma produced by the bronchodilating drugs.

The alveolar walls usually appear to be normal in younger patients (Fig. 5). In older persons dying of asthma, emphysema of variable degree is seen, with the characteristic thinning, fibrosis and rupture of the alveolar walls. Thickening of the adventitia and the muscular layers of blood vessels is much less frequently seen in young children than in adults. Mast cells are decreased in the bronchi of asthmatics dying in status asthmaticus (Connell, 1971) and show marked degranulation of the remaining cells (Salvato, 1968).

The majority of pathologic studies have utilized autopsy material. The sections from asthmatic lung illustrated in Figure 6, however, were taken from surgical specimens obtained at lobectomy. They do not differ in any essential features from the autopsy material, except that the cilia seem to be more intact.

No characteristic gross or microscopic pathologic changes have been reported in other organs in autopsy material, although right-sided cardiac hypertrophy has been present in some patients. In one child who suffered a fatal paroxysm of asthma, we noted considerable eosinophilic infiltration of tissues and cerebral edema, with eosinophils clustered around the cerebral blood vessels.

Since most severe asthmatics who die in acute asthmatic attacks have usually undergone extensive, long-term corticosteroid treatment, some of the pathologic changes encountered have been

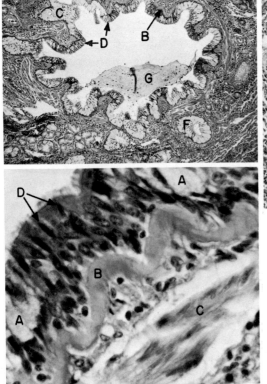

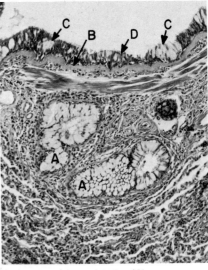

Figure 6. Sections of asthmatic lung. *Top left,* Cross section of bronchus (× 66) showing *(A)* cartilage, *(B)* basement membrane which is thickened, *(C)* epithelium containing many goblet cells, *(D)* area of many ciliated epithelial cells, *(F)* mucous gland, *(G)* mucous plug. *Top right,* Bronchial epithelium (× 136) showing *(A)* mucous glands, *(B)* hyaline basement membrane, *(C)* goblet cells, *(D)* ciliated cells. *Bottom left,* Bronchial epithelium (× 700) showing *(A)* goblet cell, *(B)* basement membrane, *(C)* connective tissue, *(D)* ciliated respiratory epithelial cells.

attributed to prolonged steroid therapy (Keeney, 1965).

Pathophysiology

The concept that allergic antibodies are fixed to lung tissue and mucous membranes and that the antigen-antibody interaction releases enzymes or substances that can produce tissue damage has evolved over the years as the explanation for the pathophysiology of asthma and allergic reactions. The substances that are thought to act as mediators of immediate hypersensitivity in humans are histamine (H-substance), acetylcholine, eosinophil chemotactic factor of anaphylaxis (ECF–A), slow-reacting substance (SRS–A) and possibly prostaglandin $F_{2\alpha}$. Various animals have serotonin (5-hydroxytryptamine), bradykinin, other kinins, anaphylotoxin, and heparin released in anaphylaxis; thus far the role of these latter substances has not been demonstrated to be that of an active mediator in human beings. The histamine present during an immediate hypersensitivity reaction in humans is thought both to come from the actual union of antigen and antibody protein and to originate from mast cells. The granules of mast cells contain large amounts of histamine, which is liberated with their disruption; this occurs as the mast cells degranulate during the allergic reaction. Histamine produces capillary dilatation, which increases the permeability of blood vessel walls, contracts smooth muscle and stimulates mucous gland secretions. The lungs and bronchi of allergic persons hyperreact to a smaller amount of histamine, methacholine and acetylcholine aerosol than do those of normal persons.

Acetylcholine can duplicate many of the effects of histamine. It has been shown in sensitized guinea pigs that acetylcholine concentration rises after injection of specific antigens. In humans the use of atropine and anticholinergic agents has exhibited some effect in decreasing asthma and other allergic reactions. It has been suggested that these two substances, histamine and acetylcholine, act as mediators by way of the autonomic nervous system, and that the autonomic state of the end-organ at the time of their release determines the clinical picture of asthma (Eppinger and Hess, 1917).

SRS–A (slow-reacting substance A of Brocklehurst) was first identified in 1956 as causing contraction of bronchial smooth muscle in human and guinea pig lung at antigen-antibody union. Since SRS–A is a relative newcomer, less is known about its properties than about those of the other mediators, but it is antagonized by atropine, epinephrine and theophylline, and increases in Ca^{++} ion concentration minimize its effect in vitro on guinea pig ileum.

The chemical nature of SRS–A is not yet established. It is a soluble substance, acidic, associated with lipid and proteins, resistant to proteolysis, but precipitated by trichloroacetic acid. It is found in rat leukocytes, in the lungs of various allergic animals after antigenic challenge, and in asthmatic human lungs. These intriguing observations suggest its potential significance in some, if not all, cases of human asthma.

Among the secondary mediators or modulators of the immediate type I, IgE anaphylactic response that are present in small amounts in normal human lung are the prostaglandins $PGF_{2\alpha}$, which produce bronchoconstriction, and PGE_1 and PGE_2, which produce bronchodilation. Serum levels of both $PGF_{2\alpha}$ and PGE_2 are higher in asthmatics than in normal subjects, and the PGF/PGE ratio was found to be higher in asthmatics than in normal subjects (Nemoto and coworkers, 1976). When $PFG_{2\alpha}$ is given by aerosol, asthmatics are 8000 times more sensitive to its bronchoconstricting effect than are normal subjects. Using a guinea pig model, it has been shown that $PFG_{2\alpha}$ has a biphasic effect on airways, producing an immediate brief constriction of large and small airways, then a late contraction of large airways that can be completely blocked by atropine (Drazen, 1975) and by analgesic anti-inflammatory drugs (aspirin, fenamates, and the like). It has been suggested that there is either an over-production of $PFG_{2\alpha}$ in asthmatics, or a defect in production or release of PGE. Cyclic AMP is elevated by PGE, and this may be the route by which this prostaglandin causes bronchodilation.

In 1948, Ahlquist's studies of the pharmacologic effect of catecholamines on the autonomic nervous system gave rise to the concept of two types of end-organ receptors, designated alpha (α) and beta (β), with opposing reactions when stimulated by catecholamines. The alpha receptors react to norepinephrine, and result in peripheral vasoconstriction, coronary vasodilation and decreased intestinal motility. The beta receptors are affected by isoproterenol, resulting in bronchodilation, myocardial stimulation and peripheral vasodilation. Epinephrine acts on both alpha and beta receptors.

The beta adrenergic receptors have been divided into two types. The β_1 type receptors found in heart and adipose tissue respond with increased heart contractility and rate and with adipose lipolysis to isoproterenol, to norepinephrine, which is about one-third to one-fourth as potent in this respect as isoproterenol, and less well to epinephrine; all three drugs are antagonized by practolol. The β_2 type adrenergic receptors are found in vascular and smooth muscle, and in liver and skeletal muscle. Stimulation with isoproterenol, epinephrine and norepinephrine—effective in that order—produces liver and muscle glycogenolysis, bronchial smooth muscle dilation, and uterine and vascular smooth muscle relaxation. A number of compounds recently developed have been shown to have selective β_2 stimulation. These are isoetharine, metaproterenol, terbutaline, hexoprenaline and salbutamol, and for them a selective antagonist is butoxamine; a nonselective antagonist is propranolol.

The beta adrenergic theory of bronchial asthma proposed by Szentivanyi (1968) states that excessive irritability of the bronchial tree is due to diminished responsiveness of beta receptors in the bronchial glands, smooth muscle and mucosal blood vessels. (The bronchioles contain primarily beta receptors.) Some of the evidence for this mechanism is based on extensive animal experiments, chiefly with pertussis-sensitized mice, and mice treated with beta adrenergic blocking agents in whom a hyperreactivity to histamine and serotonin develops. Turning to human reactions, experience has shown that nonspecific as well as immunologic factors often heighten or produce asthma and other allergic reactions. Among these are exercise, chilling, emotional stress, fatigue, bacterial infections, inhalation of irritating dust or fumes, and certain drugs.

The beta adrenergic theory proposes that the failure of beta receptors to respond normally at a cellular level to these stimuli is the final common pathway for these diverse causes to result in asthma. Furthermore, it is postulated that the beta receptor is the enzyme adenylcyclase, which is defective, decreased or malfunctioning in asthma. This, then, does not produce its catalytic conversion of ATP (adenosine triphosphate) to cyclic $3'5'$ adenosine monophosphate (cyclic $3'5'$ AMP). Thus, the metabolic effect of $3'5'$ AMP to produce glycogenolysis and lipolysis and smooth muscle relaxation does not occur normally. This is in effect a beta blockade with resulting bronchial constriction. There are various different types of evidence to support this idea: the direct stimulation of beta receptors by epinephrine and isoproterenol, the potentiating effect of corticosteroids on epinephrine, the blocking of phosphodiesterase by theophylline, which prevents breakdown of cyclic $3'5'$ AMP, and the effect of sodium lactate and bicarbonate in restoring epinephrine responsiveness in asthma.

The beta adrenergic blocking theory is consistent with many, in fact most, of the observed features of asthma. It does relate in a logical fashion many diverse observations, and opens up new avenues of investigation into the pathophysiology of asthma and the atopic state.

Clinical Features

SYMPTOMS. The symptoms of asthma reflect the major component of bronchial and bronchiolar obstruction and are directly due to interference in air exchange. Hacking and paroxysmal, irritative, nonproductive cough marks the *first stage*, i.e., bronchial edema. The tenacious mucus that accumulates may also act somewhat like a foreign body in stimulating cough.

As secretion becomes more profuse in the *second stage* of asthma, the cough becomes more rattling and productive of frothy, clear, gelatinous sputum. At this stage the patient begins to feel slightly short of breath, he attempts to breathe more deeply, his expiration becomes prolonged, and exhalation produces a high-pitched musical wheeze. He is seen to have retraction of the soft tissue of the neck and retraction of the intercostal spaces, and his facial expression is anxious. He speaks in short, panting, broken phrases, and he sits in a hunched-over position, hands on the edge of the bed or chair, his braced arms supporting his chest to facilitate the use of accessory muscles of respiration. He is often pale, although some children have a rosy malar flush and bright red ears. The lips assume a deep, dark red hue, but later they may become cyanotic, as may the nailbeds and the skin, especially about the mouth. The chest becomes overdistended and rounded and moves relatively little with each breath. The younger children revert to abdominal breathing, with suprasternal and intercostal retraction and flaring of the rib margins at each breath. Young infants and children become very restless during this second stage and cannot be made comfortable in any position in bed, often resting only briefly upright in an attendant's arms. The cough becomes less effective, the respiratory rate

increases, breathing becomes shallow, panting or grunting, and cyanosis rapidly increases.

The *third stage* is that of severe bronchial obstruction or spasm, when so little air is moved per breath that breath sounds and rales become almost inaudible. This is a dangerous stage of asthma, and one that is often misinterpreted as improvement by those unfamiliar with the disorder. The absence of rales is taken to represent clearing, whereas in actuality no sound is being made because no air is moving; even cough seems to be suppressed at this point. Shallow or irregular respirations and sudden rise in respiratory rate are ominous signs indicating that asphyxia may be imminent.

In some children the order of these groups of symptoms is reversed, and the attack may be initiated by a sudden acute, severe, generalized bronchospasm that may follow one or two harsh, sharp coughs. Some instances of sudden death from asthma have occurred with this sequence of events, and the bronchospasm has been so severe and generalized that an adequate airway could not be established rapidly enough to maintain life. Fortunately, in most instances the bronchospasm is neither so rapid in onset nor so extensive, and even though respiration is seriously embarrased, there is sufficient time for the child to effect some adjustment to this and for relief measures to be instituted.

It has been suggested that this sudden bronchospasm is an anaphylactic-like reaction, the challenging agent reaching all the bronchi simultaneously by way of the blood stream and not by inhalation. The validity of this hypothesis in spontaneously occurring asthma cannot easily be tested in human patients because the emergency situation is not suitable for such direct study. By inference from data involving penicillin and other drug reactions, serum reactions after insect stings and anaphylactic accidents during skin testing, however, this challenge by blood stream appears to occur occasionally. In addition, a

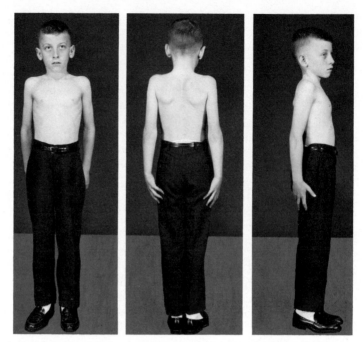

Figure 7. Asthmatic habitus, showing typical posture of 12-year-old boy with chronic grade III asthma. Note flattened malar bones, circles beneath eyes, narrow nose, and protruding upper teeth. Shoulders are squared, supraclavicular area is retracted, neck muscles are tense, scapulae are prominent and anteroposterior chest diameter is increased.

few instances of anaphylactic-like reactions to foods suggesting blood stream challenge have been reported in children (Crawford and coworkers, 1958).

PHYSICAL SIGNS. The principal physical findings in asthma are rapid, labored respiration, paroxysmal cough and prolonged expiration. It has already been noted that the chest is emphysematous or overdistended, the shoulders tend to be held high, the sternocleidomastoid and upper chest muscles are taut, and the ribs are widely spaced with the rib margins flared. The anteroposterior diameter of the chest is increased. The supraclavicular and suprasternal areas retract with inspiration, and the intercostal spaces may also retract. The angle made by the margin of the rib cage and the sternum becomes obtuse (Fig. 7).

Percussion is hyperresonant over the entire chest, especially over the lower posterior part of the chest. The excursion of the diaphragms may be decreased to 1 to 2 cm. The cardiac borders are difficult to outline because of the overlying inflated lungs. Tactile fremitus is usually normal, although it may be decreased.

Breath sounds are distant, with a prolongation of expiration. There are musical rales of inconstant nature over the entire chest, changing in intensity after cough or deep breathing. In latent asthma, compression of the chest wall between the stethoscope and the examiner's hand may elicit wheezing rales. In addition, sibilant and coarse, moist, sonorous rales may be present over the larger bronchi. Spoken voice sounds are normal or increased.

The pulse rate is accelerated, and the volume may become weak and thready. Paradoxical pulse and slowing and diminution of pulse volume with inspiration may be present. The heart may show signs of right-sided failure in acute episodes of asthma that are severe and protracted. This condition should be suspected when the pulse rate increases without good cause, the

basilar rales take on a moist or wet nature, the liver enlarges or becomes
tender, and the eyelids have a puffy appearance.

In young infants and toddlers the
prolongation of expiration is not as apparent as in older children because of
the more pliable chest and more rapid
respiratory rate. Unfortunately, the
distinction between expiratory and inspiratory dyspnea is less clear at this
age when it would be most helpful in
differentiating the nonasthmatic causes
of dyspnea.

Many asthmatics have the so-called
adenoidal or allergic facies, with narrow maxilla and nose, high palate and
malocclusion, but there seems to be no
particular type seen in asthma, nor is
there necessarily any alteration in
growth pattern. Spock (1965) has reviewed the growth patterns in 200 asthmatic children from our clinic and reports that they have a tendency to be a
little below the mean in both height
and weight. A few children are chronically ill and show the decreased height
and weight expected for their degree
of illness. Others are short because of
steroid therapy. Clubbing of fingers
and toes is not characteristic even for
severe chronic asthma, unless it is complicated by some other chronic lung or
heart disease; even then it may be absent.

Generalized slight enlargement of superficial lymph nodes is common in
asthmatic children, tonsils often appear
large and cryptic, and adenoids may be
palpated or seen extending into the
nasopharynx. When removed surgically, adenoids tend to recur rapidly as
bits or clusters of lymphoid tissue over
the posterior pharyngeal wall. The soft
palate ordinarily has a peculiar "goose
flesh" appearance owing to the prominence of minute lymphoid follicles.

Clinical Types

Classification of asthma by clinical
type (Table 4) has obvious limitations
and exceptions, but it does serve one
significant and useful purpose: it

**TABLE 4. CLINICAL TYPES OF
ASTHMA IN CHILDREN**

Allergic (atopic)
　Dermal-respiratory syndrome (Ratner)
　　Eczema-asthma-prurigo (Bray)
　　Spasmodic
　　Continuous
　　Intractable
　Allergic rhinitis–asthma
　　Seasonal (hay fever)
　　Nonseasonal (inhalant)

Nonallergic (nonatopic)
　Infectious—lung damage
　Mechanical obstruction
　Exercise-induced
　Aspirin-induced

Status asthmaticus

directs the physician to the most likely
causes and therefore to the most suitable treatment programs. At the same
time it emphasizes that asthma has
many origins and, like headache, cannot be expected to run the same course
in all patients.

ALLERGIC (ATOPIC) ASTHMA. *Dermal-
Respiratory Syndrome.* "Dermal-respiratory syndrome" (Ratner and coworkers,
1956) or "eczema-prurigo-asthma syndrome" (Bray, 1937) describes the truly
"allergic child" who has atopic eczema
in infancy with respiratory symptoms or
coryza (allergic rhinitis) and who later
suffers asthma with persistent neurodermatitis continuing into childhood
and adult life. The classic findings of
atopy are present here: vasomotor
lability with white dermographism,
strong sensitivites with positive immediate skin test results to protein allergens,
and blood and tissue eosinophilia.
Other family members are likely to have
allergic disorders, and many nonspecific factors may precipitate symptoms.

The infant's asthmatic breathing may
be first noted with respiratory infections that last longer and seem more
prostrating than expected. Attacks are
often recurrent, with only a few days of
normal breathing before a second episode begins. Asthma follows eczema in
about one-half to two-thirds of true

atopic eczema patients, regardless of the severity of the eczema (Dees, 1957). The respiratory symptoms become more prominent by about two years of age. These babies are likely to have strongly positive immediate skin test results to egg, although egg may not be a major or primary cause of symptoms. Buffum (1963) felt that this positive reaction is significant in that it indicates that allergic sensitization is present, and it may herald the persistence of asthma beyond ten years of age.

In this group of patients one sees the emergence of a stereotyped set of symptoms. As the child reaches three to five years of age, definite "attacks" of asthma occur. They frequently come on abruptly at night, with little or no warning, or they may be preceded by a few hours or a whole day of coryza, nasal obstruction and hacking cough. Dyspnea and cough of increasing severity finally culminate in hard wheezing and labored breathing. The cough may be so severe that vomiting results, and this in turn is often followed by improvement in dyspnea.

If untreated, such an attack will last several hours or days, until the child appears completely exhausted. Then there may be sudden, rapid improvement, all symptoms quickly subsiding, and the child returns to his normal state in a relatively short time. During the attack he often loses five to ten pounds in weight, which is rapidly regained thereafter. If treated with an adequate bronchodilator, the attack is shorter and milder. The eczema usually improves when asthma begins, but small patches may "flare up" just before the asthma attack and may serve as a warning of impending trouble. In other children whose eczema has remained active, there may be a remission during asthma with prompt recurrence on recovery from asthma. Each child tends to follow a repetitive pattern of the same antecedent symptoms, exhibiting these each time he has asthma. In some children mild to severe cramping midabdominal pain is the premonitory complaint. Other chil-

dren may have one or more of the following: constipation or diarrhea, abnormal appetite, darkening of the periocular skin (aptly termed "allergic shiners" by Marks, 1963), a glassy-eyed appearance, and allergic tension-fatigue (Crook, 1963) consisting of a change in disposition usually associated with irritability, whining, listlessness or hyperactivity. Occasionally the hyperactivity extends to insomnia and nightmares. Some mothers report that the child sweats excessively at night or has enuresis in the prodromal stage. Others may have a peculiar type of throat-clearing or itching of the throat.

Between attacks these children are apt to wheeze briefly if they laugh suddenly or overexert themselves. They are also very susceptible to weather and temperature changes, and they frequently sneeze, cough and wheeze when exposed to a draft or sudden chilling. Many other nonspecific irritants and stresses also appear to act as immediate causes of symptoms.

A variety of factors may determine whether the asthma occurs intermittently in attacks, with symptom-free intervals gradually decreasing in duration until finally the wheezing is mild, constant and punctuated by more severe symptoms. Variation in the individual asthmatic pattern is partly related to the nature of the specific causes and to the degree of sensitivity of the particular child, as well as to the amount of exposure he has to his particular allergens. In some children whose asthma becomes intractable despite apparently complete and efficient removal of noxious agents from the environment, the reason for worsening is obscure. In these cases one usually finds considerably decreased pulmonary function, abnormal bronchi (when tissue is available for study), and the nonspecific factors of emotional tension, fatigue, and hyperreaction to temperature change, all operating in an important way. These are the children who are destined to become pulmonary cripples, and every effort should be made to detect them early and to institute vigorous antiallergic treatment with the hope of arresting or reversing the process. Unfortunately, much still remains to be explained about the various causes of intractable asthma.

ALLERGIC RHINITIS–ASTHMA. Another clinical type of allergic asthma is that associated with hay fever or perennial allergic rhinitis. Asthma may appear after several years of upper respiratory tract allergic symptoms, or both may develop about the same time. Specific causes are usually air-borne allergens, either pollen, dusts or animal danders. Sensitization can be regularly demonstrated by direct and indirect skin tests or other conventional allergy tests and can be confirmed by provocative tests. If hay fever is the antecedent, patients are usually five to six years of age or older at the onset of asthma. If perennial allergic rhinitis is present, the age at onset is usually much younger, even as early as one to two years.

The severity of symptoms in the upper and lower airways varies directly with the level of the patient's sensitivities and with the frequency, duration and amount of exposure to the inciting allergen(s). Nonspecific factors that aggravate symptoms are the presence of vasomotor rhinitis or intercurrent infection, anatomic malconfiguration of the upper airway, inclement weather, and other provocative environmental conditions. These factors all contribute to produce a variable clinical picture, ranging from the mildest infrequent attack to intractable asthma and, rarely, to status asthmaticus. This allergic rhinitis–asthma group of patients consists of those in whom response to specific etiologic treatment and improvement after medication are the most clear-cut. Allergic rhinitis, both seasonal and perennial, may persist after asthma has been controlled. From the foregoing it is obvious that the ultimate prognosis for both the improvement and control of asthma symptoms can be better in this group than in the preceding dermal-respiratory type, or in the lung-damage type to be described below.

NONALLERGIC (NONATOPIC) ASTHMA.

Infectious or Lung-Damage Asthma. Lung-damage type of asthma, as it has been designated by Bray and others, is a type of asthma in which hereditary features are lacking or are minor and which may have originated so soon after an attack of measles, bronchiolitis, influenza or some other viral disease affecting the lung that this appears to have been the initial insult. From then on an infection of any kind seems to precipitate an asthmatic attack. There is fever with the attack, leukocytosis is higher than with other types of asthma, and pathogenic bacteria are often cultured from the sputum, paranasal sinuses or nasopharynx. Although elimination of these bacteria does not completely prevent attacks, the symptoms always seem worse when they are present. There is much fibrosis and more emphysema of an irreversible type in these children than in those of the atopic group; the skin tests to allergens are likely to yield unimpressive results, but they may show strong immediate and delayed reactions to bacterial vaccines and extracts.

Some of these children will suffer sufficient pulmonary insult from the initial illness that they are never well thereafter, becoming pulmonary cripples with a poor prognosis for both health and life and exhibiting a course comparable to that in adults with the "vanishing lung syndrome."

In some instances of uncomplicated "infectious asthma" the outlook becomes less gloomy as the child grows older and he seems to handle the respiratory infections better and with decreasing bronchospasm. If extensive damage has not occurred within the first few years of the disease, the prospects brighten as the child improves and eventually remains well except for rare sporadic asthma with respiratory infection. Asthma of this type is then considered to have been "outgrown." Children with this form of asthma present diagnostic problems and are difficult to classify. As refinements in both viral isolation and immunologic methods become available and exercise challenge has more general clinical use, and as the techniques of bronchial and lung biopsy become less formidable, some of this confusion in differentiation may disappear.

EXERCISE-INDUCED ASTHMA. Physical exercise is among the most frequently mentioned immediate events that precipitate wheezing in children. This is reiterated by parents of small children and noted by teenage would-be athletes. Active research interest in this aspect of hyperreactive airway disease has focused attention on the condition. This has done much to clarify the responsible mechanisms, has added new dimensions to the management of this phase of asthma, has provided us with a model whereby the pharmacologic effects of various drugs can be measured with some precision, and has demonstrated that this is a tendency which also occurs with greater frequency in the families of such asthmatics than in normal persons.

At a Symposium on Exercise and Asthma, held at Seattle, Washington, July 2, 1974 (Bierman and Pierson, 1975), it was reported that exercise-induced asthma (EIA) as judged by a fall of peak respiratory flow rate (PEFR) of 15 per cent was present in 65 to 70 per cent of asthmatics, in 41 per cent of atopic nonasthmatics, and in 7 per cent of control subjects, as determined by free running standardized exercise tests. Godfrey and König (1975) found that 58 per cent of children who had been wheezy babies still had an abnormal degree of bronchial lability, even if asymptomatic. Their performance closely resembled that of the children who had continued to wheeze. Also, 38 per cent of the relatives of atopics, including twin studies, had a high incidence of bronchial lability, atopic disease and positive skin tests, as did the relatives of wheezy babies, all findings that were different from the normal controls. This strongly suggests that bronchial lability is a genetic trait. Exercise-induced bronchospasm (EIB) can be used to differentiate the so-called extrinsic asthmatic from the intrinsic, since the extrinsic responds with a greater de-

gree of bronchospasm than does the intrinsic, and the incidence of EIB is greater in the extrinsic asthmatic.

The physiologic changes noted in EIB after a standard exercise test (running, treadmill or bicycle ergometer) for 6 to 8 minutes to induce a pulse rate of 170 to 180 (200) beats per minute cause mild bronchodilation during and for possibly two minutes after exercise, followed by bronchoconstriction 5 to 10 minutes later lasting up to 30 minutes, occasionally requiring bronchodilator medication to resolve. The following changes occur (Bierman and Pierson, 1975):

1. Decrease in forced expiratory volume at 1 second (FEV_1).

2. Decrease in peak expiratory flow rate (PEFR).

3. Decrease in forced expiratory flow rate at 25 to 75 per cent of vital capacity ($FEF_{25-75\%}$) or midmaximal expiratory flow (MMEF).

4. Increase in airway resistance (R_{aw}) and decrease in specific airway conductance (SG_{aw}).

5. Decrease in forced vital capacity (FVC).

6. Increase in functional residual capacity (FRC).

It was noted that the most sensitive tests for measuring EIB were specific airway conductance (SG_{aw} and $FEF_{25-50\%}$), with the least sensitive test being FVC. Responses showed that the major component of EIB is large airway obstruction, with small airway obstruction developing in some patients who show a degree of hyperinflation and decreased FVC. The major blood gas alteration in asthmatics with EIB was an immediate and sustained increase in the alveolar-arterial oxygen gradient (in contrast to normals, who show a decrease in this value), which is interpreted as an exaggeration after exercise of pre-existing perfusion-ventilation abnormalities. In some cases of asthma, EIB is related to hypocapnia, hypoxemia and acidosis, but atopic children do not develop as abnormal Pa_{CO_2}, Pa_{O_2} or pH levels as have been reported in adults (Katz and coworkers, 1975).

The methylxanthines (theophylline, diphylline, choline theophyllinate), the beta adrenergic stimulants (epinephrine, isoproterenol, metaproterenol, terbutaline, salbutamol), atropine by aerosol in some patients, and cromolyn all were effective in reducing exercise-induced bronchospasm (EIB). All of these drugs except cromolyn produced bronchodilation at rest and more during exercise, and inhibited EIB after exercise. Cromolyn differs in that it does not produce bronchodilation at rest, but does inhibit EIB. In one study a combination of theophylline, ephedrine and hydroxyzine taken one hour before exercise had an additive effect in reducing EIB (Bierman and coworkers, 1975), in contrast to a clinical study of Weinberger and Bronsky (1974), which showed no advantage of a similar combination over theophylline alone in control of clinical symptoms of asthma. The corticosteroids were not effective in relieving postexercise bronchospasm, and aerosolized atropine caused bronchodilation and effectively reduced bronchospasm in Godfrey's study, whereas other investigators were unable to demonstrate any protection by atropine in their patients. Variation in the route of administration, the dose, and the type of exercise test used might account for the discrepancies. The importance of this point is in its place in establishing the degree of vagal activity in EIB and asthma. If atropine does prove to be the potent bronchodilator that some investigators find it to be, then we have one more drug to add to our selection for asthma, and one more possible mechanism for the production of attacks.

ASPIRIN-INDUCED ASTHMA. Asthma following the ingestion of aspirin has been recognized in adults for many years and has been associated with rhinitis, nasal polyps, and at times high eosinophilia, urticaria and/or angioedema (Samter, 1973; Farr, 1970). The asthma is characteristically very severe and of rapid onset after taking aspirin, and fatalities have been reported. Asthma has followed the use of indomethacin, pyrazoline, and tartrazine (FDC yellow No. 5 food dye) in patients with aspirin asthma. The latter reacts in 15 per cent of aspirin-induced asthma patients (Settipane and Pudapakkan, 1975). An IgE-mediated reaction has been demonstrated in a very few persons with aspirin urticaria by positive skin tests to aspirin polylysine conjugates. This has not been the case in aspirin asthma, where all evidence points to an interference in prostaglandin (PGE) metabolism as the most likely basis for the syndrome, since aspirin and all the other drugs implicated are ones that inhibit prostaglandin biosynthesis (Szczeklik and associates, 1976).

While most of the reports of aspirin asthma have dealt with adults and have stressed the increased incidence with advancing years (Chaffee and Settipane, 1974), the condition does occur in children and probably is often overlooked. We have encountered several families in whom young children as well as older generations were affected. It is important to ask routinely about the use of aspirin, since it is a drug frequently given to children, and it can be replaced by acetaminophen, which is free of this hazard. Falliers (1973) analyzed a series of 1298 asthmatic children and found 25 (1.9 per cent) with aspirin intolerance. They had the following risk factors: sudden and late onset of asthma (mean 11 years), a negative history of atopy, frequent nasal polyps, and a high percentage of incidence among girls. Yunginger and coworkers (1973) reported on five children with aspirin asthma, four boys and one girl, all of whom were over 12 years of age. Families in whom aspirin-induced asthma has occurred in children and adults have shown that some have only asthma or urticaria, while others have both conditions. The mode of inheritance is not established (von Mauer and coworkers, 1974; Settipane and Pudapakkan, 1975).

STATUS ASTHMATICUS. Many of the children who suffer status asthmaticus, defined as asthma unresponsive to sympathomimetic bronchodilators, come from the "infectious asthma" as well as the atopic group. We have noted that many of our patients subject to recurrent episodes of status asthmaticus have had evidence of very marked gastroesophageal reflux. This can be demonstrated radiographically with the barium swallow water-siphon test. In these children we feel that aspiration of stomach contents at times may trigger intractable attacks and that this can often be prevented by taking precautions to prevent aspiration, particularly at night (Dees, 1974). The children with "infectious asthma" present with signs of severe asthma within a short time after the initial onset of an apparently minor respiratory infection. The asthma does not improve until acidosis and ventilatory abnormalities are corrected and the infection is controlled. Clinical evidence suggests that these children often have immunologic deficiencies, and they usually suffer more frequent complications of asthma than children with the strong atopic trait. (See section on Treatment, p. 650.)

Laboratory Findings

SPUTUM. The sputum in asthma is a peculiar clear to whitish gelatinous, glairy material, very tenacious and sticky, which is coughed up in stringy casts or molds of the bronchioles (Curschmann spirals). Sometimes small, firm, pelletlike matter is present; these are similar rolled-up casts that are twisted and convoluted and often contain air bubbles. The chemical composition has not been completely established, but mucopolysaccharides, serum albumin and globulins (IgA) are present, the last in higher concentration than is found in serum or saliva. The sputum lacks a proteolytic enzyme found in nonasthmatic, purulent sputum (Mendes and coworkers, 1963; Dennis and coworkers, 1964). Determination of neuraminic acid/fucose ratios suggests that bronchial fluid in asthma arises mainly from the secretory structures, rather than as tissue fluid transudate. It also appears that stasis following mild shearing of sputum, which could occur in bronchoconstriction, results in an 80-fold increase in viscosity, which along with dehydration may contribute to bronchial cast formation (Keal and Reid, 1975).

The sputum consists largely of an amorphous eosinophilic-staining mucus, eosinophils and polymorphonuclear cells, with few bacteria. The Charcot-Leyden crystals are also a unique feature of asthmatic sputum and are seen in specimens several hours old. *The unmistakable appearance of asthmatic sputum is a useful and neglected diagnostic aid in recognizing asthma.* Even when there is some degree of complicating infection, the casts retain their shape, although they may become an opaque yellow. In more extensive infections this may be overshadowed by an excess of purulent secretion, but asthmatic sputum rarely has the homogeneous appearance seen in other pulmonary conditions. In children too young to cough on command, tracheal aspirate will yield the same characteristic secretion.

NASAL SECRETION. Nasal secretion has been the object of much interest in asthma, particularly in nasal allergy, since Hansel (1936) popularized the use of staining for eosinophils as a diagnostic test. He describes the secretion as alkaline and nonirritating to nasal mucosa and skin, in contrast to infectious exudate, which is acid and irritating. IgA and IgE globulins have been isolated from the nasal secretion, as from other body fluids.

BLOOD. Most asthmatic children tend to have hematocrit values and hemoglobin concentrations above average, findings which are related directly to the degree of hypoxia and its duration. In very young children during an attack of asthma it is not uncommon to see values of 14 to 15 gm. per 100 ml. or higher, which then fall 2 to 3 gm. (to 12 to 13 gm. per 100 ml.) when the dyspnea is relieved. Dehydration may contribute to this, as the white blood cell count may rise without demonstrable infection. Eosinophils are frequently present in concentrations over 5 per cent, and values may reach 30 to 40 per cent in severe, long-standing asthma or in drug- or parasite-induced asthma. Although Cooke (1947) believed that infectious asthma was characterized by a higher eosinophilia than that seen in asthma due to allergens, this opinion is not universally shared. During the peak of an asthmatic attack, eosinophils may virtually disappear from the blood smear and then reappear with improvement. Basophils may be found in either increased or decreased concentration in chronic or acute allergic states (Shelley, 1963). This has been related to the mast cell degranulation of anaphylaxis (Selye, 1965). In some children, neutropenia and decrease in platelets occur during an asthmatic attack. Various theories as to their transient disappearance have been offered, among them one hypothesis that sequestration in the lung or other shock organ is responsible, and another that their dissolution is brought about by the products of antigen-antibody union.

Much has been written about the gamma globulin levels in asthmatic children, but no conclusive proof has been presented that there is any constant quantitative or qualitative alteration in gamma globulin. There appears, however, to be a small percentage of young children and an almost minute percentage of older children in whom gamma globulin level is low and features of both allergic disorders and collagen diseases are present. In addition, these children have a high family incidence of arthritis and collagen diseases and are found to have a dysgammaglobulinemia, often with reduction or absence of one portion of the gamma globulin component, commonly the IgA globulin. This condition may be suspected on clinical grounds if there are severe recurrent purulent sinopulmonary infections. There is no reason to give gamma globulin injections to asthmatics except for the currently accepted therapeutic uses, prophylaxis of hepatitis and measles, and the absence of IgG.

The development of sensitization to gamma globulin after repeated injections makes it imperative to restrict its therapeutic use to unequivocal necessity (Allen and Kunkel, 1963).

The sedimentation rate is slow in allergic diseases, including asthma; 0 to 2 mm. per hour, Wintrobe, uncorrected, is a usual range. When infection supervenes, more rapid rates are found, but they are frequently slower than in nonallergic patients with comparable active infections.

There are no specific changes or trends seen in asthma in the various other blood tests used for detecting the presence of infection, such as C-reactive protein, latex fixation, antistreptolysin O, and cold and heterophil agglutinins. Also, the various chemical constituents of the blood do not show any characteristic changes or trends in asthma except that beta adrenergic drugs produce less rise in blood sugar or lactate and less eosinopenia in asthmatics than in normal persons.

SWEAT. Sweat chloride levels are normal or low in asthmatics. Values above 40 mEq. per liter are present in cystic fibrosis, whereas normal and allergic children do not reach this concentration if sweating is normal. Thus, the sweat test for chlorides is an aid in differentiating the two conditions.

GASTRIC SECRETION. Gastric secretion tends to have a low hydrochloric acid content in allergic children. It has been suggested that this condition may be a predisposition to food sensitization, since protein is not subjected to normal amounts of the acid for digestion and thus may reach the absorption areas of the small bowel in an incompletely degraded state, with antigenic potential. This possible mechanism needs reexamination with current methods for studying intestinal physiologic processes before it can be accepted as the explanation for food sensitization, however.

Dynamics of Respiration

The dynamics of respiration are discussed in detail by Comroe (1962) and by Bates, Macklem and Christie (1971), and in various other studies of special aspects of lung physiology. (See also the section on The Functional Basis of Respiratory Pathology, page 3.) The consensus of these investigators regarding the abnormalities in asthma is that bilateral obstructive inflation is produced by a decrease in the caliber of the bronchi and bronchioles. The extra effort required to inhale and expel air through a narrowed airway, in order to accommodate to increased resistance to outflow, produces an abnormal breathing pattern with prolonged expiration. As this abnormal pattern continues, the rate increases, the fatigue that results from inefficient respiratory movements deepens, expiration becomes more prolonged, and inspiration becomes shallow and panting until finally the chest is almost fixed in an overdistended inspiratory position. This, in turn, results in the distention of alveoli, inadequate and uneven alveolar ventilation, pulmonary hypertension, and loss of lung elasticity and compliance.

The ventilating capacity for static lung volumes and forced vital capacity in 21 asthmatic children from attack to symptom-free status has been studied by Engström (1964) by means of a closed-circuit helium-dilution technique. The mechanics of breathing, tidal volume, flow rate and changes in intraesophageal pressure were measured simultaneously to calculate lung compliance and pulmonary flow resistance. A reverse body plethysmograph was used for measuring tidal volume.

During an asthmatic attack, Engström found increased inspiratory and expiratory pulmonary flow resistance to be the characteristic expression of bronchial obstruction, with

$$\frac{E}{I} = 1.6$$

where E represents expiratory and I inspiratory resistance; vital capacity and dynamic compliance were low. Five days after the asthma attack, all parameters had reverted toward normal, but

TABLE 5. SUMMARY OF TRENDS IN VENTILATORY CAPACITY IN 21 ASTHMATIC CHILDREN

	Attack	Symptom-free Interval
Pulmonary flow resistance (R)	↑	N* or ↑
Functional residual capacity (V_{FRC})	↑	↓
Residual volume (V_R)	↑	↓
Dynamic compliance (C)	↓	↑ or N
Vital capacity (V_{VC})	↓	↑
Forced expiratory 1-second volume ($FEV_{1.0}$)	↓	↑
Total lung capacity (V_{TLC})	↓	↑

Modified from Engström, I.: *Acta Paediatr.*, Suppl. 155, 1964, pp. 49–50.
*N = normal.

hyperinflation and reduced ventilatory ability persisted. In the symptom-free interval, forced expiratory 1-second volume ($FEV_{1.0}$) was always lower than would have been expected for the amount of pulmonary resistance found (Table 5).

Previous study (Kraepelien, Engström and Karlberg, 1958) suggested that accelerated growth of the lung occurred in those asthmatic children in whom vital capacity (VC) was greater than normal at symptom-free status. Normal growth of the lung is consistent with widening of the alveoli and airways. During an asthmatic attack, expansion of alveoli also occurs; this is reversed when bronchial obstruction is removed. Engström's recent study suggests that after repeated attacks the expansion no longer reverses completely, and airways seem to expand in proportion to alveoli. By assuming an inspiratory position in the thorax, the lungs may be aided in maintaining a hyperventilated state without bronchial obstruction, thus hampering expiratory movement. This, in turn, implies that there may be increased distensibility of the lung, with air-trapping in addition to bronchial obstruction, to explain hyperinflation at normal pulmonary flow resistance in symptom-free periods. Pecora and Bernstein (1964) reported that pulmonary diffusing capacity in eight children with intractable asthma without hyperinflation was slightly lower than the normal range, whereas it was normal in 17 others with hyperinflation.

In addition to the measurement of various parameters in asthma, the changes in vital capacity (V_{vc}), forced expiratory 1-second volume ($FEV_{1.0}$), maximum voluntary ventilation (MVV), peak flow (PF) and pulmonary resistance (R) after the inhalation of a bronchodilator (such as isoproterenol) provide a good estimate of the degree of bronchospasm in asthma and aid in the detection of emphysema and air trapping.

Status asthmaticus is the term used to designate the extreme stage of refractory asthma when so little air is exchanged with each breath that carbon dioxide retention, respiratory acidosis, loss of chloride and constantly deepening hypoxia result. The disturbed acid-base balance of respiratory acidosis may be complicated by metabolic acidosis, or may be compensated by respiratory alkalosis if assisted ventilation is used, with carbon dioxide narcosis as the final stage of respiratory failure. Examples of the change in pH, P_{CO_2}, base excess and oxygen saturation, ranging from those seen in respiratory acidosis, which develops first as the result of various combinations of partial decompensation, through those due to respiratory alkalosis are shown in Table 6.

The measurement of plasma bicarbonate and blood pH is crucial in determining the amount of carbon dioxide retention. This information is essential for correction of the metabolic derangement in severe status asthmaticus, particularly in the very young child, in whom fatigue may develop so rapidly that his appearance may not accurately reflect the seriousness of his condition. When facilities for the direct measurement of P_{CO_2}, P_{O_2}, oxygen saturation and total base in plasma are not available, but when blood pH value can be obtained, a formula for deriving an estimated P_{CO_2} can be applied (Kassirer and Bleich, 1965). This now makes it possible for any physician who can obtain blood pH and total carbon dioxide content to follow this crucial parameter of his patient's metabolism. Kassirer and Bleich described their method as follows:

Estimation of Blood [H^+] from pH

Hydrogen ion concentration in nanomoles (10^{-9} moles) per liter can readily be estimated from blood pH over a wide range of pH values. Two fortuitous relations form the basis of this empirical conversion.

The two digits that follow the decimal point in the normal blood pH of 7.40 and the normal value for blood hydrogen ion concentration of 40 nanomoles per liter are numerically identical.

Over a wide range of values, each deviation in pH of 0.01 unit from the normal value corresponds to a deviation in [H^+] of 1 nanomole per liter.

Estimation of Plasma P_{CO_2} from [H^+] and Total Carbon Dioxide Content.

The blood pH of 7.16 is 0.24 unit more acid than normal, and thus

blood [H^+] $\approx$ 40 + 24, or 64 nanomoles per liter;

$$\text{blood } P_{CO_2} \approx [H^+] \times \frac{\text{total } CO_2 \text{ content}}{25}$$

$$= 64 \times \frac{20}{25}, \text{ or } 51 \text{ mm. Hg}$$

The actual value for P_{CO_2}, calculated from the Henderson-Hasselbalch equation with the aid of a table of logarithms, is 53 mm. of mercury (Kassirer and Bleich).

TABLE 6. SUMMARY OF METABOLIC DERANGEMENTS IN SEVERE ASTHMA

	pH	P_{CO_2}	HCO_3^-	BE*
Respiratory acidosis, acute	7.20	74	28	−2
Respiratory acidosis, chronic	7.40	66	31	+8
Mixed respiratory and metabolic acidosis	7.10	80	23	−8
Metabolic acidosis	7.25	40	17	−10
Metabolic alkalosis	7.55	36	31	+9
Respiratory alkalosis	7.60	20	18	0

*BE = base excess.

Wood (1969) calls attention to the value of the ratio of physiologic dead space to total volume (Vd/Vt) in evaluating children with impending respiratory failure. The expired gas is collected over a measured period of time while counting respirations. The volume of gas is measured and corrected for temperature, barometric pressure and vapor pressure, and the P_{CO_2} of the gas is measured Pe_{CO_2}. Vt is calculated by dividing minute volume by the respiratory frequency per minute (F). During the collection time, arterial blood is drawn for Pa_{CO_2}. The formula is (Comroe, 1965)

$$Vd/Vt = \frac{Pa_{CO_2} - Pe_{CO_2}}{Pa_{CO_2}}$$

The normal value for adults and children is 0.3. Wood has found that a Vd/Vt value of 0.7 or greater is an ominous sign in status asthmaticus.

Differential Diagnosis

Each of the characteristic features of asthma—the tight cough, rapid respiration, dyspnea, obstructive emphysema and wheezing—may be found to some degree in a wide variety of different chest conditions and general systemic diseases. Furthermore, many very young asthmatic children, under four years of age, do not respond typically to skin tests or exhibit other characteristic features of atopic asthma, thus making it essential for the physician to be informed enough to rule out the nonallergic causes of wheezing and cough (Table 7). Most frequent among these are croup, asthmatic bronchitis, acute respiratory disease frequently due to rhinovirus or respiratory syncytial virus, and bronchiolitis. Croup is characterized by the sudden onset of a harsh, barking cough, but differs from asthma in its inspiratory stridor. All the rest diffusely involve the bronchioles in inflammatory edema and bronchospasm and are characterized by some fever, wheezing and dyspnea. Emphysema and prostration are especially marked in bronchiolitis occurring in young infants, and are much more severe than in asthma. Since most cases of bronchiolitis are due to viral infections, and since tests for antiviral an-

---

TABLE 7. DIFFERENTIAL DIAGNOSIS OF ASTHMA IN INFANTS AND YOUNG CHILDREN*

Foreign body, any part of airway

Upper airway
  Nose: enlarged adenoids, choanal atresia, polyps
  Throat: retropharyngeal or peritonsillar abscess, *flaccid epiglottis, short neck*
  Larynx: *croup, infection*, structural anomalies, paralysis of vocal cord, polyps, allergic edema, tetany

Lower airway
  Trachea: *tracheomalacia, infection*, external compression by nodes, tumor, vascular ring, or foreign body in esophagus
  Bronchus: infection, such as *asthmatic bronchitis, bronchiolitis, bronchitis* or bronchiectasis; obstruction due to endobronchial disease, stenosis or *external compression*
  Lungs: *pneumonias, cystic fibrosis*, tuberculosis, histoplasmosis, pertussis, aspiration pneumonia, pneumothorax, *Pneumocystis carinii, atelectasis*, compression from lung or enteric cysts, intralobar emphysema, sequestration of lung, anomalies of lung such as agenesis of a lobe, Loeffler's syndrome

Extrarespiratory disorders
  Cardiovascular: congenital heart disease of various types, vascular ring, anomalies of great vessels
  Central nervous system: hyperventilation, encephalitis, hysteria, cerebral palsy, palate paralysis, myasthenia gravis, drug intoxication (e.g., salicylism)
  Alpha$_1$-antitrypsin deficiency

Modified from Dees, S. C.: *J.A.M.A., 175*:365, 1961.
*Italicized conditions are most common.

tibodies and direct viral cultures as yet are too time-consuming to make them diagnostically feasible, one must rely on finding evidence of infection and on observing the response to bronchodilating drugs. This response will be much less impressive, if detectable, in bronchiolitis than in asthma.

The presence of a foreign body in either the trachea or esophagus must be considered in *every* child who shows difficulty in breathing. Removal of this cause for wheezing requires prompt and often emergency treatment. Small children, of course, present with this condition much more often than older children and the parents characteristically report that symptoms began abruptly (often the exact moment can be recalled long afterward), describing some degree of respiratory difficulty or dysphagia, usually accompanied by harsh, barking, irritative cough and varying amounts of persistent wheezing. If the foreign body is lodged in one or the other main stem bronchus, unilateral wheezing is often heard. If the object is freely movable, one may hear a "click" or "slap" as it moves up and down the airway with breathing. If the object nearly but not completely obstructs the bronchus, a ball-valve effect results, with emphysema occurring in the lung distal to the foreign body. With complete obstruction of a bronchus, atelectasis of the lobe supplied by that bronchus results. It is important to bear in mind that a foreign body may produce reflex bronchospasm with generalized signs that may easily obscure localizing ones.

An important cause of wheezing and paroxysmal cough frequently mistaken for asthma is cystic fibrosis (mucoviscidosis). Here a sweat test with chloride greater than 40 to 70 mEq. per liter is diagnostic. Formerly, pertussis was frequently mistaken for asthma; a leukocytosis with lymphocytosis is characteristic of pertussis. Atelectasis, usually of the right middle lobe, may be associated with a wheezing, irritative cough, and may be suspected from the clinical signs of respiratory infection and the nature of the sputum. Roentgenographically, it can be recognized by a characteristic wedge-shaped area of increased density on lateral view or by blurring of the right cardiac border and obliteration of the right cardiophrenic angle. Other frequent causes of wheezy cough are flaccid epiglottis, tracheomalacia and laryngeal stridor. These abnormalities occur in early infancy, and are primarily heard in inspiration. The signs of respiratory difficulty can be corrected or greatly decreased by change of position and by other maneuvers such as advancing the mandible; they diminish with age.

Less common but not less important and correctable causes of cough and wheeze are vascular rings and other anomalies of blood vessels that compromise tracheal or bronchial function. Also, hilar lymph nodes enlarged from any cause, but especially from tuberculosis, may compress the trachea or bronchus and cause wheezing.

ALPHA₁-ANTITRYPSIN DEFICIENCY. (SEE CHAPTER 39.) An inherent abnormality in serum protein alpha₁-antitrypsin deficiency presenting with severe cough, dyspnea and wheezing was first reported from Sweden by Laurell and Eriksson (1963) and shown to be associated with early onset of severe emphysema in several kindreds. Subsequent studies have reported this dysgammaglobulinemia with early adult bronchitis and with liver disease in infants. A system for determining genetic types has been evolved based on electrophoretic mobility of alpha₁-antitrypsin. This designates Pi types (protease inhibitor) as F (fast), M (medium), S (slow) and Z (very slow), with 21 or 23 codominant alleles active as autosomal recessives in the inheritance of this trait. The homozygous ZZ individuals have early emphysema or the potential for it. The heterozygotes have an intermediate deficiency, and less severe or later onset or a clinically unexpressed condition. It is estimated that 5 per cent of the United States population are heterozygotes for alpha₁-antitrypsin deficiency. A community study of the relation of alpha₁-antitrypsin levels to obstructive lung disease indicates that intermediate levels do not represent either an important risk factor or a predictor for this disease (Morse and coworkers, 1975).

A survey of "normal" and asthmatic children (Katz and associates, 1976) showed the same incidence of alpha₁-antitrypsin deficiency and 3 per cent phenotype Z variants in both groups. Pulmonary function tests were done in the asthmatics, not in the controls, and family history of emphysema was not obtained from the "normals." The asthmatics were divided into non-steroid-dependent and steroid-dependent. The steroid-dependent individuals had an increased but not statistically significant difference in the number of Pi variants, but Z variants occurred in a greater number of the steroid-dependent asthmatics (6 per cent).

Two recent reports of affected persons describe evidence of impaired pulmonary function tests in asymptomatic heterozygous relatives (Dunand and coworkers, 1976; Johnson and coworkers, 1976). These authors stress the importance of wheezing as well as dyspnea and emphysematous changes in the clinical course of their patients' condition. This has been observed by others, whose patients also presented as intractable "asthmatics." It is important to test for this abnormality in such children.

Clinical Course and Complications

The clinical course of asthma assumes many variations in different patients; many different factors influence it. In addition to the degree of allergic sensitivity and the amount, duration and frequency of exposure to allergens, a number of nonspecific factors are influential; among these are infections, chilling, fatigue, exercise, emotional stress, physical debility, and predisposition by age and sex. Allowing for these many variables, the natural history of a representative (hypothetical) case of asthma may be described as follows.

A four-year-old boy with a feeding problem, mild transient facial eczema in infancy, and frequent "colds" accompanied by much mucus in the postpharynx and trachea all his life suddenly has acute, moderately severe nocturnal wheezing two days after the onset of his first fall "cold." The attack improves after treatment with steam, cough medicine and an antibiotic. Two weeks later there is a recurrence, more severe than the first, which is refractory to the previous treatment and progresses to severe respiratory distress with accompanying cyanosis; this improves promptly after treatment with a bronchodilator such as epinephrine or aminophylline. During the next year he appears to have less trouble when milk and peanuts are removed from his diet.

In the two ensuing years, wheezing of varying severity accompanies every respiratory infection. At seven years of age he has asthma attacks without infection, and although by nine years of age foods no longer seem to disagree with him, his respiratory difficulties are obviously worse at particular seasons of the year. He also finds that he cannot ride horseback without wheezing, nor can he handle his dog without mild symptoms. His health remains about the same until he is 14 years old, when he begins to improve, and by 17 years of age he no longer has asthma attacks, except for mild wheezing with strenuous exertion. He continues to have hay fever and perennial nasal obstruction made bearable by an occasional dose of antihistamine. For the next two decades he has so little trouble that he forgets he ever had any allergy. At 35 years of age, however, he has become an avid gardener and golfer, and while he is engaged in these hobbies his hay fever recurs. Several months later, on a cool damp evening in the fall, he has an attack of asthma. From then on he notices increasing dyspnea on exertion; there is also coughing and wheezing. Asthma attacks become more and more frequent, so that by the time he is 50 years old he is emphysematous and has almost continuous mild asthma with severe attacks associated with respiratory tract infection.

Contrary to the usual pattern described above, asthma may begin abruptly in some children; in these cases, food sensitivity seldom appears to play a significant role in producing symptoms. Asthma attacks may merely show a gradual increase in severity and frequency. These children are almost invariably sensitive to air-borne allergens and have some associated nasal symptoms, with either perennial allergic rhinitis or hay fever. Also, many of them react to changes in temperature and humidity, worsening with every spell of cold, damp weather; sometimes their parents can even predict inclement weather by the child's heightened symptoms. These are children whose chronic nasal obstruction leads to changes in the structure of the mouth and nasal passages, producing malocclusion of the jaws and a detrimental cosmetic effect, often improperly termed the "adenoid facies." The narrowing of the upper jaw, with high palate, causes the upper teeth to protrude, and the nasal passage becomes narrow and elongated. The tendency to mouth-breathe directs the flow of air upward against the hard palate. This constant mild pressure on the hard palate may further aggravate the tendency toward elevation in the central part, which, in turn, decreases the size of the nasal passage above. In bypassing the normal cleaning and warming function of the nose, the air that reaches the lungs is also prevented from being in the more or less "steady state" provided by constant humidification. Children with asthma previously associated with perennial allergic rhinitis are more likely to have sinus complications in later years. They also are more apt to have serous otitis media than are the children with the dermal-respiratory syndrome. It appears, however, that serous otitis media is seen less often in the children who have asthma combined with perennial allergic rhinitis than in those with allergic rhinitis alone.

Although there seems to be no demonstrable reason for it, the asthmatic girl has only half as good a chance of "outgrowing" her ailment around puberty as has the asthmatic boy. The dermal-respiratory syndrome may occur a little more frequently in boys than in girls, and in our series more girls had persistent eczema or neurodermatitis at puberty than did the boys, but the severity and persistence of asthma appeared to be the same in both sexes. Among a very small group of patients (30) with right middle lobe syndrome and complicated asthma, the girls outnumbered the boys two to one. This group is too small to permit conclusions, but the incidence in girls appeared to be predominant only in this instance.

The various complications seen in asthma could be woven into the hypothetical asthmatic story, but for brevity they are listed as follows:

1. Other allergic disorders—hay fever, perennial allergic rhinitis, eczema, urticaria, serous otitis media, gastrointestinal allergy, and so on.
2. Infection—sinusitis, bronchitis, bronchiolitis, pneumonias (all types), otitis media, tuberculosis.
3. Atelectasis—partial, recurrent or chronic with bronchiectasis involving one or more lobes (usually the right middle lobe).
4. Massive collapse of the entire lung.
5. Pneumothorax—pneumomediastinum, subcutaneous emphysema.
6. Status asthmaticus.
7. Emphysema.
8. Right-sided cardiac failure.
9. Emotional and behavior problems.
10. "Adenoid" or "allergic" facies—malformation of the nose and dental arches due to chronic mouth-breathing caused by associated chronic nasal allergy.
11. Immunologic disorders, dysgammaglobulinemia.

Certain of these complications deserve special emphasis, but all warrant the same warning—that it is a grave mistake to attribute all respiratory symptoms to asthma and not constantly bear in mind that other lung conditions may be marked by overt wheezing.

Hyperinflation, ultimately culminating in the emphysematous chest with

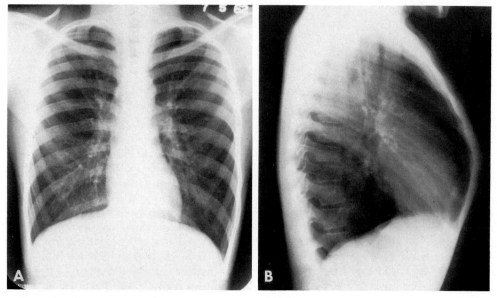

Figure 8.   Roentgenogram of asthmatic chest. *A,* Posteroanterior projection showing radiolucent lungs, low diaphragm, wide interspaces between ribs, and small, centrally placed heart. *B,* Lateral projection. Note the increased radiolucent lung anterior to the heart.

depressed diaphragms and increased anteroposterior chest diameter, is illustrated radiographically in Figure 8. Atelectasis, complete or partial, and usually involving the right middle lobe (Fig. 9), is often the cause of persistent and severe refractory wheezing; this may arise in connection with pneumonia and last long after the pneumonia has cleared. It may also arise from other causes of compression of the right middle lobe (or other) bronchus,

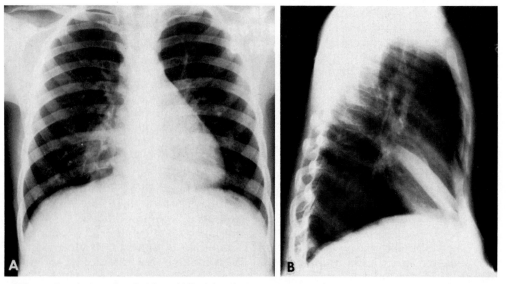

Figure 9.   Atelectasis of right middle lobe during asthma attack. *A,* Posteroanterior roentgenogram shows only an indistinctly outlined infiltration along the right cardiac border. *B,* Lateral projection shows a dense area of infiltration representing complete atelectasis of the right middle lobe.

or it may be due to endobronchial obstruction by a foreign body, accumulated secretion (mucous plug) or bronchostenosis, sometimes congenital. Endobronchial masses are rarely found in children, although one boy with atelectasis recently had a polypoid fold of mucosa extensively infiltrated with lymphocytic cells obstructing the bronchus. To date, no endobronchial malignancies in children have been seen in our clinic, but obviously this is a main cause of wheezing and atelectasis in older persons.

Massive collapse rarely occurs in asthma, but is a critical emergency when it does occur. When complete obstruction of a main bronchus is responsible, good intrapulmonary circulation will cause the air to be rapidly absorbed so that the lung becomes atelectatic (Fig. 10). On the other hand, a tiny rupture of an alveolar wall may result in the slow accumulation of air in the extrapleural space, producing pneumothorax and lung collapse. Incessant cough, shift of the mediastinum and its contents, rapid, shallow respirations with no movement of the affected side,

deviation of the trachea away from the affected side, hyperresonance and absence of breath sounds are the most frequent findings in pneumothorax. If the process is gradual in the older child whose mediastinum is a little more stable, respiratory embarrassment will be present, but may not be severe. Often the alveolar rupture will close spontaneously, and the intrapleural air already present will be slowly resorbed with consequent spontaneous reexpansion of the lung. The air may dissect along the fascial planes into the mediastinum, causing varying degrees of cardiac embarrassment. Other common pathways for extrapleural air are the cervical fascial planes leading to subcutaneous emphysema in the neck and over the chest.

The most dangerous kind of massive collapse is that associated with tension pneumothorax, which occurs when a large amount of air enters the pleural space at one time and continues to be drawn into the thorax with each breath. Such collapse often occurs as a complication of staphylococcal pneumonia, and we have seen it three times in asth-

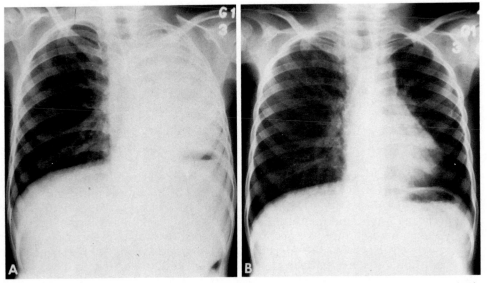

Figure 10. Massive collapse of the left lung during an asthmatic attack. *A,* Posteroanterior projection roentgenogram showing trachea deviated to the affected left side, with the heart and mediastinum shifted to the left. Note the elevated left diaphragm as shown by air in the stomach. *B,* Resolution of density in the left lung, with reexpansion. Note that the trachea is nearer the midline.

matic children who were receiving treatment with intermittent positive pressure breathing apparatus (IPPB). It may also occur in asthmatics during the height of a paroxysm of coughing. Prompt thoracotomy with continuous drainage of the pneumothorax is necessary to permit reexpansion of the lung and relieve the respiratory embarrassment.

Status asthmaticus has been described previously in respect to the deranged respiratory metabolism, and treatment will be discussed later. Its frequency in asthmatic children is difficult to estimate. Children who have once suffered status asthmaticus tend to become repeaters; these children almost invariably react in this way to apparently minor respiratory tract infections. To date, no one has offered an entirely satisfactory explanation for the development of status asthmaticus and atelectasis. Although Kravis and Lecks (1965) have suggested lack of surfactant or an abnormality in the substance as the causative factor, this attractive hypothesis has not been proved. Although this condition is fortunately infrequent, it accounts for many of the hospital admissions for asthma. A basic emergency routine for such patients should be established in each hospital so that prompt treatment can be instituted and properly monitored by the blood gas and pH determinations to correct metabolic derangements and to prevent irreversible changes.

Prognosis

The various reports on the prognosis of asthma are generally characterized by confusion and discrepancies due largely to the lack of uniformity of methods of sampling, the use of divergent classifications, and the inconsistencies in data inherent in retrospective studies. It is obvious from the preceding discussion of the variables in asthma that the prognosis for either control of symptoms or the eventual disappearance of symptoms ("cure") will differ among children with rare

infrequent attacks, those with constant wheezing, and those who are subject to episodes of status asthmaticus. Thus it is inaccurate to base the prognosis on sex, age, duration of disease, or prior treatment. Furthermore, none of the reported studies use uniform criteria for the selection of patients; nor do they separate like kinds of asthma in every respect. Ryssing and Flensborg (1963) attempted this, but did not clearly differentiate the types of therapy. Also, in almost all reports some sort of therapy is superimposed on the entire group, thereby coloring the prognosis for the natural course of the illness. An untreated child population is described in Smith's (1971) recently reported five-year survey of rural Iowa families. It was found that among 95 asthmatic children, 75 per cent were limited in activity by asthma at the time of the first interview, and only 7 per cent were still limited five years later. A total of 29 children were considered to have "outgrown" their attacks. Four of 33 children under ten years of age and 23 of 27 over ten years of age at the time of the first visit still had asthma when reinterviewed after five years. The severity, frequency and duration of attacks appeared unrelated to ultimate improvement.

Although recognizing these problems and the capricious nature of asthma, one can nevertheless conclude that an impressive number of asthmatic children lose their symptoms at puberty. This is borne out by the well established observation that boys with asthma outnumber girls two to one under the age of 15 years, while after that age the sex ratio is nearly equal, and in early and later adulthood women asthmatics slightly outnumber men. Williams and McNicol's (1969) survey of school children in Melbourne, Australia, using a sample of 401 seven-year-olds from a population of 30,000 showed that 62 per cent of those wheezing at the beginning of the study were no longer wheezing at ten years of age and had not wheezed in two years; 6 per cent had experienced

TABLE 8. PROGNOSIS IN ASTHMA*

Author	Date	Place	Number of Patients	Cured	Percentage Improved	Un-changed†
Ryssing and Flensborg	1963	Copenhagen	442	37	9	54
Aas	1963	Oslo	174	44	17	39
Wilken-Jensen	1963	Copenhagen	625	65	29	6
Kraepelien	1963	Stockholm	528	29	65	6
Freeman et al.	1964	Colorado	608	57	–	–‡
Dees	1957	North Carolina	236	44	36	20
Rackemann	1952	Massachusetts	449 < 13 yrs.§	31	56	13
			239 > 13 yrs.	22	26	52

*Based on evaluation of asthmatic patients, both treated and untreated, between adolescence and young adulthood (see text).

†Includes mortalities from asthma or other causes.

‡Not stated.

§Asthma began before 13 years (<13 yrs.), after 13 years (>13 yrs.).

the last attack one to two years previously. On the other hand, the 32 per cent who still wheezed were having regular attacks. In the milder wheezing group the preponderance were girls. In the group whose wheezing stopped at ten years there were more boys. In those who continued to wheeze at ten years, the ratio of boys to girls was 7:3. There is no mention as to whether children received any treatment.

The data from the Scandinavian countries, reported in *Acta Paediatrica* (1963), probably represent the largest and most nearly comparable series of asthmatics to date, but even here significant differences exist in the selection and grouping of patients, making it impossible to summarize the results and compare them in all respects (Table 8). Nevertheless, in each series (Ryssing and Flensborg, 1963; Aas, 1963; Kraepelien, 1963) the percentage of untreated or minimally treated patients reported as asthma-free ("cured") at puberty or after a ten-year follow-up ranged from 30 to 44 per cent. Wilken-Jensen (1963) analyzed a series of 625 treated patients and reported 65 per cent to be asthma-free. Investigators concur that prognosis for "cure" or improvement depends on the severity of the asthma (Table 9), multiplicity of allergic diseases, multiple sensitivity, positive family history of allergy, and duration of disease before the onset of treatment. The more severe and numerous the symptoms, the longer they

TABLE 9. CORRELATION BETWEEN SEVERITY AND PROGNOSIS IN ASTHMA

Grade of Disease	Attacks/Year	Percentage CURED	IMPROVED	Author
Grade I	0–5	73	82	Aas
Grade II	5–10	30	30	
Grade III	10 or more	Less than 30		
Grade I		–	–	Ryssing and Flensborg
Grade II		0	49	
Grade III		0	27	
Grade I		–	–	Wilken-Jensen
Grade II		–	33	
Grade III		–	37	

have been present, and the more allergic the family, the poorer is the prognosis for improvement. Wilken-Jensen, however, found a slightly higher rate of improvement among his patients with a positive family history. He suggests that the increased enlightenment in the patient's family regarding allergy may be a possible explanation.

However comforting it may be for the parents of young asthmatic boys to hear that asthma is largely a preadolescent phenomenon, the statistics do not reveal which particular child may "outgrow" asthma, nor do they tell which boy may merely enjoy a free interval between adolescence and early adulthood, only to relapse into wheezing and chronic emphysema in later years (Freeman and coworkers, 1964). An attempt to characterize and identify these children is found in a ten-year follow-up on 518 asthmatic children reported by Buffum and Settipane (1966), who found 41 per cent asymptomatic, 52.4 per cent slightly or occasionally asthmatic, and 5.6 per cent still handicapped. Mortality was 1 per cent. The intractable cases were characterized by having had eczema, onset of asthma before two years of age, and a positive scratch test to egg.

In fact, when the evaluation of "cure" is based on examination and pulmonary function studies and not just on the patient's statement, one finds a far higher number of adolescent boys with asthma than predicted by the alleged "outgrowing" phenomenon that is supposed to occur at puberty. An interesting small series of 12 males who had had childhood asthma after an average symptom-free period of 11 years were studied with ventilatory function studies by Blackhall (1970). She found an increase in residual volume (RV) in the majority of subjects, and while relative levels of FEV_1 and FEV_1/FVC ratio were normal in most cases, an abnormal degree of bronchial lability in response to isoproterenol inhalation was found in seven subjects. One also finds that upper respiratory

and other forms of allergy do not decline in these so-called cured patients and may indeed become more severe at this age. It would appear, then, that there may be a shift in the major shock organ at this age (from bronchi to nose), rather than true loss of allergy — just as a shift from skin to bronchi is often seen at the end of infancy.

The attempts to separate those children who will "outgrow" their sensitivity from those who will not have not been successful.

Treatment

LONG-RANGE TREATMENT.   The foregoing discussion of the prognosis in asthma has already alluded to the long-range treatment of asthma. The keystone of this kind of "allergy program" is an evaluation of the patient's general health combined with an accurate assessment of both the specific allergic factors and the nonspecific factors that precipitate symptoms. Specific allergens may be detected by skin, conjunctival or other mucous membrane tests with protein allergy extracts; direct skin tests by scratch or intradermal technique are most frequently used. Indirect skin tests by Prausnitz-Küstner reaction are performed by injection of the serum of the patient's blood into the recipient's skin and the testing of these sites with allergens. Sensitivities can also be detected by inhalation testing (bronchial challenge) or by controlled exposure (such as diet trial). In vitro testing for serum IgE antibodies by RAST (radioallergosorbent test) is now available for many different antigens.

After the identification of significant allergens and the confirmation by provocative tests, the first step in therapy is the avoidance of the noxious substances. If avoidance is impossible (as in allergies to air-borne pollen), a hyposensitization (immunotherapy) program may be initiated. A series of injections of allergens of gradually increasing potency are administered at intervals to cause the increasing production of blocking antibodies in the allergic patients; sensitivity to the particular antigen is thereby minimized.

Although this form of treatment has been used for more than 50 years, the mechanism invoked in the process is incompletely understood (Noon, 1911) and is now the subject of active reinvestigation in many laboratories and clinics (Norman and coworkers, 1968). It is thought that such injections stimulate the production of a thermostable IgG antibody, called a "blocking" antibody since it blocks skin tests, in some cases with a concurrent fall in IgE antibody. It has been shown that IgE antibody response requires the presence of both T and B lymphocytes. These B lymphocytes are different from those that are precursors of IgG antibody–forming cells. Ishizaka (1976) suggests that if the important factor in immunization is the suppression of T cells and their helper effect in IgE production, thus favoring IgG response, then theoretically one might improve the effects of injection treatment of allergy by using denatured antigens or polypeptide chains that react with T cells and not with B cells. Some studies in progress support this idea. It has therefore been postulated that antigen-antibody union is consummated by the "blocking" antibody, thereby protecting cells from the damage caused by the mediators of an allergic reaction that would otherwise have taken place in some vulnerable tissue, such as the bronchial tree or the lungs. There are, however, many experimental and clinical observations that cannot be reconciled with this oversimplified explanation. For details of these controversial points, as well as the relative merits of aqueous, oil emulsion repository (Loveless, 1957) and alum-precipitated pyridine (Allpyral) (Fuchs and Strauss, 1959) extracts, and of various treatment schedules — preseasonal, coseasonal, perennial — the reader is referred to the various texts and specialty journals of allergy.

In some instances the removal of environmental factors will suffice as a pre-ventive measure, as evidenced by the improvement noted when a child who is dog- or cat-sensitive no longer has exposure to the animal, or when egg is removed from the diet of an egg-sensitive child. Since most allergic persons are sensitive to house dust (a substance produced by the aging of cotton linters and other household furnishings), use of precautions to decrease household dust exposure, particularly by setting up a "dust-free" bedroom,* is one of the most common treatment measures. This is accomplished by removing excess room appointments and bric-a-brac, by encasing pillows, mattresses, box springs and similar furnishings in airtight plastic covers, or by the substitution of synthetic or rubber foam products for these furnishings. These rearrangements and modifications, plus frequent scrupulous cleaning, often supply immediate and significant relief to dust-sensitive children.

Voorhorst and coworkers (1969) called attention to the dust mite, *Dermatophagoides pteronyssinus,* as the major allergen in house dust. This claim has been disputed on both immunologic and clinical grounds for dusts collected in the United States and Canada by investigators in these countries. Since the mite population is higher in damp environments, and higher in mattress dust than in other areas in a home, these factors may have some bearing on the discordant findings. Skin tests on children clinically sensitive to house dust will sometimes show a close correlation between the size of reaction to dust extract and that to mite extract, whereas at other times there is no correlation in apparent degree of skin sensitivity. Since house dust is such a heterogeneous substance, it is difficult to evaluate which of its many components is the significant factor for a given patient. Allergy to mites is an attractive hypothesis to explain the differences that some

---

*Specific instructions for preparing a dust-free bedroom for the patient can be obtained from manufacturers of nonallergic bedding.

patients notice in certain homes and not in others.

Treatment directed toward the non-specific factors that often trigger allergic symptoms is also important. This includes provision for adequate humidity in the house (especially in winter), protection of the child from temperature extremes, with simultaneous and systematic exposure of the child to temperature differences so that he will develop greater tolerance, and the decrease of exposure to air-borne irritants such as dust, pollens and chemicals by the installation of an air conditioner equipped with a high efficiency particulate air (HEPA) or an electronic air cleaner. For special problems in which emotional stress plays a leading role, psychotherapy, change of environment, and separation from the family with temporary residence in a foster home or special asthma residence are often utilized with much benefit.

For the child with exercise-induced asthma, there are several approaches to minimize the handicap it imposes. These are (1) a gradual systematic program of increasing exercise, selecting an activity such as swimming, which has been found most suitable, since it provokes less bronchospasm than those activities involving much running; (2) a "warm-up" period before starting a sport; and (3) use of premedication just before the exercise with a beta adrenergic drug, xanthine or cromolyn (Bierman and Pierson, 1975).

For some years, aerosol therapy for the inhalation of a bronchodilating drug, originally epinephrine and more recently isoproterenol, isoetharine and metaproterenol, has been extensively used not only for relief of acute asthma symptoms but as a prelude to a breathing exercise or postural drainage program. The first devices were glass inhalers delivering a particle of 3 to 9 microns in size, such as the de Vilbiss #40 and #640, propelled by hand bulb, compressor or bicycle pump (Halpern and coworkers, 1964). Then intermittent positive pressure breathing (IPPB) was introduced to propel the aerosol into the lungs with more force. This has proved useful in treating some patients with acute severe bronchospasm. Within the last twenty years, the pressurized aerosol "bomb" type dispensers with the active drug packaged under pressure and propelled by Freon (fluoroalkane) have skyrocketed in popularity. Epinephrine, isoproterenol and isoetharine and steroids are marketed for nebulization in this form. Unfortunately, with this quick, though brief, relief so attractive to patients has come the inevitable overuse and misuse of these potent drugs. Their effectiveness necessitates perfect timing of the mist with inhalation, which is almost an impossibility with small children. Therefore, their usefulness and suitability are very limited in pediatrics.

Many patients have become "spray addicts," and it has become apparent that these aerosols may be associated with an increase in sudden death in asthmatics, as has been discussed in a previous section of this chapter dealing with mortality from asthma (Caplin and Haynes, 1969). Some additional reactions to the catecholamines that may be involved in this adverse reaction are the following: in about 50 per cent of asthmatic patients the hypoxemia is aggravated by epinephrine, isoproterenol and aminophylline, with a decrease of Pa_{O_2} of 5 mm. Hg or more. Paradoxical delayed severe bronchoconstriction has been observed by Keighley (1966) and also by Van Metre (1969), who aptly called this the "locked lung syndrome." The circumstantial evidence is such that these potent drugs should be under more careful supervision than they are at present in order to keep their benefits and avoid risk in asthmatics.

Corrective breathing and posture exercises, plus general physical fitness programs, are helpful in improving the asthmatic child's exercise tolerance. Certain children can be taught to control their breathing so that they can use exercises designed to relieve shortness of breath and thereby abort the kind of asthmatic attack triggered by a sudden laugh or overexertion. Postural drainage for all or certain lung areas is frequently helpful for the "wet" asthmatic child who has excessive bronchial secretions, and for the patient with copious secretion and cough in the phase of asthma after bronchospasm has been relieved. The child with asthma and concomitant bronchitis, bronchiectasis or atelectasis also benefits from postural drainage. The aid of a physical therapist for instruction and assistance is invaluable, but, lacking this, one may obtain an instructive pamphlet which illustrates and describes various helpful exercises.* (See Chapter 4, Diagnostic and Therapeutic Procedures, page 105).

The use of bacterial vaccines in treating asthmatic patients is a controversial subject which, although practiced for many years, has not been scrutinized and evaluated by standards for safety and efficacy presently considered acceptable for other forms of therapy. Sometimes respiratory bacterial vaccines and extracts were also used for "nonspecific protein effect," as were typhoid and pertussis vaccines, sterile milk, snake venom and autohemotherapy injections some years ago. The efficacy of these agents has never been proved by controlled studies. The same is true for injections of precipitated sulfur, extracts of *Rhus quercifolia* (Anergex), bacterial pyrogens (Piromen) and ethylene disulfonate. Other forms of therapy not generally accepted, but still with enthusiastic advocates, are hypnosis, glomectomy (surgical removal of the carotid body), sympathectomy, the Gay treatment (potassium iodide and Fowler's solution), ultraviolet light treatment, inhalation of negative ionized air, ozone and fumes of "asthma powders," and even sleeping with a chihuahua dog to "take" the

asthma, or the wearing of amber beads.

The association of a bacterial or viral respiratory infection with the onset of acute asthma or the continuation of prolonged asthmatic attacks is too frequent an observation to be relegated to folklore. Regardless of the mechanism involved, these children are frequently given antibiotics, and when needed the drug should be used in full therapeutic doses for a full therapeutic course. Parents should understand the importance of maintaining an effective drug level by proper administration in order to achieve eradication of infection, to prevent emergence of drug-resistant bacteria, and to minimize the development of drug sensitivity from repeated, often inadequate courses. Many physicians hesitate to give penicillin to allergic children for fear of sensitization. Although this may be wise in theory, this useful drug should not be denied asthmatics when it is the drug of choice for significant infection unless there is reason to suspect intolerance to it.

Tonsillectomy and adenoidectomy were once almost routine procedures for asthmatics before falling into disfavor because of an alleged increase in the incidence and severity of asthma after surgery. While this is still the most frequently performed operation in all children, the present consensus among many pediatricians and allergists and some nose and throat surgeons is that there are very few indications for tonsillectomy and adenoidectomy and these should be the same for allergic as for nonallergic children. Pollen-sensitive children should not have nasopharyngeal surgery during a period when pollen to which they are sensitive is prevalent. Tonsil and adenoid tissue has been found to contain cells that stain positively for IgE and IgA, and these globulins have been isolated from nasal washings, saliva and parotid ducts. Since this lymphatic tissue is active immunologically, this constitutes a valid

---

*Breathing Exercises for Asthmatic Children, American Academy of Pediatrics, Evanston, Illinois, 1969.

reason for not allowing indiscriminate tonsillectomy and adenoidectomy, particularly in infection-prone children.

We have been so impressed with the high incidence of family epidemics of infection and with family carriers of pathogens, usually either beta-hemolytic streptococci or coagulase-positive staphylococci, among the infection-prone allergic and asthmatic children (Dees, 1960) that we now consider a search for such carriers an integral part of the child's treatment. If it were practical to do similar samplings for respiratory viruses among family members, one would undoubtedly find an even higher incidence of infection, and possibly of carriers. Until such testing is possible, however, and until a satisfactory vaccine is generally available for unusually susceptible children, this very important aspect of respiratory illness will continue to be undocumented and without specific treatment.

Regardless of the importance of the specific and nonspecific factors discussed in the foregoing, the pressing need for the patient with chronic asthma or frequently recurring attacks is relief of difficulty in breathing. Since it has been clearly demonstrated that a large percentage of asymptomatic asthmatics have a significant degree of airway obstruction, the long-term use of some type of bronchodilator, either a beta adrenergic drug or xanthine, is currently advised even in relatively asymptomatic periods. The various drugs that are now available are discussed in detail in the following section on Acute Treatment.

In addition to the use of bronchodilators, the prophylaxis of asthma has been augmented in recent years by the introduction, first in England, of a new drug, disodium cromoglycate (Intal) (Intal, Aarane in the United States; Lomudal in Europe). It was derived from an analog of khellin by Altounyan in 1967. It is a bis-chromone, entirely different from any previously devised antiallergic drugs. When inhaled as a powder prior to an inhalation challenge of pollen, the experimental asthma was blocked.

While its mode of action as an antiallergic drug is not entirely clear, since it does not block antigen-antibody union, it appears to exert its effect by stabilizing the mast cell membrane, and preventing degranulation and release of chemical mediators of the allergic reaction. One mechanism appears to be by increasing intracellular cyclic AMP through inhibition of CAMP phosphodiesterase (Lavin and coworkers, 1976). This could account for its effectiveness in preventing type I, IgE-mediated immediate reactions, for which it is experimentally and clinically effective. This does not account for its effectiveness in preventing exercise-induced bronchospasm, or hyperventilation bronchospasm, or the reaction to certain inhaled chemical irritants, or certain type III delayed forms of bronchospasm. Cromolyn has no anti-inflammatory or bronchodilating properties. It does not antagonize histamine, methacholine, SRS–A, bradykinin or serotonin.

There have now been over 300 clinical trials of cromolyn (disodium cromoglycate) involving more than 10,000 patients (Smith and Devey, 1968; Jones and Blackhall, 1970; Pepys and Frankland, 1970; Poppius and coworkers, 1970; Mascia and coworkers, 1976). From this experience it has been shown that cromolyn is most effective in treating extrinsic asthma, but is also effective in some patients with intrinsic asthma. It has a steroid "sparing" effect, allowing some steroid-dependent patients to discontinue steroids. It prevents exercise-induced asthma when inhaled just prior to exercise. It does not lose effectiveness for most patients even after long use.

Relatively few side-effects are reported; these have been chiefly skin rashes (Sheffer and coworkers, 1975) and pneumonitis (Hermance and Brown, 1976), which have been reversible on discontinuing the drug. The results in children over five years of age are usually good, provided the child is properly instructed and supervised in the correct use of the spinhaler, the device from which the finely powdered drug is inhaled. The recommended dose is 20 mg. inhaled at six-hour intervals, at least until symptoms are controlled, which may take a week to a month. When improvement occurs, a more flexible schedule with fewer doses sometimes can be used. In our experience, the major cause of failure of the drug is failure to pay careful attention to the technique for inhalation, and spacing the doses at longer than recommended intervals, especially at night. If the patient is mildly wheezy, a pretreatment with Isuprel aerosol may allow cromolyn to be inhaled without provoking excessive cough or wheezing. Again, it must be stressed that cromolyn is *not* the treatment for an acute attack of asthma and should not be used in such circumstances.

The disadvantages of cromolyn are those inherent in any medicine that must be taken regularly even when "well," the inconvenience of doses during school time and at night, and the cost of the drug, all of which may seem either trivial or significant, depending on the patient's condition and personality.

ACUTE TREATMENT. Acute attacks of asthma are a medical emergency. It is imperative for physicians, nurses and parents to learn that the more promptly bronchospasm is relieved, the less medication will be required, the less heroic will treatment need to be, and the greater likelihood that relief will be complete. It is almost impossible for one who has not experienced acute severe air hunger to appreciate the anxiety and panic this produces. When this physiologic reaction is recognized and appreciated, asthmatics receive better care, and some of their demanding, anxious, clinging behavior is more easily understood and dispelled.

The objectives in treating acute asthma are the relief of bronchial obstruction (1) by bronchodilation, (2) by reduction of the edema of the mucous membranes and (3) by the removal of excess bronchial secretions, and the prevention and relief of fatigue. The drugs that serve these objectives—bronchodilators, expectorants and sedatives—are listed individually with 24-hour dosage instruction in Table 10.

Rapidly acting bronchodilators are the beta adrenergic catecholamines epinephrine (Adrenalin), isoetharine and isoproterenol. Another adrenergic drug that has been synthesized by substitution of the catechol group is metaproterenol (Metaprel, Alupent), which is a resorcinol derivative of isoproterenol. Terbutaline and fenoterol are derived from metaproterenol. Fenoterol, salbutamol (a saligenin derivative), and hexoprenaline (formed from two modified noradrenalin molecules) are not yet available for clinical use in the United States. There is much research activity in developing β_2-adrenergic compounds that will have enhanced rapidity of action, prolonged effect and minimal side-effects on tissues other than the bronchi, which are responsive to beta stimulation.

Ephedrine for many years was the only orally effective sympathomimetic bronchodilator that had any prolonged action. It is thought to act as a direct stimulator of beta receptors, displacing norepinephrine from neuronal stores. This accounts for its effect on blood vessels and its stimulation on the central nervous system. In some way its prolonged use tends to block the effect of epinephrine. It rates as a less potent bronchodilator than other beta adrenergic drugs or theophylline. Studies by Weinberger and others have emphasized the adverse effects of ephedrine combined with theophylline, citing animal studies of increased intoxication from the combination, and increased side-effects clinically. Many asthmatics who have obtained good relief from these combinations for years would disagree with these conclusions. These drugs are often supplemented or used in conjunction with xanthines, theophylline and theophylline ethylenediamine (aminophylline) because the latter are equally potent and have a longer-lasting bronchodilating effect. Tables 11 and 12 list some commonly used individual compounds with their trade

**TABLE 10. DOSAGES OF DRUGS COMMONLY USED FOR
ALLERGIC CHILDREN*†**

Drug		Dose	Warning
Bronchodilators			
Epinephrine hydrochloride (Adrenalin chloride)	USP	1:1000 aq. 0.01 ml./kg./*DOSE* (Max. 0.5 ml.) Repeat every 4 hrs. as necessary 1:100 aq. nebulizer as necessary 0.1 ml./dose/4 hrs. 1:200 aq. suspension 0.1–0.25 ml./dose/12 hrs. 1:500 oil 0.01–0.02 ml./kg. Daily or every 12 hrs. im.	*Vasopressor*
Ephedrine sulfate	USP NF	3 mg./kg./24 hrs. (max. 30 mg./dose) Divide in 4–6 doses (o., sq., or iv.) Syrup—4 mg./ml.	*Excitation*
Isoproterenol	USP, NNR	1:100 0.3 ml.; 1:200 0.5 ml.; 10%, 25% powder for inhalation, 3 × day 0.4 mg./kg./24 hrs. (o.), divide in 3 doses	*Palpitation*
Aminophylline (Theophylline ethylenediamine)	USP	15 mg./kg./24 hrs. Divide in 4 doses (iv., im., or o.) Rectal 2 × above	*Poisoning overdose*
Expectorants			
Iodides (saturated solution) potassium iodide	USP	1 drop/yr. of age (up to 15 yrs.)§ 3 × day in milk or water	*Nausea*
Guaiphenesin (Robitussin Syrup,‡ Glycotuss)		10 mg./kg./24 hrs. (o.), divide in 3–4 doses 20 mg./ml.	
Ipecac syrup	USP	5 drops first year of age§ 1 drop per year thereafter per dose May repeat in 2 hrs. (max. 0.5–2 ml.)	*Vomiting Poisoning*
Ammonium chloride	USP	75 mg./kg./24 hrs. Divide in 4 doses (o.) Give 1 glass water per dose	*Acidosis*
Sedatives			
Phenobarbital	USP	6 mg./kg./24 hrs. Divide in 3 doses (o., iv., or im.)	*Habituation Poisoning*
Chloral hydrate (Noctec)‡	USP	50 mg./kg./24 hrs. (max. 1 gm./dose) Divide 3–4 doses (o. or r.)	*Liver*

Key: o., oral; sq., subcutaneous; im., intramuscular; iv., intravenous; r., rectal.

*Vaughan, V. C., III, and McKay, R. J.: *Nelson Textbook of Pediatrics.* 10th ed. Philadelphia, W. B. Saunders Company, 1975, pp. 1755 and 1776.

†Goodman, L. S., and Gilman, A.: *Pharmacologic Basis of Therapeutics.* 5th Ed. New York, Macmillan, 1975.

‡From *Physician's Desk Reference.* Oradell, N. J., Medical Economics, Inc., 1976.

§Speer, F.: *The Allergic Child.* New York, Paul B. Hoeber, Inc., 1963.

names. (It is not feasible to list the prescription or over-the-counter antiasthmatic combinations of these drugs, since *Physician's Desk Reference* lists more than 250 now on the market.)

Subcutaneous doses of 0.1 ml. of epinephrine 1:1000 in aqueous solution will rapidly relieve most uncomplicated severe acute asthma; aminophylline (3 mg. per pound) given orally, rectally or

TABLE 11. DRUGS USED AS BRONCHODILATORS

Generic Name	Trade Name
Sympathicomimetic amines	
Epinephrine hydrochloride USP	Adrenalin
	Sus-Phrine
Ethyl-norepinephrine hydrochloride	Bronkephrine
Isoproterenol hydrochloride USP (14)*	Isuprel
	Aludrin (Aerolone)
	Proternol
Isoproterenol sulfate NNR	Medihaler-iso
	Norisodrine
Ephedrine hydrochloride NF	Ephedrine hydrochloride
Ephedrine sulfate USP (65)*	Isofedrol
	Ephedresol
Racephedrine hydrochloride NF	Ephoxamine
Phenylephrine hydrochloride USP (73)*	Neo-Synephrine
	Isophrine
Phenylpropanolamine NNR (42)*	Propadrine
Methoxyphenamine hydrochloride NNR	Orthoxine hydrochloride
Xanthines	
Theophylline USP (34)*	
Theophylline ethylenediamine USP (14)*	Aminophylline, Elixophyllin
Choline theophyllinate (oxtriphylline)	Choledyl
Theophylline monoethanolamine	Fleet-Theophylline
Theophylline sodium glycinate NF	Synophylate
Dyphylline	Dilor, Lufyllin, Neothylline

*( ) = Number of commercial preparations containing this drug as listed in *Physician's Desk Reference* (Oradell, N. J., Medical Economics, Inc., 1976).

intravenously as a single dose is equally effective. Isoproterenol either in solution (1:100 or 1:200) or as a dry powder is used by inhalation, and is also effective when absorbed sublingually. Oral administration of metaproterenol, terbutaline or ephedrine or one of their derivatives will usually relieve an attack of asthma at its onset or will control one that is moderate or mild. These drugs are also useful to maintain the brief relaxation effected by more potent and rapidly active bronchodilators such as epinephrine, aminophylline or isoproterenol. To counteract the stimulation and excitation that ephedrine may produce, it is usually combined with a sedative. One should never give morphine for a severe asthmatic attack, since this suppresses the respiratory center and has apparently supplied the coup de grâce in many reported fatal attacks of asthma. For the same reason and because of the ease of addiction, meperidine (Demerol) and the repeated use of other opiates, such as codeine, should be avoided.

The side-effects of all these bronchodilating compounds are excitation, nervousness, wakefulness, headache, tremor and tachycardia. Epinephrine and ephedrine raise blood pressure, and isoproterenol tends to produce flushing, palpitation and dizziness. The xanthines act as diuretics and gastric irritants, and they may cause vomiting and diarrhea. Since their effect is cumulative, intoxication from overdose may result in convulsions, in coma and sometimes in fatality (White and Daeschner, 1956).

Interest in and the use of xanthines as bronchodilators have increased in the past decade, after the period between 1955–1965, when reports of aminophylline toxicity and fatalities, particularly in children, made physicians hesitant to use the drugs at all or to use them in doses that were lower than those recommended when

TABLE 12.   NEW DRUGS FOR ASTHMA

Generic Name	Trade Name
Sympathicomimetic	
Beta adrenergic agonists	
Isoetharine	Bronkosol, Bronkometer
Metaproterenol	Alupent
	Metaprel
Terbutaline	Bricanyl
	Brethine
Salbutamol*	
Xanthines	
Theophylline (USP anhydrous)	Aerolate
	Theolair
	Slo-Phyllin
Theophylline ethylenediamine	Somophyllin
Oxtriphylline	Brondecon
Cromolyn sodium	Aarane
	Intal
	Lomudal†
Corticosteroid	
Beclomethasone	Vanceril
	Becotide†

*Not currently available for prescription in the United States. Others under investigation are soterenol, fenoterol and hexoprenaline.
†Trade names in Europe.

they were introduced for this purpose. Some of the observed adverse side-effects of nervousness, abdominal discomfort and nausea may have been due to their combination with ephedrine as noted in the study of Weinberger and Bronsky (1974). The rationale for combining these drugs was undoubtedly the clinical observation that theophylline would restore responsiveness to epinephrine in many "adrenalin-fast" patients. Theophylline is thought to act as a phosphodiesterase inhibitor in preventing the conversion of cyclic AMP to $3',5'$-AMP, thus increasing the intracellular concentration of cyclic AMP.

Average oral doses of the xanthines calculated as theophylline base are 5 mg. per kilogram every six hours (aminophylline equivalent is 85 per cent theophylline base) (Ellis and Eddy, 1974). These doses will usually result in a safe therapeutic blood level between 10 and 20 micrograms. Levels below this are apt to be ineffective; above this,

side-effects and toxic reactions are common. Since the advent of available methods for measuring theophylline serum and plasma levels, it has been shown that there is great individual variation in the blood levels and the duration of level from a given dose. Some persons metabolize the drug more rapidly or slowly than the average, and children metabolize 60 per cent more rapidly than adults. The average peak from a single oral dose occurs between 30 minutes and one hour (Welling and associates, 1976), and the half-life varies between four and seven hours (Maselli and coworkers, 1970; Ellis, 1975, Jenne, 1975).

Ellis (1975) has used 4 mg. aminophylline per kilogram of body weight as an intravenous bolus over four to five minutes in a study to compare the effect on airway obstruction of the same dose given over an eight-hour period. This showed superiority in relief of symptoms and the attainment of plasma theophylline levels of 10 micrograms per milliliter within five minutes, with a mean plasma half-life of 2½ hours. When given too rapidly or in too small a volume of fluid, aminophylline may cause an alarming drop in systolic blood pressure, and instances of sudden death due to cardiac arrest have been reported after rapid injection.

Jenne (1975) recommends injection of the loading dose in 50 ml. intravenous solute over a 15-minute period. We believe the dose of 2 to 2.5 mg. per pound should be given in a sufficient volume of fluid (5 per cent dextrose in ½ N saline) to require one-half hour for administration (in rare emergencies, as rapidly as 15 minutes). This should be followed by a continuous intravenous drip with 2 to 2.5 mg. aminophylline per pound of body weight added every six to eight hours, depending on the patient's clinical condition and blood theophylline levels. When rectal suppositories (Dees, 1943) or instillation is used, care must be taken that the rectum is empty in order for the drug to be absorbed promptly. Rectal doses of 3 mg. per pound every eight hours in children over four years of age are recommended; this usually affords effective and long-lasting relief. Rarely, a child will complain of local burning or pain in the legs after the use of suppositories.

Water, as steam and by mouth, is the most effective means of liquefying secretions. This must be constantly kept in mind, especially when the child is ill with acute, severe asthma, or when there has been a severe attack of asthma of several days' duration and he has become dehydrated. Expectorants are the usual type of drug used in both acute and chronic asthma to assist in the liquefying of secretions; the patient is thus more readily able to rid himself of these secretions by coughing them up. Those most useful are potassium iodide or other iodides, glyceryl guaiacolate (Guaiphenesin) and syrup of ipecac.

The variation and combination of proprietary antiasthmatic preparations is bewildering in number and complexity. Many pharmaceutical companies have added sedatives (chiefly barbiturates), antihistamines, and occasionally salicylates and corticosteroids. None of these offers any real, basic advantage over the simple drugs used alone or compounded to order, however, except possibly a minor economic one. Furthermore, they invite the hazard of prescribing by "name" and the danger of ordering an inflexible combination with possible excess of certain ingredients. If combined therapy is used, one should thoroughly familiarize himself with one or two combinations and use these whenever practical (Ellis and Eddy, 1974).

Relief of the symptoms of severe asthma was one of the first recognized clinical applications for the adrenal corticosteroid compounds. After the first flush of enthusiasm, however, there has been increased recognition of the occurrence of steroid dependency and undesirable side-effects; these include cushingoid changes, increased susceptibility to infection, arrest or retardation in growth, and rarely pseudotumor cerebri — all features that seriously detract from the general usefulness and safety of steroids for children (Dees and McKay, 1959).

The corticosteroids have almost completely supplanted the use of adrenocorticotropic hormone (ACTH) in the treatment of severe asthma. Many synthetic derivatives have been produced since compound E was identified and cortisone and hydrocortisone became available for clinical use (Table 13). These are prednisone, prednisolone and methyl prednisolone, which are preferable in asthma because they are short-acting in terms of adrenal suppression. Triamcinolone, betamethasone and dexamethasone are used in some instances because of their longer action, but this detracts from their usefulness when prolonged alternate-day therapy is required to control severe unremitting asthmatic disease, and growth suppression is undesirable.

Beclomethasone dipropionate (Van-

TABLE 13.   EQUIVALENT DOSES OF CORTICOSTEROIDS
USED IN ASTHMA*

Generic Name	Trade Name	Manufacturer
Cortisone acetate	Cortisone Acetate	Upjohn
25 mg.	Cortone Acetate	Merck Sharp & Dohme
Hydrocortisone	Hydrocortone	Merck Sharp & Dohme
20 mg.	Cortef	Upjohn
	Cortril	Pfizer
Prednisone	Meticorten	Schering
5 mg.	Deltasone	Upjohn
	Deltra	Merck Sharp & Dohme
	Delta-Dome	Dome Chemical
	Paracort	Parke Davis
	Prednisone	USV, Rexall
Prednisolone	Meticortelone	Schering
5 mg.	Delta-Cortef	Upjohn
	Sterane	Pfizer
	Hydeltra	Merck Sharp & Dohme
	Predne-Dome	Dome Chemical
	Prednisolone	USV, McKesson, Rexall
	Paracortol	Parke Davis
	Sterolone	Rowell
Methyl prednisolone	Medrol	Upjohn
4 mg.		
Triamcinolone	Aristocort	Lederle
4 mg.	Kenacort	Squibb
Betamethasone	Celestone	Schering
0.6 mg.		
Dexamethasone	Decadron	Merck Sharp & Dohme
0.75 mg.	Deronil	Schering
	Dexameth	USV
	Gammacorten	Ciba
	Hexadrol	Organon
Paramethasone acetate	Haldrone	Lilly
2 mg.		
Beclomethasone,	Vanceril	Schering
50 micrograms		

*From *Physician's Desk Reference*. Oradell, N. J., Medical Economics, Inc., 1976.

ceril, Becotide in England) is a halogenated corticosteroid recently released in the United States. It has a high degree of topical activity that allows a dose effective for asthma but that is insufficient to allow adrenal suppression from the swallowed or absorbed portion. The drug is not recommended for children under six years of age. For children six to 12 years of age, a dose of 50 to 100 micrograms in one to two inhalations from a pressurized nebulizer, three to four times daily, is used. Special warning and precautions are given to steroid-dependent patients for the maintenance of an adequate supportive level of systemic steroid while changing to beclomethasone; there should be slow gradual weaning, and large additional systemic steroid for stress periods, such as acute asthma, may be needed to prevent adrenal insufficiency. Deaths have occurred in patients in whom these precautions were not taken because inhaled beclomethasone has no appreciable systemic steroid effect. Oral and tracheal moniliasis has developed in some patients, and the long-term effect on airways and lungs and the immunologic response of these structures are not known. Unless these or other as yet unrecognized side-effects prove to be serious, the drug would appear to have an area of usefulness in certain pediatric patients (Francis, 1976).

The physiologic daily dose of cortisone, 25 mg., or 37.5 mg. of hydrocortisone, is equivalent to the biologic activity of 5 mg. of prednisone. In acute or chronic asthma an amount much larger than this is needed, and the dosage level should be whatever is required to control symptoms. We have employed the schedule used at the National Asthma Center, Denver (Chai, 1975), with a few slight modifications in children with severe acute asthma unresponsive to other therapy. This protocol begins with 20 to 40 mg. of prednisone per 24 hours, divided into two to four doses; rarely, some patients will require a larger initial dose. Once control is achieved, the dose is decreased 5 mg. twice daily every five to seven days, depending on the child's condition, until 20 mg. is reached. This amount is given at 8:00 A.M. once per day. Every three to five days thereafter, one decreases the dose by 5 mg. until the minimum effective level is reached.

An attempt to convert to alternate-day therapy is then made. This is done by tripling the minimum effective dose, which is given at 8:00 A.M. Once control on alternate-day treatment is achieved, one again tries to decrease this dose at two-week intervals to the minimum effective level. If breakthrough occurs during this process, it is necessary to return to the original 20 to 40 mg. per day for one to two days, rarely longer, to control asthma. When the child is symptom-free, one resumes the lowest previously effective alternate dose level. Further reduction should be tried periodically at monthly or longer intervals, depending on the stability of the patient's condition.

In such a program, the physician must remember that he not only is dealing with the problem of restoration of adrenal function, but is still faced with the need to control asthma, for which the steroids were prescribed in the first place. He must simultaneously insist on the use of bronchodilators and allergen control to the fullest extent. Many parents tend to forget all about the relief these measures can give or have given a child, and abandon them to rely solely on steroids. It is not uncommon to find that asthma is not as well controlled on the off-day as on the medication day, but this is not a reason to give up alternate-day therapy, since this does permit a normal growth rate in most children.

The mode of action of the corticosteroids in asthma is still unclear because of a multiplicity of hormonal effects, although much has been learned about their anti-inflammatory action. Some of those actions that relate to asthma are an increase in adenyl cyclase activity, a decrease in ATPase activity, and, questionably, a decrease in guanylate cyclase activity. Thus, in smooth muscle they increase sensitivity to alpha adrenergic stimulation in vascular tissue, while in bronchial tissue beta adrenergic stimulation is increased. In vivo they induce a decrease in phosphodiesterase activity in tissues, presumably allowing accumulation of cyclic AMP in cells. Other effects are an immediate leukopenia and fall in T and B lymphocytes, and decrease in mitogen response following a dose of corticosteroids. No direct effect on IgE production in humans has been established, but they may have a role in histamine and SRS–A metabolism. The corticosteroids may be implicated in prostaglandin metabolism, since some of their effects are similar. They may possibly interfere with replacement of prostaglandin synthetase, since prostaglandin $PGF_{2\alpha}$ causes bronchoconstriction, and with PGE_2 bronchodilation as well as cause a decrease in immunologic chemical mediators and lysozomal enzymes (Middleton, 1975).

STATUS ASTHMATICUS. The treatment of status asthmaticus must be individualized, since some patients are more acutely ill and refractory than are others because of complicating conditions, duration of the attack and previous medication. This must be ascertained at once from a brief history and physical examination. By definition, status asthmaticus is a continuous state of severe asthma, resistant to vigorous therapeutic measures and particularly to epinephrine injections. Therefore, it is usually useless to give more epinephrine or similar preparations, which may even have the paradoxical effect of increasing bronchospasm (Downes and coworkers, 1966; Lecks and coworkers, 1966; Wood and coworkers, 1968; Richards and Siegel, 1969). In the past few years much has been written about the management of status asthmaticus and acute respiratory failure in both children and adults (Downes and coworkers, 1966; Wood and coworkers, 1968; Reisman, 1968; Richards and Siegel, 1969; Cotton and Parry, 1975).

Criteria for respiratory failure have been stated to be any *two* of the following:

1. decreased or absent inspiratory breath sounds,
2. severe inspiratory retraction and use of accessory muscles,
3. cyanosis in 40 per cent oxygen,
4. depressed level of consciousness and response to pain,
5. poor skeletal muscle tone, plus an arterial P_{CO_2} of 65 mm. Hg or higher (Wood, 1969).

In most, if not all, of these patients, assisted ventilation is necessary to maintain life until the hypercapnia, hypoxia and acidosis can be corrected and epinephrine responsiveness is restored.

It has been found that volume type respirators (Emerson*; Engstrom†) are usually more satisfactory for children in status asthmaticus than pressure-cycled (Bird‡; Bennett§), since the volume-cycled machine ensures proper alveolar ventilation without overinflation of

---

*J. H. Emerson Company, Cambridge, Massachusetts.
†Schick X-ray Company, Chicago, Illinois.
‡Bird Corp., Palm Springs, California.
§Puritan-Bennett Company, Kansas City, Missouri.

open alveoli at periods of low resistance, and guards against high pressure caused by sudden obstruction.

In treating a child in status asthmaticus, it is imperative to monitor the arterial pH, P_{CO_2}, P_{O_2} and buffer base levels frequently, since it is now recognized that the clinical signs of cyanosis and respiratory rate disturbance may be misleading in not reflecting the gravity of the patient's condition. Cyanosis cannot be reliably detected until Pa_{O_2} falls below 50 mm. Hg, which is very near the critical level of Pa_{O_2} 30 to 40 mm. Hg, where irreversible damage from hypoxia will occur.

It is equally urgent to correct respiratory acidosis; this is done by alkalinization and, if necessary, by assisted ventilation. In so doing, "epinephrine-fastness" may be reversed in most patients. The increasing use of alkalis in status asthmaticus has undoubtedly saved many lives. Originally sodium lactate was used for this purpose, but at present sodium bicarbonate is preferred.

In desperate situations, the buffer THAM (tromethamine *tris* hydroxymethyl aminomethane) may be used to correct acidosis. Because of its potential to depress respiration, assisted ventilation should have been started or be instantly available. THAM (0.3 M) 1.5 mEq. per kilogram is given intravenously in the first ten minutes at a rate not over 10 ml. per minute, or slowly for one hour. This solution is prepared by dissolving one bottle in 1000 ml. distilled water or 5 per cent dextrose (0.3 mEq. per 1 ml.). The arterial blood pH must be monitored every 15 to 20 minutes, and THAM discontinued at pH 7.3 to avoid overalkalinizing the patient. The drug may cause respiratory depression, hypoglycemia, oliguria and tissue slough if extravasated. In spite of these drawbacks and the precautions necessary for its use, it is a most effective alkalinizing agent when the desired result has not been accomplished by bicarbonate.

The formula generally selected for calculating the dose of alkalinizing agents to raise the pH above 7.25 is:

BE (base excess) × body weight (kg.) × 0.3
= mEq. alkalinizing agent

This is then followed by additional bicarbonate at the rate of 1 mEq. per kilogram per day in the intravenous fluid to keep the pH at 7.25 to 7.45 (Wood and coworkers, 1968).

Richards and Siegel (1969) prefer Kaplan's (1962) formula because patients with acute respiratory acidosis may have a normal base excess. This formula is:

1.5 × body weight (kg.) =
mEq. alkalinizing agent/hour,

with the initial dose given rapidly in ten minutes or over one hour, depending on the patient's condition. Additional alkali is given based on the response and conditions.

Isoproterenol administered by continuous intravenous infusion has been established as an additional step in the medical management of impending respiratory failure in status asthmaticus not responding to aminophylline, steroids or alkalinization, and may prevent the need for assisted ventilation (Wood and Downes, 1973). The infusion is administered by slow infusion pump (Harvard, Holter, Sigma motor) as a solution of 10 micrograms per milliliter isoproterenol, at an initial dose of 0.1 microgram per kilogram per minute, and is increased by 0.1 to 0.2 microgram per kilogram per minute every 15 to 20 minutes to the maximum dose recommended by Downes (3.5 micrograms per kilogram per minute). The increases are determined by Pa_{CO_2} changes, by the pulse rate, which should not rise above 200 per minute, or by the development of arrhythmias, which require reduction or discontinuation of the medication. The electrocardiogram, Pa_{CO_2} Pa_{O_2} and pH must be continuously monitored, and the infusion usually must be maintained for an average of 48 hours, or at least 12 hours, and has been used as long as six days. When the Pa_{CO_2} has stabilized at 36 to 40 mm. Hg, the Pa_{O_2} has stabilized at 80 to 100 mg. Hg and the pH is at a normal range, the process of weaning off the isoproterenol infusion is started by lowering the dose by 0.1 microgram per kilogram per minute every one to two hours. In the series of Wood and

---

TABLE 14. PROGRAM FOR DIAGNOSTIC AND MONITORING PROCEDURES IN STATUS ASTHMATICUS

Brief history: Medications used for this attack.
Aminophylline, theophylline, amount? On steroids? Which? Amount? How long? On antibiotics? Fluids? Vomiting? Any drug allergy?

Brief physical examination: Type, depth of respiration, breath sounds, include eye grounds for papilledema, note sensorium, muscle tone.

Immediate hospitalization: Attendant continuously; vital signs (T.P.R., BP, weight if possible). Repeat T.P.R., BP at least hourly. Fluid intake and output recorded.

Laboratory tests on admission:
Blood count, urinalysis.
Arterial blood gases and pH *stat* and hourly or at less frequent intervals as indicated by condition.
Blood electrolytes *stat* and as indicated, usually every four to eight hours while acutely ill.
Culture (Gram stain) nasopharynx, or sputum. **Caution:** tracheal aspiration may increase acute laryngospasm.
Stool specimen for blood if steroids used.

Chest roentgenogram, posteroanterior and lateral (portable, if necessary).

EKG if cardiac strain suspected, continuous recording if intravenous isoproterenol used.

Defer any optional tests or procedures while patient is acutely ill.

Downes, intravenous isoproterenol effectively reversed respiratory failure of status asthmaticus in 90 per cent of the patients treated; in another series it was successful in 27 of 35 patients who otherwise would have required assisted ventilation (Cotton and Parry, 1975). The toxic effects of isoproterenol, chiefly arrhythmias and cardiac arrest, have occurred most often in adolescents and adults.

When respirator therapy is necessary, the patient must be prevented from "fighting" the respirator. An endotracheal or nasotracheal intubation or tracheostomy is carried out, and muscle paralysis is usually obtained by tubocurare or succinyl-choline chloride. For this procedure one must have not only the proper blood gas–pH monitoring but also an experienced team consisting of anesthetist, inhalation therapist, and nurse as well as the primary physician, all of whom must be in constant attendance until the attack is controlled.

The procedures for monitoring and treating a child with status asthmaticus and respiratory failure have been evolved from the bitter experience of many physicians. In brief outline, to be used as a guide, these are shown in Tables 14 and 15.

We have gained the impression in the past few years that there is a general increase in understanding and familiarity among physicians and hospital staffs of danger signals in status asthmaticus, and of the methods for combating them. That this may be effecting a more favorable outcome for some severely ill patients is indicated by some recent reports analyzing death from asthma, and in our own experience (Palm and associates, 1970; Buranakul and coworkers, 1974).

As the attack subsides, one may change to oral administration of fluids and medication, utilize postural drainage and breathing exercises to help remove secretion, and discontinue steroids and other heroic treatment as rapidly as feasible. No attempt should be made to perform diagnostic allergy tests immediately after an episode of status asthmaticus, since the results will probably be unreliable, owing to unreactive skin. There seems to be a tendency for certain children to have repeated attacks of status asthmaticus; in some no obvious irritating cause can be found, and in others localized lung disease is discovered after careful investigation.

At the earliest opportune time, these children should undergo a thorough allergic study and be started on appropriate treatment to prevent recurrence. There is no more alarming situation than status asthmaticus, nor one which calls for more prompt, persistent, coordinated treatment or constant vigilance from medical personnel, who must conceal their own anxiety from the frightened child and family in order to be effective.

Summary

It should be apparent at this point that asthma embraces more than one disease and that the gamut of the clinical syndrome — its pathophysiology, etiology and immunology — embraces many different disciplines. The various approaches to comprehensive treatment and management, about which we know a great deal without fully understanding the fundamental causes of allergy, are complex. The physician dealing with asthma must be a "jack-of-all-trades," able to change tempo in a moment from the considered atmosphere of the consultation room to the supercharged tension of emergency surgery.

Fresh approaches in research into the nature of asthma must be found. Parents must be encouraged to take a middle course in their attitudes between overprotection and freedom. The severely involved child must be treated supportively with relief from his anxiety, while he is simultaneously being taught to care for himself within his limitations. Finally, the general public, educators and public health officials must be educated about asthma and its

TABLE 15. TREATMENT OF STATUS ASTHMATICUS

A. *Moderately severe* (P_{O_2} above 60 mm. Hg, P_{CO_2} below 65 mm. Hg, arterial pH 7.38 or above)
1. Nothing by mouth except clear liquid, if condition permits. Immediate intravenous fluid to correct dehydration, to liquefy secretion, and to provide route for medication, 5 per cent dextrose in ½ N saline. (See B for alkalinizing agents.)
2. Administer moist oxygen by tent 8 liters per minute, by plastic face mask 4 liters per minute, by nasal cannula 8 to 10 liters per minute.
3. Bronchodilator
    a. Aminophylline intravenously 4 mg. per kg. body weight in 100 ml. of 5 per cent dextrose in ½ N saline in 15 to 30 minutes. Repeat in 6 to 8 hours. (If patient has had aminophylline in previous 8 hours, use 2 mg. per kg.) Omit if there are any toxic symptoms.
    b. Isoproterenol (1:200) 0.25 to 0.5 ml. in 1.5 ml. saline aerosol by face mask or IPPB every 4 hours.
4. Corticosteroids
    a. Solu-Cortef, 100 mg., intravenously every 4 to 6 hours as needed, or equivalent amount of other corticosteroids (less desirable).
5. Mild sedation for agitation *not* due to hypoxia
    a. Chloral hydrate, 15 mg. per kg., orally or rectally or
    b. Librium, 10 mg., intramuscularly, or dose appropriate to age, for children over six years.
6. Antibiotics—selection as indicated for infection
7. Expectorants
    a. Sodium iodide intravenously, 25 mg. per kg. per 24 hours; give over 4-hour period once daily.
    b. Syrup of ipecac, 5 drops age 1 year, over 1 year add 1 drop per year of age to maximum of 10 drops. May repeat in 2 hours if patient is not vomiting.

B. *Severe* (not improved by the above treatment) (P_{O_2} 60 mm. Hg or less, P_{CO_2} 65 mm. Hg or above, arterial pH 7.28 to 7.38. Clinical condition: restless, mental confusion, respiration irregular, decreasing breath sounds, cyanosis)
1. Correct acidosis
    General formula: amount alkalinizing agent in mEq. =
    (a) $1.5 \times$ body weight (kg.) *per hour*
                                      or
    (b)   B.E. (base excess) $\times$ body weight (kg.) $\times 0.3$
    a. Na bicarbonate intravenously, calculate dose by (a) or (b) above, give in first 10 minutes to 1 hour. Continue with same amount in next 1 to 4 hours, maximum 7 mEq. per kg. per 24 hours. (Na bicarbonate 7.5 per cent solution equals 0.9 mEq. per 1 ml.)
2. Correct hypoxia
    Clean airway with gentle suction, use continuous moist O_2
    b. IPPB with saline—see part A-3 for isoproterenol.

C. *Respiratory failure* (P_{O_2} below 50 mm. Hg, P_{CO_2} above 65 mm. Hg, arterial pH below 7.2 to 7.25. Clinical state: as in B plus patient is unresponsive to pain and has poor muscle tone)
1. Intravenous isoproterenol infusion
    Dosage 0.1 microgram/kg./min. initial dose; increased by 0.1–0.2 microgram/kg./min. every 15–20 minutes, to maximum of 3.5 micrograms/kg./min. (Isuprel 0.5 mg. per 50 ml. fluid Voluset equals 10 micrograms/ml.). Monitor EKG, pulse > 200, arrhythmia, discontinue. If Pa_{CO_2} increases, increase dose (see text).
    Be ready to start assisted ventilation at once if respirations are depressed.
2. Controlled or assisted ventilation
    Intubate or do tracheostomy, give 100 per cent moist O_2 during preceding 3 to 5 minutes, preferably done in operating room if unresponsive to action suggested above.
    Obtain complete muscle relaxation in 3 to 4 minutes with one of the following:
    (a) succinylcholine Cl 2 mg. per kg. intramuscularly, or
    (b) tubocurare Cl 0.4 mg. per kg. intramuscularly, or
    (c) gallamine 1 mg. per kg. intramuscularly
    Attach endotracheal, nasotracheal, or tracheostomy tube to respirator, preferably volume-controlled. Check patient's tolerance for unassisted ventilation hourly.
3. Digitalis
    If cardiac failure or strain is present, EKG changes, liver is enlarged or tender, tachycardia is increased.

problems and informed of the heavy toll that illness from asthma takes from school children and young adults in their most productive years.

REFERENCES

Aas, K.: Prognosis for allergic children. *Acta Paediatr. (Stockholm)*, 87 (Suppl. 140):81, 1963; *Pediatrics*, 21:980, 1958.

Ahlquist, R. P.: Study of adrenotropic receptors, *J. Physiol.*, 153:586, 1948.

Alexander, H. L.: A historical account of deaths from asthma. *J. Allergy*, 34:305, 1963.

Allen, J. C., and Kunkel, H. G.: Antibodies to genetic types of gamma globulin after multiple transfusions. *Science*, 139:419, 1963.

Altounyan, R. E. C.: Inhibition of experimental asthma by a new compound—disodium cromoglycate "Intal." *Acta. Allerg.*, 22:485, 1967.

Bates, D. V., Macklem, P. T., and Christie, R. V.: *Respiratory Function in Disease*. 2nd Ed. Philadelphia, W. B. Saunders Company, 1971.

Bierman, C. W., and Pierson, W.E.: Symposium on exercise and asthma. *Pediatrics*, 56(Suppl. 2):843, 950, 1975.

Bierman, C. W., Pierson, W. E., and Shapiro, G. G.: The pharmacological assessment of single drugs and drug combinations in exercise-induced asthma. *Pediatrics*, 56 (Suppl. 2):919, 1975.

Blackhall, M. I.: Ventilatory function in subjects with childhood asthma who have become symptom free. *Arch. Dis. Child.*, 45:363, 1970.

Bray, G. W.: *Recent Advances in Allergy*. 3rd Ed. Philadelphia, Blakiston, 1937.

Brocklehurst, W. E.: A slow-reacting substance in anaphylaxis—"SRS-A." In Wolstenholme, G. E. W., and O'Connor, C. A., (Eds.): *Ciba Foundation Symposium: Jointly with the Physiological Society and the British Pharmacological Society on Histamine: Honouring Sir Henry Dale*. Boston, Little, Brown & Company, 1956.

Brocklehurst, W. E.: Histamine and other mediators in hypersensitivity reactions. In Halpern, B. N., and Holtzer, A. (Eds.): *Reports of the Third International Congress of Allergology*. Paris, Flammarion, 1958.

Broder, L., Higgins, M. W., Mathews, K. P., and Kelles, J. B.: Epidemiology of asthma and allergic rhinitis in a total community, Tecumseh, Michigan. III. Second survey of the community. *J. Allergy Clin. Immunol.*, 53:127, 1974.

Buffum, W. P.: The prognosis of asthma in infancy. *Pediatrics*, 32:453, 1963.

Buffum, W. P., and Settipane, G. A.: Prognosis of asthma in childhood. *Am. J. Dis. Child.*, 112:214, 1966.

Buranakul, B., Washington, J., Hillman, B., Mancuso, J., and Sly, R. M.: Causes of death during acute asthma in children. *Am. J. Dis. Child.*, 128:343, 1974.

Caplin, I., and Haynes, J. T.: Complications of aerosol therapy in asthma. *Ann. Allergy*, 27:65, 1969.

Chaffee, F. H., and Settipane, G. A.: Aspirin intolerance. I. Frequency in an allergy population. *J. Allergy Clin. Immunol.*, 53:193, 1974.

Chai, H.: Management of severe chronic perennial asthma in children. *Adv. Asthma Allergy*, 2:1, 1975.

Coca, A. F., and Cooke, R. A.: On the classification of the phenomena of hypersensitiveness. *J. Immunol.*, 8:163, 1923.

Comroe, J. H.: *Physiology of Respiration*. Chicago, Year Book Publishers, Inc., 1965.

Comroe, J. H., and others: *The Lung*. 2nd Ed. Chicago, Year Book Publishers, Inc., 1962.

Connell, J. T.: Asthmatic deaths, role of the mast cell. *J.A.M.A.*, 215:769, 1971.

Cooke, R. A.: *Allergy in Theory and Practice*. Philadelphia, W. B. Saunders Company, 1947, p. 139.

Cooke, R. A., and Vander Veer, A.: Human sensitization. *J. Immunol.*, 1:201, 1916.

Cooke, R. A., Barnard, J. H., Hebald, S., and Stull, A.: Serological evidence of immunity with coexisting sensitization in a type of human allergy (hay fever). *J. Exp. Med.*, 62:733, 1935.

Cotton, E. K., and Parry, W.: Treatment of status asthmaticus and respiratory failure. *Pediatr. Clin. North Am.*, 22:163, 1975.

Crawford, J. D., and others: Observations of a metabolic lesion in cow's milk allergy. *Pediatrics*, 22:122, 1958.

Crook, W. G.: The allergic tension-fatigue syndrome. In Speer, F. (Ed.): *The Allergic Child*. New York, Paul B. Hoeber, Inc., 1963, Chapter 21.

Dees, S. C.: The use of aminophylline rectal suppositories in treatment of bronchial asthma. *J. Allergy*, 14:492, 1943.

Dees, S. C.: Development and course of asthma in children. *Am. J. Dis. Child.*, 93:228, 1957.

Dees, S. C.: Infection and the allergic child. *Va. Med. Mon.*, 87:607, 1960.

Dees, S. C.: Asthma in infants and young children. *J.A.M.A.*, 175:362, 1961.

Dees, S. C.: The role of gastroesophageal reflux in nocturnal asthma in children. *N. C. Med. J.*, 35:230, 1974.

Dees, S. C., and McKay, H. W.: Occurrence of pseudotumor cerebri (benign intracranial hypertension) during treatment of children with asthma by adrenal steroids. *Pediatrics*, 23:1143, 1959.

Dennis, E. V., Hornbrook, M. M., and Ishizaka, K.: Serum proteins in sputum of patients with asthma. *J. Allergy*, 35:464, 1964.

Downes, J. J., Wood, D. W., Striker, T. W., and Lecks, H. I.: Diagnosis and treatment: advances in the management of status asthmaticus in children. *Pediatrics*, 38:286, 1966.

Drazen, J. M.: In vivo effect of humoral mediators. In Stein, M. (Ed.): *New Directions in Asthma*. Park Ridge, Ill., American College of Chest Physicians, 1975, pp. 251–260.

Dunand, P., Cropp, G. J. A., and Middleton, E.,

Jr.: Severe obstructive lung disease in a 14 year old girl with alpha-1-antitrypsin deficiency. *J. Allergy Clin. Immunol., 57*:615, 1976.

Dunnill, M. S., Massarallo, G. R., and Anderson, J.: A comparison of the quantitative anatomy of the bronchi in normal subjects, in status asthmaticus, in chronic bronchitis and emphysema. *Thorax, 24*:176, 1969.

Ellis, E. F.: Asthma in childhood: clinical pharmacology of theophylline in asthmatic children. In Stein, M. (Ed.): *New Directions in Asthma.* Park Ridge, Ill., American College of Chest Physicians, 1975, pp. 317–324.

Ellis, E. F., and Eddy, E. D.: Anhydrous theophylline equivalents of commercial theophylline formulations. *J. Allergy Clin. Immunol., 53*:116, 1974.

Engström, I.: Respiratory studies in children. XI. Mechanics of breathing, lung volumes and ventilatory capacity in asthmatic children from attack to symptom-free status. *Acta Paediatr.,* Suppl. 155, 1964.

Engström, I.: Respiratory studies in children. XII. Serial studies of mechanics, breathing, lung volumes and ventilatory capacity in provoked asthmatic attacks. *Acta Paediatr., 53*:345, 1964.

Eppinger, H., and Hess, L.: *Vagotonia; a Clinical Study in Vegetative Neurology.* 2nd Ed. New York, Nervous and Mental Diseases Publishing Co., 1917. (Nervous and mental disease monograph series, No. 20.).

Eriksson, S.: Pulmonary emphysema and alpha-1-antitrypsin deficiency. *Acta Med. Scand., 175*:197, 1964; Suppl. 177, 1965.

Falliers, C. J.: Corticosteroids and anabolic hormones for childhood asthma. *Clin. Pediatr., 4*:441, 1965.

Falliers, C. J.: Aspirin and subtypes of asthma: risk factor analysis. *J. Allergy Clin. Immunol., 52*:141, 1973.

Farr, R. S.: The need to reevaluate acetylsalicylic acid (aspirin): *J. Allergy, 45*:321, 1970.

Francis, R. S.: Long-term beclomethasone dipropionate aerosol therapy in juvenile asthma. *Thorax, 31*:309, 1976.

Freeman, G. L., and others: Allergic diseases in adolescents. I. Description of survey; prevalence of allergy. *Am. J. Dis. Child., 107*:548, 1964.

Freeman, G. L., and others: Allergic diseases in adolescents. II. Changes in allergic manifestations during adolescence. *Am. J. Dis. Child., 107*:560, 1964.

Fuchs, A. M., and Strauss, M. B.: The clinical evaluation and the preparation and standardization of suspension of a new water-insoluble whole ragweed pollen complex. *J. Allergy, 30*:66, 1959.

Godfrey, S., and König, P.: Exercise-induced bronchial lability in wheezy children and their families. *Pediatrics, 56* (Suppl. 2):851, 1975.

Graff-Lonnevig, V., and Kraepelien, S.: Asthma mortality in Sweden among children and adolescents during the period 1952–1972. *Acta Allergol., 31*:159, 1976.

Grieco, M. H.: Current concepts of the pathogenesis and management of asthma. *Bull. N. Y. Acad. Med., 46*:597, 1970.

Halpern, S., and others: Practical tips on aerosol therapy in asthma. *Am. J. Dis. Child., 107*:280, 1964.

Hamman, R. F., Halil, T., and Holland, W. W.: Asthma in school children. *Br. J. Prev. Soc. Med., 29*:228, 1975.

Hansel, F. K.: *Allergy of the Nose and Paranasal Sinuses.* St. Louis, C. V. Mosby Company, 1936.

Hermance, W. E., and Brown, E. A.: Long-term use of disodium cromoglycate in bronchial asthma. *Ann. Allergy, 36*:423, 1976.

Ishizaka, K., and Ishizaka, T.: Human reaginic antibodies and immunoglobulin E. *J. Allergy, 42*:330, 1968.

Ishizaka, K., and Ishizaka, T.: The significance of immunoglobulin E in reaginic hypersensitivity. *Ann. Allergy, 28*:189, 1970.

Ishizaka, K., and Ishizaka, T.: Immunoglobulin E. Current studies and clinical laboratory applications. *Arch. Pathol. Lab. Med., 100*:289, 1976.

Jenne, J. W.: Rationale for methylxanthines in asthma. In Stein, M. (Ed.): *New Directions in Asthma.* Park Ridge, Ill., American College of Chest Physicians, 1975, pp. 391–414.

Johansson, S. G. O.: Immunological studies of an atypical (myeloma) globulin. *Immunology, 13*:381, 1967.

Johnson, T. F., Reismann, R. E., Arbesman, C. E., Mattar, A. G., and Murphey, W. H.: Obstructive airway disease associated with heterozygous alpha-1-antitrypsin deficiency. *J. Allergy Clin. Immunol., 58*:69, 1976.

Jones, R. S., and Blackhall, M. I.: Role of disodium cromoglycate ("Intal") in treatment of childhood asthma. *Arch. Dis. Child., 45*:49, 1970.

Kallós, P., and Waksman, B. H. (Eds.): *Progress in Allergy,* Vols. I–XIV. Basel, S. Karger, 1965.

Kaplan, S., Fox, P. P., and Clark, L.: Aminobuffers in the management of acidosis. *Am. J. Dis. Child., 103*:4, 1962.

Kassirer, J. P., and Bleich, H. L.: Rapid estimation of plasma carbon dioxide tension from pH and total carbon dioxide content. *N. Engl. J. Med., 272*:1067, 1965.

Katz, R. M., Lieberman, J., and Siegel, S. C.: Alpha-1-antitrypsin levels and prevalence of Pi variant phenotypes in asthmatic children. *J. Allergy Clin. Immunol., 57*:41, 1976.

Katz, R. M., Siegel, S. C., and Rachelefsky, G. S.: Blood gas in exercise-induced bronchospasm: a review. *Pediatrics, 56* (Suppl. 2):880, 1975.

Keal, E. E., and Reid, L.: Pathologic alterations in mucus in asthma within and without the cell. In Stein, M. (Ed.): *New Directions in Asthma.* Park Ridge, Ill., American College of Chest Physicians, 1975, pp. 223–240.

Keeney, E. L.: The pathology of corticosteroid-treated asthma. *J. Allergy, 36*:97, 1965.

Kieghley, J. F.: Iatrogenic asthma associated with adrenergic aerosols. *Ann. Intern. Med., 65*:985, 1966.

Kraepelien, S.: Prognosis of asthma in childhood,

with special reference to pulmonary function and the value of specific hyposensitization. *Acta Paediatr.*, 87(Suppl 140):92, 1963.

Kraepelien, S., Engström, I., and Karlberg, P.: Respiratory studies in children. II. Lung volumes in symptom-free asthmatic children, 6–14 years of age. *Acta Paediatr.*, 47:399, 1958.

Kravis, L. P., and Lecks, H. I.: Therapeutic aerosols in childhood asthma. A review with clinical observations on two new preparations. *Clin. Pediatr.*, 4:193, 1965.

Laurell, C. B., and Eriksson, S.: The electrophoretic alpha-1 globulin pattern of serum in alpha-1-antitrypsin deficiency. *Scand. J. Clin. Lab. Invest.*, 15:132, 1963.

Lavin, N., Rachelefsky, G. S., and Kaplan, S. A.: An action of disodium cromoglycate: inhibition of cyclic 3′,5′-AMP phosphodiesterase. *J. Allergy Clin. Immunol.*, 57:80, 1976.

Lecks, H. I., Wood, D. W., and Kravis, L.: Childhood status asthmaticus, recent clinical and laboratory observations and their application in treatment. *Clin. Pediatr.*, 5:209, 1966.

Logan, G. B.: Mechanism of the immediate allergic reaction and some therapeutic implications, *Am. J. Dis. Child.*, 97:163, 1959.

Logan, G. B.: Steps toward a better understanding of the acute allergic reaction. *Ann. Allergy*, 18:17, 1960.

Loveless, M. H.: Repository injections in pollen allergy, *J. Immunol.*, 79:68, 1957.

Macdonald, J. B., Seaton, A., and Williams, D. A.: Asthma deaths in Cardiff 1963–1974: 90 deaths outside hospital. *Br. Med. J.*, 1:1493, 1976.

Marks, M. B.: Significance of discoloration in the lower orbitopalpebral grooves in allergic children (allergic shiners). *Ann. Allergy.* 21:26, 1963.

Mascia, A. V., Friedman, E. A., Jr., and Kornfield, M. A.: Clinical experience with long-term cromolyn sodium administration in 53 asthmatic children. *Ann. Allergy*, 37:1, 1976.

Maselli, R., Casel, G. L., and Ellis, E. F.: Pharmacologic effects of intravenously administered aminophylline in asthmatic children. *J. Pediatr.*, 76:777, 1970.

Mendes, E., and others: Immunochemical studies of the asthmatic sputum. *Acta Allergol.*, 18:17, 1963.

Mercer, T. T., and others: Output characteristics of several commercial nebulizers. *Ann. Allergy*, 23:314, 1965.

Middleton, E., Jr.: Mechanism of action of corticosteroids. In Stein, M. (Ed.): *New Directions in Asthma.* Park Ridge, Ill., American College of Chest Physicians, 1975, pp. 433–447.

Miller, F. F.: Eosinophilia in the allergic population. *Ann. Allergy*, 23:177, 1965.

Morse, J. O., Lebowitz, M. D., Knudson, R. J., and Burrows, B.: A community study of the relation of alpha-1-antitrypsin levels to obstructive lung disease. *N. Engl. J. Med.*, 292:278, 1975.

Nathanson, C. A., and Rhyne, M. B.: Social and cultural factors associated with asthmatic symptoms in children. *Soc. Sci. Med.*, 4:293, 1970.

Nemoto, T., Aoki, H., Ike, A., Yamada, K., Kondo, T., Kobayski, S., and Inagawa, I.: Serum prostaglandin levels in asthmatic patients. *J. Allergy Clin. Immunol.*, 57:89, 1976.

Noon, L.: Prophylactic inoculation against hayfever. *Lancet*, 1:1572, 1911.

Norman, P. S., Winkenwerder, W. L., and Lichtenstein, L. M.: Immunotherapy of hay fever with ragweed antigen E: comparison with whole pollen extract and placebos. *J. Allergy*, 42:93, 1968.

Palm, C. R., et al.: A review of asthma admissions and deaths at children's hospital of Pittsburgh from 1935–1968. *J. Allergy*, 46:257, 1970.

Patterson, J. W., et al.: Isoprenaline resistance and the use of pressurized aerosols in asthma. *Lancet*, 2:426, 1968.

Pecora, L. J., and Bernstein, I. L.: Pulmonary diffusing capacity in children with intractable asthma with and without chronic hyperinflation of the lung. *J. Allergy*, 35:479, 1964.

Pepys, J., and Frankland, A. W.: *Disodium Cromoglycate in Allergic Airway Disease.* London, Butterworth & Company, 1970.

Poppius, H., et al.: Exercise asthma and disodium chromoglycate. *Br. Med. J.*, 4:337, 1970.

Rackemann, F. M.: Intrinsic asthma. *J. Allergy*, 11:147, 1940.

Rackemann, F. M., and Edwards, M. C.: Medical progress; asthma in children; follow-up study of 688 patients after interval of 20 years. *N. Engl. J. Med.*, 246:815; 858, 1952.

Rapaport, H. G., Appel, S. J., and Szanton, V. L.: Incidence of allergy in a pediatric population. Pilot survey of 2169 children. *Ann. Allergy*, 18:45, 1960.

Ratner, B., Crawford, L. V., and Flynn, J. A.: Allergy in the infant and preschool child. *Am. J. Dis. Child.*, 91:593, 1956.

Reisman, R. E.: Asthma induced by adrenergic aerosols. *J. Allergy*, 46:162, 1970.

Reisman, R. E., Friedman, I., and Arbesman, C. E.: Severe status asthmaticus; prolonged treatment with assisted ventilation. *J. Allergy*, 41:37, 1968.

Richards, W., and Patrick, J. R.: Death from asthma in children. *Am. J. Dis. Child.*, 110:4, 1965.

Richards, W., and Siegel, S. C.: Status asthmaticus. *Pediatr. Clin. North Am.*, 16:9, 1969.

Ryssing, E., and Flensborg, E. W.: Prognosis after puberty for 442 asthmatic children examined and treated on specific allergologic principles. *Acta Paediatr.*, 52:97, 1963.

Salvato, G.: Some histological changes in chronic bronchitis and asthma. *Thorax*, 23:168, 1968.

Samter, M.: Intolerance to aspirin. *Hosp. Pract.*, 8:85, 1973.

Sanerkin, N. G.: Causes and consequences of airways obstruction in bronchial asthma. *Ann. Allergy*, 28:528, 1970.

Schiffer, C. G., and Hunt, E. P.: Illness among children (data from U. S. National Health Survey). Children's Bureau Publ. No. 405. Washington, D. C., U. S. Dept. of Health, Education and Welfare, 1963.

Selye, H.: *The Mast Cells*. London, Butterworth & Company, 1965.

Settipane, G. A., and Pudapakkan, R. K.: Aspirin intolerance. III. Subtypes, familial occurrence and cross reaction with tartrazine. *J. Allergy Clin. Immunol.*, 56:215, 1975.

Sheffer, A. L., Rocklin, R. E., and Goetzl, E. J.: Immunologic components of hypersensitivity reaction to cromolyn sodium. *N. Engl. J. Med.*, 293:1220, 1975.

Shelley, W. B.: The circulating basophile as an indicator of hypersensitivity in man. *Arch. Dermatol. Syph.*, 88:759, 1963.

Smith, J. M.: A five-year prospective survey of rural children with asthma and hay fever. *J. Allergy*, 47:23, 1971.

Smith, J. M.: Incidence of atopic disease. *Med. Clin. North Am.*, 58:3, 1974.

Smith, J. M., and Devey, G. F.: Clinical trial of disodium cromoglycate in the treatment of children with asthma. *Br. Med. J.*, 2:340, 1968.

Spain, W. C., and Cooke, R. A.: Studies in specific hypersensitiveness. II. The familial occurrence of hay fever and bronchial asthma. *J. Immunol.*, 9:521, 1924.

Speizer, F. E.: Deaths from asthma. *Rev. Allergy*, 23:132, 1969.

Speizer, F., Doll, R., and Heaf, P.: Investigations into the use of drugs preceding death from asthma. *Br. Med. J.*, 1:339, 1968.

Spock, A.: Growth patterns in 200 asthmatic children. *Ann. Allergy*, 23:608, 1965.

Stiehm, E. R., and Fudenberg, H. H.: Antibodies to gamma globulin in infants and children exposed to isologous gamma globulin. *Pediatrics*, 35:229, 1965.

Stolley, P. D.: Asthma mortality. *Am. Rev. Resp. Dis.*, 105:883, 1972.

Szczeklik, A., Gryglewski, R. J., Czermawska-Mysik, G., and Zmuda, A.: Aspirin-induced asthma. *J. Allergy Clin. Immunol.*, 58:10, 1976.

Szentivanyi, A.: The beta adrenergic theory of the atopic abnormality in bronchial asthma. *J. Allergy*, 42:203, 1968.

Taylor, G. J., IV, and Harris, W. S.: Cardiac toxicity of aerosol propellants. *J.A.M.A.*, 2414:136, 1970.

U. S. Dept. of Health, Education and Welfare: Vital statistics of the United States. Vol. IIA. Washington, D. C., 1967, 1972.

Van Metre, T. E., Jr.: Adverse effects of inhaling excessive amounts of nebulized isoproterenol in status asthmaticus. *J. Allergy*, 43:101, 1969.

Van Metre, T. E., and Pinkerton, H. L., Jr.: Growth suppression in asthmatic children receiving prolonged therapy with prednisone or methylprednisone. *J. Allergy*, 30:103, 1959.

von Mauer, K., Adkinson, N. F., Van Metre, T. E., Jr., Marsh, D., and Norman, P. S.: Aspirin intolerance in a family. *J. Allergy Clin. Immunol.*, 54:380, 1974.

Voorhorst, R.: *Basic Facts of Allergy*. Leiden, H. E. Stenfert, Kroese N. V., 1962.

Voorhorst, R., Spieksma, F., Th. M., and Varekamp, H.: *House Dust Atopy and the House Dust Mite*, Dermatophagoides pternyssinus. Leiden, Staflen, 1969.

Weinberger, M. M., and Bronsky, E. A.: Oral bronchodilator therapy. *J. Allergy Clin. Immunol.*, 53:78, 1974.

Welling, P. G., Domeradzki, J., Sims, J. A., and Reed, C. E.: Influence of formulation on bioavailability of theophylline. *J. Clin. Pharmacol.*, 16:43, 1976.

White, B. H., and Daeschner, C. W.: Aminophylline poisoning in children. *J. Pediatr.*, 49:262, 1956.

Wilken-Jensen, K.: Prognosis of asthma in childhood. *Acta Paediatr.*, 87(Suppl. 140):90, 1963.

Williams, H., and McNicol, K. N.: Prevalence, natural history, and relationship of wheezing bronchitis and asthma in children. *Br. Med. J.*, 4:321, 1969.

Wood, D. W.: Pulmonary function testing in children. *Pediatr. Clin. North Am.*, 16:139, 1969.

Wood, D. W., and Downes, J. J.: Intravenous isoproterenol in the treatment of respiratory failure in childhood status asthmaticus. *Ann. Allergy*, 31:607, 1973.

Wood, D. W., Downes, J. J., and Lecks, H. I.: The management of respiratory failure in childhood status asthmaticus. Experience with 30 episodes and evolution of technique. *J. Allergy*, 42:261, 1968.

Yunginger, J..W., O'Connell, E. J., and Logan, G. B.: Aspirin-induced asthma in children. *J. Pediatr.*, 82:218, 1973.

CHAPTER FORTY-TWO

NONASTHMATIC ALLERGIC PULMONARY DISEASE

C. Warren Bierman, M.D., William E. Pierson, M.D., and F. Stanford Massie, M.D.

An increasing number of substances associated with home, hobbies, vocations and medications are capable of inducing non–IgE-mediated allergic pneumonitides, which may be subdivided into three major categories based upon pathophysiologic features, mechanism of tissue injury and etiologic agent. Hypersensitivity pneumonitis, or extrinsic allergic alveolitis, is the most common and best characterized of these diseases, and occurs primarily in nonatopic individuals. Allergic bronchopulmonary disease, by contrast, occurs exclusively in allergic patients who usually have chronic asthma; it has characteristics of both IgE-mediated allergy and hypersensitivity pneumonitis. Pulmonary reactions to chemicals or drugs may resemble asthma, hypersensitivity pneumonitis or allergic bronchopulmonary disease and may occur with equal frequency in "nonallergic" and "allergic" individuals.

In all of these diseases, symptoms of severe, nonwheezing dyspnea, coughing, fever and malaise may occur hours to days after exposure to the allergen. Because symptoms are delayed, neither physician nor patient may relate them to the causative agent. Yet early diagnosis is the physician's obligation, since early recognition and prompt therapy may prevent the development of such irreversible lung damage as pulmonary fibrosis or saccular bronchiectasis.

The number of substances and agents capable of causing such lung disease has been steadily increasing since the first of these disease states was recognized shortly over a decade ago. Undoubtedly, many additional causes of "idiopathic" chronic lung disease have yet to be identified. In patients with such symptoms, a detailed history of home, school, occupation or hobbies may identify the cause. Only early recognition and prompt therapy may avoid years of disability and ultimate death from respiratory failure.

HYPERSENSITIVITY PNEUMONITIS OR EXTRINSIC ALLERGIC ALVEOLITIS

"Hypersensitivity pneumonitis"* is a term that was introduced by Fink and coworkers in 1968 to characterize a group of pulmonary diseases resulting from the inhalation of organic dust particles of less than 10 microns in diameter, which include mold spores, bacterial products, avian droppings and other proteins of animal origin. It is the term most frequently employed in the United States. Extrinsic allergic alveolitis* was introduced by Pepys in 1969

---

*For purposes of this chapter, extrinsic allergic alveolitis and hypersensitivity pneumonitis will be used interchangeably.

in England. While the term is not anatomically appropriate, because these diseases are associated with bronchiolar as well as alveolar involvement and occasionally with sarcoid-like granulomas (Gandevia, 1973), it has become a generally accepted term in the European literature. Table 1 lists those diseases that can result from a variety of inhaled organic dusts.

Clinical Features

Extrinsic allergic alveolitis, or hypersensitivity pneumonitis, can occur as an acute intermittent systemic and respiratory illness or as an insidious and progressive respiratory disease. The characteristics of these two forms are shown in Table 2 (Fink and coworkers, 1976).

THE ACUTE FORM. On intermittent exposure, symptoms usually occur between four and eight hours after inhalation of the offending substance and consist of chills, fever, malaise, cough, dyspnea and even cyanosis. Physical findings during the acute episodes include temperatures as high as 40° C. (104° F.), rapid respirations, moist basilar crepitant rales with minimal hyperinflation and no wheezes.

The clinical abnormalities usually re-

TABLE 1. CLASSIFICATION OF HYPERSENSITIVITY PNEUMONITIS

Type of Exposure	Disease	Source	Antigen
Dietary	Heiner's syndrome	Ingestion	Cow's milk
	Chronic respiratory infection with milk precipitins	Ingestion Aspiration (?)	Cow's milk
Environmental	Humidifier lung	Home humidifiers and air conditioning systems	Thermophilic actinomycetes
	Humidity tent lung	Home humidity tents	*Bacillus subtilis* enzymes (?)
Hobbies — pets	Pigeon breeder's disease	Pigeon, parakeet or parrot droppings (infrequently chicken)	Avian protein antigen
Occupational	Bagassosis	Moldy sugar cane	*Micropolyspora faeni*
	Cheese worker's disease	Cheese mold spores	*Penicillium casei*
	Enzyme worker's lung	Bacterial products inhalation	*B. subtilis* enzymes
	Farmer's lung Mushroom worker's disease	Moldy hay Compost	*Thermoactinomyces vulgaris*
	Malt worker's lung	Germinating barley	*Aspergillus clavatus*
	Maple bark disease	Moldy maple bark	*Coniosporium corticale*
	Mill worker's disease	Mill dust	*Sitophilus granarius*
	Poultry worker's disease	Poultry sheds	Chicken dander
	Sequoiosis	Moldy redwood sawdust	*Graphium pullularia*
	Suberosis	Moldy cork dust	*M. faeni, T. vulgaris*
Medication	Pancreatic extract lung	Pancreatic enzymes inhalation	Pig pancreatic protein
	Pituitary snuff-taker's lung	Pituitary powder inhalation	Ox or pig protein

TABLE 2. DIAGNOSTIC CLINICAL AND LABORATORY FEATURES IN 8 PATIENTS WITH INTERSTITIAL LUNG DISEASE

	Acute Form	Insidious Form
Dyspnea	4/4	4/4
Cough	4/4	3/4
Weight loss	3/4	2/4
Abnormal chest roentgenogram	4/4	4/4
Abnormal pulmonary functions	4/4	4/4
Thermophiles in environment	3/4	2/4
Serum precipitins to thermophiles	4/4	4/4
Serum precipitins to other dusts	4/4	2/4
Biopsy evidence of interstitial lung disease	4/4	3/4
Thermophiles detected in biopsy	ND	3/3
Response to challenge with antigen	4/4	ND
Relief by environmental alteration	4/4	2/4
Intermittent respiratory symptoms related to environmental exposure	4/4	0/4
Intermittent chills and fever	4/4	0/4
Progressive respiratory symptoms without acute episodes	0/4	4/4

From Fink, J. N., et al. *Ann. Intern. Med.,* 84:410, 1976.

solve within 12 to 18 hours after onset, although occasionally they may last up to three to four days unless terminated by the administration of corticosteroids.

THE INSIDIOUS FORM. When exposure to the offending substance is prolonged and continuous, the disease may present with progressive respiratory symptoms without acute episodes. The course is marked by progressive symptoms of cough and exertional dyspnea without chills or fever. In severe stages,

anorexia and weight loss are prominent, especially in the pediatric age group (Fig. 1).

On physical examination, fine basilar rales may be the only abnormality present, and clubbing of the fingers is rare.

Laboratory Features

During the acute phase, there may be a leukocytosis as high as 25,000 white

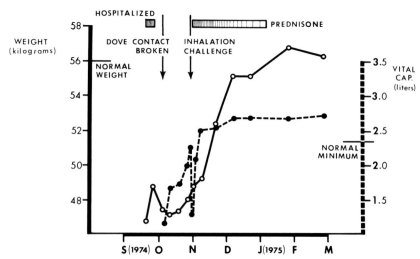

Figure 1. Clinical course of child with hypersensitivity pneumonitis due to exposure to dove antigens. (From Cunningham, A. S., Fink, J. N., and Schlueter, D. P.: *Pediatrics,* 58:441, 1976.)

blood cells per mm.[3], with a predominance of segmented forms of polymorphonuclear leukocytes and up to 10 per cent eosinophils associated with chills and fever. These findings return to normal when the acute symptoms subside. In the chronic form, the blood count is usually normal. As in other chronic pediatric pulmonary disorders, such as cystic fibrosis and chronic granulomatous disease, all the immunoglobulins may be elevated. The exception is a normal serum total IgE, except in the coincidentally allergic person with this disease. Nonspecific changes such as rheumatoid factor and a positive mononucleosis spot test may be found in the acute illness. The erythrocyte sedimentation rate may be elevated, but is usually normal. Smears and cultures of the throat, sputum and blood are negative. These nonspecific, abnormal findings usually return to normal in the chronic intermittent-exposure form of the disease (Fink, 1976).

Radiographic Studies

In the acute form, the chest roentgenogram (Fig. 2) shows a diffuse, interstitial infiltrate of the alevolar walls and adjacent lobular septa, fine reticular densities with multiple small nodules and patchy infiltration at the lung bases (Marinkovich 1975; Fink review, 1976). Chronic disease is manifested radiographically as a diffuse interstitial fibrosis with coarsening of the bronchovascular markings that is particularly prominent in the upper lobes. Hyperinflation is rare. Since none of these findings is specific for hypersensitivity pneumonitis, the chest roentgenogram must be correlated with the clinical features (Zylak and coworkers, 1975).

Pulmonary Function Tests

Restrictive impairment to ventilation is the primary abnormality of hypersensitivity pneumonitis. Forced vital capacity (FVC) is reduced in acute episodes and may return to normal during remissions. It is irreversibly reduced because of pulmonary fibrosis in the chronic phase of the disease. Pulmonary compliance is decreased owing to increased stiffness of the lung, and carbon monoxide diffusion is diminished, indicating an alveolar-capillary blockade with reduced gas transfer. Func-

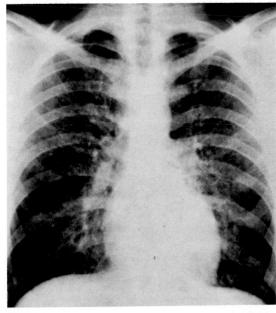

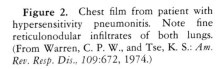

Figure 2. Chest film from patient with hypersensitivity pneumonitis. Note fine reticulonodular infiltrates of both lungs. (From Warren, C. P. W., and Tse, K. S.: *Am. Rev. Resp. Dis., 109*:672, 1974.)

tional residual capacity and total lung capacity are low. Arterial blood gases reveal diminished Pa_{O_2} and decreased oxygen saturation, which fall further with exercise.

Arterial P_{CO_2} is usually diminished, and the pH is slightly elevated with a mild to moderate respiratory alkalosis during acute episodes. Renal compensation allows the pH to return to normal (Schlueter and coworkers, 1969; Slavin, 1976; Fink, 1976). Airways resistance by plethysmography, forced expiratory volume at one second (FEV_1) and midmaximal flow rates are usually normal unless the patient is atopic and has superimposed asthma.

In insidious hypersensitivity pneumonitis, some patients also have increased residual volumes, decreased flow rates and loss of pulmonary elasticity as found in emphysema (Fink review, 1976).

Immunologic Responses

SEROLOGIC STUDIES. Precipitating IgG antibodies to suspect organic dusts containing fungal antigens, thermophilic actinomycetes or avian proteins are characteristically found in the serum of patients with hypersensitivity pneumonitis (Fig. 3). These antibodies may also be detected in a significant number

(up to 50 per cent) of asymptomatic, similarly exposed individuals, and thus do not indicate the presence of disease (Fink review, 1976; Slavin, 1976). Early studies postulated that they were responsible for a type III or Arthus hypersensitivity pulmonary reaction. Recent experimental and human studies implicate monocytes as the cause of the pulmonary reaction. Precipitating antibodies are now believed to play a protective role.

Although precipitating antibody titers are generally greater in symptomatic versus asymptomatic exposed individuals, there are marked intersubject variations (Hansen and Penny, 1974a, b; Moore and Fink, 1975). Cross reactions have also been noted between various organic dust antigens (Flaherty and coworkers, 1974a; Moore and Fink, 1975; Kurup and coworkers, 1975).

Epidemiologic studies have employed serum precipitating antibodies in screening patients with possible or existing disease, and are useful (Roberts and associates, 1976; doPico and colleagues, 1976) in detecting exposure to the antigens. Further historical, radiographic and immunologic information is necessary to diagnose hypersensitivity pneumonitis.

Serum hemolytic complement

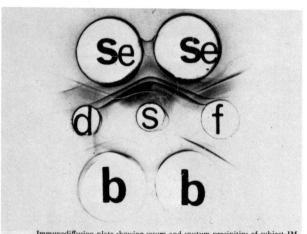

Figure 3. Serum and bronchial precipitins to chicken proteins in patient with hypersensitivity pneumonitis. (From Warren, C. P. W., Tse, K. S.: *Am. Rev. Resp. Dis., 109*: 672, 1974.)

Immunodiffusion plate showing serum and sputum precipitins of subject JM. Se = subject's serum, b = subject's bronchial washing, d = chicken droppings extract, S = chicken serum, and f = chicken feather extract.

(C_{H50}) activity falls in asymptomatic but not in symptomatic pigeon breeders upon inhalation challenge with pigeon antigens (Moore and Fink, 1975; Marx and Flaherty, 1976; Olenchock and Burrell, 1976). This difference has been attributed to the handling of inhaled antigens. In asymptomatic pigeon breeders with precipitating antibodies, inhaled antigen is absorbed from the lungs and eliminated by complement activation. In symptomatic pigeon breeders with lung disease, the inflammation impedes systemic absorption so that serum complement does not fall. Extracts of *Micropolyspora faeni*, important in farmer's lung disease, have also been found to consume complement in vitro in the absence of detectable antibodies (Marx and Flaherty, 1976; Olenchock and Burrell, 1976).

CELLULAR IMMUNE STUDIES. In patients with hypersensitivity pneumonitis, peripheral blood lymphocytes undergo blast transformation or migration inhibition factor (MIF) production, or both, on in vitro culture with the appropriate fungal or avian antigens. Lymphocytes from asymptomatic individuals with precipitating antibodies to these agents fail to show this response (Schatz, 1976). In animal models, lymphocytes are of equal importance. Animals infused with sensitized lymphocytes develop pulmonary lesions on antigenic inhalation challenge, whereas those receiving only serum do not (Bice and coworkers, 1976; Slavin, 1976; Fink, 1976). In human disease, both bone marrow–derived B cells, which produce precipitating antibody, and thymic-derived helper T cells, which induce cellular hypersensitivity, are important in modulating hypersensitivity pneumonitis (Moore and Fink, 1975). This response appears to be linked to genetic control by an immune response gene closely linked to the major histocompatibility locus (Allen and coworkers, 1976). Thus, the pulmonary damage appears to result from a combination of hu-moral and cellular factors, which include complement activation in the lung, the release of lymphokines from mononuclear cells and the irritant effects of thermophilic agents.

SKIN TESTS. Scratch, prick or intracutaneous skin tests are useful with pigeon-derived antigens (pigeon serum and dropping extracts) in pigeon breeder's disease, as are other bird proteins in chicken sensitivity lung disease (Pepys, 1974; Fink, 1976). Skin testing may also be helpful in pituitary snuff lung and pancreatin sensitivity to pig and cow protein. It cannot be used satisfactorily in hypersensitivity pneumonitis from thermophilic actinomycetes because extracts of these agents are irritating and may give nonspecific, false-positive reactions.

Rarely, an immediate wheal and flare reaction occurs 20 minutes after skin testing. The usual reaction is an erythematous, occasionally ecchymotic reaction that occurs four to eight hours later. Biopsy of the skin test site shows a mild infiltration of polymorphonuclear leukocytes and plasma cells surrounding the vessels consistent with an Arthus type of response (Pepys, 1969; Fink, 1976).

Inhalation Challenge Studies

On inhalation challenge with extracts of causative agents (Pepys, 1974; Fink, 1976), patients with hypersensitivity pneumonitis develop chills, fever, malaise, leukocytosis, restrictive pulmonary changes and a fall in Pa_{O_2} four to eight hours after exposure. Because these reactions may be severe, inhalation challenge must be done with great caution in the hospital, and a severe reaction should be terminated with corticosteroids. Challenge material must be pure, since extracts contaminated with endotoxin can produce a nonspecific response (Slavin, 1976). In some patients, careful re-exposure to areas suspected of containing offending antigens, such as a pigeon coop, barn or place of employment, may be necessary.

Histologic Studies

As with serologic, radiologic and pulmonary function tests, tissue histology in patients with hypersensitivity pneumonitis varies between the acute and chronic phases of the disease (Fink review, 1976). Lung biopsies from patients with acute hypersensitivity pneumonitis reveal interstitial pneumonia, with involvement of the alveolar walls and spaces and bronchioles, with positive fluorescent staining for immunoglobulin and complement (Wenzel and coworkers, 1971). Infiltrations with lymphocytes, plasma cells and occasional clusters of histiocytes containing foamy cytoplasm may be seen, associated with intra-alveolar proteinaceous fluids with increased numbers of alveolar macrophages. Focal sarcoid-type, noncaseating granulomas with Langhans-type giant cells, bronchiolitis and minimal vasculitis may also be present (Seal and coworkers, 1968; Hensley, 1974; Fink and Sosman, 1974).

In chronic hypersensitivity pneumonitis, fibrosis and destruction of lung parenchyma may be seen, with lymphocyte and plasma infiltration of alveolar walls being less prominent (Fig. 4). Obliteration of bronchioles by collagen deposition and granulation tissue and honeycombing cystic changes are associated with severe fibrosis (Fink, 1976).

None of these findings is specific for hypersensitivity pneumonitis, and biopsy material must be correlated with other clinical and laboratory features.

Experimental Studies

Experimental hypersensitivity pneumonitis has been induced in many animal models, including rats, guinea pigs, rabbits, horses and monkeys, to a number of antigens, including extracts of pigeon guano, bagasse, thermophilic actinomycetes and Aspergillus spores.

All features of human disease have been reproduced in rabbits (Moore and coworkers, 1975). Rabbits exposed by

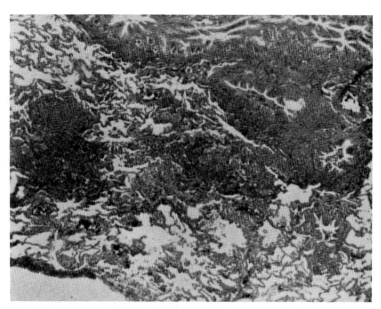

Figure 4.   Appearance of a typical section of biopsied lung obtained from a patient with "pigeon fancier's disease." Note the diffuse involvement as well as the large nodular cellular aggregates. At higher magnification, these were seen to contain chronic inflammatory cells, including plasma cells, lymphocytes, rare multinucleated giant cells, and large sheets of finely vacuolated histiocytes. Most of the alveolar septa were thickened by similar cells. (From Van Arsdel, P. P., Jr.: *Yale J. Biol. Med.*, 40:501, 1967.)

aerosol to large quantities of pigeon antigens developed a humoral, but not cellular, immunologic response, and their lungs remained normal histologically. A single intravenous injection of killed BCG vaccine in oil facilitated the induction of pulmonary cell-mediated hypersensitivity to the inhaled antigen as well as the development of pulmonary lesions. Further, animals with normal lung examined histologically had a fall in complement levels after aerosolized pigeon antigen challenge, whereas the BCG-treated animals did not. Transfer of sensitivity by lymphoid cells in rabbits also resulted in alveolar, interstitial and peribronchial lesions (Bice and coworkers, 1976).

Diagnosis

The diagnosis of hypersensitivity pneumonitis depends on a high index of suspicion and on a good history, with particular attention to the patient's home environment, hobbies and work. In the acute form, the physician may be misled by the fever, leukocytosis and pulmonary infiltrates, and may attribute clinical improvement to antibiotics rather than to hospitalization and change in environment. The recurrence of symptoms on returning to the previous environment should be the key to the diagnosis.

Patients with insidious onset disease do not relate their symptoms to an exposure to antigen. Some may smoke and have chronic bronchitis so that the diagnosis may easily be missed. These patients are at risk of progressing to chronic pulmonary fibrosis. In these patients, the insidious onset and progressive nature of dyspnea without other systemic symptoms should encourage the physician to examine the patient's environment, culturing for air-borne fungi when appropriate, and performing serologic tests for precipitins to these fungi. Inhalation challenge or open lung biopsy with specific immunologic studies may be necessary to confirm the diagnosis.

Therapy

Management depends on avoiding further exposure and on corticosteroid therapy. If steroids are necessary, the therapeutic aim should be to achieve a maximum improvement in lung function by administering 40 mg. prednisone daily as a single morning dose, gradually reducing the dose until the drug has been discontinued or lung function decreases. If long-term steroids appear necessary, alternate day steroids should be tried. When exposure can be avoided, most patients do not require long-term steroids. Accordingly, it is a clinical challenge to the physician to convince the patient or his parents to change homes, occupations, hobbies or life styles, depending on the etiologic agent of the hypersensitivity lung disease.

SPECIFIC SYNDROMES

Dietary Proteins

Pulmonary Disease Associated with Serum Milk Precipitins

Two types of chronic lung disease in children have been related to the ingestion of milk. The first, hemosiderosis associated with milk precipitins, is described by Dr. Douglas Heiner in Chapter 36. Patients with this form of disease appear to benefit from the elimination of cow's milk from their diet.

The second form, though less clearcut, appears to be a separate entity. In the 1960s, a group of children with chronic respiratory "infections" were described (Heiner and Sears, 1960; Heiner and coworkers, 1962) who had precipitating antibody to milk detectable with ordinary gel diffusion (Ouchterlony technique). These patients improved substantially when milk was removed from their diets. Population screens for precipitating antibodies in normal children, on the other hand, revealed many children with milk precipitins who were well, casting doubt on the significance of the precipitins in children who were ill. Further studies have not been done.

Symptomatic patients with milk precipitins may have a form of hypersensitivity pneumonitis of which precipitating antibodies to milk may be a marker but not the cause. Young children with recurrent pulmonary disease should be tested for serum precipitating antibodies to milk, and if such antibodies are present, the children should receive a trial of a milk-free diet.

Diseases Related to Home Environment

Interstitial Lung Disease Due to Contamination of Forced Air Systems

In the home and office environment, humidifiers and air conditioning systems present specific hazards of hypersensitivity pneumonitis. In 1970, Banaszak and associates recognized hypersensitivity pneumonitis in four patients as a result of a home air conditioner that was contaminated with thermophilic fungi. Since then, many patients have been reported who have had either chronic or acute hypersensitivity pneumonitis secondary to either home or office heating or air conditioning systems. The etiologic antigens identified to date are *Thermoactinomyces candidus*, *T. vulgaris*, *T. sacchari* and *Mucor faeni*. Table 3 lists the reported cases and the sources of contamination.

In an epidemiologic survey of 272 subjects, Banaszak and coworkers (1974) cultured the homes for thermophilic fungi, performed pulmonary function tests, took chest roentgenograms and performed serum studies for precipitating antibodies to a group of fungi. Thermophilic fungi were recovered in culture from 74 per cent of the homes. Substantially higher concentrations were found in homes with symptomatic subjects. There were substantially more precipitating antibodies identified among the symptomatic group, although there was not good correlation between precipitating antibodies, degree of pulmonary involvement and chest roentgenogram abnormalities. Of eight subjects whose disease resulted from chronic exposure to actinomycetes-contaminated home humidifiers, three had persistent lung disease in spite of recognition and therapy (Fink, 1976). In the child with persistent respiratory problems, the chronic use of humidifiers or vaporizers should be suspected as the cause of his disease (Hodges and coworkers, 1974; Seabury and associates, 1976).

TABLE 3.   HYPERSENSITIVITY PNEUMONITIS RESULTING FROM EXPOSURE TO THERMOPHILIC FUNGI IN AIR CONTROL SYSTEMS

Number of Cases	Source of Contamination	Authors
4	Office air conditioner	Banaszak (1970)
1	Home furnace humidifier	Fink (1970)
1	Home furnace humidifier	Sweet (1971)
1	Home humidifier	Tomville (1970)
1	Air conditioner	Weiss (1971)
5	Room humidifier	Koller (1972)
1	Cool mist vaporizer	Hodges (1974)
1	Home air conditioner	Marinkovich (1975)
8	Home furnace humidifiers (4)	Fink (1976)
	Air conditioners (2)	
	Unknown exposure (2)	

Lung Disease Due to Contamination of Humidifying Tents in the Home

In 1972, Motoyama and coworkers studied the effects of prolonged environmental humidification on patients with cystic fibrosis. Lung function tests were obtained during a six-week period when the child slept in mist tents, and during the same period of time when the child was no longer in a mist tent. Simultaneously, cultures obtained from the water in the mist tents were found to be heavily contaminated with *Bacillus subtilis* organisms. A substantial number of the patients showed improved pulmonary function when removed from such tents. While cultures for Thermoactinomyces or other thermophilic fungi and precipitin tests for the thermophilic fungi were not carried out in this group of patients, it is probable that products of *B. subtilis* contamination* were responsible for increased pulmonary disease in these children. The physician prescribing prolonged humidification for children with chronic pulmonary disease has an obligation to measure pulmonary function regularly and to culture such tents both for thermophilic fungi and for *B. subtilis* (Kohler and coworkers, 1976).

Diseases Due to Hobbies

Pigeon Breeder's Disease

In 1960, Pearsall and coworkers reported a patient with pulmonary infiltrates, fever, basilar rhonchi, and a pleural effusion that cleared on admission to the hospital, recurred on discharge home and was identified as a hypersensitivity reaction to the 200 parakeets that she had in her home. The relationship to the parakeets was established by the presence in the serum of precipitating antibodies specific for the extract of parakeet dander, as well as by an exacerbation of the disease on re-exposure to parakeet dander. Since then, hypersensitivity pneumonitis has been related to a variety of avian antigens, including those of pigeons, parrots, doves, parakeets (budgerigars) and chickens.

Younger children who have these birds as pets are at risk, as are adolescents who raise the birds as a hobby. The youngest children reported to date with hypersensitivity pneumonitis from avian antigens were both eight years of age. The clinical features of these reported cases are noted in Table 4.

In children, hypersensitivity pneumonitis due to avian antigen has an insidious onset with a prolonged course over a period of months to years. In addition, children have weight loss more commonly than do adults. In several reported children, an initial diagnosis has been anorexia nervosa. The recent demonstration of celiac disease–like duodenal villous atrophy in patients with pigeon breeder's disease (Berrill and coworkers, 1975) suggests that this weight loss is related to an anatomical lesion in the gastrointestinal tract, possibly secondary to swallowing inhaled antigens.

Diagnosis is suggested by the clinical course, a typical chest roentgenogram (Fig. 5), detection of serum precipitating antibodies to pigeon, parakeet, dove or chicken serum or guano extracts, an Arthus-like skin test to the intradermal injection of avian serum or plasma, and the demonstration of lymphocyte transformation and migratory inhibition factor production in response to the specific avian antigens. It may be confirmed by inhalation challenge performed in the hospital (Hargreave and Pepys, 1972; Hansen and Penny, 1974b).

As in other forms of hypersensitivity pneumonitis, therapy consists of elimination of the birds and administration of corticosteroids. The course of one such patient is seen in Figure 1, and chest roentgenograms obtained before and after therapy are noted in Figure 5.

---

*See Enzyme Worker's Lung, page 682.

TABLE 4. CLINICAL FEATURES IN THE LITERATURE ON CHILDREN WITH PIGEON BREEDER'S DISEASE

Literature Reports*

Clinical Features	Stiehm et al. (1967)					Shannon et al. (1969)	Chandra and Jones (1972)			Reiss et al. (1974)	Purtilo et al. (1975)	Cunningham et al. (1976)
	1	2	3	4	5	15	1	2	3	8	14	13
Age (yr.)	10	13	8	15	15	15	10	12	14	8	14	13
Sex	M	M	M	M	M	M	M	M	M	F	M	F
Presenting complaints												
Cough	+	+	+	+	+	+	0	0	+	+	+	+
Dyspnea	+	+	+	+	+	+	+	+	+	+	+	+
Weight loss	+	+	0	+	0	+	+	0	0	0	+	+
Exposure-symptom relationship												
Duration of exposure	5 mo.	SY	SY	3 yr.	3 yr.	7 yr.	U	U	U	6 wk.	7 yr.	2 yr.
Duration of symptoms	4 mo.	>4 mo.	4 mo.	>1 mo.	3 yr.	5 mo.	6 wk.	3 wk.	5 wk.	2 wk.	1 mo.	>3 mo.
History of acute episodes	0	+	0	+	+	0	0	0	0	0	0	0
Objective findings												
Basilar rales	+	0	0	0	NS	+	+	0	+	0	+	+
Wheezing	0	0	0	0	NS	0	0	0	0	0	0	0
Abnormal chest x-ray film	+	+	+	+	0	0	+	+	+	+	+	+
Immunoglobulins												
IgG	I	I	I	I	N	N	NS	NS	NS	I	N	I
IgM	I	I	N	I	N	N	NS	NS	NS	N	N	I
IgA	I	N	N	N	N	N	NS	NS	NS	D	N	I
Eosinophilia	+	0	NS	0	0	+	0	0	0	+	0	+
Precipitins to avian antigens	+	+	+	+	+	+	+	+	+	+	+	+
Skin test reactions												
Immediate	+	NS	NS	NS	NS	NS	0	NS	NS	0	0	+
Late onset	+	NS	NS	NS	NS	NS	0	NS	NS	0	0	+
Abnormal lung biopsy	+	NS	NS	NS	+	NS	NS	NS	NS	NS	+	NS
Pulmonary functions†												
FVC	D	D	D	N	NS	D	D	NS	NS	D	D	D
FEV/FVC	NS	N	N	N	NS	N	N	N	N	N	N	N
Peak flow rate	D	NS	NS	NS	NS	N	N	D	NS	NS	NS	NS
RV/TLC	I	N	N	N	NS	I	N	N	N	NS	NS	NS
D,co	D	D	N	NS	NS	N	D	NS	D	D	NS	D
P_{O_2}	D	NS	NS	NS	NS	D	D	NS	0	D	D	N

From Cunningham, A. S., Fink, J. N., and Schlueter, D. P.: *Pediatrics*, 58:436, 1976.

*SY = several years; U = unknown; NS = not studied; N = normal; I = increased; D = decreased.

†FVC = forced vital capacity; FEV/FVC = forced expiratory volume divided by forced vital capacity; RV/TLC = residual volume divided by total lung capacity; D_{CO} = carbon monoxide diffusion capacity; P_{O_2} = arterial oxygen tension.

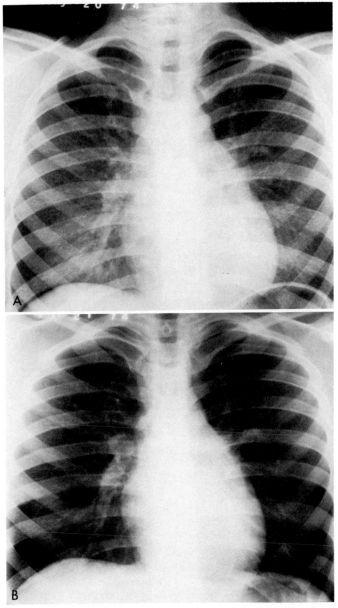

Figure 5. Acute (*A*) and convalescent (*B*) chest films of child with hypersensitivity pneumonitis due to exposure to doves in the home. (From Cunningham, A. S., Fink, J. N., and Schlueter, D. P.: *Pediatrics*, 58:436, 1976.)

Occupational Lung Disease

Bagassosis

This form of hypersensitivity pneumonitis develops four to five hours after exposure to moldy sugar cane (Salvaggio and coworkers, 1966). The etiologic agent is *Thermoactinomyces vulgaris.* The diagnosis can be made by a history of exposure to moldy sugar cane in poorly ventilated buildings and by bronchial challenge if necessary (Kawai and coworkers, 1972).

Cheese Worker's Lung

Hypersensitivity pneumonitis of cheese workers results from exposure to the spores of *Penicillium casei.* The diagnosis and therapy are essentially the same as those noted above for other forms of hypersensitivity pneumonitis (Molina and coworkers, 1974).

Enzyme Worker's Lung

In the late 1960s, the introduction of enzymes derived from *Bacillus subtilis* into laundry detergents was identified as a source of chronic pulmonary problems in some workers in factories where these enzyme proteins were produced. In a study of the factory workers exposed to these enzymes (Pepys, 1973), two-thirds of the workers had IgE and IgA antienzyme antibodies. Although atopic workers were much more likely to have an IgE antibody response to enzymes, some nonatopic workers developed delayed symptoms four to eight hours after exposure; these symptoms persisted for prolonged periods. The risk of respiratory disease has prompted the removal of these enzymes from the U.S. market.

Farmer's Lung

This disease of workers exposed to moldy hay can occur as an acute form with symptoms of coughing, wheezing, chills, fever and dyspnea four to eight

hours following exposure, or as an insidious form with symptoms of progressive dyspnea, weight loss and decreased exercise tolerance with restrictive changes in lung function. The etiologic agents are thermophilic actinomycetes, including Micropolyspora. Diagnosis is made by a history of exposure. Serum precipitating antibodies to the offending antigen may be helpful but are not diagnostic owing to cross reactivity and nonspecificity of some antibody responses. Lymphocyte transformation and MIF inhibition appear to be more helpful immunologic tests in patients with symptomatic farmer's lung. Bronchial challenge to the antigen reproduces clinical symptoms four to eight hours later. Skin testing is not helpful because antigens from thermophilic organisms are irritating and induce nonspecific reaction. Treatment includes avoidance of the offending agent and systemic corticosteroid therapy until lung function returns to normal (Dicki and coworkers, 1958; Patterson and colleagues, 1976).

Malt Worker's Disease

This disease of malt workers in Scotland is due to spores from *Aspergillus clavatus* that contaminate malting (sprouting) barley on open floors (the first step of making scotch whiskey) (Grant and coworkers, 1976). Typical symptoms occur four to eight hours after exposure. Diagnosis is suggested by history. Serum precipitating antibodies may not be diagnostic because of cross reactivity with other Aspergillus species. Bronchial challenge confirms the diagnosis of this disorder. The disease can be avoided by utilizing a closed malting technique and employing barley free of Aspergillus contamination.

Maple Bark Disease

Maple bark disease occurs among workers who strip bark infected with *Coniosporium (Cryptostroma) corticale* from maple logs. Clinical manifestations are typical of hypersensitivity pneumonitis after exposure to maple logs. The identification of precipitating antibody and the isolation of *Coniosporium corticale* from the nostrils are helpful diagnostic procedures (Emanuel and coworkers, 1966).

Mill Worker's Disease

This disorder is characterized by either acute wheezing and dyspnea or insidious progressive dyspnea, productive coughing, fever and malaise. It is caused by *Sitophilus granarius*, a mite found in flour mills (Warren and coworkers, 1974).

Mushroom Worker's Disease

The etiologic agent is *Micropolyspora faeni*, which is a gram-positive thermophilic organism isolated from mushroom compost (Bringhurst and coworkers, 1959). Clinical manifestations include cough, dyspnea, and sometimes chills and fever approximately four to eight hours after exposure to the mushroom compost. In the insidious form it presents as progressive pulmonary obstruction and decreasing exercise tolerance. The diagnosis is made by history of exposure, identification of the organism by culture and identification of precipitating antibodies by counterelectrophoresis (Moller and Halberg, 1976).

Poultry Worker's Disease

This disease has been described among a few young poultry workers, the youngest being 16 years old (Warren and Tse, 1974). The etiologic agent appears to be an antigen derived from epithelial cells shed with the down as young chickens acquire feathers, in contrast to pigeon breeder's disease, in which the major offending antigen can be found in serum or guano extracts. Signs and symptoms are typical of hypersensitivity pneumonitis. Precipitating antibodies to chicken dander found in sputum may be diagnostic.

Sequoiosis

Sequoia wood workers may have hypersensitivity pneumonitis from the mold *Graphium pullularia* found in moldy redwood sawdust. The clinical manifestations are typical for hypersensitivity pneumonitis. The diagnosis is made by a history of exposure to redwood sawdust in poorly ventilated saw mills, identification of precipitating antibody and a positive bronchial challenge test (Cohen and coworkers, 1967).

Suberosis

This disorder of hypersensitivity pneumonitis results from exposure to oak bark, or cork dust. Etiologic agents are *Micropolyspora faeni* or *Thermoactinomyces vulgaris*, or both (Kaltreider, 1973). The clinical manifestations, diagnosis and therapy are similar to other diseases caused by thermophilic agents.

Diseases Related to Medication

Pancreatic Enzyme Lung

The inhalation of desiccated pancreatic powder by parents of children with cystic fibrosis who add powdered pancreatic enzymes to their children's food may induce profuse nasal congestion, rhinorrhea, cough and wheezing shortly after exposure. This may be followed by a second reaction four to six hours later consisting of dyspnea, cough, chest "tightness" and fever. Pulmonary function studies show that obstructive changes predominate in the immediate reaction, and restrictive changes predominate in the second response. Therapy is avoidance of pancreatic powder inhalation by using either tablets (Viokase) or pancreatic powder in capsules (Cotazym) (Bergner and Bergner, 1975).

Pituitary Snuff Taker's Lung

This syndrome is due to inhaling porcine or ox pituitary snuff for therapy of diabetes insipidus. The clinical features are similar to those of pancreatic enzyme lung. The introduction of synthetic Pitressin has virtually eliminated this form of hypersensitivity pneumonitis (Pepys and coworkers, 1966).

ALLERGIC BRONCHOPULMONARY DISEASE

Allergic bronchopulmonary disease occurs in individuals who are atopic and who have chronic asthma; it is characterized by high serum IgE levels, in contrast to hypersensitivity pneumonitis, in which IgE is usually normal. Bronchial challenge elicits a biphasic response, the initial response modified by isoproterenol but not by corticosteroids, and the secondary response modified by corticosteroids but not by adrenergic agents. Although initially recognized as due to Aspergillus, other organisms, such as *Candida albicans* and alternaria (Fink, 1974), have been implicated. While this discussion relates primarily to Aspergillus-associated allergic bronchopulmonary disease, additional etiologic agents will undoubtedly be identified as more sensitive investigative techniques are developed.

Aspergillus, especially *A. fumigatus,* may be responsible for at least five types of human disease:

1. Disseminated aspergillosis: an invasive infection occurring in some patients with immune deficiency states or artificially suppressed immunity.

2. Solitary aspergilloma: an Aspergillus infection that occurs in a congenital pulmonary cyst or bronchiectatic cavity.

3. IgE-mediated asthma: asthma occurring on inhalation of Aspergillus spores by patients with type I sensitivity to Aspergillus.

4. Malt worker's lung: an extrinsic allergic alveolitis or hypersensitivity pneumonitis occurring in brewery and distillery workers who inhale the spores of *Aspergillus clavatus,* which contaminate malting barley.

5. Allergic bronchopulmonary aspergillosis: a disease occurring in patients with chronic asthma whose respiratory tracts are colonized by *Aspergillus fumigatus.*

Clinical Features

The comparison of extrinsic allergic alveolitis and allergic bronchopulmonary aspergillosis is noted in Table 5.

Patients with allergic bronchopulmonary aspergillosis are atopic and

TABLE 5. COMPARISON OF HYPERSENSITIVITY PNEUMONITIS AND ALLERGIC BRONCHOPULMONARY DISEASE

Manifestation	Hypersensitivity Pneumonitis	Allergic Bronchopulmonary Disease
Physical findings	Rales or rhonchi	Wheezing
Chest roentgenograms	Interstitial infiltrates	Lobular infiltrates
Pulmonary function	Restrictive	Restrictive and obstructive
Blood count	Elevated with increased polymorphonuclear leukocytes	Eosinophilia
Sputum findings	Normal	Eosinophils and mycelia
Skin test	Delayed	Immediate and delayed
IgE	Normal	Elevated
Specific antibodies agent	IgG precipitating	IgE skin sensitizing IgG precipitating

Modified from Slavin, R. G.: *Postgrad. Med.,* 59:137, 1976.

usually have a long-standing history of bronchial asthma. In children, the onset is frequently insidious and characterized by low-grade fever, progressive fatigue, moderate to marked weight loss, night sweats and an increasingly productive cough (Jordan and coworkers, 1971). On physical examination, signs of chronic asthma with hyperinflation, prolonged expiration and generalized expiratory wheezing are found in association with basilar rales and rhonchi in subjects who appear chronically ill. In the more chronically ill patients, clubbing of the fingers may occur. The untreated patient may progress to bronchiectasis, which is unique to this condition in that it is saccular and involves proximal bronchi, sparing the peripheral or distal airways (McCarthy and coworkers, 1970).

Laboratory Features

General laboratory features include eosinophilia in peripheral blood and sputum plus marked IgE elevation (Patterson and coworkers, 1973). Expectorated sputum frequently contains brownish plugs from which fungal mycelia and *Aspergillus fumigatus* grow readily on culture.

Radiographic Features

Radiographic features are variable, depending on the severity of asthma and the degree of tissue damage resulting from the disease. The initial chest roentgenogram of a child with allergic bronchopulmonary aspergillosis and a follow-up film seven years later are shown in Figure 6.

Acute changes may vary from small areas of consolidation with patchy areas of atelectasis to large areas of consolidation with atelectasis of an entire lobe. There are frequently homogeneous shadows 2 to 3 cm. in length, which are due to bronchi filled with secretions, and "tramlines" or parallel hairline shadows extending from the hilum, which are due to dilated bronchi. The

atelectasis resulting from mucus plugs may result in a mediastinal shift to the affected side. *Chronic changes* consist of ring shadows 1 to 2 cm. in diameter due to dilated bronchi; circular shadows 2 to 3 cm. in diameter representing cavities; and tubular shadows, parallel lines wider than a bronchus separated by a translucent zone, due to saccular bronchiectasis, which is characteristically proximal and frequently involves the upper lobes (McCarthy and coworkers, 1970).

Lung scans with strontium-87M are characteristic, with localization of the radionuclide in radiographic abnormalities. The presence of a positive scan in a patient with chronic pulmonary disease should suggest occult allergic bronchopulmonary aspergillosis (Adiseshan and Oliver, 1973).

Pulmonary Function Studies

Like chest roentgenograms, pulmonary function studies vary with the activity and severity of the disease. Values range from mild obstructive airway changes to severe airway obstruction that is not reversed by isoproterenol, hyperinflation, increased total lung capacity and decreased diffusing capacity (Safirstein and coworkers, 1973).

Immunologic Studies

SEROLOGIC STUDIES. Precipitin tests performed by immunodiffusion or radioimmunoelectrophoresis revealed the presence of IgG precipitating antibodies in the majority of patients (Safirstein and coworkers, 1973), and up to three arcs have been found in over 90 per cent. By contrast, in aspergillosis with tissue invasion, a broader humoral response occurs, with up to eight precipitin arcs (Citron, 1975; Bardana and coworkers, 1975).

Marked elevations of serum IgE (10,000 to 30,000 I.U./ml.) are characteristic of allergic bronchopulmonary aspergillosis during acute pulmonary

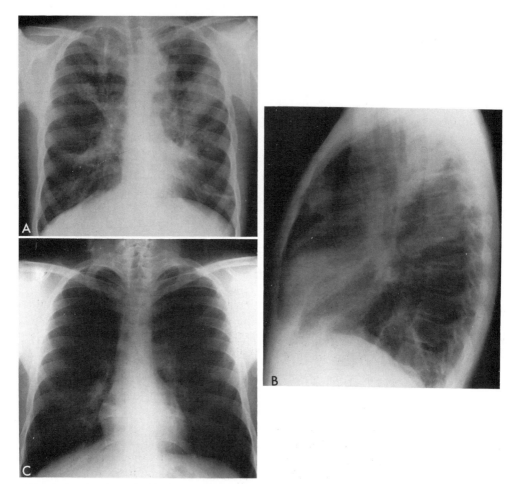

Figure 6. *A* and *B,* Roentgenograms of 13-year-old boy with allergic bronchopulmonary aspergillosis. Note atelectasis in left base and left lingula. There is consolidation of right upper lobe and both midlungs with dilated bronchi in apical segments of both upper lobes. Note bullous lesion of right suprahilar area. *C,* At age 19 years, lungs are clear except for enlarged inferior right hilar density and lobe linear streaking (probable fibrosis) in left lower lobe. (Courtesy of Dr. Byron H. Ward, Department of Radiology, Children's Orthopedic Hospital and Medical Center, Seattle.)

infiltrations (Patterson and coworkers, 1973). Some, but not all, of the IgE is specific for Aspergillus antigens (Patterson and Roberts, 1974).

Histamine release studies have suggested that both IgE and IgG, anti-Aspergillus antibodies, may be cytophilic for human basophils (Citron, 1975; Bardana and coworkers, 1975).

CELLULAR IMMUNE STUDIES. Aspergillus-induced blast transformation in vitro and the presence of granulomas in pathologic sections of the lung in some patients with allergic bronchopulmonary aspergillosis have suggested a role for cell-mediated immune responses. In-depth studies have not yet been done (Bardana, 1974; Turner-Warwick and coworkers, 1975).

SKIN TESTING. Skin tests with *A. fumigatus* antigen frequently induce a dual response, with an immediate IgE-mediated wheal and flare at 12 to 20 minutes followed by a late four- to six-hour IgG-mediated Arthus-type reaction. Skin tests correlate well with bronchial inhalation challenge studies with *A. fumigatus* extracts.

Inhalation Challenge Studies

Inhalation studies with *A. fumigatus* result in a dual reaction, an immediate and a delayed reaction, in contrast to only a delayed reaction in hypersensitivity pneumonitis (McCarthy and Pepys, 1971).

The immediate reaction occurs within minutes and consists of "tickling" in the throat, eyes or ears, dry repetitive coughing and tightness of the chest with wheezing. Lung function testing shows asthma or increased asthma with a fall of 500 ml. or more in the $FEV_{1.0}$. The "late" reaction occurs after about three to eight hours and consists of a productive cough, wheezing, dyspnea, malaise, headache, anorexia and "flu-like" sensation and an inability to sleep. Signs of airway ob-

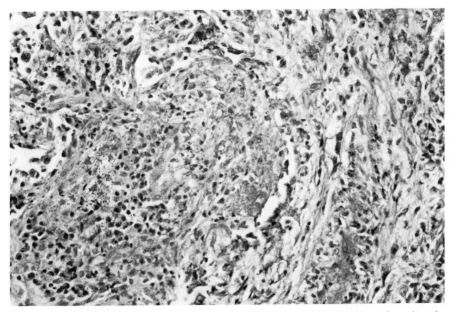

Figure 7. Appearance of a typical section of biopsied lung from a child with allergic bronchopulmonary aspergillosis. The bronchial wall on the right is severely involved, with total destruction of the epithelial lining and only remnants of smooth muscle. The alveolar lumens are filled with inflammatory exudate and cellular debris. Other areas of this biopsy contained some multinucleated giant cells, eosinophils and mononuclear cells. (Courtesy of Dr. Joel E. Hass, Department of Pathology, Children's Orthopedic Hospital and Medical Center, Seattle.)

struction reappear or become worse on clinical examination in association with a fall of 500 ml. or more in $FEV_{1.0}$ after initial recovery. Pyrexia and leukocytosis are maximal 24 hours after the test.

The early reaction may be prevented by pretreatment with cromolyn, or reversed by isoproterenol; the late reaction is less frequently prevented by cromolyn, is infrequently reversed by isoproterenol and may require corticosteroid treatment. Inhalation challenge should be performed only when the patient is in the hospital for 48 hours, with concentrations of inhaled antigens determined by quantitative skin testing.

Histologic Studies

Pathologic changes may be seen in conducting bronchi and alveoli (Fig. 7) and consist of dilated bronchi with inspissated mucus containing noninvasive fungal hyphae. The bronchial mucosa exhibits squamous metaplasia, and the walls have a cellular infiltrate of eosinophils, lymphocytes and plasma cells. Focal eosinophilic pneumonia and bronchiolitis obliterans may accompany necrotic parenchymal granulomas and vasculitis (Katz and Kniker, 1973; Katzenstein and coworkers, 1975). The end result of saccular bronchiectasis of the proximal bronchi occurs because the antigenic source, growing in the bronchial lumen, continually sheds antigens into the tissues, where a chain immunologic reaction causes bronchial wall damage and surrounding pulmonary consolidation.

Diagnosis

Any child or adolescent with bronchial asthma who develops progressive weight loss, fatigue, chronic low-grade fever or night sweats should be suspected of having allergic bronchopulmonary disease. Chest roentgenograms show transient pulmonary infiltrates with areas of hyperinflation and atelec-

tasis. The causative fungus can be found in sputum cultures. Skin tests usually show positive immediate wheal and flare reaction as well as a "late" response six to eight hours later. IgE levels are uniformly and markedly elevated (Patterson and coworkers, 1973), and most patients also possess serum IgG precipitating antibodies. Inhalation challenge with Aspergillus antigen results in a dual response, with immediate bronchospasm followed by late bronchospasm four to six hours later, but should be performed with caution, since severe reactions may occur.

Therapy

Therapy with corticosteroids is necessary in addition to appropriate bronchodilator therapy for asthma and intensive respiratory therapy with postural drainage and clapping (frappage) to eliminate viscid secretions and mucus plugs in which the fungus is lodged. Steroids decrease the inflammatory response and relieve obstructed airways, thereby enhancing removal of the fungus. Prolonged corticosteroid therapy may be necessary for months to years, and must be continued as long as allergic bronchopulmonary signs and symptoms continue. Antifungal agents are ineffective because they are unable to reach the fungus, which is surrounded by thick viscid secretions.

PULMONARY HYPERSENSITIVITY STATES DUE TO CHEMICAL AGENTS AND DRUGS

An increasing number and variety of chemical agents and drugs induce such diverse pulmonary hypersensitivity reactions as bronchospasm and obstructive airway disease, restrictive pulmonary disease or both. These varied pulmonary hypersensitivity states are

TABLE 6. CAUSES OF CHEMICAL AND DRUG-INDUCED HYPERSENSITIVITY LUNG DISEASE

	Chemicals		
NAME	SOURCE	SUBSTANCE	TYPE REACTION
Cedar worker's disease	Western red cedar sawdust	Plicatic acid	Obstructive, restrictive or both
Coffee worker's disease	Coffee bean dust	Chlorogenic acid	Restrictive
Meat-wrapper's asthma	Plastic wrap	Organic copolymers of polyvinyl chloride	Obstructive
Metal fume fever	Plastic wrap	Zinc salts	Restrictive and obstructive
Polymer fume fever	Industrial exposure	Polytetrafluoro-ethylene	Obstructive
TDI diseases	Polyurethane plastics	Toluene diisocyanate	Obstructive
Others (see text)			
	Drugs		
Aspirin asthma	Oral medication	Acetylsalicylic acid	Obstructive
Blood transfusion lung	Multiple transfusions	Donor HLA antigens	Restrictive
Cromolyn sodium	Inhaled medication	Cromolyn sodium	Restrictive and obstructive
Pulmonary drug reaction	Ingested medication	Nitrofurantoin	Restrictive
Others (see text)			

included in this section, although they mimic asthma, hypersensitivity pneumonitis or allergic bronchopulmonary disease, because in most cases either the antigen, antibody or mechanism of tissue damage has not been identified. Only a small portion of the persons exposed actually develops symptoms; the reactions appear to be specifically acquired. The major diseases are noted in Table 6.

The development of pulmonary hypersensitivity to chemicals has become an increasing problem in our chemical-based society. Although these chemical pneumonopathies have not been considered of importance in children and adolescents, an increasing number of young adults with overt pulmonary disease have had their initial exposure to the offending agent in childhood or adolescence. Children and adolescents may be unknowingly exposed to potentially serious chemical agents in their hobbies after receiving far more intense exposure than do industrial workers, whose exposures are carefully controlled and monitored.

Clinical Features

As noted in Table 5, the clinical manifestations of chemical and pulmonary drug reactions vary from acute bronchospasm, as in meat-wrapper's asthma and polymer fume fever, to restrictive pulmonary disease with interstitial pneumonitis, as in nitrofurantoin pulmonary hypersensitivity, or both, as in sawmill workers who inhale western red cedar sawdust. Because these reactions may take such diverse forms and because the number of chemical agents capable of inducing such reactions is growing steadily, the physician must be increasingly aware of the environmental chemicals to which his patients are exposed.

Laboratory Features

In vitro tests are available for a few drugs. Cellular and humoral immune responses to cromolyn sodium have been demonstrated in a few patients with allergic reactions to the drug (Sheffer and coworkers, 1975). Immunopathologic mechanisms have not been delineated, however, in the majority of drug-induced pulmonary reactions (Rosenow, 1976).

Inhalation bronchial challenge is used in diagnosing immediate and late pulmonary reactions to a number of occupational antigens, such as chemical vapors, drugs and enzymes (Butcher and coworkers, 1976).

SPECIFIC SYNDROMES

Chemicals

Cedar Worker's Disease

The induction of an asthma-like syndrome and rhinitis or hypersensitivity pneumonitis following exposure to the dust of western red cedar (*Thuja plicata*) is due to plicatic acid, a small molecular weight, simple chemical occurring in the dust. Cedar worker's disease is frequently characterized by a dual response to inhalation challenge. The initial airway obstruction 3 to 15 minutes after inhalation of plicatic acid may be followed by chest pain, chills, fever and marked lassitude four to eight hours later. Some patients may show only a single reaction, however. Diagnosis is by bronchial challenge. Therapy necessitates avoidance of cedar dust, and may require a change of occupation (Chan-Yeung and coworkers, 1973).

Coffee Worker's Disease

This disease, a hypersensitivity pneumonitis usually of insidious onset, is associated with progressive cough, dyspnea, fever, malaise and a maculopapular skin eruption. The roentgenogram is characteristic, with infiltrative and noduloreticular lesions. The etiologic agent of coffee worker's disease is believed to be chlorogenic acid, a small organic acid found in coffee bean dust. Treatment includes avoidance and the short-term use of glucocorticoid for the relief of symptoms.

Meat-Wrapper's Asthma

This disorder has been described in people who wrap meat in plastic film and is characterized by sneezing, rhinorrhea, nasal congestion and coughing following exposure to the pyrolysates of polyvinyl chloride (PVC) or heat-activated price labels (Sokol and coworkers, 1973). Tobacco smokers have more severe symptoms than nonsmokers do. Pulmonary function studies usually reveal diffuse obstructive large airway disease with decreased FEV_1, and an increase in alveolar-arteriolar oxygen gradient. The etiologic agent appears to be the organic copolymers of fumes from both the wrapping material and the heat-activated price labels (Andrasch and Bardana, 1976).

Metal Fume Fever

Metal fume fever results from the inhalation of high particulate metallic oxide fumes with content of zinc, copper, iron, magnesium, cadmium and antimony. Zinc oxide, in particles of 0.05 to 0.5 micron, is the most common offender. The fumes induce bronchiolar, respiratory duct and alveolar inflammation, with interstitial edema and inflammatory cellular infiltrates. Clinically, it is characterized by paroxysms of acute influenza-like attacks, with fever, chills, cough and marked fatigue occurring four to eight hours after exposure. In metal fume fever, a tolerance may be acquired with prolonged daily exposure, which is lost when the patient avoids contact for at least 48 hours. Bronchodilating drugs and corticosteroids have been useful in temporary management, but avoidance of exposure is mandatory to prevent progressive lung disease (McConnell and coworkers, 1973).

Polymer Fume Fever

This syndrome is produced by two different chemicals: polytetrafluoroethylene (Teflon) and polyvinyl fluoride. These chemicals are widely used in the coating of cookingware, chemical vessels, wires, gaskets, bearings and medical instruments (Kuntz, 1974).

Following the inhalation of pyrolysis products, the patients develop "gripping chest pain," chills and fever, along with moderate wheezing. Pulmonary function studies show a mild pulmonary restrictive disorder. Pathologically, the lesion is primarily pulmonary edema and necrosis of bronchiolar mucosa. The disagnosis of polymer fume fever is made by history and confirmed by re-exposure.

Toluene diisocyanate

Toluene diisocyanate workers exposed to toluene diisocyanate (TDI) over prolonged periods may develop a diverse immunologic and pulmonary hypersensitivity response. Either the 2,4 or the 2,6 monomer of toluene diisocyanate may combine with proteins of the bronchiolar and alveolar cellular lining to form a conjugate tissue antigen, which may induce a reaction from IgE or IgG antibodies or both (Butcher and coworkers, 1976). In some patients there is also a complement-dependent agglutination response. The result is a diffuse obstructive lung disease manifested by a significant decrease in the forced expiratory volume in one second (FEV_1) and in pulmonary flow rates.

Clinical features vary greatly. Some patients have immediate coughing, sneezing and tightness of the chest, which can be relieved by bronchodilating agents such as aerosolized epinephrine. Others have a delayed response, and symptoms of coughing and chest tightness, wheezing and low-grade fever do not occur for four to 12 hours after exposure. Patients with delayed responses have positive agglutination tests that are complement-dependent, as opposed to those with the immediate reaction. A third population of subjects who are initially symptomatic become asymptomatic on continued exposure to low concentrations. This tolerance or anergy corresponds to the development of IgG precipitating antibodies in their serum. The diagnosis is made by bronchial challenge. Immunologic tests include identification of specific IgE antibodies and IgG precipitating antibodies. Agglutination tests using latex-fixed TDI will identify late responders. Therapy consists of avoidance of the offending antigen (TDI) or a reduction of the TDI exposure to a level below 2.02 parts per million. In certain patients with acute immediate reactions, treatment with adrenergic agents such as epinephrine or isoproterenol is helpful.

Other Chemicals

An increasing list of other chemicals that can induce pulmonary reactions includes phenylglycine acid hydrochloride (penicillin manufacturing), tannic acid (leather tanning), tartrazine (yellow food coloring), salts of nickel, platinum, vanadium and tungsten, formaldehyde, and piperazine hydrochloride.

Drugs

Aspirin Asthma

In adults with intrinsic asthma, the triad of aspirin intolerance, nasal polyps and sinusitis is well known to internists. In such patients, aspirin intolerance is manifested by severe asthma or anaphylaxis or both. Until recently, such reactions were rarely recognized in children. A double-blind study of 50 children with chronic asthma showed 14 (28 per cent) had similar aspirin reactions in the absence of nasal polyps or sinusitis (Rachaelefsky and coworkers, 1975). Although the mechanism is not fully known, it is not IgE-mediated, and current evidence suggests that it may be due to a prostaglandin imbalance accentuated not only by acetylsalicylic acid but also by indomethacin and/or tartrazine (a yellow dye used in coloring many medications) in some patients. Ironically, patients intolerant to aspirin can tolerate sodium salicylate (Samter and Beers, 1968).

Children and adolescents with chronic asthma should avoid aspirin and should be warned about the many over-the-counter preparations that contain aspirin. Acetaminophen should be prescribed as an appropriate alternative.

Pulmonary Hypersensitivity Reactions to Blood Transfusions

Patients who receive multiple blood transfusions may develop lymphocytotoxic antibodies for specific donor leukocyte antigens of the HLA system. A further transfusion of the incompatible HLA blood may induce a fatal pulmonary reaction, with chills, fever, cough, tachycardia and marked dyspnea unresponsive to beta adrenergic agents. Several fatal reactions have been reported in which autopsy revealed massive hemorrhagic pulmonary edema with focal aggregates of hemosiderin-laden phagocytes, dilated veins and capillaries engorged with aggregates of erythrocytes, and many granulocytes in alveolar spaces.

Diagnosis is made by the demonstration of marked pulmonary edema following blood transfusion in contrast to hyperinflation of the lungs seen in acute anaphylaxis. Therapy consists of respiratory support, treatment of pulmonary edema, digitalization, diuretics and systemic corticosteroids. Adrenergic drugs appear to be of only minimal aid. The use of red blood cells as free of extraneous antigen as possible may prevent or minimize this reaction.

Cromolyn Sodium

A few patients inhaling cromolyn sodium for asthma have developed more severe disease because of allergy to cromolyn. Chest roentgenograms reveal diffuse shifting pulmonary infiltrates. Lung biopsy shows both interstitial and alveolar eosinophilic infiltrates. Both humoral and lymphocytic (in vitro MIF production) antibodies have been identified. Discontinuation of cromolyn and a short course of steroids reverse these lesions (Sheffer and coworkers, 1975).

Nitrofurantoin-induced Lung Disease

In the acute form, the chest roentgenogram reveals noncardiac pulmonary edema and pleural effusion. When bronchospasm is present, there may be hyperinflation. Eosinophilia may be seen, and pulmonary function tests reveal obstructive abnormalities. In the chronic form, the chest roentgenogram reveals basilar interstitial pneumonitis with fibrosis. Eosinophilia is absent, and pulmonary function tests are primarily restrictive, with decreased alveolar gas diffusion. On lung biopsy, interstitial pneumonitis with fibrosis predominates (Rosenow, 1976). In some biopsies, the changes have been consistent with desquamative interstitial pneumonitis (Bone and coworkers, 1976). Pearsall and coworkers (1974) have reported increasing lymphocyte sensitivity with blast transformation and MIF production in vitro in a patient with the chronic form. They described a cell layer model in which sensitized lymphocytes interacted with alveolar cell explants with cytotoxicity to fibroblasts and macrophage activation. This in vitro model appears promising in unraveling the immunologic mechanisms in drug-induced pulmonary reactions.

Other Drugs

Pharmacologic agents that have been reported to cause pulmonary hypersensitivity include spiramycin, chymotrypsin, hydrochlorothiazide, gold, methotrexate, methysergide and bleomycin. Although the mechanism by which they cause tissue damage has not been elucidated, the clinical and roentgenographic changes resemble hypersensitivity pneumonitis response.

REFERENCES

Adiseshan, N., and Oliver, W. A.: Strontium lung scans in the diagnosis of pulmonary aspergillosis. *Am. Rev. Resp. Dis., 108*:441, 1973.

Allen, D. H., Basten, A., and Woolcock, A. J.: Family studies in hypersensitivity pneumonitis. *Chest, 69*(Suppl. 2):283, 1976.

Andrasch, R. H., and Bardana, E. J., Jr.: Thermoactivated price-labeled fume intolerance. *J.A.M.A., 235*:937, 1976.

Banaszak, E. F., Barboriak, J., Fink, J., et al.: Epidemiologic studies relating thermophilic fungi and hypersensitivity lung syndromes. *Am. Rev. Resp. Dis., 110*:585, 1974.

Banaszak, E. F., Thiede, W. H., and Fink, J. N.: Hypersensitivity pneumonitis due to contamination of an air-conditioner. *N. Engl. J. Med., 283*:271, 1970.

Bardana, E. J., Jr.: Measurement of humoral antibodies to aspergilli. *Ann. N.Y. Acad. Sci., 221*:64, 1974.

Bardana, E. J., Jr., Gerber, J. D., Graig, S., and Cianciulli, F. D.: The general and specific immune response to pulmonary aspergillosis. *Am. Rev. Resp. Dis., 112*:799, 1975.

Bergner, A., and Bergner, R.: Pulmonary hypersensitivity associated with pancreatin powder exposure. *Pediatrics, 55*:814, 1975.

Berrill, W. T., Fitzpatrick, P. F., Macleod, W., et al.: Bird fancier's lung and jejunal villous atrophy. *Lancet, 2*:1006, 1975.

Bice, D. E., Salvaggio, J., and Hoffman, E.: Passive transfer of experimental hypersensitivity pneumonitis with lymphoid cells in the rabbit. *J. Allergy Clin. Immunol., 58*:250, 1976.

Bone, R. C., Wolfe, J. Sobonya, R. E., Kerby, G. R., Stechschulte, D., Ruth, W. E., and Welch, M.: Desquamative interstitial pneumonia following chronic nitrofurantoin therapy. *Chest, 69*(Suppl. 2):296, 1976.

Booth, B. H., LeFoldt, R. H., and Moffitt, E. M.: Wood dust hypersensitivity. *J. Allergy Clin. Immunol., 57*:352, 1976.

Bringhurst, L. S., Byrne, R. N., and Gashon-Cohen, J.: Respiratory disease of mushroom workers. *J.A.M.A., 171*:15, 1959.

Butcher, B. T., Salvaggio, J. E., Weill, H., and Ziskind, M. M.: Toluene diisocyanate (TDI) pulmonary disease: immunologic and inhalation challenge studies. *J. Allergy Clin. Immunol., 58*:89, 1976.

Chan-Yeung, M.: Maximal expiratory flow and airway resistance during induced bronchoconstriction in patients with asthma due to western red cedar *(Thuja plicata). Am. Rev. Resp. Dis., 108*:1103, 1973.

Chan-Yeung, M., Barton, G. M., MacLean, L., and Grzybowski, S.: Occupational asthma and rhinitis due to western cedar *(Thuja plicata). Am. Rev. Resp. Dis., 108*:1094, 1973.

Chandra S., and Jones, H. E.: Pigeon fancier's lung in children. *Arch. Dis. Child., 47*:716, 1972.

Citron, K. M.: Respiratory fungus allergy and infection. *Proc. R. Soc. Med., 68*:587, 1975.

Cohen, H., Merigan, T. C., Losek, J. C., and Eldridge, F.: Sequoiosis, a granulomatous pneumonitis associated with redwood sawdust inhalation. *Am. J. Med., 43*:785, 1967.

Cunningham, A. S., Fink, J. N., and Schlueter, D. P.: Childhood hypersensitivity pneumonitis due to dove antigens. *Pediatrics, 58*:436, 1976.

Dicki, H. A., and Rankin, J.: Farmer's lung: an acute granulomatous interstitial pneumonitis. *J.A.M.A., 167*:1069, 1958.

doPico, G. A., Reddan, W. G., Chmelik, F., Peters, M. E., Reed, C. E., and Rankin, J.: Value of precipitating antibodies in screening for hypersensitivity pneumonitis. *Am. Rev. Resp. Dis., 113*:451, 1976.

Emanuel, D., Lawton, B. R., and Wenzel, F. J.: Pneumonitis due to *Cryptostroma corticale. N. Engl. J. Med., 274*:1413, 1966.

Fink, J. N.: Hypersensitivity pneumonitis: a case of mistaken identity. *Hosp. Pract.*, March 1974, p. 119.

Fink, J.: Hypersensitivity pneumonitis. In Kirkpatrick, C. E., and Reynolds, H. Y. (Eds.): *Lung Biology and Health Disease.* Vol. 1. Immunologic and Infectious Reactions in the Lung. New York, Marcel Dekker, Publisher, 1976, pp. 229–241.

Fink, J. N., and Sosman, A. J.: Allergic lung disease not mediated by IgE. *Med. Clin. N. Am., 58*:157, 1974.

Fink, J. N., and Sosman, A. J., Barboriak, J. J., et al.: Pigeon breeder's disease. A clinical study of a hypersensitivity pneumonitis. *Ann. Intern. Med., 68*:1205, 1968.

Fink, J. N., Banaszak, E. F., Barboriak, J. J., Hensley, G. T., Kurup, V. P., Scanlon, G. T., Schlueter, D. P., Sosman, A. J., Thiede, W. H., and Unger, G. F.: Interstitial lung disease due to contamination of forced air systems. *Ann. Intern. Med., 84*:406, 1976.

Flaherty, D. K., Murray, H. D., and Reed, C. E.: Cross reactions to antigens causing hypersensitivity pneumonitis. *J. Allergy Clin. Immunol., 53*:329, 1974a.

Flaherty, D. K., Barboriak, J., Emanuel, D., Fink, J., Marx, J., Moore, V., Reed, C. E., and Roberts, R.: Multilaboratory comparison of three immunodiffusion methods used for detection of precipitating antibodies in hypersensitivity pneumonitis. *J. Lab. Clin. Med., 84*:293, 1974b.

Gandevia, B.: Hypersensitivity disorders of the lungs and bronchi. *Ann. Clin. Lab. Sci., 3*:386, 1973.

Grant, J. W. B., Blackadder, E. S., and Greenberg, M. B.: Extrinsic allergic alveolitis in Scottish malt workers. *Br. Med. J., 1*:490, 1976.

Hansen, P. J., and Penny, R.: Pigeon breeder's disease. Study of the cell-mediated immune response to pigeon antigens by the lymphocyte culture technique. *Int. Arch. Allergy Appl. Immunol., 47*:498, 1974a.

Hansen, P. J., and Penny, R.: The immune mechanisms and diagnosis of pigeon breeder's disease. *Med. J. Aust., 1*:984, 1974b.

Hargreave, F. E., and Pepys, J.: Allergic respiratory reactions in bird fanciers provoked by allergen inhalation provocation tests. *J. Allergy Clin. Immunol., 50*:157, 1972.

Heiner, D. C., and Sears, J. W.: Chronic respiratory disease associated with multiple circulating precipitins to cow's milk. *Am. J. Dis. Child., 100*:500, 1960.

Heiner, D. C., Sears, J. W., and Kniker, W. T.: Multiple precipitins to cow's milk in chronic respiratory disease: syndrome including poor growth, gastrointestinal symptoms, evidence of allergy, iron deficiency anemia, and pulmonary hemosiderosis. *Am. J. Dis. Child., 103*:634, 1962.

Hensley, G. T., Fink, J. N., and Barboriak, J. J.: Hypersensitivity pneumonitis in the monkey. *Arch. Pathol., 97*:33, 1974.

Hodges, G. R., Fink, J. N., and Schlueter, D. P.: Hypersensitivity pneumonitis caused by a contaminated cool mist vaporizer. *Ann. Intern. Med., 80*:501, 1974.

Johnson, K. J., and Ward, P. A.: Acute immunologic pulmonary vasculitis. *Am. J. Clin. Invest., 54*:349, 1974.

Jordan, M. C., Bierman, C. W., and Van Arsdel, P. P., Jr.: Allergic bronchopulmonary aspergillosis. *Arch. Intern. Med., 128*:56, 1971.

Kaltreider, H. B.: Hypersensitivity pneumonitis. *J. Occup. Med., 15*:949, 1973.

Katz, R. M., and Kniker, W. T.: Infantile hypersensitivity pneumonitis as a reaction to organic antigens. *N. Engl. J. Med., 288*:233, 1973.

Katzenstein, A. L., Liebow, A. A., and Friedman, P. J.: Bronchocentric granulomatosis, mucoid impaction, and hypersensitivity reactions to fungi. *Am. Rev. Resp. Dis., 111*:497, 1975.

Kawai, T., Salvaggio, J., Lake, W., and Harris, J. O.: Experimental production of hypersensitivity pneumonitis with bagasse and thermophilic actinomycete antigen. *J. Allergy Clin. Immunol., 50*:276, 1972.

Kohler, P. F., Gross, G., Salvaggio, J., and Hawkins, J.: Humidifier lung: hypersensitivity pneumonitis related to thermotolerant bacterial aerosols. *Chest, 69*(Suppl. 2):294, 1976.

Kuntz, W.: Polymer fume fever. *J. Occup. Med., 16*:480, 1974.

Kurup, V. P., Barboriak, J. J., Fink, J. N., and Lechevalier, M. P.: *Thermoactinomyces candidus,* a new species of thermophilic actinomycetes. *Int. J. Syst. Bacteriol., 25*:150, 1975.

Marinkovich, V. A.: Hypersensitivity alveolitis. *J.A.M.A., 321*:944, 1975.

Marx, J. J., and Flaherty, D. K.: Activation of the complement sequence by extracts of bacteria and fungi associated with hypersensitivity pneumonitis. *J. Allergy Clin. Immunol., 57*:328, 1976.

McCarthy, D. S., and Pepys, J.: Allergic bronchopulmonary aspergillosis. *Clin. Allergy, 1*:414, 1971.

McCarthy, D. S., Simon, G., and Hargreaves, F. E.: Radiological appearances in allergic bronchopulmonary aspergillosis. *Clin. Radiol., 21*:366, 1970.

McConnell, L. H., Fink, J. N.: Schlueter, D. P., and Schmidt, M. G., Jr.: Asthma caused by nickel sensitivity. *Ann. Intern. Med., 78*:808, 1973.

Molina, C., Aiache, A., Tourreau, A. J., et al.: Les troubles respiratoires des fromagers. *Nouv. Presse Med., 3*:1603, 1974.

Moller, B. B., Halberg, P., Gravesen, S., and Weeke, B.: Precipitating antibody against *Micropolyspora phaeni* in sera from mushroom workers. *Acta Allergol., 31*:61, 1976.

Moore, V. L., and Fink, J. N.: Immunologic studies in hypersensitivity pneumonitis—quantitative precipitins and complement fixing antibodies in symptomatic and asymptomatic pigeon breeders. *J. Lab. Clin. Med., 85*:540, 1975.

Moore, V. L., Fink, J. N., Barboriak, J. J., Ruff, L. L., and Schlueter, D. P.: Immunologic events in pigeon breeders' disease. *J. Allergy Clin. Immunol.*, 53:319, 1974.

Moore, V. L., Hensley, G. T., and Fink, J. N.: An animal model of hypersensitivity pneumonitis in the rabbit. *J. Clin. Invest.*, 56:937, 1975.

Motoyama, E. K., Gibson, L. E., and Vegas, C. J.: Evaluation of mist-tent therapy in cystic fibrosis using maximum expiratory flow volume curves. *Pediatrics*, 50:299, 1972.

Olechock, S. A., and Burrell, B.: The role of precipitins and complement activation in the etiology of allergic lung disease. *J. Allergy Clin. Immunol.*, 58:76, 1976.

Parish, W. E.: Short-term anaphylactic IgG antibodies in human sera. *Lancet*, 1:591, 1970.

Patterson, R., and Roberts, M.: IgE and IgG antibodies against *Aspergillus fumigatus* in sera of patient with bronchopulmonary allergic aspergillosis. *Int. Arch. Allergy*, 46:150, 1974.

Patterson, R., Fink, J. N., Pruzansky, J. J., Reed, C., Roberts, M., Salvin, R., and Zeiss, C. R.: Serum immunoglobulin levels in pulmonary allergic aspergillosis and certain other lung diseases with special reference to immunoglobulin E. *Am. J. Med.*, 54:16, 1973.

Patterson, R., Roberts, M., Roberts, R. C., Emanuel, D. A., and Fink, J. N.: Antibodies of different immunoglobulin classes against antigens causing farmer's lung. *Am. Rev. Resp. Dis.*, 114:315, 1976.

Pearsall, H. R., Morgan, E. H., Tesluk, H., and Beggs, D.: Parakeet dander pneumonitis. Acute psittaco-kerato-pneumonitis. Report of a case. *Bull. Mason Clin.*, 14:127, 1960.

Pearsall, H. R., Ewalt, J., Tsoi, M., Sumida, S., and Backus, D.: Nitrofurantoin lung sensitivity. *J. Lab. Clin. Med.*, 83:728, 1974.

Pepys, J.: Hypersensitivity disease of the lungs due to fungi and other organic dusts. In Monographs in Allergy, No. 4. Basel, Switzerland, S. Karger, 1969.

Pepys, J.: Immunological and clinical findings in workers and consumers exposed to the enzymes of *Bacillus subtilis*. *Proc. R. Soc. Med.*, 66:930, 1973.

Pepys, J.: Immunologic approaches in pulmonary disease caused by inhaled materials. *Ann. N.Y. Acad. Sci.*, 221:27, 1974.

Pepys, J., Jenkins, P. A., Lackman, P. J., et al.: An iatrogenic autoantibody response to pituitary snuff in patients with diabetes insipidus. *Clin. Exp. Immunol.*, 1:377, 1966.

Purtilo, D. T., Brem, J., Ceccaci, L., et al.: A family study of pigeon breeder's disease. *J. Pediatr.*, 86:569, 1975.

Rachaelefsky, G. S., Conlson, A., Siegel, S. C., and Stiehm, F. R.: Aspirin intolerance in chronic childhood asthma: detected by oral challenge. *Pediatrics*, 56:443, 1975.

Reiss, J. S., Weiss, N. S., Payetter, K. M., and Strimas, J.: Childhood pigeon breeder's disease. *Ann. Allergy*, 32:208, 1974.

Richerson, H. B., Cheng, F. H., and Bauserman, S. C.: Acute experimental hypersensitivity pneumonitis in rabbits. *Resp. Dis.*, 104:586, 1971.

Roberts, R. C., Wenzel, F. J., and Emanuel, M. D.: Precipitating antibodies in a midwest dairy farming population toward the antigens associated with farmer's lung disease. *J. Allergy Clin. Immunol.*, 57:518, 1976.

Rosenow, E. C., III: Drug-induced hypersensitivity disease of the lung. In Kirkpatrick, C. E., and Reynolds, H. Y. (Eds.): *Lung Biology and Health Disease*. Vol. 1. Immunologic and Infectious Reactions in the Lung. New York, Marcel Dekker, Publisher, 1976, pp. 261–287.

Safirstein, B. H., D'Souza, M. F., Simon, G., Tai, E. H. C., and Pepys, J.: Five-year follow-up of allergic bronchopulmonary aspergillosis. *Am. Rev. Resp. Dis.*, 108:450, 1973.

Salvaggio, J. E., Buechner, H. A., Seabury, J. H., and Arguembourg, P. Bagassosis. I. Precipitins against extracts of crude bagasse in the serum of patients. *Ann. Intern. Med.*, 64:748, 1966.

Samter, M., and Beers, R. F., Jr.: Intolerance to aspirin: clinical studies and consideration of its pathogenesis. *Ann. Intern. Med.*, 68:975, 1968.

Schatz, M., Patterson, R., Fink, J., and Moore, V.: Pigeon breeder's disease. *Clin. Allergy*, 6:7, 1976.

Schlueter, D. P., Fink, J. N., and Sosman, A. J.: Pulmonary functions in pigeon breeders' disease. *Ann. Intern. Med.*, 70:457, 1969.

Seabury, J., Becker, B., and Salvaggio, J.: Home humidifier thermophilic actinomycete isolates. *J. Allergy Clin. Immunol.*, 57:174, 1976.

Seal, R. M. E., Hapke, E. J., Thomas, G. O., Meek, J. C., and Hayes, M.: The pathology of acute and chronic stages of farmer's lung. *Thorax*, 23:469, 1968.

Shannon, D. C., Andrews, J. L., Recavarren, S., and Kazemi, H.: Pigeon breeder's lung disease and interstitial pulmonary fibrosis. *Am. J. Dis. Child.*, 117:504, 1969.

Sheffer, A. L., Rocklin, R. E., and Goetzl, E. J.: Immunologic components of hypersensitivity reactions to cromolyn sodium. *N. Engl. J. Med.*, 293:1220, 1975.

Slavin, R. G.: Immunologically mediated lung diseases, extrinsic allergic alveolitis and allergic bronchopulmonary aspergillosis. *Postgrad. Med.*, 59:137, 1976.

Sokol, W. N., Aelony, Y., and Beall, G. N.: Meat-wrapper's asthma. *J.A.M.A.*, 226:639, 1973.

Spector, S. L., and Farr, R. S.: Comments on bronchial inhalation provocation tests. *J. Allergy Clin. Immunol.*, 48:120, 1971.

Stiehm, E. R., Reed, C. E., and Tooley, W. H.: Pigeon breeder's lung in children. *Pediatrics*, 39:904, 1967.

Sweet, L. C., Anderson, J. A., Callies, Q. C., et al.: Hypersensitivity pneumonitis related to a home furnace humidifier. *J. Allergy. Clin. Immunol.*, 48:171, 1971.

Turner-Warwick, M., Haslam, P., and Weeks, J.: Antibodies in some chronic fibrosing lung diseases. *Clin. Allergy*, 1:209, 1971.

Turner-Warwick, M., Citron, K. M., Carroll, K. B., Heard, G. E., Mitchell, D. N., Pepys, J., Scadding, J. D., and Sontar, C. A.: Immunologic lung disease due to Aspergillus. *Chest, 68*:3; 346, 1975.

Warren, C. P. W., and Tse, K. S.: Extrinsic allergic alveolitis owing to hypersensitivity to chickens. *Am. Rev. Resp. Dis., 109*:672, 1974.

Warren, P., Cherniack, R. M., and Tse, K. S.: Hypersensitivity reactions to grain dust. *J. Allergy Clin. Immunol., 53*:139, 1974.

Wenzel, F. J., Emanuel, D. A., and Gary, R. L.: Immunofluorescent studies in patients with farmer's lung. *J. Allergy Clin. Immunol., 48*:224, 1971.

Zylak, C. J., Dyck, D. R., Warren, P., and Tse, K. S.: Hypersensitivity lung disease due to avian antigens. *Radiology, 114*:45, 1975.

CHAPTER FORTY-THREE

TUMORS OF THE CHEST

JAMES W. BROOKS, M.D.

Neoplasms of the chest in children may be divided into the following categories:

1. Pulmonary
   a. Benign
   b. Malignant
   c. Metastatic
2. Mediastinal
   a. Cysts
   b. Solid tumors
   c. Lymphatic
   d. Vascular
3. Cardiac
4. Diaphragmatic
5. Chest wall

PULMONARY TUMORS

In the pediatric age group, all forms of primary pulmonary tumors are unusual.

BENIGN PULMONARY TUMORS

Hamartoma

The term "hamartoma" was coined in 1904 by Albrecht, who defined it as a tumor-like malformation formed by an abnormal mixing of the normal components of the organ. Hamartomas of the lung consist largely of cartilage and also include variable quantities of epithelium, fat and muscle (Fig. 1). They are usually located in the periphery of the lung, but involvement of intermediate and primary bronchi has been reported. Developmental derangement is apparently responsible for their occurrence.

The incidence of hamartoma in all patients is 0.25 per cent (Lindskog and Liebow, 1962), but only six have been reported in the pediatric age group; four of these were discovered at autopsy, and two were successfully removed.

Although 53 cases of endobronchial hamartoma have been reported in adults, none has been seen in children.

Unlike hamartomas in adults, which are usually asymptomatic and small, the rare case found in infancy has been large and symptomatic and has contributed to the death of the infant (prematurity combined with respiratory inadequacy). At least four of the six reported hamartomas had obvious progressive intrauterine development and had attained considerable size at the time of birth.

Recognition and prompt removal of such large intrapulmonic tumors is nec-

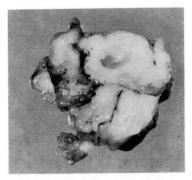

Figure 1. Hamartoma removed from right upper lobe of an adult. Note predominance of cartilage.

697

essary for survival. Difficult resuscitation or early demise, however, makes this difficult.

Although solid masses seen on chest roentgenograms in infants may cause one to suspect hamartoma, the diagnosis cannot be substantiated without thoracotomy. Surgical removal is the treatment of choice.

Holder and Christy (1964) have collected from the literature 32 cases of cystic adenomatoid malformation of the lung in newborn infants. These authors suggest that the entity be designated "adenomatoid hamartoma"; although this is a form of congenital cystic disease of the lung resulting from abnormal growth of normal lung components, it is not a true hamartoma.

Polypoid Intrabronchial Mesodermal Tumors

As far as can be determined, chondromas, granular cell myoblastomas and mesenchymomas have not been reported in the pediatric age group.

Benign Parenchymal Tumors of Mesodermal Origin

Plasma cell granuloma of the lung has been reported in approximately 20 pediatric patients, with the greatest number between eight and 12 years of age. Many patients are asymptomatic; others show signs of pulmonary infection. Roentgenograms are frequently interpreted as tumor. Calcification is frequent. Regional lymph nodes may be enlarged. Since the lesion is benign, surgical removal should conserve pulmonary tissue.

Study of the literature has revealed no case of sclerosing hemangioma in the pediatric age group.

Bronchial Adenoma

Bronchial adenoma is a neoplasm arising from either the cells of the mucous glands of the bronchi or the cells lining the excretory ducts of these glands.

Two histologic types are defined.

The *carcinoid type* (90 per cent) has histologic resemblance to carcinoid tumors of the small bowel; it is composed of somewhat oval cells filled almost entirely by nucleus. The cells, which have barely detectable lumens, are arranged in a quasiacinar fashion and are piled up in several layers. The tumor is very vascular and is surrounded by a thin capsule of fibrous tissue that is not invaded by the tumor cells. Metaplastic epithelium of the bronchial mucosa covers the intrabronchial component. The tumor is frequently shaped like a dumbbell, with the smaller component intrabronchial and the larger one intrapulmonic. Though considered a benign tumor, bronchial adenomas have a definite malignant potential; lymph node metastasis (15 per cent) is more frequent than distant blood-borne metastasis.

The *cylindromatous type* (10 per cent) is made up of cuboidal or flattened epithelial cells, arranged in two layers, which form corelike structures of the cylinders. Histologically, it closely resembles mixed tumors of the salivary glands and basal cell carcinoma of the skin. There is a 40 per cent chance of malignancy.

Twenty-one cases of bronchial adenoma, all apparently of the carcinoid type, have been reported in the pediatric age group. There were no metastases, and the carcinoid syndrome was not described.

The most prominent symptoms and signs are recurrent and refractory pneumonitis, elevated temperature, cough, and chest pain due to bronchial obstruction with associated distal infection. Hemoptysis and wheeze are not as common in children as in adults. The right main bronchus is most commonly involved, and the diagnosis can usually be made by biopsy obtained at bronchoscopy. The tumor occurs five times more commonly in males. Although the youngest recorded patient was a ten-month-old infant, all the others were seen in children at least eight years of age (Fig. 2).

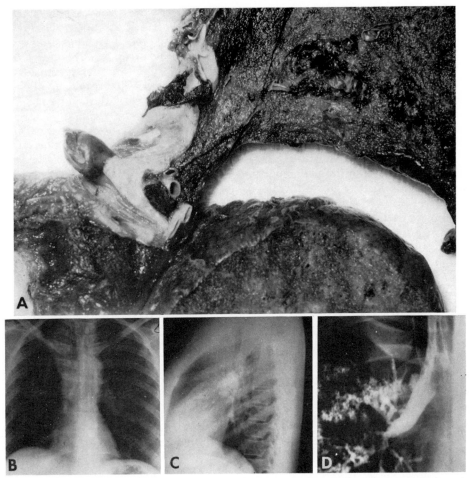

Figure 2. Bronchial adenoma (carcinoid type) and (*A*) total obstruction of the right upper lobe bronchus and distal atelectasis (*B* and *C*). Recurrent pneumonitis, cough and hemoptysis had occurred. Diagnosis of biopsy at the time of bronchoscopy. *D*, Obstruction of right upper lobe bronchus demonstrated with bronchograms. Treated by right upper lobectomy.

No case of peripheral bronchial adenoma has come to our attention.

Thoracotomy and resection of a segment, lobe or total lung according to the degree of involvement is indicated. Treatment by bronchoscopy is not effective, since complete removal of the tumor cannot be thus carried out. Rarely, a bronchial adenoma can be removed by bronchial resection.

Papilloma of the Trachea and Bronchi

Twenty-three cases of papilloma of the trachea and bronchi have been re-corded in children (Fishman, 1962). These lesions, the cause of which is not known, may be single, but are more frequently multiple. The tendency for these tumors to disappear spontaneously at puberty has suggested a hormonal relationship.

Symptoms depend on the location and size of the tumor. The lesions may be attached by a pedicle and oscillate in and out of orifices during inspiration and expiration (flutter valve). Single, slow-growing, high lesions within the trachea may be asymptomatic for years. Dyspnea and stridor are the most common symptoms, occurring in 63 per cent of the cases. Cough, at first dry and later productive, is another frequent symptom.

Wheeze, audible at the open mouth, is the earliest sign of papilloma of the trachea. This eventually develops into stridor and is associated with slowly increasing dyspnea. Such secondary changes as obstructive emphysema, atelectasis, pneumonia, lung abscess and bronchiectasis may result in the distal parts of the tracheobronchial tree; empyema may also occur. Unless diverted, the usual course is one of increasing dyspnea that terminates in asphyxia.

These tumors should be removed because of their tendency to obstruction. Distal pulmonary infection or death from asphyxia may result. Ogilvie (1953) has reported two instances of malignancy arising from tracheobronchial papillomas.

Excision is the treatment of choice. Owing to the frequent multiplicity of the papillomas, treatment may be difficult and tedious, requiring numerous endoscopic procedures. Electrocoagulation can be used, and x-ray therapy has been most beneficial when there are multiple papillomas. The prognosis is good, but there is a tendency to recurrence, and constant vigilance with repeat bronchoscopic follow-up is indicated.

Fibroma of the Trachea

Nine cases of fibroma of the trachea have been recorded in infants (Gilbert and coworkers, 1953).

Angioma of the Trachea

Six children with benign angioma have been reported by Gilbert and colleagues (1953). Congenital hemangioma of the trachea may cause death by the compromise of a vital structure, bleeding complications, intractable cardiac failure from atrioventricular shunting of blood within the tumor, or malignant change. In infants and children these tumors are usually

below the vocal cords, sessile, flat, and associated with dyspnea. Ninety per cent of the recorded patients have been six months of age at the time of the onset of symptoms, and females predominate over males two to one. Fifty per cent of the infants have hemangiomas elsewhere.

The onset is insidious, with symptoms of respiratory obstruction such as stridor, retraction, dyspnea, wheezing, and sometimes cyanosis and cough. The symptoms tend to be intermittent and labile. Usually fever and leukocytosis are absent, but superimposed infection may produce fever and an elevated white blood cell count. The best diagnostic tools are roentgenogram and endoscopy. Biopsy is not advisable at the time of endoscopy, since bleeding may cause asphyxia or an exsanguinating hemorrhage. Tracheostomy with x-ray therapy is probably the best form of therapy.

Leiomyoma of the Lung

Grossly, these tumors cannot be differentiated from other benign tumors of the lung. Leiomyomas of the lung are usually asymptomatic unless there is partial or complete bronchial obstruction. In a review of the world literature, Guida and coworkers (1965) found only one case in a child. This six-year-old had a tumor in the right lower lobe, successfully treated by lobectomy.

Lipoma

Review of the literature reveals no case of lipoma of the bronchus or lung in the pediatric age group.

Neurogenic Tumors

Primary intrapulmonic neurogenic tumors have been recorded in three children out of 32 proved cases in the world literature. One was a neurofibroma, and the other two were neurilemomas.

MALIGNANT PULMONARY TUMORS

Bronchogenic Carcinoma

Only 17 cases of primary bronchogenic carcinoma of the lung in children have been reported. In three of these, congenital malformations of the lung were present; two had cystic disease, and one had congenital atelectasis. The cases were equally distributed between males and females. The youngest patient was a five-month-old female infant with cystic lung disease and malignancy in the left lung reported by Schwyter in 1928. Every cell type except alveolar cell carcinoma, giant cell carcinoma, mucoepidermoid and carcinosarcoma has been seen in the pediatric age group.

1. Carcinoma.................................. 4
2. Adenocarcinoma 4
3. Squamous cell epithelioma.......... 6
4. Oat cell carcinoma..................... 2
5. Undifferentiated carcinoma......... 1

All patients have had widespread disease at the time when diagnosis was made. None has been resected. The longest recorded survival was seven years in a patient treated by irradiation (Wasch and coworkers, 1940). At the time of death there were widespread metastases.

Fibrosarcoma of the Bronchus

Review of the literature reveals only five cases of primary fibrosarcoma of the bronchus in the pediatric age group. Three were in girls and two in boys.

Fever, probably due to bronchial obstruction and distal infection, is the most common symptom; hemoptysis is relatively uncommon. Diagnosis in these cases should be established by bronchoscopy. Resection is the treatment of choice, since recurrence is frequent when any other mode of therapy is used. As a rule, metastasis occurs by way of the blood stream, but lymph node involvement is possible.

Leiomyosarcoma

There have been three cases of primary leiomyosarcoma and four cases of nonspecific primary sarcoma of the lung reported in children. Cough, dyspnea and signs of obstructive pneumonitis are usually present. Surgery is indicated (Fig. 3).

Multiple Myeloma

Multiple myeloma is usually limited to the medullary space. Extramedullary plasma cell tumors are relatively uncommon (myeloma or solitary plasmacytoma of the lung parenchyma). In a

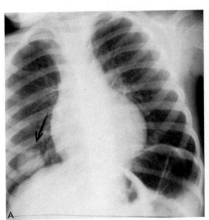
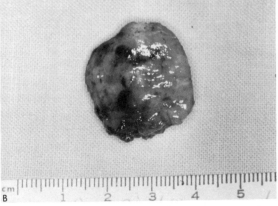

Figure 3. A, Three-year-old white male with increasing mass in right lower lobe of lung. B, Shelled-out leiomyosarcoma after lower lobectomy. No recurrence after one year.

review of the literature, Sekulich and coworkers (1965) found only 19 cases since 1911; one of these was a plasmacytoma in a three-year-old girl. Cytologic examination of sputum may be diagnostic.

Chorioepithelioma

A case of chorioepithelioma of the lung in a seven-month-old white female infant has been reported by Kay and Reed (1953). The presenting symptoms were fever, dyspnea and anorexia; massive hemoptysis then occurred. Roentgenogram showed almost complete opacity of the right side of the chest. Pneumonectomy was performed, but the child died several hours postoperatively.

Systemic Neoplasms Affecting the Lung

Myeloid and lymphatic leukemia may have a pulmonary component, but isolated pulmonary disease has not been recorded. Similarly, Hodgkin's disease and lymphosarcoma may involve the lung during the course of the disease, but neither occurs as an isolated pulmonary lesion.

METASTATIC PULMONARY TUMORS

Primary sarcomas occur much more frequently in children than do primary carcinomas. The literature does not contain a report of a primary carcinoma in an infant with metastases to the lung; however, there are a number of references to primary sarcomas with pulmonary involvement by metastases. Primary sarcoma of the kidney (Wilms'), primary malignant skeletal tumors (chondrosarcoma and osteogenic sarcoma), Ewing's tumor, reticulum cell sarcoma, and soft tissue sarcomas (fibrosarcoma, rhabdomyosarcoma, liposarcoma, malignant neurilemoma and synovioma) may metastasize to the lung. In general, the indications for resection of metastatic pulmonary disease should be based on the following criteria: (1) unilateral pulmonary involvement, and (2) evidence of local control of the primary malig-

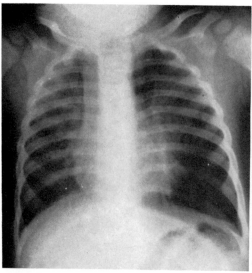
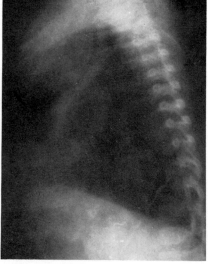

Figure 4. Obstructive emphysema of left lower lobe bronchus caused by partial occlusion of lumen. Left diaphragm is flattened, mediastinal and cardiac shadows are displaced toward right, left upper lobe is compressed, and there is increased radiolucency of left lower lobe.

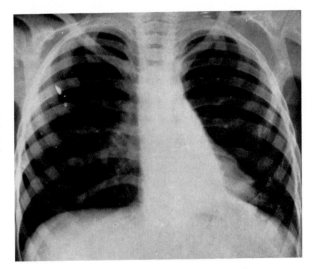

Figure 5. Total atelectasis of left lower lobe secondary to inflammatory stricture of left lower lobe bronchus. Retrocardiac position tends to confuse diagnosis in some cases.

nancy for a period of one year before pulmonary resection.

If the lesion is thought to be unilateral, planograms of the opposite lung should be obtained before resection is carried out. Pneumonectomy may be necessary for the removal of multiple unilateral lesions.

Bilateral pulmonary resections for metastatic disease are seldom indicated.

DISCUSSION

Children who have symptoms of pulmonary involvement that do not disappear promptly when treated in the

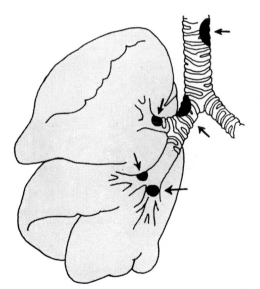

Figure 6. Diagram illustrating locations of lesions within the lumen of major bronchi. Location of such lesions will dictate area of pulmonary involvement, unilateral or bilateral, and extent of signs and symptoms.

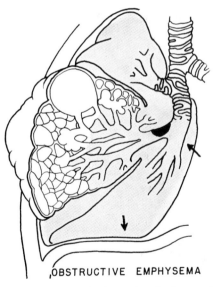

OBSTRUCTIVE EMPHYSEMA

Figure 7. Partial obstruction leads to retention of air in pulmonary parenchyma distal to obstructed bronchus. This will cause ipsilateral compression of adjacent normally aerated lung tissue, widening of intercostal spaces, descent of diaphragm, shift of mediastinum away from lung with partially obstructing lesion, and wheeze accompanied by decreased breath sounds over affected pulmonary tissue.

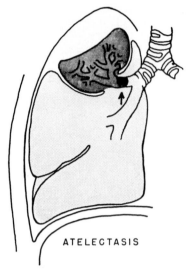

ATELECTASIS

Figure 8. Persistence of the lesion with ultimate total obstruction gives rise to atelectasis, absent breath sounds over affected lung tissue, overexpansion of surrounding lung tissue, and shift of diaphragm to more normal position, with return of mediastinum to midline. Bronchial secretions may actually decrease in amount.

usual manner by expectorants and antibiotics must be suspected of having a space-occupying lesion. Posteroanterior and lateral chest roentgenograms are

mandatory whenever respiratory symptoms persist.

Indeed, it would seem logical that all children should have a routine chest roentgenogram within the first six months of life. Certainly a physical examination in the adult patient is no longer considered complete without a chest roentgenogram. Why should the child be excluded from this advanced form of diagnosis? Without such refinement, how can we expect to help those with potentially curable lesions? Only by such techniques can obstructive emphysema (Fig. 4), atelectasis (Fig. 5) or actual solid masses be seen at a stage of development when active resectional surgery may have some hope of cure (Figs. 6 to 10).

In addition to a probing history and complete physical examination, children with respiratory symptoms should have other studies.

SPUTUM. It is impossible to obtain sputum voluntarily from the infant, but swabs from the posterior portion of the pharynx may be studied. In older children, however, sputum can be col-

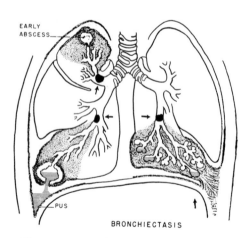

EARLY
ABSCESS

PUS

BRONCHIECTASIS

Figure 9. Continuing persistence of obstructing lesion leads to permanent destructive changes in pulmonary parenchyma distal to the lesion, such as abscess formation, chronic pneumonitis with fibrosis, pleurisy, empyema, and bronchiectasis with parenchymal contracture secondary to fibrosis.

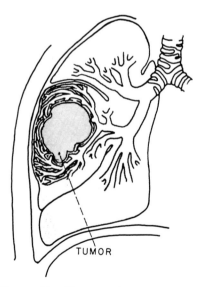

TUMOR

Figure 10. If tumor is within pulmonary parenchyma, pressure on adjacent lung and bronchi will give surrounding zone of pneumonitis that may actually show incomplete, temporary improvement on conservative management.

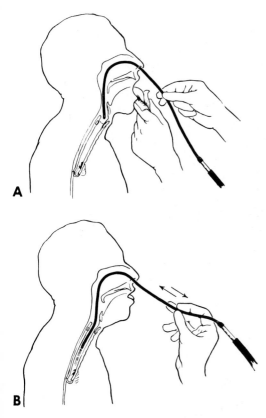

A

B

Figure 11. Diagram illustrating placement of rubber catheter through nose into posterior pharynx (*A*), followed by insertion into the trachea (*B*) through opened epiglottis at time of deep inspiration or cough to obtain bronchial secretions.

lected. A small catheter placed through the nose and adjusted into the trachea, thereby producing cough, will allow one to collect sputum through the catheter (Fig. 11). Any sputum thus collected should be studied by smear and culture for routine bacteria, acid-fast bacilli and fungi; bacteria should be tested for *antibiotic* sensitivity. Cytologic analysis for tumor cells should be carried out.

SKIN TESTS. The tuberculin (PPD or tine) skin test should be applied. Coccidioidin, blastomycin and histoplasmin* skin tests may be applied, although they are not as accurate as complement-fixation studies.

BLOOD TESTS. Protein electro-

*Histoplasmin skin test not available at present.

phoresis may show hypogammaglobulinemia to be a primary or secondary etiologic factor in recurrent pulmonary infectious processes. Complement-fixation studies for fungal infections are generally more reliable than the skin tests. Pulmonary complications of hematologic disorders, such as leukemia, Hodgkin's disease or lymphosarcoma, may be properly identified by examination of the peripheral blood smear.

BONE MARROW. Examination of the bone marrow may give diagnostic evidence of blood dyscrasias, such as leukemia or myeloma, or even metastatic malignancy.

SWEAT CHLORIDES. Cystic fibrosis as a cause of chronic recurrent pulmonary inflammatory disease may be suggested or ruled out by sweat chloride determination. (See Chapter 45, Cystic Fibrosis.)

ROENTGENOLOGIC EXAMINATION. Roentgenologic examination of the chest with fluoroscopy and cinefluoroscopy, special views such as apical lordotic, right and left oblique, and planograms may be necessary for final definition. Cinefluoroscopy allows repeated examination of the thoracic organs in motion (function) without subjecting the infant to excessive radiation exposure. During this examination and at the time of fluoroscopy, studies with barium in the esophagus will aid in determining any displacement of the posterior mediastinum.

PNEUMOPERITONEUM. The introduction of air into the peritoneal cavity, outlining the diaphragm, may aid in the diagnosis of abnormalities adjacent to the diaphragm; congenital diaphragmatic hernias may also be visualized (Fig. 12).

ANGIOGRAPHY. Angiocardiograms, outlining the cardiac chambers, will point up any displacement due to masses in the lung, mediastinum or pericardium. Certain lesions may be studied better by venous angiography outlining the major veins of the mediastinum. The use of aortograms will assist in ruling out such vascular causes for symptoms as vascular ring, congeni-

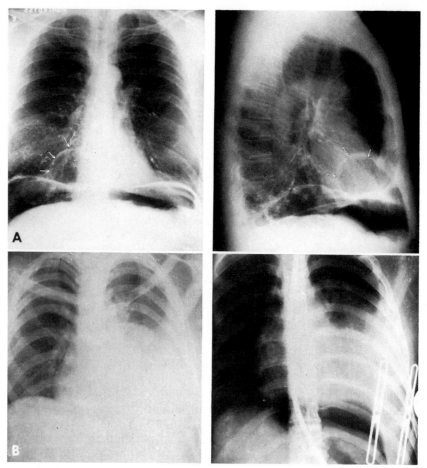

Figure 12. *A*, Diagnostic pneumoperitoneum showing congenital diaphragmatic hernia of Morgagni; *B*, outlining normal diaphragm with intrapleural or pneumonic density above.

tal aneurysm, or congenital vascular malformations of the pulmonary tree.

BRONCHOGRAMS. Bronchograms are extremely useful in the study of the trachea, major bronchi, and lobar and segmental bronchi. Intraluminal lesions, obstructive lesions and those causing displacement of bronchial segments may be identified (Fig. 13). Air bronchograms may give detail sufficient to dispense with contrast liquid materials (Fig. 14).

BRONCHOSCOPY. Bronchoscopy is the best available procedure for the study of tracheobronchial and pulmonary disease. This procedure enables visual study of the vocal cords, larynx, trachea, major bronchi and their important segmental orifices. Congenital anatomic abnormalities may be visualized; lesions within the lumen can be biopsied for a definitive diagnosis; prognosis in extensive lesions is evaluated by study of the carina and trachea. Aspiration of secretions is an important therapeutic contribution. Study of secretions and washings must include cytologic studies for malignant cells, routine bacterial smear, culture, and sensitivity studies, acid-fast smear and cultures, and fungal smear and cultures. (See Bronchoscopy, Chapter 4.)

LYMPH NODE BIOPSY. Biopsy of palpable lymph nodes may be of aid in the diagnosis of abnormal processes in the lung. Most important are the scalene

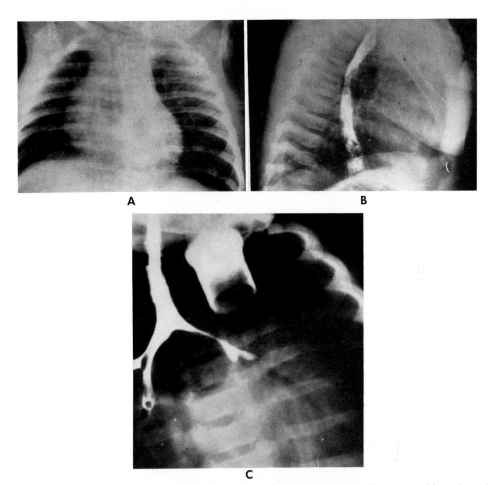

Figure 13. *A* and *B*, Anterior and lateral chest roentgenograms in infant with congenital bronchogenic cyst at carina and clinical respiratory distress. *C*, Contrast tracheobronchogram delineates narrowing of left main bronchus and displacement of right main bronchus.

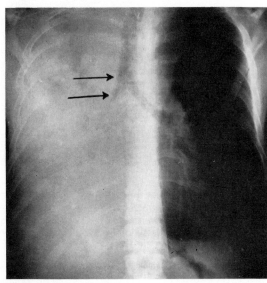

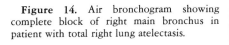

Figure 14. Air bronchogram showing complete block of right main bronchus in patient with total right lung atelectasis.

lymph nodes, which drain the pulmonary parenchyma. Regardless of palpability, these nodes should be biopsied in those cases of pulmonary disease in which the diagnosis is uncertain and thoracotomy is contemplated. Scalene lymph node biopsy and mediastinoscopy with biopsy of mediastinal nodes available as distal as the carina are of great help in the diagnosis of sarcoi-

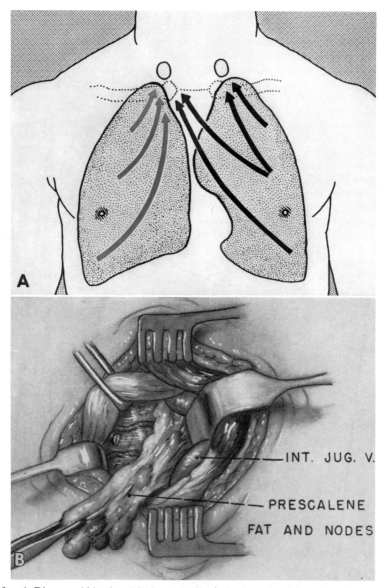

Figure 15. *A,* Disease within the right lung usually drains into the right scalene lymph node group, while that in the left lung may drain to either scalene node group in a pattern similar to that indicated on the illustration. Generally, left lung disease requires bilateral scalene node biopsy, while right lung disease requires only right scalene node biopsy. Regardless of the side of lung disease, all palpable nodes in the scalene node area should be biopsied. *B,* The scalene group of nodes is contained in the fat pad bounded medially by the internal jugular vein, inferiorly by the subclavian vein and superiorly by the posterior belly of the omohyoid muscle. The base of the triangle is formed by the anterior scalene muscle. Retraction of the internal jugular vein is essential in order to get all nodes in this group.

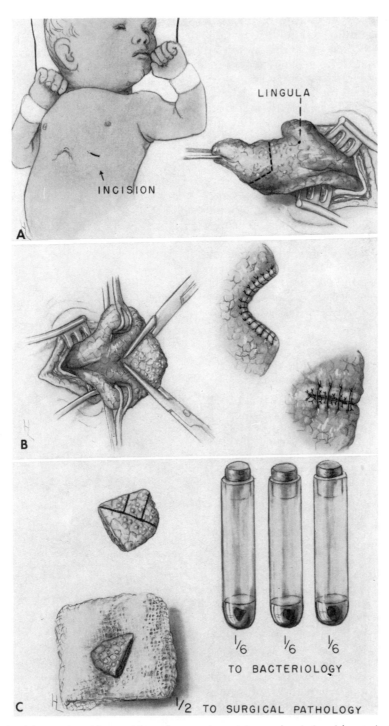

Figure 16. Adequate lung biopsy with specimens to bacteriology and pathology laboratories is essential. In general, a small open thoracotomy has many advantages over the blind needle biopsy technique.

dosis, in lymphatic malignancy such as Hodgkin's disease and lymphosarcoma, and in primary neoplasms of the lung and mediastinum. Lymph nodes obtained at the time of biopsy should be subjected to histologic study, and a portion sent to the bacteriology laboratory for routine bacterial smear and culture, studies for sensitivity of the organism to antibiotics, acid-fast smear and culture, and fungal smear and culture (Fig. 15).

LUNG BIOPSY AND THORACOTOMY. When all other methods have failed to produce a definitive diagnosis, thoracotomy should be considered. A limited incision may first be made, and biopsy of the lung obtained. If the situation appears to be an inoperable problem, biopsy may afford useful information (Fig. 16). Thoracotomy should not be unnecessarily delayed when definitive diagnosis has not been made.

MEDIASTINAL TUMORS

The mediastinum, the portion of the body that lies between both lungs, is bounded anteriorly by the sternum and posteriorly by the vertebrae. Superiorly, it extends from the suprasternal notch and terminates inferiorly at the diaphragm. Cysts or tumors that arise within the mediastinum may originate from any of the structures contained therein, or may be the result of developmental abnormalities. The mediastinum is lined on both sides by parietal pleura, and contains all structures of the thoracic cavities except the lungs. At times the lungs may herniate into the mediastinum. For ease of definition of sites of disease, the mediastinum may be divided into four arbitrary compartments (Fig. 17): (1) the superior mediastinum—that portion of the mediastinum above a hypothetical line drawn from the junction of the manubrium and gladiolus of the sternum (angle) to the intervertebral disk between the fourth and fifth thoracic vertebrae; (2) the anterior medias-

tinum—that portion of the mediastinum which lies anterior to the anterior plane of the trachea; (3) the middle mediastinum—that portion containing the heart and pericardium, the ascending aorta, the lower segment of the superior vena cava bifurcation of the pulmonary artery, the trachea, the two main bronchi and bronchial lymph nodes; (4) the posterior mediastinum—that portion which lies posterior to the anterior plane of the trachea.

A great number of lesions (even very large ones) in the mediastinum will remain asymptomatic for a considerable period of time and will be discov-

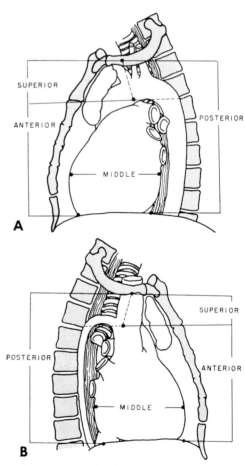

Figure 17. *A,* Mediastinal compartments as seen from left hemithorax. *B,* Mediastinal compartments as seen from right hemithorax.

ered only through the use of routine chest roentgenograms. The patient becomes aware of lesions within the mediastinum only when pressure is exerted upon sensitive structures of the mediastinum or the structures are displaced; therefore, the severity of symptoms depends upon the size and location of the tumor, the rapidity of growth, and the presence or absence of the actual invasion of organs. Symptoms resulting from mediastinal lesions may become manifest according to the disturbance of function of the various organs in the mediastinum.

RESPIRATORY SYMPTOMS. In mediastinal lesions of children, respiratory symptoms are the most important. These symptoms are the result of direct pressure on some portion of the respiratory tract. This pressure causes narrowing of the trachea or the bronchi, or compression of the lung parenchyma (Fig. 18). Dry cough may be present; stridor or wheeze may occur at the same time or may precede it. The compression may be sufficient to produce enough occlusion so that there is distal obstructive emphysema or atelectasis, pneumonitis or chronic recurrent lower respiratory tract infections with

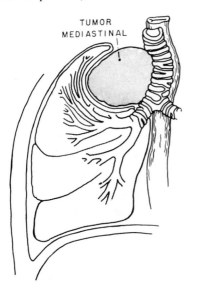

TUMOR
MEDIASTINAL

Figure 18. Diagram illustrating large mediastinal tumor or cyst with pressure on tracheobronchial tree as well as pulmonary parenchyma, thus possibly giving rise to pulmonary symptoms.

associated fever and leukocytosis. The dry cough may be replaced by a productive one with mucoid sputum; if infection occurs, the secretion will become purulent. The unilateral nature of the wheezing and respiratory complaints serves to rule out asthma, bronchiolitis or chronic recurrent infections secondary to cystic fibrosis or hypogammaglobulinemia, but will not eliminate the possibility of endobronchial or endotracheal lesions; nor can the possibility of a foreign body in the tracheobronchial tree be discarded. Bronchoscopy is necessary in order to make this differentiation.

If the lesion in the mediastinum exerts pressure on the recurrent laryngeal nerve, hoarseness and a brassy cough will result. Dyspnea, which may be progressive, is a common symptom of mediastinal tumors. Acute episodes of dyspnea with associated pneumonitis may occur when there is tracheal or bronchial obstruction, leading to distal infection. Hemoptysis occurs in less than 10 per cent of mediastinal tumors in children.

GASTROINTESTINAL SYMPTOMS. Symptoms referable to the gastrointestinal tract result primarily from pressure on the esophagus. Regurgitation of food, and dysphagia with a slight sensation of sticking in the lower esophagus, are common. Displacement of the esophagus usually does not cause dysphagia; however, if there is fixation of the mass secondary to infection, hemorrhage or malignant degeneration, thereby causing interference with the peristaltic activity of the esophagus, dysphagia will occur. Vomiting is rare when the tumor is benign, but may occur when it is malignant; this is the result of the systemic effects of the malignancy.

NEUROLOGIC SYMPTOMS. In older children there is often a feeling of vague intrathoracic discomfort, fullness or ache caused by pressure on the sensitive intercostal nerves. Such pain may be mild or severe and is common in tumors of neurogenic origin. The appearance of herpes zoster indicates involvement of an intercostal nerve, but this is not common in the pediatric age group. When lesions impinge on the pleura, the pain may be of pleuritic nature. Erosion of vertebrae causes a boring pain located in the interscapular area. A malignant lesion that invades the brachial plexus causes severe pain in the upper extremities; Horner's syndrome indicates involvement of the cervical sympathetics. Inflammation, intracystic hemorrhage, or malignant degeneration causing pressure on the phrenic nerve may result in hiccups. Certain dumbbell tumors of the spinal cord and mediastinum may exhibit symptoms referable to spinal cord pressure.

VASCULAR SYMPTOMS. Benign lesions of the mediastinum rarely cause obstruction of the great vessels in the mediastinum; however, obstruction is a common finding in malignant mediastinal tumors and carries a poor prognosis. Superior vena caval involvement gives rise to a dilatation of veins in the upper extremity, head and neck. As the obstruction progresses, there is cyanosis of the head and neck area associated with bounding headaches and tinnitus. Either innominate vein may be involved, causing unilateral venous distention and edema of the upper extremity, head and neck (ipsilateral). Pressure on the inferior vena cava is less common, but when present there may be associated edema of the lower extremities.

MISCELLANEOUS SYMPTOMS. Fever is uncommon in mediastinal lesions unless there is secondary infection in the tracheobronchial tree; it may also be present with Hodgkin's disease, lymphosarcoma, or breakdown of malignant disease. Weight loss, malaise, anemia and anorexia are uncommon unless there is malignancy.

PHYSICAL FINDINGS. Physical findings are frequently absent; wheeze, rhonchi or rales may be present. There may be dullness to percussion over the area of mediastinal enlargement; this extends laterally from each sternal border or posteriorly between the scapulae and above the diaphragm. Occasionally, there is tenderness over the chest wall when a mediastinal tumor exerts pressure on the parietal pleura in that area.

DIAGNOSTIC PROCEDURES. The same diagnostic procedures apply in cases of lung lesions and mediastinal tumors. Certain situations unique to mediastinal tumors will be mentioned.

A tumor or lesion of the mediastinum should never be aspirated preoperatively when operation is clearly indicated. If a neoplasm is present, such needle aspiration may cause spread of the tumor cells. Needle aspiration of lesions of the mediastinum should be reserved for the inoperable tumor, or the acute emergency when tremendous cystic enlargement may jeopardize the child's life or may interfere with a good course of induction at the time of anesthesia.

The use of trial x-ray therapy for undiagnosed mediastinal lesions is not warranted. Deep x-ray therapy can be administered in dosage sufficient to produce shrinkage of hyperplasia of the thymus, mediastinal nodes in Hodgkin's disease and lymphosarcoma. The danger of radiation-induced thyroid carcinoma makes the use of deep x-ray therapy for the shrinkage of hyperplasia of the thymus inadvisable. Peripheral lymph node biopsy is preferable in suspected cases of Hodgkin's disease or lymphosarcoma. If such lymph nodes are not diagnostic, thoracotomy is then indicated.

Hydatid disease is not common in the United States, and only when it is present in the lung adjacent to the mediastinum can mediastinal tumor be simulated. The precipitin and skin test results are positive in hydatid disease with an active hydatid cyst. Often hooklets may be found in the sputum of patients so affected.

Mediastinal abscess will rarely be confused with a neoplasm of the mediastinum. Usually there is a history of trauma, foreign body in the esophagus, or instrumentation. High fever, tachycardia, dyspnea, extreme weakness, and prostration usually come on rapidly; thus, the signs and symptoms of acute infection are paramount. The development of a fluid level in the mediastinum is diagnostic of mediastinal abscess if the above-mentioned physical findings are also present. Intensive antibiotic therapy and prompt surgical drainage are indicated. There may be masses in the neck secondary to extension from lesions within the mediastinum.

PRIMARY MEDIASTINAL CYSTS

Lesions occurring within the mediastinum may be predominantly cystic or predominantly solid. Those in the cystic group are usually benign, while the solid group has a more malignant potential.

Primary mediastinal cysts probably represent abnormalities in embryologic development at the site of the foregut just when separation of esophageal and lung bud occurs (Fig. 19).

Structures that arise from the foregut are the pharynx, thyroid, parathyroid, thymus, respiratory tract, esophagus, stomach, upper part of the duodenum, liver and pancreas; thus, abnormal development at this stage

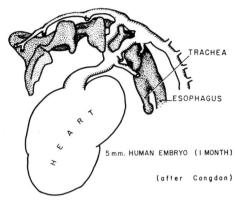

Figure 19. Foregut lying between tracheal and esophageal buds is probable site of embryologic maldevelopment, which gives rise to foregut cyst development.

may give rise to (1) bronchogenic cysts, (2) esophageal duplication cysts, and (3) gastroenteric cysts.

Bronchogenic Cysts

Maier (1948) has classified bronchogenic cysts according to location (Fig. 20) as (1) tracheal, (2) hilar (Fig. 21), (3) carinal (Fig. 22), (4) esophageal, and (5) miscellaneous (Fig. 23).

Bronchogenic cysts are usually located in the midmediastinum, but have been described in all mediastinal sub-

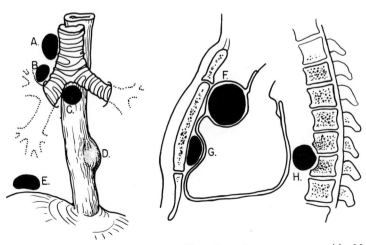

Figure 20. Diagrammatic illustration of location of bronchogenic cysts as suggested by Maier; B and C are the most common sites recorded.

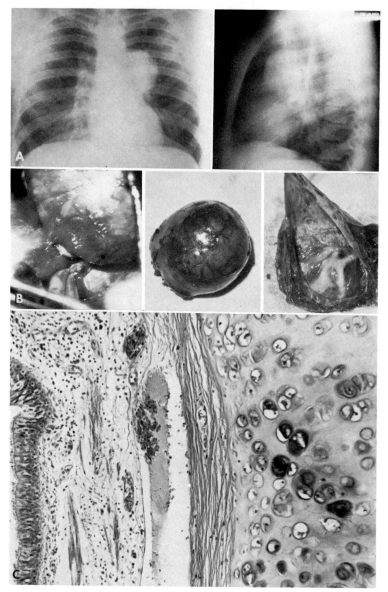

Figure 21. *A,* Typical left hilar bronchogenic cyst with rounded, smooth border, and density similar to cardiac density. *B,* At the time of thoracotomy, solid stalk was found attached to left main bronchus. Cyst was unilocular, containing thick, yellowish mucoid material. The wall was thin with typical trabeculations. *C,* Microscopic study revealed cartilage, smooth muscle and pseudostratified, ciliated, columnar epithelium.

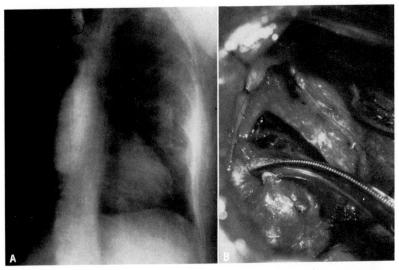

Figure 22. *A*, Overexposed posteroanterior chest film showing a carinal bronchogenic cyst. *B*, At operation, the location is clearly seen at the carina with a solid fibrous stalk attached at the carina and separated just beneath the instrument dissector.

divisions. Under microscopic examination, bronchogenic cysts may contain any or all of the tissues normally present in the trachea and bronchi (fibrous connective tissue, mucous glands, cartilage, smooth muscle, and a lining formed by ciliated pseudostratified columnar epithelium or stratified squamous epithelium). The fluid inside the

cyst is either clear, water-like liquid, or viscous, gelatinous material. The amylase content of the fluid is very high.

Bronchogenic cysts are usually asymptomatic. There may, however, be frequent upper respiratory tract infections, vague feelings of substernal discomfort, and respiratory difficulty (cough, noisy breathing, dyspnea, and

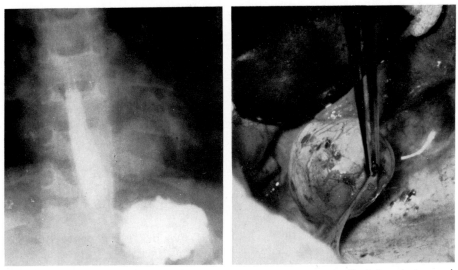

Figure 23. Bronchogenic cyst in child located retropleurally, overlying the distal thoracic aorta and not attached to the respiratory tract or esophagus.

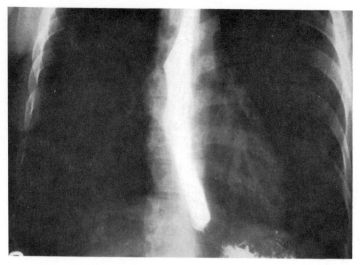

Figure 24.   Hilar bronchogenic cyst with esophageal indentation seen on esophagogram.

possibly cyanosis). Bronchogenic cysts may communicate with the tracheobronchial tree and show varying airfluid levels accompanied by the expectoration of purulent material. If communication with the tracheobronchial tree is present, this may be visualized by bronchoscopy and by bronchograms. Hemoptysis may occur when there is infection and communication of the cyst with the tracheobronchial tree.

On x-ray examination, the bronchogenic cyst is usually a single, smooth-bordered, spherical mass (Fig. 24). It has a uniform density similar to the cardiac shadow. Calcification is unusual. Fluoroscopic examination of the cyst may demonstrate that it moves with respiration, since it is attached to the tracheobronchial tree; its shape may be altered during the cycles of respiration. Evidence of bone erosion with bronchogenic cysts is not recorded.

When the bronchogenic cyst is located at the carina, it may cause severe respiratory distress owing to compression of either one or both major bronchi (Figs. 13 and 25). Early diagnosis and prompt removal are necessary.

The recorded incidence of bronchogenic cysts varies greatly. For exam-

ple, Gross (1953) found one bronchogenic cyst out of a total of 33 cysts and tumors of the mediastinum, while Heimburger and Battersby (1965) found seven cases (20 per cent) in their series of 36 cysts and tumors. When the latter combined five series from the literature, bronchogenic cysts were found in 10 per cent of the cases.

In a review of the literature by Dobbs and coworkers (1957), there were ten cases of intrapericardial bronchogenic cysts.

Bronchogenic cysts should be treated by surgical removal. Their exact diagnosis can rarely be confirmed prior to thoracotomy. Removal is indicated because the lesion represents an undiagnosed thoracic mass; inflammation and intracystic hemorrhage may cause symptoms of severe respiratory distress and complicate removal; and finally, continued growth will embarrass surrounding vital structures.

Esophageal Cysts (Duplication)

Esophageal cysts are located in the posterior mediastinum; they are usually on the right side, and are intimately associated in the wall of the esophagus

(Fig. 26). They occur more frequently in males than in females.

There are two types of esophageal cysts; the more characteristic type resembles adult esophagus with the cyst lined by noncornified, stratified squamous epithelium having a well defined muscularis mucosae and striated muscle in the wall. Intimate association in the muscular wall of the esophagus is not accompanied by communication with the lumen of the esophagus.

The second type is lined by ciliated mucosa, thus resembling that of the fetal esophagus. Esophageal cysts may be associated with mild dysphagia and regurgitation, but most frequently are asymptomatic. Barium esophagogram shows smooth indentation of the esophagus. On esophagoscopy there is indentation of the normal mucosa by a pliable, movable, soft, extramucosal mass. Removal by thoracotomy is indicated for the same reasons as noted in discussion of the therapy of bronchogenic cysts.

Gastroenteric Cysts

The third type of cyst arising from the foregut is the gastroenteric. This group of cysts lies against the verte-

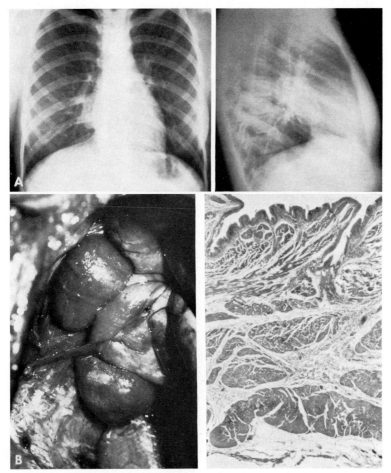

Figure 25. *A*, Bronchogenic cyst in a child whose mother had tuberculosis. The child was treated with antituberculous drugs for one year without change. *B*, At operation, a dumbbell-shaped bronchogenic cyst was found in the region of the inferior pulmonary vein. Microscopic section shows a wall with ciliated epithelium, but no cartilage, and smooth muscle wall of two layers.

brae, posterior or lateral to and usually free of the esophagus, and usually in the posterior mediastinum with the main attachment posteriorly. It may be recalled that the early esophagus is lined by columnar epithelium, much of which is ciliated, and this is only gradually converted to the stratified epithelium of the definitive organ. The change is generally complete or almost complete at birth (Arey, 1965). Thus, if a cyst arises from the embryonic esophagus, the ciliated lining is expected.

The enteric nature of a posterior mediastinal cyst is presumably certain if microscopic examination reveals a frank gastric or intestinal type of epithelium, but in general a better index of the nature and origin of such a cyst is the presence of well developed muscularis mucosae, tela submucosa, and two or even three main muscle coats. Gastric glands are most frequent, but esophageal, duodenal or small intestinal glands may be found. At operation, the cyst sometimes seems grossly "stomach-like" or "bowel-like." The significant fact is that cysts encountered in the posterior mediastinum show a highly developed mesodermal wall and even

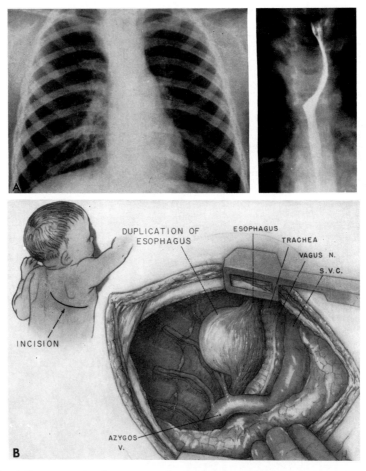

Figure 26.   *A,* Posteroanterior chest roentgenogram taken in a child with an upper respiratory tract infection. A mass is seen in the posterior superior mediastinum and presenting into the right hemithorax. At the time of an esophagogram, the esophagus is seen displaced toward the left by a smooth mass. *B, C* and *D,* Artist's drawings of findings at operation. Note the plane of separation from the mucosa of the esophagus and lack of communication with the esophageal lumen. *E,* Opened operative specimen, cavity of which was filled with mucoid fluid. Lining of duplication was typical squamous cell.

Illustration continued on opposite page

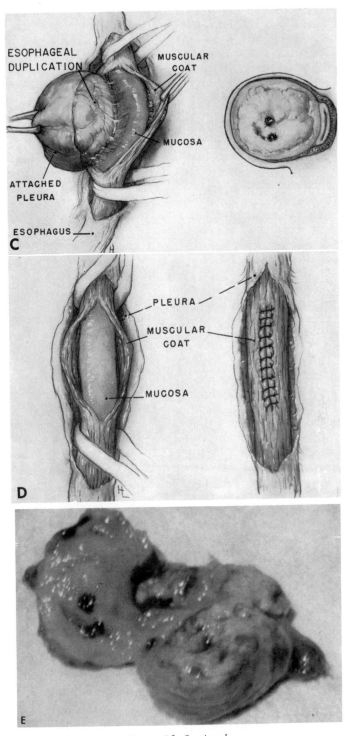

Figure 26. *Continued.*

the presence of Meissner's and Auerbach's plexuses, whereas the lining epithelium from case to case may range from columnar ciliated epithelium to a typical small intestinal type.

Two types of gastroenteric cysts have been described: (1) acid-secreting cysts, which are functionally active; and (2) cysts in which the mucosa has no functional activity.

Males are predominantly affected with this abnormality. In contrast with other foregut cysts, the posterior gastroenteric cyst is usually symptomatic. The symptoms are usually due to pressure on thoracic structures or rupture into bronchi with massive hemoptysis and death. Calcification also is frequent. Ossification has been reported by Steele and Schmitz (1945) in a cyst from a 15-year-old girl.

If the lining is gastric, dyspnea is the usual presenting symptom and occurs early. Actual peptic perforation of the lung with hemorrhage has been recorded.

Hemoptysis in young infants is difficult to distinguish from hematemesis; it may follow ulceration of a gastroenteric cyst (with gastric lining) of the mediastinum, with subsequent erosion into the lung. Gastric epithelium associated with intestinal or respiratory epithelium is apparently less secretory. Many functional cysts may lose their functional activity when the secretive areas of the mucosa are destroyed. Renin, pepsin, chlorides and free hydrochloric acid have been demonstrated in the contents of some of the cysts.

Posterior gastroenteric foregut cysts of the mediastinum are frequently associated with two other types of congenital anomalies; (1) mesenteric and (2) vertebral abnormalities. Both types may occur in the same case. In the embryo, the notocord and the entoderm are at one time in intimate contact; thus, this combined developmental anomaly may result from abnormal embryonic development.

Penetration of the diaphragm by a cyst arising primarily from the thorax may occur; conversely, penetration of the diaphragm by the free end of an intramesenteric intestinal duplication is also possible.

A survey of the literature on mediastinal cysts combined with vertebral anomalies reveals that hemivertebra, spina bifida anterior or infantile scoliosis has been reported in 61 per cent of 18 cases. Most of these vertebral lesions involve the upper thoracic and lower cervical vertebrae, and the cyst tends to be caudad to the vertebral lesion. Planograms may be necessary for diagnosis.

The presence of spina bifida anterior, congenital scoliosis, Klippel-Feil syndrome or similar but less defined lesions in the cervical or dorsal vertebra suggests the possibility that enteric cysts may be present in the mediastinum or in the abdomen.

In a survey by Abell (1956), four such gastroenteric cysts (3 per cent) were present in a series of 133 tumors of the mediastinum; they composed 10 per cent of the mediastinal cysts in this series. All produced symptoms, were present in patients whose ages ranged from seven months to five years, were located in the posterior mediastinum, had abnormalities of the cervical or dorsal spine, and were resected successfully.

Pericardial Celomic Cysts

These mesothelial cysts are developmental in origin, and formal genesis is related to the pericardial celom. The primitive pericardial cavity forms by the fusion of celomic spaces on each side of the embryo. During the process, dorsal and ventral parietal recesses are formed. Dorsal recesses communicate with the pleuroperitoneal celom, while the ventral recesses end blindly at the septum transversum. Persistence of segments of the ventral parietal recess accounts for most pericardial celomic cysts.

The cysts are usually located anteriorly in the cardiophrenic angles, more frequently on the right, and occasionally on or in the diaphragm (Fig.

27). They are usually asymptomatic and are discovered by routine chest roentgenogram. Rarely do they reach sufficient size to cause displacement of the heart or produce pressure upon the pulmonary tissue. Infection is unusual.

Pericardial cysts are usually unilocular. The walls are thin and the intersurfaces smooth and glistening, lined by a single layer of flat mesothelial cells. The mesothelium is supported by fibrous tissue with attached adipose tissue.

These cysts are usually not diagnosed in the pediatric age group. There are no recorded cases of symptomatic pericardial celomic cysts in children.

Intrathoracic Meningoceles

Intrathoracic meningoceles are not true mediastinal tumors or cysts; they are diverticuli of the spinal meninges that protrude through the neuroforamen adjacent to an intercostal nerve and present beneath the pleura in the posterior medial thoracic gutter. The wall represents an extension of the leptomeninges, and the content is cerebrospinal fluid. Enlargement of the intervertebral foramen is common; vertebral or rib anomalies adjacent to the meningocele are also frequent. The most commonly associated anomalies are kyphosis, scoliosis, and bone ero-

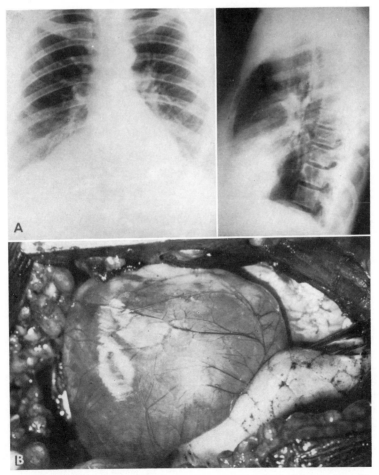

Figure 27. *A,* Typical location of pericardial cyst in posteroanterior and lateral chest films at the right cardiophrenic angle. *B,* Large cyst seen at the time of thoracotomy.

sion or destruction. The wall of these cysts is formed by two distinct components; these are the dura mater and the arachnoidea spinalis, with small nerve trunks and ganglia occasionally incorporated in the wall.

Of the 46 reported cases of intrathoracic meningocele, four were in the pediatric age group.

A threefold syndrome with generalized neurofibromatosis (von Recklinghausen's disease), kyphoscoliosis and intrathoracic meningocele may occur, but thoracic meningocele as an isolated defect is much less frequent. This lesion is usually asymptomatic; it occurs on the right side approximately three times as often as on the left. Rarely, the lesion may be bilateral. In patients with neurofibromatosis, posterior sulcus tumors are more likely to be meningoceles and are rarely neurofibromas.

On x-ray examination the lesion is a regular, well demarcated, intrathoracic density located in the posterior sulcus; there are associated congenital anomalies of the spine and thorax. On fluoroscopic examination, pulsations may be noted in the sac. Diagnosis may be confirmed by myelograms.

When diagnosis is established, no therapy is indicated unless the lesion is symptomatic.

Operative complications such as empyema, meninigits and spinal fluid fistula have been greatly reduced since the advent of the antibiotics.

THYMUS

Normally the thymus is located in the anterior superior mediastinum, but abnormalities of the thymus have been reported in all areas of the mediastinum. Abnormalities of the thymus in children are (1) hyperplasia of the thymus, (2) thymic neoplasms, (3) benign thymomas, (4) thymic cysts, (5) teratoma in the thymus, and (6) tuberculosis of the thymus.

Hyperplasia of the Thymus

Thymic masses are the most common of the mediastinal masses in children; of these, hyperplasia of the thymus is most frequent.

The function of the thymus is still not clear, but recent studies suggest that it may in some way be involved in the determination of immunologic individuality. The thymus varies greatly in size. Steroids, infection, androgens and irradiation may make the thymus smaller; those stimuli that cause it to increase in size are not understood. Local variations in size are, as in other ductless glands, probably related to chance.

In a reveiw of normal chest roentgenograms, Ellis and coworkers (1955b) found that there was almost always a recognizable thymic shadow present during the first month of life; there was great variation in the size and shape. The mediastinal shadow in this age group seemed to be proportionally wider than in older children and adults because of the proportionally larger heart and thymic shadow. In the age group from one to 12 months, the thymic shadow was still present if it had been seen earlier. Between one year and three years, very little of the thymic shadow remained. Two per cent of children over four years of age still have a recognizable thymus on x-ray examination. It does not contain calcium, and there are transmitted pulsations on fluoroscopy. Noback, in a study of the thymus in both live and stillborn infants, found a cervical extension of the thymus gland in 80 per cent of the cases. If located in the superior thoracic inlet, enlargement of the thymus may cause tracheal compression (Fig. 28).

The diagnosis of obstruction from an enlarged gland is established by good x-ray films, made in full inspiration with the child's head in a neutral position when the lateral film is made. Both esophageal and angiographic studies can be used to exclude a vascular ring.

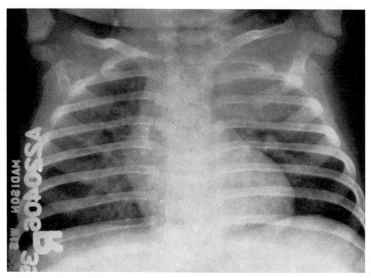

Figure 28. Mild respiratory distress in an infant with an enlarged thymus. Gradual improvement with age and no specific therapy.

Figure 29. *A*, Enlarged thymus in an infant with (*B*) reduction in size after seven days of steroid therapy.

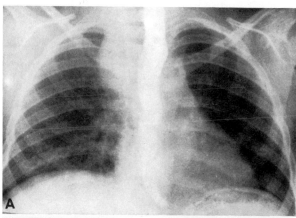

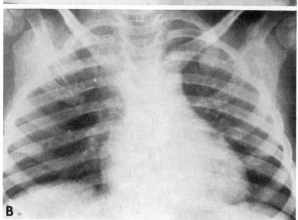

In cases of vascular ring obstruction, most patients find that their distress is relieved by hyperextension of the head.

Treatment of an enlarged thymus causing respiratory obstruction may be carried out in one of three ways.

First, the thymus responds rapidly to small doses (70 to 150 r) of irradiation; however, the danger of carcinogenic effect has caused this method of treatment to be abandoned.

Second, corticosteroids cause a rapid decrease in the size of the thymus, usually within a period of five to seven days. After cessation of corticosteroid therapy, the gland may reach a size greater than that before treatment was instituted. Such a response may also be used in distinguishing between a physiologic enlargement of the thymus and a neoplasm (Fig. 29).

Third, surgery may be indicated both for the treatment of respiratory obstruction and for diagnosis.

Neoplasm of the Thymus

Malignant thymic tumors in children are quite rare. Lymphosarcoma is by far the most frequent; primary Hodgkin's disease of the thymus and carcinoma have been described. In none has there been an associated myasthenia gravis.

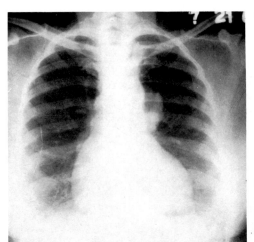
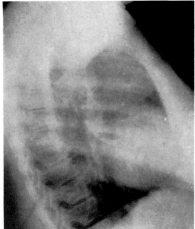
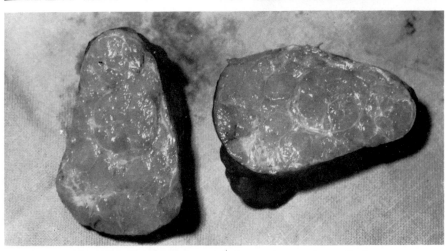

Figure 30.   Benign thymoma located in the anterior superior mediastinum.

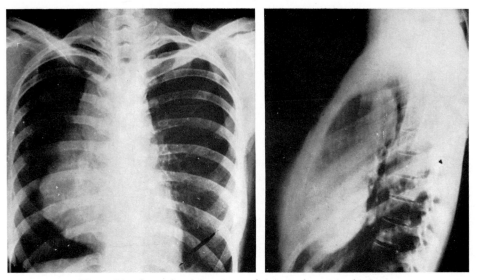

Figure 31. Large thymic cyst in an adult located near the diaphragm.

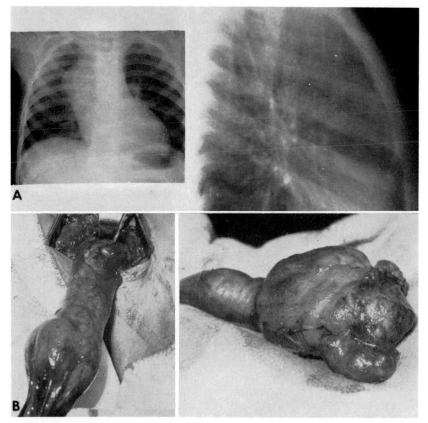

Figure 32. *A*, Large thymic cyst in four-year-old boy which presented in the right side of the neck as well as by chest roentgenogram. Removal required thoracotomy and supraclavicular incision. *B*, Thymic cyst as seen after thoracotomy and at time of removal through neck incision.

Benign Thymoma

Only six benign thymic tumors have been reported in children (Fig. 30).

Thymic Cysts

Multiple small cysts of the thymus are frequently observed in necropsy material, but large thymic cysts are rare (Fig. 31). Fridjon (1943) described a large cyst in the thymus of a one-day-old infant. Thymic cysts have been resected from the neck (Fig. 32).

Teratoma of the Thymus

Teratoma of the thymus in a two-day-old white female infant has been described by Sealy and coworkers (1965); there was progressive respiratory distress, and she underwent operation at seven weeks of age.

Tuberculosis of the Thymus Gland

A single case of tuberculosis involving only the thymus gland has been described in a stillborn infant.

TERATOID TUMORS

Teratoid tumors of the mediastinum may be classified as (1) benign cystic teratomas, (2) benign teratoids (solid), or (3) teratoids (carcinoma).

Benign Cystic Teratoma

Teratoma of the anterior mediastinum probably results from faulty embryogenesis of the thymus or from local dislocation of tissue during embryogenesis.

Benign cystic teratoma (mediastinal dermoid cyst) contains such elements of ectodermal tissue as hair, sweat glands, sebaceous cysts and teeth. Other elements, including mesodermal and entodermal tissue, may also be found when benign cystic teratoid lesions are subjected to comprehensive examination; thus, such tumors are more properly classified as teratoid than dermoid cysts.

Cystic teratomas are more common than solid ones. These lesions are predominantly located in the anterior mediastinum and may project into either hemithorax, more commonly the right. In children, females are affected more often than males. Malignant degeneration is less common than in the solid form of teratoid tumor.

It seems reasonable to assume that most, perhaps all, mediastinal teratomas are present at birth; however, Edge and Glennie (1960) have reported two adult patients from whom large teratoid tumors were removed two and four years after a routine chest roentgenogram was normal.

These cystic masses usually cause symptoms because of pressure on or erosion into the adjacent respiratory system. Symptoms are usually those of vague chest discomfort associated with cough, dyspnea and pneumonitis. Infection may cause a sudden exacerbation of symptoms, and rupture into the lung may occur with expectoration of hair; rupture into the pleura or pericardium may also occur.

The lesion is usually in the anterior mediastinum. On x-ray film, the lesion is well outlined with sharp borders; definite diagnosis is not possible unless teeth can be demonstrated in the mass. Calcification is not unusual, and appears as scattered masses rather than as diffuse, small densities. Cystic swelling in the suprasternal notch may occur.

Benign cystic teratomas should be removed. In cases in which infection, perforation, intracystic hemorrhage or malignant degeneration has occurred, complete removal may be difficult or impossible, owing to adherence to surrounding vital structures.

Benign Solid and Malignant Teratoid Tumors

Teratoma is the most common tumor occurring in the anterior mediastinum

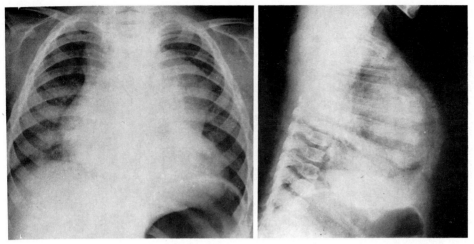

Figure 33. Large solid teratoid, benign, in an infant. Note anterior mediastinal position and forward displacement of the sternum.

of infants and children (Fig. 33). The solid tumors in the teratoid group are much more complex and have a greater propensity for malignant change (Fig. 34). The incidence of malignancy is about 20 per cent.

In the benign solid teratoid tumors, there are well differentiated structures that are rarely observed in the malignant group. Whereas the connective tissue stroma of malignant teratoma is usually poorly arranged, that of benign teratoma is dense and of the adult type. In the benign type, nerve tissue, skin and teeth may be found. Skin and its appendages are usually present and remarkably well formed. Hair follicles preserve their normal slightly oblique position relative to the free surface and are always accompanied by well developed sebaceous glands. Sweat glands, often of the apocrine type, are frequently located near the sebaceous glands. Smooth muscle, closely resembling arrectores pilorum, is occasionally encountered.

Mesodermal derivatives, such as connective tissue, bone, cartilage and muscle arranged in organoid pattern, are frequently found. When present, hematopoietic tissue is found only in asso-

ciation with cancellous bone. Smooth muscle is most often observed as longitudinal or circular bundles in organoid alimentary structures. Occasionally it is also seen in bronchial walls.

Entodermal derivatives, representing such structures as intestine, and respiratory and pancreatic tissue are also present.

In a review of mediastinal tumors, Ellis and DuShane (1956) found 27.6 per cent teratomatous tumors in infants. Of this group of 16 teratomatous tumors, eight were benign teratomas, five were teratoid cysts, and three were teratoid carcinoma.

The symptoms, signs and roentgenographic findings in these cases are identical with those found in teratoid cysts unless malignant spread has occurred.

The final decision as to malignancy can be determined only after removal and histologic study of the tumor. Malignant degeneration usually involves only one of the cellular components.

Heuer and Andrus (1940) reviewed 217 cases of teratoid tumors and found that only 5.5 per cent were discovered under the age of 12 years. Both benign and malignant teratoid tumors may occur within the pericardial sac.

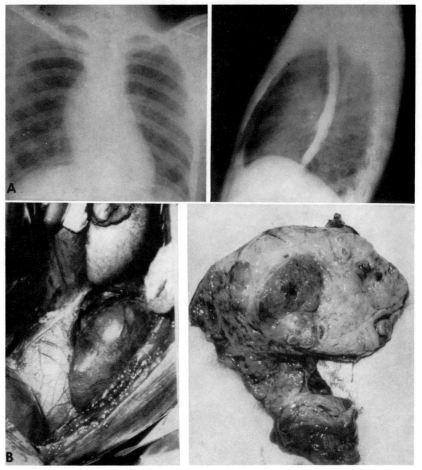

Figure 34. *A,* Posteroanterior and lateral x-ray films of anterior malignant teratoid in an older child. *B,* Note the anterior mediastinal position with teratoid wedged between the heart and sternum.

NEUROGENIC TUMORS

Neurogenic tumors, by far the most common of posterior mediastinal origin, may be classified as follows:
1. Neurofibroma and neurilemoma
   a. Malignant schwannoma
2. Tumors of sympathetic origin
   a. Neuroblastoma
   b. Ganglioneuroma
   c. Ganglioneuroblastoma
   d. Pheochromocytoma
3. Chemodectoma

Benign neurofibromas, neurilemoma and malignant schwannomas are extremely unusual in the pediatric age group, and when present are most often asymptomatic (Fig. 35).

The neuroblastoma is a malignant tumor arising from the adrenal medulla and occasionally from ganglia of the sympathetic nervous system; it consists of uniform cell layers with or without pseudorosettes. The cells have a dark nucleus and scant cytoplasm, and are separated by an eosinophilic fibrillar stroma. Cellular differentiation is sometimes very poor. Although the primary neuroblastoma may cause the first clinical signs or symptoms, metastases in the bone, skin or lymph nodes may be the first indication of its presence.

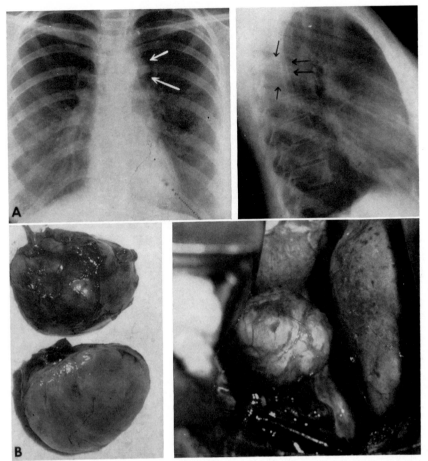

Figure 35. *A,* Neurofibroma seen posteriorly located in posteroanterior and lateral films. *B,* Note solid nature of lesion, round, smooth outline and attachment to intercostal nerve.

The ganglioneuroma is a benign tumor made up of mature ganglion cells, few or many in number, in a stroma of nerve fibers.

Ganglioneuroblastoma is a tumor composed of various proportions of neuroblastoma and ganglioneuroma.

Ganglioneuroma and ganglioneuroblastoma are more likely to occur after the age of two years. The more malignant forms, such as neuroblastoma, frequently occur before the age of two years. Ganglioneuroma is more common in children than in adults; respiratory symptoms are rare (Fig. 36).

Tumors of nerve origin usually occur in the upper two-thirds of the hemithorax and tend to extend locally. They may grow into the lower part of the neck, across the midline through the posterior mediastinum to the opposite hemithorax, descend through the diaphragm into the upper part of the abdomen or into the intercostal spaces posteriorly, and involve one or several of the vertebral foramina. Ganglioneuroblastoma rarely metastasizes to lymph nodes.

A large number of neurogenic tumors, more often the benign type, may be asymptomatic. Symptoms such as radicular pain, paraplegia, motor disturbances or Horner's syndrome may occur.

Upper respiratory tract infections, dyspnea, elevated temperature, weight

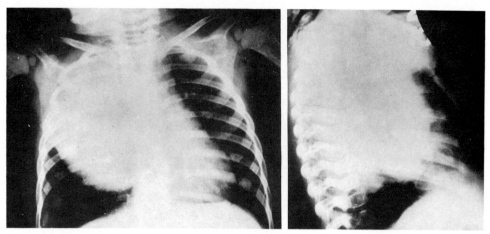

Figure 36.   Large ganglioneuroma in infant. Benign lesion was removed with good follow-up result.

loss and asthenia may occur. Neurogenic tumors of the neuroblastoma group usually occur in younger children, and respiratory symptoms, thoracic pain and fever are more common (Fig. 37).

On x-ray examination, neurogenic tumors are round, oval or spindle-shaped, and are characteristically located posteriorly in the paravertebral gutter. On thoracic roentgenograms, the ganglioneuroma appears as an elongated lesion and may extend over a distance of several vertebrae. Typically, a neurofibroma tends to be more rounded in outline. Calcifications within the tumor may be seen, more commonly in the malignant forms. Even though not demonstrated on x-ray examination, calcification may be found at the time of histologic examination. Bone lesions, such as intercostal space widening, costal deformation, vertebral involvement and metastatic bone disease, are not unusual with neurogenic tumors.

The therapy for neurogenic tumors of the thoracic cavity is surgery. Every case of ganglioneuroma reported in a study by Schweisguth and coworkers (1959) was amenable to resection. In malignant neurogenic tumor, all possi-

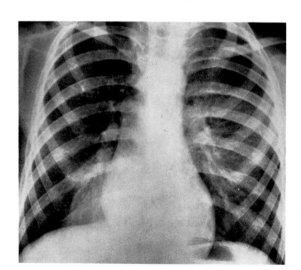

Figure 37.   Neuroblastoma in a six-year-old boy.

ble tumor growth should be excised and postoperative irradiation therapy instituted. X-ray therapy must be given judiciously, since growth disturbances, pulmonary fibrosis and other sequelae may develop. In the hourglass type of tumor, laminectomy must precede thoracotomy.

Mediastinal chemodectomas are usually located anteriorly; they are likely to be associated with similar tumors in the carotid body and elsewhere. There is a tendency for these tumors to be multiple.

Mediastinal pheochromocytomas are extremely rare and have not been recorded in the pediatric age group.

In Heimburger and Battersby's series of mediastinal tumors in childhood, 25 per cent of 36 tumors were of the neurogenic type. Ellis and DuShane reported 32 per cent neurogenic tumors in a review of primary mediastinal cysts and neoplasms in infants.

LYMPH NODES

Abnormalities of the lymph nodes in the mediastinum may be classified as follows:
1. Leukemia
2. Hodgkin's disease
3. Lymphosarcoma
4. Sarcoidosis
5. Inflammatory
   a. Tuberculosis
   b. Fungus
   c. Nonspecific

Any lymph node enlargement in a child should be viewed with suspicion. Lymphatic tumors are one of the more frequently observed malignant growths in childhood. The diagnosis is made by biopsy. Tumors of the Hodgkin's lymphosarcoma and reticulum cell sarcoma group are found primarily in children over three years of age, with a peak incidence from eight to 14 years. Over 95 per cent of children with primary lymphatic malignancy will have lymph node enlargement as the presenting sign. Tonsillar hypertrophy and ade-noidal hyperplasia, pulmonary hilar enlargement, splenomegaly, bone pain, unexplained fever, anemia, infiltrative skin lesions, and rarely central nervous system symptoms may also be present. The diagnosis should be sought through the study of peripheral blood smears, lymph node biopsy or bone marrow examination.

Surgery has limited value in lymphosarcoma, since the disease is usually widespread. When, however, the lesions are apparently isolated in the neck, axilla, mediastinum or gastrointestinal tract, surgery may be of great benefit. With few exceptions, all the tumors in this group are radiosensitive; however, they are not curable by x-ray therapy.

In most cases of mediastinal malignancy, bilateral hilar enlargement, as well as bilateral mediastinal enlargement, will be present. The lymph node enlargement may rarely be unilateral and relatively localized. In such cases, routine study of the blood smear, scalene lymph node biopsy and bone marrow studies may not provide the diagnosis, and open thoracotomy may be necessary. In such cases, complete lymph node removal should be carried out if technically feasible.

Inflammatory

Lymph node enlargement in the hilus of the lung or mediastinum may be secondary to tuberculous, fungal or bacterial lung disease. Diagnosis is usually confirmed by means of sputum culture, washings from the tracheobronchial tree at the time of bronchoscopy, scalene node biopsy, and skin tests correlated with the general clinical picture. The same is true in sarcoidosis. In sarcoidosis there may be involvement of the eye, skin, peripheral lymph nodes, mediastinal or hilar lymph nodes, and the lung parenchyma. It is possible to establish the diagnosis with this clinical picture and scalene node biopsy in approximately 80 to 85 per cent of the cases of sarcoidosis.

Although nonspecific symptomatic or asymptomatic enlargement of the mediastinal lymph nodes may occur, a cause can usually be found. For example, histoplasmosis may produce the clinical picture outlined.

Veneziale and coworkers (1964) have described angiofloccular hyperplasia of the mediastinal lymph nodes. Although this rare, benign localized lymph node enlargement may occur in extrathoracic locations, it most often occurs as an isolated asymptomatic mediastinal or pulmonary hilar tumor. Grossly, the tumors are moderately firm and usually well encapsulated. Calcification may occur, but is unusual. On microscopic examination, the two main features of these lymphoid masses are a diffuse follicular replacement of the lymph node architecture and much follicular and interfollicular vascular proliferation. Sixty per cent of patients with this entity are asymptomatic. When symptoms occur, they may include cough, fatigue, chest pain and fever. Surgical excision is the treatment of choice and is usually successful.

VASCULAR AND LYMPHATIC ABNORMALITIES

Vascular and lymphatic abnormalities of the mediastinum may be classified as (1) cavernous hemangioma, (2) hemangiopericytoma, (3) angiosarcoma or (4) cystic hygroma.

Vascular tumors of the mediastinum in children are rare, and preoperative diagnosis is unusual. Vascular tumors may occur at any level in the mediastinum, but are more frequently seen in the upper portion of the thorax and in the anterior mediastinum. They are uniformly rounded in appearance and are moderately dense. Calcification within the tumor is unusual. They are usually asymptomatic.

Cystic hygromas are relatively rare, but occur more often in infants and children than in adults. These tumors consist of masses of dilated lymphatic channels containing clear, watery fluid; they are lined with flat endothelium and are usually multilocular. They may appear to be isolated in the mediastinum (Fig. 38), but more often have an

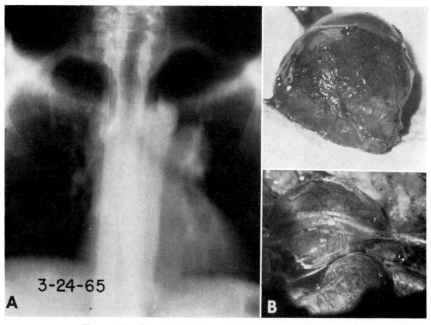

Figure 38.   Large lymphatic cyst in anterior mediastinum.

associated continuation into the neck. They may be rather large and unilateral, with lateral masses in the superior mediastinum. In 1948, Gross and Hurwitt reported 21 cases of cervical mediastinal hygromas and only eight cases of isolated mediastinal hygromas.

Diagnosis of a cervicomediastinal hygroma is made by physical examination of the cervical swelling and x-ray examination of the chest. Periodic fluctuation in size frequently occurs in cervical hygromas. This is even more characteristic of the combined cervicomediastinal lesions; in these, the cervical component may increase in size during inspiratory movements. X-ray films and fluoroscopic examination may show descent of the mass into the mediastinum on inspiration with a prominence in the neck during expiration.

Cystic hygromas confined to the mediastinum are usually discovered at autopsy or as an unanticipated finding on x-ray examination. The soft and yielding nature of the cysts allows them to attain considerable size without producing symptoms. On x-ray film there is a somewhat lobulated, smoothly outlined mass; however, it is usually not possible to distinguish hygromas from other benign tumors or cysts of the mediastinum by this method.

When respiratory infections occur, hygromas often become infected. Such infections are usually controlled by chemotherapy or by incision and drainage. A mediastinal or blood stream infection may result, however, or infection may be followed by local fibrosis and the disappearance of the mass. Spontaneous or post-traumatic hemorrhage into a cyst may result in extension of the cyst; this may cause sudden tracheal compression, a surgical emergency. Malignant change in hygroma has not been reported.

Surgical excision is the treatment of choice. Mediastinal hygromas can usually be excised with little difficulty because tissue planes around the cysts are well developed.

Chylothorax may result when there is cervical hygroma with involvement of the thoracic duct.

MEDIASTINAL LIPOMA AND LIPOSARCOMA

Intrathoracic lipoma is rare in children. Lipomas of the mediastinum have been divided into three groups according to their location and form: (1) tumors confined within the thoracic cage; (2) intrathoracic lipomas that extend upward into the neck; and (3) intrathoracic lipomas with an extrathoracic extension, forming a dumbbell configuration.

Of the 80 cases of lipoma reported in the world literature, 61 were intrathoracic, 8 cervicomediastinal, and 11 of the dumbbell type. Only two occurred in the pediatric age group, and these were intrathoracic. There have been three cases of liposarcoma of the mediastinum in children. Although these tumors usually do not metastasize, their invasiveness and tendency to recur place them in the malignant group.

In general, lipomas of the subcutaneous tissue are benign, while those of the retroperitoneal area and deep somatic soft tissue are usually malignant. The tumors of the mediastinum seem to have an incidence and behavior similar to those of lipomas in the peritoneal region.

Radical surgical excision is the procedure of choice. Repeated surgical attacks may serve as a method of extended control, and x-ray therapy may be added for palliative use.

THYROID AND PARATHYROID

Substernal thyroid is a common anterior superior mediastinal tumor in the adult age group, but apparently does not occur before puberty. Ectopic thyroid in the mediastinum does occur in children, and in such cases blood supply is derived from a mediastinal vessel.

Parathyroid adenoma with a typical syndrome of hyperparathyroidism does not occur before puberty.

PRIMARY CARDIAC AND PERICARDIAL TUMORS

Primary tumors of the heart in infants may cause cardiac enlargement or enlargement of the cardiac silhouette, giving rise to symptoms in the lungs or esophagus. Most frequently, the signs and symptoms of congestive heart failure are much more prominent than those of the respiratory system or esophagus.

Rhabdomyoma appears to be the only cardiac tumor showing a definite predilection for the younger age groups. This is particularly true in children with tuberous sclerosis, in whom rhabdomyoma of the heart is prone to occur. Such tumors are not considered true neoplasms, but probably represent an area of developmental arrest in the fetal myocardium. It is not unusual for rhabdomyoma to regress spontaneously without causing any appreciable impairment of cardiac function.

Myxoma is by far the most frequent primary tumor of the heart; this accounts for slightly more than 50 per cent of all primary cardiac tumors. It may be encountered at almost any age. The signs and symptoms vary widely, but ultimately lead to cardiac failure that does not respond to the usual medical management. Most myxomas are located in the atria, more frequently on the left than on the right. They tend to proliferate and project into the chambers of the heart, preventing normal cardiac filling by obstruction to the mitral or tricuspid valve. The origin appears to be in the atrial septa.

Primary sarcoma of the heart is less common than myxoma, but may occur at any age. It does not, as a rule, proliferate into the lumens of the heart; it infiltrates the wall of the myocardium and frequently extends into the pericardial cavity.

Other primary tumors of the heart are angioma, fibroma, lipoma and hamartoma. All are rare and usually produce prominent circulatory symptoms.

Primary neoplasms of the pericardium are rare. On histologic examination, the predominant tumors are mesotheliomas (endothelioma) and sarcomas, but occasionally leiomyomas, hemangiomas and lipomas may occur.

A single instance of a large cavernous hemangioma of the pericardium has been described; this occurred in an eight-year-old girl and was successfully removed.

TUMORS OF THE DIAPHRAGM

Tumors involving the diaphragm may cause chest pain and discomfort or pulmonary compression; thus, they may simulate mediastinal or primary pulmonary neoplasms. Primary tumors of the diaphragm are extremely rare in the pediatric age group.

Benign tumors of the diaphragm that have been reported, though not necessarily in children, are lipoma, fibroma, chondroma, angiofibroma, lymphangioma, neurofibroma, rhabdomyofibroma, fibromyoma and primary diaphragmatic cysts.

Malignant tumors of the diaphragm that have been reported are fibrosarcoma, rhabdomyosarcoma, myosarcoma, leiomyosarcoma and fibromyosarcoma. None of these tumors appears to have been reported in children.

PRIMARY TUMORS OF THE CHEST WALL

Figures 39 and 40 illustrate findings seen in two forms of chest wall tumors.

Lipoma of the chest wall is frequent

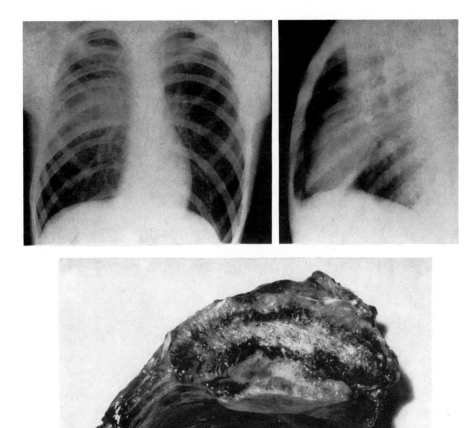

Figure 39. Reticulum cell sarcoma in chest wall of eight-year-old white boy. Survival longer than 18 months.

in adults, but rare in the pediatric age group. As noted previously, these may be dumbbell in shape, presenting on the chest wall with a large component intrathoracically. Chest roentgenogram will aid in its definition.

Extensive cavernous hemangiomas of the thoracic wall are seen in infancy or childhood. They may be isolated or associated with similar lesions in other tissues, including the lung. In these cases, the diagnosis of Osler-Weber-Rendu syndrome is suggested. Intrathoracic extension of these lesions may occur.

In von Recklinghausen's disease, multiple cutaneous and subcutaneous nodules are present. These patients should be carefully studied for the pos-

sible coexistence of mediastinal neurofibromas or intrathoracic meningocele.

Chondroma and chondrosarcoma are the principal bony tumors of the chest wall; 80 per cent of these occur in the ribs or sternum, usually in the anterior extremity of a rib near the costochondral junction. They may also occur in the sternum, scapula, clavicle or vertebral bodies. There may be few, if any, symptoms. X-ray examination reveals a discrete expansion of the bone with an intact, thinned-out cortex.

Chondrosarcoma of the rib occurs more frequently in males; it is usually seen in the posterior half and paravertebral portion of the rib, but sometimes involves the transverse process and the

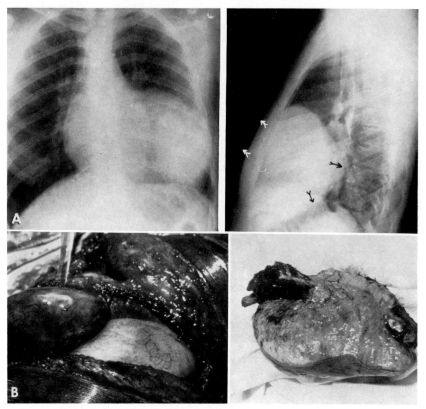

Figure 40.   Desmoid tumor of chest wall in a child 18 months after patent ductus surgery. The desmoid was in the line of the posterior lateral incision.

vertebral body either primarily or secondarily. Occasionally the direction of growth appears to be entirely internal, thus simulating the radiologic appearance of a primary pleural or mediastinal tumor. Usually, however, there is an externally visible and palpable tumefaction. This usually occurs during the middle decades of life.

Solitary plasmacytoma, a lesion histologically similar to multiple myeloma, but localized to a single bone, may involve any part of the thoracic cage; it may involve the vertebrae, rarely attacks the ribs, and may involve the lung itself. In solitary plasmacytoma, the bone is thinned and can be greatly expanded.

Ewing's tumor is sometimes primary in a rib, and is unusual before the second decade of life.

REFERENCES

General

Ackerman, L. V., and del Regato, J. A.: *Cancer: Diagnosis, Treatment and Prognosis.* 2nd Ed. St. Louis, C. V. Mosby Company, 1954.

Arey, L. B.: *Developmental Anatomy.* 7th Ed. Philadelphia, W. B. Saunders Company, 1965.

Ariel, I. M., and Pack, G. T.: *Cancer and Allied Diseases of Infancy and Childhood.* Boston, Little, Brown and Company, 1960.

Banyai, A. L.: *Nontuberculous Diseases of the Chest.* Springfield, Illinois, Charles C Thomas, 1954.

Benedict, E. B., and Nardi, G. L.: *The Esophagus: Medical and Surgical Management.* Boston, Little, Brown and Company, 1958.

Benson, C. D., Mustard, W. T., Ravitch, M. M., Snyder, W. H., Jr., and Welch, K. J.: *Pediatric Surgery.* Vol. I. Chicago, Year Book Medical Publishers, Inc., 1962.

Blades, B.: *Surgical Diseases of the Chest.* St. Louis, C. V. Mosby Company, 1961.

Clinical Pathologic Conference, Children's Medical Center, Boston, Mass. *J. Pediatr., 54:*529, 1959.

Felson, B.: *Fundamentals of Chest Roentgenology.* Philadelphia, W. B. Saunders Company, 1960.

Flavell, G.: *The Oesophagus.* London, Butterworth, 1963.

Fried, B. M.: *Tumors of the Lungs and Mediastinum.* Philadelphia, Lea & Febiger, 1958.

Gilbert, J. G., Mazzarella, L. A., and Feit, L. J.: Primary tracheal tumors in the infant and adult. *Arch. Otolaryngol., 58*:1, 1953.

Gross, R. E.: *The Surgery of Infancy and Childhood.* Philadelphia, W. B. Saunders Company, 1953.

Hinshaw, H. C.: *Diseases of the Chest.* 3rd Ed. Philadelphia, W. B. Saunders Company, 1969.

Hollinger, P. H., Slaughter, D. P., and Novak, F. J., III: Unusual tumors obstructing the lower respiratory tract of infants and children. *Trans. Am. Acad. Ophthalmol. Otolaryngol.,* 54th Session: 223, 1949.

Hopkins, A. M., and Freitas, E. L.: Bilateral osteochondroma of the ribs in an infant: an unusual cause of cyanosis. *J. Thorac. Cardiovasc. Surg., 49*:247, 1965.

Jones, P. G., and Campbell, P. E.: *Tumours of Infancy and Childhood.* London, Blackwell Scientific Publications; Philadelphia, J. B. Lippincott Company, 1976.

Keith, A.: *Human Embryology and Morphology.* 6th Ed. Baltimore, Williams & Wilkins Company, 1948.

Leigh, T. F., and Weens, H. S.: *The Mediastinum.* Springfield, Illinois, Charles C Thomas, 1959.

Lindskog, G. E., Liebow, A. A., and Glenn, W. W. L.: *Thoracic and Cardiovascular Surgery with Related Pathology.* Des Moines, Iowa, Meredith Publishing Company, 1962.

Myers, J. A.: *Diseases of the Chest—Including the Heart.* Springfield, Illinois, Charles C Thomas, 1959.

Naclerio, E. A.: *Bronchopulmonary Diseases, Basic Aspects, Diagnosis and Treatment.* New York, Paul B. Hoeber, Inc., 1957.

Ochsner, A., Jr., Lucas, G. L., and McFarland, G. B., Jr.: Tumors of the thoracic skleleton, Review of 134 cases. *J. Thorac. Cardiovasc. Surg., 52*:311, 1966.

Odom, J. A., De Muth, W. E., and Blakemore, W. S.: Chest wall chondrosarcoma in youth. *J. Thorac. Cardiovasc. Surg., 50*:550, 1965.

Pack, G. T., and Ariel, I. M.: *Treatment of Cancer and Allied Diseases.* 2nd Ed. Vol. IV, Tumors of the Breast, Chest and Esophagus. New York, Paul B. Hoeber, Inc., 1960.

Perry, K. M. A., and Sellors, T. H.: *Chest Diseases.* Vol. 2. London, Butterworth, 1963.

Postlethwait, R. W., and Sealy, W. C.: *Surgery of the Esophagus.* Springfield, Illinois, Charles C Thomas, 1961.

Potts, W. J.: *The Surgeon and the Child.* Philadelphia, W. B. Saunders Company, 1959.

Rubin, E. H.: *The Lung as a Mirror of Systemic Disease.* Springfield, Illinois, Charles C Thomas, 1956.

Rubin, E. H., and Rubin, M.: *Thoracic Diseases, Emphasizing Cardiopulmonary Relationships.* Philadelphia, W. B. Saunders Company, 1961.

Sabiston, D. C., and Spencer, F. C.: *Gibbon's*

Surgery of the Chest. 3rd Ed. Philadelphia, W. B. Saunders Company, 1976.

Schaffer, A. J., and Avery, M. E.: *Diseases of the Newborn.* 4th Ed. Philadelphia, W. B. Saunders Company, 1977.

Shaw, R. R., and Paulson, D. L.: *The Treatment of Bronchial Neoplasms.* Springfield, Illinois, Charles C Thomas, 1959.

Smithers, S. W., and Bignall, J. R.: *Neoplastic Diseases at Various Sites.* Vol. I, Carcinoma of the Lung. London, E. & S. Livingstone, Ltd., 1958.

Spain, D. M.: *Diagnosis and Treatment of Tumors of the Chest.* New York, Grune & Stratton, Inc., 1960.

Stout, A. P.: Tumors of the peripheral nervous system. In *Atlas of Tumor Pathology.* Washington, D.C., 1949.

Sweet, R. H.: *Thoracic Surgery.* 2nd Ed. Philadelphia, W. B. Saunders Company, 1954.

Symposium on Certain Tumors of the Bronchi and on Tumors of the Trachea. *Proc. Staff Meet. Mayo Clin., 21*:409, 1946.

Terracol, J., and Sweet, R. H.: *Diseases of the Esophagus.* Philadelphia, W. B. Saunders Company, 1958.

Unin, J.: *Neoplastic Diseases.* 4th Ed. Philadelphia, W. B. Saunders Company, 1940.

Benign Pulmonary Tumors

Albrecht, E. E.: *Verh. Dtsch. Ges. Pathol., 7*:153, 1904.

Archer, F. L., Harrison, R. W., and Moulder, P. V.: Granular cell myoblastoma of the trachea and carina treated by resection and reconstruction. *J. Thorac. Surg., 45*:539, 1963.

Baker, D. C., and Pemington, C. L.: Congenital hemangioma of the larynx. *Trans. Am. Laryngol., Rhinol. Otol. Soc.,* 60th Meeting: 84, 1956.

Barrett, N. R., and Barnard, W. G.: Some usual thoracic tumors. *Br. J. Surg., 32*:447, 1945.

Blackman, J., Cantril, S. T., Lund, T. K., and Sparkman, D.: Tracheobronchial papillomatosis, treated by roentgen irradiation. *Radiology, 73*:598, 1959.

Campbell, J. S., Wiglesworth, F.W., Latarroca, R., and Wilde, H.: Congenital subglottic hemangiomas of the larynx and trachea in infants. *Pediatrics, 22*:727, 1958.

Cavin, E., Masters, J. H., and Moody, J.: Hamartoma of the lung. *J. Thorac. Surg., 35*:816, 1958.

Doermann, P., Lunseth, J., and Segnitz, R. H.: Obstructing subglottic hemangioma of the larynx in infancy, review of the literature and report of a deceptive case. *N. Engl. J. Med., 258*:68, 1958.

Ferguson, C. F., and Flake, C. G.: Subglottic hemangioma as a cause of respiratory obstruction in infants. *Trans. Am. Bronchoesoph. A., 41*:27, 1961.

Fishman, L.: Papilloma of the trachea. *J. Thorac. Cardiovasc. Surg., 44*:264, 1962.

Graham, G. G., and Singleton, J. W.: Diffuse hamartoma of the upper lobe in an infant: report of a successful surgical removal. *J. Dis. Child., 89*:609, 1955.

Guida, P. N., Fultcher, T., and Moore, S. W.:

Leiomyoma of the lung. *J. Thorac. Surg.*, 49:1058, 1965.

Holder, T. M., and Christy, M. G.: Cystic adenomatoid malformation of the lung. *J. Thorac. Surg.*, 47:590, 1964.

Jackson, C. L., Konzelmann, F. W., and Norris, C. M.: Bronchial adenoma. *J. Thorac. Surg.*, 14:98, 1945.

Jones, C. J.: Unusual hamartoma of the lung in the newborn infant. *Arch. Pathol.*, 48:150, 1949.

Jones, R., MacKenzie, K. W., and Biddle, E.: Bronchial adenoma, a case report. *Br. J. Tuber.*, 37:113, 1943.

Kauffman, S. L., and Stout, A. P.: Histiocytic tumors (fibrous xanthoma and histiocytoma) in children. *Cancer*, 14:469, 1961.

Kramer, R., and Som, M. L.: Further study of adenoma of the bronchus. *Ann. Otol. Rhinol. Laryngol.*, 44:861, 1935.

Kumis, F. D., and Conn, J. H.: Endobronchial hamartoma, *J. Thorac. Surg.*, 50:138, 1965.

Littler, E. R.: Asphyxia due to hemangioma in the trachea. *J. Thorac. Cardiovasc. Surg.*, 45:552, 1963.

Lukens, R. M.: Papilloma of the trachea. *Ann. Otol. Rhinol. Laryngol.*, 45:872, 1936.

Ogilvie, O. E.: Multiple papillomas of the trachea with malignant degeneration. *Arch. Otolaryngol.*, 58:10, 1953.

Pearl, M., and Woolley, M. W.: Pulmonary xanthomatous postinflammatory pseudotumors in children. *J. Pediatr. Surg.*, 8:255, 1973.

Peterson, H. O.: Benign adenoma of the bronchus. *Am. J. Roentgenol.*, 36:836, 1936.

Rosenblum, P., and Klein, R. I.: Adenomatous polyp of the right main bronchus producing atelectasis. *J. Pediatr.*, 7:791, 1935.

Smoller, S., and Maynard, A. DeL.: Adenoma of the bronchus in a nine year old child. *Am. J. Dis. Child.*, 82:587, 1951.

Som, M. L.: Adenoma of the bronchus: endoscopic treatment in selected cases. *J. Thorac. Surg.*, 18:462, 1949.

Souders, C. R., and Kingsley, J. W.: Bronchial adenoma. *N. Engl. J. Med.*, 239:459, 1948.

Stein, A. S., and Volk, B. M.: Papillomatosis of the trachea and lung. *Arch. Pathol.*, 124:127, 1959.

Taraska, J. J.: Case report of a postinflammatory pseudotumor of the trachea. *J. Thorac. Cardiovasc. Surg.*, 51:279, 1966.

Taylor, T. L., and Miller, D. R.: Leiomyoma of the bronchus. *J. Thorac. Cardiovasc. Surg.*, 57:284, 1969.

Thomas, M. R.: Cystic hamartoma of the lung in a newborn infant. *J. Pathol. Bacteriol.*, 61:599, 1949.

Verska, J. J., and Connolly, J. E.: Bronchial adenomas in children. *J. Thorac. Cardiovasc. Surg.*, 55:411, 1968.

Walcott, C. C.: Bronchial adenoma. *Laryngoscope*, 72:1952.

Ward, D. E., Jr., Bradshaw, H. H., and Prince, T. C.: Bronchial adenoma in children. *J. Thorac. Surg.*, 27:295, 1954.

Wilkins, E. W., Darling, R. C., Soutter, L., and

Sniffen, R. C.: A continuing clinical survey of adenomas of the trachea and bronchus in a general hospital. *J. Thorac. Cardiovasc. Surg.*, 46:279, 1963.

Womack, H., and Graham, E. A.: Mixed tumors of the lung. *Arch. Pathol.*, 26:165, 1938.

Primary and Metastatic Malignant Pulmonary Tumors

Bartley, J. D., and Arean, V. M.: Intrapulmonic neurogenic tumors. *J. Thorac. Surg.*, 50:114, 1965.

Beardsley, J. M.: Primary carcinoma of the lung in a child. *Can. Med. Assoc. J.*, 29:257, 1933.

Berman, L.: Extragenital chorionepithelioma with report of a case. *Am. J. Cancer*, 38:23, 1940.

Bogardus, G. M., Knudston, K. P., and Mills, W. H.: Pleural mesothelioma. *Am. Rev. Tuberc.*, 71:280, 1955.

Breton, A., Gaudier, R., and Ponte, C.: Tumeurs bronchiques chez l'enfant. *Pediatrie (Lyon)*, 13:43, 1958.

Breton, A., Gaudier, B., Delacroiz, R., Dupont, A., and Poingt, O.: Neurinomes intrapulmonaires primitives. *Arch. Fr. Pediatr.*, 18:26, 1961.

Cayley, C. K., Mersheimer, W., and Caez, H. J.: Primary bronchogenic carcinoma of the lung in children. *J. Dis. Child.*, 82:49, 1951.

Cliffton, E. E., and Pool, J. L.: Treatment of lung metastasis in children with combined therapy. *J. Thorac. Cardiovasc. Surg.*, 54:403, 1967.

Curry, J. J., and Fuchs, J.: Expectoration of a fibrosarcoma. *J. Thorac. Surg.*, 19:135, 1950.

de Parades, C. G., Pierce, W. S., Groff, D. B., and Waldhausen, J. A.: Bronchogenic tumors in children. *Arch. Surg.*, 100:574, 1970.

Doesel, H.: Intrabronchioles psammöses neurofibroma. *Thoraxchirurgie*, 8:657, 1961.

Donahue, F. E., Anderson, H. A., and McDonald, J. B.: Unusual bronchial tumor. *Ann. Otol. Rhinol. Laryngol.*, 65:820, 1956.

Dooley, B. N., Beckman, C., and Hood, R. H.: Primary mesothelioma of the pericardium. *J. Thorac. Cardiovasc. Surg.*, 55:719, 1968.

Dowell, A. R.: Primary pulmonary leiomyosarcoma. *Ann. Thorac. Surg.*, 17:384, 1974.

Drews, G. A., and Willman, K. H.: Das primare Lungensarkom. *Langenbecks Arch. Klin. Chir.*, 274:95, 1953.

Dyson, B. C., and Trentalance, A. E.: Resection of primary pulmonary sarcoma. *J. Thorac. Surg.*, 47:577, 1964.

Feldman, P. A.: Sarcoma of the lungs, a report of three cases. *Br. J. Tuberc. Chest Dis.*, 51:331, 1957.

Gerber, I. E.: Ectopic chorioepithelioma. *J. Mt. Sinai Hosp.*, 2:135, 1935.

Gray, F. W., and Tom, B. C. K.: Diffuse pleural mesothelioma: a survival of one year following nitrogen mustard therapy. *J. Thorac. Cardiovasc. Surg.*, 44:73, 1962.

Harris, W. H., and Schattenberg, H. H.: Anlagen and rest tumors of the lung. *Am. J. Pathol.* 18:955, 1942.

Herring, N., Templeton, J. Y., III, Haup, G. J.,

and Theodos, P. A.: Primary sarcoma of the lung. *Dis. Chest,* 42:315, 1962.

Hill, L. D., and White, M. L., Jr.: Plasmacytoma of the lung. *J. Thorac. Surg.,* 25:187, 1953.

Hirsch, E. F.: Extragenital choriocarcinoma, with comments on the male origin of trophoblastic tissues. *Arch. Pathol.,* 48:516, 1949.

Hochberg, L. A.: Endothelioma of the pleura. *Am. Rev. Tuberc.,* 63:150, 1951.

Hollinger, P. H., Johnston, K. C., Gosswiller, N., and Hirsch, E. C.: Primary fibrosarcoma of the bronchus. *Dis. Chest,* 37:137, 1960.

Kay, S., and Reed, W. G.: Chorioepithelioma of the lung in a female infant seven months old. *Am. J. Pathol.,* 29:555, 1953.

Killingsworth, W. P., McReynolds, G. S., and Harrison, A. W.: Pulmonary leiomysarcomas in a child. *J. Pediatr.,* 42:466, 1963.

Kyriakos, M., and Webber, B.: Cancer of the lung in young men. *J. Thorac. Cardiovasc. Surg.,* 67:634, 1974.

Lewis, J.: Sarcoma of the bronchus. *Proc. R. Soc. Med.,* 40:119, 1947.

McNamara, J. J., Paulson, D. L., Kingsley, W. B., Salinas-Izaquirre, S. F., and Urschel, H. C.: Primary leiomyosarcoma of the lung. *J. Thorac. Cardiovasc. Surg.,* 57:635, 1969.

Mallory, T. B.: Cabot case, N. R. 20202. *N. Engl. J. Med.,* 218:843, 1938.

Mallory, T. B.: Case record 24202, Mass. Gen. Hosp. *N. Engl. J. Med.,* 218:845, 1938.

Merrit, J. W., and Parker, K. R.: Intrathoracic leiomyosarcoma. *Can. Med. Assoc. J.,* 77:1031, 1957.

Noehren, T. H., and McKee, F. W.: Sarcoma of the lung. *Dis. Chest,* 25:633, 1954.

Ochsner, S., and Ochsner, A.: Primary sarcoma of the lung. *Ochsner Clinic Reports,* 3:105, 1957.

Randell, W. S., and Blades, B.: Primary bronchogenic leiomyosarcoma. *Arch. Pathol.,* 42:543, 1946.

Sekulich, M., Pandola, G., and Simon, T.: A solitary pulmonary mass in multiple myeloma: report of a case. *Dis. Chest,* 48:100, 1965.

Shaw, R. R., Paulson, D. L., Kee, J. L., and Lovett, V. F.: Primary pulmonary leiomyosarcomas. *J. Thorac. Cardiovasc. Surg.,* 41:430, 1961.

Sherman, R. S., and Malone, B. H.: A study of muscle tumors primary in the lung. *Radiology,* 54:507, 1950.

Simpson, J. A., Smith, F., et al.: Bronchial adenoma: a review of 26 cases. *Aust. N. Z. J. Surg.,* 44:110, 1974.

Stout, A. P., and Himidi, G. M.: Solitary (localized) mesothelioma of the pleura. *Ann. Surg.,* 133:50, 1951.

Verska, J. J., and Connolly, J. E.: Bronchial adenomas in children. *J. Thorac. Cardiovasc. Surg.,* 55:411, 1968.

Wasch, M. G., Lederer, M., and Epstein, B. S.: Bronchogenic carcinoma of seven years' duration in an 11-year-old boy. *J. Pediatr.,* 17:521, 1940.

Watson, W. L., and Anlyan, A. J.: Primary leiomyosarcoma of the lung. *Cancer,* 7:250, 1954.

Mediastinal Tumors

Abell, M. R.: Mediastinal cysts. *Arch. Pathol.,* 61: 360, 1956.

Ackerman, L. R., and Taylor, F. H.: Neurogenic tumors within the thorax. *Cancer,* 4:669, 1951.

Adams, F. H.: Unusual case for bronchogenic lung cyst simulating dextrocardia. *J. Pediatr.,* 39:483, 1951.

Adams, W. E., and Thornton, T. F., Jr.: Bronchogenic cysts of the mediastinum: with report of three cases. *J. Thorac. Surg.,* 12:503, 1943.

Adler, R. H., Taheri, S. A., and Waintraub, D. G.: Mediastinal teratoma in infancy. *J. Thorac. Surg.,* 39:394, 1960.

Andrus, W. D. W., and Foote, N. C.: Report of a large thymic tumor successfully removed by operation. *J. Thorac. Surg.,* 6:648, 1937.

Archer, O., Pierce, J. C., and Good, R. A.: Role of the thymus in the development of the immune response. *Fed. Proc.,* 20:26, 1961.

Arcomand, J. P., and Azzoni, A. A.: Intralobar pulmonary sequestration and intralobar enteric sequestration associated with vertebral anomalies. *J. Thorac. Cardiovasc. Surg.,* 53:470, 1967.

Arnason, B. G., Jankovic, B. D., and Wadsman, B. H.: A survey of the thymus and its relation to lymphocytes and immune reactions. *Blood,* 20:617, 1962.

Arnheim, E. E.: Cervicomediastinal lymphangioma (cystic hydroma). *J. Mt. Sinai Hosp.,* 10:404, 1943.

Arnheim, E. E., and Gemson, B. L.: Persistent cervical thymus gland: thymectomy. *Surgery,* 27:603, 1950.

Bale, P. M.: A congenital intraspinal gastroenterogenous cyst in diastematomyelia. *J. Neurol. Neurosurg. Psychiatry,* 36:1011, 1973.

Bednav, B.: Malignant intrapericardial tumor of heart. (Translation.) *Cas. Lek.,* 48:1355, 1950.

Bernard, E. D., and James, L. S.: The newborn cardiac silhouette in newborn infants: a cinematographic study of the normal range. *Pediatrics,* 27:13, 1961.

Bernatz, P. E., Harrison, E. G., and Clagett, O. T.: Thymoma: a clinicopathologic study. *J. Thorac. Cardiovasc. Surg.,* 42:424, 1961.

Bill, A. H., Jr. Sentrill, S. T., and Creighton, S. A.: The spectrum of malignancy in childhood compared with that seen in adults. Personal communication.

Bill, A. H., Jr., and others: Common malignant tumors of infancy and childhood. *Pediatr. Clin. North Am.,* 6:1197, 1959.

Bjorn, T., and Hayes, L. L.: Duplication of the stomach. *Surgery,* 44:585, 1958.

Blades, B.: Mediastinal tumors: report of cases treated at Army thoracic surgery centers in the U.S. *Ann. Surg.,* 123:749, 1946.

Bremmer, J. L.: Diverticuli and duplications of the intestinal tract. *Arch. Pathol.,* 38:132, 1944.

Brescia, M. A.: Chylothorax, report of a case in an infant. *Arch. Pediatr.,* 58:345, 1941.

Brewer, L. A., III, and Dolley, F. S.: Tumors of the mediastinum: a discussion of diagnostic procedure and surgical treatment based on experience with 44 operated cases. *Am. Rev. Tuberc.*, *60*:419, 1949.

Burkell, C. C., Cross, J. M., Kent, H. P., and Manson, E. M.: Mass lesions of the mediastinum. *Curr. Probl. Surg.*, June 1969.

Burnett, W. E., Rosemond, G. P., and Bucher, R. M.: The diagnosis of mediastinal tumors. *Surg. Clin. North Am.*, *32*:1673, 1952.

Caffey, J., and Silbey, R.: Regrowth and overgrowth of the thymus after atrophy induced by oral administration of adrenocorticosteroids to human infants. *Pediatrics*, *26*:762, 1960.

Callahan, W. J., and Simon, A. L.: Posterior mediastinal hemangioma associated with vertebral body hemangioma. *J. Thorac. Cardiovasc. Surg.*, *51*:283, 1966.

Cicciarelli, E. H., Soule, E. H., and McGoon, D. C.: Lipoma and liposarcoma of the mediastinum, a report of fourteen tumors including one lipoma of the thymus. *J. Thorac. Surg.*, *47*:411, 1964.

Claireaux, A. E.: An intrapericardial teratoma in a newborn infant. *J. Pathol. Bacteriol.*, *63*:743, 1951.

Clark, D. E.: Association of irradiation with cancer of the thyroid in children in adolescence. *J.A.M.A.*, *157*:107, 1955.

Conklin, W. S.: Tumors and cysts of the mediastinum. *Dis. Chest*, *17*:715, 1950.

Conti, E. A., Patton, G. D., Conti, J. E., and Hempelmann, L. H.: The present health of children given x-ray treatment to the anterior mediastinum in infancy. *Radiology*, *74*:386, 1960.

Cruickshank, D. B.: Primary intrathoracic neurogenic tumors. *J. Fac. Radiol.*, *8*:369, 1957.

Curreri, A. R., and Gale, J. W.: Mediastinal tumors. *Arch. Surg.*, *58*:797, 1949.

Dameshek, W.: The thymus and lymphoid proliferation. (Editorial.) *Blood*, *20*:629, 1962.

Davidson, L. R., and Brown, L.: Gastrogenous mediastinal cyst. *J. Thorac. Surg.*, *16*:458, 1947.

Dieter, R. A., Jr., Riker, W. L., and Hollinger, P.: Pedunculated esophageal hamartoma in a child. *J. Thorac. Cardiovasc. Surg.*, *59*:851, 1970.

Dobbs, C. H., Berg, R., Jr., and Pierce, E. C., II: Intrapericardial bronchogenic cysts. *J. Thorac. Surg.*, *34*:718, 1957.

Dowd, C. N.: Hygroma cysticum colli, its structure and etiology. *Ann. Surg.*, *58*:112, 1913.

Drash, E. C., and Hyer, H. J.: Mesothelial mediastinal cysts: pericardial celomic cysts of Lambert. *J. Thorac. Surg.*, *19*:755, 1950.

Duffy, B. J., Jr., and Fitzgerald, P. J.: Thyroid cancer in childhood and adolescence: report of 28 cases. *Cancer*, *3*:1018, 1950.

Duprez, A., Corlier, R., and Schmidt, P.: Tuberculoma of the thymus. *J. Thorac. Cardiovasc. Surg.*, *44*:115, 1962.

Edge, J. R., and Glennie, J. S.: Teratoid tumors of the mediastinum found despite previous normal chest radiography. *J. Thorac. Cardiovasc. Surg.*, *40*:172, 1960.

Ellis, F. H., Jr., and DuShane, J. W.: Primary mediastinal cysts and neoplasms in infants and children. *Am. Rev. Tuberc. Pulmonary Dis.*, *74*:940, 1956.

Ellis, F. H., Jr., Kirklin, J. W., and Woolner, L.

B.: Hemangioma of the mediastinum: review of literature and report of case. *J. Thorac. Surg.*, *30*:181, 1955a.

Ellis, F. H. Jr., Kirklin, J. W., Hodgson, J. R., Woolner, L. B., and DuShane, J. W.: Surgical implications of the mediastinal shadow in thoracic roentgenograms of infants and children. *Surg. Gynecol. Obstet.*, *100*:532, 1955b.

Emerson, G. L.: Supradiaphragmatic thoracic duct cysts. *N. Engl. J. Med.*, *242*:575, 1950.

Evans, A.: Developmental enterogenous cysts and diverticula. *Br. J. Surg.*, *17*:34, 1929.

Fallon, M., Gordon, A. R. G., and Lendrum, A. C.: Mediastinal cysts of fore-gut origin associated with vertebral abnormalities. *Br. J. Surg.*, *41*:520, 1954.

Ferguson, J. O., Clagett, O. T., and McDonald, J. R.: Hemangiopericytoma (glomus tumor) of the mediastinum: review of the literature and report of case. *Surgery*, *36*:320, 1954.

Filler, R. M., Traggis, D. G., Jaffe, N., and Vawter, G. F.: Favourable outlook for children with mediastinal neuroblastoma. *J. Pediatr. Surg.*, *7*:136, 1972.

Flege, J. B., Jr., Valencia, A. G., and Zimmerman, G.: Obstruction of a child's trachea by polypoid hemangioendothelioma. *J. Thorac. Cardiovasc. Surg.*, *56*:144, 1968.

Forsee, J. H., and Blake, H. A.: Pericardial celomic cyst. *Surgery*, *31*:753, 1952.

Fridjon, M. H.: Cysts of the thymus in a newborn baby. *Br. Med. J.*, *2*:553, 1943.

Friedman, N. B.: Tumors of the thymus. *J. Thorac. Cardiovasc. Surg.*, *53*:163, 1967.

Garland, H. L.: Cancer of the thyroid and previous radiation. *Surg. Gynecol. Obstet.*, *112*:564, 1961.

Gebauer, P. W.: Case of intrapericardial teratoma. *J. Thorac. Surg.*, *12*:458, 1953.

Gerami, S., Richardson, R., Harrington, B., and Pate, J. W.: Obstructive emphysema due to mediastinal bronchogenic cysts in infancy. *J. Thorac. Cardiovasc. Surg.*, *58*:432, 1969.

Gledhill, E. Y., and Marrow, A. G.: Ciliated epithelial cyst of the esophagus: report of case. *J. Thorac. Surg.*, *20*:923, 1950.

Godwin, J. T., Watson, W. L., Pool, J. L., Cahan, W. G., and Nardiello, V. A.: Primary intrathoracic neurogenic tumors. *J. Thorac. Surg.*, *20*:169, 1950.

Gondos, B., and Reingold, I. M.: Mediastinal ganglioneuroblastoma. *J. Thorac. Surg.*, *47*:430, 1964.

Greenfield, E., Steinberg, I., and Touroff, A. S. W.: "Spring water" cyst of the mediastinum: case report. *J. Thorac. Surg.*, *12*:495, 1943.

Griffiths, S. P., Levine, O. R., Baker, D. H., and Blumenthal, S.: Evaluation of an enlarged cardiothymic image in infancy: thymolytic effect of steroid administration. *Am. J. Cardiol.*, *8*:311, 1961.

Grosfeld, J. L., Ballatine, T. V. N., Lowe, D., and Baehner, R. L.: Benign and malignant teratomas in children: analysis of 85 patients. *Surgery*, *80*:297, 1976.

Gross, R. E.: Thoracic sugery for infants. *J. Thorac. Surg.*, *48*:152, 1964.

Gross, R. E., and Hurwitt, E. S.: Cervical mediastinal cystic hygromas. *Surg. Gynecol. Obstet.*, 87:599, 1948.

Gross, R. E., Holcomb, G. W., and Farber, S.: Duplications of the alimentary tract. *Pediatrics*, 9:449, 1952.

Grutezner, P.: *Ein Fall von mediastinal Tumor durch ein lymphosarcom Bedingt.* Berlin, G. Lang, 1869.

Guinn, H.: Mediastinal teratoma. *Radiology*, 8:438, 1927.

Haller, J. A., Mazur, D. O., and Morgan, W. W.: Diagnosis and management of mediastinal masses in children. *J. Thorac. Cardiovasc. Surg.*, 58:385, 1969.

Hardy, L. M.: Bronchogenic cysts of the mediastinum. *Pediatrics*, 4:108, 1949.

Hedblom, C. A.: Intrathoracic dermoid cysts and teratomata, with report of six personal cases and 185 cases collected from the literature. *J. Thorac. Surg.*, 3:22, 1933.

Heimburger, I. L., and Battersby, J. S.: Primary mediastinal tumors of childhood. *J. Thorac. Cardiovasc. Surg.*, 50:92, 1965.

Herlitzka, H. A., and Gayle, J. W.: Tumor and cysts of the mediastinum. *Arch. Surg.*, 76:697, 1958.

Heuer, G. J.: The thoracic lipomas. *Ann. Surg.*, 98:801, 1933.

Heuer, J., and Andrus, W.: The surgery of mediastinal tumors. *Am. J. Surg.*, 50:146, 1940.

Hollingsworth, R. K.: Intrathoracic tumors of the sympathetic nervous system. *Surg. Gynecol. Obstet.*, 82:682, 1946.

Hopkins, S. M., and Freitas, E. L.: Bilateral osteochondroma of the ribs in an infant, an unusual cause of cyanosis. *J. Thorac. Surg.*, 49:247, 1965.

Hurwitz, A., Conrad, R., Selvage, I. L., and Oberton, E. A.: Hypertrophic lobar emphysema secondary to a paratracheal cyst in an infant. *J. Thorac. Cardiovasc. Surg.*, 57:412, 1966.

Jackson, C.: Thymic tracheostenosis, tracheoscopy, thymectomy, cure. *J.A.M.A.*, 48:1753, 1907.

Jellen, J., and Fisher, W. B.: Intrapericardial teratoma. *Am. J. Dis. Child.*, 51:1397, 1936.

Joel, J.: Ein Teratom auf der Artena Pulmonalio innerhalb des Herzbeutals. *Arch. Pathol. Anat.*, 122:381, 1890.

Jones, J. C.: Esophageal duplications or mediastinal cysts of enteric origin. *West. J. Surg.*, 55:610, 1947.

Kauffman, S. L., and Stout, A. P.: Lipoblastic tumors of children. *Cancer*, 12:912, 1959.

Kennedy, R. L. J., and New, G. B.: Chronic stridor in children sometimes erroneously attributed to enlargement of the thymus gland. *J.A.M.A.*, 96:1286, 1931.

Kent, E. M., Blades, B., Valle, A. R., and Graham, E. A.: Intrathoracic neurogenic tumors. *J. Thorac. Surg.*, 13:116, 1944.

Kessel, A. W. L.: Intrathoracic meningocele, spinal deformity and multiple neurofibromatosis. *J. Bone Joint Surg.*, 33B:87, 1951.

Key, J. A.: Mediastinal tumors. *Surg. Clin. North Am.*, 34:959, 1954.

Kirwan, W. O., Walbaum, P. R., and McCormack, R. J. M.: Cystic intrathoracic derivatives of the pregut and their complications. *Thorax*, 28:424, 1973.

Koop, C. P., Kiesewetter, W. B., and Horn, R. C.: Neuroblastoma in childhood: an evaluation of surgical management. *Pediatrics*, 16:652, 1955.

Kuipers, F., and Wieberdink, J.: An intrathoracic cyst of enterogenic origin in a young infant. *J. Pediatr.*, 42:603, 1953.

Ladd, W. E., and Scott, H. W., Jr.: Esophageal duplications or mediastinal cysts of enteric origin. *Surgery*, 6:815, 1944.

Laipply, T. C.: Cysts and cystic tumors of the mediastinum. *Arch. Pathol.*, 39:153, 1945.

Lambert, A. V.: Etiology of thin-walled thoracic cysts. *J. Thorac. Surg.*, 10:1, 1940.

Leagus, C. J., Gregorski, R. F., Crittenden, J. J., Johnson, W. D., and Lepley, D.: Giant intrapericardial bronchogenic cyst. *J. Thorac. Cardiovasc. Surg.*, 52:581, 1966.

Lillie, W. E., McDonald, J. R., and Clagett, O. T.: Pericardial celomic cysts and pericardial diverticula: Concept of etiology and report of cases. *J. Thorac. Surg.*, 20:494, 1950.

Longino, L. A., and Meeker, E., Jr.: Primary cardiac tumors in infancy. *J. Pediatr.*, 43:724, 1953.

McLetchie, N. G. B., Purves, J. K., and Saunders, R. L.: Genesis of gastric and certain intestinal diverticula. *Surg. Gynecol. Obstet.*, 99:135, 1954.

Maksim, G., Henthorne, J. C., and Allebach, H. K.: Neurofibromatosis with malignant thoracic tumor and metastasis in a child. *Am. J. Dis. Child.*, 57:381, 1939.

Maier, H. C.: Bronchogenic cysts of the mediastinum. *Ann. Surg.*, 127:476, 1948.

Marsten, J. L., Cooper, A. G., and Ankeney, J. L.: Acute cardiac tamponade due to perforation of a benign mediastinal teratoma into the pericardial sac. *J. Thorac. Cardiovasc. Surg.*, 51:700, 1966.

Mason, C. B.: Intrathoracic lymph nodes. *J. Thorac. Surg.*, 37:251, 1959.

Mayo, P.: Intrathoracic neuroblastoma in a newborn infant. *J. Thorac. Surg.*, 45:720, 1963.

Meltzer, J.: Tumorformige nebenlunge in Herzbeutal. *Virchows Arch. [Pathol. Anat.]*, 308:199, 1941.

Miscall, L.: Cited by H. P. Goldberg and I. Steinberg: Primary tumors of the heart. *Circulation*, 11:936, 1955.

Mixter, C. G., and Clifford, S. H.: Congenital mediastinal cysts of gastrogenic and bronchogenic origin. *Ann. Surg.*, 90:714, 1929.

Myers, R. T., and Bradshaw, H. H.: Benign intramural tumors and cysts of the esophagus. *J. Thorac. Surg.*, 21:470, 1951.

Nanson, E. M.: Thoracic meningocele associated with neurofibromatosis. *J. Thorac. Surg.*, 33:650, 1957.

Neal, A. E., and Menten, M. L.: Tumors of the thymus in children. *Am. J. Dis. Child.*, 76:102, 1948.

Nicholls, M. F.: Intrathoracic cyst of intestinal structure. *Br. J. Surg.*, 28:137, 1940.

Olken, H. G.: Congenital gastroenteric cysts of

the mediastinum, review and report of a case. *Am. J. Pathol., 20*:997, 1944.

Page, U. S., and Bigelow, J. C.: A mediastinal gastric duplication leading to pneumonectomy. *J. Thorac. Cardiovasc. Surg., 54* 291, 1967.

Patcher, M. R.: Mediastinal non-chromaffin para ganglioma. *J. Thorac. Surg., 45*:152, 1963.

Perry, T. M., and Smith, W. A.: Rhabdomyosarcoma of the diaphragm, a case report. *Am. J. Cancer, 35*:416, 1939.

Pickardt, O. C.: Pleuro-diaphragmatic cyst. *Ann. Surg., 99*:814, 1934.

Pirawoon, A. M., and Abbassioun, K.: Mediastinal enterogenous cyst with spinal cord compression. *J. Pediatr. Surg., 9*:543, 1974.

Pohl, R.: Meningokele im Brustraum unter dem Bilde eines intrathorakalen Rundschattens. *Röntgenpraxis, 5*:747, 1933.

Raeburn, C.: Columnar ciliated epithelium in the adult oesophagus. *J. Pathol. Bacteriol., 63*:157, 1951.

Ranström, S.: Congenital cysts of the esophagus. *Acta Otolaryngol., 33*:486, 1945.

Rath, J., and Touloukian, R. J.: Infarction of a mediastinal neuroblastoma with hemorrhagic pleural effusion. *Ann. Thorac. Surg., 10*:552, 1970.

Reiquam, C. W., Beatty, E. C., and Allen, R. P.: Neuroblastoma in infancy and childhood. *Am. J. Dis. Child., 91*:588, 1956.

Reuben, S., and Stratemeier, E. H.: Intrathoracic meningocele, a case report. *Radiology, 58*:552, 1952.

Richards, G. E., Jr., and Reaves, R. W.: Mediastinal tumors and cysts in children. *J. Dis. Child., 95*:284, 1958.

Sabiston, D. C., and Scott, H. W.: Primary neoplasms and cysts of the mediastinum. *Ann. Surg., 135*:777, 1952.

Saini, V. K., and Wahi, P. L.: Hour glass transmural type of intrathoracic lipoma. *J. Thorac. Surg., 47*:600, 1964.

Sakulsky, S. B., Harrison, E. G., Dines, D. E., and Payne, W. S.: Mediastinal granuloma. *J. Thorac. Cardiovasc. Surg., 54*:279, 1967.

Schowengerdt, C. G., Suyemoto, R., and Main, F. B.: Granulomatous and fibrous mediastinitis. *J. Thorac. Cardiovasc. Surg., 57*:365, 1969.

Schwarz, H., II, and Williams, C. S.: Thoracic gastric cysts, report of two cases with review of the literature. *J. Thorac. Surg., 12*:117, 1942.

Schweisguth, O., Mathey, J., Renault, P., and Binet, J. P.: Intrathoracic neurogenic tumors in infants and children: a study of forty cases. *Ann. Surg., 150*:29, 1959.

Scott, O. B., and Morton, D. R.: Primary cystic tumor of the diaphragm. *Arch. Pathol., 41*:645, 1946.

Sealy, W. C., Weaver, W. L., and Young, W. G., Jr.: Severe airway obstruction in infancy due to the thymus gland. *Ann. Thorac. Surg., 1*:389, 1965.

Seybold, W. D., McDonald, J. R., Clagget, O. T., and Harrington, S. W.: Mediastinal tumors of blood vascular origin. *J. Thorac. Surg., 18*:503, 1949.

Seydel, G. N., Valle, E. R., and White, M. L., Jr.: Thoracic gastric cysts. *Ann. Surg., 123*:377, 1946.

Shackelford, G. D., and MacAlister, W. H.: The aberrant positioned thymus. *Am. J. Roentgenol., 120*:291, 1974.

Skinner, G. E., and Hobbs, M. E.: Intrathoracic cystic lymphangioma, report of two cases in infants. *J. Thorac. Surg., 6*:98, 1936.

Singleton, A. O.: Congenital lymphatic disease—lymphangiomata. *Ann. Surg., 105*:952, 1937.

Smid, A. D., Ellis, F. H., Logan, G. B., and Olson, A. M.: Partial respiratory obstruction in an infant due to a bronchogenic cyst, report of a case. *Proc. Staff Meet. Mayo Clin., 30*:282, 1955.

Smith, R. E.: Case of mediastinal dermoid cyst in an infant. *Guy's Hosp. Rep., 80*:466, 1930.

Sochberg, L. A., and Robinson, A. L.: Primary tumor of the pericardium involving the myocardium, surgical removal. *J. Circulation, 1*:805, 1950.

Soloman, R. D.: Malignant teratoma of the heart: report of a case with necropsy. *Arch. Pathol., 52*:561, 1951.

Soto, M. V.: Un caso de lipoma de la cara toracica del diafragma. *J. Int. Coll. Surg., 6*:146, 1943.

Starer, F.: Successful removal of an anterior mediastinal teratoma from an infant. *Arch. Dis. Child., 27*:371, 1952.

Steel, J. D., and Schmitz, J.: Mediastinal cyst of gastric origin. *J. Thorac. Surg., 14*:403, 1945.

Stich, M. H., Rubinstein, J., Freidman, A. B., and Morrison, M.: Mediastinal lymphosarcoma in an infant. *J. Pediatr., 42*:235, 1953.

Stout, A. P.: Ganglioneuroma of the sympathetic nervous system. *Surg. Gynecol. Obstet., 84*:101, 1947.

Stowens, D.: Neuroblastomas and related tumors. *Arch. Pathol., 63*:451, 1957.

Svien, H. J., Seybold, W. D., and Thelen, E. P.: Intraspinal and intrathoracic tumor with paraplegia in a child; report of case. *Proc. Staff Meet. Mayo Clin., 25*:715, 1950.

Swift, W. A., and Neuhof, H.: Cervicomediastinal lymph angioma with chylothorax. *J. Thorac. Surg., 15*:173, 1946.

Tarney, T. J., Chang, C. H., Nugent, R. G., and Warden, H. E.: Esophageal duplication (foregut cyst) with spinal malformation. *J. Thorac. Cardiovasc. Surg., 59*:293, 1970.

Touroff, A. S. W., and Sealey, H. P.: Chronic chylothorax associated with hygroma of the mediastinum. *J. Thorac. Surg., 26*:318, 1953.

Thompson, D. P., and Moore, T. C.: Acute thoracic distress in childhood due to spontaneous rupture of a large mediastinal teratoma. *J. Pediatr. Surg., 4*:416, 1969.

Veneziale, C. M., Sheridan, L. A., Payne, W. S., and Harrison, E. G., Jr.: Angiofollicular lymph node hyperplasia of the mediastinum. *J. Thorac. Surg., 47*:111, 1964.

Ware, G. W.: Thoracic neuroblastoma. *J. Pediatr., 49*:765, 1956.

Weichert, R. F., III, Lindsey, E. S., Pearce, C. W., and Waring, W. W.: Bronchogenic cyst with unilateral obstructive emphysema. *J. Thorac. Cardiovasc. Surg.,* 59:287, 1970.

Weimann, R. B., Hallman, G. L., Bahar, D., and Greenberg, S. D.: Intrathoracic meningocele. *J. Thorac. Surg.,* 46:40, 1963.

Weinstein, E. C., Payne, W. S., and Soule, E. H.: Surgical treatment of desmoid tumor of the chest wall. *J. Thorac. Surg.,* 46:242, 1963.

Welch, C. S., Ettinger, A., and Hecht, P. L.: Recklinghausen's neurofibromatosis associated with intrathoracic meningocele: report of case. *N. Engl. J. Med.,* 238:622, 1948.

White, J. J., Kaback, M. M., and Haller, J. A.: Diagnosis and excision of an intrapericardial teratoma in an infant. *J. Thorac. Cardiovasc. Surg.,* 55:704, 1968.

Williams, K. R., and Burgord, T. H.: Surgical treatment of granulomatous paratracheal lymphadenopathy. *J. Thorac. Surg.,* 48:13, 1964.

Williams, M. H., and Johnson, J. F.: Mediastinal gastric cysts, successful excision in an eight week old infant. *Arch. Surg.,* 64:138, 1952.

Willis, R. A.: An intrapericardial teratoma in an infant. *J. Pathol. Bacteriol.,* 58:284, 1946.

Wilson, J. R., and Bartley, T. D.: Liposarcoma of the mediastinum. *J. Thorac. Surg.,* 48:486, 1964.

Wilson, J. R., Wheat, M. W., Jr., and Arean, V. M.: Pericardial teratoma. *J. Thorac. Surg.,* 45:670, 1963.

Wyllie, W. G.: Myasthenia gravis. *Proc. R. Soc. Med.,* 39:591, 1946.

Ya Deau, R. E., Clagett, O. T., and Divertie, M. B.: Intrathoracic meningocele. *J. Thorac. Surg.,* 49:202, 1965.

Yater, W. M.: Cyst of the pericardium. *Am. Heart J.,* 6:710, 1931.

Cardiac Tumors

Kilman, J. W., Craenen, J., and Hoiser, D. M.: Replacement of entire atrial wall in an infant with a cardiac rhabdomyoma. *J. Pediatr. Surg.,* 8:317, 1973.

Simcha, A., Wells, B. G., Tynan, M. J., and Waterston, D. J.: Primary cardiac tumors in childhood. *Arch. Dis. Child.,* 46:508, 1971.

Van De Hauwaert, L. G.: Cardiac tumours in infancy and childhood. *Br. Heart J.,* 33:125, 1971.

Diaphragm and Chest Wall Tumors

Anderson, L. S., and Forrest, J. V.: Tumors of the diaphragm. *Am. J. Roentgenol.,* 119:259, 1973.

Bolanowski, P. J. P., and Groff, D. B.: Thoracic wall desmoid tumor in a child. *Ann. Thorac. Surg.,* 15:632, 1973.

Grundy, G. W., and Miller, R. W.: Malignant mesothelioma in childhood. Report of 13 cases. *Cancer,* 30:1216, 1972.

OTHER DISEASES WITH A PROMINENT RESPIRATORY COMPONENT

CHAPTER FORTY-FOUR

COR PULMONALE

Jacqueline A. Noonan, M.D.

Pulmonary heart disease, also termed cor pulmonale, may complicate pulmonary disorders in children. Cor pulmonale is defined as right ventricular hypertrophy secondary to disease of the lung parenchyma or of the pulmonary vasculature, or resulting from abnormalities of pulmonary function. The basic component of cor pulmonale is pulmonary artery hypertension, which is responsible for the development of right ventricular hypertrophy. In most children, pulmonary hypertension results from pulmonary vasoconstriction as a response to hypoxia. Anatomic changes in the pulmonary vessels may be absent or limited to medial hypertrophy of the small pulmonary arteries, and if the underlying cause of the hypoxia can be corrected, the pulmonary hypertension is reversible. In some forms of diffuse progressive lung disease, interstitial fibrosis, with destruction of the alveolar wall and capillaries, may occur, leading to restriction of the pulmonary vascular bed. In such cases, pulmonary artery hypertension may not be completely reversible. When pulmonary hypertension results from pulmonary vascular disease due to multiple pulmonary emboli or from so-called primary pulmonary hypertension, there is little chance for reversibility. In Table 1, a simple classification of the causation of cor pulmonale is presented.

PARENCHYMAL LUNG DISEASE

OBSTRUCTIVE AIRWAY DISEASE

Asthma, chronic bronchitis and fibrocystic disease are common causes of obstructive airway disease in children. Wheezing, prolonged expiration and overexpanded lungs usually allow ready clinical recognition of obstructive airway disease. Pulmonary function studies show a decrease in vital capacity with an increase in residual volume and an increase in the functional residual capacity. The obstruction of the small airways may occur because of inflammation of the mucosa, constriction of the bronchiolar smooth muscle, edema of the bronchial tissue or plugging of the lumen by mucus. In any event, the degree of narrowing is variable among the many small airways, and the distribution of inspired gases is not uniform. This results in an abnormal ratio between pulmonary blood flow and ventilation and leads to hypoxemia with a

TABLE 1. CLASSIFICATION OF COR PULMONALE IN CHILDREN

Hypoxia
 Parenchymal lung disease
  Obstructive airway, e.g., with fibrocystic disease
  Restrictive lung disease, e.g., diffuse interstitial fibrosis
  Other lung disease, e.g., lymphangiectasis
 Extrinsic factors
  Upper airway obstruction
  Neuromuscular disorders
  Thoracic cage deformity
  Respiratory center dysfunction
  High altitude

Pulmonary Vascular Disease
 Thromboembolism
 Primary pulmonary hypertension
 Pulmonary veno-occlusive disease

decreased arterial P_{O_2}. Since the uninvolved, relatively normal portion of the lungs may hyperventilate as a response to hypoxia, the P_{CO_2} may remain quite normal until, with increasing severity of airway obstruction, there is overall alveolar hypoventilation.

Cor pulmonale is a recognized complication, particularly in fibrocystic disease. From many clinical reports, there is good evidence to support the concept that hypoxia is the major factor leading to pulmonary artery hypertension. The clinical diagnosis of cor pulmonale in children with obstructive airway disease is sometimes difficult. The electrocardiogram as a tool to diagnose early right ventricular hypertrophy in patients with obstructive airway disease has been disappointing. The overexpanded lungs apparently cause an alteration in electrical conduction. Liebman and coworkers (1967) have shown that the Frank system of the vectorcardiogram is quite reliable and superior to the conventional electrocardiogram in the diagnosis of right ventricular hypertrophy. Moss and associates (1965) have found that the vital capacity was very helpful in predicting pulmonary hypertension, which was likely to be present in patients with fibrocystic disease when the vital capacity was reduced to less than 60 per cent of the predicted normal. Serial chest roentgenograms demonstrating progressive enlargement of the pulmonary artery is a useful diagnostic tool, but the heart size may appear within normal limits because of the overall increase in chest size. More recently, a study of right ventricular thickness by echocardiogram has shown a good correlation with the clinical severity of cystic fibrosis. With more clinical experience, this new, noninvasive tool may prove to be the most reliable method of determining right ventricular hypertrophy in this group of patients.

Physical examination is also of importance in diagnosing cor pulmonale in children with obstructive airway disease. The development of a systolic murmur along the lower left sternal border, indicating tricuspid insufficiency, is strong evidence of pulmonary hypertension. A right-sided gallop is often present when right heart failure occurs. Fluid retention and hepatomegaly are expected when heart failure results as a complication of cor pulmonale. The marked overexpansion of the lungs makes auscultation of the heart sounds less reliable in obstructive airway disease than in other pulmonary disorders.

Bronchiectasis may be a complication of obstructive airway disease, such as chronic bronchitis or fibrocystic disease, but so far, in the author's experience, cor pulmonale has not been a problem in children with severe bronchiectasis. Only mild pulmonary hypertension has been noted at cardiac catheterization, and there is surprisingly little decrease in the arterial P_{O_2}. Liebow and coworkers (1949) have demonstrated bronchial artery to pulmonary artery communications in bronchiectasis, and we were able to confirm their findings in several of our patients. Because pulmonary blood flow to the destroyed lung segment is generally markedly reduced, the pulmonary flow and ventilation are fairly well matched and little hypoxemia results. A significant left to right shunt, however, may be noted at the pulmonary artery level from the bronchopulmonary anastomoses. Should there be extensive diffuse lung disease in addition to localized bronchiectasis, pulmonary artery hypertension would be expected. In such patients, the presence of a left to right shunt would impose an increased burden on the left ventricle, and both right- and left-sided heart failure might result.

Vigorous treatment of the underlying pulmonary disease is an essential part of therapy. In addition, correction of the hypoxia and oxygen or the use of vasodilating agents, such as tolazoline, may reduce pulmonary artery pressure. Digitalis should be used, if there is evidence of congestive cardiac failure. Diuretics are of particular value in the overall management of such patients, since fluid retention is an important component of the complicating right-sided heart failure.

RESTRICTIVE LUNG DISEASE

In restrictive lung disease, there is impairment of diffusion because of thickening of the alveolar or capillary membrane by transudate, exudate, fibrosis or granulomatous tissue. This results in an increased diffusion pattern for oxygen from the alveoli to capillary blood. The distribution of gas is uneven and results in a low P_{O_2}. The resulting hypoxemia stimulates hyperventilation, and since the relatively normal lung segments are then overventilated, the P_{CO_2} is usually significantly decreased. The low P_{O_2} causes pulmonary vasoconstriction, which may result in pulmonary artery hypertension. Unfortunately, diffuse pulmonary fibrosis (Hamman-Rich syndrome), chronic pneumonia of various types, sarcoidosis, hemosiderosis and Wilson-Mikity disease, to name a few of the conditions resulting in restrictive lung disease, may, with increasing severity of the lung process, cause an actual reduction in the total pulmonary capillary bed. Pulmonary artery hypertension, in this group of patients, may result from two factors, namely (1) pulmonary vasoconstriction from hypoxia and (2) actual destruction of part of the pulmonary vascular bed from fibrosis.

Patients with restrictive lung disease have effort dyspnea, fatigue, vague chest pain, and often an irritating, nonproductive cough. On physical examination, respirations are generally shallow and rapid. The lungs may be clear, although some patients will have fine, dry rales. Clubbing is often present. Cyanosis is noted on exertion or with crying, but in severe cases may be present even at rest. The presence of cyanosis and the absence of striking lung findings by physical examination may lead to a mistaken diagnosis of cyanotic heart disease. The chest roentgenogram usually shows a diffuse infiltrative process but varies, depending on the underlying disease process. If significant pulmonary artery hypertension is present, there is usually definite right ventricular hypertrophy indicated by the electrocardiogram.

As mentioned elsewhere in this text, it is very important to diagnose the underlying pathologic condition in the lung, since some forms of restrictive lung disease are reversible by proper therapy. If routine laboratory studies and cultures are not productive in es-

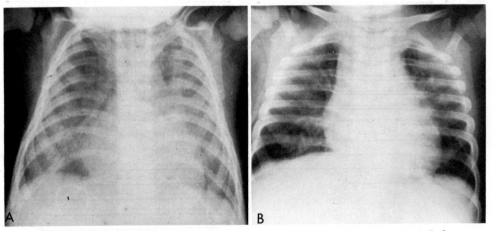

Figure 1. Chest roentgenograms of infant with desquamative interstitial pneumonitis. *A,* Before treatment. *B,* After treatment with steroids.

tablishing a clear-cut, definitive diagnosis, a lung biopsy should be considered early in the course of the disease in order to arrive at a proper diagnosis. Hamman-Rich syndrome, eosinophilic granuloma, desquamative interstitial pneumonitis and collagen disease are all entities that may respond to steroid therapy, whereas chronic granulomatous disease, such as tuberculosis, histoplasmosis or other fungal infections, require specific therapy. Establishing a definite diagnosis and instituting proper therapy offer the best chance of reversing the cor pulmonale. Figure 1 shows the roentgenogram of a patient with desquamative interstitial pneumonia before and after successful treatment with steroid therapy. Digitalis and diuretics should be used in the presence of suspected or overt congestive heart failure.

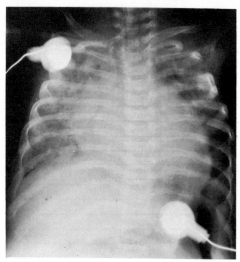

Figure 2. Infant six months of age with bronchopulmonary dysplasia shortly before death from cor pulmonale.

roentgenogram of an infant shortly before death at age six months from cor pulmonale, resulting from bronchopulmonary dysplasia.

OTHER LUNG DISEASE

It is not always possible to classify the pulmonary disease as purely obstructive or restrictive, since some conditions result in the combination of these two physiologic derangements. One such entity is pulmonary lymphangiectasis, which is discussed elsewhere in this text. Wilson-Mikity disease and bronchopulmonary dysplasia have elements of both obstructive and restrictive lung disease. It is important to remember that in the newborn the pulmonary blood vessels have not yet lost their thick, medial muscle layer and that the pulmonary vessels are especially reactive to hypoxia. Resulting pulmonary vasoconstriction may cause severe pulmonary artery hypertension and lead to the very rapid development of cor pulmonale. Unfortunately, the newborn lung also seems to be quite susceptible to the toxic effects of oxygen, so that the clinical management of the young infant requires a delicate balance between enough and not too much supplemental oxygen. Serial blood gases and careful monitoring of inspired oxygen are essential. Figure 2 is a

EXTRINSIC FACTORS RESULTING IN HYPOVENTILATION

UPPER AIRWAY OBSTRUCTION

Upper airway obstruction causing cor pulmonale is a very important condition to recognize, since it may be reversed and thereby promote relief of the obstruction. The clinical picture includes noisy respirations with stridor, particularly in the supine position. In addition, somnolence, congestive cardiac failure and roentgenographic evidence of pulmonary edema are common findings. Although hypertrophied tonsils and adenoids have been the most common cause of upper airway obstruction, micrognathia, glossoptosis, macroglossia, Crouzon's disease, Hurler's disease, laryngeal web, laryngotracheomalacia and Pierre Robin syndrome have all been reported to cause this interesting syndrome. It is significant that many patients reported in the literature have had evidence of mental retardation. It is possible that a central nervous system factor may predispose to this condition, as has been proposed in the Pickwickian syndrome.

With upper airway obstruction, generalized hypoventilation of both lungs results. Therefore, there is not only a decreased P_{O_2} but also an elevated P_{CO_2} and, eventually, respiratory acidosis with a lowered pH. In all our patients with this syndrome, severe pulmonary hypertension was demonstrated at cardiac catheterization and was reflected by right ventricular hypertrophy and P pulmonale on the electrocardiogram. In addition, there was marked cardiac enlargement and pulmonary congestion on x-ray examination. Severe pulmonary hypertension present during hypoxia and hypercapnia can be promptly reversed with relief of the upper airway obstruction. It was interesting to note that in our patients with upper airway obstruction, an elevated wedge or left atrial pressure was found at cardiac catheterization, and in several patients studied there was also an elevation of the end diastolic pressure in the left ventricle. Hypoxia alone has little effect on left ventricular function. However, the combination of hypoxia plus acidosis has been shown experimentally to be quite detrimental to left ventricular function. It is possible that the pulmonary edema noted on the roentgenogram and the elevated pulmonary wedge pressure reflect left ventricular failure. The exact pathogenesis of the pulmonary edema noted in this syndrome has not yet been clearly defined.

It is essential that this syndrome be considered in any patient presenting with unexplained heart failure, particularly when somnolence is a clinical feature. Many patients reported in the literature were moribund at the time of admission, and four patients have been reported to have died before a correct diagnosis was made. Relief of the upper airway obstruction by removal of the tonsils and adenoids, tracheotomy or insertion of an endotracheal tube should be done promptly. It is very important to be cautious in the use of supplemental oxygen in patients with an elevated P_{CO_2} who are hypoxic, since severe respiratory acidosis will quickly result if the hypoxic respiratory drive is inhibited by oxygen therapy. Use of sedation should be avoided until the upper airway obstruction has been relieved. Digitalis and diuretic therapy are recommended in addition to prompt relief of the upper airway obstruction.

NEUROMUSCULAR DISEASES

Inadequate respiration may result in weakness of the respiratory muscles. Werdnig Hoffmann syndrome, Guillain-Barré syndrome, myasthenia gravis or poliomyelitis are but a few of the conditions that may result in alveolar hypoventilation, which may, in turn, lead to hypoxemia and hypercapnia and eventually cause pulmonary hypertension and cor pulmonale. It is important to follow serial blood gases in patients with neuromuscular diseases and to employ assisted ventilation as soon as it is indicated. Acute respiratory failure and death are probably more common in neuromuscular disease than cor pulmonale.

DEFORMITIES OF THE THORACIC CHEST

A small immobile or deformed chest from any cause that fails as a chest "bellows" may lead to cor pulmonale. Kyphoscoliosis is the most common thoracic deformity causing cor pulmonale, but since this condition is slowly progressive, symptoms are delayed until adult life and it is seldom a problem in childhood. Pectus excavatum is a very frequent thoracic deformity, but it rarely results in severe pulmonary dysfunction. There are, however, a number of severe congenital defects that may result in pulmonary insufficiency from so-called "asphyxiating" thoracic dystrophy. Vigorous physiotherapy and chest exercises should be employed to improve pulmonary function and to prevent or at least postpone the development of cor pulmonale. An associated respiratory infection will often result in respiratory failure. If serial blood gases indicate deterioration, treatment with artificial ventilation should be instituted promptly to prevent the development of cor pulmonale or severe respiratory insufficiency.

Diaphragmatic paralysis, usually well tolerated in an older child or adult, may be very poorly tolerated in the newborn. One infant with a paralyzed right diaphragm developed cor pulmonale and marked wasting. Surgical plication of the right diaphragm brought marked clinical improvement. The electrocardiogram returned to normal, as did the pulmonary artery pressure and blood gases. Although an Erb's palsy associated with diaphragmatic paralysis is usually transient, in its severe form it may lead to cor pulmonale, which can be reversed by proper treatment.

RESPIRATORY CENTER DYSFUNCTION

The Pickwickian syndrome is a term that has been applied to obese patients who hypoventilate and develop cor pulmonale. Although obesity itself does interfere with chest expansion because of the marked increase in work required to enlarge the thoracic cavity in the presence of excess weight, only a moderate reduction of vital capacity is expected. It is estimated that about 10 per cent of markedly obese adults actually hypoventilate and are at risk of developing the Pickwickian syndrome. There is good evidence to implicate a depression of the respiratory center as an important factor in the development of the Pickwickian syndrome. A decreased sensitivity of the central nervous system to carbon dioxide inhalation, which does return to normal after weight reduction, has been demonstrated. This is a relatively uncommon syndrome in childhood, but several well documented cases have been reported. It is interesting that mental retardation has been present in several of the obese children reported with Pickwickian syndrome. Weight reduction is an essential part of the treatment planned for such patients.

Primary alveolar hypoventilation due to central nervous system disease is a rare cause of cor pulmonale. Both brain stem disease and hypothalamic lesions have been associated with hypoventilation. Unfortunately, primary apnea or hypoventilation due to respiratory center dysfunction (Ondine's curse) is rather poorly understood and very difficult to treat. Our recent experience with such a patient has been quite frustrating. Respiratory stimulants, in general, are not effective in this syndrome. Mechanical ventilation was necessary to reverse cor pulmonale in our patient on many occasions. Although progesterone therapy has been helpful in the treatment of some adults with a depressed respiratory center, this therapy was not effective in our patient. Ondine's curse is fortunately a rare disease, but one that should be kept in mind when an infant develops unexplained cyanosis and deep somnolence. If careful observation of the respiratory pattern and blood gas determinations demonstrate the presence of hypoventilation, mechanical ventilation should be instituted at once to reverse the symptoms. If the central nervous system problem is temporary, such as with drug intoxication, recovery should be expected. In the case of Ondine's curse, the prognosis is more guarded. Fortunately, our patient has improved with increasing age but his future prognosis is still in doubt. He has a tracheostomy but has not required assisted ventilation for nearly a year.

HIGH ALTITUDE

It is well documented that altitudes above 10,000 feet result in hypoxia and lead to pulmonary hypertension, which can be reversed upon descent to sea level. Children living at high altitudes frequently have abnormal rightward shift in the mean QRS axis on the electrocardiogram and a raised pulmonary artery pressure at rest, which may in some cases increase markedly with exercise. Most children are asymptomatic in spite of increased pulmonary artery pressure. There is, however, an increased incidence of primary pulmonary hypertension among patients living at high altitude, and it is well known that patients with congenital heart disease, particularly those with left to right shunts, have a higher pulmonary vascular resistance and smaller left to right shunt when studied at high altitude as compared with those studied at sea level.

PULMONARY VASCULAR DISEASE

THROMBOEMBOLISM

Pulmonary emboli are uncommon in children but may complicate sickle cell anemia, rheumatic fever, bacterial endocarditis and schistosomiasis. Chronic cor pulmonale as a complication of multiple pulmonary emboli is even rarer but has been well documented as a complication of ventriculovenous shunt for the treatment of hydrocephalus. Although the causation and pathogenesis of this interesting complication are unknown, several factors have been proposed, such as infection, periarteritis of the pulmonary vessels as an autoimmune reaction of the pulmonary vessels to cerebrospinal fluid, or the presence of brain thromboplastin in the circulation predisposing to repeated thromboembolization. Thrombosis of the superior vena cava and right atrium as a complication of the

foreign body in the cardiovascular system might well serve as a source for repeated thromboemboli.

Early recognition of the complication of thromboembolism before severe pulmonary hypertension has developed is necessary to reverse the process. The most important part of therapy would be to remove the shunt from the cardiovascular system and substitute a peritoneal or other similar shunt in its place.

Acute cor pulmonale has been reported in children from the development of primary thrombosis of the pulmonary artery, particularly in patients with the nephrotic syndrome. Multiple pulmonary emboli may also occur as a complication of sepsis or severe dehydration. The use of foreign bodies for deep intravenous hyperalimentation increases the risk of thromboembolism in children, particularly if infection occurs.

PRIMARY PULMONARY HYPERTENSION

Primary pulmonary hypertension is a rare but important cause of cor pulmonale in children. In Wagenvoort's series (1970) of 110 patients with primary pulmonary hypertension, over one-third were under 15 years of age. The symptoms develop insidiously and may begin in early infancy. Fatigue, dyspnea on exertion, syncope and convulsions are common complaints, and congestive cardiac failure is a frequent complication. Because loss of consciousness described as fainting or convulsion may be a predominant presenting symptom, it is not uncommon for the patient to be misdiagnosed as having a convulsive disorder. On physical examination, cyanosis may or may not be present. Typically, there is evidence of right ventricular hypertrophy with a right ventricular lift and a markedly increased pulmonary second sound, often without a significant murmur. An ejection click, systolic ejection murmur and parasternal diastolic blow as well as a murmur of tricuspid insufficiency have all been described, however. On chest roentgenogram, a prominent pulmonary artery, moderate cardiac enlargement and decrease in the pulmonary vascularity in the peripheral lung fields are classic findings. Electrocardiogram usually shows evidence of severe right ventricular hypertrophy. Cardiac catheterization and angiocardiography will usually exclude congenital heart disease as the cause of the pulmonary hypertension. A normal wedge pressure helps to exclude left-sided obstructive lesions such as congenital mitral stenosis, cor triatriatum or stenosis of the pulmonary veins, all of which may mimic primary pulmonary hypertension. Blood gases may show some reduction in the P_{O_2}. The P_{CO_2} is usually quite low, since these patients tend to hyperventilate. Pulmonary artery pressure is markedly elevated and frequently at or near systemic level. End diastolic pressure in the right ventricle and the right atrial pressure are elevated if congestive heart failure is present. Cardiac output is generally quite low and fixed, and angiograms will show dilated pulmonary vessels with a "pruned" appearance and a slow passage of dye through the lungs. The etiologic factor of this serious disease is unknown. There is, however, a fairly high familial incidence, suggesting that there is some genetic predisposition for the development of this disease. Wagenvoort (1970) suggests that increased vasomotor tone is the initial factor in primary pulmonary hypertension. Microscopic examinations of the lungs reveal medial hypertrophy of the small pulmonary arteries, with intimal lesions and plexiform lesions becoming more frequent with increasing age. Wagenvoort feels that the vascular lesions in primary pulmonary hypertension show the same range of vascular alterations as that noted in patients with severe pulmonary hypertension resulting from other causes. He suggests that patients with primary pulmonary hypertension have extreme hyperactivity of their pulmonary vasculature, but what initiates the initial vasoconstriction is unknown.

At the present time, there is no specific treatment. Digitalis and diuretics are helpful in treating the complications of congestive failure. Intermittent oxygen therapy may improve symptoms. A variety of drugs have been tried without real success. Anticoagulants are worthwhile if one cannot exclude the possibility of multiple pulmonary emboli. Acetylcholine, tolazoline, isoproterenol, and hexamethonium have been given by short-term intravenous or interpulmonary arterial administration with occasionally some drop in pulmonary artery pressure. Oral administration of isoproterenol has been used in a few patients with symptomatic improvement, but unfortunately has not prevented progression of the disease process.

When symptoms appear and a definite diagnosis is made, the prognosis is very poor, especially in children; in this age group, death usually occurs within one year. Death is frequently sudden and may be precipitated by diagnostic procedures such as cardiac catheterization or even bone marrow aspiration.

PULMONARY VENO-OCCLUSIVE DISEASE

A rare disorder that may be confused with primary pulmonary hypertension is intrapulmonary veno-occlusive disease. This condition is associated with pathologic changes and obstruction of the small pulmonary veins and venules. The clinical features are similar to other forms of primary pulmonary hypertension and include dyspnea on effort, easy fatigue, chest pain and syncopal episodes. An occasional patient may present with orthopnea and paroxysmal nocturnal dyspnea, which are rare in patients with primary pulmonary hypertension. Mild arterial unsaturation is frequent.

On physical examination, these patients resemble other patients with severe pulmonary hypertension and demonstrate a loud pulmonary second sound and occasionally the murmur of tricuspid insufficiency or pulmonary insufficiency. Some patients may have fine rales heard in the lungs, unlike the patient with primary pulmonary hypertension whose lungs are clear. The chest roentgenogram is most useful in distinguishing clinically between primary pulmonary artery hypertension and pulmonary veno-occlusive disease (Fig. 3). In both, there is evidence of right ventricular enlargement and a dilated main pulmonary artery. In intrapulmonary veno-occlusive disease, there is a fine and diffuse increase in the interstitial and vascular marking associated with Kerley B lines and visualization of the interlobar fissures. Occasionally, there may be pleural thickening or an effusion. The radiographic findings are suggestive of pulmonary venous hypertension, secondary to a left-sided obstructive lesion of the heart. The roentgenogram may resemble that of a patient with severe mitral stenosis, but there is no evidence of enlargement of the left atrium.

The electrocardiogram is similar to that seen in primary pulmonary hypertension, showing right ventricular hypertrophy. An echocardiogram may be very helpful in ruling out obstructive left-sided heart disease as the cause of pulmonary venous congestion. This shows enlargement of the right ventricle, but the left atrium and the left ventricle are normal in size and there is a normal mitral valve.

Cardiac catheterization reveals severe pulmonary artery hypertension with a normal wedge and is not distinct from that in a patient with primary pulmonary hypertension, except that there is usually some pulmonary venous unsaturation present.

On histologic examination, the small pulmonary veins show intimal fibrosis as expected with pulmonary venous congestion. There are varying degrees of obstruction of the small veins by thrombi and multiple foci of interstitial fibrosis. There are also capillary congestion and hemosiderosis, and often an increase in inflammatory cells.

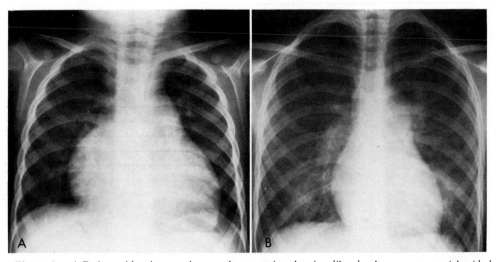

Figure 3. *A*, Patient with primary pulmonary hypertension showing dilated pulmonary artery, right-sided enlargement with clear lung fields. *B*, Patient with pulmonary veno-occlusive disease showing an increase in interstitial and vascular markings with Kerley B lines at both bases.

Illustration continued on following page

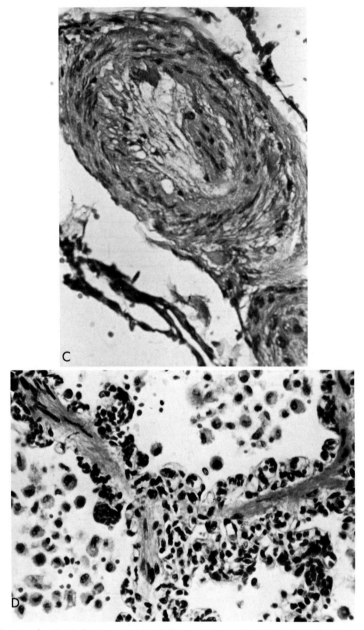

Figure 3 *Continued.*   *C,* Medial hypertrophy and severe internal proliferation of pulmonary artery characteristic of primary pulmonary hypertension. *D,* Capillary congestion, interstitial fibrosis, and increase in inflammatory and heart failure cells characteristic of pulmonary veno-occlusive disease.

Changes in the pulmonary arteries are always less extensive and more recent than those of the veins. The causation of this interesting entity is unknown, although an infectious origin has been proposed in some cases. Most patients, however, have no constitutional symptoms, and in the great majority, the etiologic factor remains obscure. In the patient reported by Rosenthal and coworkers (1973), a genetic factor could be implicated. The prognosis is poor, and all treatment has been ineffective. Of the reported cases, survival after diagnosis was usually under two years, but our patient shown in Figure 3 was dead within two months of the onset of clinical symptoms.

SUMMARY

The causation of cor pulmonale in children is varied and in some cases may be reversed by prompt recognition and therapy. In general, treatment of the underlying lung disease with relief of hypoxia is the most important part of management. Digitalis is helpful and should be used. Care must be taken to avoid toxicity by careful attention to the potassium level. Diuretics are of great value in relieving the fluid retention of right-sided heart failure. Lasix may be of particular value in reducing the pulmonary congestion that often accompanies pulmonary disease. Oxygen to relieve hypoxia is important but should be administered with care if there is significant CO_2 retention. Mechanical respiratory assistance to correct respiratory insufficiency may be necessary to reverse cor pulmonale in some patients. Cor pulmonale should be considered a serious complication of respiratory disease, and care should be taken to prevent this problem whenever possible.

REFERENCES

Ainger, L. E.: Large tonsils and adenoids in small children with cor pulmonale. *Br. Heart J.*, *30*: 356, 1968.

Avery, M. E., Riley, M. C., and Weiss, A.: The course of bronchiectasis in childhood. *Bull. Johns Hopkins Hosp.*, *109*:20, 1961.

Bergofsky, E. H.: Cor pulmonale in the syndrome of alveolar hypoventilation. *Prog. Cardiovasc. Dis.*, *9*:414, 1967.

Bingham, J. A. W.: Two cases of unilateral paralysis of the diaphragm in the newborn treated surgically. *Thorax*, *9*:248, 1954.

Bland, J. W., Edwards, F. K., and Brinsfield, D.: Pulmonary hypertension and congestive heart failure in children with chronic upper airway obstruction. New concepts of etiologic factors. *Am. J. Cardiol.*, *23*:830, 1969.

Bove, K. E., and Scott, R. C.: The anatomy of chronic cor pulmonale secondary to intrinsic lung disease. *Prog. Cardiovasc. Dis.*, *9*:227, 1966.

Bristow, J. D., Morris, J. F., and Kloster, F. E.: Hemodynamics of cor pulmonale. *Prog. Cardiovasc. Dis.*, *9*:239, 1966.

Buchta, R. M., Park, S., and Giammona, S. T.: Desquamative interstitial pneumonia in a seven-week old infant. *Am. J. Dis. Child.*, *120*:341, 1970.

Cayler, G. G., Mays, J., and Riley, H. D.: Cardiorespiratory syndrome of obesity (Pickwickian syndrome) in children. *Pediatrics*, *27*:237, 1961.

Cox, M. A., Schiebler, G. L., Taylor, W. J., Wheat, M. W., and Krovetz, L. J.: Reversible pulmonary hypertension in a child with respiratory obstruction and cor pulmonale. *J. Pediatr.*, *67*:192, 1965.

Cronje, R. E., Human, G. P., and Simson, I. W.: Hypoxaemic pulmonary hypertension in children. *S. Afr. Med. J.*, *40*:2, 1966.

Emery, J. L., and Hilton, H. B.: Lung and heart complications of treatment of hydrocephalus by ventriculoauriculostomy. *Surgery*, *50*:309, 1961.

Enson, Y., Giuntini, C., Lebois, M. L., Morris, T. Q., Ferrer, M. I., and Harvey, R. M.: The influence of hydrogen ion concentration and hypoxia on the pulmonary circulation. *J. Clin. Invest.*, *43*:1146, 1964.

Favara, B. E., and Paul, R. N.: Thromboembolism and cor pulmonale complicating ventriculovenous shunts. *J.A.M.A.*, *199*:668, 1967.

Finkelstein, J. W., and Avery, M. E.: The Pickwickian syndrome. Studies on ventilation and carbohydrate metabolism: case report of a child who recovered. *Am. J. Dis. Child.*, *106*:251, 1963.

Fishman, L. S., Samson, J. H., and Sperling, D. R.: Primary alveolar hypoventilation syndrome (Ondine's curse). *Am. J. Dis. Child.*, *110*:155, 1965.

Gerald, B., and Dungan, W. T.: Cor pulmonale and pulmonary edema in children secondary to chronic upper airway obstruction. *Radiology*, *90*:679, 1968.

Gilroy, J., Cahalan, J. L., Berman, R., and Newman, M.: Cardiac and pulmonary complications in Duchenne's progressive muscular dystrophy. *Circulation*, *27*:484, 1963.

Goldring, R. M., Fishman, A. P., Turino, G. M., Cohen, H. I., Denning, C. R., and Anderson, D. H.: Pulmonary hypertension and cor pulmonale in cystic fibrosis of the pancreas. *J. Pediatr.*, *65*:501, 1964.

Gootman, N., Gross, J., and Mensch, A.: Pulmonary artery thrombosis; a complication occurring with prednisone and chlorothiazide therapy in two nephrotic patients. *Pediatrics*, *34*:861, 1964.

Griffin, J. T., Kass, I., and Hoffman, M. S.: Cor pulmonale associated with symptoms and signs of asthma in children. *Pediatrics*, *24*:54, 1959.

Heath, D.: Pulmonary hypertension in pulmonary parenchymal disease. *Cardiovas. Clin.*, *4*:80, 1972.

Herbert, F. A., Nahmias, B. B., Gaensler, E. A., and MacMahon, H. E.: Pathophysiology of interstitial pulmonary fibrosis: report of 19 cases and follow-up with corticosteroids. *Arch. Intern. Med.*, *110*:628, 1962.

Hilton, H. B., and Rendle-Short, J.: Diffuse progressive interstitial fibrosis of the lungs in childhood (Hamman-Rich syndrome). *Arch. Dis. Child.*, *36*:102, 1961.

Hodgman, J. E., Mikity, V. G., Tatter, D., and

Cleland, R. S.: Chronic respiratory distress in the premature infant. Wilson-Mikity syndrome. *Pediatrics, 44*:179, 1969.

Hood, W. B., Spencer, H., Lass, R. W., and Daly, R.: Primary pulmonary hypertension: familial occurrence. *Br. Heart J., 30*:336, 1968.

Husson, G. S., and Wyatt, T. C.: Primary pulmonary vascular obstruction in children. *Pediatrics, 36*:75, 1965.

Javett, S. N., Webster, I., and Braudo, J. L.: Congenital dilatation of the pulmonary lymphatics. *Pediatrics, 31*:416, 1963.

Jersetz, R. M., Huszar, R. J., and Basu, S.: Pierre Robin syndrome. Cause of respiratory obstruction, cor pulmonale, and pulmonary edema. *Am. J. Dis. Child., 117*:710, 1969.

Jeune, M., Carron, R., Berard, C., and Loaec, Y.: Polychondradystrophie avec blocage thoracique d'evolution fatale. *Pediatrie, 9*:390, 1954.

Jordan, J. D., and Snyder, C. H.: Rheumatoid disease of the lung and cor pulmonale: observations in a child. *Am. J. Dis. Child., 108*:174, 1964.

Kass, H., Hanson, V., and Patrick, J.: Scleroderma in childhood. J. Pediatr., 68:243, 1966.

Kelminson, L. L., Cotton, E. K., and Vogel, J. H. K.: The reversibility of pulmonary hypertension in patients with cystic fibrosis: observations on the effects of tolazoline hydrochloride. *Pediatrics, 39*:24, 1967.

Khoury, G. H., and Howes, C. R.: Primary pulmonary hypertension in children living at high altitude. *J. Pediatr., 62*:177, 1963.

Levin, S. E., Zamet, R., and Schamman, A.: Thrombosis of the pulmonary arteries and the nephrotic syndrome. *Br. Med. J., 1*:153, 1967.

Levy, A. M., Tabakin, B. S., Hanson, J. S., and Markewicz, R. M.: Hypertrophied adenoids causing pulmonary hypertension and heart failure. *N. Engl. J. Med., 277*:506, 1967.

Liebman, J., Doershuk, C. F., Rapp, C., and Matthews, L.: The vectorcardiogram in cystic fibrosis. Diagnostic significance and correlation with pulmonary function tests. *Circulation, 35*:552, 1967.

Liebow, A. A., Hales, M. R., and Lindskog, G. E.: Enlargement of the bronchial arteries, and their anastomoses with the pulmonary arteries in bronchiectasis. *Am. J. Pathol., 25*:211, 1949.

Liebow, A. A., Steer, A., and Billingsley, J. G.: Desquamative interstitial pneumonia. *Am. J. Med., 36*:369, 1965.

Luke, M. J., Mehrizi, A., Folger, G. M., and Rowe, R. D.: Chronic nasopharyngeal obstruction as a cause of cardiomegaly, cor pulmonale, and pulmonary edema. *Pediatrics, 37*:762, 1966.

Melmon, K. L., and Braunwald, E.: Familial pulmonary hypertension. *N. Engl. J. Med., 269*:770, 1963.

Menashe, V. D., Farrehi, C., and Miller, M.: Hypoventilation and cor pulmonale due to chronic upper airway obstruction. *J. Pediatr., 67*:198, 1965.

Morgan, A. D.: Cor pulmonale in children: re-

view and etiological classification. *Am. Heart J., 73*:550, 1967.

Moss, A. J., Harper, W. H., Dooley, R. R., Murray, J. F., and Mack, J. R.: Cor pulmonale in cystic fibrosis of the pancreas. *J. Pediatr., 67*:797, 1965.

Noonan, J. A.: Pulmonary heart disease. *Pediatr. Clin. North Am., 18*:1255, 1971.

Noonan, J. A.: Pulmonary thromboembolism in children. In Mobbin-Uddin, K. (Ed.): *Pulmonary Thromboembolism.* Springfield, Illinois, Charles C Thomas, 1975.

Noonan, J. A., and Ehmke, D. A.: Complications of ventriculovenous shunts for control of hydrocephalus. Report of three cases with thromboemboli to the lungs. *N. Engl. J. Med., 269*:70, 1963.

Noonan, J. A., Walters, L R., and Reeves, J. T.: Congenital pulmonary lymphangiectasis. *Am. J. Dis. Child., 120*:314, 1970.

Northway, W. H., Rosan, R. C., and Porter, D. Y.: Pulmonary disease following respiratory therapy of hyaline-membrane disease. *N. Engl. J. Med., 276*:357, 1967.

Penaloza, D., Gamboa, R., Dyer, J., Echevarria, M., and Marticorena, E.: The influence of high altitudes on the electrical activity of the heart. I. Electrocardiographic and vectorcardiographic observations in the newborn infants and children. *Am. Heart J., 59*:111, 1960.

Pirnar, T., and Neuhauser, E. B. D.: Asphyxiating thoracic dystrophy of the newborn. *Am. J. Roentgenol., 98*:358, 1966.

Rao, B. N. S., Moller, J. H., and Edwards, J. E.: Primary pulmonary hypertension in a child: response to pharmacologic agents. *Circulation, 40*:583, 1969.

Rodman, T., Resnick, M. E., Berkowitz, R. D., Fennelly, J. F., and Olivia, J.: Alveolar hypoventilation due to involvement of the respiratory center by obscure disease of the central nervous system. *Am. J. Med., 32*:208, 1962.

Rosenow, E. C., O'Connell, E. J., and Harrison, E. G.: Desquamative interstitial pneumonia in children. *Am. J. Dis. Child., 120*:344, 1970.

Rosenthal, A., Vawten, G., and Wagenvoort, C. A.: Intrapulmonary veno-occlusive disease. *Am. J. Cardiol., 31*:78, 1973.

Rubin, E. H., and Rubin, M.: Lung biopsy for diffuse pulmonary lesions: value and limitations. *Dis. Chest, 46*:635, 1964.

Shettigar, U. R., Hultgren, H. N., Specter, M., Martin, R., and Davies, D. H.: Primary pulmonary hypertension: favorable effect of isoproterenol. *N. Engl. J. Med., 295*:1414, 1976.

Staub, N. G.: Alveolar-arterial oxygen tension gradient due to diffusion. *J. Appl. Physiol., 18*:673, 1963.

Talner, N. S., Liu, H. Y., Oberman, H. A., and Schmidt, R. W.: Thromboembolism complicating holter valve shunt. A clinicopathologic study of four patients treated with this procedure for hydrocephalus. *Am. J. Dis. Child., 101*:602, 1961.

Thilenius, O. G., Nadas, A. S., and Jockin, H.: Primary pulmonary vascular obstruction in children. *Pediatrics, 36*:75, 1965.

Vogel, J. H. K., Pryor, R., and Blount, S. G.: The cardiovascular system in children from high altitude. *J. Pediatr., 64*:315, 1964.

Vogel, J. H. K., McNamara, D. G., Rosenberg, H. S., Hallman, G. L., McGrady, J. D., Grover, R. F., and Blount, S. G.: Influence of altitude on the pulmonary circulation in experimental animals and patients with ventricular septal defects. *Clin. Res., 13*:113, 1965.

Wagenvoort, C. A., and Wagenvoort, N.: Primary pulmonary hypertension: a pathologic study of the lung vessels in 156 clinically diagnosed cases. *Circulation, 42*:1163, 1970.

Wagenvoort, C. A.: Vasoconstrictive primary pulmonary hypertension and pulmonary veno-occlusive disease. *Cardiovasc. Clin., 4*:98, 1972.

Whitman, V., Stern, R. C., Bellet, P., Doershuk, C. F., Liebman, J., Boat, T. F., Borkat, G., and Matthews, L. W.: Studies on cor pulmonale in cystic fibrosis. *Pediatrics, 55*:83, 1975.

Yater, W. M., and Hansmann, G. H.: Sickle cell anemia: a new cause of cor pulmonale. Report of two cases with numerous disseminated occlusions of the small pulmonary arteries. *Am. J. Med. Sci., 191*:474, 1936.

CHAPTER FORTY-FIVE

CYSTIC FIBROSIS

HARRY SHWACHMAN, M.D.

Cystic fibrosis is a new clinical entity first reported in 1936. In 1938 it was considered a rare pancreatic disorder uniformly fatal and affecting only small infants. Although this disease is not limited to the pancreas, many of the designations refer to the pancreas such as fibrocystic disease of the pancreas, pancreatic fibrosis, pancreatic infantilism or cystic fibrosis of the pancreas. Farber first pointed out the generalized nature of the disease with involvement of many of the mucus-secreting glands and later (1945) suggested the name "mucoviscidosis." Bodian (1953) subsequently used the designation "mucosis." Eccrinosis has been suggested by Kagan (1955) to indicate a widespread involvement of the exocrine glands. A very early name that did not attain widespread usage for obvious reasons is dysporia enterobronchopancreatica congenita familiaris. There is no satisfactory name for this disease.

Numerous advances have been made in the past 25 years which indicate that:

① this is not a disease limited to the pancreas; for that matter, it may occur without evidence of pancreatic insufficiency;

② this is no longer a rare disease—it is 10 to 20 times as frequent as phenylketonuria, with an incidence of approximately one per 1600.

③ survival into adulthood and even parenthood can be achieved; however, 97 per cent of males are sterile as a result of an anatomic defect in wolffian-derived structures, namely, the epididymis, the seminal vesicles and the vas deferens;

④ the diagnosis can be made with ease, even in the neonatal period;

⑤ it is a hereditary disease transmitted as a mendelian recessive;

⑥ it is a serious disease with protean manifestations and complications affecting the respiratory system in nearly all cases; and

⑦ the cause of death is most often related to the pulmonary involvement.

It is appropriate, therefore, to consider this disease in a text dealing with pulmonary disease in childhood.

Incidence

Accurate incidence figures are not available because reliable diagnostic methods have been in use only a short time. Estimates range from one in 500 to one in 3500 live births. Our own estimate is between one in 1000 and one in 1600 live births. Many patients with mild symptoms escape diagnosis in early childhood because the physician may not be familiar with such a benign course. In a recent study of 70 patients over 25 years of age, 16 per cent were first diagnosed after the age of 15 years. On the the other hand, in 85 newly diagnosed cases in our clinic in a one-year period, nearly 50 per cent of the patients were diagnosed under one year of age. There is a high incidence of disease in the Caucasian race and a low one in the Negro. It occurs infrequently in the Oriental, the Puerto Rican and the American Indian. The clinical and pathologic findings appear the same in cases reported from various racial groups as well as from different parts of the world. The disease occurs equally in both sexes and in all levels of social and economic groups.

The family background of patients seen in the New England area suggests a wide ethnic source with a predominant Canadian and European origin. The affected families have the following ancestry: French-Canadian, English, Irish, Scottish, Russian, German, Polish, Spanish, Portuguese and Dutch — not unlike the rest of the population in this area. Cystic fibrosis occurs in approximately 3 per cent of the post-mortem examinations performed in children's hospitals. The incidence in the Ashkenazi Jews in Israel is the same as in other countries and approximates the incidence in the Caucasian.

Etiology

Cystic fibrosis is a disease of obscure origin. Etiologic considerations include the following:

(1) Cystic fibrosis is inherited as a mendelian recessive trait.

(2) The disease cannot be reproduced in animals.

(3) Theories based on blood incom-patibilities, maternal health in pregnancy, failure of secretin formation, vitamin A deficiency and viral infection are most unlikely.

(4) Dysautonomia, altered cell membrane permeability or cell metabolism with inadequate function of lysosomal enzymes involving mucoprotein, "sodium pump" defect, or altered salt crystal structural formation may be responsible for the primary defect resulting in increased viscosity of many body secretions and increased salt content or eccrine and salivary glandular secretions.

Pathogenesis

Cystic fibrosis is a generalized disease involving eccrine and mucous secretory glands. The increase in viscosity of mucus suggested the name "mucoviscidosis." In view of the almost constant functional abnormality of the sweat glands, this name no longer applies.

The pathogenetic mechanisms may be depicted as shown at the bottom of this page.

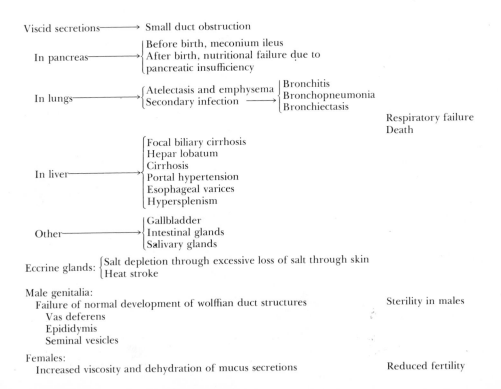

Genetics

Cystic fibrosis is transmitted as a mendelian recessive disorder. The affected patient is the homozygote, and his healthy parents are the heterozygotes. His brothers and sisters may appear healthy or may also have the disease either in the same severe form or in a milder degree. Figure 1 illustrates a theoretical family of four children, one of whom has cystic fibrosis. Of the three healthy children, one does not carry the gene, and the other two are carriers of the gene or heterozygotes. By definition, all healthy siblings have normal sweat electrolyte levels. In any one family it is impossible to predict the incidence or the outcome of future pregnancies. The same one-to-four chance of cystic fibrosis exists regardless of the number of previously affected children. We have seen one family with five of six children affected and another family of 11 children with only one affected child. The parents of our patients do not present abnormal clinical or laboratory findings that

would segregate them from the rest of a healthy adult population (see Fig. 2).

Figure 1 also illustrates the results of the union of a heterozygote and a noncarrier as well as the union of a female homozygote with a noncarrier. We have estimated that approximately 1 per cent of our female population of cystic fibrosis patients attains parenthood. This figure may increase as a result of improved therapy and better recognition of the disease. As indicated previously, homozygote males do not reproduce (with rare exception).

Definite progress has been made in identifying the heterozygote. Investigations in which the test individual is subjected to a stress condition prior to collecting sweat have not been successful in detecting the heterozygote. The analysis of certain tissues such as fingernail and toenail clippings for sodium and potassium content may segregate the carrier state in childhood, but not in the adult. Preliminary data indicate that approximately one-third of the healthy siblings of children with cystic fibrosis have a distinct elevation of the sodium and potassium content in their nails. Tests for the detection of the heterozygote in identifying a specific serum factor are at present complicated and have limited practical application. We have employed such a test based on sodium transport in the presence of glucose across the rat intestinal membrane using the Ussing chamber and measuring short circuit current at five-minute intervals. Serum from homozygotes and heterozygotes inhibits sodium transport under the experimental conditions, whereas serum from healthy controls does not. Since serum from other disease states also inhibits sodium transport, this test is not specific for cystic fibrosis and is similar to other nonspecific methods for heterozygote detection. Tissue culture techniques for this purpose are still in the experimental stage. The incidence of the heterozygote in the adult population is calculated after the frequency of the disease has been established or estimated. If the incidence of the dis-

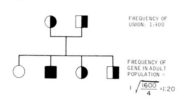

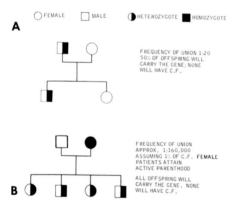

Figure 1. Recessive inheritance in cystic fibrosis, based on an estimated incidence of one in 1600 live births.

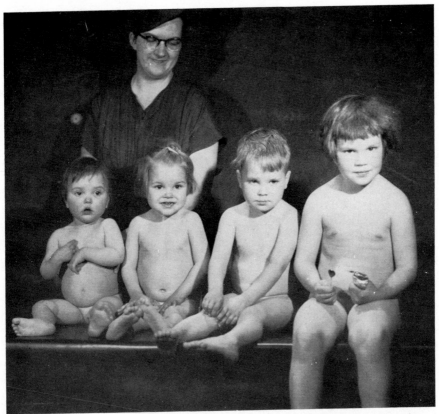

Figure 2. M. family. The proband case is the second girl on the left. She had typical pulmonary and gastrointestinal symptoms of cystic fibrosis. As soon as the diagnosis was made in November 1953, her three siblings were studied. The eldest girl was found to be healthy, and her duodenal fluid showed normal enzymes. The other two siblings were found to have the disease, but with milder clinical manifestations. Duodenal intubation on each showed increased viscosity with absent trypsin, lipase and amylase. The sweat test had not yet been discovered, but when available the following year (1954), it confirmed the clinical diagnosis. The mother was pregnant when the photograph was taken, and shortly after delivery her baby was found to be healthy.

The photograph is included to point out (1) the testing of all children in a family as soon as one child is discovered to have cystic fibrosis, and (2) the familial incidence with healthy first and fifth children and three affected. There were three subsequently healthy children. Two of the three children with cystic fibrosis have succumbed, the boy at age 14 years (August 1964) and the proband patient at age 12 years (November 1963).

ease is one in 1600, then the frequency of the gene in the adult population is one in 20. Prenatal diagnosis by examination of amniotic fluid has not yet been accomplished.

Pathology

The name of the disease is derived from the initial description of the changes noted in the pancreas. Farber (1944) pointed out that the morphologic changes in this disease are not limited to the pancreas, but occur in many mucus-secreting cells in the body.

The demonstration of altered function of eccrine sweat glands is not reflected in a morphologic or histochemical change in these glands. The changes noted in the pancreas are not fixed; i.e., the lesion may evolve gradually, and the appearance may vary according to the age of the patient or the severity of the disease. The end stage of the pancreatic lesion that may occur in the older patient is fat replacement and fibrosis with a few clusters of islet cells.

When this occurs, the diagnosis of cystic fibrosis cannot be made on a morphologic basis. This progressive change probably explains the increasing incidence of diabetes mellitus in the older patients.

The most characteristic lesion of the pancreas is seen in the first few years and consists in a dilatation of the ducts, a flattening of the epithelium, enlargement of the acini to form cysts, the presence of eosinophilic concretions and a diffuse fibrosis with varying degrees of leukocytic infiltration (Fig. 3). Grossly, the pancreas is firm, irregular and shrunken. The lesion need not be uniform in all areas. In such cases, functional tests of the pancreas reveal varying degrees of enzyme insufficiencies. In some cases the pancreatic lesion is minimal. The progressive morphologic and chemical changes in the pancreas have been described by Kopito and coworkers (1976).

INTESTINE. The earliest lesion and the one responsible for approximately 15 per cent of all cases of cystic fibrosis occurs in the intestine in the form of meconium ileus. The obstruction is generally in the region of the terminal ileum and is due to the abnormal nature of the meconium. The degree of obstruction may vary, and in a pediatric hospital practice one is more likely to see the severe cases requiring surgical correction. In a small number of patients, however, the meconium obstruction is relieved spontaneously or by means of pancreatin enemas. The meconium is tarry and very sticky, contains a large amount of serum proteins and can readily be liquefied by proteolytic enzymes. In patients with meconium ileus, the absence of pancreatic enzymes helps explain the persistence of the large amount of protein found in the meconium. The intestinal wall in the region proximal to the obstruction may be thin, and the lumen large. The intestinal glands at the site of obstruction are flattened and show evidence of hyperactivity. Complications are frequent and include perforation with meconium peritonitis, volvulus and secondary atresia (see Table 1). On occasion the surgeon may be unable to provide an accurate etiologic diagnosis of intestinal obstruction in the newborn. It is recommended that all newborns with intestinal obstruction be

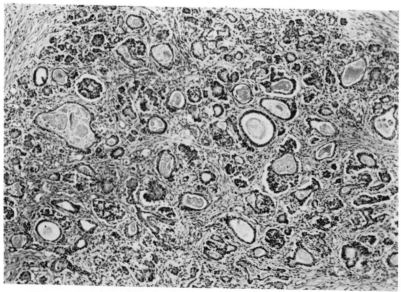

Figure 3. Microscopic appearance of the pancreas. (×140). This shows the typical changes with inspissation of secretions, dilatation of ducts and acini, as well as increased fibrosis.

TABLE 1. COMPLICATIONS OF MECONIUM ILEUS IN 127 INFANTS REQUIRING SURGERY (1940 to 1965)

	Total	Surgical Survivals (Beyond 2 Months)	Dead Before Reaching 2 Months
Meconium ileus only	68	31	37
Meconium ileus + peritonitis	14	1	13
Meconium ileus + peritonitis + atresia	9	3	6
Meconium ileus + atresia	9	6	3
Meconium ileus + peritonitis + volvulus	12	5	7
Meconium ileus + volvulus	4	–	4
Meconium ileus + peritonitis + volvulus + atresia	3	2	1
Meconium ileus + peritonitis + perforated colon	8	4	4
Birth weight below 5 pounds	10	1	9
Birth trauma	3	–	3
Septicemia	7	1	6
Rh incompatibility	1	1	–
Meningitis	1	–	1
Kernicterus due to prematurity	1	–	1
Convulsion	1	–	1
Subarachnoid hemorrhage	4	1	3
Bleeding? Hypoprothrombinemia	4		4
Hyaline membrane disease	1	–	1
Epidermolysis bullosa	1	–	1
Acute duodenal ulcer	1	–	1
Congenital abnormalities	9	–	9
Hirschsprung's aganglionic colon and congenital short bowel			
Herniation of bowel through mesenteric defect – 2 patients			
Meckel's diverticulum in 3 patients			
Atypical lobulation of left lung			
Absent left testis			
Polycystic kidneys			
Mesenteric pseudocyst			

subjected to a sweat test. An attempt to clarify the diagnosis is justified by recent experiences and forms the basis of providing proper therapeutic, prophylactic, prognostic and genetic information to the parents. Ileal atresia may be a complication of meconium ileus.

Morphologic changes in mucus-secreting glands may be found in various regions of the intestinal tract. Duodenal mucosal biopsy specimens may on occasion reveal a lesion of diagnostic value, but a biopsy of the rectal mucosa may also suggest the disease. The morphologic criteria include the appearance of the surface epithelium, lamina propria and glandular structures. In a typical example, the surface epithelium is denuded and disorgan-

ized with tortuous disordered glands and a decrease in the number of crypts; these show dilatation with gaping of the crypt mouths. Special stains may reveal an increase in the acid mucopolysaccharides. The appendix may provide a clue, since it may be firm with a thick wall, revealing active mucus secretion with inspissation and even extrusion of casts. In older patients, intestinal obstruction may result from the inspissation of secretions with the formation of firm intraluminal masses. Intussusception is another complication that is occasionally seen in the older child.

LIVER. The basic changes in the liver include cell atrophy, fatty metamorphosis, periportal fibrosis, and proliferation of the bile ducts, often distended by obstruction. The initial lesion in the liver is analogous to the changes noted in the pancreas. Focal obstructive lesions resulting from the bile-containing mucous plugs have suggested the name "focal biliary cirrhosis." This lesion is present in less than one-fifth of the cases examined at autopsy. Adjacent to the areas of proliferation of bile ducts with dilated obstructed lumens, the portal areas are broad and fibrosed. When these areas grossly distort the lobule and join one another, the appearance is that of a multilobular cirrhosis or "hepar lobatum." Such advanced changes occur in less than 5 per cent of the cases and may result in the production of clinical symptoms of portal vein obstruction. Hypersplenism and hemorrhage from esophageal varices may occur as a result of the increased portal pressure, and shunting procedures with splenectomy may be necessary. Jaundice is rarely noted in spite of extensive liver involvement. Some of the commonly used liver function tests may give normal results. However, the prothrombin time may be prolonged and the alkaline phosphatase may be elevated. The total serum protein may remain the same, with a gradual increase of globulins at the expense of albumin. The transaminases may also be abnormal.

The fatty changes noted in the liver are common and do not appear to be related to the nutritional status of the patient and are not specific.

The gallbladder is often shrunken and contains a small amount of viscid bile.

RESPIRATORY TRACT. Most deaths are due to chronic pulmonary infection and pulmonary insufficiency. At autopsy, the trachea and bronchi are generally filled with a mucopurulent material. The thorax is rounded, and the lungs are emphysematous. Pleural adhesions, congestion, emphysematous blebs, subpleural hemorrhage and areas of pneumonic consolidation and abscesses may be seen. When dissected, the bronchi may be found dilated and

filled with purulent exudate. Lung section reveals areas of bronchopneumonia, emphysema and atelectasis, with widespread dilatation of bronchi, which ooze purulent exudate upon pressure (Fig. 4). The bronchiectasis is usually tubular and generally involves all lobes. The hilar lymph nodes are enlarged. The bacteria grown from the exudate are generally *Staphylococcus aureus* or *Pseudomonas aeruginosa*, or both.

The initial lesion in the lung is obstruction of the smaller bronchi and bronchioles, which leads to irregular aeration with collapse of some alveoli and overdistention of others. Infection supervenes, and a chronic inflammatory process occurs in which the *S. aureus* predominates initially. The bronchial and tracheal glands appear active and secrete a viscid material (Fig. 5). The sticky sputum or mucopurulent secretion is the combined product of the mucus-secreting glands and the infectious process. The infection contributes cellular debris, bacteria and their products, and necrotic leukocytes. The bronchial walls become thick, and adjacent alveoli are involved in a chronic pneumonia. Focal areas of atelectasis occur when the bronchiolar obstruction is complete. This process is noted more

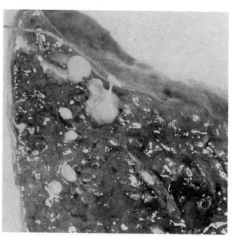

Figure 4. Section of a resected lung from a child with cystic fibrosis to show the thick, sticky, mucopurulent exudate that oozes from many of the bronchi. A culture revealed mucoid Pseudomonas.

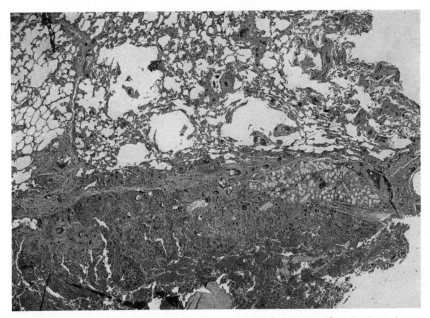

Figure 5. Microscopic appearance of lung showing bronchus and tracheal glands.

frequently in the smaller infant. Larger segments of the bronchial tree may also obstruct and cause segmental and even lobar collapse. The atelectatic segment may become a seat of abscess cavities. Surgical removal of such areas is feasible, provided the remaining lung tissue is in relatively good condition. The persistence of the chronic bronchial infection results in a cylindrical bronchiectasis. The chest becomes rounded. Digital clubbing occurs. Some of the pulmonary complications include hemoptysis, pneumothorax and cor pulmonale. The chronic infection may result in a granulomatous lesion resembling an actinomycosis and is more properly described as botryomycosis. The degree of pulmonary involvement can be estimated clinically as well as by chest films, lung scans and pulmonary function tests.

The upper respiratory tract is usually affected. Chronic sinus infection is present in almost all patients with this disease. The mucus-secreting cells may be hyperactive, and the membrane edematous and hypertrophied. The turbinates are often swollen. Nasal polyps may occur as early as two years

of age, and there is an incidence of nearly 10 per cent in patients over ten years of age; they may occur at almost any age. Nasal polyps are generally multiple, occur bilaterally and often recur after polypectomy.

OTHER CHANGES. The eccrine sweat glands are histologically normal and produce an abnormal secretion with a high sodium, potassium and chloride concentration. Other serous glands, especially the salivary and parotid glands, likewise may appear normal, yet produce a secretion that may be slightly abnormal. The concentration of electrolytes is normal in the secretions of the lacrimal glands.

Lesions secondary to pancreatic insufficiency and malabsorption may occur. Failure to absorb fat and fat-soluble vitamins has led to vitamin A, vitamin E and vitamin K deficiency, hypolipemia and hypocholesterolemia.

Diagnosis

A high degree of clinical suspicion is essential in making a diagnosis of cystic fibrosis. Some years ago, physicians commonly remarked that the appearance of the patient was so good that the diagnosis of cystic fibrosis could be discarded. This statement implies that patients with this disease are necessarily severely malnourished and stunted. Perhaps it is for this reason that many cases today are not diagnosed, and only when advanced changes take place does the diagnosis suggest itself.

The disease should be suspected in any child having chronic or recurrent symptoms involving the upper or lower respiratory tract. Some of these symptoms are found in over 90 per cent of the patients at one time or another and may include chronic cough, asthma-like symptoms in infancy, recurrent pneumonitis, bronchitis or pneumonia, atelectasis (focal or lobar), nasal polyposis (see Fig. 6) and chronic sinusitis, empyema and bronchiectasis.

The diagnosis should be suspected in any child with symptoms suggesting pancreatic insufficiency or malabsorption. These symptoms are present in approximately 80 per cent of the patients and include slow growth or failure to thrive, a good to huge appetite, frequent large, foul movements, a protuberant abdomen, rectal prolapse (usually recurrent), intestinal obstruction in the newborn, fecal impaction in older children, infants with vitamin K deficiency, infants with hypoproteinemic edema (see Fig. 12), infants suspected of having milk allergy (see Fig. 12), and infants suspected of having celiac disease.

The diagnosis should also be suspected in children with cirrhosis of the liver presenting with portal hypertension with or without hypersplenism. A small number of patients may have this complication, and in some cases these symptoms may be the ones for which initial medical attention is sought.

The diagnosis should also be suspected in patients with "heat stroke." The climate as well as diet may influence the occurrence of this complication. In some patients, "heat stroke" has been the initial complaint. Conditions causing excess sweating with loss of salt and water result in circulatory collapse.

Whenever the diagnosis is firmly established in any one patient, it is essential to examine and test all siblings. Inquiry should be made about the health of first cousins, noting that the incidence in such persons is approximately ten times as great as in a randomly selected or control group.

The symptoms may vary widely in se-

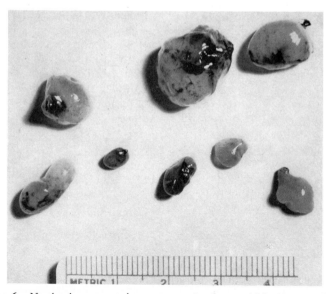

Figure 6.   Nasal polyps removed at one operation from a child with cystic fibrosis.

TABLE 2. AGE AT DIAGNOSIS OF 85 NEW PATIENTS SEEN IN 1963

Age at Diagnosis	No. of Patients	(%)	Accumulated % of Patients
Meconium ileus	8	(9)	
1 week — 11 months	34	(41)	50
1 year — 3 years	20	(24)	74
4 years — 7 years	15	(18)	91
8 years — 9 years	2	(2)	
10 years — 12 years	1	(1)	
13 years — 16 years	2	(2)	
17 years — 20 years	2	(2)	
Over 21 years	1	(1)	100
Total	85	100	

verity as well as in the age at onset. Some infants have severe manifestations from the first weeks of life and show a rapid downhill course. Others with an early onset of symptoms may respond to therapy and survive to adulthood. Still others have their first symptoms at two years of age or even later. In some cases there is pulmonary disease without any digestive or pancreatic involvement. On the other hand, the gastrointestinal manifestations may predominate for months or years before signs of chronic pulmonary disease appear. By far the largest number of infants and children with this disease have symptoms of pulmonary involvement and pancreatic insufficiency. In recent years, most of the newly diagnosed older patients appear to have predominantly the respiratory features with no evidence of pancreatic insufficiency. We have also seen a number of patients whose first symptoms appeared in late adolescence or early adulthood.

It may be of interest to show the age at diagnosis of all new patients seen in our clinic in 1963 (Table 2). The total number was 85. Eight had intestinal obstruction at birth, and at the other end of the scale, five were first correctly diagnosed after the age of 13. It should be noted that approximately 50 per cent of all patients were diagnosed under the age of one year (see also Table 3).

MECONIUM ILEUS. The earliest manifestation of cystic fibrosis is intestinal obstruction of the newborn (meconium ileus). This manifestation of cystic fibrosis (noted in approximately 15 per cent of all patients with cystic fibrosis) actually begins in utero and may be associated with a number of complications such as volvulus, perforation of the bowel with meconium peritonitis and secondary atresia. There appears to be a higher incidence of prematurity than in children with cystic fibrosis born without this complication. The mortality rate in this group is high, partly owing to the presence of associated conditions at birth and to the high risk of development of pulmonary symptoms with secondary bronchopneumonia. Many infants with mecon-

TABLE 3. DIFFERENTIAL DIAGNOSIS

1) Chronic bronchitis
2) Recurrent respiratory infection
3) Bronchopneumonia
4) Staphylococcal pneumonia
5) Pertussis
6) Bronchiectasis
7) Asthma
8) Pulmonary tuberculosis
9) Familial dysautonomia
10) Agammaglobulinemia
11) Celiac disease
12) Milk allergy in early infancy
13) Protein-losing enteropathy
14) Intestinal atresia in newborn
15) Pancreatic insufficiency and bone marrow hypoplasia
16) Cirrhosis — portal hypertension may be present
17) Heat stroke — encephalitis

ium obstruction require surgical correction. A variety of surgical approaches are currently in vogue, and the one favored by Gross (1953) is the Mikulicz ileostomy. It appears that the Bishop-Koop procedure is more popular among pediatric surgeons. The overall mortality rate in surgically treated cases is in the vicinity of 20 to 30 per cent by two months of age. The survivors of meconium ileus may exhibit the other symptoms of cystic fibrosis, and their subsequent course depends in general on the same factors that determine survival in any other child with the disease. Our oldest patients with this disease are now young adults gainfully employed. We have noted a high incidence of meconium ileus in certain families, and this may suggest the operation of environmental factors in determining the genetic mode of expression of the disease.

In a number of infants, the meconium may be delayed in passing or may be passed with difficulty. The neonatologist suspects cystic fibrosis in such patients. This form of mild obstruction generally is not reported, and the number of cases falling in this category is unknown. Recent attempts at nonsurgical efforts to overcome the obstruction have met with success. The use of N-acetylcysteine and, more recently, Gastrografin by enema has proved successful. These agents should be administered in a proper setting by the surgeon with the assistance of the radiologist. The N-acetylcysteine appears to separate the sticky meconium from the wall of the intestine. Gastrografin is effective because of its high osmotic activity; it draws fluid into the gut and liquefies the meconium, which can be expelled. This latter procedure should be tried in all uncomplicated cases of meconium ileus. An intravenous line is essential when the latter method is employed.

The meconium in these infants is usually viscid and contains serum protein. Normal meconium, by contrast, has very little protein. The abnormal meconium can be readily digested by a variety of proteolytic enzymes. The lack of pancreatic function explains the persistence of protein in the meconium. There are many other abnormalities in the meconium, such as the presence of high concentration of disaccharidase, the presence of other serum proteins besides albumin, and the presence of high concentration of lysosomal enzymes. A popular but not yet totally proved method for screening newborns for cystic fibrosis involves a test for the presence of albumin. In meconium from healthy babies, the concentration of albumin is negligible. The signs of intestinal obstruction in the newborn do not distinguish this form from many others, although the roentgenographic appearance may be suggestive of meconium ileus. The appearance of air bubbles entrapped in the meconium provides a clue. One can also perform a pilocarpine iontophoresis sweat test, and if this reveals the characteristic elevation of sodium and chloride, the diagnosis of cystic fibrosis can be made.

——PULMONARY MANIFESTATIONS. The earliest pulmonary symptom is usually cough. At first this may attract little attention, but it soon becomes chronic and even paroxysmal, at times suggesting pertussis. Feeding or sudden changes of environmental temperature may induce coughing, and in the older child an emotional response may initiate a paroxysm of coughing. Vomiting associated with coughing is not uncommon in young patients. An observant mother may detect the presence of thick mucus that the baby is unable to expel. In severely affected babies, "strings of mucus" can be pulled from the oropharynx. The mother may also note that the respiratory rate is rapid and that the baby breathes noisily. These symptoms may begin as early as two or three weeks of age, but are more common a few months later. The development of frank pneumonia generally ascribed to S. aureus is not uncommon. By two years of age, over 75 per cent of children with cystic fibrosis have already had some of the foregoing symptoms.

The auscultatory findings may be normal in the early stages, and even with advanced changes may not be striking. Roentgenograms of the chest may reveal the characteristic early changes, namely, evidences of irregular aeration with scattered areas of atelectasis. The lungs are hyperinflated, and the diaphragm may be depressed. The heart size may be small or unaffected. On occasion one may note segmental or lobar atelectasis, a finding more commonly observed on the right side than on the left. On occasion large atelectatic areas may re-expand, but they are more likely to persist and present challenging therapeutic problems. Eventually the peribronchial markings become pronounced, and the diagnosis may be readily suspected from the roentgenographic appearance of the chest (see Fig. 7). In addition to the cough and elevated respiratory rate, the pulmonary findings in the infant may include intercostal and suprasternal retraction as well as a rounding of the chest; wheezing respiration may occur as a result of bronchospasm and does not necessarily indicate an asthmatic state. Actual measurements of the lateral and anteroposterior dimensions with calipers will establish this abnormal relationship. Digital clubbing is noted frequently, and in our experience is not a very good index of the degree of pulmonary involvement and may occur as early as six months of age. I always examine the hand carefully for digital clubbing, since its presence may be a good clue for the diagnosis of cystic fibrosis. Fever is usually absent; when present, it signifies frank pulmonary infection. Persistent rales confirm the clinical impression of bronchiectasis. Right-sided cardiac failure may be a terminal event, although extensive bronchiectasis with respiratory failure is more often the cause of death.

Only a small number of patients escape pulmonary involvement in infancy. It is estimated that less than 10 per cent of the recognized patients are free of pulmonary signs or symptoms and have clear lung fields on the roentgenogram by two years of age. (See Tables 4 and 5.)

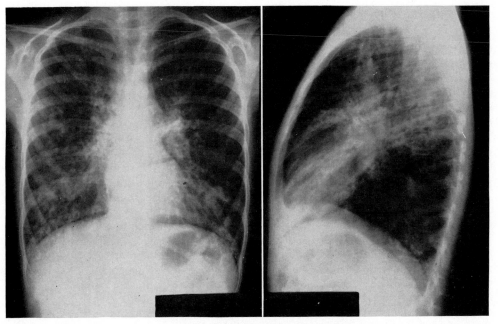

Figure 7. Chest roentgenogram of a child with severe pulmonary involvement.

TABLE 4.   CLINICAL FEATURES OF PULMONARY INVOLVEMENT

1. Manifestation of widespread bronchial obstruction and infection
2. Often confused with "asthma" in small infants
3. Onset in infancy in majority of patients
4. May present in infancy as lobar or lobular atelectasis or in later childhood as bronchiectasis

Symptoms

Cough, initially infrequent, later persistent and often paroxysmal. May initiate vomiting and interfere with sleep

Wheezing is common. The bronchospasm may be secondary to infection, or the patient may also be an atopic individual

Respiratory rates of over 70 per minute may be noted in small babies

Easy fatigue and reduced exercise tolerance

As pulmonary disease progresses
Cough becomes productive
Fever may be present
Poor to fair appetite in a child formerly a good eater
Weight loss
Cyanosis

Findings

Irregular aeration with increased markings noted by x-ray film

Atelectasis, lobular or lobar. Lobar atelectasis is more common in small infants and occurs more commonly on the right side. It is often transient and responds to vigorous therapy. If persistent, prognosis is worsened

Rounding of chest, increased AP dimension

Intercostal and suprasternal retraction

Stooped shoulders

Digital clubbing

Auscultatory changes

Right-sided failure

Abnormal pulmonary function tests

Clinical Evaluation

A system of clinical evaluation has been devised to aid in determining the severity of the disease and the patient's response to therapy (Table 6). The evaluation is derived from an appraisal of each of four categories: ① general activity, ② physical findings, ③ nutritional status, and ④ findings on chest roentgenograms. Each category is given the equal weight of 25 points, 100 points representing a perfect score. The status of the patient is considered excellent when the score is over 85, good when the score is between 71 and 85, mild between 56 and 70, moderate between 41 and 55, and severe when 40 or below. The scoring is made without consideration of the therapeutic regimen in use at the time. This system of scoring, which does not involve complicated laboratory procedures, has been used in assessing the effect of therapeutic programs.

Diagnostic Tests

The most reliable diagnostic test for cystic fibrosis is the quantitative analysis of sweat for both sodium and chloride. In no disease that can be confused with cystic fibrosis is there so great an elevation of electrolyte levels. A positive sweat test result in the absence of symptoms does not establish the diagnosis, however. The only exception to this rule may be made in the study of newborn siblings of patients with cystic fibrosis during the first weeks of life. The sweat test result may be positive long before clinical symptoms appear.

The sweat test is carried out in three stages: ① stimulation of sweat glands, ② collection of the sweat sample, and

TABLE 5. PULMONARY FUNCTION STUDIES

These tests confirm in general the impressions gathered from the clinical and roentgenographic examinations. In patients with minimal pulmonary involvement, the tidal volume, respiratory rate, lung volumes, lung compliance and resistance are normal. In the severely ill child the changes are striking, as shown in the following data taken from studies of Cook and coworkers (1959). Patient 1 is compared with patient 2. Patient 1 is a 14-year-old girl with minimal pulmonary involvement, and her pulmonary function test results are normal. This patient is well nine years after these studies were carried out. Patient 2 is a severely ill child of 13 years with extensive pulmonary involvement. She had pronounced changes by roentgenogram and grossly abnormal tests. She died approximately five months after the tests were done.

Respiratory Data in Patients 1 and 2

	PATIENT 1	PATIENT 2
Clinical rating	Excellent	Severe
Chest film rating	Excellent	Severe
Respiratory rate/minute	21	30
Tidal volume (ml.)	414	186
Minute ventilation (1)	8.7	5.6
Residual volume*	+ 1	+153
Functional residual capacity	+ 1	+ 59
Vital capacity*	− 9	− 43
Total lung capacity*	− 7	+ 10
Compliance*	− 10	− 76
Resistance*	+ 25	+112
RV/TLC %	25	61
FRC/TLC %	56	72

*Volumes expressed in terms of per cent above or below the predicted value for a normal child of the same height.

The expiratory peak flow can be readily determined with a Wright Peak Flow Meter in the office and is a good indication of pulmonary obstruction. Results are expressed in liters per minute and in per cent of the predicted normal. Serial measurements provide an additional method of assessing progress of the patient.

(3) analysis of the sweat. A variety of procedures have been used for each of these steps. To minimize errors, it is strongly urged that one person, usually a trained technician, be responsible for the entire procedure. Each laboratory must use a standard procedure that yields reliable and reproducible results and must establish a range of normal in healthy and sick controls. We prefer the painless pilocarpine iontophoresis method of stimulating local sweat production (Fig. 8), which takes five minutes, collection of the sweat produced over a 30-minute period into a weighed gauze pad, and determination of the chloride concentration by a titration procedure and the sodium and potassium with the flame photometer. A sample of less than 50 mg. is too small for accurate assay by our methods. In such instances we stimulate two separate areas of the skin with pilocarpine and combine the samples. This test can be performed on babies one day of age, in patients acutely ill and even in patients sleeping in mist tents. The entire procedure can be done in less than an hour. The chloride value is known immediately, and the physician knows the test results before the patient leaves the laboratory.

Two other methods are in wide use— the conductivity measurement and the direct chloride ion electrode applied to the skin. These methods are reliable in the hands of experts, but have yielded disappointing results in the hands of the average laboratory technician. Many factors influence the level of electrolytes in sweat, and a number are listed below (see Table 7).

TABLE 6. CLINICAL EVALUATION—
SYSTEM OF RATING SEVERITY OF DISEASE

Grading	Points	General Activity	Physical Examination	Nutrition	Roentgenogram Findings
Excellent (86–100)	25	Full normal activity; plays ball, goes to school regularly, and so on	Normal; no cough; pulse and respirations normal; clear lungs; good posture	Maintains weight and height above 25th percentile; well formed stools, almost normal; fair muscle tone and mass	Clear lung fields
Good (71–85)	20	Lacks endurance and tires at end of day; good school attendance	Resting pulse and respirations normal; rare coughing or clearing of throat; no clubbing; clear lungs; minimal emphysema	Weight and height at approximately 15th to 20th percentile; stools slightly abnormal; fair muscle tone and mass	Minimal accentuation of bronchovascular markings; early emphysema
Mild (56–70)	15	May rest voluntarily during the day; tires easily after exertion; fair school attendance	Occasional cough, perhaps in morning upon rising; respirations slightly elevated; mild emphysema; coarse breath sounds; rarely localized rales; early clubbing	Weight and height above 3rd percentile; stools usually abnormal, large and poorly formed; very little, if any, abdominal distention; poor muscle tone with reduced muscle mass	Mild emphysema with patchy atelectasis; increased bronchovascular markings
Moderate (41–55)	10	Home teacher; dyspneic after short walk; rests a great deal	Frequent cough usually productive; chest retraction; moderate emphysema; may have chest deformity; rales usually present; clubbing 2 to 3+	Weight and height below 3rd percentile; poorly formed, bulky, fatty, offensive stools; flabby muscles and reduced mass; abdominal distention, mild to moderate	Moderate emphysema; widespread areas of atelectasis with superimposed areas of infection; minimal bronchial ectasia
Severe (40 or below)	5	Orthopneic, confined to bed or chair	Severe coughing spells; tachypnea with tachycardia and extensive pulmonary changes; may show signs of right-sided cardiac failure; clubbing 3 to 4+	Malnutrition marked; large protuberant abdomen; rectal prolapse; large, foul, frequent, fatty movements	Extensive changes with pulmonary obstructive phenomena and infection; lobar atelectasis and bronchiectasis

Elevated values may be obtained in patients with adrenal insufficiency, ectodermal dysplasia or diabetes insipidus, in some patients with glycogen storage disease as well as in some rarely occurring metabolic diseases. An important factor is age. In the first two to three days of life, the values are higher than after the first week of life. By about 16 or 17 years the values for sodium and chloride gradually increase to adult levels, which may be nearly twice the value in childhood. There is no other disease that can be compared with cystic fibrosis that gives a persistent positive sweat test. The practicing physician should be aware of the inadequacy of the performance of sweat tests and question the technique. In our experience, approximately 50 per cent of

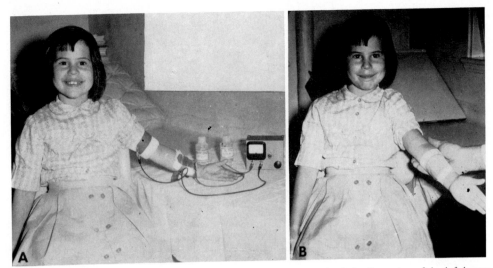

Figure 8. Pilocarpine iontophoresis. *A,* Stimulation of local sweat glands in the region of the left lower part of the forearm. *B,* Collection of sweat sample.

sweat tests performed outside our center have yielded the wrong answer.

Figure 9 shows the results of 4231 sweat tests carried out in our laboratory. The end of the bar indicates the mean value, and the numbers in the bar indicate the range of values. Note that in 745 patients with cystic fibrosis tested, the lowest values recorded are 77 mEq. per liter for chloride and 72 mEq. per liter for sodium. We have omitted from the chart seven patients we believe have cystic fibrosis, since they have incomplete expression of the disease and borderline sweat electrolysis on repeated testing. Except for this

TABLE 7. SWEAT TEST: FACTORS INFLUENCING LEVEL OF ELECTROLYTES

The Patient
  Nature of the disease
  Genetic stock
  Age
  Sex: no difference noted in childhood; adult females sweat less than males with heat stimulus
  Individual variation: minimal on repeated testing; may be of considerable magnitude in rare individuals
  Condition of patient: dehydration, circulatory failure, respiratory distress, hypothyroidism, malnutrition, edema, adrenal insufficiency, and so on
  Diet, especially salt intake
  Time of day and season of year
  Exhaustion of glands
  Acclimatization
  Activity of patient
  Unknown or unrecognized factors
Sweat Induction and Collection
  Heat vs. drug or combination
  Environmental and body temperature; humidity and effect of evaporation

  Rate of sweating
  Duration of sweat period
  Area of body
  Total body sweat vs. local collection
Drug Used and Application
  Pilocarpine, Furmethide, Mecholyl
  Method of application of drug: intradermal injection or by iontophoresis
Analytical Factors
  Size of sample
  Weight determined on analytical balance by weighing sweat absorbed on gauze pads, cotton or filter paper
  Volume measured directly with volumetric pipet
  Method of determining chloride: semiquantitative, electrometric, titrimetric, polarographic
  Flame-photometric analysis for sodium and potassium
  Dilution factor
  Contamination
  Technical: personal factor

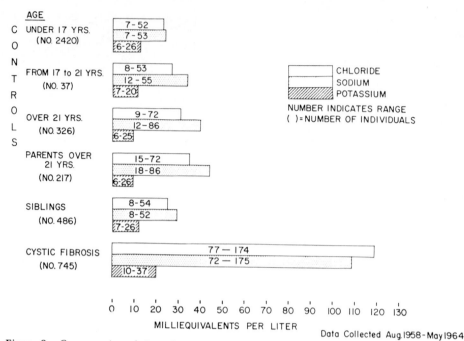

Figure 9. Concentration of electrolytes in the sweat after pilocarpine stimulation in 4231 patients. The end of the bar in each case represents the mean value. There is little overlapping between the patients with cystic fibrosis and all the others tested except in a small number of subjects over 21 years of age.

special and small group of patients, repeat testing of healthy patients as well as of those patients with cystic fibrosis shows a remarkable constancy of the sweat electrolyte findings. The chart also shows the increase with age as noted in the control group; the findings in siblings correspond to the findings in the healthy controls under 17 years of age, and the results of the sweat test in parents correspond to the results in the older control group. The mean sodium value exceeds the chloride in all groups except in the patients with cystic fibrosis, in whom the mean chloride value exceeds the mean sodium. The potassium concentration decreases with increasing age and has no diagnostic value, although the mean value in patients with cystic fibrosis is nearly twice as high as in the control group.

We have not been able to confirm the observation of others that the sweat electrolyte levels are elevated in the heterozygote. In our hands the administration of 9α-fluorohydrocortisone did not alter the sweat electrolytes so that one could distinguish the patient with cystic fibrosis from the heterozygote or others with high or borderline values. The sweat test is rarely difficult to interpret even though a few adults in good health have values that exceed the upper limits of normal in children. (See Fig. 10.) We feel strongly that the pilocarpine iontophoresis sweat test is a reliable diagnostic test in the adult.

The reliability of the sweat test in childhood and adolescence is close to 99 per cent; this is indeed a remarkable laboratory finding, since this test reflects on the function of one type of gland that is not known to contribute to the main features of the disease. The level of the salt concentration is not a measure of the severity of the disease. In a small number of patients with cystic fibrosis, the values tend to be in the borderline zone or even in the high normal region. The diagnosis is, in such cases, most difficult to establish, and a variety of other procedures are justified. Sweat tests are advised for all

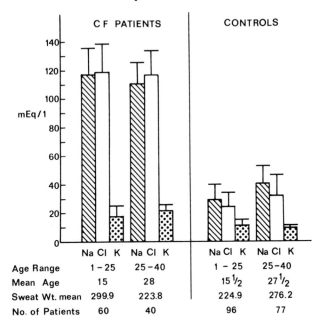

Figure 10. Quantitative pilocarpine iontophoresis.

		CF PATIENTS		CONTROLS	
		Na Cl K	Na Cl K	Na Cl K	Na Cl K
Age Range		1 – 25	25 – 40	1 – 25	25 – 40
Mean Age		15	28	15 1/2	27 1/2
Sweat Wt. mean		299.9	223.8	224.9	276.2
No. of Patients		60	40	96	77

siblings; a positive finding may provide supportive data. In children, the analysis of fingernail and toenail clippings for the sodium and potassium content may help establish the diagnosis in doubtful cases. Repeated sweat tests as well as careful clinical observations are indicated when equivocal results are obtained. The assay for a "serum factor" is still in the experimental stage but should be carried out if available. Parents of such children should also be tested, since both should be positive for the serum factor. All assays for the heterozygote should be considered still experimental and not used as a guide in genetic counseling.

Screening tests for sweat chloride levels are helpful, especially when properly done. These tests, of which there are many, should not be regarded as a final diagnostic procedure. We have seen serious errors made with such tests, especially when too much reliance was placed on a single negative result. In our clinic the most reliable procedure (a quantitative pilocarpine iontophoresis measuring sodium and chloride concentrations) is performed on any patient suspected of having cystic fibrosis. In our report we include the amount of sweat collected, and if the weight is less than 50 mg., we indicate that this is an inadequate amount. The test is then repeated in the hope of obtaining a larger sample. Two sites may be combined, if necessary. We generally perform two sweat tests on all patients who yield a positive test on the first occasion.

PANCREATIC FUNCTION. The most direct method of studying pancreatic function is to obtain duodenal fluid and determine the activity of pancreatic enzymes. The viscosity measurement of the duodenal aspirate is of considerable value in patients with cystic fibrosis, since this is significantly increased in approximately 90 per cent of patients. The volume of fluid is also reduced, and the pH is lower than in healthy controls. The bicarbonate concentration is reduced. The enzyme assay includes measurement of trypsin, chymotrypsin, lipase and amylase. There is a rough parallelism in enzyme activity in the healthy gland or in the case of complete pancreatic achylia. In the former case all enzyme values are normal, and in the latter all are virtually absent. Under these circumstances, assay for trypsin alone is sufficient. In patients with partial involvement of the pancreas, however, a dissociation of enzyme activity may be noted. Complete pancreatic enzyme insufficiency is not indicated by finding low to absent enzyme values in the fasting state, but must include the measurement of enzyme activity following intravenous secretin or intraduodenal stimulation with olive oil.

Indirect tests for pancreatic function are numerous, and one we have developed as a simple test is the gelatin film technique of testing feces. In infants and small children, the normal stool contains considerable proteolytic activity; in patients with complete pancreatic insufficiency, the stool trypsin is markedly reduced or absent. We have also used a quantitative technique for measuring trypsin and chymotrypsin feces, using synthetic substrates. The measurement of fecal fat by determining the total free fatty acids is a practical one and can be readily performed in most clinical laboratories. Patients with pancreatic insufficiency may excrete as much as 30 gm. or more of fat a day. They also excrete excess nitrogen. Nearly all infants and children with pancreatic insufficiency have cystic fibrosis. The small number who do not may have either a congenital anomaly or dysplasia of the pancreas or a syndrome we recently described. Initially the first three patients with this syndrome were regarded as atypical examples of cystic fibrosis because pulmonary manifestations failed to develop, and the patients had normal sweat test results. These cases, which now number 20 in our series, include the following clinical and laboratory features: pancreatic insufficiency, failure to thrive, bone marrow hypoplasia, neutropenia, thrombocytopenia or anemia, and transient galactosuria. Nearly one-third have metaphyseal dysplasia.

It is a familial disorder, and cases have recently been reported from Australia, Switzerland, and various parts of this country. Familial pancreatic calcification is a rare condition with late onset of mild symptoms and is easily distinguishable from cystic fibrosis.

A variety of oral absorptive tests have been proposed, such as gelatin or casein for measuring protein digestion, vitamin A and Lipiodol for measuring fat absorption, and glucose or xylose for measuring glucose absorption. In patients with pancreatic insufficiency, the xylose and glucose absorption test results are normal, whereas protein and fat absorption test results are abnormal.

The clinical response to dietary modifications has often been used to assess pancreatic function. These tests, although helpful, should never be regarded as conclusive evidence unless balance studies are made.

DIAGNOSTIC TESTS IN ADULTS.   The sweat test in adults is as reliable as in children, with a wider range of values in healthy adults. Rarely will a healthy adult have values above the diagnostic range, i.e., above 60 mEq. per liter. The presence of diabetes, ulcers or other complications seen in cystic fibrosis does not necessarily point to the disease when these features are first noted in adults. We have seen the appearance of diabetes mellitus in one patient prior to the diagnosis of cystic fibrosis. However, other complications, such as nasal polyps, cirrhosis of the liver or chronic obstructive pulmonary disease, should lead the physician to perform a diagnostic sweat test. We have seen only one patient in whom diabetes occurred prior to the correct diagnosis of cystic fibrosis. The clinical picture must be consistent with the disease and usually includes a history of illness beginning in childhood. Roentgenograms of the chest may be helpful, and the family history must also be taken into account. However, some adults in whom the diagnosis is made will deny any history of either pulmonary or gastrointestinal disorders until shortly before they seek medical attention.

Treatment

The nature of the basic disorder remains unknown; hence therapy, although effective, must be considered nonspecific or empiric. Treatment is given to relieve the presenting complaints and to prevent complications. Although prophylactic therapy is the most important aspect of managing the child with cystic fibrosis, it is least understood. Three examples of prophylactic therapy, each affecting a different system, follow:

1. The *eccrine sweat glands.* The use of salt in a warm climate or when the patient sweats excessively even in cold weather may prevent "salt depletion" or "heat stroke."

2. *Respiratory system.* Measles may be a serious disease and may precipitate a downward course; hence, measles prophylaxis should be advised in all children with cystic fibrosis.

3. *Gastrointestinal.* Dietary and pancreatic therapy, when given to patients diagnosed in early infancy, will reduce the incidence of rectal prolapse to nearly zero from an incidence of over 20 per cent in untreated patients. Proper nutrition in infants will also prevent hypoproteinemia or vitamin K deficiency. (See Figs. 11 and 12.) Proper dietary therapy will usually permit normal growth and development in infancy.

In many communities, patients suspected of having cystic fibrosis are hospitalized for study, and if the diagnosis is confirmed, the therapeutic program is instituted and education of parents undertaken. In a center where facilities and personnel are available, hospitalization is reserved for the very sick and in many cases is avoided. The amount of time and effort needed to provide parents with an understanding of the disease, the training in methods of physical therapy, the consultation with social workers, nurses and dietitians, and the evaluation of all siblings is considerable. In our clinic, relatively few patients are hospitalized for diagnostic study. The patients have ready access to our staff at all times and are seen regularly at periodic intervals. These intervals vary from once a week to once every three months, depending on the individual situation.

PULMONARY SYSTEM. In the last three to four years we have instituted a new type of elective hospitalization for children with cystic fibrosis. These are patients who lose weight and fatigue more readily and who may have a more persistent cough. A ten-day hospital stay with an intensive therapeutic program that includes intravenous antibiotics, postural drainage three times a day, aerosol antibiotics and bronchodilators is instituted. Also included is a high calorie, low fat diet supplemented with a potent pancreatic preparation and MCT oil and vitamins. This approach has produced a beneficial effect. This is judged not only by clinical criteria, but also by quantitative data derived by pulmonary function testing at the time of admission and again prior to discharge. This feeling of improvement and well-being may persist for one to more than six months.

The chief considerations are the prevention of bronchial obstruction and the accompanying infection. When these already exist, the therapeutic program must be vigorous and include the following measures.

Antibiotic Therapy. Oral therapy is preferred, and the antibiotics may be selected from a fairly large list. The study of sputum or throat cultures and the testing of the microorganisms to a variety of antibiotics may be of help in determining which agent to use. The most common organism recovered in the initial cultures is penicillin-resistant *Staphylococcus aureus.* Chlortetracycline, oxytetracycline, erythromycin, oxacillin, cephalosporin or Lincocin may be administered in a dosage of approximately 25 to 60 mg. per kilogram per day, depending on the severity of the disease and the clinical response of the

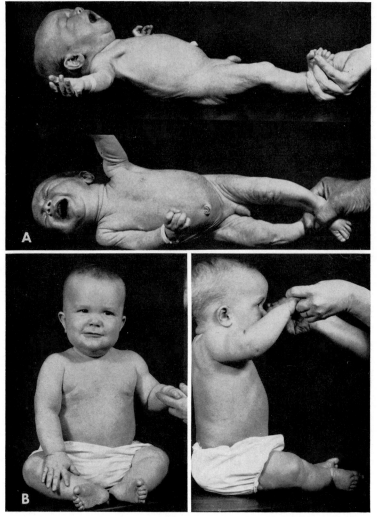

Figure 11. *A,* Patient when first seen at two months of age; *B,* after eight months of therapy.

patient. We frequently employ Gantrisin in combination with one of the above antistaphylococcal drugs. Gram-negative bacteria such as *aerogenes, Klebsiella pneumoniae* and *P. aeruginosa* may be predominant; chloramphenicol may be a clinically effective drug, although the bacteria isolated may be resistant. In patients with persistent infection, continuous antibiotic therapy may be necessary, and when the clinical and radiologic condition deteriorates, the combination of chloramphenicol and oxacillin or erythromycin may be used for long periods. Close observation is essential when chloramphenicol is used, since there may be hematologic, ophthalmologic and neurotoxic complications. In patients with no or minimal pulmonary disease, continuous antibiotic therapy is not necessary. Aerosol antibiotic therapy is a useful adjunct to systemic therapy. Neomycin solution, 50 mg. per ml., or colistin, 5 to 10 mg. per ml., plus isoproterenol may be used as often as two or three times daily for prolonged periods of time.

Relief of Bronchial Obstruction. The removal of viscid mucus and the exudate produced as a result of infection is

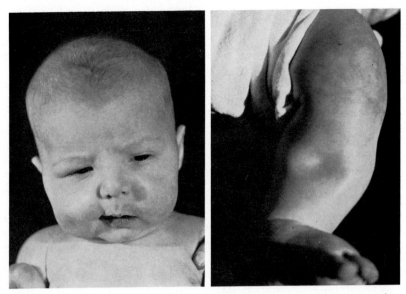

Figure 12. Patient presenting at 2½ months of age with edema, hypoproteinemia and anemia. The anemia was due to a deficiency in metal-binding globulin. The edema and hypoproteinemia cleared rapidly with changes in formula from a soybean preparation to an evaporated milk formula and the addition of pancreatin. This is an unusual manifestation of cystic fibrosis noted in early infancy.

the main aim of the following therapeutic measures.

Mist tent therapy. The provision of a water-saturated atmosphere makes it easier for the patient to mobilize his secretions. The tent is set up in the home, and the patient sleeps in this tent throughout the night. A variety of effective pieces of equipment are commercially available to provide a mist. A 10 per cent solution of propylene glycol or distilled water is placed in the nebulizer, and a fine mist with a particle size of less than 5 microns can be achieved. When first placed in a tent, many patients with moderate pulmonary involvement will report that they slept comfortably for the first time in many a night, that they no longer awoke through the night coughing. They also find it easier to cough up sputum.

Until five years ago, the majority of our patients slept in mist tents. Most of our patients have discontinued this form of therapy, since withdrawal has not resulted in any detectable deterioration. However, a small number of patients feel that they are more comfortable and cough less, and find it easier

to expectorate. A rare individual will claim that the noise and vibration of the machine puts him to sleep. Under these circumstances we find no objection to use of the ultrasonic mist tent.

Postural drainage. The use of mechanical means to assist expulsion of pulmonary secretions is advocated. The patient is placed in the appropriate position, i.e., with the bronchus from the area to be drained perpendicular to the ground; by clapping and vibrating, the secretions from the affected area are loosened and expelled. Parents are instructed by the physical therapist and may be advised to drain the affected lobes once or more times a day.

Breathing exercises. As in most types of obstructive bronchopulmonary disease, the expiratory phase is relatively ineffective and the residual air is increased. Breathing exercises are instituted to improve this defect.

Other measures include the use of expectorant drugs and mucolytic agents. These drugs may be used for prolonged periods of time and are often beneficial, but in no way affect the basic disorder. Steroid therapy may relieve the bronchospasm in the severely ill infant or may be used in an attempt to prevent the regrowth of nasal polyps, which is usually ineffective.

Pulmonary resection may provide a palliative form of therapy in selected patients who have long-standing areas of persistent atelectasis with underlying abscess formation or bronchiectasis. The areas resected and the results of the first 29 resections performed in our hospital are given in Table 8. At present (May 1976), 50 patients have undergone pulmonary resection. Two common and serious pulmonary complications are pneumothorax and hemoptysis.

DIGESTIVE SYSTEM. No special dietary considerations are needed in patients with good pancreatic function. The majority of patients, however, have either complete or partial insufficiency. The aim of therapy in these patients is to satisfy hunger by providing an adequate diet and vitamin supplementation, and to replace missing pancreatic enzymes. The total caloric intake in untreated patients may be surprisingly high, and as soon as proper dietary therapy is begun, hunger is less intense and the caloric

intake diminished to a nearly normal level. The diet consists of food generally consumed by the family with emphasis on restricting the fat and increasing the protein intake. The weight change and the nature and frequency of the stool will in most cases serve as a guide. Many parents are not aware of the stool abnormality, and an inspection by the physician is urged. Commercial pancreatin preparations are effective and best administered with each meal. We have found the powder suitable for infants and small children, and tablets or capsules for older patients. We have had considerable experience with Viokase powder and tablets, and find these products effective. Other available commercial products are Cotazym and Pancreatic granules. The effective dose may vary with each child and is determined by the nature of the response. At present, nearly all commercially available multivitamin preparations are in water-soluble form. We recommend twice the usual dose and also the addition of vitamin B complex in patients receiving antibiotics orally. Vitamin K is given to all small infants, since they are more prone to develop hypoprothrombinemia.

TREATMENT OF COEXISTING CONDI-

TABLE 8.   RESULTS OF PULMONARY RESECTIONS IN 29 PATIENTS WITH CYSTIC FIBROSIS

Excellent	4 (14%)	Symptom-free and full activity
Good	15 (51.5%)	Definite decrease in symptoms with increased sense of well-being
Fair	4 (14%)	Mild decrease in symptoms with increased sense of well-being
Unsatisfactory	1 (3.5%)	Unchanged
Poor	5 (17%)	Patient either died as result of operation or is worse

Area Resected

RIGHT SIDE	No. OF PATIENTS	LEFT SIDE	No. OF PATIENTS
Pneumonectomy	1	Pneumonectomy	1
Upper lobe	3	Left upper	2
Middle lobe	4	Lingula	1
Upper and middle lobes	4	Left lower	4
Anterior segment of upper lobe	1	Left lower lobe and lingula	2
Middle and lower lobes	4	Total	10
Lower lobe	1		
Superior segment of lower lobe	1		
Total	19		

From Schuster, S., Shwachman, H., and Khaw, K. T.: *J. Thorac. Cardiovasc. Surg., 48*:5, 1964.

TIONS. Patients with cystic fibrosis are subject to all conditions that appear in the general population. Congenital anomalies that need correction should be dealt with. Associated conditions such as allergies are treated in the accepted manner. The incidence of allergic disorders is no more frequent in patients with cystic fibrosis than in the child population. We have encountered two patients who had an associated lactase deficiency and two who had a gluten enteropathy. These children responded to the appropriate dietary exclusion therapy, i.e., a gluten-free diet, a low fat diet, water-miscible vitamins and pancreatin with each meal.

Complications

It is difficult to determine what constitutes a complication or a symptom. When one diagnoses an infant newly born into a family with other cystic fibrosis children, there are usually no symptoms or complaints. The only positive finding is the elevation of sodium and chloride in his sweat (above 70 or 80 mEq. per liter). If one observes such an infant carefully, the stools may become abnormal. The baby develops a large appetite and fails to gain, or he may begin to cough or breathe rapidly. Some of these early symptoms can be prevented, and when prophylactic therapy accomplishes this, one is clearly left with a baby symptom-free yet labeled as having cystic fibrosis. Our ultimate aim is to establish the diagnosis very early and prevent the complications, many of which are now considered symptoms of the disease. Table 9 lists the complications, and the frequency with which they occur is indicated by the letters R for rarely, O for occasionally and C for commonly. Some of the complications are iatrogenic.

Conclusion

Cystic fibrosis is a frequent cause of chronic pulmonary disease in childhood. Although the cause of the hereditary disorder is unknown, considerable progress has been made in diagnostic methods and in therapeutic management. Early detection and prompt treatment will favorably affect the outcome. The enormous economic and psychologic burden borne by the parents cannot be overemphasized, and successful management cannot be carried out without the cooperation of the parents. Consultation with experts at treatment centers is recommended to assure that the diagnosis is correct and that proper prophylactic therapy is available, and to provide genetic counseling and financial and other assistance. The knowledge that a number of patients have reached adulthood, have graduated from college, have married and are leading productive lives should encourage us to continue to search for a better understanding of the underlying disorder with the hope of providing a more specific type of therapy.

Prognosis

The outlook for patients with cystic fibrosis has improved a great deal in the past 30 years. Before 1945 most patients diagnosed succumbed to this disease within a few years. At that time the survival of a child beyond ten years of age was unusual. Death was due to the extensive pulmonary involvement, infection playing a large role. With the advent of broad-spectrum antibiotics in 1948, a striking improvement in the course of the disease was noted. As new antibiotics appeared, many were found to be effective in combating the pulmonary infection. Other therapeutic advances included home therapy, aerosols combining antibiotics with bronchodilators or mucolytic agents, mist tent therapy, physical therapy with breathing exercises, and postural drainage. Emphasis on therapy shifted from pancreatic and dietary management to a variety of measures designed to prevent and control pulmonary infection or complications initiated by the process of diffuse bronchiolar plug-

TABLE 9.   COMPLICATIONS VERSUS FEATURES OF DISEASE

Emphysema	C		Right-sided heart failure	O
Atelectasis	C		Pulmonary hypertension	O
Bronchiectasis	C			
Hemoptysis	O		Botryomycosis	R
Sinusitis	C		Osteomyelitis	R
Nasal polyposis	C			
			Ocular changes	R
Empyema	R		Salt depletion syndrome	R
Pneumothorax	R		Calcification of pancreas	R
Growth retardation	C		Intestinal obstruction	C
Delayed sexual development	C		Meconium ileus (see Table 1)	
Gynecomastia	R		Atresia	
Diabetes mellitus	R		Fecal impactions	
Osteoarthropathy	C		Intussusception	R
Parotitis	R		Duodenitis	O
Osteoporosis	O		Duodenal ulcerations	R
Hypoproteinemia*	R		Pancreatitis	R
Edema,* generalized	R		Portal hypertension	O
Anemia secondary to blood loss	R		Hypersplenism	R
Deficient metal-binding globulin*	R		Cirrhosis of liver	C
Vitamin K deficiency	O		Hypergammaglobulinemia	R
Vitamin A deficiency	O		Ascites	R
Vitamin E deficiency	O		Pneumatosis intestinalis	R
Sterility in male	C		Rectal prolapse	O
			Inguinal hernia	C

Complications – Iatrogenic

Iodides: goiter
        hypothyroidism
Pancreatic replacement: constipation
        Pork allergy: diarrhea
Antibiotics†
    Tetracyclines: discoloration of teeth
             deposition in bone
             photosensitivity
             "growth factor"
             bulging fontanel
             vomiting
             diarrhea
    Novobiocin: fever, dermatitis
    Chloramphenicol: ocular changes, loss of vision
                pancytopenia
                toxic neuritis
Anabolic agents: androgenic effects
IPPB: pneumothorax
      extension of infection

R = rare; *O* = occasional; *C* = common.
*Figure 12 illustrates infant with hypoproteinemia, generalized edema, and anemia.
†See packet literature; only a few examples are given.

ging. Measles vaccination as well as protection against influenza is widely practiced.

The extent to which we are effective in applying measures to prevent the progress of the pulmonary lesion will in large measure determine the prognosis. Unfortunately, in the past, many pa-tients presented with advanced and irreversible pulmonary lesions. The advent of more reliable and easily performed diagnostic tests plus a greater awareness of the varied clinical manifestations makes it possible to recognize the disease in its earliest stages. Today, many cystic fibrosis clinics can boast of a mortality rate of less than 4 per cent per year of all newly diagnosed cases, excluding meconium ileus. In our clinic, 100 patients are over 25 years of age, whereas fifteen years ago no patients were over 25 years of age. Many have completed college, and at least 50 have married. A current survey of babies born to mothers with documented cystic fibrosis revealed 17 mothers and 20 deliveries. Two of the babies and three of the mothers succumbed. In our series of older patients, the males outnumber females. These observations point to a much better prognosis today than was possible at any previous time.

REFERENCES

Andersen, D. H.: Cystic fibrosis of the pancreas and its relation to celiac disease. *Am. J. Dis. Child.*, 56:344, 1938.

Anderson, D. H.: Pathology of cystic fibrosis; in problems in cystic fibrosis. *Ann. N. Y. Acad. Sci.*, 93:500, 1962.

Bodian, M.: *Fibrocystic Disease of the Pancreas: A Congenital Disorder of Mucus Production — Mucosis.* London, Heinemann, 1953.

Cook, C. D., Shwachman, H., and others: Studies of respiratory physiology in children. II. Lung volumes and mechanics of respiration in 64 patients with cystic fibrosis of the pancreas. *Pediatrics*, 24:2, 1959.

Craig, J. M., Haddad, H., and Shwachman, H.: The pathological changes in the liver in cystic fibrosis of the pancreas. *Am. J. Dis. Child.*, 93:357, 1957.

di Sant'Agnese, P. A., and Talamo, R. C.: Pathogenesis and physiopathology of cystic fibrosis of the pancreas. *N. Engl. J. Med.*, 277:1287; 1343; 1399, 1967.

Doershuk, C. F., Matthews, L. W., Tucker, A. S., and Spector, S.: Prophylactic and therapeutic program for cystic fibrosis. *Pediatrics*, 36:675, 1965.

Donnison, A. B., Shwachman, H., and Gross, R. E.: A review of 164 children with meconium ileus. *Pediatrics*, 37:833, 1966.

Fanconi, G., and Uehlinger, E., and Knauer, C.: Das Coeliakiesyndrom bei angeborener zystischer Pankreasfibromatose und Bronchiektasien. *Wien. Med. Wochenschr.*, 86:753, 1936.

Farber, S.: Pancreatic function and disease in early life. V. Pathologic changes associated with pancreatic insufficiency in early life. *Arch. Pathol.*, 37:238, 1944.

Farber, S.: Some organic digestive disturbances in early life. *J. Mich. Med. Soc.*, 44:587, 1945.

Featherby, E. A., Weng, T. R., Crozier, D. N., Duic, A., Reilly, B. J., and Levison, H.: *Dynamic and Static Lung Volumes, Blood-Gas Tensions and Diffusing Capacity in Patients With Cystic Fibrosis.* Proc. 5th International Cystic Fibrosis Conference. Published by C. F. Research Trust, Stuart House, 1 Tudor St., London, E. C., 4, 1969, pp. 232–254.

Glanzmann, E.: Dysporia enterobronchopancreatica congenital familiaris, zystische Pankreasfibrose, *Ann. Paediatr.*, 166:289, 1946.

Grand, R. A., and di Sant' Agnese, P. A.: Personal communication.

Gross, R. E.: *The Surgery of Infancy and Childhood.* Philadelphia, W. B. Saunders Company, 1953.

Guide to Diagnosis and Management of Cystic Fibrosis. National Cystic Fibrosis Research Foundation, 521 Fifth Ave., N. Y., March 1963.

Holsclaw, D. S., Perlmutter, A. D., Jockin, H., and Shwachman, H.: Genital abnormalities in male patients with cystic fibrosis. *J. Urol.*, 106:568, 1971.

Kagan, B. M.: Cystic fibrosis of the pancreas. Eccrinosis. *Ill. Med. J.*, 107:120, 1955.

Kaplan, E., Shwachman, H., Perlmutter, A. D., Rule, A., Khaw, K. T., and Holsclaw, D. S.: Reproductive failure in males with cystic fibrosis. *N. Engl. J. Med.*, 279:65, 1968.

Katznelson, D., Vawter, G. F., Foley, G. E., and Shwachman, H.: Botryomycosis, a complication in cystic fibrosis. *J. Pediatr.*, 65:525, 1964.

Kobayashi, Y.: Autopsied case of cystic fibrosis of the pancreas. *Acta Paediat. Jap.*, 65:597, 1961.

Kopito, L., Khaw, K. T., Townley, R. R. W., and Shwachman, H.: Studies in cystic fibrosis — analysis of nail clippings for sodium and potassium. *N. Engl. J. Med.*, 272:504, 1965.

Kopito, L. E., Shwachman, H., Vawter, G. F., and Edlow, J.: The pancreases in cystic fibrosis: chemical composition and comparative morphology. *Pediatr. Res.*, 10:742, 1976.

Matthews, L. W., Doershule, C. F., and Spector, S.: Mist tent therapy of the obstructive pulmonary lesion in cystic fibrosis. *Pediatrics*, 39:176, 1967.

Murray, A. B., and Cook, C. D.: Measurement of peak expiratory flow rates in 220 normal children from 4.5 to 18.5 years of age. *J. Pediatr.*, 62:186, 1963.

Orzalesi, M. M., Kohner, D., Cook, C. D., and Shwachman, H.: Anamnesis, sweat electrolyte and pulmonary function studies in parents of patients with cystic fibrosis of the pancreas. *Acta Paediatr.*, 52:267, 1963.

Rosan, R. C., Shwachman, H., and Kulzycki, L. L.: Diabetes and cystic fibrosis of the pancreas. *Am. J. Dis. Child.*, 104:265, 1962.

Salam, M. Z.: Cystic fibrosis of the pancreas in Middle East. *J. Med. Liban.*, 15:61, 1962.

Schuster, S., Shwachman, H., and Khaw, K. T.: Pulmonary surgery in cystic fibrosis. *J. Thorac. Cardiovasc. Surg.*, 48:5, 1964.

Shwachman, H., and Kulczycki, L. L.: A report

of 105 patients with cystic fibrosis of the pancreas studied over a five to fourteen year period. *Am. J. Dis. Child., 96*:6, 1958.

Shwachman, H., Diamond, L. K., Oski, F. A., and Khaw, K. T.: The syndrome of pancreatic insufficiency and bone marrow dysfunction. *J. Pediatr., 65*:645, 1964.

Shwachman, H., Kulczycki, L. L., and Khaw, K. T.: Studies in cystic fibrosis. A report of 65 patients over 17 years of age. *Pediatrics, 36*:689, 1965.

Shwachman, H., Redmond, A., and Khaw, K. T.: Studies in cystic fibrosis: report of 130 patients diagnosed under 3 months of age over a 20-year period. *Pediatrics, 46*:335, 1970.

Shwachman, H., Kowalsi, M., and Khaw, K. T.: Cystic fibrosis: a new outlook; 70 patients above 25 years of age. *Medicine* (in press).

CHAPTER FORTY-SIX

TUBERCULOSIS

Edwin L. Kendig, Jr., M.D.

General Considerations

From the beginnings of history, tuberculosis has created a major health problem throughout the civilized world. This disease has been a serious and constant threat, and although great strides toward its eradication have been made in many countries, there are other areas in which it is still largely uncontrolled.

Prior to 1882 there was sharp difference of opinion as to the infectiousness of the disease. In that year, however, Koch announced discovery of the causative agent of tuberculosis, and a more unified and enlightened approach to the problem ensued.

This identification of the tubercle bacillus led subsequently to community action, and finally to organized public health measures aimed at control and eradication of the disease. That these measures, in addition to a far better standard of living, have been effective in the United States, though less so in some parts of the world, is evinced by the sharp drop in mortality from the disease, from 200 per 100,000 population in 1900 to less than 50 per 100,000 in 1940. The advent of the antimicrobial agents, particularly streptomycin in 1944 and isoniazid in 1952, has resulted in an even more precipitate drop, so that mortality from tuberculosis in the United States in 1974 was 1.8 per 100,000 population.

Further evidence of the effectiveness of the campaign against tuberculosis in the United States is the great decrease in the number of persons sensitive to tuberculin. Whereas 40 years ago the rate of sensitivity among youths of high school age (15 to 19 years) was approximately 32 per cent, a 1958–1969 survey of more than a million Navy recruits of 17 to 21 years of age showed that only slightly more than 5 per cent were positive reactors.

It is apparent, then, that there has been significant progress toward control of tuberculosis in the United States, but the optimistic feeling engendered by these figures that this disease will soon be eradicated is misleading. In 1974 there were more than 30,000 new active cases of tuberculosis in the United States, and approximately 1200 of these were under five years of age. Diagnosis was made at autopsy in 1100 (4 per cent) of these new cases.

Another indication of the high incidence of tuberculosis in infants and young children in certain segments of the population is evident in the results of a ten-year study on BCG vaccine conducted in the Child Chest Clinic at the Medical College of Virginia and involving more than 1500 infants less than six months of age. In this study it was found that 12 per cent of the unvaccinated or control group became infected with tuberculosis, as determined by a positive tuberculin reaction (Mantoux).

That tuberculosis can ever be controlled solely by antimicrobial agents seems extremely doubtful. Certainly this cannot be accomplished with the drugs now available. The present-day approach must still be aimed at early diagnosis, isolation of infected persons, and the judicious use of BCG vaccine (prophylaxis) and available antituberculosis drugs.

Etiology

In 1882 Koch demonstrated that *Mycobacterium tuberculosis* is the causative agent of tuberculosis in humans. This agent is a member of the family Mycobacteriaceae, the chief characteristic of which is acid fastness, a property which may be defined as resistance to acid decoloration displayed by organisms that have been stained with aniline dyes. Although it is an oversimplification to state that the lipid content is the sole cause of this characteristic of acid fastness, mycolic acid is thought to play a role, perhaps a large one. Lipids also appear to be a factor in the formation of tubercles. Tuberculoproteins, the cause of the hypersensitivity that occurs after infection has taken place, are also important in antibody production.

There is no chemical constituent of the tubercle bacillus that has any demonstrable toxic effect for tissues not sensitized to tuberculin.

When stained with acid-fast stain, and examined under the oil-immersion lens of a microscope, tubercle bacilli appear as slender, bright, refractile red rods, about 4 microns in length and 0.5 micron in width. They are often

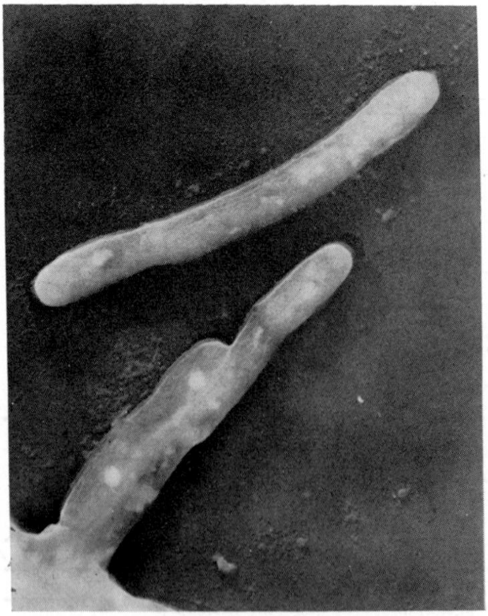

Figure 1. Virulent tubercle bacilli (H 37 Rv × 38,000). (From NTA Bulletin, June 1961. Courtesy of the American Lung Association, 1740 Broadway, New York, New York 10019.)

slightly curved and may be of various sizes and shapes, and may appear to be beaded or segmented (Fig. 1).

Dried tubercle bacilli kept in the dark may survive and remain virulent for many months, but they can be killed by exposure to direct sunlight or ultraviolet rays. In a fluid suspension they are killed by one minute of boiling or by a temperature of 60° C. (140° F.) within 15 or 20 minutes. One of the most effective household and hospital disinfectants is 70 per cent isopropyl alcohol.

Epidemiology

Because of the great decrease in mortality and the closure of many sanatoriums, there has been widespread propaganda to the effect that tuberculosis is no longer a serious problem in the United States. This is hardly an accurate estimate of the present status of this disease. As noted previously, figures indicating a large reduction in the death rate from tuberculosis do not reflect the seriousness of the problem. The number of newly reported cases is a more accurate measure of the widespread nature of the disease, but even these tell only part of the story.

It should be kept clearly in mind that an adult, adolescent or older child who has active pulmonary tuberculosis has a contagious disease. Spread of the infection is usually accomplished by droplets containing viable tubercle bacilli, and household contacts, particularly children, are extremely susceptible to this danger. In general, those children with nonprogressive primary pulmonary tuberculosis should not be considered contagious.

In a study carried out at the Medical College of Virginia, it appears that contact of an infant with a mother who has supposedly inactive tuberculous disease and sputum negative for tubercle bacilli may not be as safe as expected. Thirty-eight of 73 infants in this category became infected with tuberculosis, and three died with tuberculous meningitis. No other tuberculous adult contact could be demonstrated (Table 1). Al-

TABLE 1. INFANTS BORN OF TUBERCULOUS MOTHERS WITH SUPPOSEDLY INACTIVE DISEASE

Infected	38
Noninfected	35
Total	73

though contact of the child with other adults in the household may not be as intimate as that with the mother, the risk does not appear inconsequential. It should be noted, however, that there is evidence that there is much less risk of tuberculous infection in that period during which the tuberculous adult receives adequate antimicrobial therapy.

Among the more common sources of tuberculous disease in the child are the more elderly members of the family, such as grandparents, aunts or uncles, or other older relatives. Baby sitters, household servants, boarders and frequent visitors in the home are often the tuberculosis contact. A one-year-old child in our practice had a positive reaction in a routine tuberculin test. Careful search of family contacts, household servants and frequent visitors to the home was not productive, but six months later the gardener, with whom the little boy often played, announced that he had been to the clinic and found that he had tuberculosis. The possibilities of contact with tuberculosis are numerous, and none should be overlooked.

That epidemic spread may occur in population groups largely unexposed to tuberculosis has been stressed by Mande and coworkers (1958), who reported 25 such epidemics in schools in France. In 1965, Lincoln collected and reviewed the reports of 84 epidemics of tuberculosis in school children from 12 countries. The source case is usually a student or one of the school personnel, more often a teacher.

Predisposing Factors

Most persons who are infected by *Mycobacterium tuberculosis* do not acquire so-called clinical disease. Some persons have a greater resistance than do others, and the resistance of a given person may vary from time to time. Important, too, is the relative virulence of the invading organisms and the number of bacilli in the inoculum.

Chronic illness, malnutrition and chronic fatigue may increase susceptibility to tuberculous disease. A quiescent tuberculous lesion may be activated by nontuberculous infections, such as measles, varicella and pertussis, by conditions of stress created by surgery, by smallpox vaccination, by severe viral pulmonary infection, and by adrenocorticosteroid therapy. It should be noted, however, that the Medical College of Virginia studies show that measles exerts no deleterious effect on either primary tuberculosis or such serious forms of the disease as tuberculous meningitis when the patient is receiving isoniazid therapy at that time. Many studies have also shown that there is no deleterious effect from adrenocorticosteroid therapy when the patient is under treatment with isoniazid.

Heredity

Although the higher incidence of tuberculosis in some families is usually the result of more intimate contact with the disease, Lurie and coworkers (1955) have presented studies with rabbits showing good evidence for the importance of hereditary factors. Congenital infection is rare.

Age, Race and Sex

The mortality rate from tuberculosis is higher during infancy and again at adolescence; it is not so high during the intervening years of childhood. There is a higher death rate from tuberculosis in the United States among nonwhites than among the white population, but differences in racial immunity are not that easily determined. It seems likely that the higher mortality rate among the nonwhite population may be largely the result of social and environmental stress and greater opportunity for infection.

During the latter part of childhood and during adolescence, girls have a higher incidence of and mortality from tuberculosis than do boys. Except for the higher incidence of disease in older males, there is no such difference between the sexes at other age levels.

Allergy and Immunity

After tuberculous infection there is a two- to ten-week period of incubation. At the close of this period, the presence of allergy is manifested by a positive reaction to the tuberculin test. With the appearance of this allergic state there is alteration in the host response to tubercle bacilli, now manifested by exudation and a tendency for the infection to become localized. At some less definite time some immunity also develops. This immunity is a relative one, and the infecting organisms may be so many in number or of such virulence that this partial resistance will be overcome; or, on the other hand, the immunity may be sufficient to withstand and protect against the infection.

Neither the mechanism that produces immunity nor the correlation between allergy and immunity is clear.

Pathogenesis and Pathology

Since the usual mode of tuberculous infection is by inhalation, the primary lesion occurs in the lung parenchyma in more than 95 per cent of the cases. It may, of course, occur elsewhere. In a previously uninfected person there is first an accumulation of polymorphonuclear leukocytes; this is followed by epithelioid cell proliferation, producing the typical tubercle. Giant cells appear, and the entire area is surrounded by lymphocytes.

Almost as soon as infection takes place, tubercle bacilli are carried by macrophages from the primary focus and travel to the regional lymph nodes. When the primary focus is in the lung parenchyma, the bronchopulmonary glands are usually involved, but an apical focus may drain into the paratracheal lymph nodes.

Hypersensitivity of body tissues to tuberculin does not take place immediately, but makes its appearance only after a period varying from two to ten weeks. During this period the primary focus may grow larger, but does not become encapsulated. When hypersensitivity develops, the perifocal reaction becomes much more prominent, and the regional lymph nodes enlarge. The primary focus may become caseous, but with the development of acquired resistance, it usually becomes walled off. This caseous material gradually becomes inspissated and later calcified. The lesion may completely disappear.

Primary foci are usually single, but the occurrence of two or more such lesions is not rare in our experience (Fig. 2). After hypersensitivity has developed, however, the typical primary complex (parenchymal focus and regional gland involvement) does not occur.

Although the usual tendency in primary pulmonary tuberculosis is toward healing, there may be progression of the primary parenchymal focus. The lesion continues to enlarge, the surrounding tissue becomes pneumonic in nature, and the overlying pleura may be thickened. Under these conditions the caseous center may liquefy and empty into one or more of the bronchi, thereby resulting in a residual cavity and one or more new areas of tuberculous pneumonia (cavitating primary).

It is during the stage of caseation, too, that acute hematogenous dissemination is most likely to occur. This may result in widespread miliary lesions throughout some or all of the viscera, or in isolated foci in such parts of the body as the eye, lungs, bones, brain, kidneys, liver or spleen. Although these isolated foci may occur under these conditions, they are more apt to result from the few tubercle bacilli that may reach the blood stream before hypersensitivity develops. This bacillemia

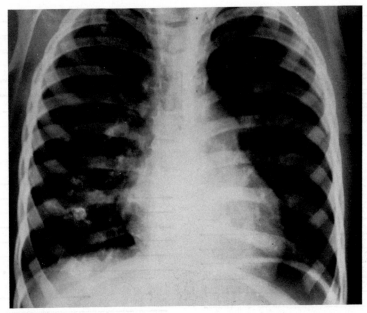

Figure 2. Multiple calcified primary foci.

may occur either directly or by way of the regional lymph nodes and the thoracic duct.

As a rule, progression of the metastatic lesions occurs as a result of seeding from the blood stream. This may be direct, as in miliary or renal tuberculosis. On the other hand, late progression resulting from a previous hematogenous seeding may occur by contiguity. For example, Rich and Mc-Cordock (1933) have demonstrated that tuberculous meningitis is more likely to result from a tuberculoma contiguous to the meninges.

The involved regional lymph nodes also have a tendency to heal, but less so than does the primary parenchymal focus. Tubercle bacilli may persist for years, even though demonstrable areas of calcification indicate that at least partial healing has occurred.

Because of their location, the hyperemic, edematous hilar lymph nodes may be the cause of considerable pathologic change, primarily of an obstructive nature. The nodes may encroach on the bronchi, causing occlusion of the lumen with resultant atelectasis of that area of the lung distal to the obstruction. Or,

more often, a caseous node or mass of nodes may become attached to the wall of the bronchus by inflammatory reaction. Infection may progress through the wall and create a fistulous tract. Disease may thus be transmitted through the bronchus to that area of the lung served by that bronchus. Similarly, too, the extrusion of the caseous contents from an affected node into the bronchus may produce complete obstruction, with atelectasis of the distal lung parenchyma. A lesion thus created is often a combination of atelectasis and pneumonia, however, and not atelectasis alone.

When obstruction of the bronchus is incomplete, a check-valve type of mechanism may result. There may be less hindrance to inspired air than to the exit of respired air, thus resulting in hyperaeration due to the obstruction.

Obstruction of a portion of the wall of a bronchus may lead to a fibrous stricture with resultant partial or complete lack of aeration to that portion of the lung. Tuberculous lymph nodes may also occasionally invade or compress adjacent structures.

Most complications of primary tuberculosis occur during the first year following the onset of the infection. After this time complications are relatively infrequent until the period of adolescence, when pulmonary tuberculosis ("adult or reinfection tuberculosis") becomes a major problem. This occurs twice as often in girls as in boys. In Hsu's (1974) report of 1881 children with subclinical tuberculous infection who were given isoniazid (INH) chemoprophylaxis, pulmonary tuberculosis developed in only six instances, a morbidity of 3.2 per 1000. There were no deaths. These results are in marked contrast with two earlier studies (Brailey, 1944; Lincoln, 1950) carried out before INH became available. Lincoln noted reactivation of pulmonary tuberculosis in 8 per cent of her cases, with 23.9 per cent mortality. Brailey's study showed a mortality of 8.4 per cent in white children and 16 per cent in black children.

It can rarely be determined whether the chronic pulmonary tuberculosis that appears years after primary tuberculosis has healed is the result of activation of the healed primary lesion or the development of a new infection. The presence of an increased resistance toward a new infection that follows the primary infection would seem to favor the endogenous theory.

Diagnosis

THE TUBERCULIN TEST. A positive reaction to the tuberculin test indicates the presence of tuberculous infection, and the test is, therefore, of great aid in the diagnosis of the disease. The degree of activity, if any, or the severity of the disease process cannot be thus determined. There are other limitations of the test, and these, including the various causes of false-positive and false-negative reactions, will be discussed later.

Tuberculin solution, utilized in skin testing, is available in two forms: purified protein derivative (PPD) and old tuberculin (OT) solution.

PPD is the tuberculin solution now recommended because it is a more specific product. It is the protein of the tubercle bacillus obtained from filtrates of heat-killed cultures of tubercle bacilli that have been grown on a synthetic medium and then precipitated by either trichloroacetic acid or neutral ammonium sulfate. The latter precipitant is used in the United States. The World Health Organization has designated one large batch of PPD (No. 49608, manufactured by Dr. Florence Seibert in 1939) as the international standard tuberculin (PPD–S). PPD is available commercially; it was formerly dispensed in tablet form and dissolved in a measured amount of diluent before use. Because tuberculoprotein, when diluted in a buffered diluent, is adsorbed in varying amounts by glass and plastics, it is now required that a small amount of polysorbate (e.g., Tween 80 at 5 ppm) be added by the manufacturer to the diluent to reduce adsorption.* In order to minimize reduction in potency by adsorption, tuberculin should never be transferred from one container to another, and skin tests should be administered as soon as practicable after the syringe has been filled.

OT solution, which has been known since the time of Koch, has some variation of potency in different batches. When kept in a refrigerator, OT is satisfactory for skin testing for at least two weeks and probably for a one-month period.†

The most accurate and reliable method of tuberculin testing is the

---

*Polysorbate-containing tuberculins are now marketed as Aplisol (5 international tuberculin units [TU] in 10-dose vials) (Parke-Davis) and as Connaught Tuberculin Purified Protein Derivative 5 TU in 10- and 50-dose vials and 1 TU in 10-dose vials (Panray Division, Ormont Drug and Chemical Company, Inc.). Polysorbate-containing PPD is said to be stable up to 12 months when refrigerated between 34 and 46° F. in the original container (Connaught).

†OT is available as a stable liquid concentrate and the diluent is a special buffered isotonic fluid available commercially (Parke-Davis). A dilution of one part concentrated tuberculin to 10,000 parts diluent supplies approximately 1 TU.

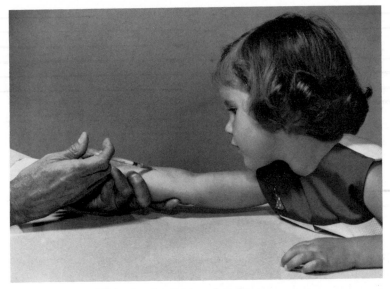

Figure 3. Application of the Mantoux test.

Mantoux (intracutaneous) test (Figs. 3 and 4). A measured amount of tuberculin solution of known concentration is injected intracutaneously. For this test, a syringe so graduated that fractional parts of a milliliter may be measured and a short-bevel 26- or 27-gauge needle should be used. Tuberculin is thermostable, and traces of it remain on syringes and glassware after ordinary cleansing methods. A syringe for tuberculin testing should, therefore, not be utilized for other skin tests. A separate needle is used for each patient. If the needle and the syringe are not of the disposable variety, they

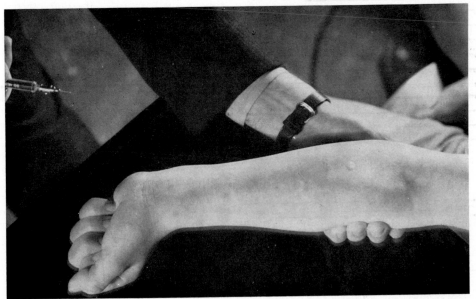

Figure 4. Demonstration of wheal produced by intracutaneous injection of tuberculin solution (Mantoux test). (Courtesy of the American Lung Association, 1740 Broadway, New York, New York 10019.)

should be sterilized by autoclaving. If this is not posssible, they should be boiled for 30 minutes.

The test must be carefully prepared, and exactly 0.1 ml. of the testing material is injected into the skin on the volar surface of the forearm. Unless a definite wheal follows injection, the test is not satisfactory and a false-negative reaction may result. This is particularly true if the material is injected subcutaneously or there is leakage at the site.

While PPD is the tuberculin solution now recommended, either PPD or OT may be utilized in the Mantoux test. In the Child Chest Clinic at the Medical College of Virginia, OT (10 TU) and PPD (5 TU) have been used concomitantly, and the former has been shown to be only slightly more sensitive. Either, therefore, may be used for routine tuberculin testing.

The test is read 48 to 72 hours later, and the area of induration should be measured at its greatest transverse diameter. An induration less than 5 mm. in diameter constitutes a negative reaction. If the area of induration measures between 5 and 9 mm. in diameter, the reaction must be considered doubtful, and the test should be repeated with the same dosage of tuberculin. The second test result may be negative, but if it shows the same degree of reaction, an attempt should be made to arrange for simultaneous testing with tuberculin solution (PPD, 5 TU) and the antigens of the atypical (unclassified) mycobacteria, when such antigens are available. Since the greatest amount of research and experience has been with PPD Battey (PPD–B), prepared from a Group III strain, and since high cross reactivity (low specificity) is exhibited by these antigens, PPD–B is recommended at present as the companion for PPD–tuberculin for comparative skin testing. Such tests often result in a small tuberculin reaction (5 to 9 mm. in diameter of induration) and a much larger reaction to one of the antigens of the atypical mycobacteria (15 to 20 mm. in diameter of induration), thereby

suggesting that the response to tuberculin is a heterologous reaction. If the tuberculin test, utilizing either OT (10 TU) or PPD (5 TU), produces an area of induration measuring 10 mm. or more, the result is considered positive (Figs. 5 and 6).

A Mantoux test may produce a severe local reaction. There may be much erythema and induration or even vesiculation or ulceration at the site of the injection in persons with a high degree of sensitivity to tuberculin, sometimes requiring the local use of hydrocortisone ointment. There may be associated lymphangitis or regional lymphadenopathy. Phlyctenular conjunctivitis is an uncommon complication, and a constitutional reaction with fever is rare.

As noted previously, the dosage of tuberculin suggested for routine skin testing and for mass immunization programs is 5 TU. This test presumably detects almost all of the persons infected with tuberculosis. Nonspecific reactions may occur when the amount of tuberculin is increased beyond 10 TU.

The other tuberculin tests (Heaf, tuberculin tine, Aplitest, Mono-Vacc) do not have the advantage of quantitative tuberculin testing afforded by the Mantoux test.

The *Heaf test*, devised in England and now utilized to some extent in this country, requires special apparatus for its use. The so-called Heaf gun makes six simultaneous skin punctures 1 mm. deep through a layer of concentrated PPD (100,000 TU per ml.) (Fig. 7). The test is read three to seven days later, and the presence of four or more papules constitutes a positive reaction (Fig. 8). However, unless vesiculation occurs, a positive reaction should in all instances be corroborated by a Mantoux test. The apparatus for this test is now available with disposable needle cartridges, and these may be resterilized and used again if so desired (Fig. 9).

The *tuberculin tine test* (Rosenthal) is

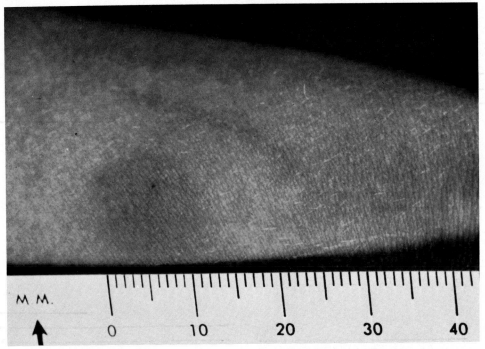

Figure 5. Positive reaction in the Mantoux test, measuring 10 mm. in diameter of induration.

one of the most practical tuberculin tests now in use (Fig. 10). The sterilized disposable unit consists of four tines that have been predipped in an old tuberculin concentrate (four times the standard strength of old tuberculin). In a strongly positive reaction, a rosette consisting of four confluent areas of induration may result (Fig. 11). Fusion of at least two papules is necessary for the result to be considered positive. Such mild reactions (2 mm. or more in diam-

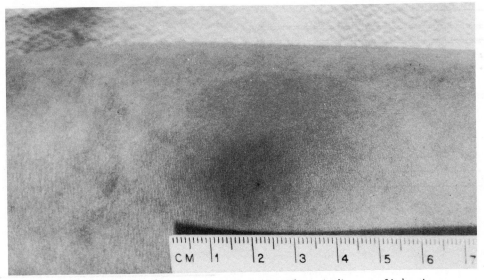

Figure 6. Mantoux test with reaction measuring 56 mm. in diameter of induration.

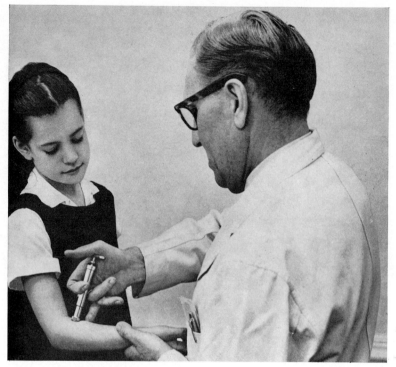

Figure 7.   Application of the Heaf test. (Courtesy of Panray-Parlam Corp., Englewood, N. J., 07631.)

eter) must be corroborated by a Mantoux test. The test is inexpensive, sterile, disposable and simple to apply.

The *Aplitest* is a recently introduced modification of the tuberculin tine test with the tines impregnated with PPD instead of OT. The test result is interpreted in the same way as the tuberculin tine test. The Aplitest has not yet been in use for a sufficient period of time so that its efficacy can be adequately evaluated, but there seems little

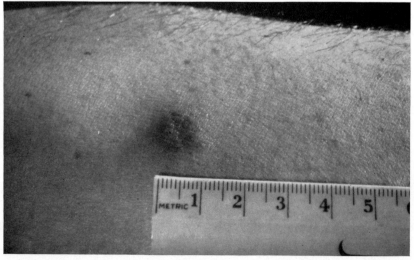

Figure 8.   Strongly positive (4+) reaction in the Heaf test. (Courtesy of Panray-Parlam Corp., Englewood, N.J. 07631.)

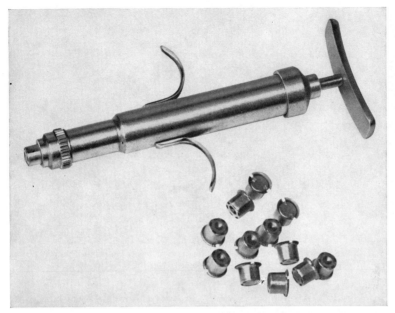

Figure 9. The Heaf gun with disposable cartridges. (Courtesy of Panray-Parlam Corp., Englewood, N. J. 07631.)

reason to believe that it differs greatly from the tuberculin tine test.

The *Mono-Vacc test* utilizes a device consisting of a nine-point plastic scarifier mounted on the outer side of a ring that fits on the thumb. A plastic tube containing old tuberculin solution is sealed around the points. The tube is removed just before application, and the tuberculin solution is squeezed onto the points. The material is then applied by pressing the points into the skin of

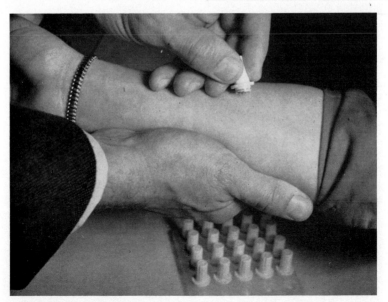

Figure 10. Application of the tine test. (Courtesy of Lederle Laboratories, A Division of American Cyanamid Co., Pearl River, N.Y. 10965.)

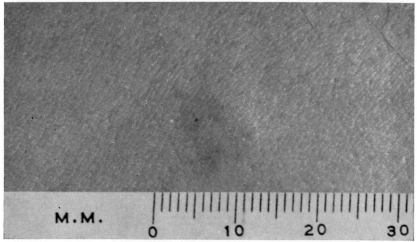

Figure 11.   The tine test. Positive reaction with four confluent areas of induration. (Courtesy of Lederle Laboratories, A Division of American Cyanamid Co., Pearl River, N.Y. 10965.)

the forearm (Fig. 12). An area of induration measuring 2 mm. in diameter constitutes a doubtful reaction and must be corroborated by a Mantoux test. An area of induration measuring 5 mm. in diameter is considered positive, but corroboration by a Mantoux test is advisable. If vesiculation occurs, the reaction is positive (Fig. 13).

False-positive tuberculin reactions may occur. As noted previously, it has been suggested (Palmer and Edwards,

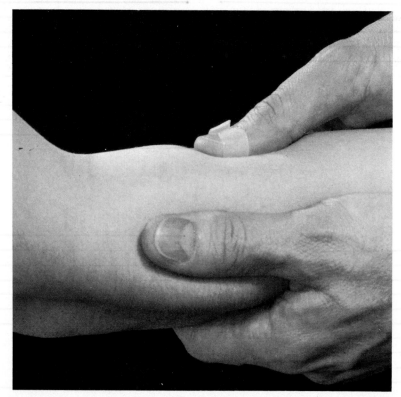

Figure 12.   Application of the Mono-Vacc test. (Courtesy of Lincoln Laboratories, Inc., Decatur, Illinois 62526.)

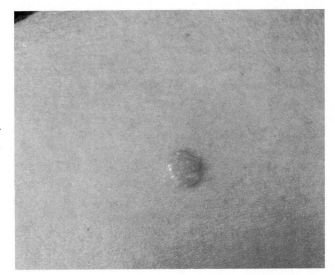

Figure 13. The Mono-Vacc test positive reaction (× 4). (Courtesy of Lincoln Laboratories, Inc., Decatur, Illinois 62526.)

1962) that the tuberculin reaction measuring between 5 and 9 mm. in diameter of induration is suspect, and they have pointed out that in certain sections of the United States the number of such reactions is abnormally large. The suggestion has been made that many of these nonspecific reactions may be the result of infection with the so-called atypical (unclassified) mycobacteria. The incidence of infection with these mycobacteria appears to be much greater in some areas of the country than in others. As determined by skin testing, there appears to be a high incidence of infection with atypical mycobacteria among children in Virginia, and it has been shown that not infrequently such infections may, by heterologous reaction, be the cause of a false-positive tuberculin reaction, such as that described above.

Other causes of a false-positive tuberculin reaction are not of great frequency. Hypersensitivity to the phenol, glycerin or bouillon in old tuberculin solution may be productive of redness and induration within the first 24 to 48 hours after application of the test. If the reading is done 48 to 72 hours after the test has been performed, the local response produced by such hypersensitivity has practically always disappeared.

It has been our experience that BCG vaccination is usually productive of a tuberculin reaction measuring 5 to 9 mm. in diameter of induration.* If a patient who has received BCG vaccine shows a reaction to PPD (5 TU) measuring 15 mm. or more in diameter of induration, the likelihood of superinfection with virulent tubercle bacilli must be considered (Fig. 14).

There are a certain number of false-negative tuberculin reactions, also; the most important of these occurs after the time when infection takes place and before allergy sets in, as manifested by a positive tuberculin reaction. It is important to remember than an infant or child who is known to have been exposed to a tuberculous adult must not be adjudged free of infection, as far as that particular contact is concerned, until he has a negative tuberculin reaction at least ten weeks after contact with the tuberculous person has ceased.

The next most important false-negative reaction may occur in those with overwhelming tuberculous disease, such as an infant moribund with tuber-

---

*This statement refers to the use of vaccine manufactured by the Research Institute, Chicago. This condition does not necessarily obtain when the BCG vaccine is manufactured outside of the United States.

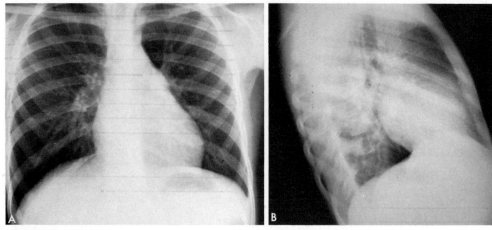

Figure 14. BCG-vaccinated patient in whom tuberculous infection developed later. Roentgenograms show multiple hilar calcifications. Tuberculin reaction (PPD 5TU) measured 12 mm. in diameter of induration three months after BCG vaccination. At time of subsequent testing, three years later, tuberculin reaction was 52 mm. Roentgenograms taken at that time (A, B) indicate presence of healed primary tuberculosis. There had been no evidence of clinical disease.

culous meningitis. This does occur, but in our experience is not nearly so frequent as was generally believed.

Certain cases of malnutrition, dehydration and inanition may show a false-negative tuberculin reaction.

During the course of measles, the tuberculin reaction will be partially or completely depressed, but hypersensitivity again becomes manifest ten days to six weeks later. Tuberculous children vaccinated against measles may have a depressed tuberculin reaction for the same period of time, and those with severe rubella may have a depressed reaction for one to three weeks. Suppression of the tuberculin reaction is also said to occur with varicella, mumps, severe viral pulmonary infection (especially influenza), infectious mononucleosis, primary atypical pneumonia, and sarcoidosis, and following the injection of live and killed viral vaccine.

Adrenocorticosteroid therapy may be the cause of a false-negative tuberculin reaction, and it is said that antihistaminics also tend to reduce tuberculin sensitivity. Although the latter may be true, our own experience has failed to corroborate the impression that such does occur to any important degree.

False-negative reactions relating to the tuberculin itself may occur. In addition to improper dilutions, bacterial contamination and exposure to heat or light, there may be adsorption of tuberculoprotein to container walls. It has been demonstrated that about 25 per cent of tuberculin in solution is lost 20 minutes after the syringe has been filled, and 80 per cent at 24 hours. Much of this adsorption is eliminated by the required addition of a surface-active agent such as Tween 80.

Faulty administration and improper reading of the reaction may also give false-negative results.

In the presence of phlyctenular conjunctivitis or erythema nodosum, or if there is a history of intimate exposure to infectious tuberculosis, a lower strength of PPD or OT solution or the use of the tine or Mono-Vacc test is indicated. Failure to observe this precaution may lead to worsening of the disease process and may be especially harmful to the diseased eye.

A routine tuberculin test should be performed between six and eight months of age, and annually thereafter (Table 2). It is, of course, always indicated when there has been known contact with a tuberculous adult. In the latter instance, if the tuberculin reac-

TABLE 2. USE OF THE ROUTINE
TUBERCULIN TEST

Test	Age at Administration
Mantoux (PPD) (5 TU)	6 to 8 months and
Mantoux (OT) (10 TU)	Annually thereafter
Tine	
Heaf	
Mono-Vacc	
Aplitest	

tion is negative, the test should be repeated ten weeks after the removal of the contact. If the child remains in contact with a tuberculous adult, the tuberculin test should be repeated at three-month intervals.

The routine tuberculin test is apparently not utilized to the extent that might be desired. A survey conducted among 2500 practicing pediatricians in the United States showed that among 1480 who answered the questionnaire, 821 (55.5 per cent) used the tuberculin test routinely, and of these, 174 (21 per cent) used the test only after three years of age, too late to be of maximum case-finding value (Table 3).

HISTORY AND PHYSICAL EXAMINATION. History of contact with a tuberculous adult is most important, and should lead immediately to the tuberculin testing routine outlined above.

The so-called tuberculosis symptom complex consisting of chronic cough, anorexia and failure to gain weight or even the loss of weight may sometimes be helpful in the diagnosis of progressive tuberculous disease, but is of little value in early diagnosis.

TABLE 3. UTILIZATION OF THE
ROUTINE TUBERCULIN TEST
BY PEDIATRICIANS

Pediatricians	1480
Use	821*
Do not use	659

*Of 821 using the test, 174 used it only after three years of age.

Expiratory stridor and bitonal cough, presumably caused by nodal compression of the bronchi, is of rare occurrence, and again is of little value in early diagnosis. Persistent fever of one to two weeks' duration often accompanies the development of primary tuberculosis, and the presence of such fever should arouse suspicion of tuberculosis. Rarely, erythema nodosum may be the first sign of tuberculous disease.

As a rule, the onset of primary tuberculosis is symptomless, and even those with progressive disease present symptoms that are far less prominent than might be expected from the associated disease process. In the Child Chest Clinic of the Medical College of Virginia, review was made of 200 children with tuberculosis infection, which ranged from a positive tuberculin reaction without other demonstrable evidence of disease to widespread pulmonary tuberculosis. Not one of these patients exhibited a single symptom or sign that could be associated with any disease process. All were diagnosed by means of a routine tuberculin test or by a tuberculin test performed because of known contact with tuberculosis.

Even in progressive tuberculous disease, symptoms and signs may not be as helpful as might be expected. A three-year-old black girl was referred to the Medical College of Virginia Hospital with a diagnosis of pulmonary tuberculosis. There was no history of contact with tuberculosis. The only symptoms were questionable failure to gain weight during the preceding year and a tendency to cough when taking violent exercise. Although physical examination yielded negative results, a chest roentgenogram showed atelectasis of the right upper lobe, a thin-walled cavity in the right lower lobe and miliary tuberculosis (Fig. 15).

Although the clinician should not overlook symptoms and signs that suggest the presence of tuberculosis, it must be stressed that the use of the tuberculin test is by far the most useful diagnostic tool.

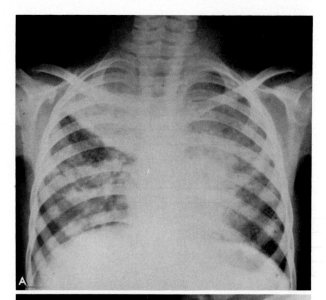

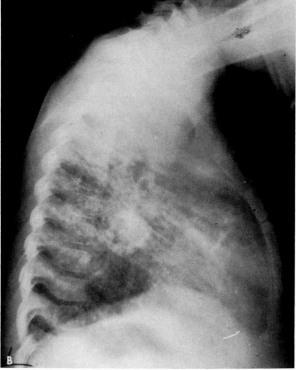

Figure 15. Negative physical examination in a child with atelectasis of the right upper lobe, cavity in the right lower lobe, and miliary tuberculosis. (Courtesy of *Am. J. Dis. Child.*, 92:558, 1956.)

ROENTGENOGRAM EXAMINATION. Once the presence of tuberculosis has been established by means of a positive tuberculin reaction, further procedures must be carried out in order to determine the location and the degree of severity of the infection. Since most primary tuberculous infections occur in the lung parenchyma (over 95 per cent), a chest roentgenogram, including both anteroposterior and lateral views, is always indicated and should be taken promptly (Fig. 16).

A primary complex, occurring after

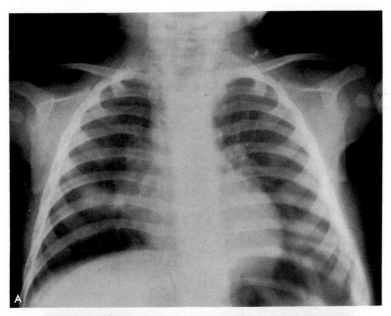

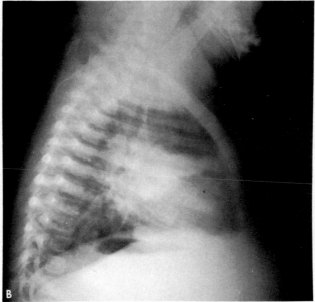

Figure 16. Roentgenograms showing the value of a lateral view. Extensive infiltration and hilar adenopathy in the lateral view (primary pulmonary tuberculosis). (See also Fig. 20.)

conversion of the tuberculin reaction from negative to positive, is more likely to be demonstrable on a roentgenogram in infants and small children. The incidence decreases with age. The primary parenchymal focus is usually small in comparison with the involved lymph nodes, and is more often not demonstrable on a roentgenogram.

Care should be exercised in positioning the patient for a roentgenogram, since relatively minor rotations of the body may result in distortions of the hilar or mediastinal areas. Braids of

hair should be pinned up, and all radiopaque objects, such as identification
tags or medals, should be removed
from the field prior to the roentgenogram.

Most important of all, films should be
made on maximal inspiration. During
expiration there will be widening of the
mediastinum, increase in the transverse
diameter of the heart and often suffusion of the lung parenchyma. Figure 17
is an illustration of this. The first film
was taken when the child was crying
loudly and was in a marked expiratory
phase. The second roentgenogram was
taken immediately thereafter. The

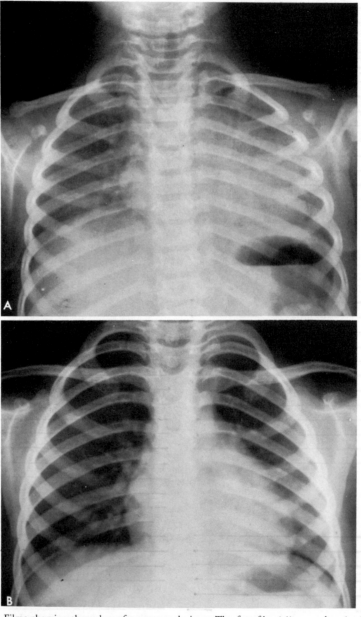

Figure 17. Films showing the value of proper technique. The first film (*A*) was taken in the expiratory phase, and the second (*B*) in the inspiratory phase. (Same patient a few minutes later.)

diaphragm should be at least as low as the eighth rib posteriorly, even in the smallest infant.

Care should be taken to avoid unnecessary exposure to radiation, and should always include a protective shield over the lower part of the abdomen.

RECOVERY OF TUBERCLE BACILLI. The diagnosis of tuberculosis is established with certainty by the finding of tubercle bacilli. Careful search for these organisms should always be made.

In infants and children, organisms reaching the pharynx from lung lesions are promptly swallowed. Examination of the gastric contents thus provides a useful way by which the diagnosis of tuberculosis may be proved. Yet the number of bacilli and the frequency of positive cultures recovered by gastric lavage are usually small, and it is, therefore, recommended that this procedure be carried out each day for three successive days. In the Child Chest Clinic of the Medical College of Virginia, single gastric cultures of children with a positive tuberculin reaction and little or no roentgenographic evidence of disease are productive of tubercle bacilli in only about 6 per cent of the cases. The infrequency of positive gastric cultures lessens the value of this procedure as a diagnostic aid.

Gastric lavage should be performed early in the morning after an overnight fast. The contents of the stomach are aspirated and placed in a sterile container. After this the stomach may be irrigated with 60 ml. of sterile water, and this is aspirated and added to the material in the container. Not all workers believe this second step is necessary, but if this is done, only sterile water should be used, since atypical mycobacteria may often be present in tap water. Direct examination of gastric contents of children with primary pulmonary tuberculosis is of little value, and the material should be promptly cultured on special media for at least two months.

Bronchial secretions for both direct examination and culture may be obtained at the time of bronchoscopy. Fluids obtained from the drainage of abscesses, by paracentesis, and especially cerebrospinal fluid, should have direct examination and culture. All cultures should be done immediately.

BIOPSY. Under satisfactory antimicrobial coverage, biopsy of the pleura and lymph nodes can now be safely performed. Some of the material obtained should be cultured and the rest submitted for histopathologic examination.

BRONCHOSCOPY. Bronchoscopy is indicated in many patients whose roentgenograms show an area of increased density suggestive of segmental obstruction. This procedure should be carried out only under optimum conditions, however. Both the bronchoscopist and the anesthesiologist should be experienced in the management of children, and satisfactory hospital arrangements should be provided.

PULMONARY FUNCTION. Although the majority of children with pulmonary tuberculosis suffer no impairment of lung function, pulmonary function tests may be of help in assessing the possible risks and benefits of surgery.

The Story of Tuberculosis

After tuberculous infection has taken place, there is a two- to ten-week period of incubation during which tubercle bacilli are conveyed from the portal of entry by way of the lymphatics to the regional lymph nodes. The lymph nodes become hyperemic and edematous and may later contain areas of caseation. In over 95 per cent of the cases, the primary focus is in the lung parenchyma.

At the close of this incubation period, allergy appears, as manifested by a positive tuberculin reaction. At this time, then, the patient has primary pulmonary tuberculosis. There are few, if any, symptoms, and the diagnosis is usually made by means of a routine tuberculin test or by one performed because of known contact with tuberculosis.

Most patients with tuberculous infection seen at the Medical College of Virginia have a negative chest roentgenogram and no physical evidence of tuberculous disease. The positive reaction to the tuberculin test is the only clue to the presence of tuberculous infection (tuberculous infection, without disease). A smaller number of children have roentgenographic evidence of disease (primary pulmonary tuberculosis). Most of these have no demonstrable primary parenchymal focus, but the chest roentgenogram shows an area of increased density in the region of the hilus, caused by the edematous lymph nodes. A still smaller group has roentgenographic evidence of a primary parenchymal focus as well as enlarged regional lymph nodes.

In a rare case the primary lesion is not in the lung parenchyma, and physical examination may reveal evidence of tuberculous disease elsewhere.

Primary tuberculosis tends to heal, but the process may become progressive. It may cause progressive destruction at the initial site, or there may be erosion of a bronchus with intrabronchial dissemination and other pulmonary lesions. If there is a massive hematogenous distribution, there will be a widespread formation of tubercles. In any of these instances, the patient will usually give some symptomatic evidence of the worsening of the disease process.

Near the close of the incubation period, there is usually a transient bacillemia. In this way, too, tuberculous foci may be set up throughout the body and remain quiescent for many years. The heaviest distribution of hematogenous seeding is likely to be in the lung, but any of the viscera may be involved. Most of the complications that result later from these foci are not immediately blood-borne. Tuberculous meningitis, for example, is likely to result from the breakdown of a contiguous tuberculoma, previously seeded.

Treatment

Isoniazid and streptomycin have been largely responsible for the drastic reduction in mortality from tuberculosis that has occurred during the past 35 years. The present-day approach to the management of this serious disease must include early diagnosis, isolation of infected persons, judicious use of BCG vaccine (prophylaxis) and the utilization of the available effective antituberculosis drugs.

An optimum therapeutic result can be achieved only when the diagnosis is established early. Since little reliance can be placed on symptoms, a routine tuberculin test is necessary in order to establish the early diagnosis of tuberculosis in childhood. An intradermal tuberculin test (Mantoux), utilizing PPD (5 TU), old tuberculin solution (10 TU), the tuberculin tine test or the Mono-Vacc skin test, should be performed on all children between six and eight months of age and annually thereafter. In those areas of the country where the incidence of tuberculosis is very low, biennial testing may suffice. The importance of the tuberculin test properly done, measured and recorded represents a major diagnostic tool in the recognition and control of tuberculosis. As indicated earlier, the tuberculin test is, of course, always indicated when there has been known contact with a tuberculous adult. In the latter instance, if the tuberculin reaction is negative, the test should be repeated ten weeks after the removal of the contact. If the child remains in contact with a tuberculous adult, the tuberculin test should be repeated at three-month intervals.

PREVENTIVE THERAPY. When the diagnosis has been established, proper therapy for the patient can be promptly instituted and precautions arranged for the prevention of infection of those in contact with the patient. Results from the United States Public Health Service Isoniazid Prophylaxis Study among household contacts suggest that the use of isoniazid is effective in reducing the incidence of tuberculous disease in this group.

A group of 117 infants born of mothers who had tuberculosis at the time of delivery, shortly beforehand or soon afterward was evaluated in Richmond. The most significant finding was the fact that the removal of the infant or child from the mother was not always enough to prevent later infection in the child. Even though 73 of the children were isolated from their respective mothers until the mother was sputum-negative, 38, or more than 50 per cent, became infected with tuberculosis when returned to the home environment. It is advised that infants born of tuberculous mothers receive BCG vaccine as soon as practicable in order to prevent infection.

GENERAL THERAPY. Whenever a child has been found to be tuberculin-positive, location and removal of the tuberculosis contact must be accomplished as soon as possible. This search entails tuberculin testing and a chest roentgenogram of all adult contacts, including parents, grandparents, baby sitters, household servants and any others who may have been in contact with the child.

An adequate diet (high protein) and the usual vitamin supplement for a growing child are necessary, but the question of bed rest varies with the type of disease. The child with asymptomatic primary tuberculosis requires no limitation of activity, and even those who are acutely ill should be allowed some activity as soon as possible, since it is recognized that complete bed rest may result in undesirable negative calcium and nitrogen balance.

The child should be protected from intercurrent infection, since not only measles, but also any acute infection, may lower resistance. The tuberculin-positive child who has measles while not then receiving therapy should be given isoniazid for a period of about six to eight weeks. The tuberculin-positive child who has not had measles should be protected against this disease by the use of measles vaccine, but he should receive isoniazid therapy for at least six to eight weeks when the vaccine is administered. Protection of the child from a source of tuberculous infection in the home is a necessity.

Sharp restriction of activity may be necessary (although today less often and for a shorter time) with certain types of tuberculous disease. Such restriction of activity has psychologic implications that may handicap the child. The child so affected should have a room of his own that is comfortable, well lighted, well ventilated and sufficiently accessible that his care can be easily managed. He should be made as self-sufficient as possible and should have a daily schedule of work and play. A Sadler footrest provides additional comfort for the child propped in a sitting position in bed.

The greatest problem is presented by children between two and six years of age. Interest may be promoted for these by picture books, unpainted blocks, housekeeping toys, dolls with numerous changes in costume, crayon color books, clay, simple wooden puzzles, "matching" games, and an occasional grab-bag consisting of a dozen ten to 25 cent toys.

Older children are more easily amused and may find pleasure in reading, drawing or crayon-coloring; weaving, knitting, soap carving and construction sets may also be useful. Carefully selected radio and television programs and phonograph records are entertaining and, indeed, may be helpful for the younger children, too.

Although restlessness and dissatisfaction will occasionally occur in the younger children, the older children, especially those approaching puberty, are the ones most prone to episodes of deep mental depression. These should be carefully watched for, and remedied promptly.

During the convalescent period, the older child may find enjoyment in photography or painting, and as soon as possible, arrangements should be made for the school child to keep up with his school work.

Chest roentgenograms at appropriate intervals are necessary.

ANTIMICROBIAL AGENTS. Isoniazid (INH), streptomycin (SM), para-aminosalicylic acid (PAS), ethambutol, and rifampin are the antimicrobial agents of greatest efficacy in the treatment of tuberculosis in childhood. Other drugs, including pyrazinamide, viomycin, cycloserine and kanamycin, have limited value.

Isoniazid (INH). Isoniazid is the most effective antituberculosis agent yet available. After oral administration of the drug, a plasma concentration 20 to 80 times the usual inhibiting concentration of the drug (0.05 microgram per milliliter) may be attained within a few hours, and effective high concentrations persist for six to eight hours. Isoniazid penetrates the cell membrane and moves freely into the cerebrospinal fluid and into caseous tissue. The drug may be found in the breast milk of those mothers receiving INH therapy and may also cross the placental barrier. INH is excreted mainly in the urine. The principal side-effects of the drug are neurotoxic, manifested as either convulsions or peripheral neuritis, and probably result from competitive inhibition of pyridoxine metabolism. Such side-effects have been noted mainly in adults, however, and pyridoxine deficiency does not appear to be a problem in children, although precautions must be exercised during adolescence. Pyridoxine, 25 to 50 mg. daily (10 mg. for each 100 mg. of isoniazid), should be added to the treatment schedule during this period. Other side-effects include gastrointestinal dysfunction and allergic reactions. Rarely, isoniazid may be hepatotoxic. Since he-

patic dysfunction is now reported more frequently (mainly in adults) than was the case in previous years, the parent of the patient for whom INH is prescribed should be questioned carefully at monthly intervals for any symptoms or signs of the toxic effects of isoniazid. Indeed, some clinics include serum bilirubin and serum glutamic oxaloacetic transaminase determinations at the time of institution of therapy, again after 6 to 12 weeks of INH therapy, and finally at the time of termination of therapy. When diphenylhydantoin (Dilantin) is given with isoniazid, interaction of the drugs may produce central nervous system symptoms, excessive sedation and incoordination. Careful observation of patients receiving diphenylhydantoin is indicated.

The question of adequate dosage may be approached in one of two ways. Since children tolerate isoniazid much better than do adults, the dosage may be increased to 20 mg. per kilogram of body weight per day, with a maximum daily dosage of 500 mg. On the other hand, combined therapy with PAS may be utilized. Since para-aminosalicylic acid apparently competes with isoniazid for acetylation in the liver, this competitive effect results in a higher blood level of isoniazid. The present trend in the treatment of tuberculosis is the simultaneous use of isoniazid and para-aminosalicylic acid or another antimicrobial agent (streptomycin, rifampin, or ethambutol). In the treatment of pulmonary tuberculosis in adults, ethambutol has largely replaced PAS. Although triple drug therapy has been shown to have little statistical advantage over treatment by two drugs (if one of the drugs is isoniazid), it is nevertheless preferred by many investigators in the treatment of such serious forms of the disease as tuberculous meningitis and miliary tuberculosis.

Although primary isoniazid-resistant tuberculosis has been reported in children, the significance has not yet been determined. Certainly, the recommendation (Steiner and coworkers, 1974) that initial therapy in children be based on the drug-susceptibility pattern of the source case strain should be heeded. If this information is not available, patients with life-threatening forms of tuberculosis should be treated with at least three antimicrobial agents.

Isoniazid is available for oral administration in tablets of 50 mg., 100 mg., and 300 mg. or in a flavored syrup containing 10 mg. per milliliter. A preparation for parenteral administration (intramuscular or intrathecal) is also available. A chemical test for the presence of INH in the urine may be of help in the determination of patient compliance.

Streptomycin (SM). Streptomycin was isolated from *Streptomyces griseus* in 1944, and became the first effective antibiotic agent against tuberculosis. The drug inhibits growth of the tubercle bacillus in a concentration of 1.6 micrograms per milliliter. After parenteral administration, the drug rapidly appears in the blood stream, reaching a peak value in two hours. It diffuses into the pleural fluid, but does not pass the cerebrospinal fluid barrier to any appreciable extent unless there is inflammation of the meninges. Streptomycin is largely excreted in the urine, with an 80 per cent recovery within 24 hours after administration.

The principal toxic effect of streptomycin is involvement of the eighth cranial nerve. Although loss of vestibular function may be permanent, children usually adjust to this defect without symptoms. Involvement of the auditory branch constitutes a real danger, but this effect is much less frequent now than it was in the days of prolonged streptomycin therapy. Allergic manifestations, such as fever and dermatitis, may occur, and agranulocytosis has been reported.

Streptomycin is administered by intramuscular injection in a suggested dosage of 20 to 40 mg. per kilogram of body weight per day, with a maximal daily dosage of 1 gm. Dosage is at the lower level (20 mg.) except in meningitis and other fulminating forms of tuberculosis. Although a single daily injection of the drug is usually given, the daily dose may be divided into two injections for a small or emaciated patient.

Streptomycin is never used as the sole therapeutic agent because of the rapid development of drug resistance. It is routinely given with at least one other tuberculostatic agent.

Experience has not proved the value of the intrathecal administration of streptomycin, and use of the drug in this manner has been largely discontinued.

Streptomycin is supplied in crystalline form, usually as a sulfate, in vials containing 1 gm. and 5 gm.

Para-aminosalicylic Acid (PAS). Para-aminosalicylic acid has some bacteriostatic activity against the tubercle bacillus, and also acts to delay the emergence of microbial resistance to streptomycin. Thus it was of great value when streptomycin was the most effective antimicrobial agent. It also delays bacterial resistance to isoniazid.

As mentioned earlier, the chief value of PAS lies in the fact that it apparently competes with isoniazid for acetylation in the liver, thereby increasing the amount of free isoniazid in the blood.

PAS is administered orally and is readily absorbed. The drug diffuses to some extent into serous surfaces and reaches the cerebrospinal fluid in small amounts. PAS has no intracellular activity. It is rapidly excreted in the urine.

Gastrointestinal disturbances constitute the principal toxic manifestations, but hypokalemia, goitrogenic effect, jaundice and leukopenia may occur. PAS may also be the cause of severe allergic reactions, including dermatoses and an otherwise unexplained fever.

Children usually have a much better tolerance for all forms of PAS than do adults. The drug should be prescribed in a dosage of 200 mg. per kilogram of body weight per day in three or four divided doses. PAS is better tolerated after meals. When salts of para-aminosalicylic acid (sodium, potassium, calcium) are used, the dosage should be correspondingly higher, 250 to 300 mg. per kilogram of body weight per day (maximum daily dose 12 gm.). PAS is supplied in 0.5 gm. tablets, as a powder, or as a solution of the sodium salt. The solution is stable for only 24 hours, and then only if kept in the dark and refrigerated.

Ethambutol. Ethambutol is an effective antimicrobial agent that acts by delaying the multiplication of bacteria through interference with RNA synthesis. It is rapidly excreted in the urine. Like PAS, when it is given in combination with other antimicrobial agents, it delays the onset of microbial resistance. It is also better tolerated and has less tendency to produce toxic effects than does PAS. So far, the drug has been used mostly in adults, where it appears to have largely replaced PAS. The dosage utilized for children at the Medical College of Virginia is 20 mg. per kilogram of body weight per day for four to six weeks, and 10 to 15 mg. per kilogram of body weight per day thereafter. With higher dosage, a few instances of retrobulbar neuritis with resultant loss of vision have been noted in adults. At the recommended dose and with precautions that include a preliminary study prior to the institution of therapy, monthly studies of visual acuity and visual fields and tests for color vision, there appears to be much less danger of this complication. The drug should be discontinued if there is a two-line loss of visual acuity as measured on a Snellen eye chart, if there is contraction of visual fields or if there is loss of color vision. In view of the foregoing, ethambutol is rarely used in young children and only when a severe form of tuberculosis exists. Ethambutol is supplied in 100 mg. and 400 mg. tablets and is administered in a single daily oral dose.

Rifampin. Rifampin is the newest and one of the most promising of the antituberculosis chemotherapeutic agents. It is a semisynthetic, orally administered derivative of rifamycin SV, and thus far appears to be relatively nontoxic, although occasional liver toxicity has been noted. Gastrointestinal disturbances, dermatosis and reversible leukopenia may occur. Action of the drug is by inhibition of DNA-dependent RNA polymerase. It is absorbed in all tissues but crosses the cerebrospinal fluid barrier only when there is infection. Elimination is by way of the urine and bile. Rifampin is recommended for use in combination with at least one other antituberculosis drug. Suggested dosage is 10 to 20 mg. per kilogram of body weight per day (maximum daily dose 600 mg.). Rifampin is administered in a single daily dose and is supplied in 300 mg. capsules.

Ethionamide. Ethionamide is also available for use in combination with one or more antituberculosis agents when bacterial resistance to isoniazid and streptomycin exists. Dosage for children has not yet been established, but a suggested dosage is 10 to 20 mg. per kilogram of body weight per day in two or three divided doses. The maximum daily dose is 750 mg. Ethionamide may be hepatotoxic and is a frequent cause of gastrointestinal dysfunction. The drug is administered orally and is supplied in 250 mg. tablets. The drug may also be given rectally.

Pyrazinamide. Although pyrazinamide has been found to be an effective drug for a short time, its ensuing ineffectiveness cannot be correlated with the emergence of pyrazinamide-resistant tubercle bacilli. There has also been much evidence of hepatic toxicity. The Committee on Therapy of the American Thoracic Society (1957) concluded that when used alone, pyrazinamide had only a limited beneficial effect, and that its serious hepatotoxic action tends to outweigh its therapeutic value. The drug is administered orally in a dosage of 20 to 30 mg. per kilogram of body weight per day (maximum 2 gm.) in three divided doses. It is supplied in tablets containing 0.5 gm. of the drug.

Viomycin. Viomycin is another drug derived from a fungus of the Streptomyces group. It has tuberculostatic properties that make it available for the treatment of tuberculosis, but it is less potent than streptomycin and is not devoid of toxicity. Such toxic manifestations include depletion of plasma electrolytes, increased blood urea nitrogen level, the appearance of albumin, casts, and white and red blood cells in the urine, acoustic nerve damage, unexplained fever, eosinophilia and urticaria. The drug is rarely used in children, therefore, and is indicated only when other therapy is not effective. It is administered intramuscularly twice weekly in a dosage of 30 mg. per kilogram of body weight and should always be utilized in combination with another antituberculosis agent. It is supplied as a sulfate in vials containing 1 gm. and 5 gm.

Cycloserine. Also derived from a member of the Streptomyces group, cycloserine is not as effective as isoniazid or streptomycin. It has also shown a number of toxic effects, the tendency toward convulsions being the most important. Cycloserine is given orally in a dosage of 5 to 15 mg. per kilogram of body weight per day in two divided doses (less in renal tuberculosis). Maximum daily dosage is 500 mg. It is supplied in 250 mg. capsules.

Kanamycin. Kanamycin is a streptomycin-like drug, which may have all the toxic effects of streptomycin and, in addition, may show renal toxicity. It is rarely used in the treatment of tuberculosis in children. Dosage is 10 to 15 mg. per kilogram of body weight per day.

Capreomycin. Capreomycin, a derivative of *Streptomyces capreolus*, is rarely used in the treatment of tuberculosis in children. Side effects include nephrotoxicity and eighth cranial nerve involvement.

Adrenocorticosteroids. Apparently, cortisone acts to suppress the usual inflammatory response of the body with impairment of granulation tissue formation, macrophage activity and fibroblastic repair. From the nature of this mechanism, it appears likely that cortisone promotes progression of tuberculous disease in the lung. This deleterious effect can be overcome, however, by specific effective antimicrobial treatment. Indications for the use of adrenocorticosteroids in specific forms of tuberculosis will be presented under individual headings.

GENERAL PRINCIPLES OF ANTIMICROBIAL THERAPY. Isoniazid is at present the most effective antituberculosis drug known. Not only is it the most effective therapeutic agent, but also it is the only drug that tends to prevent complications of tuberculous disease. Accordingly, it must be included in every therapeutic regimen, unless contraindicated because of the patient's intolerance to the drug (allergy or hepatic dysfunction) or because the causative organism is isoniazid-resistant.

Isoniazid is used alone in the treatment of a positive tuberculin reaction and primary tuberculosis. In progressive primary tuberculosis, isoniazid is used in conjunction with para-aminosalicylic acid. In such severe forms of tuberculosis as miliary tuberculosis and tuberculous meningitis, a triple drug regimen with isoniazid, streptomycin and rifampin should be utilized. Steiner's report of primary isoniazid-resistant tuberculosis in children substantiates the need for therapy in children to be based on the drug-susceptibility pattern of the source case strain. If this information is unavailable, children with life-threatening forms of tuberculosis should be treated with at least three antimicrobial agents.

CLASSIFICATION OF TUBERCULOSIS

The new classification of tuberculosis as determined by the Committee on

Diagnostic Standards of the American Thoracic Society (1974) is as follows:

0. No tuberculosis exposure, not infected (no history of exposure, negative tuberculin skin test).

I. Tuberculosis exposure, no evidence of infection (history of exposure, negative tuberculin skin test).

II. Tuberculous infection, without disease (positive tuberculin skin test, negative bacteriologic studies [if done], no roentgenographic findings compatible with tuberculosis, no symptoms due to tuberculosis).

III. Tuberculosis: infected, with disease.

    A. Location of disease (predominant site; other sites if significant).

    B. Bacteriologic status.

    C. Chemotherapy status.

    D. Roentgenogram findings.

    E. Tuberculin skin test.

Tuberculosis Suspect: may be used until diagnostic procedures are complete but not for more than three months.

POSITIVE TUBERCULIN REACTION

As noted above, the Committee on Diagnostic Standards of the American Thoracic Society classifies the patient who has a positive tuberculin reaction with no evidence of disease elsewhere as "tuberculous infection, without disease." However, it has been established that in more than 95 per cent of the cases, the initial lesion of primary tuberculosis is in the lung parenchyma. If, therefore, there is a positive tuberculin reaction with no evidence of tuberculous disease elsewhere, it must be assumed that there is a primary focus in the lung parenchyma, too small to be visible on roentgenogram, with associated regional gland involvement. At

the Medical College of Virginia this is the most common form of tuberculous infection.

Treatment

As far as is known, no available antimicrobial agent will eradicate tubercle bacilli. The aim of antimicrobial therapy, therefore, is not only the arrest of the existing tuberculous condition, but also the prevention of the complications of the disease. So far, sufficient evidence is not available for the assumption that antimicrobial therapy is effective in the treatment of primary tuberculosis itself. No drug, other than isoniazid, has shown the capability to prevent the more serious forms of the disease, such as tuberculous meningitis, miliary tuberculosis and Pott's disease.

Whenever a patient less than six years of age has a positive tuberculin reaction, with no physical or roentgenographic evidence of disease, he should be given isoniazid in a dosage of 10 to 15 mg. per kilogram of body weight per day for one year (Table 4). The drug is administered orally in a single daily dose or in two divided doses at the time of the morning and evening meals. It has been our experience that a crushed tablet in jam, preserves or applesauce constitutes the most practical method of administration. This is preferable to the use of the available flavored syrup, the potency of which may be variable. Such a child is not considered infectious, and his activity is not curtailed. Unless complications arise, it is necessary for the patient to be seen by the attending physician only once each month during the period in which he receives medication and annually thereafter. Follow-up roentgenograms, one to three months after diagnosis and again at the completion of one year of therapy, are suggested. Naturally, if there is symptomatic evidence of worsening of the disease process during that period, such a routine must be correspondingly altered. After the first year, an annual or bien-

TABLE 4. TREATMENT OF PATIENT WITH POSITIVE TUBERCULIN REACTION

	Drug	Daily Dosage	Number of Daily Doses	Maximum Daily Dose	Duration of Therapy
Positive tuberculin reaction	INH	10–15 mg./kg.	1 or 2	300 mg.	12 months

nial chest roentgenogram is indicated. This annual or biennial roentgenogram should be continued through puberty and adolescence, particularly in girls, who merit special attention during that period of life. The tuberculous adult is removed from contact with the patient as soon as possible.

Brailey's (1944) work indicates that the first year after infection with tuberculosis is the most dangerous period, and it is recommended that any child who converts from a negative to a positive tuberculin reaction within a one-year period be given the same treatment as that outlined above. This, of course, accentuates the value of the routine annual tuberculin test (Table 4).

Although it is not nearly so certain that a child over the age of six years with a positive tuberculin reaction and no physical or roentgenographic evidence of tuberculous disease benefits from isoniazid therapy, there is now general agreement that *any* child with a positive tuberculin reaction and no other evidence of disease should receive isoniazid for a one-year period. If such a child does not receive antimicrobial therapy—and most of them *do*—he should have a careful follow-up, with routine monthly examinations, an occasional roentgenogram through the ensuing year and an annual chest roentgenogram thereafter.

All children, particularly girls, with a positive tuberculin reaction merit special attention during puberty and adolescence. At present, it is our policy to institute a one-year course of isoniazid therapy in those adolescents who have been demonstrated to have a positive tuberculin reaction and who have not received a previous course of isoniazid

therapy. For those pregnant adolescents with a positive tuberculin reaction, it may be preferable to delay INH prophylaxis until delivery has been effected.

PRIMARY PULMONARY TUBERCULOSIS

The primary complex is composed of the primary focus, the involved regional lymph nodes and the lymphatics between them. Primary tuberculosis includes the primary complex and the progression of any of its components.

After tuberculous infection there is a two- to ten-week period of incubation. During this time there is an accumulation of polymorphonuclear leukocytes and then epithelioid cell proliferation, producing a typical tubercle; giant cells make their appearance, and the area is surrounded by lymphocytes. These organisms are carried by the lymphatics to the regional lymph nodes, and the lymphatics contained in the area between the primary parenchymal focus and the regional lymph nodes constitute the interfocal zone. At the end of the incubation period, the presence of allergy is manifested by a positive tuberculin reaction. The patient, who is usually asymptomatic, has primary pulmonary tuberculosis.

Before the body tissues develop hypersensitivity to tuberculin, the primary focus may become larger, but does not become encapsulated. When hypersensitivity develops, the perifocal reaction becomes much more prominent, and the regional lymph nodes enlarge. The primary focus may become caseous; however, with the development of acquired resistance, it is usually walled off. The caseous material gradually becomes inspissated and later calcified or may completely disappear. The lesion, of course, may become progressive.

Patients with uncomplicated primary tuberculosis may be divided into three groups: those with roentgenographic evidence of mediastinal gland enlargement, but without evidence of a primary parenchymal focus; those with a demonstrable primary complex; and those with evidence of extrapulmonary primary tuberculosis.

The most common form of primary tuberculosis (excluding the positive tuberculin reaction with no evidence of disease elsewhere) is the patient whose chest roentgenogram shows enlarged mediastinal lymph nodes with no demonstrable primary parenchymal focus (Fig. 18). In such instances, when the disease process has healed, demonstrable calcific deposits will often be present at one or more sites in the lung parenchyma as well as in the hilus (Ghon complex). This calcification in the lung parenchyma is indicative of a healed primary focus that had never been visible on roentgenogram (Fig. 19). Less common is the primary complex with both a demonstrable primary parenchymal focus and enlarged hilar lymph nodes. Figure 20 shows a primary complex with demonstrable involvement of the interfocal zone in the lateral view.

Finally, there is a small group of patients who have a positive tuberculin reaction and no roentgenographic evidence of disease, but in whom there is an extrapulmonary tuberculous lesion demonstrable on physical examination, e.g., enlargement of a superficial cervical lymph node.

If the primary complex appears on the roentgenogram at all, it appears at the time of the onset of the disease. It may show progression for one to two months and does not begin to diminish for three to four months. It may remain visible for six to 12 months, or even longer. Resolution of the primary complex is apparently not hastened by antimicrobial therapy.

As far as can be determined, no patient with a primary parenchymal focus without enlarged regional lymph nodes has ever been seen at the Medical College of Virginia. Because of the lymphatic drainage in the mediastinum, a primary focus in the left lung parenchyma may be associated with enlarged lymph nodes on both the left and right sides. In our experience, a focus in the right lung has not been the cause of enlarged lymph nodes on the left.

Calcification is more often seen in the regional lymph nodes than in the

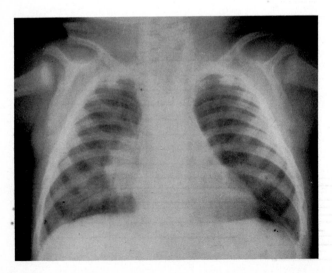

Figure 18. Primary pulmonary tuberculosis, with enlarged mediastinal lymph nodes, right. (Courtesy of *Am. J. Dis. Child.*, 88:148, 1954.)

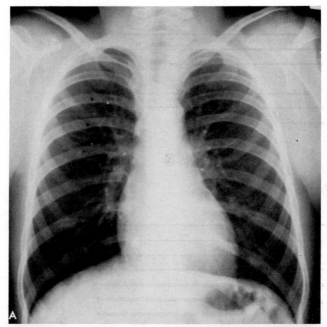

Figure 19. Calcific densities indicating the presence and location of the healed primary complex (Ghon complex). The primary parenchymal focus was not visible on the roentgenogram taken during the acute phase of the disease.

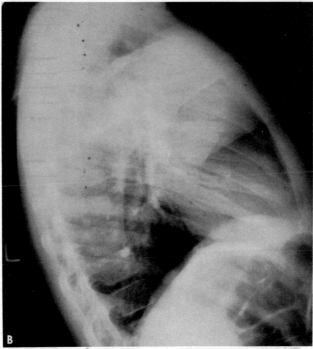

parenchymal foci, probably because there is early migration of the tubercle bacilli from the parenchymal focus to the regional lymph nodes. The first sign of calcification may appear within six months after the diagnosis of pri-

mary tuberculosis in an infant, or somewhat later in an older child.

As previously stressed, the diagnosis of primary tuberculosis is practically always accomplished by means of the tuberculin test, performed either rou-

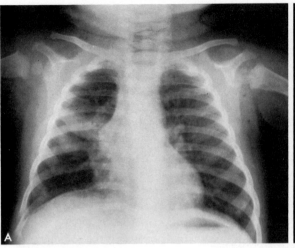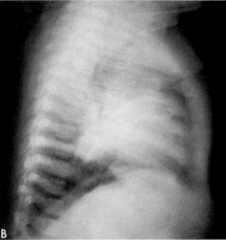

Figure 20. Primary complex with demonstrable involvement of the interfocal zone (visible on lateral view, *B*).

tinely or because of the history of contact with a tuberculous adult. Symptoms and signs are rarely of benefit.

Whenever a positive reaction occurs in the tuberculin test, a chest roentgenogram is indicated, and this should include both an anteroposterior and a lateral view.

The prognosis of unhealed primary tuberculosis depends largely on the age of the patient, on the duration of infection, and to some degree on the extent of the primary lesion. Whenever calcification is seen on the roentgenogram, it may be assumed that the infection is at least six months old. Thus, the presence of calcification is of good prognostic import, but the amount of calcification and the persistence of roentgenographic evidence of the primary infection are important, too (Fig. 21).

Treatment

The child of any age with roentgenographic evidence of primary pulmonary tuberculosis should be treated in exactly the same manner (Table 5) as that utilized in the treatment of a child with a positive tuberculin reaction, except that INH dosage is 10 to 20 mg. per kilogram of body weight per day, and the maximum daily dose is 400 mg.

PROGRESSIVE PRIMARY PULMONARY TUBERCULOSIS

Local progression of the pulmonary component of the primary complex occasionally occurs, but at the Medical College of Virginia it is a rarity. When this does occur, the area of caseation enlarges and then liquefies, and the contents are disseminated into the bronchi, thereby setting up new pulmonary foci of disease. This is a severe form of tuberculosis that occurs much more often in young children, and when it is untreated, the mortality rate

TABLE 5. TREATMENT OF ASYMPTOMATIC PRIMARY TUBERCULOSIS

Drug	Daily Dosage	Number of Daily Doses	Maximum Daily Dose	Duration of Therapy
Isoniazid	10–20 mg./kg.	1 or 2	400 mg.	12 months

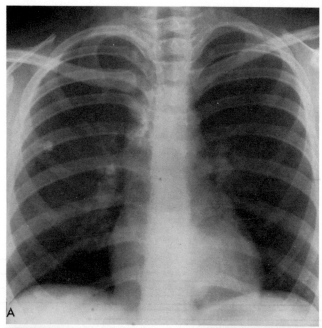

Figure 21. Calcified primary complex with no evidence of active tuberculous disease.

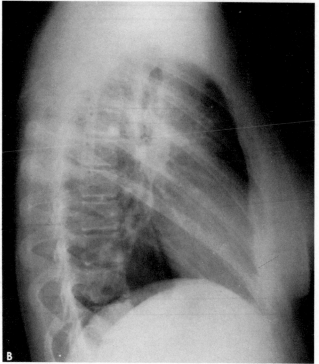

TABLE 6.   TREATMENT OF PROGRESSIVE PRIMARY
(PULMONARY) TUBERCULOSIS

Drug	Daily Dosage	Number of Daily Doses	Maximum Daily Dose	Duration of Therapy
Isoniazid	15–20 mg./kg.	1 or 2	500 mg.	12 months or longer
PAS	200 mg./kg.	3 or 4	12 gm.	12 months or longer
If response is unsatisfactory, add streptomycin	20 mg./kg.	1 (2)	1 gm.	One month after satisfactory clinical response
For endobronchial disease, add prednisone	1 mg./kg.	4	60 mg.	6–12 weeks

is high (above 50 per cent). Symptoms of progressive disease are persistent fever, anorexia, apathy and loss of weight. Physical examination of the chest is most often noncontributory, but there may be moist rales over the diseased area.

Prompt antimicrobial therapy of primary pulmonary tuberculosis is practically always successful in preventing this form of tuberculous disease. When the diagnosis of tuberculosis is not made until the disease has reached this stage, the prognosis is less favorable.

Treatment

Pulmonary progression of primary tuberculosis requires an intense therapeutic approach. Antimicrobial therapy consists of isoniazid, 15 to 20 mg. per kilogram of body weight, with a maximum daily dose of 500 mg., and para-aminosalicylic acid, 200 mg. per kilogram of body weight, with a maximum daily dose of 12 gm. Isoniazid is given in a single daily dose or in two daily divided doses, and PAS is given in three or four divided doses. If the child does not respond satisfactorily to this treatment, it will be necessary to add streptomycin, 20 mg. per kilogram of body weight per day, with a maximum daily dose of 1 gm. Streptomycin is given once each day by the intramuscular route, although for a small or emaciated patient the daily dose may be divided into two injections. Streptomycin therapy is continued for one month after satisfactory clinical response, but

isoniazid and PAS therapy should be carried out for at least one year, and sometimes longer (Table 6). Rarely, rifampin or ethambutol may be necessary.

When irreversible damage has occurred, surgical resection of the diseased area of the lung may be necessary.

TUBERCULOUS PNEUMONIA (HEMATOGENOUS)

Tuberculous pneumonia of hematogenous origin may also occur. This makes its appearance near the close of the incubation period and is usually accompanied by few, if any, symptoms. On roentgenogram, the lesion itself is indistinguishable from that of a primary parenchymal focus (Fig. 22).

OBSTRUCTIVE LESIONS OF THE BRONCHI (TUBERCULOUS BRONCHITIS OR LYMPH NODE– BRONCHIAL TUBERCULOSIS)

The regional lymph nodes draining the primary parenchymal focus are tuberculous. They become hyperemic

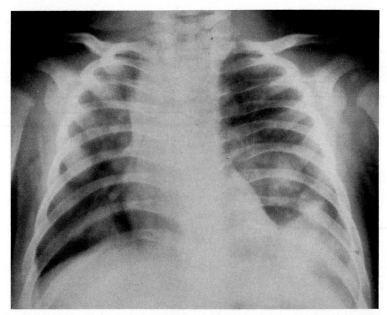

Figure 22. Roentgenogram of infant whose diagnosis was made at 23 days of age, showing several lesions that may be either primary foci or pneumonia of hematogenous origin (indistinguishable on x-ray film). (Courtesy of *Am. Rev. Tuberc.*, 70:161, 1954.)

and edematous and may contain areas of caseation. These nodes may be so placed that they impinge upon the wall of a bronchus, causing occlusion of the lumen and atelectasis of that area of the lung distal to the obstruction (extrabronchial or extraluminal tuberculosis).

Much more often, the infected nodes adhere to the adjacent bronchus. This infection may progress no further than the outer wall of the bronchus, but often penetrates to the mucosa. There may be even further progress of the disease process with ulceration of the mucosa and formation of granulation tissue, which may completely obstruct the lumen of the bronchus. Occasionally, too, a tuberculous node penetrates the wall of the bronchus, creating a sinus tract through which caseous material is extruded into the bronchus. When the lumen of the bronchus is thus occluded, there is atelectasis of

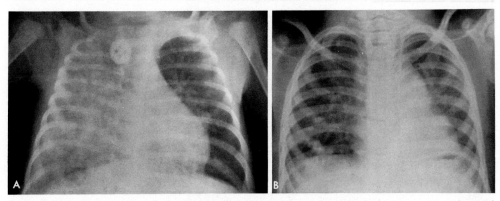

Figure 23. Roentgenograms of infant whose diagnosis was made at 19 days of age, with widespread pulmonary tuberculosis. Patient recovered from the disease. (Courtesy of *Am. Rev. Tuberc.*, 61:747, 1950.)

that area of the lung served by the bronchus (Fig. 24). Under these conditions there may also be an associated pneumonia (Fig. 25). Obviously, tuberculous bronchitis must exist whenever this type of tuberculous pneumonia occurs. Tuberculous bronchitis, however, can be present without an accompanying tuberculous pneumonia.

Bronchoscopy is desirable, but should be carried out only if there is available an experienced bronchoscopist and an anesthesiologist, and the hospital is suitably equipped for the study of infants. If the lesion is extraluminal or if there is no obvious obstructive lesion within the lumen, nothing will be accomplished. In due time, however, the

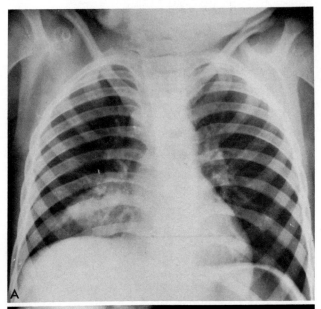

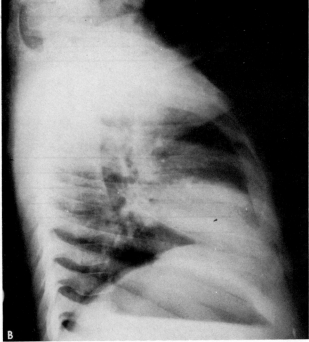

Figure 24. Atelectasis of the right middle lobe. Convex borders also suggest either early atelectasis or an associated pneumonic process.

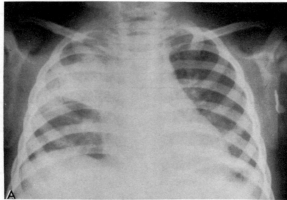

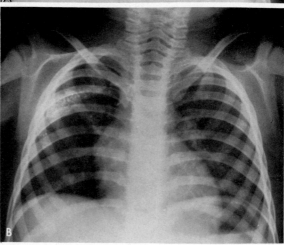

Figure 25. Roentgenograms illustrating tuberculous pneumonia associated with atelectasis. *B* shows heavy calcium deposits in lung parenchyma after clearing of atelectasis and pneumonia. (Courtesy of *Am. J. Dis. Child.*, 88:148, 1954.)

edematous nodes will recede, the lumen of the bronchus will again become patent, and that area of the lung which has been atelectatic will usually become re-aerated. On the other hand, if the lesion is an endobronchial (intraluminal) one, some of the caseous material can be removed and the patency of the lumen often reestablished. Incomplete obstruction of the lumen with a check-valve mechanism, often associated with an intrabronchial polyp, may occur in the same manner and result in hyperaeration (so-called obstructive emphysema) instead of atelectasis (Fig. 26).

Other complications that may occur include the retention of normal secretions, causing edema and congestion of that area of the lung involved, and rarely suffocation as a result of the extrusion of large masses of caseous material into the bronchus with complete obstruction of the airway.

In our experience, atelectasis is seen more often in the right lung, with the middle lobe most often involved and the upper lobe next in frequency.

Treatment

Although the antimicrobial therapy of tuberculous bronchitis is essentially the same as that for other progressive primary tuberculosis, results with this mode of therapy alone have not been satisfactory. For some time there has been a feeling that the use of adrenocorticosteroids, in conjunction with antimicrobial therapy, may be of value in such instances. In an excellent double-blind study involving 100 patients, Nemir and her associates (1963) have concluded that prednisone as an ad-

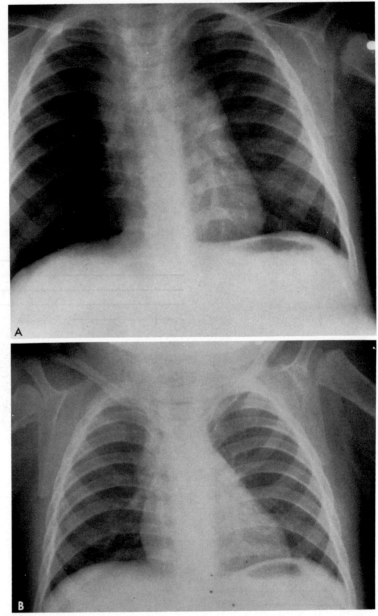

Figure 26. *A,* Hyperaeration (so-called obstructive emphysema) of right lung. *B,* Nineteen days after the addition of prednisone to the therapeutic regimen (INH and PAS), the roentgenogram showed complete clearing of the process.

junct to antimicrobial therapy is most successful when given early in the course of lymph node–bronchial disease, i.e., when there is compression of the bronchus as seen by bronchoscopic examination. In her series, when there was a more advanced stage of lymph node–bronchial tuberculosis (evidence

of rupture of a caseous lymph node into the bronchus), the difference in results obtained with prednisone and placebo was not conclusive.

The response in those patients treated early in the course of disease may be explained on the basis of the lesion in the lymph node. Since sufficient time has not elapsed for occurrence of fibrosis, the anti-inflammatory action of prednisone may pave the way for greater penetration of the lymph node by effective antimicrobial agents.

Experience at the Medical College of Virginia, although not as definitive as that contained in Nemir's material, tends to corroborate her results.

Prednisone in a dosage of 1 mg. per kilogram of body weight should be continued for six to 12 weeks.

J. S., a six-month-old black female infant, was admitted to a study on the therapy of primary tuberculosis conducted at the Medical College of Virginia. Chest roentgenogram showed right hilar adenopathy, and the patient was without symptoms. Isoniazid, 15 mg. per kilogram of body weight, was prescribed, and she was seen each month thereafter for follow-up examination. At the time of her visit five months later (11 months of age) there was a history of anorexia. Physical examination at that time revealed diminished breath sounds and hyperresonance over the entire right side of the chest. Diagnosis of hyperaeration of the right lung (so-called obstructive emphysema) was corroborated by chest roentgenogram. The patient was hospitalized, and bronchoscopy revealed the lumen of the right main bronchus to be almost completely occluded by caseous material. A portion of this material was removed, and para-aminosalicylic acid, 200 mg. per kilogram, and prednisone, 1 mg. per kilogram

of body weight, per day, were added to the therapeutic regimen. Within ten days there was clinical improvement, and within three weeks the hyperaeration was no longer apparent on the chest roentgenogram. Prednisone was continued for 12 weeks, with gradual reduction in dosage before the drug was discontinued. Bronchoscopy before discharge from the hospital showed no evidence of disease (Fig. 26).

TUBERCULOSIS IN THE NEWBORN

Congenital tuberculosis is a rarity, and tuberculosis in the newborn period is relatively uncommon. When the mother is known to have pulmonary tuberculosis, the newborn infant should be isolated from the mother immediately after delivery. However, evaluation of 117 infants in Richmond, Virginia, born of mothers who had tuberculosis at the time of delivery, shortly beforehand, or soon afterward revealed that removal of the infant from the mother was not always enough to prevent later infection in the child. Even though 75 of the children were isolated from their mothers until the mother was sputum-negative, 38 became infected with tuberculosis when returned to the home environment (Table 7).

TABLE 7. EFFECTS OF BCG VACCINATION OF INFANTS OF TUBERCULOUS MOTHERS

Vaccination Status	Maternal Tuberculosis Diagnosed Before Delivery (Number of Infants)	Maternal Tuberculosis Diagnosed After Delivery (Number of Infants)	Total
BCG vaccine			
Infected infants	0	0	0
Noninfected infants	30	0	30
No BCG vaccine			
Infected infants	38 (3 deaths)	8 (1 death)	46
Noninfected infants	37*	4	41
Total Infants	105	12	117

From Kendig, E. L.: *N. Engl. J. Med.*, *281*:520, 1969. Reprinted, by permission, from The New England Journal of Medicine.

*Three patients died, two with pneumonia (no contact with mother) and one at two months of age of undetermined cause.

Nevertheless, when the mother is known to have pulmonary tuberculosis, the newborn infant should be isolated from the mother immediately after delivery. In addition, it is suggested that BCG vaccine be promptly administered to the newborn infant; if the vaccine is administered when the infant is two weeks of age or more, a tuberculin test and chest roentgenogram must be performed prior to vaccination. A negative result should be obtained in both studies before the infant is vaccinated.

After BCG vaccination, the infant's isolation from the mother should be continued for a period of at least six weeks and until the mother's tuberculous disease is so controlled that contact with the infant is deemed advisable.

If the mother has evidence of hematogenous tuberculosis or far advanced pulmonary disease with sputum positive for tubercle bacilli, the infant should be isolated from the mother and should receive INH (15 to 20 mg. per kilogram) for a period of three months. The infant should have a tuberculin test and chest roentgenogram at the end of that period; if these are negative, BCG vaccination is performed. The infant should, of course, be isolated from the mother for an additional six-week period and until the mother is no longer considered infectious (Table 8).

Isoniazid prophylaxis for a one-year period in all children born of tuberculous mothers has also been recommended. However, attention has been called to the fact that despite the absence of neurotoxicity noted among infants treated with INH, neither the pharmacology of this drug nor its efficacy in chemoprophylaxis for the newborn infant has been systematically studied. More important, Sweet (1968) reviewed the records of 25 infants of low socioeconomic background who were born into a tuberculous household. All infants were referred to a special follow-up clinic when discharged from the newborn nursery. Sixteen babies were lost to follow-up observations, all but one before 12 months of age. Only two of the ten patients followed had completed the planned 12 months of isoniazid prophylaxis.

The obvious dangers of this approach seem to make BCG the logical choice for prevention of tuberculosis in infants born of tuberculous mothers.

TABLE 8.   PROPHYLACTIC REGIMEN FOR INFANTS OF TUBERCULOUS MOTHERS

Mother	Infant	Treatment of Infant
Known tuberculosis	Newborn	Maternal isolation (if active disease present)
		BCG vaccine
		Maternal isolation for 6 weeks
	>2 weeks of age	Maternal isolation (if active disease present)
		Tuberculin test and x-ray examination of chest (both negative)
		BCG vaccine
		Maternal isolation for 6 weeks
Miliary or far advanced pulmonary disease	Any age	Maternal isolation
		INH (15–20 mg./kg.) for 3 months
		Tuberculin test and x-ray examination of chest (both negative)
		BCG vaccine
		Maternal isolation for at least 6 weeks and until maternal disease inactive

From Kendig, E. L.: *N. Engl. J. Med.*, *281*:520, 1969. Reprinted, by permission, from The New England Journal of Medicine.

Decision as to the breast-feeding of infants born of tuberculous mothers must be individualized.

If the infant has already acquired tuberculous infection, isoniazid (15 to 20 mg. per kilogram of body weight per day) should be administered for at least one year; if there has been progressive tuberculous involvement, a more radical therapeutic approach is required.

ACUTE MILIARY TUBERCULOSIS

Acute miliary tuberculosis is a generalized hematogenous disease, with multiple tubercle formation and manifestations that are more often pulmonary. It is an early complication of primary tuberculosis and usually occurs within the first six months after the onset of the disease. It is more frequent in infants and young children, but may be seen at any age.

The tubercles, which are of relatively uniform size, result from the lodgment of tubercle bacilli in small capillaries. Necrosis tends to develop in spite of an epithelioid response. The size of the lesions may in part be determined by host resistance. Practically all the organs of the body may be affected, and the lungs are prominently involved.

The onset of miliary tuberculosis is usually acute with high fever, most often remittent. The patient appears acutely ill, but symptoms and signs of respiratory disease may be absent. Enlargement of the spleen, the liver or the superficial lymph nodes may be present in about half of the cases. Initially, in rare instances, there are pulmonary manifestations of acute nature.

About one to two weeks after the onset of the disease, the mottled lesions, resembling snowflakes, make their appearance on the roentgenogram (Fig. 27). Shortly thereafter, fine crepitant rales may be present over the lung fields.

In the untreated cases, the mortality rate is almost 100 per cent. Death occurs within four to 12 weeks, usually as the result of tuberculous meningitis. In the successfully treated cases, subsidence of the fever is slow, the temperature usually reaching a normal level in 14 to 21 days after the institution of therapy. Improvement of the lesions on the roentgenogram is usually demonstrable within five to ten weeks, but the lesions do not disappear until later.

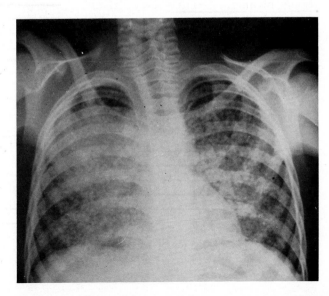

Figure 27. Miliary tuberculosis.

TABLE 9.   TREATMENT OF MILIARY TUBERCULOSIS

Drug	Daily Dosage	Number of Daily Doses	Maximum Daily Dose	Duration of Therapy
INH	20 mg./kg.	1 or 2	500 mg.	12 months or longer
Rifampin*	10–20 mg./kg.	1	600 mg.	12 months or longer
Streptomycin	20–40 mg./kg.	1 (2)	1 gm.	1 month after satisfactory clinical response
Prednisone	1 mg./kg.	4	60 mg.	Used only during period of extreme dyspnea

*After a few months, PAS, 200 mg./kg. (maximum daily dose 12 gm.), may be substituted for rifampin.

Treatment

Therapy consists of a triple drug regimen with isoniazid, 20 mg. per kilogram of body weight per day, rifampin, 10 to 20 mg. per kilogram per day, and streptomycin, 20 to 40 mg. per kilogram per day. After a few months, PAS may be substituted for rifampin. Isoniazid and para-aminosalicylic acid are continued for at least one year, but streptomycin is given for one month after satisfactory clinical response. Adrenocorticosteroids have been recommended for extreme dyspnea, but are used only for the period necessary to control the dyspnea (Table 9). Cerebrospinal fluid examinations should be performed at regular intervals in order to make an early diagnosis should meningitis occur. These examinations should be carried out at weekly intervals during the early stages of treatment and less often thereafter.

PLEURISY WITH EFFUSION

Tuberculosis pleurisy with effusion is a relatively common early complication of primary pulmonary tuberculosis. It occurs much more often during school age, but is not rare even in young infants. In a group of 303 infants infected with tuberculosis when less than two years of age, reviewed at Johns Hopkins Hospital, Hardy and Kendig (1945) found that 3.3 per cent showed roentgenographic evidence of pleurisy with effusion. Approximately twice as many males as females have this complication.

According to Rich (1951), most of the cases of tuberculous pleurisy with effusion result from extension of the infection from a subpleural focus. Hypersensitivity to tuberculin, too, appears to be a factor (Fig. 28).

The onset is usually acute, with high fever and chest pain that is worse on deep inspiration. There may be limitation of respirations on the affected side. Dyspnea and tachycardia may be present when the effusion is massive, and, rarely, there may be bulging of the intercostal spaces.

Fever usually persists for two to three weeks. Although much of the fluid is usually absorbed by the end of this period, some fluid may persist for considerably longer.

Any patient with a serous pleural effusion and a positive reaction to the tuberculin test must be assumed to have tuberculous pleurisy with effusion until proved otherwise. A diagnostic thoracentesis should always be done promptly. No more than 30 ml. of fluid should be withdrawn unless the effusion is so massive that there is respiratory embarrassment. The fluid shows elevation of protein, and the cellular content, predominantly lymphocytes except in the very early stages, varies from 200 to 10,000 per cubic millimeter. Culture of the fluid should be done, but the result will be useful only

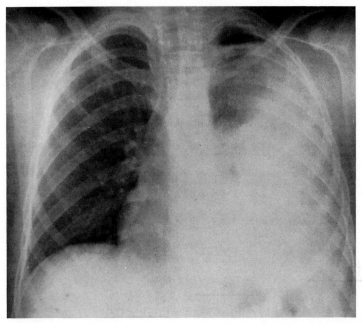

Figure 28. Tuberculous pleurisy with effusion.

as a corroborative measure. Pleural biopsy may also be helpful.

The prognosis depends on the underlying tuberculous disease.

Spontaneous pneumothorax and caseous pleuritis may occur. Tuberculous empyema is rare now, and no case has been seen at the Medical College of Virginia in recent years.

Scoliosis, presumably due to pleural adhesions, is a rare later result of tuberculous pleurisy with effusion, and contraction of a hemithorax is even more rare.

Treatment

Isoniazid, 15 to 20 mg. per kilogram, and para-aminosalicylic acid, 200 mg.

per kilogram of body weight per day, should be given for at least a 12-month period (Table 10). Antimicrobial therapy is thus utilized in order to reduce the danger of progressive tuberculous disease and complications such as tuberculous meningitis. There is also evidence that such therapy promotes a reduction in the incidence of later pulmonary tuberculosis. Specific antimicrobial therapy appears to have no direct effect on the pleurisy with effusion.

Although the study of Filler and Porter (1963) indicates that subsequent pulmonary function is not improved by the use of adrenocorticosteroids, it does appear that they exert an immediately favorable effect on the pleurisy with ef-

TABLE 10. TREATMENT OF TUBERCULOUS PLEURISY WITH EFFUSION

Drug	Daily Dosage	Number of Daily Doses	Maximum Daily Dose	Duration of Therapy
Isoniazid	15–20 mg./kg.	1 or 2	500 mg.	12 months or longer
PAS	200 mg./kg.	3 or 4	12 gm.	12 months or longer
Prednisone	1 mg./kg.	4	60 mg.	Until pleurisy with effusion is controlled

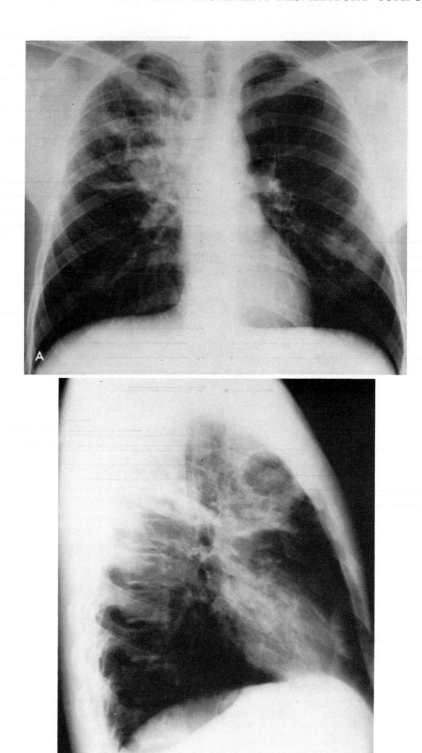

Figure 29.   Chronic pulmonary tuberculosis with cavitation in a 16-year-old male.

fusion, promoting a rapid control of fever and the disappearance of the fluid. The dosage of prednisone is 1 mg. per kilogram of body weight per day in three or four divided doses. This drug is continued until the effusion is controlled. The dosage is then gradually reduced before discontinuation.

CHRONIC PULMONARY TUBERCULOSIS

Chronic pulmonary tuberculosis occurs as a late involvement in those persons who earlier became infected with tubercle bacilli. The interval between the first infection and chronic pulmonary tuberculosis may be short, but the latter is usually a late complication. In our experience, chronic pulmonary tuberculosis is not common in childhood.

Although it has been established that chronic pulmonary tuberculosis can occur as a result of superinfection (exogenous), the presence of the increased resistance to a second infection which follows the primary infection favors the theory that the majority of the cases of chronic pulmonary tuberculosis in children are endogenous in origin.

The lesion of chronic pulmonary tuberculosis usually appears in the apical or subapical portion of the lung (Fig. 29). Since chronic pulmonary tuberculosis occurs when the tissues have already been sensitized to tuberculin, there is a tendency toward localization of the bacilli and not toward spread by way of the lymphatics. After multiplication of the bacilli has occurred, the lesion ulcerates, and the liquefied material is disseminated through the bronchi. The disease, if untreated, will continue to progress, often causing destruction of large areas of lung tissue. At this stage, too, there is occasionally tuberculous enteritis and laryngitis.

Healing occurs by fibrosis and, not nearly so often at this age, by calcification. In addition to the usual closure and obliteration of cavities, there may be re-epithelialization of the bronchocavitary junction, frequently after antimicrobial therapy. This is the so-called open healing (Fig. 30).

The best approach to the early diagnosis of chronic pulmonary tuberculosis is the routine use of the tuberculin test, between six and eight months of age and annually thereafter (biennially in areas of low incidence of tuberculous infection). If a child has a positive tuberculin reaction, an annual or biennial

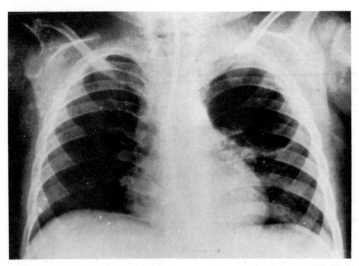

Figure 30.   "Open healing" in a 16-month-old Negro male infant with tuberculous meningitis. Diagnosis corroborated at necrospy. (Courtesy of *Am. Rev. Tuberc. Pulmonary Dis., 73:99, 1956.*)

TABLE 11.   TREATMENT OF CHRONIC PULMONARY TUBERCULOSIS

Drug	Daily Dosage	Number of Daily Doses	Maximum Daily Dose	Duration of Therapy
INH	10 mg./kg.	1 or 2	300 mg.	2 years after sputum is negative
PAS	200 mg./kg.	3 or 4	12 gm.	2 years after sputum is negative
(or) Ethambutol	10–15 mg./kg.	1		2 years after sputum is negative
Surgical resection may be necessary				

roentgenogram is indicated. During puberty and early adolescence, girls are more likely to experience activation of disease. The year of menarche is an extremely unstable period, and some workers feel that more frequent chest roentgenograms are necessary during that time.

Although symptoms are not a reliable aid to early diagnosis, lassitude, cough, loss of weight, anemia and the suppression of menses are indications for the application of a tuberculin test. If the tuberculin reaction is positive, a chest roentgenogram should be done.

Whenever an older child with a positive tuberculin reaction shows a persistent density on roentgenogram, diagnosis of active tuberculosis should be made unless proved otherwise.

Treatment

Since the lesions of chronic pulmonary tuberculosis in children are extremely unstable, prompt therapy should be instituted. The patient should be hospitalized. If the lesion is a minimal one, prolonged hospitalization may be unnecessary, but the patient will be properly instructed in the necessary measures of hygiene and in his future care. If the lesion is advanced, a longer stay in the hospital will be necessary. Isoniazid, 10 mg. per kilogram of body weight per day (maximum daily dose 300 mg.), and either para-aminosalicylic acid, 200 mg. per kilogram of body weight (maximum daily dose 12 gm.), or ethambutol, 10 to 15

mg. per kilogram of body weight, should be given for two years after the sputum has become negative for tubercle bacilli (Table 11). Rifampin may be substituted for ethambutol.

If the disease is advanced and there is a great deal of caseation necrosis, surgical resection may be necessary. Pulmonary function studies may be of help in assessing the possible risks and benefits of surgery.

OTHER TUBERCULOUS INVOLVEMENT OF THE RESPIRATORY TRACT

In the past, primary tuberculous infection of the tonsils was not uncommon, but with the advent of the pasteurization of milk and the tuberculin testing of cows, such involvement has become a rarity.

That there may be a retropharyngeal abscess accompanying tuberculosis of the cervical vertebrae in a young child is well recognized. Nevertheless, a tuberculous retropharyngeal abscess arising from caseous lymph nodes in the retropharynx must be rare, and no case has been seen at the Medical College of Virginia in recent years.

Tracheoesophageal fistula may be a rare complication of tuberculous infection. A 16-month-old black female was admitted to the Medical College of Virginia Hospital with diagnosis of pri-

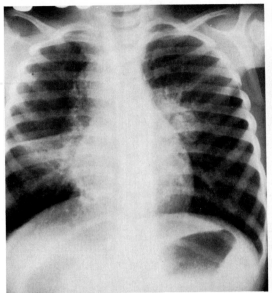

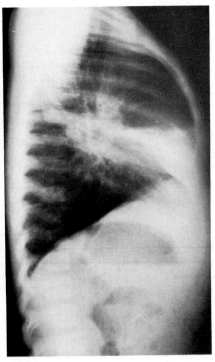

Figure 31. Aspiration pneumonia resulting from tracheoesophageal fistula, presumably of tuberculous origin.

mary pulmonary tuberculosis and early miliary tuberculosis. On isoniazid and para-aminosalicylic acid therapy, she appeared to make satisfactory progress, and after three months was transferred to the Sanatorium Division of the Medical College of Virginia for continued therapy. About three weeks after transfer, she vomited and developed fever. X-ray examination at that time showed pneumonic involvement of the right middle lobe (Fig. 31). Roentgenograms utilizing contrast medium swallow demonstrated the fistula (Fig. 32). On INH and PAS therapy, recovery was uneventful.

There may be tuberculous involvement of the larynx, middle ear, and mastoid and salivary glands.

EXTRAPULMONARY TUBERCULOSIS

Since this is a discussion of respiratory disease in children, little space will be allotted to the extrapulmonary man-ifestations of tuberculosis. There are several, however, that merit brief discussion.

TUBERCULOSIS OF THE SUPERFICIAL LYMPH NODES

Tuberculosis of the superficial lymph nodes does not occur as frequently as it did in the days before routine tuberculin testing of cows and pasteurization of milk, but the disease is still important.

Involvement of the superficial lymph nodes occurs at the time of the bacillemia (near the close of the incubation period) when tubercle bacilli are deposited in foci, where they usually remain quiescent unless activated by some trigger mechanism.

There is usually involvement of more than one lymph node. At first there is lymphoid hyperplasia and tubercle formation; later the lesion is that of a chronic granuloma. Caseation and necrosis produce a confluent caseous mass, which, when untreated, will eventuate in a sinus tract. Calcification is

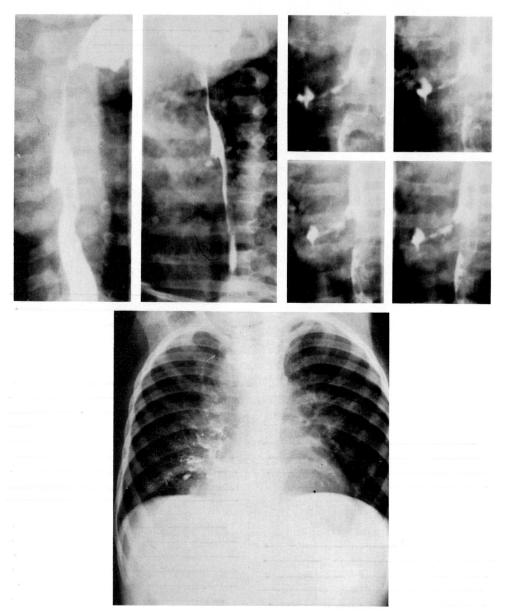

Figure 32. Contrast medium swallow demonstrating tracheoesophageal fistula.

often present in a healed tuberculous lymph node.

Since a trigger mechanism is usually required for activation, the disease process often occurs in the superficial cervical lymph nodes. Here quiescent tubercle bacilli are usually activated by acute tonsillitis or adenoiditis. The bacterial infection is controlled by appropriate antibiotics, but the lymphadenop-

athy persists, and, indeed, the lymph nodes continue to enlarge. There is usually no associated pain. Later the affected lymph nodes adhere to each other, then to the skin, which becomes discolored, and the caseous material ruptures into the surrounding tissues. Eventually the caseous material drains externally through a sinus tract (Fig. 33).

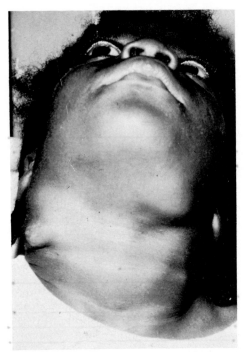

Figure 33. Multiple areas of suppurative lymphadenitis. (Courtesy of *J. Pediatr.,* 47:607, 1955.)

Tuberculosis of the superficial lymph nodes may also result from direct lymphatic drainage from an extrapulmonary primary tuberculosis focus. This mode of involvement is uncommon.

Other diseases that must be ruled out as a cause of chronic suppurative lymphadenitis are: acute pyogenic infections, coccidioidomycosis, blastomycosis, histoplasmosis, actinomycosis, brucellosis, infectious mononucleosis, leukemia, lymphoma, Hodgkin's dis-

ease, catscratch fever and infection with the atypical mycobacteria.

Infection with one of the atypical (unclassified) mycobacteria may produce a picture identical with that caused by tuberculous infection. If the positive tuberculin reaction measures less than 10 mm. in diameter of induration, it is probable that infection with one of the atypical (unclassified) mycobacteria exists. Skin testing with both tuberculin solution and the antigens of the atypical mycobacteria (when available) may be helpful, too. (See Chapter 47, Infections with the Atypical Mycobacteria.)

Treatment

Lymphadenitis should be first treated with one of the wide-spectrum antibiotics or with penicillin. The latter is usually the most effective agent in the treatment of lymphadenitis of bacterial origin.

If there is a positive tuberculin reaction, and if the lymph nodes measure 2 by 2 cm. or more in diameter, and, in spite of therapy with a wide-spectrum antibiotic or penicillin, are increasing in size, or show early signs of suppuration, prompt excision and the use of isoniazid and para-aminosalicylic acid therapy for a full year are indicated (Table 12). If the mass of nodes is too great, or if complete liquefaction of the node has already occurred and excision cannot be carried out, the completely liquefied node should be aspirated. Tonsillectomy is advised only if there are indications for it.

TABLE 12.   TREATMENT OF TUBERCULOSIS OF THE
SUPERFICIAL LYMPH NODES

1. Excision and

> INH   15–20 mg./kg. (maximum daily dose 500 mg.) for 12 months or longer
> PAS   200 mg./kg. (maximum daily dose 12 gm.) for 12 months or longer

or, if excision is not feasible,
2. Aspiration (when liquefied) and

> INH   15–20 mg./kg. (maximum daily dose 500 mg.) for 12 months or longer
> PAS   200 mg./kg. (maximum daily dose 12 gm.) for 12 months or longer

TUBERCULOUS MENINGITIS

This is the most serious form of tuberculosis. Before the advent of streptomycin, it was presumably 100 per cent fatal. At present, with the use of isoniazid and two of the other antituberculosis chemotherapeutic agents, more than 90 per cent of such patients admitted to the Medical College of Virginia Hospital survive. Some recover entirely, and others have various degrees of residual involvement. Earlier diagnosis would increase the number with complete recovery and decrease the number and severity of the residua in those who survive.

Tuberculous meningitis is caused by the direct extension of a local contiguous lesion (Rich and McCordock, 1933) and is an early complication of tuberculosis. The two principal causes of neurologic sequelae are tuberculous arteritis and obstruction to the flow of the cerebrospinal fluid caused by a thick, gelatinous exudate at the base of the brain.

The clinical course is divided into three stages: the first stage, in which the symptoms are vague and generalized; second, a transitional stage, with early meningeal symptoms and increased intracranial pressure; and third, severe central nervous system involvement, with the patient comatose.

The onset of tuberculous meningitis is usually insidious (although a convulsion may be the first sign), and the symptoms are vague. Apathy, lassitude, anorexia, sometimes irritability, low-grade fever and occasionally vomiting and constipation occur early in the course of the disease.

In the second stage, drowsiness becomes deeper, and there may be convulsions. There is nuchal resistance, often rigidity, and opisthotonos may occur. There may be bulging of the fontanel and ocular paralysis. The patient's condition steadily worsens.

In the final stage, the patient lapses into a coma with irregular respirations and high fever. There may be hyperglycemia and glycosuria.

The duration of untreated tuberculous meningitis is approximately three weeks. Early diagnosis is essential, since the disease, when untreated, is always fatal; even when it is treated, it may result in survivors with various neurologic residua.

The *diagnosis* is established by means of the tuberculin test, cerebrospinal fluid findings and chest roentgenogram. The tuberculin reaction is practically always positive, but may be negative in the last stages of the disease. Most of the patients with tuberculous meningitis have some evidence of primary tuberculosis on the chest roentgenogram. The cerebrospinal fluid is ground glass in appearance and has a cellular content of 10 to 1000 per cubic millimeter. The cells are predominantly polymorphonuclear in the early stages of disease, but lymphocytes are usually more common later. The protein is elevated above 40 mg. per 100 ml., and the sugar is usually decreased. The chlorides are normal in the early stages and frequently below normal later.

Absolute diagnosis can be made only by the isolation of tubercle bacilli from the cerebrospinal fluid. Thus, careful direct examination of the fluid should be made. Even though direct examination is unsuccessful, treatment should never be deferred until the causative agent has been identified.

Treatment should consist of a triple drug regimen (Table 13): isoniazid in a daily dosage of 20 mg. per kilogram of body weight per day (maximum 500 mg.), rifampin in a daily dosage of 10 to 20 mg. per kilogram of body weight per day (maximum 600 mg.), and streptomycin, 20 to 40 mg. per kilogram of body weight per day (maximum 1 gm.). The first two drugs are given for at least one year (PAS may be substituted for rifampin after a few months), and streptomycin is given for one month after satisfactory clinical response, as determined by the general condition of the patient, the disappearance of fever and improvement in the cerebrospinal fluid picture.

TABLE 13. TREATMENT OF TUBERCULOUS MENINGITIS

Drug	Daily Dosage	Number of Daily Doses	Maximum Daily Dose	Duration of Therapy
INH	20 mg./kg.	1 or 2	500 mg.	12 months or longer
Rifampin*	10–20 mg./kg.	1	600 mg.	12 months or longer
Streptomycin	20–40 mg./kg.	1 (2)	1 gm.	1 month after satisfactory clinical response
Prednisone	1 mg./kg.	4	60 mg.	6–12 weeks

*After a few months, PAS, 200 mg./kg. (maximum daily dose 12 gm.), may be substituted for rifampin.

Antimicrobial agents appear to be reasonably effective in the treatment of tuberculous meningitis if they can reach the organism. The use of prednisone may decrease the likelihood of cerebrospinal fluid obstruction, and, in addition, reduction of the inflammatory process may lessen the danger of irreversible thrombotic phenomena. The use of prednisone after cerebrospinal fluid block has occurred often results in dissolution, as exemplified in the accompanying case report.

Obviously, prevention of such obstruction is more desirable. The drug is usually administered for a six- to 12-week period.

CASE REPORT. During the period before the effectiveness of adrenocorticosteroid therapy in prevention and dissolution of cerebrospinal fluid obstruction had become recognized, a two-year-old black girl had such a block. Cerebrospinal fluid protein was 5600 mg. per 100 ml. when therapy with cortisone was instituted. After two weeks the cerebrospinal fluid protein was 650 mg. per 100 ml., but as dosage of the drug was decreased and finally discontinued, the cerebrospinal fluid protein level gradually rose to 5800 mg. per 100 ml. When it then became apparent that the obstruction could be controlled by cortisone, such therapy was again added to the regimen (INH, PAS, streptomycin), and the obstruction rapidly dissolved (Fig. 34).

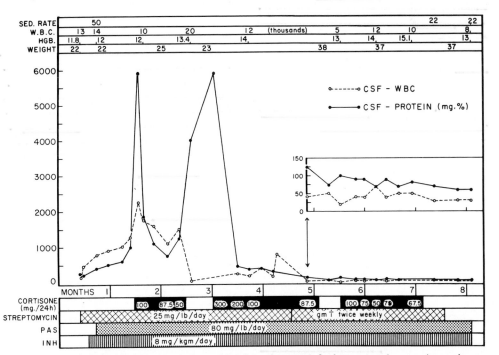

Figure 34. Diagram depicting precipitous fall of cerebrospinal fluid protein when cortisone therapy was instituted. (Courtesy of *Am. Rev. Tuberc. Pulmonary Dis.*, 73:99, 1956.)

The promptness of the response to antimicrobial therapy varies considerably. In general, the earlier the diagnosis is made, the more prompt will be the response. An affected child may lie in a stuporous, semicomatose or even comatose state for months and finally attain an almost complete or even complete recovery.

TUBERCULOSIS OF THE BONES AND JOINTS

Tuberculosis of the bones and joints usually results from the bacillemia that occurs near the close of the incubation period. Clinical disease may occur soon thereafter, or the organism may remain quiescent and reactivate months or even years later. The bones most frequently involved are the head of the femur (hip), the vertebrae and the fingers and toes. The pathologic process usually begins in the metaphyseal portions of the epiphyses.

As recommended by the Committee on Treatment of Tuberculosis in Children, American Thoracic Society (1969), treatment with isoniazid and PAS is carried out for a period of 24 months or longer. (Recent evidence suggests that rifampin may be more effective than PAS.) Dosage of these drugs is the same as that mentioned under the therapy of progressive primary tuberculosis. All superficial and accessible abscesses should be drained. Immobilization is not necessary in the non-weight-bearing structures; if, however, weight-bearing structures (vertebrae, hip and others) are involved, whatever means are necessary to prevent weight-bearing are used. For example, the treatment of tuberculosis of the spine (Pott's disease) may vary widely. Some utilize only a hard mattress and the aforementioned drug therapy; others feel that a plaster cast is advisable. Fusion is advised by some orthopedists, and others use fusion only when there appear to be special indications for it (Table 14).

RENAL TUBERCULOSIS

Tuberculosis of the kidney is blood-borne in origin, and infection occurs either at the time of the early bacillemia or as part of generalized miliary tuberculosis. Occasionally it may be a late complication.

When the patient does not have associated miliary tuberculosis and has only a positive tuberculin reaction, the most common finding is a persistent sterile pyuria. There may also be albuminuria, hematuria, dysuria and local renal tenderness. Urine culture will corroborate the diagnosis, and urograms are indicated in order to determine the area and degree of involvement.

Therapy should be carried out for at least 24 months. So-called triple drug therapy with isoniazid, PAS and streptomycin has been advocated for this period, but in those cases in which the urogram shows no abnormality, streptomycin may be discontinued after six months. One authority gives isoniazid, PAS and one other drug—cycloserine,

TABLE 14.   TREATMENT OF TUBERCULOSIS OF BONES AND JOINTS

Drug	Daily Dosage	Maximum Daily Dose	Duration of Therapy
Isoniazid	15–20 mg./kg.	500 mg.	24 months or longer
PAS	200 mg./kg.	12 gm.	24 months or longer
(or)			
Rifampin	10–20 mg./kg.	600 mg.	24 months or longer

Immobilization of involved weight-bearing structures
Drainage of all superficial accessible abscesses

TABLE 15. TREATMENT OF RENAL TUBERCULOSIS

Drug	Dosage	Maximum Daily Dose	Duration of Therapy
Isoniazid	15–20 mg./kg./day	500 mg.	2 years
PAS	200 mg./kg./day	12 gm.	2 years
Streptomycin	20 mg./kg./	1 gm.	2 years
or	3 times weekly		(6 months in very mild cases)
Cycloserine	4–5 mg./kg./day	500 mg.	2 years
or			
Ethionamide	10 mg./kg./day	750 mg.	2 years
or			
Ethambutol	10 mg./kg./day	—	2 years

ethionamide or ethambutol—for two years, usually in a single dose. Rifampin has not been adequately evaluated, but would seem a logical choice as the third drug. Dosage of isoniazid is 15 to 20 mg. per kilogram of body weight per day, of PAS 200 mg. per kilogram of body weight per day, and of streptomycin (when used) 20 mg. per kilogram of body weight three times weekly. The dosage of cycloserine (when used) is 4 to 5 mg. per kilogram, of ethionamide (when used) 10 mg. per kilogram of body weight per day, and of ethambutol (when used) 10 mg. per kilogram of body weight per day. (Maximum dose is indicated in Table 15.) Since there is a possibility that ureteral stricture may appear during therapy, an intravenous pyelogram and ureteral calibration every four months during treatment and annually thereafter for a ten-year period would seem advisable.

INTRA-ABDOMINAL TUBERCULOSIS

Intra-abdominal tuberculosis has been a rarity on the pediatric service of the Medical College of Virginia in recent years. Tuberculous enteritis may be primary, but is usually secondary to a lesion in the lungs and is nearly always combined with involvement of the mesenteric and retroperitoneal lymph nodes. The main symptoms are tenesmus and chronic diarrhea, with some associated bleeding. There may

be fever, abdominal tenderness and distention. There are also debility and anemia. In addition to the antimicrobial therapy routine outlined for progressive primary tuberculosis, the usual general measures for tuberculosis are necessary, and a low residue diet of adequate caloric and vitamin content is also helpful. Therapy is otherwise symptomatic.

When tuberculous enteritis is primary, the principal lesion is in the mesenteric and retroperitoneal lymph nodes. Symptoms are abdominal pain and tenderness. No local treatment is usually required, but rarely excision of enlarged or calcified abdominal lymph nodes may be necessary for the relief of pain.

Tuberculous peritonitis usually results from the rupture of a caseous lesion in a mesenteric lymph node, and also occasionally from an intestinal lesion that has penetrated through the outer coat. The onset is insidious, with mild abdominal pain, debilitation and low-grade fever. Later there may be vomiting and abdominal distention.

Tuberculous peritonitis is treated in the same manner as tuberculosis in general, and the addition of adrenocorticosteroid therapy may also be helpful. If an exploratory laparotomy is required to establish the diagnosis, it is essential that suitable biopsy material be obtained for tissue section and bacteriologic study. If there is an associated enteritis, a low residue diet provides some symptomatic relief.

OTHER EXTRAPULMONARY TUBERCULOSIS

There are other less common forms of extrapulmonary tuberculosis. These are tuberculosis of the skin, eye, heart and pericardium, endocrine and exocrine glands, genital tract and fistula in ano. For consideration of these entities, the reader is referred to those publications that deal with tuberculosis in its entirety.

THE PREVENTION OF TUBERCULOSIS

There are three methods that have been demonstrated to be reasonably effective in preventing tuberculous infection: the isolation of those adults with infectious tuberculosis; the use of BCG vaccine, and the administration of isoniazid to household contacts of tuberculous patients.

Results from the United States Public Health Service Isoniazid Prophylaxis Studies among tuberculin-positive household contacts indicate that isoniazid is effective in reducing the incidence of tuberculous disease in this group of children. Further studies by the United States Public Health Service have shown that extending the use of isoniazid to all household contacts results in less tuberculous disease during the year of prophylactic therapy and continuing good effect lasting at least through the ten years following discontinuation of isoniazid therapy.

BCG vaccine has been conclusively shown to increase resistance to exogenous tuberculous infection, and is mainly of use in this country to those children living in a home in which there is an adult with infectious tuberculous disease, or one with potentially infectious disease,* such as a mother who has been discharged from a sanatorium with apparently arrested tuberculosis. It is also useful in those population groups in which there is a high incidence of tuberculous infection.

*See Tuberculosis in the Newborn, p. 823.

BCG vaccination may be effected by the multiple puncture technique or by the intracutaneous route. One of the main disadvantages of BCG vaccination is said to be the positive tuberculin reaction that results. It has been our experience with the vaccine *manufactured in the United States* that the resultant positive tuberculin reaction nearly always measures 5 to 9 mm. and rarely above 12 to 14 mm. in diameter of induration. If the reaction is 15 mm. or more in diameter of induration, the physician can be reasonably sure that there has been infection with virulent tubercle bacilli, and further investigation is indicated.

In order to be eligible for BCG vaccination, the patient must have a negative tuberculin reaction (PPD 5 TU or OT 10 TU) and a negative chest roentgenogram within the previous two weeks. Eight to 12 weeks after vaccination, the same procedures should be carried out. At this time the tuberculin reaction should be, and practically always is, positive; if this is not the case, the vaccination is repeated.

The multiple puncture disk method, as described by Rosenthal (1961), is the preferable procedure. The vaccination is performed over the deltoid region, and the area should be cleansed with acetone and allowed to dry thoroughly. There should be no constriction of the arm. Three drops of BCG vaccine are placed on the skin of the deltoid area, using a syringe and a 22-gauge needle. The disk is picked up by a sterile magnet-type holder (Fig. 35), allowing the wide margin of the disk to extend beyond the magnet and away from the operator. The operator holds the disk at a 30 degree angle and distributes the vaccine over an area about 2.5 cm. square, tapping with the wide margin of the disk. The points of the disk are dipped into the vaccine, rotating the disk slightly, so that all points become moistened with BCG vaccine. The disk is placed in the center of the vaccine site, with the long axis of the holder at a right angle to the arm, and the magnet is moved to the center of the disk.

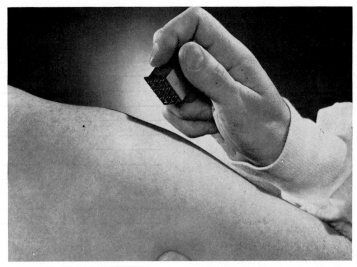

Figure 35. Multiple puncture disk and magnet-type of holder held in position before depressing for BCG vaccination. (Courtesy of S. R. Rosenthal, Research Foundation, 70 W. Hubbard Street, Chicago, Illinois 60610.)

This will avoid bending of the disk. The arm under the vaccine site is grasped with the operator's other hand, thereby tensing the skin over the vaccination area. With the butt of the magnet in the curve of the index finger, downward pressure is applied so that the points of the disk are well buried in the skin (Fig. 36). Enough pressure is applied so that penetration of the points is readily felt by the hand. With pressure still exerted as above, the disk is rocked forward and backward and from side to side twice. The grasp underneath the arm is then released. The operator slides the magnet toward himself and off the disk, maintaining a slight downward pressure. After a successful procedure, the disk remains flat on the arm, with the points still in the skin. If the points are on top of the skin, the procedure must be repeated. The disk is again picked up with the magnet, allowing the wide margin to extend beyond the magnet. By utilizing the wide margin of the disk, the vaccine

Figure 36. Multiple puncture disk being pressed in outer aspect of arm. Disk is pressed downward through drop of BCG vaccine. (Courtesy of S. R. Rosenthal, Research Foundation, 70 W. Hubbard Street, Chicago, Illinois 60610.)

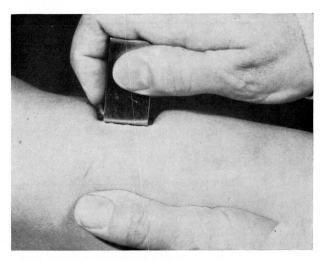

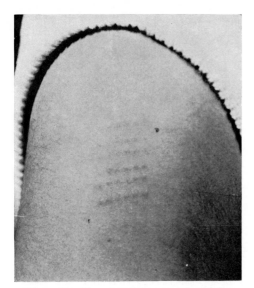

Figure 37. Size of multiple puncture BCG vaccination, 13 days after vaccination (actual photograph). (Courtesy of S. R. Rosenthal, Research Foundation, 70 W. Hubbard Street, Chicago, Illinois, 60610.)

is gently tapped so that each perforation of the skin is covered with vaccine. If too much pressure is exerted, the vaccine will be pressed out of the perforations. The vaccine is allowed to dry on the arm without a dressing. The vaccinated area should not be washed for 24 hours (Fig. 37).

Infants and children from tuberculous households (and all adults) should receive the two-site method of BCG vaccination. The procedure differs from the foregoing only in that a larger area of the deltoid region is cleansed and utilized, with one vaccination site in the upper portion and a second in the lower one.

Materials for use in BCG vaccination may be obtained from the Research Foundation, 70 West Hubbard Street, Chicago, Illinois 60610. BCG vaccine is also commercially available from the Eli Lilly Company, 740 South Alabama Street, Indianapolis, Indiana 46206.

REFERENCES

Adams, W. C.: Variations in the endurance of positive Mantoux reactions in primary childhood tuberculosis. *Am. Rev. Resp. Dis., 81*:955, 1960.

Anderson, S. R., and Smith, M. H. D.: The Heaf multiple puncture tuberculin test. *Am. J. Dis. Child., 99*:764, 1960.

Aronson, J. D.: BCG vaccination among American Indians. *Am. Rev. Tuberc., 57*:96, 1948.

Aspin, J., and O'Hara, H.: Steroid-treated tuberculous pleural effusion. *Br. J. Tuberc., 52*:81, 1958.

Barclay, W., Ebert, R. H., and Koch-Weser, D.: Mode of action of isoniazid. *Am. Rev. Tuberc., 67*:490, 1953; *70*:784, 1954.

Beaudry, P. H., Brickman, H. F., Wise, M. B., and MacDougall, D.: Liver enzyme disturbances during isoniazid chemoprophylaxis in children. Am. Rev. Resp. Dis., *110*:581, 1974.

Belsey, M. A.: Tuberculosis and varicella infection in children. *Am. J. Dis. Child., 113*:448, 1967.

Bentley, F. J., Grzybowski, S., and Benjamin, B.: *Tuberculosis in Childhood and Adolescence: With Special Reference to the Pulmonary Form of the Disease.* London, The National Association for the Prevention of Tuberculosis, 1954.

Brailey, M. E.: Prognosis in white and colored tuberculous children according to initial chest x-ray findings. *Am. J. Public Health, 33*:343, 1944.

Committee on Diagnostic Skin Testing, American Thoracic Society: *The Tuberculin Skin Test.* New York, American Lung Association, 1974.

Committee on Therapy, American Thoracic Society: A statement on pyrazinamide. *Am. Rev. Tuberc., 75*:1012, 1957.

Committee on Treatment of Tuberculosis in Children, American Thoracic Society: The treatment of tuberculosis in children. *Am. Rev. Resp. Dis., 99*:304, 1969.

Committee to Revise Diagnostic Standards, American Thoracic Society: *Diagnostic Standards and Classification of Tuberculosis and Other Mycobacterial Diseases.* New York, American Lung Association, 1974.

Comstock, G. W., Edwards, L. B., and Livesay, V. T.: Tuberculosis morbidity in the United States Navy: its distribution and decline. *Am. Rev. Resp. Dis., 110*:572, 1974.

Dahlström, G., and Difs, H.: Efficacy of BCG vaccination; study on vaccinated and tuberculin negative non-vaccinated conscripts. *Acta Tuberc. Scand.,* Suppl. 27, 1951.

Davies, D., and Glowinski, J. J., Jr.: Jaundice due to isoniazid. *Tubercle, 42*:504, 1961.

Debré, R., and Brissaud, H. E.: *Meningite Tuberculeuse et Tuberculose Miliare* de l'Enfant; Leur Traitement. Paris, Masson et Cie, 1953.

Debré, R., and Papp, K.: About the tuberculin skin test during the course of measles and rubella. *C. R. Soc. Biol., 95*:29, 1926.

de March A. P.: Tuberculosis and pregnancy. *Chest, 68*:800, 1975.

Dieu, J. C., and others: Rifampin in the treatment of lymph node and pulmonary involvement of primary tuberculosis in infants and children. *Rev. Tuberc. (Paris), 34*:320, 1970.

Doster, B., Murray, F. J., Newman, R., and Woolpert, S. F.: Ethambutol in the initial treatment of pulmonary tuberculosis. *Am. Rev. Resp. Dis., 107*:177, 1973.

Edwards, L. B., Edwards, P. Q., and Palmer, C. E.: Sources of tuberculin sensitivity in human populations. *Acta Tuberc. Scand.,* Suppl. 47, 1959.

Edwards, L. B., Palmer, C. E., Affronti, L. F., Hopwood, L., and Edwards, P. Q.: Epidemiologic studies of tuberculin sensitivity. II. Response to experimental infection with mycobacteria isolated from human sources. *Am. J. Hyg., 71*:218, 1960.

Edwards, P. Q., and Edwards, L. B.: Story of the tuberculin test from an epidemiologic viewpoint. *Am. Rev. Resp. Dis., 91* (part 2): 1, 1960.

Elmendorf, D. G., Jr., Cauthorn, W. W., Muschenheim, C., and McDermott, W.: The absorption, distribution, excretion and short term toxicity of isoniazid (Nydrazid) in man. *Am. Rev. Tuberc., 65*:429, 1952.

Ferebee, S. H.: Controlled chemoprophylaxis trials in tuberculosis. A general review. *Adv. Tuberc. Res., 17*:28, 1969.

Ferebee, S. H., and Mount, R. W.: Prophylactic effect of isoniazid on primary tuberculosis in children, a preliminary report: United States Public Health Service tuberculosis prophylaxis trial. *Am. Rev. Tuberc., 76*:942, 1957.

Filler, J., and Porter, M.: Physiologic studies of the sequelae of tuberculous pleural effusion in children treated with antimicrobial drugs and prednisone. *Am. Rev. Resp. Dis., 88*:181, 1963.

Furcolow, M. L., and Robinson, E. L.: Quantitative studies of the tuberculin reaction. II. The efficiency of a quantitative patch test in detecting reactors to low doses of tuberculin. *Public Health Rep., 56*:2405, 1941.

Gerbeaux, J.: *Primary Tuberculosis in Childhood.* Springfield, Illinois, Charles C Thomas, 1970.

Ghon, A., and Kudlich, H.: Die Eintrittspforten der Infektion vom Standpunkte der pathologischen Anatomie. In Engel, S., and Pirquet, C.: *Handbuch der Kindertuberculose.* Vol. 1. Stuttgart, Georg Thieme Verlag, 1930.

Goldstein, R. A., Ang Un Hun, Foellmer, J. W., and Janicki, B. W.: Rifampin and cell-mediated immune responses in tuberculosis. *Am. Rev. Resp. Dis., 113*:197, 1976.

Grzybowski, S., Dorken, E., and Bates, C.: Disparities of tuberculins. *Am. Rev. Resp. Dis., 100*:86, 1969.

Hanson, M. L., and Comstock, G. W.: Efficacy of hydrocortisone ointment in the treatment of local reactions to tuberculin skin tests. *Am. Rev. Resp. Dis., 97*:472, 1968.

Hardy, J. B., and Kendig, E. L., Jr.: Tuberculous pleurisy with effusion in infancy. *J. Pediatr., 26*:138, 1945.

Heimbeck, J.: Vaccination sous-cutanée et cutanée au B.C.G., 1926–1948. *Sem. Hôp. Paris, 25*:771, 1949.

Holden, M., Dubin, R. R., and Diamond, P. H. : Frequency of negative intermediate strength tuberculin sensitivity in patients with acute tuberculosis. *N. Engl. J. Med., 285*:1506, 1971.

Houck, V. N.: Tuberculin: past, present, and future. *J.A.M.A., 222*:1421, 1972.

Hsu, K. H. K.: Isoniazid in the prevention and treatment of tuberculosis. *J.A.M.A., 229*:528, 1974.

Jacobs, J.: A concept of pulmonary tuberculosis in childhood. *Br. J. Clin. Pract., 12*:778, 1958.

Jenkins, D. W., and Byrd, R. B.: The tuberculin tine and Mono-Vacc tests in the patient with active tuberculosis. *Am. Rev. Resp. Dis., 112*:140, 1975.

Johnson, J. R., and Davey, W. N.: Cortisone, corticotropin and antimicrobial therapy in tuberculosis in animals and man. *Am. Rev. Tuberc., 70*:623, 1954.

Johnson, W. J.: Biological acetylation of isoniazid. *Nature, 174*:744, 1954.

Johnston, J. A.: *Nutritional Studies in Adolescent Girls and Their Relation to Tuberculosis.* Springfield, Illinois, Charles C Thomas, 1953.

Kendig, E. L., Jr.: The effect of antihistaminic drugs on the tuberculin patch test. *J. Pediatr., 35*:750, 1949.

Kendig, E. L., Jr.: The routine tuberculin test—a neglected pediatric procedure. *J. Pediatr., 40*:813, 1952.

Kendig, E. L., Jr.: Tuberculosis in the very young. *Am. Rev. Tuberc., 70*:161, 1954.

Kendig, E. L., Jr.: Incidence of tuberculous infection in infancy. *Am. Rev. Tuberc., 74*:149, 1956a.

Kendig, E. L., Jr.: Early diagnosis of tuberculosis in childhood. *Am. J. Dis. Child., 92*:558, 1956b.

Kendig, E. L., Jr.: BCG vaccinations in Virginia. *J. Pediatr., 51*:54, 1957.

Kendig, E. L., Jr.: Prognosis of infants born of tuberculous mothers. *Pediatrics, 26*:97, 1960.

Kendig, E. L., Jr.: Unclassified mycobacteria in children: correlation of skin tests and gastric cultures. *Am. J. Dis. Child., 101*:749, 1961.

Kendig, E. L., Jr.: Unclassified mycobacteria as a causative agent in the positive tuberculin reaction. *Pediatrics, 30*:221, 1962.

Kendig, E. L., Jr.: Unclassified mycobacteria: incidence of infection and cause of a false positive tuberculin reaction. *N. Engl. J. Med., 268*:1001, 1963.

Kendig, E. L., Jr.: The place of BCG vaccine in the management of infants born of tuberculous mothers. *N. Engl. J. Med., 281*:250, 1969.

Kendig, E. L., Jr., and Brummer, D. L.: Tuberculosis. In Kagan, B. M. (Ed.): *Antimicrobial Therapy.* 2nd Ed. Philadelphia, W. B. Saunders Company, 1974.

Kendig, E. L., Jr., and Burch, C. D.: Short-term antimicrobial therapy of tuberculous meningitis. *Am. Rev. Resp., 82*:672, 1960.

Kendig, E. L., Jr., and Hudgens, R. O.: The effect of rubeola on tuberculosis under antimicrobial therapy. I. Primary tuberculosis treated with isoniazid. II. Tuberculous meningitis treated with isoniazid, Streptomycin, and para-aminosalicylic acid. *Pediatrics, 24*:616, 1959.

Kendig, E. L., Jr., and Johnson, W. B.: Short-term antimicrobial therapy of tuberculous meningitis. *N. Engl. J. Med., 258*:928, 1958.

Kendig, E. L., Jr., and Rogers, W. L.: Tuberculosis in the neonatal period. *Am. Rev. Tuberc., 77*:418, 1958.

Kendig, E. L., Jr., and Wiley, T. M.: The treatment of tuberculosis of the superficial cervical lymph nodes in children. *J. Pediatr.*, *47*:607, 1955.

Kendig, E. L., Jr., Choy, S. H., and Johnson, W. H.: Observations on the effect of cortisone in the treatment of tuberculous meningitis. *Am. Rev. Tuberc.*, *73*:99, 1956.

Kendig, E. L., Jr., Trevathan, G. E., and Ownby, R. J.: Isoniazid in treatment of tuberculosis in childhood. *J. Dis. Child.*, *88*:148, 1954.

Lanier, V. S., Russell, W. F., Jr., Heaton, A., and Robinson, A.: Concentrations of active isoniazid in serum and cerebrospinal fluid of patients with tuberculosis treated with isoniazid. *Pediatrics*, *21*:910, 1958.

Leunda, J. J., Panizza Blanco, A., and Raggio, O. V.: The tuberculous infection and the measles infection. *Arch. Ped. Uruguay*, *14*:502, 1943.

Lincoln, E. M.: Course and prognosis of tuberculosis in children. *Am. J. Med.*, *9*:623, 1950.

Lincoln, E. M.: Epidemics of tuberculosis. *Adv. Tuberc. Res.*, *14*:157, 1965.

Lincoln, E. M., and Sewell, E. M.: *Tuberculosis in Children.* New York, McGraw-Hill Book Company, Inc., 1963.

Lincoln, E. M., Davies, P. A., and Bovornkitti, S.: Tuberculous pleurisy with effusion in children: a study of 202 children, with particular reference to prognosis. *Am. Rev. Tuberc.*, *77*:271, 1958.

Long, E. R.: *The Chemistry and Chemotherapy of Tuberculosis.* 3rd Ed. Baltimore, Williams & Wilkins Company, 1958.

Lorriman, G., and Bentley, F. J.: The incidence of segmental lesions in primary tuberculosis: with special reference to the effect of chemotherapy. *Am. Rev. Tuberc.*, *79*:765, 1959.

Lurie, M. B., Zappasodi, P., and Tickner, C.: On the nature of genetic resistance to tuberculosis in the light of the host-parasite relationship in natively resistant and susceptible rabbits. *Am. Rev. Tuberc.*, *72*:297, 1955.

Mande. R., Herrault, A., Loubry, P., and Bouchet, C.: Les epidémies scolaires de tuberculose. *Sem. Hôp. Paris*, *34*:1837, 1958.

Morales, S. M., and Lincoln, E. M.: The effect of isoniazid therapy on pyridoxine metabolism in children. *Am. Rev. Tuberc.*, *75*:594, 1957.

Nemir, R. L., Cardona, J., Lacoius, A., and David, M.: Prednisone therapy as an adjunct in the treatment of lymph node–bronchial tuberculosis in childhood. *Am. Rev. Resp. Dis.*, *88*:189, 1963.

1974 Tuberculosis Statistics: States and Cities. United States Department of Health, Education, and Welfare, Public Health Service, Center for Disease Control, Bureau of State Services, Tuberculosis Control Division, Atlanta, Georgia, July 1975.

Oseasohn, R.: Current use of BCG. *Am. Rev. Resp. Dis.*, *109*:500, 1974.

Palmer, C. E., and Edwards, L. B.: Geographic variations in the prevalence of sensitivity to tuberculin (PPD-S) and to the Battey antigen (PPD-B) throughout the United States. *Bull. Int. Union Tuberc.*, *32*:373, 1962.

Renzetti, A. C., Wright, K. W., Edling, J. H., and

Bunn, P.: Clinical, bacteriologic and pharmacologic observations upon cycloserine. *Am. Rev. Tuberc.*, *74*:128, 1956.

Rich, A. R.: *The Pathogenesis of Tuberculosis.* 2nd Ed. Springfield, Illinois, Charles C Thomas, 1951.

Rich, A. R., and McCordock, H. A.: The pathogenesis of tuberculous meningitis. *Bull. Johns Hopkins Hosp.*, *52*:5, 1933.

Robinson, A., Meyer, M., and Middlebrook, G.: Tuberculin hypersensitivity in tuberculous infants treated with isoniazid. *N. Engl. J. Med.*, *252*:983, 1955.

Rosenthal, S. R.: *BCG Vaccination Against Tuberculosis.* Boston, Little, Brown & Company, 1957.

Rosenthal, S. R.: The disk-tine tuberculin test (dried tuberculin-disposable unit). *J.A.M.A.*, *177*:452, 1961.

Rosenthal, S. R., Nikurs, L., Yordy, E., Hoder, B., and Thorne, M.: Tuberculin tine and Mantoux tests. *Pediatrics*, *30*:385, 1965.

Rudoy, R., Stuemby, J., and Polay, J. R.: Isoniazid administration and liver injury. *Am. J. Dis. Child.*, *125*:733, 1973.

Schwartz, W. S., and Moyer, R. E.: The chemotherapy of pulmonary tuberculosis with pyrazinamide used alone and in conjunction with streptomycin, para-aminosalicylic acid or isoniazid. *Am. Rev. Tuberc.*, *70*:413, 1954.

Section on Diseases of the Chest, American Academy of Pediatrics: The Tuberculin Test. *Pediatrics*, *54*:650, 1974.

Sippel, J. E., Mikhail, I. A., Girgis, N. I., and Youssef, H. H.: Rifampin concentrations in cerebrospinal fluid of patients with tuberculous meningitis. *Am. Rev. Resp. Dis.*, *109*:579, 1974.

Starr, S., and Berkovich, S.: Effects of measles, gamma globulin modified measles and vaccine measles on the tuberculin test. *N. Engl. J. Med.*, *270*:386, 1964a.

Starr, S., and Berkovich, S.: The depression of tuberculin reactivity during chicken pox. *Pediatrics*, *33*:769, 1964b.

Steigman, A. J., and Kendig, E. L., Jr.: Frequency of tuberculin testing. *Pediatrics*, *56*:160, 1975.

Steiner, P., Rao, M., Goldberg, R., and Steiner, M.: Primary drug resistance in children. Drug susceptibility of strains of *M. tuberculosis* isolated from children during the years 1969 to 1972 at the Kings County Hospital Medical Center of Brooklyn. *Am. Rev. Resp. Dis.*, *110*:98, 1974.

Storey, P. B., and McLean, R. L.: Some considerations of cycloserine toxicity. *Am. Rev. Tuberc.*, *75*:514, 1956.

Strom, L.: Vaccination against tuberculosis. *Am. Rev. Tuberc.*, *75*:28, 1956.

Sweet, A. Y.: Personal communication. In *Committee on Drugs, American Academy of Pediatrics: Infants of tuberculous mothers: further thoughts.* Vol. 420, 1968, p. 393.

Tuberculosis Advisory Committee and Special Consultants to the Director, Center for Disease Control; Isoniazid-associated hepatitis. Morbid. Mortal. Weekly Rept., *23*:97, 1974.

Vanderhoof, J. A., and Ament, M. E.: Fatal hepatic necrosis due to isoniazid chemoprophylaxis in a fifteen year old girl. *J. Pediatr.*, *89*:867, 1976.

Viomycin. *Am. Rev. Tuberc.*, *63*:1, 1951.

Wallgren, A.: Pulmonary tuberculosis: relation of childhood infection to the disease in adults. *Lancet*, *1*:417, 1938.

Wallgren, A.: Pulmonary tuberculosis in children. In Miller, J. A., and Wallgren, A.: *Pulmonary Tuberculosis in Adults and Children.* New York, Thomas Nelson and Sons, 1939.

Wallgren, A.: The time table of tuberculosis. *Tubercle*, *29*:245, 1948.

Wasz-Höckert, O.: Variola vaccination as an activator of tuberculous infection. *Ann. Med. Exp. Biol. Fenn.*, *32*:26, 1954.

Wijsmuller, G., and Termini, J.: The tuberculin test: effects of storage and method of delivery on reaction size. *Am. Rev. Resp. Dis.*, *107*:267, 1973.

Zack, M. B., and Fulkerson, L. L.: Clinical reliability of stabilized and nonstabilized tuberculin-PPD. *Am. Rev. Resp. Dis.*, *102*:91, 1970.

Zumstein, P.: Des effets secondaires de l'acide para-aminosalicylique (PAS). *Praxis*, *45*:48, 1956.

CHAPTER FORTY–SEVEN

INFECTIONS WITH THE ATYPICAL MYCOBACTERIA

EDWIN L. KENDIG, JR., M.D.

It has been established by examination of resected pulmonary lesions and suppurative or granulomatous lymph nodes that human disease can be caused by mycobacteria previously considered to be harmless. These pathogenic organisms are called atypical (anonymous, unclassified) mycobacteria.

General Characteristics of Mycobacteria

These mycobacteria are species and strains of the family Mycobacteriaceae. They differ from each other and from the human and bovine tubercle bacilli in rate of growth, type of colony, temperature of optimal growth, pigment formation, enzymatic activity, phage susceptibility, and specific antigenicity. They occur in water, in vegetable matter and in the soil. For example, scotochromogens, often called the tap water bacillus, may be isolated from water coolers; the vegetable matter and soil are usually warm and moist in character. Occasionally, pathogens have been found in swimming pools and sewage.

The portal of entry remains uncertain, and the occurrence of person-to-person transmission has not yet been established.

The atypical mycobacteria are nonpathogenic for guinea pigs, although Group I organisms may produce a small abscess at the site of inoculation and sometimes in the regional lymph node; rarely, a single granuloma may be found in the lung or spleen of these animals. On the other hand, the atypical mycobacteria may be pathogenic for mice. In the laboratory, the atypical mycobacteria possess a BCG-like effect in their capacity to modify the course of subsequent infection with *M. tuberculosis.*

Specific therapy with the so-called antituberculosis chemotherapeutic agents is usually effective for infection with Group I organisms, but is much less effective in treatment of infection with Groups II, III and IV.

Whether or not these organisms are mutations of *Mycobacterium tuberculosis,* resulting from treatment with chemotherapeutic agents, may not be completely settled, but few workers support this view; certainly, since similar organisms occurred in nature prior to the advent of the chemotherapeutic agents, this must at least not be the entire answer.

Classification of Mycobacteria

The most important consideration from a clinical point of view is the differentiation of the human tubercle bacillus from the atypical mycobacteria. Although additional subclassification of these organisms is, therefore, not essential, it may be helpful. The most useful classification to date is that contained in *Diagnostic Standards and Classification of Tuberculosis and Other Mycobacterial Diseases,* published by the American Lung Association in 1974 (Table 1).

GROUP I: PHOTOCHROMOGENS *(M. kansasii, M. marinum).* These organ-

TABLE 1. MYCOBACTERIA RECOVERED FROM VERTEBRATES, INCLUDING HUMANS

RUNYON GROUP	Potentially Clinically Significant		Usually Not Significant	
	SPECIES	SYNONYMS (REMARKS)	SPECIES	SYNONYMS
	M. tuberculosis* M. bovis* M. africanum*† M. microti		M. bovis, BCG*	
I	M. kansasii* M. marinum* M. simiae	(Yellow bacillus) M. luciflavum M. balnei, M. platypoecilus M. habana		
II	M. scrofulaceum*	M. marianum, M. paraffinicum	M. gordonae*	M. aquae, tap water scotochrome
	M. szulgai*		M. flavescens*	
III	M. avium* M. intracellulare* M. ulcerans* M. xenopi*	(Battey bacillus) M. brunense M. buruli M. littorale	M. gastri* M. nonchromogenicum* M. terrae* M. triviale* M. novum*	
IV	M. fortuitum* M. chelonei* M. chelonei subsp. abscessus*	M. ranae, M. giae, M. minetti M. borstelense M. runyonii, M. abscessus	M. phlei* M. smegmatis* M. vaccae* M. diernhoferi M. thamnopheos	M. moelleri
Others	M. paratuberculosis	M. johnei (needs mycobactin for growth)		
	M. leprae*	Hansen's bacillus (no growth on lab media)		
	M. lepraemurium	Stefansky's bacillus (no growth on lab media)		

Modified from *Diagnostic Standards and Classification of Tuberculosis and Other Mycobacterial Diseases.* New York, American Lung Association, 1974. Printed with permission of the American Lung Association.
*Indicates species found in humans.
†An organism intermediate between *M. tuberculosis* and *M. bovis*; status as distinct species being evaluated.

isms grow creamy white in the dark but become bright yellow to orange when exposed to light. Growth is more rapid than that of tubercle bacilli, reaching good maturity in about two weeks (sometimes three or more). Many strains form rather rough, dry colonies.

GROUP II: SCOTOCHROMOGENS *(M. scrofulaceum, M. szulgai, M. gordonae).* These mycobacteria produce pigment in the darkness as well as in the light and are orange to brick red.* They mature in one to two weeks. Colonies are usually moist and spreading.

GROUP III: NONPHOTOCHROMOGENS *(M. avium, M. intracellulare [Battey Bacillus], M. ulcerans, M. xenopi).* No pigment is produced either in the dark or when exposed to light.* There is good maturity in one to two weeks, and growth is complete in 21 to 28 days. The small, dome-shaped, discrete nonpigmented colonies usually retain their original appearance.

GROUP IV: RAPID GROWERS *(M. fortuitum, M. chelonei, M. chelonei subsp. abcessus).* The chief characteristic of this heterogeneous group is the rapid rate of growth. They are able to produce well-formed colonies in two to seven days.

M. szulgai is scotochromogenic when grown at 37° C., but photochromogenic at 25° C.

M. xenopi: Pigment intensifies either with age or after prolonged (two weeks) exposure to light.

Incidence and Epidemiology

In the United States, disease caused by the atypical mycobacteria is seen more frequently in the southern states, particularly those bordering the Gulf of Mexico. Edwards and Palmer (1959) have noted a high incidence of infection without clinical symptoms in persons living in the southeastern states, and studies in Richmond have corroborated this observation. It has been suggested that in this warm, moist climate, infection may be acquired from the soil or from vegetation. It has been demonstrated that some cattle show a positive reaction to skin tests with the antigens of the atypical mycobacteria; also, swine may develop scrofulous cervical lymph nodes produced by infection with a modification of the avian organism identical with or similar to the Battey bacillus. As previously noted, person-to-person transmission has not been demonstrated. It is interesting to note that organisms resembling atypical mycobacteria have been isolated from lesions in patients with sarcoidosis; however, this observation is not considered to be significant.

Pathology

In the light of present knowledge, the pathology appears similar to that of tuberculosis, and only a few minor differences have been noted. In children particularly, there seems to be a greater tendency toward superficial lymph node involvement than there is in tuberculosis.

Necrosis occurs relatively early in those infected with the atypical mycobacteria, and there is a tendency more toward liquefaction than to semisolid caseation. The inflammatory reaction is generally more nonspecific than granulomatous.

For all practical purposes, however, the lesions of tuberculosis and those caused by the atypical mycobacteria are indistinguishable.

Clinical Disease

Chronic suppurative lymphadenitis following granuloma is the usual form of the disease as it occurs in children. Photochromogens, scotochromogens or the Battey bacillus may be the causative agent, and on occasion all three have been demonstrated at the Medical College of Virginia. The superficial cervical lymph nodes are much more often involved, and Chapman (1959) has cultured identical organisms from the adenoids, the tonsils and the affected lymph nodes. In our experience, the cervical lesion is usually unilateral and more often involves a node or node group at the angle of the mandible (Fig. 1); other workers have noted the frequent occurrence of submandibular and submaxillary lesions. Involvement of the superficial cervical lymph nodes usually follows one or more acute attacks of tonsillitis or adenoiditis, and when the disease involves a lymph node elsewhere, there is usually some evidence of an associated skin lesion. Chronic suppurative lymphadenitis oc-

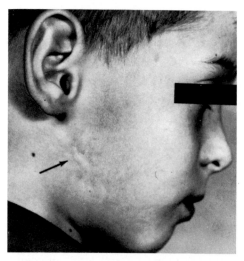

Figure 1. Chronic suppurative lymphadenitis usually involves a node or node group at the angle of the mandible. The healed lesion depicted here was caused by a scotochromogen. This mass of nodes liquefied before excision could be carried out, and aspirations were substituted. The patient fell from a bicycle, the mass ruptured, and healing ensued.

curs more frequently in young children, most often in those under five years of age.

The development of the lesion in the lymph nodes seems to be more rapid than that noted in tuberculosis, and fluctuation occurs early. Liquefaction is often complete by the time surgery is instituted.

In adults, the pulmonary form of the disease is frequently restricted to the lung and resembles tuberculosis. Symptoms in adults are relatively nonspecific and include malaise, low-grade fever, mild cough, generalized aching and occasionally slight hemoptysis. The lesion in the lung tends to remain localized and to undergo cavitation (with thin walls) and some fibrosis. Bronchogenic dissemination is rare. In a review of the world literature, Lincoln and Gilbert (1972) found mycobacteriosis of the lungs to have been infrequently reported in children. They documented 13 cases of pulmonary mycobacteriosis in children less than 17 years of age and eight cases of probable or possible mycobacteriosis. Included as proved cases were all children who had radiographic evidence of disease of the lungs and from whom organisms identified as atypical acid-fast bacilli had been obtained in pure culture from gastric* or bronchial washings, lung biopsies, surgical specimens, or material obtained at autopsy. The clinical and radiographic pictures were varied. In addition, ten of 12 patients with disseminated mycobacteriosis, two patients with chronic osteomyelitis and one with suspected meningitis had lung involvement. In all, 34 cases were found in which there was pulmonary involvement, including cases in which the evidence appeared only on postmortem examination.

CASE REPORT. T. H., an 11-week-old white girl, was admitted to the Medical College of Virginia Hospital with history of worsening respiratory infection of three days' duration. At time of admission, physical examination revealed a subacutely ill child with paroxysmal cough, tachypnea and dyspnea. Temperature was 102° F. (rectal). Routine laboratory studies were not remarkable. Roentgenogram of the chest showed right hilar adenopathy and right middle lobe infiltrate, compatible with primary tuberculosis, but the tuberculin reaction was negative (Fig. 2).

Approximately three weeks after admission, the patient appeared to be clinically well, but the chest roentgenogram showed no appreciable improvement. Culture of gastric contents, taken at the time of admission to the hospital, was reported to be productive of the Battey bacillus. In view of these developments, concomitant skin testing was carried out. The tuberculin test (PPD 5 TU) produced an area of induration measuring 8 mm. in diameter, while the Battey antigen skin test (PPD–B 5 TU) showed an area of induration measuring 26 mm. in diameter. The patient subsequently made a complete recovery.

Another form of disease is the so-called swimming pool granuloma, of which the causative agent is M. marinum (balnei). This organism, the natural reservoir for which is in fish and other cold-blooded animals, usually grows along the side of the pool, and lesions occur when the swimmer suffers abrasions of the skin when entering or leaving the pool. The lesions, which are painless, are characteristically slowly evolving granulomas in the skin that ulcerate after a time. The ulcers are shallow, with markedly thickened, irregular edges and seropurulent drainage. Regional lymph nodes are not involved.

Other reported variations of disease caused by the atypical mycobacteria include lesions of the bone, miliary and meningeal lesions, and generalized systemic involvement.

Sensitivity to Tuberculin

In children, the most important problem posed by infection with the atypical mycobacteria is that of the heterologous reaction produced on tuberculin testing, the so-called false-positive tuberculin reaction. This was first demonstrated by Edwards and Palmer

---

*It should be noted that atypical mycobacteria are not infrequently present in the gastric washings of patients who have no clinical disease.

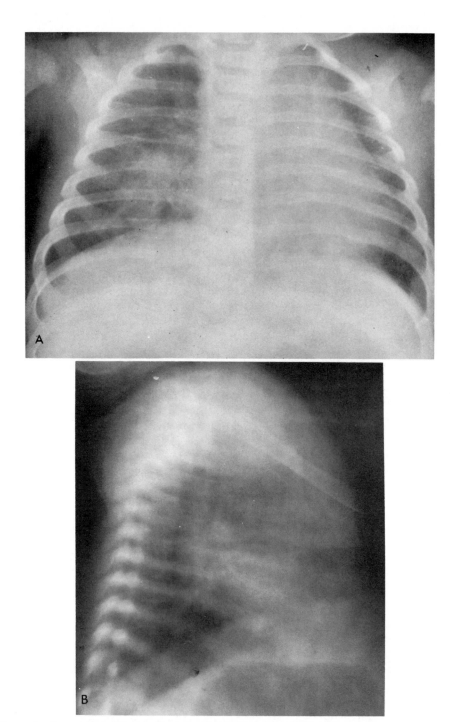

Figure 2.   Roentgenograms of an 11-week-old girl with Battey infection showing right hilar lymph-adenopathy with involvement of the right middle lobe.

(1959), who suggested that the tuberculin reaction measuring less than 10 mm. in diameter of induration is suspect. At the Medical College of Virginia, there have been three corroborative studies. Whenever there is a positive tuberculin reaction measuring 5 to 9 mm. in diameter of induration, the tuberculin test should be repeated. If the same result occurs, concomitant skin testing with tuberculin solution and the antigens of the more common atypical mycobacteria is indicated.* Such testing often results in a small tuberculin reaction (5 to 9 mm. in diameter of induration) and a much larger reaction to one of the antigens of the atypical mycobacteria (15 to 20 mm. in diameter of induration), thereby suggesting that the response is a heterologous reaction.

Since the value of such testing lies in the differentiation between infection caused by *M. tuberculosis* and that caused by the atypical mycobacteria, the fact that the antigens of the unclassified mycobacteria are apparently not sufficiently specific to distinguish between the Timpe-Runyon groups is not of foremost importance.

If the results obtained on concomitant skin testing do not clearly differentiate between tuberculosis and infection with the atypical mycobacteria, repeat skin testing two or three months later is often helpful.

Treatment

The usual antituberculosis drugs are utilized in treatment, but these agents are not always effective; they are more effective in Group I and much less effective in Group II, III and IV infections. In the treatment of Group III infections, authorities have advised the use of drug combinations, often four drugs: one injectable and three oral. In fact, all treatment consists of at least two drugs used concomitantly. The results of susceptibility studies will determine the antimicrobial agents to be utilized.

Isoniazid should be given orally in a dosage of 20 mg. per kilogram of body weight per day in a single dose or in two divided doses (maximal daily dose of 500 mg.), and para-aminosalicylic acid (PAS) in a dosage of 200 mg. per kilogram of body weight per day orally in three or four divided doses (maximal daily dose 12 gm.). If the organism is even partially sensitive, medication should be continued for one year.

Streptomycin in a single intramuscular daily dose of 20 to 40 mg. per kilogram of body weight per day (maximal daily dose 1 gm.) is continued until clinical improvement is noted, and the drug may then be administered three times each week. The duration of treatment with this drug depends on the course of the disease, but if such treatment is prolonged, the patient should be carefully watched for possible damage to the eighth cranial nerve.

Ethambutol is given orally in a suggested dosage of 20 mg. per kilogram of body weight per day for four to six weeks and 10 to 15 mg. per kilogram per day thereafter in a single daily dose. The drug appears to be an effective and relatively safe agent, although use in pediatric patients under 13 years of age is experimental. It is well tolerated, and there have been few reports of allergic reactions. So far, the drug has been used mainly in adults, and with higher dosage a few instances of retrobulbar neuritis with resultant loss of vision have been noted. At the recommended dose and with precautions that include monthly studies of visual acuity and visual fields and tests for color vision, there appears to be much less danger of this side-effect. The drug should be discontinued if there is more than a two-line loss of visual acuity as measured on a Snellen eye chart, if there is contraction of the visual fields or if there is loss of color vision.

Ethionamide, also available for use in combination with one or more drugs, is administered orally in a suggested dosage of 10 to 20 mg. per kilogram of body weight per day (dosage in children has not been established). It is

---

*See text on page 794.

given in two or three divided doses (maximum daily dose 750 mg.). The drug may be hepatotoxic.

Kanamycin, given intramuscularly in a dosage of 10 to 15 mg. per kilogram of body weight per day, is similar to streptomycin and may have all the toxic effects of streptomycin plus renal toxicity.

Reports suggest that rifampin possesses significant activity against certain strains (Group I) of the atypical mycobacteria. Indeed, four cases of atypical mycobacterial cervical adenitis have been successfully treated with rifampin (Mandell and Wright, 1975) without excision of the affected lymph nodes. In two instances, Group III mycobacteria were isolated, and in the other two cases, drainage was sterile and diagnosis was established by means of the clinical manifestations and appropriate skin tests. Suggested dosage of rifampin is 10 to 20 mg. per kilogram of body weight per day (maximum daily dose 600 mg.).

Prompt excision of suppurative lymph nodes is usually the most important part of the therapeutic approach (see above). Since there is a tendency toward early and complete liquefaction of affected lymph nodes these nodes should be completely removed as soon as possible. In adults with pulmonary disease who have localized lesions that have not responded to chemotherapy and who are in satisfactory general condition, pulmonary resection is the treatment of choice. They should continue to receive the same antimicrobial therapy as previously outlined. As noted previously, there have been a few reports of pulmonary disease in children (Lincoln and Gilbert, 1972), but such involvement in this age group appears to be rare.

Skin lesions caused by *Mycobacterium marinum (balnei)* must sometimes be excised, and the patient is given the same antimicrobial therapy.

Patients with clinical disease caused by the atypical mycobacteria should not be treated in a tuberculosis sanatorium.

REFERENCES

Bates, R. D., and Chapman, J. S.: Tuberculin test: some inherent limitations. *Tex. State J. Med., 60*:517, 1964.

Bialkin, G., Pollak, A., and Weil, A. J.: Pulmonary infection with *Mycobacterium kansasii. Am. J. Dis. Child., 101*:739, 1961.

Black, B. G., and Chapman, J. S.: Cervical adenitis in children due to human and unclassified mycobacteria. *Pediatrics, 33*:887, 1964.

Chapman, J. S.: Varieties of tuberculosis in children. *Minn. Med., 42*:1773, 1959.

Chapman, J. S.: *The Anonymous Mycobacteria in Human Disease.* Springfield, Illinois, Charles C Thomas, 1960.

Chapman, J. S.: Atypical mycobacterial infections: pathogenesis, clinical manifestations and treatment. *Med. Clin. North Am., 51*:503, 1967.

Chapman, J. S., and Guy, L. R.: Scrofula caused by atypical mycobacteria. *Pediatrics, 23*:323, 1959.

Committee on Diagnostic Skin Testing, American Thoracic Society: Current indications for the use of atypical mycobacterial skin test antigens. *Am. Rev. Resp. Dis., 102*:468, 1970.

Committee on Diagnostic Skin Testing, American Thoracic Society: *The Tuberculin Skin Test.* New York, American Lung Association, 1974.

Committee to Revise Diagnostic Standards, American Thoracic Society: *Diagnostic Standards and Classification of Tuberculosis and Other Mycobacterial Diseases.* New York, American Lung Association, 1974.

Cuttino, J. T., and McCabe, A.: Pure granulomatous nocardiosis: a new fungus disease distinguished by intracellular parasitism. *Am. J. Pathol., 25*:1, 1949.

Davis, S. D., and Comstock, G. W.: Mycobacterial cervical adenitis in children. *J. Pediatr., 58*:771, 1961.

Edwards, P. Q., and Edwards, L. B.: Story of the tuberculin test. *Am. Rev. Resp. Dis., 81*:1, part 2, 1960.

Edwards, L. B., and Palmer, C. E.: Isolation of "atypical" mycobacteria from healthy persons. *Am. Rev. Resp. Dis., 80*:747, 1959.

Edwards, L. B., Edwards, P. Q., and Palmer, C. E.: Sources of tuberculin sensitivity in human populations. *Acta Tuberc. Scand., 47*(Suppl):77, 1959.

Edwards, L. B., and others: Epidemiologic studies of tuberculin sensitivity. II. Response to experimental infection with mycobacteria isolated from human sources. *Am. J. Hyg., 71*:218, 1960.

Guy, L. R., and Chapman, J. S.: Susceptibility in vitro of unclassified mycobacteria to commonly used antimicrobials. *Am. Rev. Resp. Dis., 84*:746, 1961.

Harris, G. D., Johanson, W. B., Jr., and Nicholson, D. P.: Response to chemotherapy of pulmonary infection due to *Mycobacterium kansasii. Am. Rev. Resp. Dis., 112*:31, 1975.

Hsu, K. H. K.: Nontuberculous mycobacterial infections in children: preliminary clinical and epidemiologic study. *J. Pediatr.*, *60*:705, 1962.

Jenkins, D. E., and others: The clinical problem of infection with atypical acid-fast bacilli. *Trans. Am. Clin. Climatol. Assoc.*, *71*:21, 1959.

Kendig, E. L., Jr.: Unclassified mycobacteria in children: correlation of skin tests and gastric cultures. *Am. J. Dis. Child.*, *101*:749, 1961.

Kendig, E. L., Jr.: Unclassified mycobacteria as a causative agent in the positive tuberculin reaction. *Pediatrics*, *30*:221, 1962.

Kendig, E. L., Jr.: Unclassified mycobacteria: incidence of infection and cause of a false-positive tuberculin reaction. *N. Engl. J. Med.*, *268*:1001, 1963.

Krieger, I., Hahne, O. H., and Whitten, C. F.: Atypical mycobacteria as a probable cause of chronic bone disease. *J. Pediatr.*, *65*:340, 1964.

Lincoln, E. M., and Gilbert, L. A.: Disease in children due to mycobacteria other than *Mycobacterium tuberculosis*. *Am. Rev. Resp. Dis.*, *105*:683, 1972.

Lunn, H. F.: Mycobacterial lesions in bone. *East Afr. Med. J.*, *40*:113, 1963.

MacKellan, A., Hilton, H. B., and Masters, P. L.: Mycobacterial lymphadenitis in childhood. *Arch. Dis. Child.*, *42*:70, 1967.

Mandell, F., and Wright, P. F.: Treatment of atypical mycobacterial cervical adenitis with rifampin. *Pediatrics*, *55*:39, 1975.

Mankiewicz, E.: The relationship of sarcoidosis to anonymous mycobacteria. *Acta Med. Scand.*, *62*(Suppl.):403, 1964.

Marks, J., Jenkins, P. A., and Tsukamura, M.: *Mycobacterium szulgai*: a new pathogen. *Tubercle*, *53*:210, 1972.

McCracken, G. H., Jr., and Reynolds, R. C.: Primary lymphopenic immunologic deficiency: disseminated *mycobacterium kansasii* infection. *Am. J. Dis. Child.*, *120*:143, 1970.

Millman, W. J., and Barness, L. A.: Unclassified mycobacteria: cause of nonspecific tuberculin reactions. *Am. J. Dis. Child.*, *104*:21, 1962.

Mollohan, C. S., and Romer, M. S.: Public health significance of swimming pool granuloma. *Am. J. Public Health*, *51*:883, 1961.

Palmer, C. E., and Long, M. W.: Effects of infection with atypical mycobacteria on BCG vaccination and tuberculosis. *Am. Rev. Resp. Dis.*, *94*:553, 1966.

Prissick, F. S., and Masson, A. M.: Cervical lymphadenitis in children caused by chromogenic mycobacteria. *Can. Med. Assoc. J.*, *75*:798, 1956.

Runyon, E. H.: Anonymous mycobacteria in pulmonary disease. *Med. Clin. North Am.*, *43*:273, 1959.

Runyon, E. H., Wayne, L. G., and Kubici, G. P.: Mycobacteriaceae. In Buchanan, R. E., and Gibbons, N. E. (Eds.): *Bergey's Manual of Determinative Bacteriology.* 8th Ed. Baltimore, Williams & Wilkins Company, 1974.

Rynearson, T. L., Shronts, J. S., and Wolinsky, E.: Rifampin: in vitro effect in atypical mycobacteria. *Am. Rev. Resp. Dis.*, *104*:272, 1971.

Schaefer, W. B., and Davis, C. L.: Bacteriologic and histopathologic study of skin granuloma due to *Mycobacterium balnei*. *Am. Rev. Resp Dis.*, *84*:837, 1961.

Section on Diseases of the Chest, American Academy of Pediatrics: The tuberculin test. *Pediatrics*, *54*:650, 1974.

Siltzbach, L. E.: Sarcoidosis and mycobacteria. *Am. Rev. Resp. Dis.*, *97*:1, 1968.

Tarshis, M. S.: The impact of chemotherapy on the tubercle bacillus and its significance. *Dis. Chest*, *41*:471, 1962.

Timpe, A., and Runyon, E. H.: Relationship of "atypical" acid-fast bacteria to human disease: preliminary report. *J. Lab. Clin. Med.*, *44*:202, 1954.

Valdivia Alvarez, J., Suarez Mendez, R., and Echemendia Font, M.: *Mycobacterium habana*: probable nueva especie dentro de las microbacterias no clasfcadas. *Bol. Hig. Epid.*, *9*:65, 1971.

Van der Hoeven, L. H., Rutten, F. J., and Van der Sar, A.: An unusual acid-fast bacillus causing systemic disease and death in a child, with special reference to disseminated osteomyelitis and intracellular parasitism. *Am. J. Clin. Pathol.*, *29*:433, 1958.

Wayne, L. G., and Doubek, J. R.: Diagnostic key to mycobacteria encounterd in clinical laboratories. *Appl. Microbiol.*, *16*:925, 1968.

Weed, L. A., Karlson, A. G., Ivirs, J. C., and Miller, R. H.: Recurring migratory osteomyelitis associated with saprophytic acid-fast bacilli. *Proc. Staff Meet. Mayo Clin.*, *31*:238, 1956.

Weed, L. A., McDonald, J. R., and Needham, G. M.: The isolation of saprophytic acid-fast bacilli from lesions of caseous granulomas. *Proc. Staff Meet. Mayo Clin.*, *31*:246, 1956.

Yakovac, W. C., Baker, R., Sweigert, C., and Hope, J. W.: Fatal disseminated osteomyelitis due to an anonymous mycobacterium. *J. Pediatr.*, *59*:909, 1961.

CHAPTER FORTY-EIGHT

SARCOIDOSIS

Edwin L. Kendig, Jr., M.D.

Sarcoidosis is a chronic systemic granulomatous disease, the cause of which is unknown. The disease appears to be relatively rare among children. In a review of the world literature to February 1953, McGovern and Merritt (1956) were able to document only 104 cases in children 15 years of age and younger. To these they added nine others, all diagnosed in Washington hospitals.* Since that time, there have been only six series, consisting of a total of 99 cases, reported in the United States. In addition, North (1970) has reported six cases of sarcoid arthritis in children. In Japan, Niitu and co-workers (1976) have reported 37 cases corroborated by positive biopsy or positive Kveim test, and 32 others in which diagnosis was made on clinical findings. Mandi (1964) noted 14 cases among children in Hungary. To date, there have been 37 cases of sarcoidosis in children diagnosed at the Medical College of Virginia. It is, of course, conceded that there are undoubtedly many other cases of recognized sarcoidosis in children still unreported, but the disease must be considered relatively rare in this age group.†

The criteria for the diagnosis of sar-coidosis were outlined by James and coworkers (1976) and presented at the Seventh International Conference on Sarcoidosis in October 1975, as follows:

Sarcoidosis is a multisystem granulomatous disorder of unknown etiology most commonly affecting young adults and presenting most frequently with bilateral hilar lymphadenopathy, pulmonary infiltration, skin or eye lesions. The diagnosis is established most securely when clinicoradiographic findings are supported by histological evidence of widespread noncaseating epithelioid cell granulomas in more than one organ or a positive Kveim-Siltzbach skin test. Immunological features are depression of delayed-type hypersensitivity suggesting impaired cell-mediated immunity and raised or abnormal immunoglobulins. There may also be hypercalciuria with or without hypercalcemia. The course and prognosis may correlate with the mode of onset: an acute onset with erythema nodosum heralds a self-limiting course and spontaneous resolution, while an insidious onset may be followed by relentless progressive fibrosis. Corticosteroids relieve symptoms and suppress inflammation and granuloma formation.

History

Sarcoidosis was first described in England by Hutchinson in 1875. Contributions clarifying certain clinical and pathologic features were made by Besnier in 1889, by Boeck in 1899, and by Schaumann in 1917. Heerfordt (1909), and somewhat more recently Garland and Thompson (1933) and Longcope and Pierson (1937), have contributed further to the description of the disease.

The use of mass radiography, introduced in many countries in an effort to detect tuberculosis (about the time of

---

*The world group as referred to hereafter in this text includes the 104 cases documented from the world literature by McGovern and Merritt and the additional nine cases reported by them, a total of 113 cases.

†Siltzbach (1968) notes that silent cases are not unusual in childhood because children are not included in mass x-ray surveys. It is his feeling that childhood sarcoidosis is more common than is generally realized and that only the advanced cases are diagnosed. Niitu's report of 69 cases diagnosed by annual roentgenograms of school children in Japan appears to support this thesis.

World War II), led to a significant advance in the knowledge of sarcoidosis. This method, first used in the Armed Forces and later in the general population, led to the finding of a high incidence of presumptive asymptomatic sarcoidosis.

Age Incidence

Sarcoidosis is encountered more frequently in adults between 20 and 40 years of age, but the disease may occur at any age. Although the youngest patient reported, substantiated by biopsy, was a two-month-old infant, most of those cases reported in childhood have occurred in the preadolescent or adolescent age group. Of the patients documented from the world literature by McGovern and Merritt (including their own cases), 75 per cent were between the ages of nine and 15 years; 34 of the 37 cases at the Medical College of Virginia fell into the same age group, with two patients eight years of age and one three years old.

Race

There is a great variation in the racial incidence. In Europe, and particularly in the Scandinavian countries, where the black population is low, the disease has been found more often in the white population. In the United States, on the other hand, sarcoidosis occurs more commonly among the black race. In three radiographic surveys of the United States Armed Forces, blacks with sarcoidosis outnumbered white personnel with the disease by a ratio varying from 7:1 to 26:1. Cummings and coworkers (1956) reported the hospitalization rate for black and white World War II veterans with sarcoidosis to be 40.1 and 3.3 per 100,000, respectively.

Although Siltzbach (1960) has noted that the apparent susceptibility of the American black is not shared by the blacks of Central Africa, where the disease is apparently unknown, he also pointed out that cases of sarcoidosis are beginning to be reported in numbers among natives of North and South Africa. He suggests, however, that the latter finding is the result of better facilities now available there for the detection of sarcoidosis.

Among the children for whom the race was stated in the world literature, only 34 per cent were black, but 27 of the 37 children in the Medical College of Virginia series were black (73 per cent).

Sex Distribution

It is generally agreed that both sexes appear to be affected with equal frequency, and in the Medical College of Virginia series there were 20 females and 17 males.

Heredity

There appears to be little evidence that heredity is in any way connected with either the incidence of sarcoidosis or the predisposition toward it. It is unlikely that such reports as that of three cases among siblings under 15 years of age are an indication of hereditary involvement.

Geographic Distribution

Sarcoidosis has been observed almost everywhere in the world, and Sweden has the highest reported incidence of the disease. In that country, the prevalence in the Armed Forces, in the general population and in Stockholm was reported to be above 40 per 100,000 population, and one rural county, Jaemtlands, had a rate of 140 per 100,000.

In the United States there have been reports by Michael and coworkers (1950), Gentry and coworkers (1955), and Cummings and coworkers (1956) on the study of the birthplace and residence of persons in the Armed Forces with sarcoidosis, indicating areas with high attack rates of sarcoidosis in the South Atlantic and Gulf states, with endemic areas in New England and the

Midwest. Nansemond County, Virginia, appears to have the highest incidence of sarcoidosis, with a projected incidence of presumptive disease of 500 per 100,000 population.*

Etiology, Pathogenesis and Immunology

The cause of sarcoidosis has not been determined. The most common belief is that sarcoidosis is a single disorder and not a syndrome, but the possibility exists that the characteristic response actually may result from one or more agents in a proper host setting. If an exogenous agent is the cause of sarcoidosis, its portal of entry is unknown. The occurrence of mediastinal adenopathy suggests an air-borne route. Systemic involvement is present at the outset. It has been suggested by Siltzbach that the occurrence of erythema nodosum favors an environmental origin, since the numerous microbial and chemical sensitivities known to precipitate an attack of erythema nodosum are all of exogenous origin.

In the patient with sarcoidosis, circulating antibodies are normally produced in response to specific challenge. However, there is a defect in cellular immunity, manifested in the patient's relative insensitivity to tuberculin and other delayed hypersensitivity antigens.

*Apperson, W. E.: Unpublished data.

Clinical Manifestations

Lesions may occur in almost any tissue or organ of the body. Since symptoms are due primarily to local tissue infiltration and injury by pressure and displacement by sarcoid lesions, the clinical manifestations depend largely on the organ or system involved.

As noted earlier, sarcoidosis most commonly involves the lungs, lymph nodes, eyes, skin, phalangeal bones, liver and spleen (Table 1).

In the Medical College of Virginia series of 37 patients, there were 25 different presenting complaints, the most common being fatigability, lethargy or malaise; one of these occurred in approximately one-third of the patients. Cough, fever and dyspnea were next in frequency, and weight loss and lymphadenopathy followed in that order.

LUNGS.   Symptoms referable to the chest are usually mild and often consist of a dry, hacking cough, and children are likely to have mild to moderate dyspnea. By international convention, the pulmonary lesions of sarcoidosis seen on roentgenogram are classified as follows: Stage 0: normal chest x-ray film; Stage 1: bilateral hilar lymphadenopathy, without detectable lung changes (Fig. 1); Stage 2: bilateral hilar lymphadenopathy with pulmonary infiltrations that may be fine or coarse miliary nodulation or cotton-wool in appearance (Fig. 2); Stage 3: fibrosis with formation of bullae and without hilar lymphadenopathy (Fig. 3).

The most common roentgenographic

TABLE 1.   COMPARISON OF ORGANS AFFECTED IN THE WORLD GROUP AND MEDICAL COLLEGE OF VIRGINIA SERIES

	World Group (113)	Medical College of Virginia (37)
Lungs (parenchyma–hilar lymph nodes)	62	37
Peripheral lymphadenopathy	54	27
Skin	57	10
Eyes	55	8
Bones	33	3
Spleen	25	9
Liver	16	11

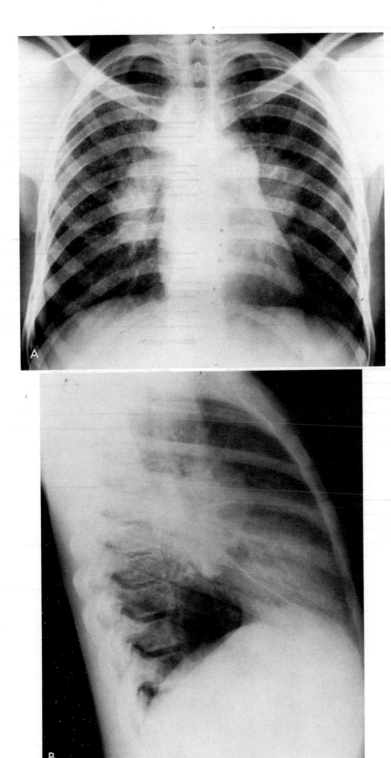

Figure 1. *A* and *B*, Bilateral hilar lymph node enlargement.

finding in children is that of bilateral hilar lymph node enlargement, with or without detectable lung changes (Figs. I and 2). In a worldwide review of sarcoidosis, James and coworkers (1976) noted involvement of the lung and hilar lymph nodes in 92 per cent of adult cases, while only 62 (55 per cent) of the 113 world cases in children were so affected; nevertheless, this 55 per cent constituted the most common finding in that series. Such involvement was noted in all 37 cases in the Medical College of Virginia group.

LYMPHATICS. Peripheral lymphadenopathy is a common feature of sarcoidosis. The nodes are discrete, painless and freely movable. The typical histologic picture is that of epithelioid cell tubercles, showing little or no necrosis (Fig. 4).

Among the reported world cases in children, there was generalized lymphadenopathy in 38 of 113 cases, with an additional 16 cases of isolated or localized lymph node involvement, a total of 48 per cent. Peripheral lymphadenopathy occurred in 27 of 37 Medical College of Virginia cases (73 per cent).

EYES. The ocular lesions have been described by a number of investigators. Uveitis and iritis constitute the most frequently observed lesions, but keratitis, retinitis, glaucoma, and involvement of the eyelids and lacrimal glands may also occur. Involvement of the eye with resultant partial or total blindness is one of the most feared lesions of sarcoidosis. Although their examination of the world literature suggests that eye lesions in children are not usually severe, McGovern and Merritt (1956) noted one case of partial blindness in their own series. This finding and a survey of the Medical College of Virginia series, in which eye involvement was noted in eight of the 37 cases, appear to refute this conception; such involvement in two patients in the latter group also resulted in partial blindness.

SKIN. Skin lesions may occur in three different forms (Longcope and Freiman, 1952): ① small, discrete, slightly elevated nodules; ② large conglomerate masses, slightly elevated and

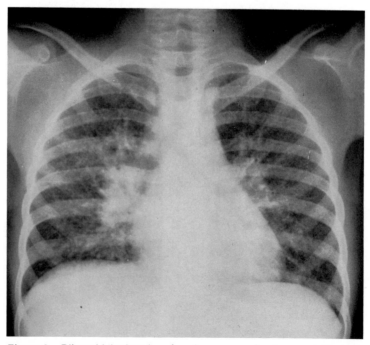

Figure 2.   Bilateral hilar lymph node enlargement and pulmonary infiltration.

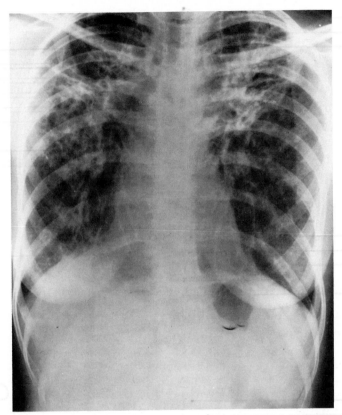

Figure 3. Sarcoidosis showing fibrosis with bullae and without hilar lymphadenopathy.

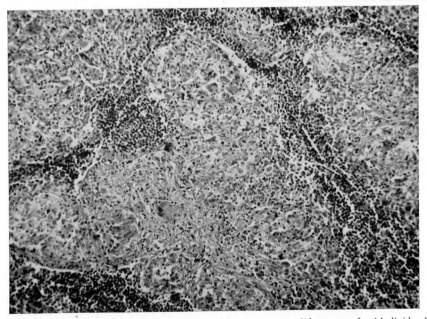

Figure 4. The architecture of the node is distorted by numerous solid masses of epithelioid cells with occasional giant cells. The masses are surrounded by lymphocytes. No necrosis or caseation is apparent. Lymphoid follicles are almost absent. (Courtesy of *N. Engl. J. Med., 260*:962, 1959.)

involving subcutaneous tissues; and ③ large flat plaques covering considerable areas of skin over the trunk or extremities. James and Siltzbach (1975) have noted that on occasion previously atrophic scars on knees or at old operative sites suddenly become purple and livid (sarcoid); this was never present in the Medical College of Virginia series.

Sarcoid skin lesions may vary in color from waxy, depigmented areas to a reddish blue or violaceous hue. They vary in size from a few millimeters to more than a centimeter in diameter. The lesions are more often seen on the face, but may occur elsewhere. Although James reported the incidence of skin lesions in adults around the world to be only 9 per cent, such lesions may be more common in children. Of the 113 reported world cases, skin lesions were present in 57, and there was involvement of the skin in ten of the 37 Medical College of Virginia cases.

UVEOPAROTID FEVER. This syndrome, consisting of ocular disturbances, parotid gland swelling and frequent facial nerve palsy, was first described by Heerfordt in 1909. Uveitis is always present at some time in the course of this syndrome. Usually, a low-grade fever, gastrointestinal symptoms and general malaise precede the eye involvement. The world group includes 28 cases (25 per cent), but there were no cases among the Medical College of Virginia group.

BONES. Osseous lesions, which are usually demonstrable as areas of decreased density and often as "punched out" areas in the metacarpals, metatarsals and distal phalanges, may be either single or multiple. Bone involvement is found in patients with chronic skin lesions. The incidence of osseous lesions in adults has been variously stated as 2 to 29 per cent; among children there was an incidence of 29 per cent in the world group, and 8 per cent in the Medical College of Virginia patients. Dunner and coworkers (1957) have suggested that bone lesions may not be as common as had been previously suspected.

LIVER. Although hepatic involvement is frequently seen at necropsy, clinical evidence of liver disease is not often apparent. Liver enlargement is the usual finding, and impairment of function is relatively uncommon unless serum protein changes are an indication of liver disease. In the world series, liver enlargement was noted 16 times (14 per cent); in the Medical College of Virginia group, there was liver enlargement in 11 of 37 patients (30 per cent). Needle biopsy of the liver is now effectively utilized as a diagnostic aid.

SPLEEN. Although splenic involvement has been demonstrated by needle biopsy, enlargement is practically the only clinical finding. The spleen was palpable in 25 of the world cases and in nine (24 per cent) of the Medical College of Virginia group.

KIDNEY. Kogut and Neumann (1961) have reviewed renal involvement in sarcoidosis and reported a case of their own. These authors point out that there have been less than ten reported cases in children; nevertheless, this would appear to place the kidney as a not uncommon site of sarcoid involvement in this age group. Renal involvement has been ascribed to one or more of the following processes: ① sarcoid granulomas infiltrating the renal parenchyma; ② glomerulitis with basement membrane changes; and ③ hypercalcemia with or without nephrolithiasis and nephrocalcinosis. Abnormal urinary findings may include proteinuria, pyuria, hematuria, granular casts, and calciuria. One of the Medical College of Virginia group had transient hematuria, and another had progressive glomerulonephritis.

HEART. Sarcoid lesions in the myocardium have been found at necropsy in a number of cases. In the 113 world cases, there was associated cardiac involvement in six instances; there was no evidence of cardiac involvement in the Medical College of Virginia group. Cardiac changes may be secondary to extensive pulmonary sarcoidosis or may be the result of conduction aberration caused by sarcoid lesions.

NERVOUS SYSTEM. Although central

nervous system involvement has been reported in adults, the most commonly noted neurologic involvement in childhood seems to be paralysis of the facial nerve. In the 113 world cases, there were four instances of facial nerve palsy. Neurologic symptoms result when sarcoid lesions cause local interruption of function, and one of the Medical College of Virginia cases had a presumptive aqueductal stenosis, probably resulting from a contiguous sarcoid lesion.

ENDOCRINE GLANDS. A definite relationship can be demonstrated with the pituitary gland. Diabetes insipidus has been reported in adults, and three of the children in the world group had some evidence of such involvement; none of the Medical College of Virginia group was so involved.

Clinical Picture

The clinical picture of sarcoidosis as reconstructed from the Medical College of Virginia patients is as follows: 27 of the 37 patients were black, and practically all were in the older age group. Hilar lymph node–lung involvement was always present, the syndrome of uveoparotid fever did not occur, eye lesions were frequently present, and serious eye lesions were noted in two instances.

Laboratory Studies

There are no detailed reports of laboratory findings in 113 world cases. Among the most frequent significant laboratory changes reported in sarcoidosis are hyperglobulinemia, eosinophilia, leukopenia, hypercalcemia, hypercalciuria and elevated alkaline phosphatase level.

HYPERGLOBULINEMIA. Salveson (1935) was the first to point out that the serum protein concentration may be abnormally high in cases of sarcoidosis. It has since been established that this hyperproteinemia is due to an absolute increase in serum globulin, so that the albumin-globulin ratio is frequently reversed. Among adult patients, abnormal globulin levels are present in 44

per cent of the cases. The Medical College of Virginia series showed hyperglobulinemia in 22 of 33 cases. Serum IgG, IgM and IgA are all elevated during the acute phase of the disease.

SERUM CALCIUM. Hypercalcemia occurs in about 11 per cent of adult patients (James and coworkers, 1976). Serum calcium concentration above 11 mg. per 100 ml. of serum was noted in five of the 30 Medical College of Virginia patients who were tested.

SERUM ALKALINE PHOSPHATASE. While elevation of serum alkaline phosphatase is not infrequently reported (Maddrey and coworkers, 1970), it is difficult to evaluate results in children. As far as can be determined, 13 of the 32 cases (40 per cent) tested at the Medical College of Virginia showed a similar increase.

EOSINOPHILIA. Next to hyperglobulinemia, the most consistent laboratory finding among the Medical College of Virginia patients was eosinophilia (4 per cent or above). This occurred in 18 of 37 cases, and in four instances there was eosinophilia above 7 per cent. This finding also occurs in adults, although apparently to a lesser degree.

LEUKOPENIA. This finding occurred in ten of the 37 Medical College of Virginia patients. In an adult series, leukopenia was found in one-fourth of the cases, but was more common among the blacks.

OTHER LABORATORY DATA. Elevation of the erythrocyte sedimentation rate will naturally be expected during the acute phase of the disease. Abnormal urinary findings will be present in those instances in which there is renal involvement; among these may be hematuria, pyuria, proteinuria, granular casts, and hypercalciuria.

Other Diagnostic Procedures

THE KVEIM TEST. This test represents an attempt to elicit a specific skin reaction by the intracutaneous injection of emulsified sarcoid tissue into patients with suspected sarcoidosis. Methods for preparing Kveim suspension have changed since Williams and

Nickerson (1935), Kveim (1941), and Danbolt (1951) first published their work, and the present method of preparation was described by Chase in 1961. The intracutaneous test is performed in the manner of a Mantoux test, with the use of 0.15 to 0.2 ml. per injection. Any nodule that appears at the injection site, no matter how small, is biopsied after 28 to 42 days. Although Siltzbach (1968) reports a positive Kveim reaction in 16 of 18 patients, scarcity of effective Kveim test material limits the usefulness of the test at this time.

BIOPSY OF LYMPH NODE OR OTHER TISSUE. Biopsy of a lymph node or other tissue with demonstration of an epithelioid cell tubercle, with little or no necrosis, is an essential in diagnosis. The diagnosis of sarcoidosis was corroborated by biopsy in all 37 Medical College of Virginia cases. Included among the biopsies were lymph node alone (31 cases); lymph node and skin (3 cases); skin (1 case) and lung (1 case); and lymph node and testis (1 case).

An enlarged peripheral lymph node is most suitable for biopsy, but if none is present, biopsy of the scalene fat pad is most likely to reveal a lesion compatible with sarcoidosis. Mediastinoscopy with biopsy of the mediastinal lymph node has also been advocated. Muscle biopsy may be indicated, and as noted above, lung biopsy is occasionally helpful. Needle aspiration of the liver appears to be particularly productive.

OTHER TESTS. The tuberculin test, the histoplasmin skin test,* and the coccidioidin skin test should be performed on each patient with suspected sarcoidosis. Although a positive reaction with one of these antigens does not necessarily controvert the diagnosis, it may be an indication that the infection is merely one which simulates sarcoidosis.

Prognosis

Sones and Israel (1960), in a review

of more than 200 adult patients in Philadelphia, have attempted to determine the prognosis of sarcoidosis. They state that sarcoidosis, as observed by them, was neither as benign as indicated in some reports, nor as malignant as in others. Sones and Israel found survival rates, calculated by the life table method, to be 88.8 per cent after five years of observation and 84.8 per cent after ten years, indicating considerable diminution of survival as the result of sarcoidosis.

Determination of the prognosis of the disease in children is not easy. Twenty-eight children, with a mean follow-up period of nine years, have been studied at the Medical College of Virginia. While none has died, five patients have sustained severe damage from the disease; two of these are blind, and three others have severe restrictive pulmonary disease.

While the presence of skin lesions suggests a guarded prognosis, a predictable outcome of any given case does not seem possible.

Treatment

Since the cause of sarcoidosis is unknown, there is no known specific therapy. Adrenocorticosteroids and corticotropin are the only agents available at present that can suppress the acute manifestations of sarcoidosis. These agents are used only during the acute and dangerous episodes.

Adrenocorticosteroid (or corticotropin) therapy is always indicated in patients with intrinsic ocular disease, with diffuse pulmonary lesions with alveolar-capillary block, with central nervous system lesions, with myocardial involvement, with hypersplenism and with persistent hypercalcemia. Relative indications for adrenocorticosteroid therapy include progressive or symptomatic pulmonary lesions, disfiguring cutaneous and lymph node lesions, constitutional symptoms and joint involvement, lesions of the nasal, laryngeal and bronchial mucosa, and persistent facial nerve palsy.

Fresh lesions are apparently more

---

*Histoplasmin skin test is currently (July 1977) unavailable in the United States. Complement fixation for histoplasmosis may be substituted.

responsive than older ones. Suppressive action is often temporary, but it is beneficial when the unremitting course of such disease will produce loss of organ function. For example, adrenocorticosteroids can reduce the level of serum calcium and may thus help prevent nephrocalcinosis and renal insufficiency and possibly band keratitis. Whether adrenocorticosteroids should be utilized in the treatment of those patients whose disease consists only of asymptomatic miliary nodules or bronchopneumonic patches in the lung fields is debatable.

The initial dose of prednisone or prednisolone is 1 mg. per kilogram of body weight per day, and of triamcinolone 0.75 mg. per kilogram of body weight per day in four divided doses. A gradual reduction in the level of dosage of adrenocorticosteroid is initiated as soon as clinical manifestations of the disease disappear. A maintenance dose of prednisone (15 mg. every other day) is continued until the patient has received a six-month total course of treatment.

Siltzbach (1968) reported the frequent occurrence of temporary relapse following the discontinuation of adrenocorticosteroid therapy, but noted that improvement usually follows even if the treatment is not resumed. In the management of ocular sarcoidosis, adrenocorticosteroids in the form of either ointment or drops (0.5 to 1 per cent) are utilized in conjunction with the systemic use of these agents. During the course of such local therapy, the pupils are kept in a state of continuous dilatation by use of an atropine ointment (1 per cent).

Adrenocorticosteroid ointment may also be utilized in the treatment of cutaneous lesions, but only in conjunction with systemic therapy, since better results are obtained with the latter.

Anderson, J., Dent, C. E., Harper, C., and Philpot, G. R.: Effect of cortisone on calcium metabolism in sarcoidosis with hypercalcaemia; possible antagonistic action of cortisone and vitamin D. *Lancet,* 2:720, 1954.

Barker, D. H. W.: Benign lymphogranulomatosis with apparent involvement of the anterior pituitary. *Br. J. Dermatol.,* 58:70, 1946.

Bauer, H. J., and Gentz, C.: The results of mass x-ray examination in Stockholm City during the years 1949–1951. *Acta Tuberc. Scand.,* 29:22, 1953.

Beier, F. R., and Lahey, M. E.: Sarcoidosis among children in Utah and Idaho. *J. Pediatr.,* 65:350, 1964.

Berger, K. W., and Relman, A. S.: Renal impairment due to sarcoid infiltration of the kidney; report of a case proved by renal biopsies before and after treatment with cortisone. *N. Engl. J. Med.,* 252:44, 1955.

Besnier, E.: Lupus pernio de la face, synovitis fongueses (scrofulotuberculeuses) symétriques des extrémités supérieures. *Ann. Dermatol. Syphiligr.,* 10:333, 1889.

Block, M.: Sarcoid diagnosed by needle biopsy of the spleen: report of a case. *J.A.M.A.,* 149:748, 1952.

Boeck, C.: Multiple benign sarcoid of skin. *J. Cutan. Genitourin. Dis.,* 17:543, 1899.

Boman, A.: Diabetes insipidus vid lymphogranulomatosis benigna. *Nord. Med.,* 47:675, 1952.

Chapman, J. S.: Notes on the secondary factors involved in the etiology of sarcoidosis. *Am. Rev. Tuberc.,* 71:459, 1955.

Chase, M. W.: The preparation and standardization of Kveim testing antigens. *Am. Rev. Resp. Dis.,* 84:86, 1961.

Committee on Therapy, American Thoracic Society: Treatment of sarcoidosis. *Am. Rev. Resp. Dis.,* 103:433, 1971.

Cummings, M. M., and Dunner, E.: Pulmonary sarcoidosis. *Med. Clin. North Am.,* 43:163, 1959.

Cummings, M. M., and Hudgins, P. C.: Chemical constituents of pine pollen and their possible relationship to sarcoidosis. *Am. J. Med. Sci.,* 236:311, 1958.

Cummings, M. M., Dunner, E., Schmidt, R. H., Jr., and Barnwell, J. B.: Concepts of epidemiology of sarcoidosis. *Postgrad. Med.,* 19:437, 1956.

Danbolt, N.: On the skin test with sarcoid-tissue-suspension (Kveim's reaction). *Acta Derm. Venereol.,* 31:184, 1951.

Davidson, C. N., and others: Nephrocalcinosis associated with sarcoidosis: a presentation and discussion of seven cases. *Radiology,* 62:203, 1954.

Deller, D. J., Brodziak, I. A., and Phillips, A. D.: Renal failure in hypercalcaemic sarcoidosis. *Br. Med. J.,* 1 1278, 1959.

Dent, C. E., Flynn, F. V., and Nabarro, J. D. N.: Hypercalcaemia and impairment of renal function in generalized sarcoidosis. *Br. Med. J.,* 2:808, 1953.

Dressler, M.: Ueber einem Fall von Splenomegalie, durch Sternalpunktion als Boecksche

Krankheit verifiziert. *Klin Wochenschr.*, 2:1467, 1938.

Dunner, E., Cummings, M. M., Williams, J. H., Jr., Schmidt, R. H., and Barnwell, J. B.: A new look at sarcoidosis, a review of clinical records of 160 patients with a diagnosis of sarcoidosis. *South. Med. J.*, 50:1141, 1957.

Essellier, A. F., and others: Die zentralnervosen Erscheinungsformen des Morbus Besnier-Boeck-Schaumann. *Schwiez. Med. Wochenschr.*, 81:376, 1951.

Fisher, A. M.: In discussion on A. M. Fisher: Some clinical and pathological features observed in sarcoidosis. *Trans. Am. Clin. Climatol. Assoc.*, 59:73, 1947.

Garland, H. G., and Thompson, J. G.: Uveoparotid tuberculosis (febris uveoparotid of Heerfordt). *Q. J. Med.*, 2:157, 1933.

Gendel, B. R., Young, J. M., and Greiner, D. J.: Sarcoidosis: a review of twenty-four additional cases. *Am. J. Med.*, 12:205, 1952.

Gentry, J. T., Nitowsky, H. M., and Michael, M. Jr.: Studies on the epidemiology of sarcoidosis in the United States; the relationship to soil areas and to urban-rural residence. *J. Clin. Invest.*, 34:1839, 1955.

Gilg, I.: Klinische undersogelser over Boeck's sarcoid (Sarcoidose): behandling og forlob. *Ugeskr. Laeger*, 118:46, 1956.

Gleckler, W. J.: Hypercalcemia and renal insufficiency due to sarcoidosis: treatment with cortisone. *Ann. Intern. Med.*, 44:174, 1956.

Heerfordt, C. F.: Ueber eine "Febris uveoparotidea subschronica," an der Glandula Parotis und der Uvea des Auges lokalisiert und haufig mit Paresen cerebrospinaler Herven kompliaiert. *Arch. Ophthalmol.*, 70:254, 1909.

Henneman, P. H., Carroll, E. L., and Dempsey, E. F.: The mechanism responsible for hypercalciuria in sarcoid. *J. Clin. Invest.*, 33:941, 1954.

Henneman, P. H., and others: The cause of hypercalciuria in sarcoid and its treatment with cortisone and sodium phytate. *J. Clin. Invest.*, 35:1229, 1956.

Holt, J. F., and Owens, W. I.: The osseous lesions of sarcoidosis. *Radiology*, 53:11, 1949.

Huchinson, J.: Cases of Mortimer's malady (lupus vulgaris multiplex nonulcerans et nonserpigeneous). *Arch. Surg. (London)*, 9:307, 1898.

Israel, H. L., and Sones, M.: Sarcoidosis: clinical observations on 160 cases. *Arch. Intern. Med.*, 102:766, 1958.

Jacques, W. E.: Sarcoidosis: a review and a proposed etiologic concept. *Arch. Pathol.*, 53:558, 1952.

James, D. G.: Ocular sarcoidosis. *Am. J. Med.*, 26:331, 1959.

James, D. G.: Quoted in L. E. Siltzbach: The Kveim test in sarcoidosis. (Editorial.) *Am. J. Med.*, 30:495, 1961.

James, D. G., and Siltzbach, L. E.: Sarcoidosis of the skin. In Madden, S.: *Current Dermatologic Management.* St. Louis, C. V. Mosby Company, 1975.

James, D. G., Carstares, L. F., and Neville, E.: Bone sarcoidosis. (Seventh International Conference on Sarcoidosis and Other Granulomatous Disorders.) *Ann. N. Y. Acad. Sci.*, 278:475, 1976.

James, D. G., Turiaf, J., Hosada, Y., Jones-Williams, W., Israel, H., Douglas, A. C., and Siltzbach, L. E.: Description of sarcoidosis: Report of the Sub-Committee on Classification and Definition. (Seventh International Conference on Sarcoidosis and Other Granulomatous Disorders.) *Ann. N. Y. Acad. Sci.*, 278:742, 1976.

James, D. G., et al.: A world wide review of sarcoidosis. (Seventh International Conference on Sarcoidosis and Other Granulomatous Disorders.) *Ann. N. Y. Acad. Sci.*, 278:321, 1976.

Johnson, J. B., and Jason, R. S.: Sarcoidosis of the heart: report of a case and review of literature. *Am. Heart J.*, 27:246, 1944.

Katz, S., Coke, C. P., and Reed, H. R.: Sarcoidosis. *N. Engl. J. Med.*, 229:498, 1943.

Kendig, E. L., Jr.: Sarcoidosis in children. *Am. Rev. Resp. Dis.*, 84:49, 1961.

Kendig, E. L., Jr.: Sarcoidosis among children. *J. Pediatr.*, 61:269, 1962.

Kendig, E. L., Jr.: The clinical picture of sarcoidosis in children. *Pediatrics*, 54:289, 1974.

Kendig, E. L., Jr., and Brummer, D. M.: The prognosis of sarcoidosis in children. *Chest*, 70:351, 1976.

Kendig, E. L., Jr., and Wiley, E. J., Jr.: Sarcoidosis in children. *Postgrad. Med. J.*, 37:590, 1961.

Kendig, E. L., Jr., Peacock, R. L., and Ryburn, S.: Sarcoidosis: report of three cases in siblings under fifteen years of age. *N. Engl. J. Med.*, 260:962, 1959.

Kennedy, A. C.: Boeck's sarcoid: report of a case with lesions detected in material obtained by sternal puncture. *Glasgow Med. J.*, 31:10, 1950.

King, D. S.: Sarcoid disease as revealed in chest roentgenograms. *Am. J. Roentgenol.*, 45:505, 1941.

Klatskin, G., and Gordon, M.: Renal complications of sarcoidosis and their relationship to hypercalcemia; with a report of two cases simulating hyperparathyroidism. *Am. J. Med.*, 15:484, 1953.

Kogut, M. D., and Neumann, L. I.: Renal involvement in Boeck's sarcoidosis. *Pediatrics*, 28:410, 1961.

Kraus, E. J.: Sarcoidosis (Boeck-Besnier-Schaumann disease) as a cause of pituitary syndrome. *J. Lab. Clin. Med.*, 28:140, 1942.

Krauss, L.: Genital sarcoidosis: case report and review of the literature. *J. Urol.*, 80:367, 1958.

Kveim, A.: Preliminary report on new and specific cutaneous reaction in Boeck's sarcoid. *Nord. Med.*, 9:169, 1941.

Lindau, A., and Lowegren, A.: Benign lymphogranulomatosis (Schaumann's disease) and the eye. *Acta Med. Scand.*, 105:242, 1940.

Longcope, W. T.: Sarcoidosis. *Veterans Admin. Tech. Bull.*, TB-10-73:1015, 1951.

Longcope, W. T., and Fisher, A. M.: Involvement of the heart in sarcoidosis. *J. Mt. Sinai Hosp.*, 8:784, 1942.

Longcope, W. T., and Freiman, D. G.: A study of

sarcoidosis; based on a combined investigation of 160 cases, including 30 autopsies, from the Johns Hopkins Hospital and Massachusetts General Hospital. *Medicine, 31*:1, 1952.

Longcope, W. T., and Pierson, J. W.: Boeck's sarcoid (sarcoidosis). *Bull. Johns Hopkins Hosp., 60*:223, 1937.

Mackensen, G.: Veranderungen am Augenhintergrund bei Besnier-Boeck-Schaumannscher Erkrankung. *Klin. Monatsbl. augenheilkd., 121*:51, 1952.

Maddrey, W. C., Johns, C. J., Boitnott, J. K., et al.: Sarcoidosis and chronic hepatic disease: a clinical and pathologic study of 20 patients. *Medicine, 49*:375, 1970.

Mandi, L.: Thoracic sarcoidosis in childhood. *Acta Tuberc. Scand., 45*:256, 1964.

Mankiewicz, E.: The relationship of sarcoidosis to anonymous mycobacteria. *Acta Med. Scand., 425*(Suppl.):68, 1964.

McCort, J. J., Wood, R. H., Hamilton, J. B., and Erlich, D. E.: Sarcoidosis: clinical and roentgenologic study of 28 proved cases. *Arch. Intern. Med., 80*:293, 1947.

McGovern, J. P., and Merritt, D. M.: Sarcoidosis in childhood. *Adv. Pediatr., 8*:97, 1956.

McSwiney, R. R., and Mills, I. H.: Hypercalcaemia due to sarcoidosis: treatment with cortisone. *Lancet, 2*:862, 1956.

Michael, J., Jr., Cole, R., Beeson, P. B., and Olson, B.: Sarcoidosis: preliminary report on a study of 350 cases with special reference to epidemiology. *Am. Rev. Tuberc., 62*:403, 1950.

Mikhail, J. R., Mitchell, D. N., Dyson, J. L., Williams, W. J., Ogunlesi, T. O. O., and Van Hein-Wallace, S. E.: Sarcoidosis with genital involvement. *Am. Rev. Resp. Dis., 106*:465, 1973.

Nagle, R.: Hypercalcemia and neophrocalcinosis in sarcoidosis. *J. Mt. Sinai Hosp., 28*:268, 1961.

Niitu, Y., Horikawa, M., Suetake, T., Hasegawa, S., and Komatsu, S.: Comparison of clinical and laboratory findings of intrathoracic sarcoidosis of children and adults. (Seventh International Conference on Sarcoidosis and Other Granulomatous Disorders.) *Ann. N. Y. Acad. Sci., 278*:532, 1976.

Niitu, Y., Watanabe, M., Suetake, T., Handia, T., Munakata, K., and Shiroishi, K.: Sixteen cases of intrathoracic sarcoidosis found among school children in Sendai in mass x-ray surveys of the chest. *Research Reports of Research Institute for Tuberculosis, Leprosy and Cancer, 12*:99, 1965.

Nitter, L.: Changes in the chest roentgenogram in Boeck's sarcoid of the lungs. *Acta Radiol., 105*(Suppl.):1, 1953.

North, A. F.: Sarcoid arthritis in children. *Am. J. Med., 48*:449, 1970.

Osterberg, G.: Iritis Boeck (sarkoid of Boeck in iris). *Br. J. Ophthalmol., 23*:145, 1939.

Pautrier, L. M.: Le syndrome de Heerfordt des ophtalmologistes n'est qu'une forme particulière de la maladie de Besnier-Boeck-Schaumann. *Ann. Dermatol. Syphiligr., 9*:161, 1938.

Pautrier, L. M.: Une Nouvelle Grande Reticuloendothéliose: La Maladie de Besnier-Boeck-Schaumann.Paris, Masson et cie, 1940.

Pennell, W. H.: Boeck's sarcoid with involvement of the central nervous system. *J. Nerv. Ment. Dis., 115*:451, 1952.

Phillips, R. W., and Fitzpatrick, D. P.: Steroid therapy of hypercalcemia and renal insufficiency in sarcoidosis. *N. Engl. J. Med., 254*:1216, 1956.

Polland, R.: Multipl benignes sarkoid bei einem Saugling. *Dermz., 61*:360, 1931.

Reed, W. G.: Sarcoidosis: a review and report of eight cases in children. *J. Tenn. Med. Assoc., 62*:27, 1969.

Refvem, O.: Pathogenesis of Boeck's disease (sarcoidosis). *Acta Med. Scand., 149*(Suppl. 294):1, 1954.

Reisner, D.: Boeck's sarcoid and systemic sarcoidosis (Besnier-Boeck-Schaumann disease): study of 35 cases. *Am. Rev. Tuberc., 49*:289, 1944.

Reisner, D.: Boeck's sarcoid and systemic sarcoidosis. *Am. Rev. Tuberc., 49*:437, 1944.

Ricker, W., and Clark, M.: Sarcoidosis: a clinico-pathologic review of 300 cases, including 22 autopsies. *Am. J. Clin. Pathol., 19*:725, 1949.

Riley. E. A.: Boeck's sarcoid. *Am. Rev. Tuberc., 62*:231, 1950.

Roos, B.: Cerebral manifestations of lymphogranulomatosis benigna (Schaumann) and uveoparotid fever (Heerfordt). *Acta Med. Scand., 104*:123, 1940.

Salveson, H. A.: Sarcoid of Boeck, a disease of importance to internal medicine; report of four cases. *Acta Med. Scand., 86*:127, 1935.

Sarcoidosis. *Stat. Navy Med., 13*:3, 1957.

Scadding, J. G.: Discussion on sarcoidosis. *Proc. R. Soc. Med., 49*:799, 1956.

Scadding, J. G.: Mycobacterium tuberculosis in the aetiology of sarcoidosis. *Br. Med. J., 2*:16, 1960.

Schaumann, J.: Etude sur le lupus pernio et ses rapports avec les sarcoides et la tuberculose. *Ann. Dermatol. Syphiliger., 6* (fifth series):357, 1916–1917.

Schmitt, E., Appleman, H., and Threatt, B.: Sarcoidosis in children. *Radiology, 106*:621, 1973.

Scholz, D. A.: Effect of steroid therapy on hypercalcemia and renal calculi and nephrocalcinosis in sarcoidosis. *J.A.M.A., 169*:682, 1959.

Scholz, D. A., and Keating, F. R., Jr.: Renal insufficiency, renal calculi and nephrocalcinosis in sarcoidosis. *Am. J. Med., 21*:75, 1956.

Scholz, D. A., Power, M. H., and Dearing, W. H.: Metabolic effects of cortisone on a case of sarcoidosis with hypercalcemia and renal insufficiency. *Proc. Staff Meet. Mayo Clin., 32*:182, 1957.

Sharma, O. P., Johnson, C. S., and Balchum, O. J.: Familial sarcoidosis. Report of four siblings with acute sarcoidosis. *Am. Rev. Resp. Dis., 104*:255, 1971.

Siltzbach, L. E.: Effect of cortisone in sarcoidosis. *Am. J. Med., 12*:139, 1952.

Siltzbach, L. E.: Sarcoidosis: prevalence and diagnosis. *Sem. Int., 9*:2, 1960.

Siltzbach, L. E.: The Kveim test in sarcoidosis. (Editorial.) *Am. J. Med., 30*:495, 1961.

Siltzbach, L. E.: Sarcoidosis: clinical features and management. *Med. Clin. North Am., 51*:483, 1967.

Siltzbach, L. E.: Sarcoidosis and mycobacteria. *Am. Rev. Resp. Dis., 97*:1, 1968.

Siltzbach, L. E., and Greenberg, G. M.: Childhood sarcoidosis. A study of eighteen cases. *N. Engl. J. Med., 279*:1239, 1968.

Sones, M., and Israel, H. L.: Course and prognosis of sarcoidosis. *Am. J. Med., 29*:84, 1960.

Stone, D. J., and Schwartz, A.: A long-term study of sarcoid and its modification by steroid therapy. *Am. J. Med., 41*:528, 1966.

Walgren, S.: Pulmonary sarcoidosis detected by photofluorographic surveys in Sweden, 1950–1957. *Nord. Med., 60*:1194, 1958.

Walsh, F. B.: Ocular importance of sarcoid; its relation to uveoparotid fever. *Arch. Ophthalmol., 21*:421, 1939.

Weekly Case Conference: Sarcoidosis. *Clin. Proc. Child. Hosp., 12*:253, 1956.

Wegelius, C., and Wijkstroem, S.: Mass radiography in Sweden. *Nord. Med., 60*:1191, 1958.

Williams, R. H., and Nickerson, D. A.: Skin reactions in sarcoid. *Proc. Soc. Exp. Biol. Med., 33*:403, 1935.

Yesner, R., and Silver, M.: Fatal myocardial sarcoidosis. *Am. Heart J., 41*:777, 1951.

CHAPTER FORTY-NINE

HISTOPLASMOSIS

Amos Christie, M. D.

Pulmonary histoplasmosis is the most prevalent systemic fungous infection. Despite this fact, the disease is still poorly understood by many. Variations in its spectrum are frequently mistaken, overlooked, or misdiagnosed as other disease processes, probably because the wide variety of manifestations caused by parasitization of tissue by *Histoplasma capsulatum* is not sufficiently appreciated by clinicians. Although the scope of this chapter must of necessity emphasize pulmonary histoplasmosis in childhood, it will be necessary to broaden the description of the disease spectrum of human histoplasmosis in order to give the student or the clinician a concept of the pathogenesis as well as the signs and symptoms of this interesting and pleomorphic disease. Its manifestations cut through each specialty and subspecialty of clinical medicine and pediatrics, and it may well be designated as the "great masquerader" of the present.

History

The organism was first described by Darling in Panama in 1906. He observed it in sections of tissue, taken at the time of postmortem examination in cases that appeared to be leishmaniasis. Consequently, the organism was thought to be a protozoan. The first case reported in North America was that by Watson and Riley in 1926, but it remained for Demonbrum at Vanderbilt University in 1934 to demonstrate conclusively the fungous origin of this disease by brilliant use of transmission and culture methods. Until 1945, histoplasmosis was thought to be a systemic fungous disease that was uniformly pro-

gressive and fatal. Since that time conclusive evidence has accumulated that there are benign or intermediate forms of the disease as well as the fatal disseminated form. A comprehensive historical review of histoplasmosis has been published by Schwarz and Baum (1957). There have been few advances in our knowledge of this disease in recent years.

General Considerations

Histoplasmosis is caused by the fungus *Histoplasma capsulatum*. This organism grows in two forms according to its environment. Although it is found free in nature in certain soils, particularly in those that have been exposed to avian excreta, it grows in its mycelial form in culture media, producing a cottony white mass at room temperature. When properly examined, the tuberculate chlamydospore will be apparent. This is the identifying feature of the fungus. It appears in the picturesque language of Demonbrum as the "Teutonic war club" (Fig. 1). No other fungi are known to have this feature. Confusion of *Histoplasma capsulatum* with any other pathogenic fungi is, therefore, impossible. There are strain differences, however, and the organism produces several antigens: e. g., there is a complement-fixing antigen and a skin test antigen.

In tissue, and when grown on certain forms of enriched culture media at 37° C., the fungus appears as a yeast cell, usually 3 to 5 microns in diameter. In pathologic sections with ordinary stains, the yeast cell has a definite border, a capsule and a crescent of deeply stained cytoplasm (Fig. 2), which

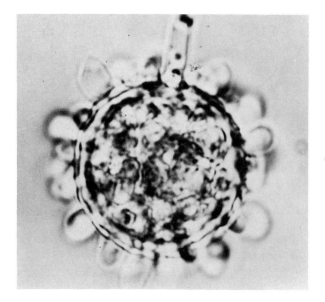

Figure 1. Tuberculate chlamydo-spore from a mycelial culture.

is the descriptive origin of the term *Histoplasma capsulatum. Histoplasma capsulatum* is not a particularly fastidious organism, although it grows slowly on any medium. It has been grown in our laboratory on Sabouraud's dextrose media between wide limits of pH. A more complete medium is that enriched with blood or plasma to which antibiotics have been added. It was originally thought that this was necessary to in-

hibit the growth of pyogenic organisms so that the rather slow-growing *Histoplasma capsulatum* could emerge. There is now evidence that adequate amounts of antibiotics and plasma may be necessary for its ideal growth requirements. This, of course, has some therapeutic implications, which will be pointed out later.

The fungus not only has been found in the soil, but also has been positively

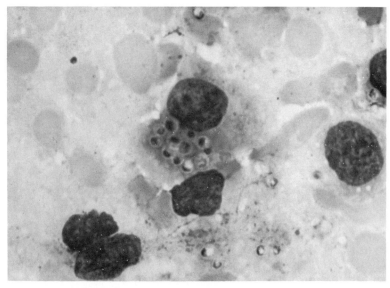

Figure 2. *H. capsulatum* as seen by Wright's stain in circulating blood or bone marrow.

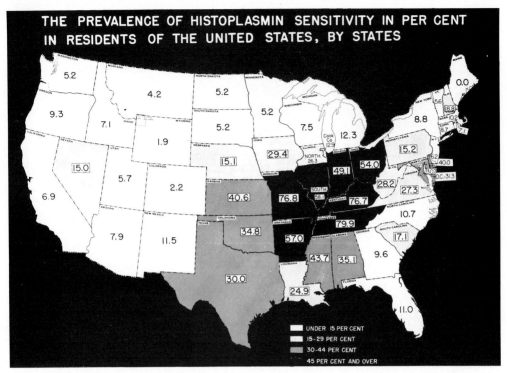

Figure 3. Prevalence of histoplasmin sensitivity in residents of the United States, by states.

identified in a wide variety of animals. There is no evidence of transmission from animal to person, animal to animal or person to person. Evidence has accumulated that there is probably contamination of the soil with an intermediate saprophytic phase. Infection of humans occurs, then, by inhalation or ingestion, or by both means.

The geographic distribution is interesting. Although histoplasmosis is worldwide, more than half of the recorded disseminated progressive cases have occurred in states that correspond to the area of the Western Appalachian slope and those bordering on the tributaries of the Ohio, Missouri and Mississippi rivers. These represent the endemic areas in this country as evidenced by sensitivity to histoplasmin (Fig. 3). This area has variously been described as avocado- or pear-shaped, the base of which is in Arkansas and Georgia, tapering off along the Western Appalachian slope with the apex in New York State. In addition, endemic foci have

been identified in other parts of the country, as far north as Minnesota and central Pennsylvania. The distribution is more worldwide than is generally appreciated. There are parts of southern Europe, Africa, and Central and South America in which histoplasmin sensitivity is relatively high, and clinical cases have been reported from these regions.

Whenever the prevalence of histoplasmin sensitivity has been demonstrated, calcification in nonreactors to tuberculin has also been shown to be prevalent (Fig. 4).

Pathology

For those who have had an opportunity to study the interesting features of this disease, it is tempting to correlate the pathologic picture with the immunologic maturity of the patient. In the young infant, the hallmark of the pathologic picture is the presence of large mononuclear phagocytes that proliferate and contain many conspicu-

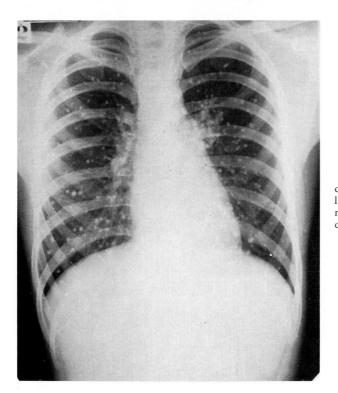

Figure 4. Healed "miliary tuberculosis" of yesteryear, now well established as healed miliary histoplasmosis. Histoplasmin-positive, tuberculin-negative.

ous intracellular parasites. There is little to be seen under gross or microscopic examination in the way of necrosis or nodular granulomatous formation (Figs. 5 and 6).

In later infancy, childhood or adult life, focal lesions occur that are often marked by caseous necrosis, granulomatous formation and a paucity of organisms, making their identification within tissue sections difficult.*

This disease, then, may be characterized pathologically by the formation of granulomatous lesions, which may be confused with those of tuberculosis. The characteristic lesion or primary complex is similar. It consists of (1) a primary focus at the site of penetration, (2) lymphangitis from this site to the regional lymph nodes, and (3) regional lymphadenitis with inflammation and tendency toward caseation. The yeast cells of the fungus tend to proliferate

---

*I am indebted to my colleague, Dr. John Shapiro, for this observation.

in the large, mononuclear phagocytic cells of the reticuloendothelial system. They multiply until the mononuclear cells are literally filled with yeast cells. Rupture apparently occurs, and the yeast cells are phagocytized by other large mononuclear cells, thus initiating new cycles. In contradistinction to tuberculosis, this reaction goes on with relatively little inflammatory response in adjacent tissues. Foci tend to become surrounded with giant cells and multinucleated cells, and these foci progress to central caseous necrosis (Fig. 7). In infants with little immunologic maturity or in debilitated adults (depending on the resistance of the host or the virulence of that particular strain of the organism), there is a tendency toward hematogenous spread or progression by postprimary complication. Just as in tuberculosis, spread of the organisms is dependent on tissue resistance of the host, and the dose (immediate or recurrent) of the inoculum. Hypersensitivity now occurs, and histo-

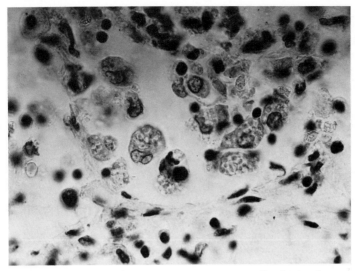

Figure 5. Large mononuclear phagocytes containing many yeast cells of *Histoplasma capsulatum* (which proliferate). No necrosis.

plasmin sensitivity is established. The time interval from the primary inoculation to this point is usually three to six weeks, similar to that in tuberculosis.

In the postprimary stage, the progressive form of the disease may occur. This is characterized by massive enlargement of the liver and spleen due to pathologic accumulations of prolifer-ative lesions. Pulmonary tissues, including the regional lymph nodes, are similarly involved, and interstitial pneumonitis may be present (Fig. 8). When there is hematogenous spread, roentgenograms of the lungs have much the same soft snowstorm appearance as that seen in miliary tuberculosis (Fig. 9). This may heal with calcifica-

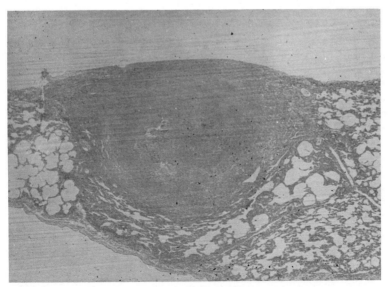

Figure 6. Proved primary histoplasmosis with granulomatous lesion in lung. Caseous necrosis and calcification present.

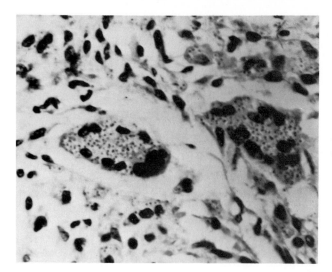

Figure 7. Multinucleated giant cells containing yeast cells of *H. capsulatum*.

tion, giving the characteristic "buck-shot" roentgenogram of the chest.

The bone marrow is commonly involved, and with this there is a proliferation of large mononuclear cells filled with the yeast cells. These cells may crowd the normal bone marrow elements and thus produce severe anemia and at times leukopenia and thrombocytopenia. Not infrequently, this clinical aspect of histoplasmosis is mistaken for aleukemic leukemia even by experienced clinicians.

In about 50 per cent of the cases there is ulceration of the skin or mucous membranes. Lesions in the oropharynx occur frequently, particularly in adults. Ulcerative lesions have been described in the bowel and colon, and a picture similar to that of tabes mesenterica of tuberculosis is well documented.

Invasion of the adrenal gland with caseous necrosis and adrenal failure produces the signs and symptoms of Addison's disease, another similarity to

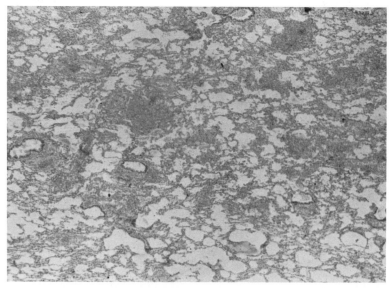

Figure 8.   Interstitial pneumonitis due to histoplasmosis.

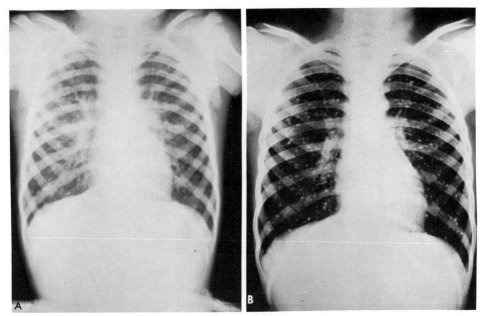

Figure 9. *A,* Multiple primary lesions simulating miliary tuberculosis. *B,* Note healing with calcification within two years.

tuberculosis. This is more commonly found in adults, however, than in children. Involvement of the nervous system is not common, but the disease process can produce signs, symptoms and laboratory findings indistinguishable from those of tuberculous meningitis.

The regional lymph nodes are frequently involved, the cervical mediastinal or mesenteric being the most common. It is not common, however, to find generalized adenopathy, such as is found in leukemia, and this may be an important differential diagnostic point.

Clinical Manifestations

Table 1 lists the clinical forms of pulmonary histoplasmosis.

Human histoplasmosis, as has been repeatedly pointed out, is a disease of protean nature. It varies with the degree of parasitization. A single primary lesion may be completely asymptomatic and appear only as acquired histoplasmin sensitivity (Fig. 10). On the other hand, infection following inhalation or ingestion of the organisms may commonly produce such symptoms as fever (101 to 103° F.), malaise and fatigue with desire to rest rather than to play after school, nonproductive cough, weight loss or failure to gain, vomiting, and diarrhea that is occasionally blood-streaked.

The physical examination, particularly of the chest, may be negative at this time. Careful effort to explain the fatigue and low-grade fever may include skin tests and result in a positive histoplasmin, but negative tuberculin,

TABLE 1. CLINICAL FORMS OF PULMONARY HISTOPLASMOSIS

1. Primary
2. Postprimary complications
   a. Intrathoracic
      (1) Miliary, "atypical" pneumonia
      (2) Mediastinal adenopathy
   b. Extrathoracic
      (1) May affect any tissue of the body: e.g., regional adenopathy; meningitis; lytic bone lesions: Addison's disease; eye, skin and mucous membrane ulcerations; myocarditis and endocarditis; ulcerative colitis; pericarditis
   c. Disseminated progressive varieties of histoplasmosis

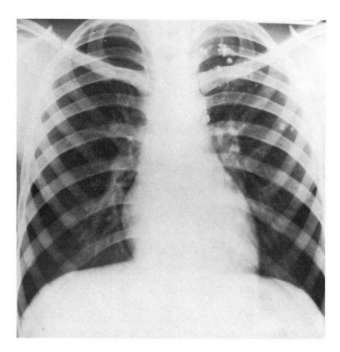

Figure 10. Healed primary histoplasmosis. Note berry-like morphology of calcification.

reaction. Roentgenograms of the chest will then reveal an infiltrative lesion with or without mediastinal adenopathy, suggesting atypical pneumonia or mediastinal malignancy (Figs. 11 and 12). A complement-fixation test of comparatively low titer (1:4) and a rapid sedimentation rate are good indices of active systemic infection and may become important in judging the prognosis or clinical course of the disease.

Gastric washing, which may be helpful, has been disappointing in the author's considerable experience with histoplasmosis.

Occasionally, a mediastinal node is of such size and location as to cause obstruction to venous return. Such instances may require bronchoscopy or exploratory thoracotomy to define the cause and relieve the obstruction (Fig. 13).

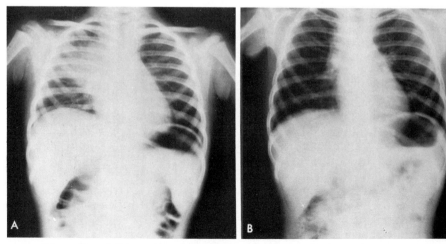

Figure 11. *A*, Primary histoplasmosis; *B*, resolution on sulfa therapy in seven months.

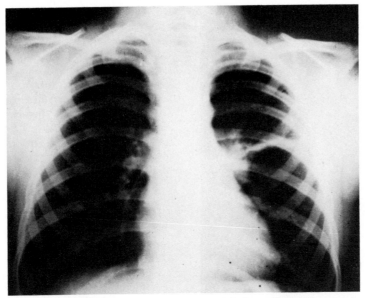

Figure 12. Primary histoplasmosis. Malaise, cough, low-grade fever of three months' duration. Positive histoplasmin and positive histoplasmin complement-fixation test results. Note peripheral lesion with mediastinal adenopathy.

If hematogenous dissemination has taken place as the result of overwhelming infection, breakdown of a primary lesion or lowered resistance of the host, the fever rises to higher levels and persists. Hepatomegaly is prominent, and the spleen may enlarge to tremendous proportions (Fig. 14). The pallor, which is due to a normochromic anemia with pancytopenia, may be the presenting clinical manifestation. Experienced house officers will admit these infants with a presumptive diagnosis of aleukemic leukemia. Adenopathy is usually regional instead of generalized as in leukemia, a finding of consider-

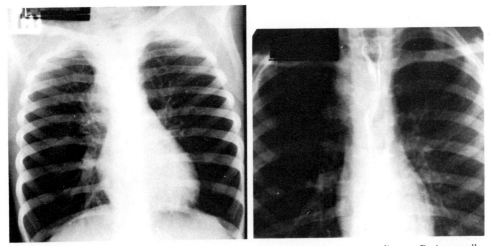

Figure 13. Mediastinal mass due to histoplasmosis with stridor and respiratory distress. Barium swallow showing narrowing of air passage. Resolution following endobronchial rupture of node (accidental). Histoplasma cultured from bronchial aspiration.

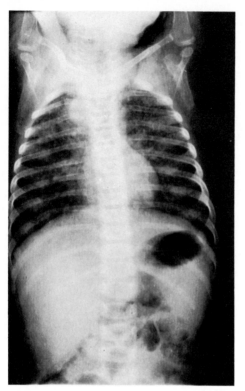

Figure 14. Postprimary dissemination of pulmonary histoplasmosis. Note fine infiltration with mediastinal adenopathy and hepatosplenomegaly.

splenomegaly, ulceration of the skin or mucous membranes (particularly of the oronasal pharynx), ulceration of the small intestine, pulmonary infiltration and atypical pneumonia. In the adult, histoplasmosis exhibits another similarity to tuberculosis by involving the adrenal gland and producing classic Addison's disease. We have also observed Histoplasma endocarditis and meningitis, the latter indistinguishable in all its clinical and laboratory manifestations from tuberculous meningitis. There are records of patients with ulcerative colitis in the Vanderbilt University files who were given the usual University Hospital workup without avail until the true definitive diagnosis was revealed in the autopsy material (Fig. 15). Pericarditis and myocarditis with endocarditis have been described, and we have seen destructive bone lesions with periosteal new bone formation.

Differential Diagnosis

It has been pointed out that acute disseminated histoplasmosis of a progressive nature must be considered whenever the diagnosis of leukemia is being considered. The absence of generalized adenopathy and of blast forms and the persistence of normal bone marrow elements are helpful. Histoplasmosis adenopathy is inclined to be regional rather than generalized. When histoplasmosis has affected the mesenteric nodes, a picture of tabes mesenterica, tuberculosis, Hodgkin's disease or other malignant lymphomatous diseases must be considered. The differential diagnosis between histoplasmosis and reticuloendothelioses of the Letterer-Siwe type is a most difficult one clinically and histologically save for the finding of yeast cells in the biopsy material or by culture of the organism. Ulcerations of the skin and mucous membranes also suggest tuberculosis, syphilis and epithelioma.

able differential diagnostic importance. As many as 50 per cent of these cases show ulceration of the skin or mucous membranes, and an equal number have evidence of pulmonary infiltration with mediastinal adenopathy.

Purpura is perhaps the commonest cutaneous lesion, and this usually means overwhelming parasitization with crowding out of the normal marrow elements. It is a poor prognostic sign.

To summarize and reemphasize, the clinical manifestations of histoplasmosis are so variable that it is wise and helpful to remember everything known about tuberculosis. The generalized reticuloendotheliosis that has been described accounts for the appearance of the disease in acute, subacute and chronic forms with systemic manifestations of irregular fever, anemia, failure to gain weight or weight loss, hepato-

Pulmonary infiltration of histoplasmosis frequently suggests virus or atypical pneumonia or tuberculosis even

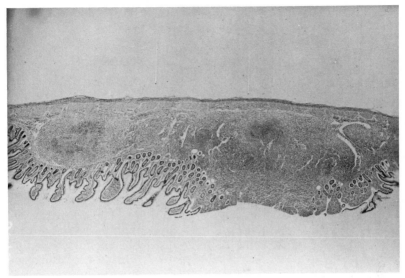

Figure 15. Ulceration of gastrointestinal mucosa due to histoplasmosis. Note submucosal proliferation suggesting granulomatous enteritis.

to the experienced clinician. We have in our files examples of atelectasis resulting from mediastinal gland enlargement due to histoplasmosis and attaining such size as to cause obstruction of the venous return, thereby suggesting a diagnosis of mediastinal malignant lymphoma. When the diagnosis of ulcerative colitis in entertained, it appears wise in endemic areas to obtain cultures and to perform other proper examinations for *Histoplasma capsulatum*. In the presence of organic heart disease with embolic phenomena, we have found *Histoplasma capsulatum* in the emboli; the typical picture of infective endocarditis caused by this fungus is well documented.

Prognosis

Histoplasmosis seems to affect most seriously the infant who is immunologically immature and the debilitated older adult who frequently is suffering from concomitant systemic disease. Several factors related to the extent of the inoculation and the virulence of the organism, as well as the resistance of the host, are also operative in determining the prognosis of histoplasmosis.

As in the primary or in the postprimary complications of tuberculosis, an opinion as to prognosis as well as the choice of the therapeutic agent is closely related to a knowledge of the natural course of this disease. In its primary form histoplasmosis is strangely benign, but in its progressive, disseminated form it is almost uniformly fatal unless adequately treated. Nevertheless, particularly in older children, in whom the disease is widely disseminated and appears to be progressive, there have been well documented spontaneous recoveries. In the intermediate forms with ulcerations of the skin and mucous membranes and extensive pulmonary infiltrative disease, patients exhibit few signs and symptoms and usually recover spontaneously or with supportive therapy in a matter of weeks to months.

The difficulty of evaluating a therapeutic agent under these varying conditions is obvious. The duration of the infection and the persistence of skin test sensitivity, as well as the presence of complement-fixing antibodies, are probably related to the degree of infection present. In some instances when the infection is a single minimal primary one, the lesion may heal completely and the patient may lose his sensitivity in a relatively short time. Calcified nodules, when taken from the lungs at autopsy, are seldom if ever associated with the presence of viable organisms. The loss of histoplasmin sensitivity occurs much more often than does loss of tuberculin sensitivity. This is probably related to the absence of viable organisms after healing or to the removal of the subject from reinfection. During childhood and early adult life, however, the opportunity for infection and reinfection is so great that there is a constantly rising level of histoplasmin sensitivity. After 30 years of age, there is a slow decline in histoplasmin sensitivity, suggesting that reinfection does not keep pace with the loss of sensitivity. Little is known about the significance of reinfection, but we have had a number of patients with caseous lesions in the lungs which have broken down and apparently served as a source of generalized dissemination of the infection. This course has been seen particularly in those patients who were receiving corticosteroid therapy.

The question is frequently raised as to whether or not there is danger of a breakdown of the lesions after they have healed to the point of calcification. There are no cases in our files suggesting that such lesions break down and result in hematogenous dissemination of the disease. The most logical explanation for this is the likelihood that the yeast cells are probably all dead or nonviable when calcification occurs, or are incapable of multiplication. As indicated previously, the disappearance of signs and symptoms and the gaining of weight are indications of inactivity of the infection. When accompanied by return of the sedimentation rate to normal and the fading out of the complement-fixing antibodies, the infection is considered to be under control or inactivated. In the disseminated form of the disease,

decrease in the size of the spleen is a good prognostic sign.

Treatment

Under the conditions described the first principle of therapeutics must be exercised. *Primum nolle nocere*, which means "to be unwilling to do harm," might be paraphrased as follows: "Try to do some good." A truly effective agent has not been found for the treatment of histoplasmosis. All means of supportive and symptomatic relief should be exercised. Anything that can be done to improve the nutrition or the general hygiene and thus increase the natural resistance of the patient is indicated. Blood transfusion is helpful in improving the general resistance and in correcting the normochromic anemia and pancytopenia frequently present. Corticosteroids appear to be contraindicated because of the danger of dissemination of the primary lesion. In vitro studies reveal that *Histoplasma capsulatum* thrives on antibiotics. It would seem, therefore, that these would be useless, perhaps contraindicated. In an early observation on biopsy material, we found that growth of the pyogenic organisms could be inhibited by penicillin and streptomycin and that a rather rapid growth of the *Histoplasma capsulatum* occurred in the presence of these antibiotics in the media.

Amphotericin B (Fungizone) has recently come into use in treatment of histoplasmosis, and favorable results have been reported from this institution and elsewhere. In its present form, however, this drug is pyrogenic, producing chills and high fever, is poorly absorbed from the gastrointestinal tract and is nephrotoxic and hepatotoxic. Its use has serious economic repercussions, since the drug should be used only in hospitals under careful observation, and the so-called course of treatment involves prolonged use. It should never be used in the benign forms (i.e., primary forms) of the disease, but rather reserved for the progressive disseminated varieties. (See section on ampho-

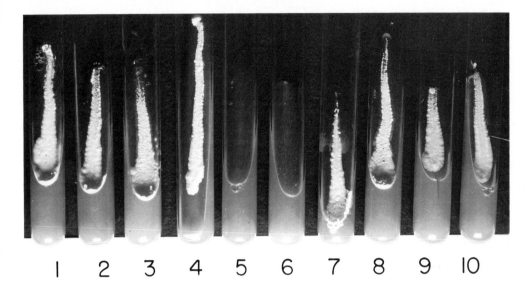

1. KANAMYCIN 45 mcg/cc 6. SULFADIAZINE 15 mg %
2. KANAMYCIN 15 mcg/cc 7. TETRACYCLINE 15 mcg/cc
3. CHLORAMPHENICOL 24 mcg/cc 8. TETRACYCLINE 5 mcg/cc
4. CHLORAMPHENICOL 8 mcg/cc 9. PEN-STREP
5. SULFADIAZINE 45 mg % 10. CONTROL

20 DAY OLD CULTURE AT 37° C.

Figure 16. Rationale for sulfa therapy. Note inability to grow *H. capsulatum* in presence of 15 mg. of sulfa. (I am indebted to Dr. William Fleet for the preparation of this illustration.)

tericin B in treatment of fungal disease, page 925.)

We have had considerable experience in studying both the natural course of the infection and in treating different forms of histoplasmosis. A triple sulfonamide suspension in a dosage that produces a level of 10 to 15 mg. per 100 ml. in the blood is our antimicrobial of choice in almost all forms of the disease, although evaluation of this or any other therapeutic agent remains a difficult problem. Sulfonamides are well tolerated by patients. The methods of regulating the drug are readily available in most laboratories, including those in private offices (blood serum levels and urinalysis). Less toxic drugs must be developed before a truly effective therapeutic agent can be made available (Fig. 16).

The Present Status of Histoplasmin Sensitivity, Serologic Tests and Other Diagnostic Methods

Histoplasmin is a dilution of a broth culture filtrate. Histoplasmin sensitivity, like old tuberculin sensitivity, is an allergic state induced by infection with *Histoplasma capsulatum*. The test quantitatively and qualitatively has no relation to the state of activity of infection with *Histoplasma capsulatum* unless recent conversion has occurred. Sensitivity to histoplasmin appears four to six weeks after infection has begun and may persist for many years after the activity of the infection has disappeared. In disseminated and progressive infection, as many as 50 per cent of the cases will demonstrate no skin test sensitivity. Re-

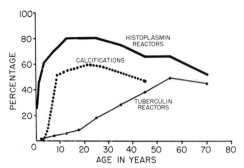

Figure 17. Pattern of histoplasmin and tuberculin sensitivity by age groups. Note relation of histoplasmin sensitivity to the development of calcification. Note also percentage of persons reacting to tuberculin and histoplasmin and percentage of calcifications, by age group.

cent known conversion of histoplasmin sensitivity has the same significance as the acquisition of tuberculin sensitivity and is of considerable clinical importance when one relates it to signs and symptoms associated with unexplained pulmonary pathologic changes or hepatosplenomegaly (Fig. 17).

In our experience, the most reliable serologic test is the complement-fixation test using the yeast cell antigen. This is because it is the yeast cell that occurs in human tissue. The mycelial form occurs on culture media. (See General Considerations.) Almost invariably, it is strongly positive in postprimary complications of the disease. The presence of complement-fixing antibodies even in low titer, i. e., 1:4, represents an acute phase reaction and is a sign of activity of the disease. The particular antibodies rapidly decrease in titer within a few weeks or months as the infection comes under control or is inactivated by therapy.

Recently, it has been shown that healthy *adults* who have positive skin tests to histoplasmin but who are serologically negative will develop complement-fixing antibodies following a single skin test. This response is to the mycelial antigen only. A rise in complement-fixing titer seldom, if ever, occurs

with the yeast phase antigen under these circumstances. Such interference, although the results have not been constant, has led internists to reexamine their use of the skin test whenever clinically active disease is suspected. No similar studies have been done on children.

As previously indicated, the skin test indicates active or current infection only when conversion from a negative to positive reaction has taken place. Therefore, particularly in early childhood, the skin test is a valuable case-finding tool. Delay in utilizing the skin test until initial serologic studies are complete may avoid their misinterpretation, although we are inclined to minimize this rather than to lose the skin test as our most valuable epidemiologic index or case-finding tool.

Adequate culture methods of biopsy or other host material will usually reveal *Histoplasma capsulatum* if that is the causative organism.

REFERENCES

Christie, A.: Histoplasmosis and pulmonary calcification. *Ann. N. Y. Acad. Sci.*, 50:1283, 1950.

Christie, A.: The disease spectrum of human histoplasmosis. *Ann. Intern. Med.*, 49:544, 1958.

Christie, A., and Peterson, J. C.: Pulmonary calcification in negative reactors to tuberculin. *Am. J. Public Health*, 35:1131, 1945. Also other articles on the same topic.

Darling, S. T.: Protozoan general infection producing pseudotubercles in the lungs and focal necrosis in the liver, spleen, and lymph nodes. *J.A.M.A.*, 46:1283, 1905.

Darling, S. T.: Notes on histoplasmosis: a fatal infectious disease resembling kala-azar found among natives of tropical America. *Arch. Intern. Med.*, 2:107, 1908.

Mayer, R. L., Eisman, P. C., Geftic, S., Konopka, E., and Tanzola, J.: Sulfonamides and experimental histoplasmosis. *Antibiot. Chemotherap.*, 6:215, 1956.

Palmer, C. E.: Nontuberculous pulmonary calcification and sensitivity to histoplasmin. *Public Health Rep.*, 60:513, 1945.

Picardi, J. L., et al.: Pericarditis caused by *Histoplasma capsulatum*. *Am. J. Cardiol.*, 37:82, 1976.

Schwarz, J., and Baum, G.: The history of histoplasmosis 1906–1956. *N. Engl. J. Med.*, 256:253, 1957.

CHAPTER FIFTY

THE MYCOSES (EXCLUDING HISTOPLASMOSIS)

John H. Seabury, M.D.

The systemic mycoses as a group are believed to occur rarely among pediatric patients. When one considers all the known factors pertinent to systemic fungous infections, this attitude is quite reasonable for infants, but much less so for children and adolescents.

Infants and children with congenital agammaglobulinemia, cystic fibrosis and other constitutional or acquired immunologic or metabolic disturbances may be expected to acquire infection from almost any agent, regardless of its usual pathogenicity. Similarly, the child with leukemia or lymphoma may acquire one or more fungous infections because of alterations produced by the disease or its treatment. This sort of infection, due to serious impairment of host resistance or iatrogenic factors (prolonged use of the same vein for infusions, cutdowns, corticosteroid treatment, or prolonged administration of antibiotics), is best termed "opportunistic." Opportunistic infections in the pediatric age group are not likely to be due to the usual pathogenic fungi, but rather to those saprophytes that are common in nature (e.g., Aspergillus) or in the normal host (e.g., Candida). Since this type of fungous infection usually occurs during management of a primary illness, recognition of mycotic superinfection may be difficult unless one thinks of such complications when the patient's course is unsatisfactory.

The common systemic mycoses, with the exception of actinomycosis, are acquired from exogenous sources in nature that usually require ambulation.

Epidemiologic studies of histoplasmosis and coccidioidomycosis indicate a low rate of infection in endemic areas until the child is freely ambulatory outside the home. Rate of infection increases during adolescence and early adult life. The epidemiology of cryptococcosis and North American blastomycosis has not been as clearly established. It appears that both are more intimately associated with restricted "point sources" of infection than is true for either histoplasmosis or coccidioidomycosis in highly endemic areas. Accordingly, the decade of maximum prevalence seems to fall in middle or later adult life. The recognition of purely pulmonary cryptococcosis and "epidemic" North American blastomycosis among pediatric patients may stimulate studies that will necessitate revision of this belief.

Fungous infection as a cause of pulmonary infiltration among pediatric patients is rarely an initial consideration. Acute inhalational histoplasmosis and the thin-walled cavitary residual of coccidioidomycosis are exceptions in areas of high endemicity. The roentgen features of these special manifestations of two mycotic diseases are sufficiently distinct to prompt comment by the experienced radiologist if he is given any clinical information. In other situations, the radiologic report should be descriptive, and perhaps suggest a differential diagnosis. The clinician should remember that there are no specific roentgenographic features for any pulmonary infection.

The diagnosis of a pulmonary mycosis, in common with all infectious diseases, depends first of all upon laboratory evidence. Isolation of the agent by culture or animal inoculation is most desirable, but one may have to rely upon microscopic and serologic examination at times. The physician's approach to the diagnosis of pulmonary disease in childhood is likely to involve a too limited differential diagnosis, and a too timid approach to securing adequate specimens for proper diagnosis. Of the two, the latter is the more serious. No one wants to inflict risk and pain, particularly when reasons for the procedure cannot be communicated to the child, but this is scarcely reason for jeopardizing his welfare. Transtracheal aspiration is simple and does not have the hazards of bronchoscopy. Direct needle aspiration of the lung carries no significant risk if pleural symphysis is present over the area of puncture. These procedures should be considered for many children who will not produce sputum. (See Chapter 4, Diagnostic and Therapeutic Procedures.)

GENERAL METHODS OF MICROBIOLOGIC DIAGNOSIS

Diagnostic methodology for fungi is grossly inferior to that for bacteria in most hospital laboratories in the United States. The fault is multilateral. There are a few simple things that the clinician can do to improve results.

First, the laboratory must be given suitable material. Swabs, 24-hour sputum collections or sputum contaminated with food or toothpaste are worthless for culture. The collection of specimens should not be left to uninstructed personnel.

If sputum can be obtained, it should be collected in the fasting state after the teeth have been cleaned with plain water only. Whatever sputum can be coughed into a sterile glass container during approximately one-half hour of effort should be taken directly to the laboratory.

When one cannot obtain sputum, transtracheal aspirates or direct needling of pneumonic or cavitary lesions is more likely to give diagnostic materials than are gastric aspirates. All are collected under as aseptic conditions as possible. Lung aspirates or cavitary washings should be transported within the original syringe so that the microbiologist can be responsible for subsequent handling with a minimum of opportunity for contamination.

Biopsy is usually performed by a surgical consultant in the operating room. The specimen should be bisected with sterile instruments; half should be sent for culture, and the other half fixed in formalin for histopathologic examination. Preliminary discussion with the surgical consultant or personal attention to the biopsy material by the clinician (or microbiologist) will prevent the common error of fixing the entire specimen in formalin.

Direct communication between clinician and laboratory worker can increase the likelihood of establishing the correct diagnosis. If the microbiologist is approached as a consultant, which he truly should be, not only can he make use of methods that are not routine, but he may also suggest sources for specimens that the clinician has not considered.

Another bonus from the close cooperation of the laboratory and physician is improved interpretation of the results of the laboratory examination. Ultimately, it is the clinician who must decide, but the counsel of a versatile microbiologist or clinical pathologist can often prevent misinterpretation of the results of serologic testing or culture. The isolation of fungi that are usually saprophytic or common laboratory contaminants may prompt additional studies if it is known that the patient has been on antibiotics or is immunologically compromised.

Aside from serologic methods, the laboratory search for fungi should begin with direct examination unless the amount of material available is so small that blind culture is necessary. Sputum or other exudate is placed in a sterile Petri dish on a black background. Granular material should be handled in a manner different from that applied to grayish or purulent flecks. A single granule may be placed on a slide in sterile saline or water and then crushed beneath the coverglass. If the granule is filamentous, suggesting Actinomyces or Nocardia, the crushed material may be allowed to dry on the slide and be stained by the Gram method.

Small flecks of grayish or purulent material are mixed with a small drop of 10 per cent hydroxide on a glass slide and covered for microscopic examination. If yeastlike forms are present, one may be able to make a diagnosis of North or South American blastomycosis, coccidioidomycosis or, rarely, cryptococcosis. Even if morphologically typical forms are not present, a finding of yeast forms is most helpful in guiding the selection of culture media and future efforts. Rarely, intracellular *Histoplasma capsulatum* may be observed in hydroxide-cleared mounts, but their morphologic characteristics are never sufficient for diagnosis. Asteroid clusters or small clumps of narrow hyphae suggest the presence of Nocardia or Actinomyces. The pseudohyphae with attached blastospores of Candida are easily recognized, but blastospores alone may be confusing. Septate hyphae can usually be distinguished from nonseptate ones, but this distinction has no clinical significance.

If the amount of exudate permits, Gram's stain should always be used on a thin smear of a selected fleck. This stain is most useful for the detection of narrow filaments suggestive of Actinomyces or Nocardia. The stain demonstrates the pseudohyphae and blastospores of Candida very well, but is not very useful for the yeastlike fungi.

A Wright's stain of thinly smeared exudate is useful in giving one a good idea of the cellular population present and of the probable source of the exudate (upper or lower respiratory tract). Hyphae and candidal blastospores are usually well delineated. Histoplasma stains well, but cannot be differentiated with certainty from Cryptococcus and other yeastlike fungi. The blastomycetes, Cryptococcus and Coccidioides may appear only as unstained negative images in many preparations. A suspicious smear stained by Wright's method can always be restained by either the periodic acid–Schiff or Gomori methenamine–silver nitrate method.

If the study of a hydroxide-cleared preparation suggests the presence of yeastlike fungi, the application of special fungous stains may be indicated. The methenamine-silver method will impregnate a wider variety of fungi than will the periodic acid–Schiff stain. Morphologic detail is better demonstrated by the periodic acid–Schiff method.

The Ziehl-Neelsen stain is useful primarily for the demonstration of *Nocardia asteroides, N. brasiliensis, N. caviae* and mycobacteria. For this purpose, destaining with acid alcohol should be shortened to three seconds or be replaced by a 1 per cent aqueous acid solution. Yeastlike fungi will often be demonstrated by the Ziehl-Neelsen stain.

Cultural isolation of pathogenic fungi may be prevented by the earlier growth of bacteria. This problem usually can be controlled by the addition of antibiotics to media at approximately neutral pH. Commercially available media (Mycosel agar, Baltimore Biological Co.; Brain-Heart cc agar, Difco Laboratories) contain chloramphenicol (0.05 mg. per milliliter) and cycloheximide (0.4 mg. per milliliter) to inhibit both bacteria and many nonpathogenic fungi. This type of medium is stable and useful for bacteria-containing specimens. Penicillin (20 units per milliliter) and streptomycin (40 micrograms per milliliter) may be added to solid media during the cooling period immediately prior to tubing, but storage life and bacterial inhibition are relatively brief. Some gram-negative bacilli (e.g., Proteus species) that are not inhibited by chloramphenicol or streptomycin can be controlled by adding polymyxin B (not to exceed 8 micrograms per milliliter), but this is not done routinely because polymyxin frequently inhibits the growth of pathogenic fungi.

Unfortunately, antibacterial substances which are added to media for the isolation of fungi may exert significant fungal inhibition. Streptomycin and chloramphenicol inhibit some strains of *Nocardia asteroides,* and cycloheximide may prevent growth of Cryptococcus. Actinomyces is completely inhibited by both penicillin and chloramphenicol. Chloramphenicol and cycloheximide have a variable de-

gree of inhibition of Blastomyces and Histoplasma when cultured at 37°C. Suggested media are shown in Table 1.

Anaerobic culture for Actinomyces is done in the author's laboratory only on purulent material from closed infections or biopsies, and on those specimens of sputum or sinus tract drainage that appear suspicious during direct examination of wet and stained preparations.

Except when Actinomyces is suspected, all the primary cultures in our laboratory are incubated at room temperature (25 to 27°C). Plates are sealed in plastic bags to prevent drying. Only screw-cap tubes 25 by 150 mm. are suitable for routine use in a general laboratory.

Conversion of the mycelial to the yeast form is a general requirement

TABLE 1. MEDIA FOR PRIMARY ISOLATION OF FUNGI PRODUCING PULMONARY DISEASE

Genus	Medium	Tube Slants (S) or Plates (P)	Temperature (°C)
Actinomyces	BHI	P	37
	BHI + 10%		
	Rabbitt blood	P	Anaerobic
	Thio broth	(Tubes)	37
Nocardia	Sab	S	
	Sab P & S	S	
	BHI	P	27
	BHI P & S	P	
Blastomyces ⎤	Sab	S	
Histoplasma ⎬	BHI P & S	S	
Coccidioides ⎦	BHI C & C	S & P	27
	BHI 5% RB C & C	P	
Cryptococcus	BHI P & S	S	
	BHI	S	27
	Sab P & S	S	
Candida ⎤	Sab	S	
Aspergillus ⎬	Sab P & S	S	27
Sporothrix ⎥	Sab C & C	P	
Mucor, Rhizopus ⎦	BHI P & S	S	

Key to abbreviations: BHI = Brain-heart infusion agar; P & S = penicillin and streptomycin; C & C = chloramphenicol and cycloheximide; RB = rabbit blood; Sab = Sabouraud's dextrose agar; Thio broth = Brewer's thioglycollate broth.

before making a *final* report of the isolation of the Blastomyces or Histoplasma, and this may apply to Sporothrix and Coccidioides (if endosporulating spherules have not been seen in the original exudate). The only practical way of converting *Coccidioides immitis* is by animal inoculation, and sometimes it is the only successful method of obtaining typical yeast forms of Histoplasma or *Blastomyces dermatitidis.* Hamsters are the most uniformly susceptible laboratory animal, but some strains of mice are suitable.

Cultural conversion of Histoplasma, Blastomyces and Sporothrix is achieved by incubation at 37°C. Brain-heart infusion agar with added rabbit blood (10 per cent), brain-heart infusion agar, and Francis's cysteine glucose blood agar are most suitable. Incubation on plates is desirable after scratch inoculation, but moisture should be conserved by sealing the plates. Cultures contaminated by bacteria may fail to convert to the yeast form despite the best cultural conditions. Repeated subculture on an antibiotic-containing medium may "purify" these cultures and permit conversion, but animal inoculation is often faster and simpler.

All cultures should be examined weekly. Unfortunately, cultural identification is rarely possible from young colonies, and slowly growing pathogenic fungi may be overgrown by saprophytes. Therefore, if several different colonies appear, and particularly if one is growing more rapidly than another, subculture of the immature colonies should be made.

Occasionally, direct examination or serologic study will indicate the probability of a fungous infection, but cultural studies will be negative. Repeated culture is certainly indicated, but animal inoculation should be done if possible. Male hamsters are the most useful laboratory animal because of both their general susceptibility to fungous infection and the ease with which intratesticular and intraperitoneal inoculations can be done. Both routes should be used in the same animal.

ACTINOMYCOSIS

The Organisms

The family Actinomycetaceae contains relatively primitive organisms that are bacteria and not fungi. The obvious morphologic resemblance to the corynebacteria and mycobacteria is thought to be phylogenetic.

Actinomyces species are all grampositive organisms, 0.5 to 1.0 micron in width; they exhibit some degree of hyphal formation and branching in young microcolonies. Improved and new methods for studying these organisms have increased the number known to be pathogens. *Actinomyces israelii* is still the most common offender in human disease; it can be separated into two serotypes. *Actinomyces naeslundii* may grow under aerobic conditions. *Actinomyces odontolyticus* has produced Pott's disease in humans and is a rare pathogen. *Bifidobacterium eriksonii (Actinomyces eriksonii)* does produce pulmonary disease in humans and is strictly anaerobic. *Arachnia propionica (Actinomyces propionicus)* is an uncommon pathogen that may be associated with chest disease. *Actinomyces bovis,* the causative agent of "lumpy jaw" in cattle, rarely, if ever, infects humans, although it was commonly used as a synonym for *A. israelii.* All of these actinomycetes are catalase-negative, whereas diphtheroids are catalase-positive. Definitive identification should be referred to the National Communicable Disease Center, where fluorescent antibody, agar gel diffusion and serotyping can be done.

A. israelii produces actinomycosis in humans and occasionally in cattle. Typically, young microcolonies show a definite hyphal configuration with branching, and mature colonies are marginally lobulated (molar tooth) with peripheral hyphal extension similar to that seen in granules in tissue. Most strains do not hydrolyze starch but do reduce nitrate to nitrite.

Actinomyces naeslundii may grow aerobically or anaerobically or both. It reduces nitrate to nitrite. It is closely related biochemically and serologically to *A. israelii*, but can be differentiated on the basis of specific fluorescent antibody staining.

Bifidobacterium eriksonii is a distinct anaerobic species that can be pathogenic for humans. It strongly hydrolyzes starch and fails to reduce nitrate. To date, it has been isolated only from a lung abscess and two different empyema fluids.

A human pathogen that produced large amounts of propionic acid from fermentation of glucose was classified as *Actinomyces propionicus*. This organism was microaerophilic and catalase-negative. However, it contains diaminopimelic acid in its cell wall, and has been reclassified. Its proper designation is *Arachnia propionica*. This organism can produce clinically typical actinomycosis.

The Clinical Disease

The early pulmonary manifestations of actinomycosis are those of bronchopneumonia or acute lung abscess. In the peribronchial pneumonic type, fever may be minor and remain so until treatment or dissemination. Cough with purulent or sanguinopurulent sputum is rare in children. Aside from weight loss, night sweats and poor tolerance for exercise, there may be little to make one suspect pulmonary disease until it is revealed by auscultation, roentgenography or obvious chest wall involvement. It is felt that lung abscess is usually aspirational and associated with early reactive bronchial occlusion. Fever, leukocytosis and evidence of acute illness are striking. Sputum is usually not produced until the bronchus has opened and a fluid level can be seen within the abscess.

Since it has become customary to prescribe antibiotics for acute pulmonary disease, neither of the two forms above is likely to be recognized unless one is pursuing a special microbiologic study. Instead, one is confronted with either an "unresolved pneumonia" with its possibility of tuberculosis or other granulomatous disease, or a "chronic lung abscess" that may require surgery unless treated properly.

Lung abscesses may be peripheral, and follow the distribution of aspirational abscesses. Pleural involvement is frequent, but may be localized if even suppressive therapy is started early. Empyema is rarely seen now unless the process has been completely neglected.

In recent years, the pulmonary actinomycosis seen by the author has consisted almost entirely of unrecognized or neglected undiagnosed pneumonias that have progressed to involvement of the pleurae and chest wall. Chest wall abscesses and sinus tracts have been present, and as in the patient shown in Figure 1, it has often been unclear whether the initial infection was pulmonary or abdominal. Transdiaphragmatic spread in either direction is different in actinomycosis than in amebiasis. The extension by contiguity in actinomycosis is accompanied by extensive fibrosis; sudden evacuation of purulent material through the bronchi and collections of free pus are not part of the usual clinical course. Neglected pulmonary actinomycosis usually extends to the chest wall, and may result in considerable deformity with or without osteomyelitis of the ribs or vertebrae. Sinus tracts are multiple as a rule, often discharging a rather watery fluid in which the sulfur granules may be found. The degree of fever and rapidity of weight loss are extremely variable, but both usually increase during chest wall involvement. Cerebral metastasis may complicate untreated pulmonary actinomycosis.

From the point of view of help in diagnosis, the description of the roentgenographic spectrum of pulmonary actinomycosis is an utter waste of time. Primary involvement of the lower lobes is more frequent than that of the upper. Pleural involvement is common, particularly in association with loculated empyema. If untreated, actinomycosis tends to produce confluent dense consolidations that suggest a suppurative pneumonitis unless obscured by organizing empyema. Acute hema-

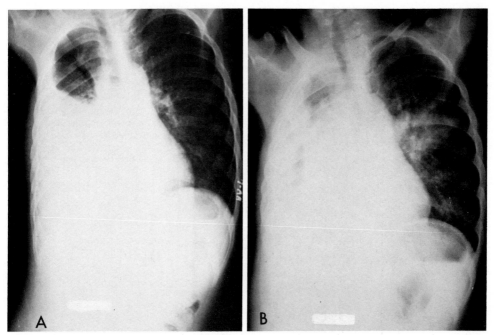

Figure 1.   A ten-year-old child with left hemiparesis and periodic convulsive seizures beginning in the first year of life. *A,* Film taken in the clinic for complaints of epigastric discomfort and constipation. She returned, complaining of an abscess of the lower right hemithorax and fever. *B,* Another film revealed a right bronchopleurocutaneous fistula and pneumonia in the left lung. Empyema fluid was culturally positive for *A. israelii.*

togenous microabscesses are rare. In the author's own experience, simultaneous bilateral involvement is rare.

Laboratory Diagnosis

The problem of early diagnosis of actinomycosis in infants and children is particularly difficult. Sputum is rarely available, and the fact that actinomycetes are found in oral secretions of many persons without actinomycosis makes gastric aspirates of doubtful value. The roentgenogram and clinical pictures often suggest the possibility of a foreign body. If bronchoscopy is done, bronchial washings should be obtained for direct study. Granules of Actinomyces usually show definite hyphal elements with branching (Fig. 2), which are rarely as well formed as in tissue sections. Inflammatory cells may be present at the periphery of the gran-

ule; these and the sheathing or "clubbing" of the hyphae that is so frequent in pus and in tissue section are not frequent in diluted bronchial washings. Small granules may fragment almost completely into clumps and clusters of what appear to be diphtheroids. In addition, Actinomyces may be present in bronchial washings as clusters of diphtheroid-like organisms without granule formation.

Any unresolved pneumonia or lung abscess that has roentgenographic evidence of definite pleuritis over the area of involvement may be safely needled for aspiration. A portion of the aspirate should be stained by Gram's method prior to utilizing the remainder for culture. Gram-positive filaments in such an aspirate always indicate the necessity of culturing for Actinomyces and Nocardia.

Pus obtained from the lung or from

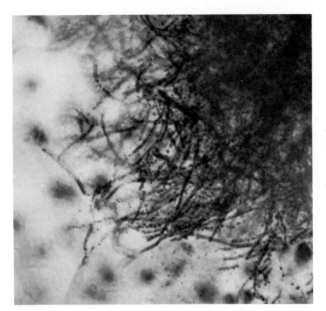

Figure 2. Gram-stained granule of *A. israelii* in sputum. The oil-immersion objective was used to magnify one margin of the granule to show the fine beading and "coccoidal bodies" that are observed frequently. True hyphal branching can be seen.

pleural fluid, pleural biopsy, or other surgical materials should be examined directly prior to culture. The exact procedure of culturing is discussed in the section under General Methods of Microbiologic Diagnosis. If so-called sulfur granules are present, they should be washed in sterile physiologic saline several times before introducing them into culture media.

Direct examination is particularly important in actinomycosis because of the necessity of correlating clinical findings with laboratory results. At present, few laboratories outside specialized medical centers appear to be qualified to make the specific identification of an actinomycete. Unless the presence of catalase is determined, it is easy to confuse cultures of anaerobic diphtheroids with Actinomyces. Such misinterpretation has occurred repeatedly. The demonstration of sulfur granules in tissue or exudates is not a sine qua non for diagnosis, but it certainly is important in doubtful circumstances.

The fluorescent antibody method is the most rapid and accurate single means of identification. At present, definitive identification should be referred to the National Center for Disease Control, where fluorescent antibody, immunodiffusion and serotyping can be done.

Epidemiology

A truly free-living form of the anaerobic actinomycetes has never been found. Their existence in the alimentary tract of humans and some other warm-blooded animals is believed to be essentially saprophytic. Noninvasive actinomycetes can be recovered from tonsillar crypts, carious teeth and the adjacent gums. In the absence of a free-living form, it is presumed that transmission is from person to person directly or through fomites.

Actinomycosis is worldwide in distribution, and is said to occur more frequently in males than in females. It is an uncommon mycosis in childhood. Better oral hygiene and dental care together with the frequent use of antimicrobials in association with exodontia, tonsillectomy and early undiagnosed bronchopulmonary infections probably account for the lessened incidence in recent years.

Pathogenesis and Pathology

It is known that many people with abnormal oral hygiene, chronic bronchial disease or chronic bronchopulmonary disease have Actinomyces in their mouths or sputum without evidence of actinomycosis. Careful study of early cases of cervicofacial actinomycosis bears out the close association of this form of the disease with significant parodontal disease, extraction or trauma. In this sense, the disease is opportunistic, and by inference a similar pathogenesis has been proposed for primary pulmonary actinomycosis.

It is also known that actinomycosis is seldom, if ever, due to infection with Actinomyces alone. Associated bacteria or the interrelations between the Actinomyces and bacteria are thought to be of primary importance in the initiation of actinomycosis. Primary pulmonary infection presumably takes place after aspiration of an infectious nidus.

Despite the fact that the bacterial flora in pulmonary actinomycosis usually contains anaerobic streptococci that are resistant to penicillin, and often contains gram-negative organisms that are similarly resistant, almost all patients respond as though the disease were due to a penicillin-sensitive organism. The same phenomenon is observed in many aspirational lung abscesses with mixed gram-negative and gram-positive flora.

Actinomycosis is characterized by a mixture of chronic and acute granulation tissue and marginal fibrosis. The Actinomyces usually occur in granules surrounded by an area of suppuration. Small and large abscesses that frequently communicate with one another are common in association with chronic granulation tissue and fibrosis. The reaction around the granules is predominantly polymorphonuclear. At the margin of the granule, the individual hyphal tips may be sheathed ("clubbed") by a host material that stains with acidophilic dyes. Multinucleate giant cells are not frequent, but may be present in the chronic granulation tissue adjacent to the area of suppuration.

Actinomycosis tends to spread by contiguity with multiple sinus tracts connecting areas of suppuration and extending through the pleurae into the chest wall or to the surface of the skin.

The individual actinomycotic granule varies greatly in size, but is usually seen easily in routine histologic preparations. The hyphal elements are colored by basophilic stains such as hematoxylin, but are best demonstrated by the Gram method. There are times when the marginal filaments can be demonstrated by either the Gomori methenamine-silver method or a periodic acid–Schiff stain with light green counter stain. Although regarded as an inferior procedure for Actinomyces and Nocardia, the latter stain can give excellent structural detail as shown in Figure 3.

A presumptive diagnosis of pulmonary actinomycosis can usually be made from resected tissue even without cultural confirmation. If a pulmonary granule contains definite hyphal filaments of approximately 1 micron in width, one can be sure that an actinomycete is present. *Nocardia asteroides* is much more commonly present in scattered filaments and loose clumps than in granules. It may, however, produce granules that are indistinguishable from Actinomyces when stained by Gram's method. Filaments and granules of *Nocardia asteroides*, *N. brasiliensis*, and *N. caviae* are usually weakly acid-fast, and this characteristic, when present, can be used for differentiating them from Actinomyces.

Treatment and Prevention

Despite the recognized importance of concomitant and mixed bacterial infection in the causation of actinomycosis, combination or broad-spectrum antimicrobial therapy is rarely necessary. The pathogenic Actinomyces species are very sensitive to penicillin, erythromycin, chloramphenicol, the tetracyclines

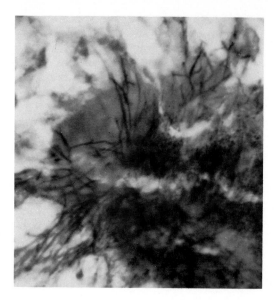

Figure 3. Actinomycotic granule in lung. The hyphae with their branchings are stained clearly by the periodic acid–Schiff method. The amorphous material surrounding the margin (sheathing) is derived from the host tissue and took the light green counterstain.

and probably most antibacterial antibiotics effective against gram-positive bacteria. Regardless of the bacterial "associates" that may be found, healing almost always occurs if penicillin is given alone for several months in a daily dose between 2 and 6 million units. Although it has been shown that the concentration of penicillin needed to suppress the growth of colonies of *A. bovis* exceeds that required to suppress loose filaments, failure of response to penicillin therapy is much more likely to be due to an unrecognized basic pathologic state (e.g., tuberculosis or penicillin-resistant staphylococcal pneumonia) than to either invasiveness of the usual bacterial "associates" of *A. israelii* or its inherent resistance to penicillin.

Penicillin in dosage sufficient to produce a plasma level between 1 and 2 Oxford units per milliliter should be effective in the treatment of pulmonary actinomycosis if given long enough. The acutely ill patient will respond more rapidly to large intravenous doses. Patients with indolent but extensive involvement may require months of treatment, which can best be given by supplementing oral medication with intermittent intramuscular injections of long-acting penicillins. All our patients are treated with parenteral administration of penicillin, unless contraindicated, until they become asymptomatic and roentgenographic regression is definite. Oral penicillin therapy in an equivalent or larger dose is then substituted and continued until recovery is evident.

Patients allergic to penicillin may be given erythromycin, a tetracycline or chloramphenicol in the usual dosage prescribed for moderate infections. The end-result is probably the same as that achieved with penicillin, but complications of therapy are more common with the broad-spectrum antibiotics.

Unless a free empyema is present, no sort of surgical drainage or exploration is indicated in the immediate treatment of pulmonary actinomycosis. The development of antimicrobial resistance during prolonged treatment for extensive disease has not been a problem. The amount of roentgenographic and functional improvement that can take place, even in the presence of extensive pleural involvement, is often amazing. Pleural decortication, resection of a destroyed portion of lung, or drainage of a subdiaphragmatic abscess may ultimately be necessary, but one may safely postpone such a decision until after four or more months of continuous and adequate antimicrobial therapy.

There is no indication for preventive measures aimed particularly at actinomycosis. Good oral and dental hygiene is an end in itself. When infected teeth and tonsils must be removed, a few days of postoperative antibiotic therapy is certainly justifiable, and is probably adequate to prevent the development of actinomycosis.

NOCARDIOSIS

The Organisms

The genus Nocardia is in the family Actinomycetaceae. Unlike Actinomyces, it is aerobic. The organisms are grampositive and exhibit similar branching of hyphae whose diameter is usually no more than 1 micron. Like Actinomyces, it is a bacterium.

Nocardia asteroides is the common causative agent of pulmonary nocardiosis, but both *N. brasiliensis* and *N. caviae* have been identified recently as agents of pulmonary (and disseminated) disease. All three are usually acid-fast or partially acid-fast in direct smears of exudates and have similar colonial morphology. Of the three, *N. brasiliensis* hydrolyzes casein and tyrosine, whereas *N. caviae* and *N. asteroides* do not. *N. caviae* decomposes xanthine, whereas *N. brasiliensis* and *N. asteroides* do not. Growth in liquid gelatin medium also differs but is more variable. Additional studies are necessary to separate Nocardia from Streptomyces, Actinomadura and *Rothia dentocariosa*, which closely resembles Nocardia.

The hyphal characteristics and branching of Nocardia are best studied in slide cultures, since aerial hyphal production may be slight. Colonies may be white, gray, or various shades of buff through orange.

In pus, sputum or tissues, Nocardia organisms are usually found in small clusters or in open hyphal strands showing various degrees of fragmentation into bacillary or coccobacillary forms. Occasionally, one may find asteroid colonies appearing in sputum or pus, such as is shown in Figure 4. Grossly, these may resemble tiny granules of *A. israelii*, but they are not

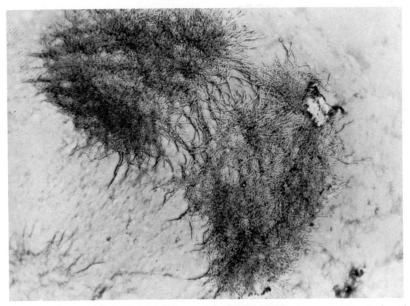

Figure 4. *Nocardia asteroides* in sputum. These two asteroid colonies were seen in a hydroxide-cleared mount of fresh sputum. The mount was fixed in alcoholic formalin before removing the coverslip and staining by a modified Ziehl-Neelsen method. The hyphae were moderately acid-fast.

sheathed, nor is there the same central mycelial mat that one finds in a true actinomycotic granule. Although 0.5 per cent aqueous sulfuric acid is usually recommended for destaining smears of sputum and pus after the application of steaming carbol-fuchsin, a three-second destain with 3 per cent hydrochloric acid in 95 per cent alcohol appears to be satisfactory, facilitating the use of standard Ziehl-Neelsen reagents. Acid-fast bacillary forms closely resembling *M. tuberculosis* may be found in abundance, but they are practically always associated with some hyphal elements.

The Clinical Disease

In the adult patient, nocardiosis may present as a subacute or chronic pulmonary illness that closely mimics the course of tuberculosis, or it may present as an acute suppurative pneumonitis that can be rapidly progressive. The number of cases reported in children is too few to establish any special features that would differentiate the childhood disease from that seen in adults.

The x-ray picture may resemble either tuberculosis or suppurative pneumonia (Fig. 5). Occasionally, bilateral, patchy pulmonary infiltration may have the appearance of a hematogenous pneumonia. Pleurisy with subsequent empyema occurs in about one-fourth of the cases, and chest wall involvement with sinus tract formation may mimic actinomycosis.

Hematogenous dissemination is much more frequent than in actinomycosis. Metastasis is particularly likely to involve the central nervous system, the kidney, and the subcutaneous tissues and bodies of the muscles of the extremities.

There are no particularly helpful symptomatic features of nocardiosis. In general, the symptoms can be said to simulate either tuberculosis or lung abscess. When sputum is being produced, it is mucopurulent and may be blood-flecked. Leukocytosis with an increase in the polymorphonuclear neutrophils is common.

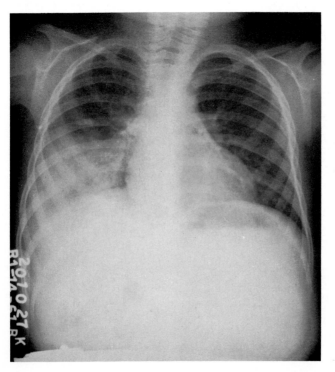

Figure 5. Pulmonary nocardiosis. This 46-month-old boy failed to improve symptomatically or radiographically during treatment with antibiotics. At thoracotomy, the right lower lobe suppurative pneumonitis contained an abscess from which *Nocardia asteroides* was recovered. (Courtesy of C. Harrison Snyder, M.D., Ochsner Clinic.)

Laboratory Diagnosis

When Nocardia occurs in clusters such as shown in Figure 4, it is difficult to overlook the fungus in potassium hydroxide wet mounts of either sputum or pus. Unfortunately, Nocardia may appear in more dispersed filaments, which are not recognized in wet mounts of sputum and are overlooked or misinterpreted in wet mounts of pus.

The thin hyphae and bacillary fragments are well seen in thin films of exudates stained by Gram's method, but may be easily overlooked if they are not numerous. If sputum or other exudate contains filaments suggestive of Nocardia, a modified Ziehl-Neelsen stain as already discussed should be done before material is planted on culture media.

The genus Nocardia is not fastidious in its growth requirements. Initial isolation may be made on any of the common solid laboratory media. Growth is usually good at room temperature or 37°C. Both should be used. The section on general microbiologic methods is applicable to the isolation of species of Nocardia with certain qualifications.

The sensitivity in vitro of N. asteroides to antibiotics is variable from strain to strain. None of the human isolates of N. asteroides studied by the author has been significantly sensitive to penicillin in vitro, although strains sensitive to penicillin have been reported. Solid media without antibiotics should always be inoculated with materials suspected of containing Nocardia, but unless no other organisms are seen on Gram's staining of the material, the usual antibiotic-containing media recommended in the section on general microbiologic methods should also be heavily inoculated. Colonial growth of N. asteroides, N. brasiliensis and N. caviae usually appears on blood agar or Sabouraud's dextrose agar between seven and ten days after inoculation, but growth may be delayed as long as three weeks. When Sabouraud's dextrose agar containing penicillin and streptomycin is the medium, colony growth is usually slow. The use of a chloramphenicol-cycloheximide–containing medium is a sometimes successful means of purifying bacterially contaminated initial isolates.

At present, there are no serologic methods that have been applied successfully to the diagnosis of nocardiosis in humans. Nocardia species appear to be poor stimulators of circulating antibody, even under experimental conditions. Serologic study has been of some value in the clarification of the taxonomic relations of Nocardia, but there is, as yet, no direct clinical application.

Epidemiology

Nocardia asteroides is a normal inhabitant of soil, where it can survive a wide range of temperature. Its distribution is probably worldwide. Nocardiosis is more frequent in males than in females.

The respiratory tract as the ordinary portal of entry is less certain for nocardiosis than for histoplasmosis, coccidioidomycosis, cryptococcosis and blastomycosis. Nevertheless, with special effort, N. asteroides can be isolated from the sputum or bronchial washings of a few hospitalized patients who have no evidence of nocardiosis. Furthermore, there appears to have been an increase in the incidence of opportunistic infections due to N. asteroides, and most of these have been pulmonary.

The possibility that nocardiosis is a common, self-limited infection has been considered, but no large-scale epidemiologic surveys are available to support this hypothesis.

Pathogenesis and Pathology

The pathogenesis of human nocardiosis is incompletely known. Critical evaluation of well documented cases during the last decade suggests that nocardiosis occurs as an opportunistic infection in about 50 per cent of the recognized cases. Whether opportunis-

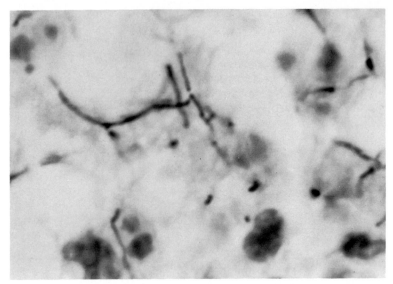

Figure 6. *N. asteroides* in the lung. The Brown and Brenn modification of the Gram stain shows the slender hyphae, branching, beading and bacillary fragmentation to good advantage. Oil-immersion magnification at the margin of a microabscess.

tic infection takes place from endogenous but inapparent sources or exogenously during the period of increased susceptibility is not known.

The most common expression of pulmonary nocardiosis is that of a suppurative pneumonitis. Acute, hematogenous dissemination may appear grossly like miliary tuberculosis. The predominant cellular response is usually that of polymorphonuclear leukocytes and plasma cells. Multiple, yellow abscesses are frequent in rapidly fatal illness, whereas cavitation and pleural involvement are common in chronic illness.

Filaments, coccobacillary forms and clusters of Nocardia can be demonstrated by the Brown and Brenn modification of the Gram stain in areas of suppuration. Small asteroid colonies may be seen, but there is no sheathing of the peripheral filaments, and no dense granule formation in the lung to suggest actinomycosis. When the filaments are sparse, whether fragmented or not, they are difficult to find and to identify microscopically except under high magnification. Filaments cannot

be seen in ordinary hematoxylin and eosin preparations.

Some patients with chronic nocardiosis have areas of cavitation and of fibrosis and chronic granulomatous reaction not unlike a mixed tuberculous and pyogenic infection. Giant cells may be found in the fibrotic areas of such chronic lesions, and few Nocardia may be found after extensive search with the best staining techniques.

The Gomori methenamine-silver stain will demonstrate Nocardia well. Hyphae of Nocardia are stained by the periodic acid–Schiff method. Nevertheless, the simpler Brown and Brenn modification of the Gram stain is the method of choice. A Brown and Brenn preparation is shown in Figure 6.

Treatment and Prevention

Sulfonamides have been the preferred drugs for the treatment of nocardiosis, especially sulfadiazine and sulfasoxazole. The daily dose of sulfadiazine should be that which yields a blood level between 10 and 15 mg. per 100 ml. Recently, the combination of sulfamethoxazole and trimethoprim has been more effective, is commercially available, and is probably the treatment of choice when tolerated. It should be given in full recommended dosage. Treatment should be continued for at least two months after all activity of the disease, clinically and radiographically, has subsided. Ampicillin is effective against a significant number of isolates of Nocardia, but minocycline and doxycycline are more effective in vitro. The latter are probably the therapeutic agents of second choice, and one can be combined with sulfamethoxazole-trimethoprim.

Surgical drainage of closed areas of infection, particularly metastases, should be accomplished soon after chemotherapy has been instituted. Pulmonary infections usually establish drainage transbronchially or through the chest wall, but soft tissue and extrathoracic visceral infections may resist treatment without surgery. If it appears likely that pulmonary resection will be necessary, it should be delayed until the full effects of chemotherapy can be evaluated.

Nocardiosis is not a public health problem, and any discussion of prevention would be meaningless except in relation to opportunistic infections.

NORTH AMERICAN BLASTOMYCOSIS

The Organism

Blastomyces dermatitidis is a dimorphic fungus whose free-living form is mycelial. It has been isolated from soils and other organic debris. The parasitic form is yeastlike and thick-walled, and has been found in the tissues of humans, dogs and horses. The perfect form has been found and is classified as *Ajellomyces dermatitidis.*

The characteristics of the parasitic form are more constant in fresh pus or sputum than in wet preparations of cultures at 37°C. Hydroxide-cleared wet mounts of exudates may be supplemen-

ted by periodic acid–Schiff stained preparations of the same material in order to study the details of budding and cytologic features. The yeastlike cells are predominantly spherical to subspherical. Form is preserved as a rule during budding, but some degree of elongation may occur. Resting cells average about 10 to 12 microns in diameter, but may vary from less than 5 to more than 25 microns. The cell wall is thick enough to be distinct, and in phase-contrast or subdued bright-field illumination, the outer and inner limiting optical surfaces may be separated by a central optical membrane producing a "doubly contoured" effect. The cells are multinucleate, whereas those of Histoplasma and Cryptococcus are uninucleate.

Budding is usually single in exudates, but may be multiple, owing to the prolonged period of attachment of the daughter cell. Evagination of the cell wall of the parent is broad, and the protoplasmic bridge is wide. As a general rule, daughter and parent are of approximately equal diameter before separation. In periodic acid–Schiff stained preparations, the broad "disjunctive" cell wall marginating the protoplasmic bridge is distinct and strikingly unlike that which one may see in similarly stained preparations of cryptococci or Histoplasma (Fig. 7).

B. dermatitidis grows less well at 37°C. than at room temperature, but primary growth of the yeast form can usually be obtained from exudates that contain sufficient organisms to be seen during direct examination. Growth on brain-heart infusion agar or blood agar at 37°C. appears within two weeks after inoculation. The colonies are grayish at first, rapidly become heaped-up and granular, and when mature, vary from light cream to dark brown in color. Pigmentation is greater on blood agar than on brain-heart infusion agar.

Cultures at 37°C. show more variation in cellular morphology than does the study of exudates. Multiple budding, giving rise to clusters or "balls" of

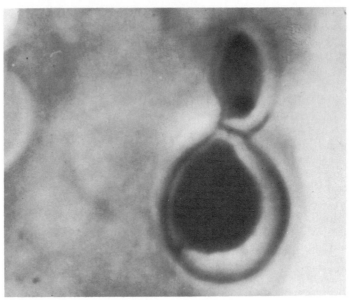

Figure 7.   Budding of *B. dermatitidis.* Periodic acid–Schiff stain of a budding organism under oil-immersion magnification to show the broad attachment and definite cross wall between mother and daughter cells. The cell wall is relatively thick. Compare with Figure 9.

yeastlike forms, is much more common, and the formation of short germ tubes or abortive hyphae is frequent.

Growth at room temperature is mycelial and more dependable than at 37°C. In the absence of bacterial contamination, growth from clinical specimens may appear within the first week of incubation, but is often delayed until the second. Initial growth may be rapidly spreading as a smooth, membranous, whitish but translucent glaze not unlike the sugar glaze on doughnuts. This growth is generally succeeded by the appearance of bristly aerial hyphae, which increase in number and length until the colony is cottony. White, cottony colonies often become tan with age and then resemble colonies of *Histoplasma capsulatum.* Some strains will not give visible growth until the fourth week of incubation, making it necessary to protect cultures against drying. Strains that grow poorly at room temperature may produce small colonies only, with little or no typical sporulation. Such strains not only may fail to convert to the yeast phase when subcultured at 37°C., but also may not

grow at this temperature. Recognition may be dependent upon heavily inoculating the mycelial culture intraperitoneally into hamsters and mice. The animals should be sacrificed, cultured, and studied histopathologically three weeks after inoculation.

The mycelial form of *B. dermatitidis* resembles the same form of *H. capsulatum* in many respects. The hyphae of mature colonies are septate and bear a variable number of spherical to ovoid, thin-walled, smooth conidia which range in size from 3 to 6 microns. Some conidia are sessile, but most are borne on slender conidiophores or at the end of hyphae. With aging of the colony, the conidia may become thick-walled. These are similar in diameter (7 to 15 microns) to the macroconidia of *Histoplasma capsulatum,* but are never tuberculate, whereas those of *H. capsulatum* are usually tuberculate.

The Clinical Disease

It is believed that the respiratory tract is the most common portal of entry for infection with *B. dermatitidis.* Nevertheless, there is no recognized clinical picture of acute inhalational blastomycosis such as exists for histoplasmosis.

The clinical spectrum of pulmonary blastomycosis is as varied as that of tuberculosis. A segmental pneumonitis is seen sufficiently often to make one believe that this may be a common expression of early disease. This kind of lesion has been seen in children. It may regress spontaneously, apparently stabilize, or progress acutely or subacutely to produce a picture of an acute suppurative pneumonitis (Fig. 8). Circumscribed mass lesions may involve rib and be confused with neoplasm. Fever, chest pain, cough and weight loss have been common symptoms in the pediatric group. Sputum, when produced, is mucopurulent and occasionally blood-streaked. Leukocytosis of mild to moderate degree is the rule in acute disease. Despite the frequency of pleuritic pain, empyema is rare. Rib and subcutaneous chest abscesses may develop without empyema.

Although any sort of radiologic picture may be seen, enlargement of the bronchial or hilar lymph nodes is frequent in all but miliary dissemination. Involvement of anterior segments of the lung is more common than in tuberculosis. The only roentgenographic feature that is particularly helpful, and common to most pulmonary mycoses, is the persistence or slow change of the lesion during treatment with antibacterial antibiotics.

Metastasis to the skin, bones or viscera is frequent during the course of recognized North American blastomycosis. Secondary foci may be more obvious than the pulmonary disease. Nevertheless, pulmonary blastomycosis not only may regress without treatment, but also may disappear roentgenographically without evidence of dissemination.

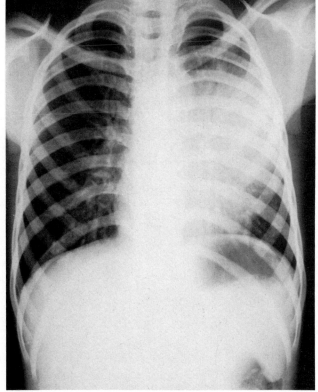

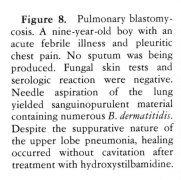

Figure 8. Pulmonary blastomycosis. A nine-year-old boy with an acute febrile illness and pleuritic chest pain. No sputum was being produced. Fungal skin tests and serologic reaction were negative. Needle aspiration of the lung yielded sanguinopurulent material containing numerous *B. dermatitidis.* Despite the suppurative nature of the upper lobe pneumonia, healing occurred without cavitation after treatment with hydroxystilbamidine.

Laboratory Diagnosis

If sputum is being produced, pulmonary blastomycosis can be diagnosed presumptively in most patients by direct examination of sputum. No single laboratory examination is so neglected. Budding yeastlike forms are characteristic to the experienced observer, but many hospital laboratory technologists have a hazy remembrance at best of the diagnostic features. Figure 9 is representative of the appearance of *B. dermatitidis* by direct examination.

The special fungous stains can be applied to fixed smears of sputum, gastric aspirates or other exudates to study morphology. Although final diagnosis must be made culturally, therapeutic considerations justify rapid methods of making a tentative diagnosis.

Sputum, bronchial washings and gastric aspirates are all suitable for culture, and should be handled according to the methodology outlined in the section on general microbiologic methods (p. 880). Pneumonic lesions extending to the pleura may be needled safely and aspirated for culture if insufficient ma-

terial is obtained for both direct examination and culture. This diagnostic approach is particularly important in children who are not producing sputum. Cultures at 27°C. are much more likely to be positive than those at 37°C. Conversion of the mycelial form to the yeastlike phase by culturing at 37°C. is usually easy, but in healing lesions this may be difficult or even impossible without animal passage. Animal inoculation may not produce macroscopic disease. It is important to sacrifice animals at approximately three weeks after inoculation and to culture homogenates of the liver, spleen, lung, testes and any visible abdominal lymph nodes. Intraperitoneal and intratesticular inoculation of hamsters seems to be as sensitive a method as the intravenous inoculation of mice.

B. dermatitidis is so easily recognized microscopically in sputum, other exudates and tissues that specific aids to diagnosis other than cultures would appear superfluous. There are times, however, when no classic budding forms are seen, and cultures, whether because of bacterial contamination or low viability, are negative. In this situa-

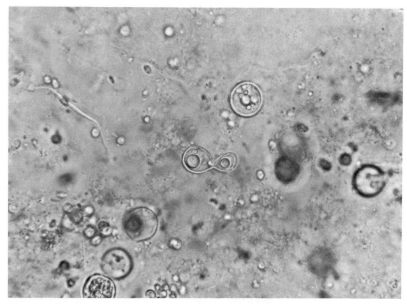

Figure 9. *B. dermatitidis* in sputum; photograph of a wet preparation of sputum containing numerous blastomycetes. Typical broad-based budding and the "double contour" of the cell wall are illustrated.

tion, fluorescent microscopy, utilizing specific antiglobulins labeled with fluorescein, may be helpful. Antiblastomyces rabbit globulin, absorbed with yeast cells of *Histoplasma capsulatum* and hyphae of *Geotrichum candidum* and conjugated with fluorescein isothiocyanate, is considered to give specific fluorescence with *B. dermatitidis*.

Recent work has shown that a specific immunodiffusion test for blastomycosis is as specific and sensitive as serologic tests for histoplasmosis. It is available only at special laboratories.

Patients with primary pulmonary histoplasmosis or coccidioidomycosis may give positive complement-fixing reactions with blastomyces antigen to a titer higher than with homologous antigen. Similarly, the patient with North American blastomycosis may give a positive complement-fixation reaction with histoplasma antigen and none with homologous antigen. The results of intradermal sensitivity tests and complement-fixation tests may be contradictory. Campbell (1960) has demonstrated the frequent occurrence of an increasing titer with homologous antigen and decreasing titer with heterologous ones in serial complement-fixation studies during the course of the primary pulmonary infections. This is of considerable immunologic interest, but scarcely helps the diagnostician in his initial contact with the patient. Of my own patients, 53 per cent had positive complement-fixing antibodies, and 26 per cent had a positive skin test result with blastomycin.

Epidemiology

North American blastomycosis is a disease of humans and some domestic animals in an area extending from Canada through Mexico. Autochthonous cases have been reported from South America and Africa; it seems likely that the increasing interest in medical mycology in all parts of the world will reveal that the character-

ization of blastomycosis as North American is inappropriate.

The organism has been isolated from soils, pigeon guano and other organic debris from old chicken coops, dilapidated houses, and outbuildings. There is a strong possibility that it may occur in association with rotting wood. Recent studies suggest that *B. dermatitidis* has a limited temporal recoverability from soils known to contain the naturally acquired fungus. Ecologic causes for this are not known. It is possible that animal reservoirs are important in bringing about soil inoculation.

Infection of children appears to be relatively infrequent in endemic areas, in contrast to the high incidence noted for other soil-inhabiting fungi such as *Histoplasma capsulatum* and *Coccidioides immitis*. Yet of ten patients with clinical illness due to *B. dermatitidis* during a five-month period in a small community, seven were 16 years of age or younger, and four of these were under seven. The actual incidence and age distribution of infection in any area is not known.

Among adults, clinical disease is more frequent in males than in females. In my own series, the ratio of males to females has been 6:1.

The portal of entry in blastomycosis is almost certainly respiratory in most instances. The clinical characteristics and course of blastomycosis from cutaneous inoculation are different from those seen in the usual cutaneous blastomycosis, which is almost certainly a manifestation of spread from an active or inactive pulmonary focus.

Pathogenesis and Pathology

Two types of primary pulmonary lesion have been recognized by roentgenographic features, but one can only infer the pathologic changes from older resected specimens and experimental infections in animals.

Bronchopneumonic lesions have been observed to clear spontaneously without cavitation or radiographic evidence of fibrosis. The histopathologic features of such lesions have not been documented in humans. In some, the disease will progress and become manifest by suppuration of draining lymph nodes or pectoral muscle extension from internal mammary nodes.

The second type of lesion seems to follow the usual evolution of mycotic "coin" granulomas, being well circumscribed and relatively dense from the time of the first roentgenographic recognition. This type of lesion is characterized by a dense fibrotic reaction within and at the margin of the granuloma. Epithelioid tissue and giant cells may predominate, or central caseation may be the outstanding feature. Differentiation from cryptococcal or histoplasmal granulomas may be difficult without culture. Unless typical budding forms and resting forms with definite multiple nuclei are present, histologic differentiation from cryptococcosis may be impossible. The mucicarmine stain does not seem to be as specific for cryptococci as has been stated by some pathologists.

A commonly recognized advanced form of blastomycotic pulmonary disease, a suppurative pneumonitis, is the result of rapid extension of primary bronchopneumonic lesions in a highly susceptible host. Blastomyces are found within areas of suppuration that are more or less circumscribed by epithelioid tissue. They are also present in the fibrinous and polymorphonuclear exudate in the alveoli and terminal bronchioles. Acute suppurative pneumonitis may be followed by cavitation, which is often multilocular. Empyema is infrequent even when suppurative pneumonitis and cavitation extend to the pleura. Rib and thoracic soft tissue involvement is not uncommon during the course of acute pulmonary blastomycosis. Extension to the bronchial and hilar lymph nodes is typical.

At the other end of the spectrum of pulmonary response to *B. dermatitidis* are those patients whose x-ray films and tissue sections are suggestive of sarcoidosis. Multiple epithelioid granulomas of varying dimensions with numerous or scanty giant cells and septal fibrosis are scattered throughout the lung. As a general rule, many of the epithelioid granulomas have some degree of central caseation necrosis, which alerts the pathologist to the probability of a fungal or mycobacterial origin. Special stains, such as the periodic acid–Schiff, will reveal Blastomyces within giant cells and areas of caseation.

Treatment

North American blastomycosis responds well to treatment with hydroxystilbamidine and amphotericin B. Patients with involvement of the central nervous system, those whose disease is severely disseminated and those critically ill should be treated with amphotericin B. Otherwise, hydroxystilbamidine is preferred because of its lesser toxicity and fewer side-effects.

Although hydroxystilbamidine can be administered intramuscularly, it is best given intravenously in a concentration no greater than 0.5 mg. per milliliter. The infusion can be given within a period of one to two hours. The dosage should be calculated on the basis of 3 to 5 mg. of hydroxystilbamidine per kilogram of body weight per day. The drug is administered daily for 21 days and every other day thereafter until the total period of treatment is between eight and 12 weeks. Treatment should not be interrupted, because resistance to hydroxystilbamidine develops more often when treatment is given in courses than when it is given continuously.

If antimicrobial resistance appears, or if the patient relapses, re-treatment should be with amphotericin B. This antibiotic can be given according to the recommendations outlined in the section on Treatment of Systemic Mycoses.

SOUTH AMERICAN BLASTOMYCOSIS (PARACOCCIDIOIDOMYCOSIS)

The Organism

Paracoccidioides brasiliensis is sometimes termed *Blastomyces brasiliensis*. Unfortunately, both generic names are used, resulting in the confusion of this organism with *B. dermatitidis*.

The free-living form grows slowly and restrictedly on Sabouraud's glucose agar at pH 7 and 27°C. Colonial morphology is variable, occasionally glabrous or cerebriform, but commonly woolly with a short nap. Colonies cannot be considered to be mature until after one month of incubation. Most colonies are pure white, but some may be gray or light brown with aging. Chlamydospores are formed by the septate, branching hyphae.

The parasitic form is diagnostic in either exudates or cultures at 37°C. when the characteristic budding can be seen. The diagnostic cell varies in size from 10 to 60 microns and is seen to have multiple buds extruded through the cell wall. The buds may be elongate, and the budding cell may resemble the wheel of a boat (*roda de leme; rueda del barco*), or the buds may be relatively large, round to spherical as in Figure 10, and four to five in number. The communication between the mother and daughter cell is narrow and tapering, unlike that seen in *B. dermatitidis*. Budding cells of diagnostic type are more easily found in cultures at 37° C. or in hydroxide-cleared mounts of exudates than in tissue sections.

Growth at 37° C. on blood agar, brain-heart infusion agar or Sabouraud's glucose agar (pH 7) appears, as a rule, earlier than at 27°C. Colonies are small, usually cerebriform, translucent to grayish, and produce large numbers of yeastlike cells. Single budding is much more common in cultures, exudates or tissue sections than the typical multiple external budding and is the basis for confusion of *P. brasiliensis* with *B. dermatitidis*. Nevertheless, direct examination of cultures at 37°C. or of hydroxide-cleared exudates will reveal the diagnostic budding forms if a diligent search is made.

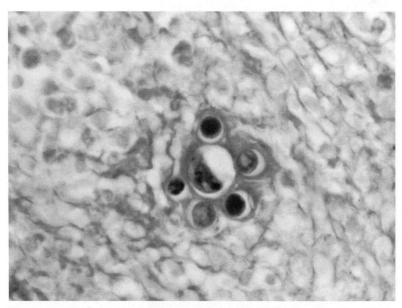

Figure 10. *Paracoccidioides brasiliensis* in lung; a periodic acid–Schiff stain of lung showing a mother cell and five daughters. The continuity of cell walls can be seen, but no cytoplasmic communication is evident at this stage.

Error is much more likely if microscopic examination of stained tissue sections is the only diagnostic method available.

The Clinical Disease

The South American literature emphasizes the primary disease, in which the portal of entry is usually considered to be the mucous membranes of the mouth or pharynx. Primary inoculation through carious teeth (apical abscesses), nasal mucous membranes, the anus and conjunctivae is considered to be much less frequent. Lacaz (1955) has suggested the respiratory tract, however, as one of the most common portals of entry. Perhaps the main fact in favor of primary oropharyngeal infection is the frequency of cervical lymph node involvement.

The most obvious manifestations of South American blastomycosis are ulcerogranulomatous lesions of the skin, mucous membranes and lymph nodes.

Involvement of the lymphatic tissue is much greater in South American blastomycosis than in the North American disease. Mucous membrane lesions are similar to those seen in North American blastomycosis, espundia, granuloma inguinale and some cases of histoplasmosis.

Whether as a primary involvement or later dissemination, pulmonary invasion is demonstrable in more than 80 per cent of autopsied cases of South American blastomycosis. Roentgenographic features are nonspecific and differ from those of tuberculosis only in that supposedly "reinfection" disease is more frequent and predominant in the lower lobes. Isolated or multiple granulomas may be seen as in histoplasmosis, cryptococcosis, North American blastomycosis and other pulmonary granulomatous diseases.

There is a recognized association of South American blastomycosis with tuberculosis (12 per cent), lymphoma and leishmaniasis; however, this relationship with tuberculosis and neoplasia is

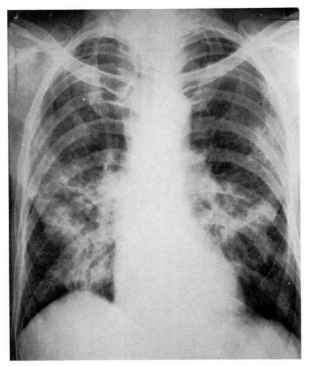

Figure 11. South American blastomycosis. The bronchopneumonic infiltration and distribution of the disease in the lungs are typical for disseminated South American blastomycosis. The characteristics of primary pulmonary complexes are not yet established. (Courtesy of Prof. Carlos de Silva Lacaz, Faculdade de Medicina da Universidade de São Paulo.)

no different from that observed for other yeastlike mycoses.

Of 1506 cases tabulated by Lacaz, less than 2 per cent occurred in children of ten years of age or younger, and less than 13 per cent were under 21 years. The patient whose x-ray film is shown in Figure 11 was an adult, but the pulmonary changes are representative of progressive disease in children.

Laboratory Diagnosis

Diagnosis of South American blastomycosis is made regularly on the basis of careful study of hydroxide-cleared mounts of material obtained from granulomatous lesions of the skin or mucous membranes, from sputum or from involved lymph nodes. Recognition of typical budding forms is sufficient for clinical diagnosis. Cultural characteristics at 37°C. and the morphology of the organisms present in the exudate when stained by the periodic acid–Schiff method are more useful for confirmation than is information gained from cultures at 27°C.

Filtrates from broth cultures, standardized by Del Negro, yield a paracoccidioidin for skin testing that is comparable in usefulness to commercial histoplasmin. Intradermal reactivity is absent during early infection and in severely disseminated disease, similar to reactivity to coccidioidin in coccidioidomycosis. Cutaneous reactivity is useful for screening, with the usual reservations about negative test results. Cross reactions occur with histoplasmin and blastomycin.

Both complement-fixation and precipitin tests have been used in the study of paracoccidioidal infections. A review of Fava Netto's (1955) serial studies with a polysaccharide antigen derived from the yeast cells suggests that there is a close parallelism between the serologic fluctuations in coccidioidomycosis and paracoccidioidal infection.

The fluorescent antibody method has been used for the diagnosis of South American blastomycosis. Rabbit antisera absorbed by the method of Silva and Kaplan (1965) appear to be specific for the yeast form of *P. brasiliensis*. Agar diffusion-precipitin reactions are of great value in special laboratories.

Epidemiology

South American blastomycosis is present in Mexico, Central and South America, and Africa (Ghana). *P. brasiliensis* has been isolated from soil in northern Brazil.

The most intensive epidemiologic studies have been in the state of São Paulo, Brazil, a highly endemic region. The disease was distinctly rural until recent years, when it became increasingly frequent in suburban and urban areas, especially in immigrant Japanese, who apparently have great susceptibility to infection by this fungus.

Clinical infection is recognized most frequently during middle life, age distribution being similar to that for North American blastomycosis. Since *P. brasiliensis* is a soil inhabitant, it is anticipated that many pediatric infections will be recognized when minor pulmonary infections are intensively studied in endemic areas and skin testing programs are introduced into the school systems.

Pathogenesis and Pathology

The gross characteristics of the ulcerogranulomatous mucosal and gingival lesions of South American blastomycosis are not distinguishable from those of the North American disease. Suppuration and drainage from the regional lymph nodes are regularly present in South American blastomycosis; lymph nodes are infrequently enlarged in North American blastomycosis. The lymphatic system is more frequently invaded by *P. brasiliensis*, whatever the site of the lesion. Cutaneous lesions are frequent, are ulcerogranulomatous or papular, and resemble those produced by *B. dermatitidis* except that central healing is not a prominent feature.

Pulmonary lesions, whether primary or secondary, are not distinctive under gross examination. The classifications that have been proposed on the basis of gross and microscopic changes are neither helpful in understanding pathogenesis nor useful in differential diagnosis. The pathologic spectrum is like that of North American blastomycosis and tuberculosis.

Under microscopic examination, *P. brasiliensis* may provoke a tissue reaction which is predominantly that of acute, chronic or mixed granulation. The pyogenic reaction is not uncommon in extensive pulmonary disease, but plasma cells are frequent, and there is little difficulty in finding large elements of chronic epithelioid granulation with multinucleate giant cells. Yeastlike cells are visible in most cases after routine hematoxylin and eosin staining, but morphology is demonstrated with greater precision by periodic acid–Schiff and methenamine-silver methods. Although the production of multiple, narrow-necked buds from the periphery of the mother cell is "characteristic" of this fungus, it may require prolonged search of several specially stained sections before they can be found.

Treatment

Clinically active infections have been treated with sulfonamides since 1940. Some patients have been cured, and many more have had prolonged suppression of the disease. Unfortunately, the development of resistance to sulfonamides is frequent.

Amphotericin B is of demonstrated value in the treatment of this disease. It has succeeded in many patients resistant to sulfonamides. Sampãio (1960), who has the largest reported experience, has had excellent results. The recommendations given in the section on treatment with amphotericin B should be followed.

Recent experience suggests that treatment with trimethoprim-sulfamethoxazole is superior to sulfonamides alone, and is perhaps as good as with amphotericin B.

COCCIDIOIDOMYCOSIS

The Organism

Coccidioides immitis is a dimorphic fungus whose free-living form inhabits soils of the Lower Sonoran Life Zone. Mycelial growth gives rise to arthrospores, which are easily dislodged and air-borne. These arthrospores are the infective units that are inhaled by humans or animals.

When arthrospores encounter a suitable tissue environment, they round up to become relatively small yeastlike spherules (sporangia); these spherules grow to a diameter between 20 and 80 microns before the protoplasm condenses peripherally and undergoes multiple cleavage (endosporulation) to produce many uninucleate endospores (sporangiospores). Growth of the endospores is followed by rupture of the sporangium, liberating the endospores, which perpetuate the cycle by differentiating into sporangia. This process is illustrated in Figure 12. Thus, both the endospore and the arthrospore differentiate similarly in susceptible tissue.

Unlike other dimorphic fungi, Coccidioides grows in the form of a mold at 37°C. on ordinary media. Some spherules may be formed rarely, but the mycelial growth predominates except for selected strains that are grown in special media. Mycelial growth is most characteristic at room temperature. Early development is characterized by an adherent, membranous growth like *B. dermatitidis* at a similar stage. Aerial hyphae usually appear, and are white at first. Colonies may remain white, become light to dark gray, or occasionally produce yellow to brown pigment. Fully virulent strains from untreated patients grow luxuriantly as a rule, and produce abun-

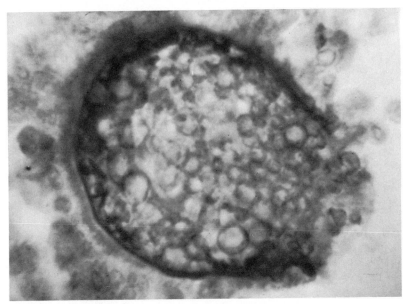

Figure 12. Mature sporangium of *Coccidioides immitis*. Multiple cleavage of the protoplasm has given rise to many sporangiospores, some of which can be seen leaving the ruptured sporangium. This is a diagnostic tissue form. Periodic acid–Schiff stain.

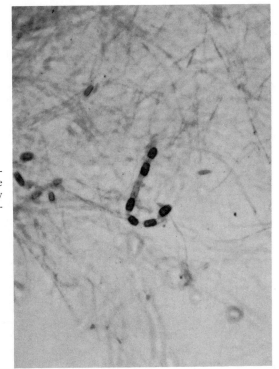

Figure 13. Arthrospores of *C. immitis*. Developing in the free-living mycelium, these ovoid spores are easily air-borne and are highly infectious. Note the empty areas of hypha adjacent to the arthrospores.

dant, loose aerial hyphae which contain arthrospores. The arthrospores are ellipsoidal or rectangular, and are usually from 4 to 6 microns in length. The arthrospores are characteristically separated one from the other by a variable length of clear, empty hypha. An arthrospore-bearing hypha is shown in Figure 13.

The Clinical Disease

In endemic areas of high prevalence, most children will acquire primary infection soon after their play activities bring them in contact with contaminated soils or dusts. Less than half have a recognized or remembered illness that might conceivably have been coccidioidomycosis. In this respect, and in most others, there is a close similarity between coccidioidomycosis, histoplasmosis and tuberculosis. Asymptomatic primary infection can be detected only by serial cutaneous and serologic testing, even though some may show a primary pulmonary complex in later roentgenograms and a very few will experience future activity of the disease.

Primary symptomatic infection may masquerade as a simple respiratory infection, the "flu" or "atypical pneumonia," or be severe. In general, there is a parallelism between the severity of the exposure, the duration of the incubation period and the height of the fever. High fever and an incubation period shorter than ten days are associated with heavy infection. The usual incubation period is from ten to 28 days. Constitutional manifestations are those common to any systemic infection. Anorexia and fatigability may persist for days or weeks even if fever has been of low grade and brief duration.

Localizing symptoms may be absent, but pleuritic or other chest pain is common, and more than half the patients have a nonproductive cough. Sputum production, with or without blood-streaking, is uncommon in children with this type of illness.

Erythema nodosum and erythema multiforme occur more frequently than in either histoplasmosis or tuberculosis, but in probably no more than 20 per cent of the symptomatic cases. Arthralgia and arthritis accompany erythema nodosum or erythema multiforme in some patients. If there is an acute febrile stage, a morbilliform exanthem may be present.

Eosinophilia is common among those exhibiting a rash or joint symptoms and is usually associated with some degree of leukocytosis. An elevated erythrocyte sedimentation rate is the most common nonspecific laboratory finding among those with symptomatic primary infection.

Although symptomatic primary disease may be either mild and transient or severe and prolonged over a number of weeks, only about 5 per cent go on to develop chronic pulmonary coccidioidomycosis. Extrapulmonary dissemination occurs in approximately 0.5 per cent of those infected, usually during the acute stage or during postprimary progression. Dissemination and chronic cavitary disease are less common in children than in adults.

Chronic pulmonary coccidioidomycosis usually manifests itself as a continuation of the symptomatic primary phase. Hemoptysis or blood-streaking of the sputum is more frequent in this type of disease and may be severe. This type of infection is best characterized by the radiologic picture.

The roentgenographic evidence of primary infection may be evanescent and invisible at the time a chest roentgenogram is taken. The primary lesion is usually similar to that of tuberculosis, North American blastomycosis and some cases of cryptococcosis. Segmental and subsegmental pneumonia are frequent. Bronchial or hilar lymph nodes are enlarged, but may be obscured by the infiltrative density, which is frequently in the form of a perihilar wedge. Extensive lesions may develop small areas of cavitation, but most primary lesions resolve completely over a period of several months. The central component of primary infections may extend to the mediastinal lymph nodes or the pericardium. The peripheral component may produce pleural thickening or frank effusion. A mycologically positive pleural fluid should prompt careful, serial serologic studies, since it is frequently part of or forerunner to dissemination.

The primary pulmonary infiltration may fail to resolve completely and may spread. During this sequence of events cavitation is frequent, and the pulmonary coccidioidomycosis becomes chronic. Cavities may persist after clearing of pneumonitis, presenting as the classic cavity without surrounding infiltration, such as is shown in Figure 14. These cavities may remain for years, may close if not too large, or may become filled with inspissated material. Occasionally, such cavities may rupture into the pleural space, producing an empyema. If a secondary intrapulmonary spread occurs, the secondary infiltrates may clear completely, remain as fibrotic infiltrates or become nodular.

Globular peripheral infiltrates, filled cavities and nodular secondary infiltrations may become radiologically dense and constitute "coccidioidomas," which are analogous to other fungal and tuberculous granulomas. Calcium may be deposited in the caseous areas of the granuloma. It may, like a tuberculoma, suddenly liquefy centrally, discharge its content into the bronchus, and become a cavity with or without secondary transbronchial spread.

Some patients with cavitary pulmonary coccidioidomycosis and a stable complement-fixation level remain asymptomatic until surgical resection of the cavitary lung is undertaken. Thereafter, new areas of infiltration and cavity formation may develop.

Laboratory Diagnosis

Hydroxide-cleared mounts of sputum or pus are usually diagnostic if many spherules are present. Endo-

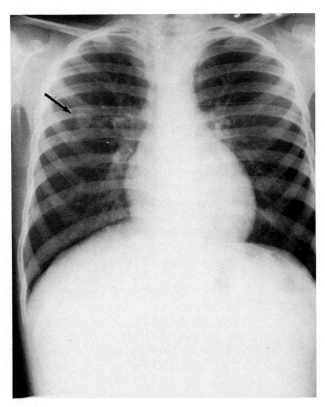

Figure 14. Cavitary pulmonary coccidioidomycosis in a six-year-old asymptomatic boy whose coccidioidin skin test result was positive. Although the right superior hilus is abnormal, there is little infiltration adjacent to the moderately thick-walled cavity in the third anterior intercostal space. Precipitins were absent, and the complement-fixation reaction was 4 + at 1:2 dilution. (Courtesy of Misha Newman, Kern County General Hospital.)

sporulating sporangia should be identified with certainty, since large yeast forms of Blastomyces may simulate Coccidioides in wet preparations. If in doubt, smears fixed in alcoholic formalin and stained by the periodic acid–Schiff method are frequently conclusive.

Cultures at 27°C. and 37°C. should be made according to the suggestions given in the section on general methods of microbiologic diagnosis, but those made at 27°C. are likely to be more characteristic. If typical sporangia have been observed in fresh clinical materials, the mycelial characteristics will be sufficient for diagnosis. Confirmation by inoculating mice, guinea pigs or hamsters intraperitoneally or intratesticularly with suspensions of the mycelial growth is helpful. Typical tissue forms of Coccidioides can be recovered from inoculated animals within two or three weeks.

Whether because of the immunologic characteristics of infection with *C. immitis* or the careful and inspired work of C. E. Smith and his colleagues (1956), no other fungous disease is as well understood serologically as coccidioidomycosis. Diagnosis by serologic methods is accurate when serial specimens can be titrated, beginning early after the onset of illness. Furthermore, the course and prognosis of clinical disease and the effects of treatment are reflected, as a rule, in serologic changes.

Primary, truly asymptomatic disease is characterized by the conversion of dermal reactivity to coccidioidin from negative to positive. Precipitins and complement-fixing antibodies in low titer (1:2, 1:4) are found in less than 10 per cent of the recognized asymptomatic infections. Some asymptomatic patients will show evidence of active disease or even dissemination at a later date.

Primary, nondisseminating, symptomatic disease is characterized by the appearance of a dermal reaction to coccidioidin (90 per cent within two weeks), precipitins and latex particle agglutinins against the same antigen. Precipitins are present in 90 per cent of the patients with this form of the disease by the fourth week and have disappeared in 60 per cent by the eighth week. Precipitins are found in no more than 5 per cent of these patients by the twenty-fourth week. Complement-fixing antibodies do not appear in many patients with nondisseminating primary disease, but can be demonstrated in approximately 50 per cent by the fourth week and in about 80 per cent between the eighth and twenty-fourth weeks. These antibodies appear later and persist longer in contrast to precipitins. The titer of complement-fixing antibodies is almost always below 1:32.

The presence of complement-fixing antibodies in a titer of 1:32 or above, and more particularly a serial rise in titers to and beyond this level, is evidence of dissemination and a guarded prognosis. Titers of 1:32 or higher, which stabilize for months or years (do not vary by more than one dilution when the test is done in the same laboratory and paired with the previously tested serum specimen), may be found in chronic disseminated disease that can ultimately heal or undergo progressive dissemination to death. Periods of renewed dissemination may be accompanied by the reappearance of precipitins. Both acutely and chronically progressive dissemination are usually associated with a negative skin reaction to coccidioidin. Nevertheless, many patients with chronic cavitary pulmonary disease may lose their dermal reactivity to 1:100 coccidioidin, and some of these maintain their low titer of complement-fixing antibodies.

Serologic cross reactions do occur to some extent between coccidioidomycosis, histoplasmosis and blastomycosis. Sera from patients with coccidioidomycosis rarely give reactions to a significant titer with other fungal antigens, however, and when this does occur, the titer will be higher with coccidioidin if the test is performed correctly.

Spherulin is now available for skin testing and tube precipitin reactions. It has definite advantages in sensitivity and specificity over coccidioidin.

Epidemiology

Coccidioidomycosis affects all ages and races, but is milder in children than in adults, and more severe in dark-skinned races. It is endemic in portions of southwest Texas, New Mexico, Arizona, small areas of Utah and Nevada, southern California, and parts of Mexico, Guatemala, Honduras, Argentina, Venezuela and Paraguay. Its distribution is limited, apparently, by the features of the Lower Sonoran Life Zone. It is a mistake to think that the environment provided by this zone is associated with widespread culturability of C. immitis from the soils.

Although C. immitis produces disease in desert rodents and can be isolated from the soil of their burrows, the factors that permit vegetative growth of the fungus in soil and widespread infection are incompletely known. Contrary to popular belief, infected soils are hard to demonstrate and seem to be much more sharply limited than the areas of high prevalence of disease. Furthermore, it has been established that there is a distinct seasonal variation in the cultural recoverability of C. immitis in soils. Culturability may be relatively high shortly after the rainy season and the appearance of warm weather and very low or absent at other times.

Coccidioidomycosis is a disease naturally acquired by the inhalation of arthrospores. It has been stated frequently that contagion does not occur, but this opinion is not biologically sound, although its statistical validity was unquestioned until recently. Arthrospores have been found in many lesions, but especially in chronic pulmonary cavities. Patients with this sort of cavity may have arthrospores in their sputum. Biologically, the possibility of infection from dried sputum of this type must be admitted. Infection of personnel caring for a patient with a plaster cast over coccidioidal involvement of an extremity has been thoroughly documented. A third item of evidence in favor of the possible contagiousness of coccidioidomycosis is the observation of the transmission of disease from an infected female rhesus monkey to its nursing offspring. One should conclude that arthrospores are capable of producing infection wherever they may be found.

Pathogenesis and Pathology

In the experimental animal, inhaled arthrospores of C. immitis provoke little immediate tissue response. The development of tissue hypersensitivity is manifested by an acute exudative reaction characterized by infiltration of neutrophils, outpouring of fibrinous fluid about the fungus cells, and a variable degree of simple necrosis. This localized lesion may be resorbed completely or partially fibrosed as immunity develops under favorable host-parasite relations.

If the infection is not quickly contained, the cycle of spherule development and release of endospores provokes a histologic picture that is dependent in large part upon host factors of immunity and hypersensitivity. If complete resolution of the initial infection does not take place early, chronic granulation tissue is produced, particularly about the sporangia. Histiocytic proliferation, epithelioid cells, Langhans' giant cells and caseation necrosis may characterize subacute and chronic pneumonitis as well as coccidioidomas.

Pneumonic lesions are likely to have areas of acute granulomatous reaction about liberated endospores interspersed with the chronic reaction. Coccidioidomas are more adynamic, and show predominantly a hyalinized fibrotic "capsule" with or without calcium deposition surrounding an area of caseation necrosis. Langhans' giant cells occur frequently subjacent to the "capsule," and it is in this region that sporangia in various degrees of degradation are likely to be seen.

The cavitary lesions vary histologically according to their age and the activity of adjacent disease. Chronic cavities are similar to those produced by tuberculosis, including associated bronchiectasis and a pseudomembranous lining of some cavities. Many have a densely fibrotic thin wall surrounded by a few to many caseous nodules.

Lymph node involvement is part of the primary infection. In this respect and in subsequent pathogenetic potentialities, the role of intrathoracic lymph node disease in coccidioidomycosis is the same as in tuberculosis. In progressive, fatal coccidioidomycosis the peribronchial and mediastinal lymph nodes may become greatly enlarged and undergo complete suppuration.

As indicated in the discussion of clinical symptoms, pleurisy is frequent during the primary infection. This may produce the characteristic signs of fibrinous pleuritis over the area of primary pulmonary involvement. In more severe primary infection, and in progressive pulmonary disease with or without cavitary rupture into the pleural space, a granulomatous pleuritis, sometimes associated with actual empyema, is present.

Active coccidioidomycosis presents no diagnostic problem histologically as a rule. Spherules with endospores can be seen by routine hematoxylin and eosin staining. In subacute and chronic pneumonic lesions and in coccidioidomas, the diagnosis may be more difficult to establish unless special stains are utilized. Periodic acid–Schiff or methenamine-silver stains of almost all lesions will give sufficient morphologic detail to be diagnostic. In both chronic cavitary lesions and coccidioidomas, hyphal elements of *C. immitis* may be seen.

Culture from active lesions should always be positive if properly done. Growth may be slow and abnormal from some lesions in patients who have been treated with amphotericin B.

Treatment and Prevention

Restriction of activity and increased bed rest are indicated for symptomatic primary and progressive primary infection, especially if complement-fixing antibodies are present and increasing in titer. Activity should be restricted until chest roentgenograms and serologic studies indicate that the infection is regressing or until it is evident that antimicrobial treatment is desirable. Restriction of activity is not indicated for asymptomatic primary and chronic disease.

The indications for therapy with amphotericin B have not been defined to the point of general acceptance. Under the circumstances, one must give great weight to the opinions and recommendations of those with experience in all manifestations of the disease.

Amphotericin B should be administered (1) to patients showing extension or exacerbation of chronic pulmonary disease, (2) to patients showing impending or actual dissemination, and (3) as coverage before and after any surgical procedure for the disease.

Clinical signs and symptoms are important in deciding when and whom to treat, but the inexperienced therapist may prefer to rely primarily on the results of serial serologic studies. These tests should be done every three or four weeks during symptomatic primary infections until a definite decline in titer is demonstrated. The titer of precipitins has not been accorded any prognostic significance, but persistence or reappearance of precipitins has a serious connotation.

In either threatened or substantiated dissemination, Winn (1962) believed that the maximum individual amphotericin B dosage of 1 to 1.5 mg. per kilogram should be given, but the duration of treatment may be tailored to the serologic and clinical responses.

Extrapulmonary coccidioidomycosis is not a concern of this chapter, but in disseminating disease, extrapulmonary considerations may determine whether or not treatment is to be given. In the presence of continued activity of pulmonary disease, one may not know whether a rising complement-fixation titer is due to intrapulmonary or extrapulmonary dissemination or both. In such circumstances, treatment would be favored.

The toxicity of amphotericin B must be weighed against the seriousness of disseminated coccidioidomycosis and the relatively poor results of treatment with amphotericin in widespread or meningeal dissemination. It seems reasonable to administer amphotericin intravenously to all infants and children with severe symptomatic primary or progressive primary disease, regardless of the serologic findings at the moment, and to all pediatric patients with active pulmonary disease and a complement-fixation titer in excess of 1:32, regardless of symptoms. There is some evidence to suggest that although the maximum tolerated individual dose should be administered, the duration of therapy necessary for suppression of acute but nondisseminated disease may be relatively short. The early administration of the antibiotic may be sufficient to permit the host to contain a potentially dangerous infection without resort to a larger or maximal dose that might produce toxic effects, a risk warranted only if the disease should progress. All severely symptomatic primary infections in members of dark-skinned races or those with metabolic diseases that are known to be associated with instability of infectious diseases should also be treated.

Progressive or disseminated coccidioidomycosis is such a serious disease and amphotericin B therapy is so marginal that means of altering or supplementing basic therapy continue to be sought. Recent literature should be consulted. Transfer factor may be of some value in patients who lack immunologic responsiveness to antigen, but it must be carefully selected and given repeatedly.

There is evidence from experimental infections (mice) that combining mino-cycline or another tetracycline with amphotericin B will increase the therapeutic index. There is evidence that some drugs in the imidazole series (e.g., miconazole, clotrimazole) may be useful in the treatment of coccidioidomycosis, but these agents are for investigationtal use only. Miconazole can be given directly into the spinal fluid as well as intravenously.

The use of amphotericin B has not eliminated the necessity for surgery in selected patients. Progressive cavitary coccidioidomycosis may fail to stabilize after treatment with amphotericin B, but may regress satisfactorily when surgical measures are combined with antibiotic therapy.

Surgical intervention is definitely indicated if a coccidioidal cavity ruptures into the pleural space or if hemoptysis is severe and persistent. Hemoptysis is rarely fatal, and it is probably wise to delay as long as possible unless the cavity is already of the chronic type. Resection of a chronic cavity is less likely to be complicated than resection of progressive primary cavities.

Chronic cavitation and fibrocavitary disease may constitute an indication for surgery, but considerable disagreement exists among physicians writing of their experiences with these problems. Postoperative exacerbation with or without the appearance of new cavities is sufficiently frequent in some series to lead to the recommendations that (1) operation should be preceded and followed by about one month of treatment with amphotericin B, and (2) thoracoplasty should accompany resection in many cases. There is evidence that thoracoplasty is helpful in preventing postoperative appearance of cavities that either were not present previously or were unrecognized. Thoracoplasty is particularly undesirable in the pediatric age group, and operation should be postponed until after full skeletal growth has been achieved, if possible.

To date, prevention of coccidioidomycosis has been directed toward modifying environmental factors associated with growth and dissemination of the fungus in soils. The application of oils to the surface of infected and agriculturally unworked soils as well as the establishment of grass coverage may be useful in relation to military encampments and village areas. These methods cannot be used to diminish infection among agricultural workers and their children, and these families remain one of the most important sources of new cases.

Experimental work in monkeys and dogs has shown that subcutaneous injection of as few as ten living arthrospores of *C. immitis* will give immunity to subsequent respiratory challenge and will not produce progressive or disseminated disease. A much greater number of arthrospores has been used to immunize dogs which were given amphotericin B orally for 21 days after injection of the spores. These dogs became immune while exhibiting no reactions to the vaccine, whereas those animals not receiving amphotericin had significant local and regional reactions, but no dissemination. Since attempts to immunize with nonliving preparations and vaccines have not been fully successful, trials with a living attenuated vaccine among children in highly endemic areas would appear to be very much in order.

PULMONARY CRYPTOCOCCOSIS

The Organism

Cryptococcus neoformans, as seen in direct examination of sputum or spinal fluid, is a spherical or oval yeast whose total diameter (including the capsule) is usually between 4 and 10 microns. Smaller forms are seen occasionally, and heavily encapsulated strains may reach a diameter of 20 microns. If the organisms are numerous, budding can be seen in most preparations, but is better studied in India ink or saline mounts from cultures. Budding may be single or multiple from any point on

the cell wall. The daughter cell is attached, before separation, by a thin cell wall arising from a small pore in the mother cell wall. Young buds are included within the mother polysaccharide capsule when it is present. During direct examination, the mucoid capsules are seen best in India ink mounts. They appear as transparent halos of variable thickness external to the cell wall. In India ink preparations, cryptococci are cleanly separated from the suspension of India ink, whereas exudative cells that may appear to have large "capsules" are encrusted with adherent ink particles around the "cell membrane." Some strains of cryptococci are unencapsulated or have capsules so thin that they cannot be recognized in direct mounts.

Cryptococci grow well on a variety of solid media commonly used in the laboratory. Brain-heart infusion agar, brain-heart infusion rabbit blood agar and Sabouraud's dextrose agar (at pH 7.0) are suitable and generally available. Only *C. neoformans* grows well at 37°C., but other species may show slight growth. Colonial growth usually appears in two to ten days, but occasionally is slower.

The colonies of initial isolation may be either mucoid or pasty. In either case they are white to cream in color and gradually darken to tan or brown. The yeast forms in pasty colonies may not show encapsulation in India ink preparations, although this is usually present after aging of the colony. If capsules cannot be demonstrated after ten days of aging, they almost always appear after subculture. The author has isolated one strain of *C. neoformans* that did not show encapsulation, except by special mucopolysaccharide stains, until after intracerebral inoculation in mice. Mucoid colonies always contain yeast forms with some degree of encapsulation.

The morphology of the cryptococci from cultural isolates is essentially the same as described for direct mounts. A few elongate cells may remain adherent, producing a short pseudomycelium. No true mycelium is formed, and the cells have the same morphology when grown at 25°C. as at 37°C. The perfect state has been found and described. It is a basidiomycete in the genus Leucosporidium *(L. neoformans).*

There are seven recognized species of the genus Cryptococcus, none of which ferments any known carbohydrate with the production of gas. All produce extracellular starch on synthetic dextrose-thiamine medium at pH 4.5. The biochemical properties of the cryptococci are used rarely for clinical laboratory diagnosis.

Within the genus Cryptococcus, only *C. neoformans* grows rapidly when subcultured and incubated at 37°C., and only *C. neoformans* is regularly pathogenic for white Swiss mice. There is considerable strain variation in the pathogenicity of *C. neoformans.* If 0.02 or 0.04 ml. of a saline suspension of the organism is injected intracerebrally into white Swiss mice, encapsulated forms can be recovered from the brain and meninges. Most strains of *C. neoformans*

kill the mice within two weeks. Intraperitoneal injection should not be relied upon for studies of pathogenicity. Central nervous system cryptococcosis is caused rarely by species other than *C. neoformans.*

The Clinical Disease

Patients with proved pulmonary cryptococcosis have fallen more or less distinctly into one of two groups. The first group, composed of those who were completely asymptomatic, could recall no significant febrile illness or pulmonary symptoms within the previous several years. Chest roentgenograms in most revealed one or several nodular lesions similar to that shown in Figure 15. Diagnosis was made after surgical resection. Others in this group were asymptomatic until the onset of central nervous system or cutaneous cryptococcosis. Many of these had negative chest roentgengrams at the time of diagnosis; the primary pulmonary lesion became evident later in the

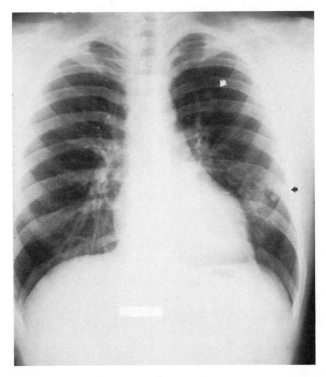

Figure 15. Asymptomatic pulmonary cryptococcosis. This 17-year-old male could recall no febrile illness or chest symptoms. The x-ray film was a routine preoperative film (pilonidal cyst). Segmental resection was followed by active pulmonary and pleural cryptococcosis.

course of illness or was discovered at autopsy.

The second group of patients, smaller in number, presented with a febrile illness accompanied by cough and sputum production. The sputum was variable in amount, mucoid or mucopurulent, and occasionally blood-streaked. Chest pain or discomfort was present in some. The chest roentgenogram in all patients in this group has shown a pneumonic infiltration of some type, often with nodular lesions as shown in Figure 16. Cryptococci were present in sputum or bronchial washings.

In addition to these two groups are patients with sputum or bronchial washings positive for *C. neoformans* or other cryptococci who have no detectable pulmonary or endobronchial disease. This may represent transient colonization, but secretions may remain positive for months.

One feature of the clinical history deserves special emphasis. When they were carefully questioned, most of the patients gave a definite history of more than casual contact with pigeons or their droppings. Such a contact history should provoke an intensive search for cryptococci in all patients with a pulmonary disease that does not follow the expected course during treatment.

Physical examination has given no important information as to the cause of the pulmonary disease unless dissemination has occurred. Acneiform or ulcerogranulomatous lesions may be found on the skin, and the peripheral lymph nodes may be enlarged in some patients with disseminated disease.

Fever, when present, varies from a daily maximum of 100°F. to 103°F.; in patients without other known disease, the fever slowly defervesces over a period of several weeks, often to normal range. The pulmonary infiltration

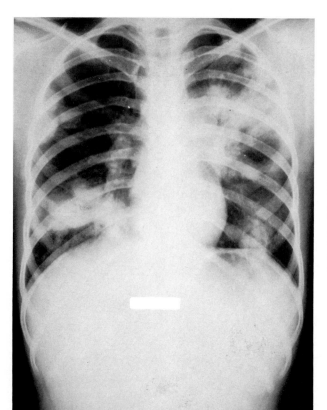

Figure 16. Active symptomatic pulmonary cryptococcosis. This 13-year-old girl experienced a sudden onset of left pleuritic pain followed by fever. The sputum contained unencapsulated and thinly encapsulated cryptococci. Note that despite the areas of confluence, the basic pattern is globular.

may stabilize or actually regress to a significant degree during hospital observation prior to diagnosis.

Although there are no radiographic features that are specific, globular lesions with fuzzy margins are sufficiently common to invite consideration of cryptococcosis. Mass pneumonic lesions tend to be dense centrally and to have irregular, hazy margins. Some globular lesions develop an air-fluid level and resemble a pyogenic lung abscess. Circumscribed nodular lesions with little or no calcification are often seen in asymptomatic patients. When this type of lesion is found in association with active pneumonic disease, postprimary progression has probably occurred.

The lower lobes, right middle lobe, and lingula are the most common sites of primary lesions, which may be either peripheral or central. The subpleural nodule, so important pathologically, may be invisible in ordinary roentgenograms. These lesions have been observed to enlarge to visibility during corticosteroid therapy for other diseases.

Active lesions may provoke sufficient pleurisy to produce roentgenographic signs, but frank effusion is uncommon. When it occurs, other causes should be sought unless cryptococci are found in the fluid.

Laboratory Diagnosis

At present, no skin test antigen is available commercially; in fact, there is no definite evidence at present that detection of cutaneous hypersensitivity is useful as a diagnostic or epidemiologic tool.

The serodiagnosis of cryptococcosis is now available at special laboratories (Center for Disease Control, Atlanta, Georgia) and is of established value. An indirect fluorescent antibody technique, a tube agglutination test for antibody, and a latex agglutination test for antigen are available, are well standardized, and should be utilized as a group. The latex agglutination test can be ap-

plied to spinal fluid when cryptococcal meningitis is suspected. Cross reactions do occur, and serodiagnosis is only presumptive.

Most patients with symptomatic pulmonary cryptococcosis have cryptococci in the sputum or bronchial washings. Unfortunately, children may not cough up sputum even with training, and bronchoscopy is a major procedure in the very young. The saprophytic habitat of cryptococci makes the evaluation of isolates of *C. neoformans* from gastric washings a matter that must be determined by the clinician rather than the laboratorian.

Although the principles for collection and study of materials for laboratory diagnosis have been discussed in the section on general methods of microbiologic diagnosis (p. 880), there are some special considerations that apply specifically to cryptococcosis. Direct examination is best accomplished with the aid of India ink. If the suspension of India ink breaks down rapidly into clumps, a second preparation with a drop of weak detergent solution (e.g., Dreft) added to the sputum before mixing with India ink may give a more stable preparation. Wet mounts should be studied promptly to prevent drying and the creation of artifacts. The detection of encapsulated yeast forms is only presumptive evidence of cryptococcosis.

Final diagnosis depends upon the isolation and identification of *Cryptococcus neoformans*. Since sputum and bronchial washings may contain rapidly growing bacteria which obscure or prevent the colonial growth of cryptococci, it is advantageous to use culture media containing antibiotics. Any of the media that have been suggested previously may be used, but cycloheximide should not be incorporated in the medium, since it is a cryptococcostatic agent.

Animal inoculation is occasionally superior to cultural methods for isolation of *C. neoformans*. The intracerebral route should be used in white Swiss mice. Direct intracerebral inoculations of bacteria-free fluids (e.g., spinal fluid) may give a diagnosis when cultures are sterile.

Lung biopsies, lymph nodes or other tissue specimens should be handled as suggested in the section on general methods of microbiologic diagnosis.

There are two staining methods that are of great help in the diagnosis of cryptococcosis. Although the mucicarmine method is simple and almost specific, a preferable method entails the use of a colloidal iron–periodic acid–Schiff stain such as that suggested by Mowry (1963) for material containing only forms with questionable capsules. These methods are applicable to formalin-fixed smears of sputum or other exudate. In our laboratory, these stains have been used on sputum smears when the specimen contained so many gram-negative bacteria and saprophytic fungi that there was uncertainty of achieving cultural isolation of the suspected cryptococcus. This difficulty is common in patients who have received several antibiotics for a number of days before a fungous infection is suspected.

The organisms shown in Figure 17 were proved to be *C. neoformans*, but no capsules could be seen in hydroxide or India ink mounts. Repeated subculturing of suspected isolates and simple aging of the primary isolate will usually yield many forms with definite encapsulation.

There are two genera of asporogenous yeasts, closely related to the cryptococci, that may be found in sputum and may cause diagnostic confusion initially. *Torulopsis glabrata* may be found in sputum and can be pathogenic for humans. Unlike the cryptococci, *T. glabrata* is an active fermenter of some carbohydrates. It produces gaseous fermentation of glucose and trehalose, but does not assimilate maltose, sucrose or cellobiose. It grows well on ordinary media, producing smooth colonies composed of spherical or ovoid cells. Rhodotorula may also be isolated from sputum. The cells are round to elongate, may produce pseudomycelium, and do not ferment carbohydrates. Pink, red or yellow pigmentation of the colony easily distinguishes it from the

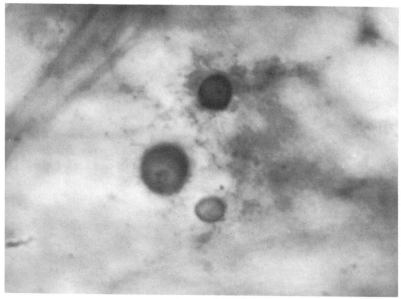

Figure 17.   Cryptococci in sputum. Periodic acid–Schiff–colloidal iron stain of sputum produced by the patient in Figure 16. The narrow, dark-staining margins of the three organisms shown took the colloidal iron and probably represent a thin layer of capsular mucopolysaccharide, which could not be seen in India ink preparations. Cultures were positive for pasty colonies. Oil-immersion magnification.

cryptococci. At least one species of Rhodotorula (mucilaginosa) has been reported to produce disseminated disease in an infant.

Epidemiology

Although the recognized incidence of cryptococcosis may vary considerably from place to place, it is worldwide in distribution. *Cryptococcus neoformans* exists as a saprophyte in nature, and has been isolated from a variety of sources, including peach juice, normal skin, human gastrointestinal tract, and the milk of cows suffering from cryptococcal mastitis. It is now known that the most important epidemiologic factor is the presence of *C. neoformans* in the excreta of pigeons and starlings, in pigeon nests, and in soils that have been contaminated with the excreta.

Animal experimentation and the contact history of patients with acute pulmonary cryptococcosis point to the respiratory tract as the most important portal of entry. Systemic cryptococcosis may be produced in marmosets by feeding large numbers of cryptococci, and it is not unreasonable to suppose that cases of cryptococcosis in association with malignant disease or the administration of immunosuppressives or corticosteroids arise from an endogenous source.

Because of the lack of a reliable antigen for skin testing, there have been no epidemiologic studies of population groups. Nevertheless, the increasing frequency of recognition of pulmonary cryptococcosis, the knowledge that pulmonary disease may be present without producing a density in the chest roentgenogram, the presence of morphologically typical but nonviable organisms in some pulmonary lesions, and the frequency with which air-borne exposure must occur in certain areas all suggest that cryptococcosis is much more common and benign than is generally thought.

Pathogenesis and Pathology

Little is known about host-parasite relations in human cryptococcosis. When factors influencing immunization and subsequent challenge were rigidly controlled, Abrahams and Gilleran (1960) were able to demonstrate a significant degree of acquired immunity in mice immunized with formalin-killed vaccine. Both specific and nonspecific immunity may be important in determining the establishment of infection after exposure to *C. neoformans*. The idea that "normal" people do not acquire cryptococcosis is inconsistent with observed data.

So far as is known, there is no systematic study of the histopathologic features and pathogenesis of experimental pulmonary cryptococcosis in anthropoids. Several different types of lesion are seen in resected and necropsied human lungs. Factors in host and parasite can be correlated with the morphologic expresson of infection only by uncertain inference.

The smallest, presumably primary, lesion observed by the author was immediately subpleural in the costophrenic sinus, was 3 mm. in diameter, and had a thin rim of calcium with a semiliquid center containing a few organisms morphologically typical of cryptococci when stained by a modification of the Rhinehart and Abul-Haj method for acid mucopolysaccharides. It was associated with pneumonic cryptococcosis extending outward from the hilus of the same lung in a girl being treated with corticosteroids for rheumatic carditis. No other calcific lesion has been seen.

Figure 18 shows a nodule, presumably early and active. Such nodules have no trace of encapsulation, very little fibrosis, and a central mucoid appearance. Under microscopic examination, the central portion of the nodule contained innumerable cryptococci of 2 to 6 microns in diameter with thin capsules. Most of the organisms were apparently free within relatively normal alveolar spaces, but some were within the cytoplasm of greatly distended and distorted histiocytes. No other inflammatory cells were present. Near the periphery of the nodule, single and clustered organisms were present, free or

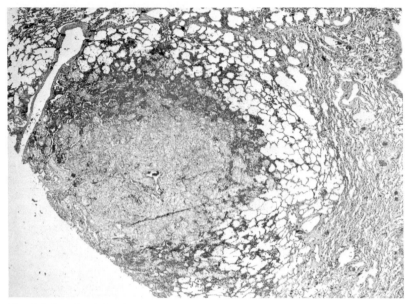

Figure 18. Subpleural nodule of cryptococcosis. This small nodule was rich in thinly encapsulated cryptococci. Heavily encapsulated forms were present at the periphery of the nodule. The pleural surface is at the right-hand margin.

in histiocytes, and had definite and often heavy encapsulation, as shown in Figure 19.

Active disseminating pulmonary lesions, nodular or pneumonic, are likely to resemble the subpleural nodule shown in Figure 18. "Coin" and mass lesions, more or less stable by roentgenographic criteria, are, in the author's experience, associated with a rubbery, neoplastic gross appearance and a relatively dense fibrotic reaction microscopically. Judging from the microscopic appearance of the cryptococci in dense-

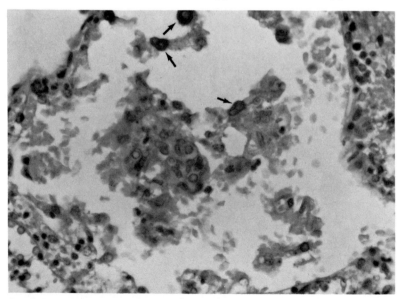

Figure 19. Cryptococci in a pulmonary nodule. The arrows point to heavily encapsulated organisms, two of which are budding. Thinly encapsulated forms are seen intracellularly in the center of the field. Mucicarmine stain.

ly fibrotic lesions and the results of a few cultural studies, it may well be that the fibrotic lesion is a manifestation of successful host response to infection.

Large pneumonic lesions may show areas of actively dividing, thinly encapsulated and relatively small cryptococci that are interspersed with larger areas of predominant fibrosis. Haugen and Baker (1954) were unable to determine any histologic criteria that they could correlate with the presence or absence of dissemination, but of nine patients with either small or "larger" subpleural nodules, only two had extrapulmonary cryptococcosis.

Multiple, small lesions containing giant cells, lymphocytes, central necrosis and many thinly encapsulated organisms may be found in acutely disseminated pulmonary cryptococcosis and in patients with presumably opportunistic infections associated with diffuse neoplasia, or its treatment. Both these lesions and the densely fibrotic lesions may escape proper recognition unless mucicarmine or, even better, Mowry acid mucopolysaccharide staining is done.

Treatment

There is significant disagreement among clinical mycologists as to the indications for treatment of pulmonary cryptococcosis. Disagreement is based primarily upon two considerations: (1) no one knows how many people with primary pulmonary cryptococcosis will get completely well spontaneously, but it is evident that some will; and (2) the toxicity of available therapeutic agents is estimated differently by those experienced in therapy. The situation is similar to that in pulmonary tuberculosis except that we have no antifungal agent as benign as isoniazid. The physician has few guidelines. I have found amphotericin B in the doses that I use to be acceptably nephrotoxic for use whenever pulmonary *disease* is associated with a positive culture for *C. neoformans*. Flucytosine, to date, appears to be of much lesser toxicity, and

is to be preferred in the treatment of pulmonary cryptococcosis when used appropriately for infections that are susceptible to this agent.

If the diagnosis has been established by lung biopsy, and cultures are negative, the patient is observed rather than treated. If cultures have not been made at biopsy, decision is based upon the morphologic appearance of the lesion and the cryptococci unless pleural or parenchymal complications appear in the early postoperative period. All patients with a cultural or histopathologic diagnosis of pulmonary cryptococcosis should have a spinal fluid examination. Asymptomatic involvement of the central nervous system may be present, and if so, the recommendations for treatment would require modification.

For uncomplicated pulmonary cryptococcosis in a patient who appears to be metabolically and immunologically normal, two to three months of treatment with amphotericin at an individual dosage level not exceeding 0.6 mg. per kilogram of body weight is probably adequate. If there is evidence of central nervous system involvement, treatment should be more intensive and extensive. Treatment with amphotericin B is discussed separately (see p. 925).

Prevention

No specific preventive measures have been developed. Although some degree of immunity can be produced experimentally by vaccines, there has been nothing to suggest that immunization would be a useful preventive measure from the public health point of view. It seems probable that children should not be closely associated with the care and raising of pigeons.

OPPORTUNISTIC FUNGUS INFECTIONS

The designation "opportunistic fungus infection" has been used for those mycotic infections developing in the presence of a major host abnormality that either predisposes to infection by fungi rarely pathogenic in normal humans or makes possible reactivation of a latent or arrested infection.

Opportunistic mycoses are the most common, clinically significant, systemic fungal infections of children. Immunosuppressive and anti-inflammatory agents, aggressive chemotherapy for neoplasms and lymphomas, and prolonged antibiotic treatment for conditions such as cystic fibrosis have made a major problem of what scarcely existed 30 years ago. The diabetic state continues to be fertile ground for fungus infections as well as tuberculosis.

The most important principle for managing the compromised host is vigilance. Pulmonary infiltrates may not be associated with constitutional symptoms or leukocytosis even when they are bacterial in origin. Laboratory study of sputum or nasopharyngeal swabs is often misleading, although direct examination is more reliable than culture. One may not be able to distinguish colonization from infection, and this may include the results of transtracheal aspiration. If immunosuppression is profound, all serologic methods may fail. Many oncologists prefer "flying blind" with shotgun therapy to pulmonary aspiration or biopsy. This approach may be justifiable as an emergency method, but the spectrum of opportunistic infection and the diversity of treatment argue for specific diagnosis. Needle aspiration of the lung or intercostal or transbronchial biopsy seem justified when diagnosis cannot be made by blood or bone marrow culture.

If one elects to "fly blind," there are some statistical findings that can be helpful. In the immunologically incompetent host, Candida, Cryptococcus, and Aspergillus are the most frequent invaders, although it is recognized that any one of hundreds of saprophytes may cause disease. Some strains of Cryptococcus and at least 50 per cent of isolates of Candida are initially resis-

tant to flucytosine. Few isolates of Aspergillus are sensitive to flucytosine or amphotericin B. Nevertheless, the tissue distribution of flucytosine is such that if there is any suspicion of central nervous system or renal parenchymal involvement, the drug should be included in a "fly blind" regimen.

Pneumocystis is believed to be a protozoon. It is an important opportunist in the compromised host and has to be considered in a "fly blind" program for pneumonitis. The best therapy at present seems to be trimethoprim-sulfamethoxazole rather than propamidine.

All of these agents have their own toxicity, and in part they are additive. The "fly blind" regimen must also include antibacterial agents for both difficult gram-negative and gram-positive bacteria. He who elects to "fly blind" as a definitive approach must weigh the hazards of multiple, cumulative toxicities against those of lung aspirate or biopsy. It is doubtful that "fly blind" or culturally guided regimens for prophylaxis are of value against fungi.

ASPERGILLOSIS

The aspergilli are ubiquitous organisms whose spores are widely airborne. They are a common source of contamination in the laboratory, and may be found on all body surfaces and in the sputum. In culture, this genus grows as a mycelium consisting of septate branching hyphae, which give rise to aerial conidiophores terminally enlarged to form a vesicle bearing specialized cells (sterigmata), which give rise to chains of small spores (conidia). Some forms are ascosporic. In solid tissue and pus from closed spaces, only the hyphae are seen, but the observation of dichotomous branching suggests the presence of this genus. Hyphal elements are usually scanty in ordinary sputum. In plugs of bronchial origin, in the content of pulmonary cavities and in cystic spaces within invaded lung, extensive hyphal elements may be seen together with spores and, occasionally, the vesicle with its sterigmata.

A number of species may be responsible for pulmonary infection, including *A. fumigatus*, *A. flavus*, *A. niveus*, *A. niger* and *A. nidulans*. Species identification is not simple, and undeniably pathogenic human isolates should be submitted for classification to a specialist in the field.

Three clinical forms of pulmonary aspergillosis are recognized: the allergic, intracavitary aspergillomatous, and invasive parenchymal varieties. It is not certain whether allergic bronchopulmonary aspergillosis arises as a disease sui generis or is always secondary to asthma or bronchitis of other origin. The consensus is that intracavitary aspergilloma is always superimposed upon some anatomic defect. Invasive parenchymal disease, pulmonary or otherwise, occurs both as an opportunistic infection and as an infection unrelated to discernible predisposition.

Allergic bronchopulmonary aspergillosis is classically characterized by episodes of fever, wheezing, transient and often migratory pulmonary infiltration, and eosinophilia in the peripheral blood or sputum, or both. Aspergilli can usually be demonstrated in the sputum, but the immediate skin reactivity to cutaneous prick tests with mixed Aspergillus antigens is more important diagnostically. The explanation for the transient pulmonary infiltrates is, at present, unknown. No definite relation exists between the allergic form of aspergillosis and invasive parenchymal disease. Precipitins may be present in allergic bronchopulmonary aspergillosis, but are not essential for the diagnosis.

Intracavitary aspergilloma occurs as a complicaton of pulmonary cavitation or infarction due to other diseases in most, perhaps all, cases. It is a real hazard in cystic fibrosis. As such, the organisms represent a purely saprophytic adaptation. Immunologic study indicates that these infections are usually accompanied by the presence of spe-cies-specific precipitins in the patient's blood and a low incidence of immediate reactivity to skin-inoculated antigen. The frequency of hemoptysis and the high incidence of serum precipitins in patients with intracavitary aspergillomas, together with the demonstration of penetration of the cavitary pseudomembrane by aspergillus hyphae, suggest the possibility that this type of infection may be the precursor of dissemination if host factors are suitable.

The *clinical picture* of intracavitary aspergilloma has only two important features: hemoptysis or blood-streaking of the sputum and the roentgenographic findings. Bloody sputum can be expected from bronchiectatic cavities, but its occurrence and recurrence are not always explainable by assuming a purely saprophytic and inert role for the aspergillus. It is possible that the superficial pericavitary vessels are made to bleed by invasion of hyphae or by the secretory products of the fungus in the cavity.

The radiographic recognition of the fungus ball is well established. The relatively uniform density, separated from the wall of the cavity by a crescentic layer of air which shifts with change of position of the patient, is evidence of a "free-ball" within the cavity. Some aspergillomas are not freely movable within the cavity. Other fungi are capable of producing the same roentgenographic appearance. The development of intracavitary fungus balls may not follow a uniform pattern. The development of the aspergilloma is not always from the dependent portion of the cavity as might be expected. At times the ball may arise on the lateral or superior wall of the cavity and become freely movable only when mature.

Pulmonary aspergillosis appearing suddenly in an apparently normal person is so unusual that some authorities would give it the special designation "primary aspergillosis." There are, as yet, no defining parameters for this type of infection. Any apparently normal person who has aspergillosis can be said to have "aspergillosis" or "primary aspergillosis," as one chooses. Figure 20 is illustrative of a pediatric patient with this disease.

Invasive aspergillosis is much more common as an opportunistic infection than as a disease in apparently normal children or adults. The most common host abnormality is leukemia, with Hodgkin's disease second in frequency. Of 20 cases of aspergillosis occurring in a cancer hospital, 30 per cent were in children under the age of ten years. It is of some interest that diabetes was also present in 15 per cent of the group. Invasive aspergillosis may be localized to a single organ, particularly as a terminal invader. Since the aspergilli tend to invade blood vessels, dissemination is frequent if the patient lives long enough.

Laboratory diagnosis may be difficult. The clinical picture, together with cu-taneous hypersensitivity, is the usual means of establishing the diagnosis of allergic aspergillosis. Aspergilli may or may not be isolated from the sputum.

Intracavitary aspergilloma is rarely seen in children without cystic fibrosis. Aspergilli may or may not be recoverable from the sputum or bronchial washings. If the cavity is accessible, culture of needle aspirates will confirm the diagnosis if the aspergilli are viable. Serum precipitins are usually present.

Aspergilli are usually present in the sputum of patients with invasive pulmonary aspergillosis. The frequent isolation of aspergilli from the sputum of patients without aspergillosis is the real source of difficulty. Unless the laboratory is aware of the problem, aspergilli may not even be reported, simply being noted as "contaminants." Whenever possible, it is advisable to isolate

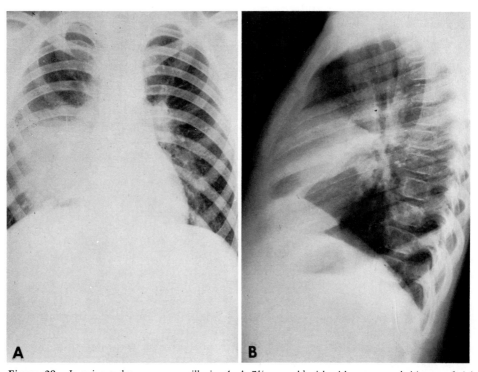

Figure 20. Invasive pulmonary aspergillosis. *A,* A 7½-year-old girl with a two-week history of right chest pain and low-grade fever presented with a small subcutaneous mass just below the nipple at the time the films were taken. The right middle lobe pneumonia was due to *A. fumigatus,* which metastasized to the brain. The child recovered. *B,* The initial pneumonia confined to the middle lobe. (Courtesy of P. E. Conen and *Dis. Chest,* 42:89, 1962.)

aspergilli from tissue, and demonstrate their presence therein by appropriate staining.

Invasive pulmonary aspergillosis is usually characterized by two types of pathologic change under microscopic examination. The aspergilli tend to occur in colonies that are surrounded by wide zones of hemorrhage and necrosis. Hyphae can often be found within the lumen of blood vessels of all sizes. The walls of such vessels are necrotic, and the lumens are filled with thrombotic material that is frequently eosinophilic, similar to the lesions produced by mucormycosis.

More diffuse lesions or tiny clusters of hyphae may provoke a predominantly pyogenic response. The lesions look like microabscesses, but the tendency for capillary hemorrhage and septal necrosis is usually obvious at the periphery. Large colonies can be seen readily with hematoxylin and eosin staining, but more diffuse lesions, and the rare lesion characterized by a chronic productive reaction with fibrosis and giant cells, may escape detection unless special stains are used.

Treatment of allergic aspergillosis has not been satisfactory. Eradication of the aspergilli from the abnormal bronchial tree is not a simple matter. Treatment with large doses of iodides may be successful, but may produce hypokalemia and hyponatremia. Aerosols of Mycostatin and amphotericin B as well as intrabronchial instillations of these antibiotics have been used with varying success. The poor response to antifungal therapy is regarded by some authors as evidence against the relationship of the aspergilli to the allergic or bronchitic state.

Intracavitary aspergilloma may not require treatment, but if the patient is diabetic or has another major host abnormality, resection of the cavity is desirable. Repeated hemoptysis is also an indication for resection. Medical treatment is not indicated unless operation is impossible or has been complicated by empyema.

Invasive pulmonary aspergillosis probably should be resected whenever possible unless dissemination has already occurred. Medical treatment is not well defined, perhaps because of the variability in sensitivity of aspergilli to therapeutic agents. There is sufficient evidence to warrant a trial of amphotericin B prior to surgical intervention. Occasionally the therapeutic response will be dramatic, making operation unnecessary. Amphotericin may be instilled directly into empyemas or pulmonary cavities. Flucytosine should be used concurrently, and clotrimazole or miconazole may be found useful.

CANDIDIASIS

Pulmonary candidiasis, with or without candidemia, is produced more often by *Candida albicans* than by other species of the genus. It is a mistake to believe that all such infections are due to *C. albicans.* Yeast forms (blastospores) may be found intracellularly or extracellularly in exudates or the blood stream. Pseudohyphae or true hyphae are usually demonstrable extracellularly. In culture, Candida gives rise to a yeast-like growth of blastospores with varying amounts of hyphae. Species identification on the basis of morphology alone is not reliable. Chlamydospore production is characteristic of *C. albicans* on special media, but chlamydospores may be produced occasionally by *C. stellatoidea* and *C. tropicalis.*

Pulmonary candidiasis is a rarity except as an opportunistic infection. In this form, it is most frequently seen in premature or debilitated infants dying in the first year or two of life. Vaginal candidiasis in the mother has been considered an important source of infection in premature and full-term infants experiencing difficult and prolonged delivery. The evidence suggests that this is strictly an aspirational infection.

The most common factors predisposing to infection in children are neoplasia, particularly the leukemia-lymphoma group; administration of multiple antibiotics, or prolonged treatment with one; treatment with adrenocorticotropic hormone or corticosteroids; severe abnormalities of the blood proteins; and prolonged use of the same needle or an intravenous catheter for infusions. Since neither the roentgenograms nor the clinical manifestions of pulmonary candidiasis are in any way specific, they are likely to be obscured by the pre-existing disease.

The signs and symptoms usually suggest either the persistence of bacterial infection or superinfection of a type not etiologically recognizable on clinical grounds. Fever is not always present, even during documented candidemia, but it is the most common sign. The appearance of fever or an increase in fever in a patient receiving antibiotic therapy for bacterial disease should always provoke consideration of opportunistic fungal infection. When pulmonary candidiasis is accompanied by fungemia, some children exhibit mental depression, psychomotor retardation, and toxic manifestations similar to those seen in typhoid fever. Pericarditis is not rare. In severely ill children, oral, cutaneous or urinary tract infection with Candida often precedes pulmonary invasion or fungemia. Such children should have frequent blood cultures so long as antibacterials or adrenocorticosteroids must be given. The pulmonary candidiasis shown in Figure 21 would have escaped proper recognition and treatment had not candidemia been present.

Although Candida species are recognized easily by direct examination or staining, species identification from cultures is best done by the methods recommended by Wickerham (1961). Candida species are found so commonly in the sputum of patients with bronchopulmonary disease and those receiving antimicrobials, corticosteroids and immunodepressive agents that even repeated isolation of Candida in freshly

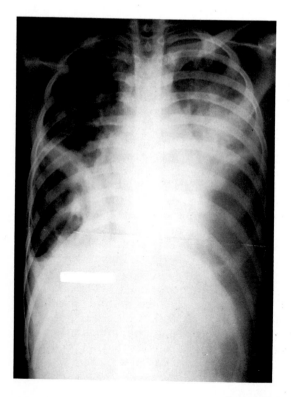

Figure 21. Opportunistic candidal pneumonia. This 12-year-old girl was being treated with multiple antibiotics for staphylococcal sepsis and pneumonia. Bilateral loculated empyemas had been converted to pyopneumothoraces by needle aspirations. The left upper lung had cleared until one day prior to the x-ray film shown here. Candidemia was present for five days. Treatment with amphotericin B controlled the candidemia and induced resolution of the pneumonia.

produced sputum is not acceptable for diagnosis. Isolation from the blood stream, from closed collections of pus or from needle aspiration of pulmonary lesions can be accepted. Circulating antibodies and cutaneous reactivity to candidal antigens are so common among well persons that serologic methods are not helpful in diagnosis.

Candida species are distributed throughout the world, and are found particularly in the alimentary tract. They are frequently present on the skin of hospitalized patients. Autopsy studies in patients with cancer suggest that the gastrointestinal tract is a common portal of entry. Candida are present frequently in the vagina in diabetic patients and in pregnant women.

Pathologically, hematogenous pulmonary candidiasis can be recognized by the presence of microabscesses or confluent lobular pneumonitis associated with thrombi containing Candida. As a general rule, the fungus will not be recognized unless periodic acid–Schiff or methenamine-silver stain is used. When the fungus is abundant, both Gram's stain and Giemsa stain will be satisfactory.

In neonatal pulmonary candidiasis, the infection is clearly bronchogenic. Hyphae and pseudohyphae with blastospores can be found within the bronchioles, often in larger bronchi, and growth can be traced out into the air sacs. In some instances there is a definite bronchopneumonia with polymorphonuclear neutrophilic reaction, considerable intra-alveolar fibrinous fluid, and some microabscesses. In other infants there may be practically no parenchymal reaction, indicating that there was aspiration shortly before death with postmortem growth of the fungus.

Although aerosolized nystatin or amphotericin B may be effective in controlling bronchial candidiasis, established pulmonary disease should be treated with intravenous administration of amphotericin B at least until sensitivity to flucytosine has been determined. If infection is recognized early and is

secondary to antimicrobial therapy, ten to 30 daily infusions may be adequate. If antibacterial antibiotics or other predisposing drugs can be discontinued, the duration of antifungal therapy is usually less. Blood cultures should be made frequently, utilizing large amounts of broth relative to the size of inoculum; these should not be discarded as negative in less than four weeks. Persistent candidemia may be associated with endocarditis requiring prolonged administration of amphotericin B in maximum tolerated dosage. Flucytosine should be given concurrently if the candida is sensitive to it. Oral clotrimazole in a dosage of 100 to 150 mg. per day may be found useful. It is still an experimental drug.

Preventive measures are applicable only to infants and children at special risk. It has been suggested that pregnant women harboring Candida in the vagina be treated with topical candicidin near term. This seems unnecessary if normal delivery is anticipated. Infants and children with thrush should be treated orally with nystatin. Diabetic children who must receive antibacterial antibiotics should be given oral nystatin concomitantly. There are no studies indicating that prophylaxis with nystatin is of value in children receiving immunodepressive therapy with drugs or x-rays, or those receiving corticosteroids with or without antibacterial antibiotics; the use of nystatin in these circumstances would seem rational.

PHYCOMYCOSIS (MUCORMYCOSIS)

This class contains some fungi that are apparently only opportunistic and others that produce subcutaneous infection in normal persons. The former are the only ones known to involve the lung. All appear in the tissue as broad, nonseptate, irregularly branching hyphae. Although septation may occur among the phycomycetes, its definite presence in tissue sections eliminates the diagnosis without cultural verification.

Too few pulmonary infections have been culturally proved to be dogmatic about the genera involved, but it is probable that most have been in the family Mucoraceae. All grow as molds with coenocytic mycelium and specialized sporangia. A text on mycology should be consulted for generic identification.

The *clinical disease* is most commonly associated with ketoacidosis, leukemia, other neoplasms, and severe burns. Although it may appear first in the lung, primary infection in the paranasal sinuses and subcutaneous tissues with subsequent metastasis is relatively common. The clinical course is usually rapid and characterized by fever, cough, hemoptysis, and signs referable to other sites of involvement. Sudden pulmonary, cerebral or orbital signs of infection in any child in acidosis or with disseminated neoplasia should lead to consideration of phycomycosis. There are no helpful roentgenologic signs. In such a clinical setting, the finding of a phycomycete in sputum, lung aspirate or other exudate should be sufficient evidence to prompt immediate therapy.

Laboratory diagnosis has been infrequent. The organisms involved are common in the environment, and merit little attention unless the laboratorian knows what is suspected. There is no difficulty in recognizing the phycomycetes in culture, but direct examination of sputum or other exudates is not likely to suggest the diagnosis except in patients with ketoacidosis. Cultural isolation of the Mucoraceae should be reported by the laboratory with the anticipation that the clinician is sufficiently informed to interpret the report.

The phycomycetes are ubiquitous in nature. It is obvious that the opportunity for infection is general. The rarity of infection is evidence of the importance of serious impairment of host resistance in pathogenesis. The portal of entry is not always found. Paranasal sinuses, the lungs and the gastrointestinal tract appear to be the common sites of entry for opportunistic infections.

The *pathologic change* produced in the lung is similar to aspergillosis. There is often more evidence of vascular invasion with thrombosis and necrosis. Suppuration is usually obvious and extensive, but coagulation necrosis predominates. The hyphae often stain well with hematoxylin and eosin, but the methenamine-silver method is more reliable.

Once the disease is recognized, *treatment* should be started with amphotericin B in the maximum tolerated dose if the underlying host abnormality is correctable. Correction of ketoacidosis may be extremely important, but treatment with amphotericin should not be delayed until after metabolic correction. Superficial infection of burns may be treated with topical amphotericin lotion to prevent deep tissue invasion or phycomycetic septicemia, but this is of limited value. Clotrimazole should be given if available.

RARE INFECTIONS

Of fungous infections that are known to involve children, but that have been reported rarely as primary pulmonary pathogens, *Sporothrix schenckii* is the most likely to be found. *Sporotrichosis* of the extremities and face occurs in children, particularly in Central and South America. Dissemination occurs rarely. The fungus is present in soil, wood and many plants. Pulmonary infection in adults may be indolent or spontaneously regressive. The fungus grows well on ordinary laboratory media, being predominantly yeastlike in its growth at 37°C. and mycelial at room temperature. Tissue diagnosis can sometimes be made with periodic acid–Schiff staining, but the fluorescent antibody method is far better. The pulmonary infections are usually asymptomatic; the roentgen findings are those of a persistent patchy bronchopneumonia, and there may be pleural involvement. If treatment with a saturated solution of potassium iodide fails, amphotericin B is effective.

Geotrichosis is reported fairly commonly as a pulmonary or bronchopulmonary disease in certain parts of the world, particularly in Brazil. Geotrichum may be recovered from the sputum of many patients with chronic bronchitis, and it sometimes forms mucosal plaques that are grossly identical with the thrush produced by Candida. Except in Brazil, there is little evidence that Geotrichum is a significant pulmonary pathogen. Lacaz considers the association with bronchopulmonary symptoms to be that of an "associate" or secondary agent. It has been isolated from the blood stream of an infant and also an elderly man. The fungus is usually recognized by direct examination of the sputum if it is present in abundance. The hyphae are septate and narrow, and form arthrospores that are rectangular or elliptical and may resemble those of *Coccidioides immitis*. It grows easily on ordinary media as a rather soft, flat, white to tawny colony that is easily picked from the surface of the agar when grown at room temperature. These colonies will show large numbers of rectangular or elliptical arthrospores together with septate branching hyphae and spherical to subspherical cells, which somewhat resemble the yeast form of Blastomyces. Oral potassium iodide therapy has been effective in eliminating the fungus from sputum in many cases. If the fungus is definitely identified in pulmonary biopsies or lung aspirates, the patient should be treated with amphotericin B.

Torulopsis glabrata is a rare cause of fungemia in humans; one case of bronchopneumonia associated with this organism has been reported in a ten-year-old boy. Its most common recovery from human sources has been in cultures of urine. *Torulopsis glabrata* grows readily on ordinary media, producing colonies that are smooth and yeastlike in form and white to brownish in color. The cells are ovoid and usually between 3 and 5 microns in dimension. It must be differentiated from Candida and yeasts that might be isolated from human sources. The work of Wickerham (1961) should be consulted for the details of identification. In experimental infections in animals, *T. glabrata* grows intracellularly and may be confused with *Histoplasma capsulatum*.

Another asporogenous yeast that has been reported to produce disseminated disease in an infant is *Rhodotorula mucilagnosa*. This yeast may resemble Cryptococcus when seen in body fluids. Cells are round to oval, occasionally elongate, and may produce a scanty amount of pseudomycelium in culture as does Cryptococcus. It reproduces by budding. Cultures may easily be differentiated from Cryptococcus or Torulopsis by means of the red or yellow pigment that colors the colonies.

One would expect that both *T. glabrata* and *R. mucilagnosa* would be sensitive to amphotericin B. At present, this antibiotic is the agent of choice in proved pulmonary infections due to either genus. Some isolates of *T. glabrata* are sensitive to flucytosine.

Fusarium sp. is a common saprophyte and laboratory contaminant. It is easily recognized by well trained medical technicians. It has become a problem in burned patients, perhaps because of the local antimicrobial therapy in vogue. It may produce systemic infection. No specific therapy is known, but sensitivity to clotrimazole should be determined.

TREATMENT OF SYSTEMIC MYCOSES

Amphotericin B is an antibiotic inhibitory to many fungi and leishmania, with maximal activity against the yeastlike fungi. Its greatest effectiveness is in the treatment of the blastomycoses, cryptococcosis, histoplasmosis, coccidioidomycosis, candidiasis and disseminated sporotrichosis. It is sometimes useful in infections due to Aspergillus, the Mucoraceae, and probably other fungi with sterols in their cell walls.

Absorption from the gastrointestinal tract is irregular and poor at best. Intramuscular injection is ineffective. The antibiotic can be administered by aerosolization, but there is no acceptable evidence that it is effective when given by this route. Amphotericin B (Fungizone) is used for intravenous administration after dilution with 5 per cent dextrose injection, U.S.P. Each ampule contains 50 mg. of amphotericin B in combination with sodium desoxycholate and phosphate buffers. When reconstituted with 10 ml. of sterile water for injection, U.S.P., a clear colloidal suspension is obtained by shaking, provided the water for injection contains no preservative. A sufficient volume of the reconstituted solution, now diluted to 5 mg. per milliliter, is added to 5 per cent dextrose injection, U.S.P., to give a final concentration of approximately 0.1 mg. of amphotericin B per milliliter.

The diluted solution should be infused over a period of one to four hours. The pediatric scalp vein needle set is satisfactory; *scalp veins should be avoided.* Close observation during the infusion is necessary to detect undesirable reactions and to prevent infiltration of the solution outside of the vein.

By careful regulation of the rate of intravenous infusion, the concentration may be doubled (to 0.2 mg. per milliliter) if the volume of infusate must be restricted.

Dose and Duration

Neither the optimum total or daily dose nor the minimal effective duration of treatment has been established for any of the deep mycoses. Dose is determined primarily by tolerance, and the duration of treatment by clinical judgment.

For disease of average severity, an initial infusion of 1 mg. is preferable. If well tolerated, the dose is increased by 1 or 2 mg. daily or every other day for infants and small children. The increments of dose may be doubled for patients weighing more than 30 kg. Whether the dose is increased daily or every other day is determined entirely by side-effects and toxic manifestations. The maintenance dose has been determined primarily by the degree of azotemia and side-effects. For patients with coccidioidomycosis, mucormycosis and aspergillosis, the maximum recommended daily dose of 1.5 mg. per kilogram should be administered if possible. A smaller maintenance dose (0.3 to 0.75 mg. per kilogram) is adequate for the treatment of other mycoses of average severity. Once maintenance dosage is achieved, one may elect to administer amphotericin on alternate days or daily. In vitro studies indicate daily treatment is preferable for candidiasis and cryptococcosis.

Dangerously ill patients may be given 0.33 mg. per kilogram of amphotericin B the first day, 0.66 mg. the second day, and 1 mg. the third day by incorporating either 2 mg. per kilogram of the sodium succinate ester of hydrocortisone or the equivalent of prednisolone sodium hemisuccinate in the infusion. Steroid dosage must be maintained for seven to ten days and then gradually reduced to the level at which mild reactions appear. Rapid achievement of maintenance dosage is accompanied by a prompt rise in the blood urea nitrogen level in most patients.

Except for opportunistic infections, treatment is maintained for several months. Two months is considered to be a minimum period for established pulmonary mycoses. Changes in the chest roentgenogram are useful as a guide to the duration of therapy only when clearing is progressive. Chronic infections with fibrosis or cavitation often stabilize without much change by x-ray film even after four months of treatment. Culture of bronchial exudate or other available material may indicate the presence of resistant organisms or inadequate dosage, but is not a good guide for the duration of treatment. Cultures usually become negative within two weeks of maintenance of adequate dosage. A significant decrease in titer of complement-fixing antibody also is of help when the pretreatment serologic reaction has been positive, but in the last analysis, it is the physician's assessment of the patient's response to treatment that determines when therapy should be stopped. As a general rule, the total dose of amphotericin should be about 50 mg. per kilogram of body weight.

Toxicity and Side Effects

The intravenous administration of amphotericin B is accompanied by a variety of side-effects and variable toxic manifestations. Flushing, diaphoresis and general malaise are common during the first week or two of treatment, but are of no consequence.

Chills and fever are usual, particularly in the early phase of treatment or whenever dosage is increased. They may be reduced by premedication with acetylsalicylic acid, and generally diminish or disappear after the maintenance dosage level has been reached. Recrudescence of chills and fever without alteration of dosage has been observed when the production lot number of amphotericin was changed. Fever of some degree usually persists if the interval between infusions is greater than two days.

Anorexia is common during prolonged or high dosage treatment. It is most intense during and for several hours after infusion. For this reason, it is advisable to infuse early in the morning or late in the evening.

Headache and nausea are usually mild and transient. Nausea and vomiting are more common during prolonged or high dosage therapy. Premedication with intramuscular trimethobenzamide (Tigan) is frequently helpful in the control of vomiting. It may become necessary to reduce the daily dose or give infusions on alternate days. If anorexia, nausea and vomiting are persistent, one should suspect the presence of hypokalemia.

Hypokalemia has appeared in approximately 25 per cent of our patients treated in the past seven years. An occasional patient offers no complaints during significant hypokalemia, but the majority complain of anorexia, nausea, vomiting and muscular weakness. Since hypokalemia may produce renal and muscular damage, prevention or prompt replacement of potassium deficit is an important adjunct to amphotericin B therapy. The serum electrolytes should be determined semiweekly. Hypokalemia may occur without nitrogen retention. Once hypokalemia occurs, large amounts of potassium may be required in order to correct it. Potassium supplementation, is usually necessary even after hypokalemia has been corrected. Oral potassium medications may be of value in some patients, but they are usually insufficient for the correction of hypokalemia. It has been necessary to give as much as 160 mEq. of potassium chloride intravenously per day to some adult patients for several days before electrolyte balance was restored. The potassium chloride solution is much more irritating to veins than is amphotericin itself, and this may present a serious problem in treatment.

Hyponatremia is an uncommon complication of therapy; it is easily corrected by increasing sodium intake orally or parenterally.

Renal toxicity is a great concern during intravenous therapy with amphotericin. The most serious effect is nephrocalcinosis, which fortunately seldom, if ever, occurs in patients treated with the average dosage. None of our patients has shown clinical evidence of impaired renal function, but several have maintained slight elevation of the blood urea nitrogen level and diminished creatinine clearance during several years of posttreatment observation. The usual changes in renal morphology are similar to the tubular changes seen in hypokalemic nephropathy; some observers have emphasized the importance of glomerular involvement.

Nitrogen retention is a common manifestation of renal toxicity. Rapid achievement of maintenance dosage is almost always accompanied by an abrupt rise in the blood urea nitrogen level. For unknown reasons, the incidence of nitrogen retention among our patients increased when the colloidal suspension of amphotericin B replaced the insoluble suspension, and there has been a further increase in incidence since 1961. The administration of amphotericin is continued without reduction of dosage unless the blood urea nitrogen level exceeds 40 mg. per 100 ml. A reduction of the daily dose by approximately 30 per cent generally results in significant lowering of the blood urea nitrogen level. If reduction in dosage does not decrease nitrogen retention satisfactorily, it may be necessary to interrupt treatment for as long as two or three weeks. Whenever dosage is interrupted for more than a week, it is advisable to resume therapy with a dose of 1 mg. The blood urea nitrogen or nonprotein nitrogen level should be determined semiweekly.

It has been suggested that the intravenous administration of mannitol before and after amphotericin B may circumvent the renal vasoconstriction produced by amphotericin and lessen renal toxicity. It has also been suggested that intravenous bicarbonate can prevent renal tubular acidosis, one of the mechanisms of renal damage.

If intravenous treatment must be interrupted for several weeks, or if relapse dictates re-treatment, therapy should be approached with caution. Initial reactions to amphotericin during re-treatment have frequently been more severe than during the first course.

Cramping abdominal pain, usually epigastric, has accompanied or followed intravenous infusion of amphotericin during a part of the therapeutic course in approximately 25 per cent of our patients. Feces may contain occult blood, and frank melena and hematemesis have been observed. Hemorrhagic gastroenteritis may occur, as is reported in dogs. If melena or hematemesis occurs, treatment should be interrupted.

Normochromic, normocytic anemia occurs routinely during the course of treatment. It usually stabilizes at a level that does not require transfusion (hematocrit level approximately 26 to 28 per cent), but an occasional patient will benefit from blood. This toxic manifestation seems to be of little clinical importance, and no patient has had persistent or progressive anemia after treatment was terminated.

Phlebitis is considered to be a frequent side-effect of intravenous infusion with amphotericin. The low incidence in our own series may be due in part to the relatively short duration of infusion, and in part to the use of dextrose solutions near neutrality. Commercially prepared dextrose solutions often have a pH less than 5.0. If the solution is allowed to infiltrate into or beyond the wall of the vein, phlebitis will occur. This is an avoidable complication.

Cyanosis may accompany severe chills and fever during the intravenous treatment of infants. It is doubtful whether this is specifically related to amphotericin B, since it has been observed with pyretotherapy with intravenous typhoid vaccine. If this side-effect occurs, 100 per cent oxygen should be administered.

Although clonic muscular contractions and convulsions have been observed during severe reactions to intravenous amphotericin therapy, these have been due to improper administration. Uneven and rapid infusion should be avoided.

Hypersensitivity, as to any antibiotic, may occur. It is apparently uncommon, and should be managed as any hypersensitivity reaction to an antibiotic. As a general rule, concomitant corticosteroid administration will be indicated.

Chills and fever may be greatly decreased or abolished by adding approximately 25 mg. (0.25 to 1.0 mg. per kilogram) of hydrocortisone sodium succinate to the infusion fluid. Headache, nausea and anorexia are decreased by corticosteroids, but are not usually abolished. Corticosteroids should not be routinely administered to patients receiving amphotericin intravenously. If reactions are severe, or if maintenance dosage must be reached rapidly, corticosteroids are given. The relatively large initial dose can be reduced gradually after seven to ten days to the level at which mild reactions appear. If at all possible, corticosteroids in any amount should be avoided for patients with coccidioidomycosis. Corticosteroids in the doses recommended have produced no deleterious effect on the course of any of our patients with systemic mycoses.

Flucytosine (5-fluorocytosine) is incorporated by some yeasts and interferes with pyrimidine metabolism. It is given orally in a usual dosage of 150 to 200 mg. per kilogram per day in four divided doses for children. It should be used only in conjunction with sensitivity determinations, since there is great variability in susceptibility of strains within the same species. For this reason, amphotericin is usually given until sensitivity to flucytosine is known. In serious infections (e.g., cryptococcal meningitis), both antimicrobials are given together if the fungus is sensitive to both.

Many isolates of Cryptococcus and approximately half of the author's disease-producing isolates of Candida are susceptible to flucytosine. Isolates of Cladosporium, Torulopsis, and occasionally Aspergillus may be sensitive.

Initial and acquired resistance to flucytosine has been a serious problem, particularly the acquired type. Resistance may develop rapidly and is total. The combination of amphotericin and flucytosine did not prevent the appearance of resistance to flucytosine in one of the author's patients with cryptococcal meningitis. This may be explained by the very low levels of amphotericin in the cerebrospinal fluid, whereas flucytosine readily passes the blood-brain barrier.

Toxic manifestations and side-effects

of flucytosine have been modest. Leukopenia, thrombocytopenia, diarrhea and nausea should be anticipated despite being uncommon. Hepatic dysfunction and intestinal perforation occur rarely.

Neither clotrimazole nor miconazole has been released for other than topical use in the United States. The oral dosage of clotrimazole has varied from 65 to 150 mg. per kilogram per day in two or three divided doses. Miconazole can be given intravenously and intrathecally for cryptococcal or coccidioidal meningitis. Although the in vitro spectrum of effectiveness of these agents is wide, the clinical value has not been determined. When desperation motivates, the manufacturers should be consulted for their recommendations.

There is laboratory evidence to justify the combining of rifampin with amphotericin, flucytosine and the sulfonamides in many mycoses. Since it is relatively innocuous, more studies of combination therapy are indicated.

REFERENCES

General Methods of Microbiologic Diagnosis

Ajello, L., Georg, L. K., Kaplan, W., and Kaufman, L.: *Laboratory Manual for Medical Mycology.* Public Health Service Publication No. 994, Washington, D.C., United States Government Printing Office, 1963.

Buechner, H. A., Seabury, J. H., Campbell, C. C., Georg, L. K., Kaufman, L., and Kaplan, W.: The current status of serologic, immunologic, and skin tests in the diagnosis of pulmonary mycoses. *Chest, 63*:259, 1973.

Campbell, C. C.: Use and interpretation of serologic and skin tests in the respiratory mycoses. *Dis. Chest, 54*(Suppl. 1):49, 1968.

Mowry, R. W.: The special value of methods that color both acidic and vicinal hydroxyl groups in the histochemical study of mucins. With revised directions for the colloidal iron stain, the use of alcian blue 8 GX, and their combinations with the periodic acid–Schiff reaction. *Ann. N.Y. Acad. Sci., 106*:402, 1963.

Seabury, J. H., Buechner, H. A., Busey, J. F., Georg, L. K., and Campbell, C. C.: The diagnosis of pulmonary mycoses. *Chest, 60*:82, 1971.

Actinomycosis

Brock, D. W., and Georg, L. K.: Characterization of *Actinomyces israelii* serotypes 1 and 2. *J. Bacteriol., 97*:589, 1969.

Brock, D. W., and Georg, L. K.: Determination

and analysis of *Actinomyces israelli* serotypes by fluorescent-antibody procedures. *J. Bacteriol.*, 97:581, 1969.

Buchanan, B. B., and Pine, L.: Characterization of a propionic acid producing actinomycete, *Actinomyces propionicus*, sp. nov. *J. Gen. Microbiol.*, 28:305, 1962.

Coleman, R. M., Georg, L. K., and Rozzell, A. R.: *Actinomyces naeslundii* as an agent of human actinomycosis. *Appl. Microbiol.*, 18:420, 1969.

Cope, V. Z.: *Actinomycosis.* London, Oxford University Press, 1938.

Georg, L. K., Coleman, R. M., and Brown, J. M.: Gel precipitin test for the serodiagnosis of actinomycosis. *J. Immunol.*, 100:1288, 1968.

Georg, L. K., Robertstad, G. W., and Brinkman, S. A.: Identification of species of *Actinomyces. J. Bacteriol.*, 88:477, 1964.

Holm, P.: Studies on the aetiology of human actinomycosis. I. The "other microbes" of actinomycosis and their importance. *Acta Pathol. Microbiol. Scand.*, 27:736, 1950.

Holm, P.: Studies on the aetiology of human actinomycosis. II. Do the "other microbes" of actinomycosis possess virulence? *Acta Pathol. Microbiol. Scand.*, 28:391, 1951.

Kaplan, W.: *The Fluorescent Antibody Technique in the Diagnosis of Mycotic Diseases.* Proceedings of the International Symposium on Mycoses. Washington, D.C., P.A.H.O. Sci. Publ. No. 205, 1970, p. 86.

Kwapinski, J. B.: Antigenic structure of the Actinomycetales. VII. Chemical and serological similarities of cell walls from 100 Actinomycetales strains. *J. Bacteriol.*, 88:1211, 1964.

Nichols, D. R., and Herrell, W. E.: Penicillin in the treatment of actinomycosis. *J. Lab. Clin. Med.*, 33:521, 1948.

Peabody, J. W., Jr., and Seabury, J. H.: Actinomycosis and nocardiosis. *J. Chron. Dis.*, 5:374, 1957.

Peabody, J. W., Jr., and Seabury, J. H.: Actinomycosis and nocardiosis: a review of basic differences in therapy. *Am. J. Med.*, 28:99, 1960.

Pine, L., and Georg, L. K.: Reclassification of *Actinomyces propionicus. Int. J. Syst. Bact.*, 19:267, 1969.

Rosebury, T., Epps, L. J., and Clark, A. R.: Study of the isolation, cultivation and pathogenicity of *Actinomyces israelii* recovered from the human mouth and from actinomycosis in man. *J. Infect. Dis.*, 74:131, 1944.

Seabury, J. H., and Dascomb, H. E.: Results of the treatment of systemic mycoses. *J.A.M.A.*, 188:509, 1964.

Weed, L. A., and Baggenstoss, A. H.: Actinomycosis: pathologic and bacteriologic study of twenty-one fatal cases. *Am. J. Clin. Pathol.*, 19:201, 1949.

Wright, J. H.: The biology of the microorganisms of actinomycosis. *J. Med. Res.*, 13:349, 1905.

Nocardiosis

Ballenger, C. N., Jr., and Goldring, D.: Nocardiosis in childhood. *J. Pediatr.*, 50:145, 1957.

Brown, J. M., Georg, L. K., and Waters, L. C.: Laboratory identification of *Rothia dentocariosa* and its occurrence in human clinical materials. *Appl. Microbiol.*, 17:150, 1969.

Carlile, W. K., Holley, K. W., and Logan, G. B.: Fatal acute disseminated nocardiosis in a child. *J.A.M.A.*, 184:477, 1963.

Causey, W. A.: *Nocardia caviae:* a report of 13 new isolations with clinical correlation. *Appl. Microbiol.*, 28:193, 1974.

Causey, W. A., and Sieger, B.: Systemic nocardiosis caused by *Nocardia brasiliensis. Am. Rev. Resp. Dis.*, 109:134, 1974.

Emmons, C. W.: The isolation from soil of fungi which cause disease in man. *Trans. N.Y. Acad. Sci.*, 14:51, 1951.

Eppinger, H.: Ueber eine neue Pathogene Cladothrix und eine durch sie hervorgerufene Pseudotuberkulosis (cladothrichica). *Beitr. Pathol. Anat. Allgem. Pathol.*, 9:287, 1891.

Hathaway, B. M., and Mason, K. M.: Nocardiosis: study of fourteen cases. *Am. J. Med.*, 32:903, 1962.

Henrici, A. T., and Gardner, E. L.: The acid-fast actinomycetes. *J. Infect. Dis.*, 28:232, 1921.

Holdaway, M. D., Kennedy, J., Ashcroft, T., and Kay-Butler, J. J.: Pulmonary nocardiosis in a 3-year-old child. *Thorax*, 22:375, 1967.

Langevin, R. W., and Katz, S.: Fulminating pulmonary nocardiosis. *Dis. Chest*, 46:310, 1964.

Murray, J. F., Finegold, S. M., Froman, S., and Will, D. W.: The changing spectrum of nocardiosis: a review and presentation of nine cases. *Am. Rev. Resp. Dis.*, 83:315, 1961.

Nocard, E.: Note sur la maladie des boeufs de la Guadeloupe connue sous le nom de farcin. *Ann. Inst. Pasteur.*, 2:293, 1888.

Peabody, J. W., Jr., and Seabury, J. H.: Actinomycosis and nocardiosis: a review of basic differences in therapy. *Am. J. Med.*, 28:99, 1960.

Raich, R. A., Casey, F., and Hall, W. H.: Pulmonary and cutaneous nocardiosis. The significance of the laboratory isolation of nocardia. *Am. Rev. Resp. Dis.*, 83:505, 1961.

Richter, R. W., Silva, M., Neu, H. C., and Silverstein, P. M.: The neurological aspects of *Nocardia asteroides* infection. *Inf. Nervous System*, 44:424, 1968.

Runyon, E. H.: *Nocardia asteroides:* studies on its pathogenicity and drug sensitivities. *J. Lab. Clin. Med.*, 37:713, 1951.

Schneidau, J. D., Jr., and Shaffer, M. F.: Studies on Nocardia and other actinomycetales. I. Cultural studies. *Am. Rev. Tuberc. Pulm. Dis.*, 76:770, 1957.

Seabury, J. H., and Dascomb, H. E.: Results of the treatment of systemic mycoses. *J.A.M.A.*, 188:509, 1964.

Stadler, H. E., Kraft, B., Weed, L. A., and Keith, H. M.: Chronic pulmonary disease due to Nocardia. *Am. J. Dis. Child.*, 88:485, 1954.

Stites, D. P., and Glezen, W. P.: Pulmonary nocardiosis in childhood. A case report. *Am. J. Dis. Child.*, 114:101, 1967.

Webster, B. H.: Pulmonary nocardiosis: a review with a report of seven cases. *Am. Rev. Tuberc.*, 73:485, 1956.

Weed, L. A., Andersen, H. A., Good, C. A., and Baggenstoss, A. H.: Nocardiosis: clinical, bacteriologic and pathological aspects. N. Engl. J. Med., 253:1137, 1955.

North American Blastomycosis

Abernathy, R. S., and Heiner, D. C.: Precipitation reactions in agar in North American blastomycosis. J. Lab. Clin. Med., 57:604, 1961.

Allison, F., Jr., Lancaster, J. G., Whitehead, A. E., and Woodbridge, H. B.: Simultaneous infection in man by Histoplasma capsulatum and Blastomyces dermatitidis. Am. J. Med., 32:476, 1962.

Baker, R. D.: Tissue reaction in human blastomycosis: an analysis of tissue from 23 cases. Am. J. Pathol., 18:479, 1942.

Boswell, W.: Roentgen aspects of blastomycosis. Am. J. Roentgenol., 81:224, 1959.

Brandsberg, J. W., Tosh, F. E., and Furcolow, M. L.: Concurrent infection with Histoplasma capsulatum and Blastomyces dermatitidis. N. Engl. J. Med., 270:874, 1964.

Busey, J. F. (Ed.): Blastomycosis. I. A review of 198 collected cases in the Veterans' Administration Hospitals. Am. Rev. Resp. Dis., 89:659, 1964.

Busey, J. F., and Hinton, P. F.: Precipitin in blastomycosis. Am. Rev. Resp. Dis., 95:112, 1967.

Campbell, C. C.: The accuracy of serologic methods in diagnosis. Ann. N.Y. Acad. Sci., 89:163, 1960.

Cherniss, E. I., and Waisbren, M. S.: North American blastomycosis: a clinical study of 40 cases. Ann. Intern. Med., 44:105, 1956.

Denton, J. F., and DiSalvo, A. F.: Isolation of Blastomyces dermatitidis from natural sites at Augusta, Georgia. Am. J. Trop. Med. Hyg., 13:716, 1964.

Denton, J. F., McDonough, E. S., Ajello, L., and Ausherman, R. J.: Isolation of Blastomyces dermatitidis from soil. Science, 133:1126, 1961.

Elson, W. O.: The antibacterial and fungistatic properties of propamidine. J. Infect. Dis., 76:193, 1945.

Emmons, C. W., and others: North American blastomycosis: two autochthonous cases from Africa. Sabouraudia, 3:306, 1964.

Foshay, L., and Madden, A. G.: The dog as a natural host for Blastomyces dermatitidis. Am. J. Trop. Med., 22:565, 1942.

Gilchrist, T. C., and Stokes, W. R.: Further observations on blastomycetic dermatitis in man. Bull. Johns Hopkins Hosp., 7:129, 1896.

Jones, R. R., and Martin, D. S.: Blastomycosis of bone: a review of 63 collected cases of which 6 recovered. Surgery, 10:931, 1941.

Kaplan, W., and Kaufman, L.: Blastomycosis and histoplasmosis — specific fluorescent antiglobulins for the detection and identification of Blastomyces dermatitidis yeast phase cells. Mycopathol. Mycol. Appl., 19:173, 1963.

Kaplan, W., and Kraft, D. E.: Demonstration of pathogenic fungi in formalin-fixed tissues by immunofluorescence. Am. J. Clin. Pathol., 52:420, 1969.

Kaufman, L., McLaughlin, D. W., Clark, M. J., and Blumer, S.: Specific immunodiffusion test for blastomycosis. Appl. Microbiol., 26:44, 1973.

Kunkel, W. M., Weed, L. A., McDonald, J. R., and Clagett, O. T.: North American blastomycosis — Gilchrist's disease: a clinicopathologic study of ninety cases. Surg. Gynecol. Obstet., 99:1, 1954.

Lockwood, W. R., Busey, J. F., Batson, B. E., and Allison, F., Jr.: Experiences in the treatment of North American blastomycosis with 2-hydroxystilbamidine. Ann. Intern. Med., 57:553, 1962.

Palmer, P. E., and McFadden, S. W.: Blastomycosis: report of an unusual case. N. Engl. J. Med., 279:979, 1968.

Ramsey, F. K., and Carter, G. R.: Canine blastomycosis in the United States. J. Am. Vet. Med. Assoc., 120:93, 1952.

Seabury, J. H., and Dascomb, H. E.: Results of the treatment of systemic mycoses. J.A.M.A., 188:509, 1964.

Smith, D. T.: Immunologic types of blastomycosis: a report on 40 cases. Ann. Intern. Med., 31:463, 1949.

Smith, J. G., Jr., Harris, J. S., Conant, N. F., and Smith, D. T.: An epidemic of North American blastomycosis. J.A.M.A., 158:641, 1955.

Stober, A. M.: Systemic blastomycosis: a report of its pathological, bacteriological and clinical features. Arch. Intern. Med., 13:509, 1914.

Turner, D. J., and Wadlington, W. B.: Blastomycosis in childhood: treatment with amphotericin B and a review of the literature. J. Pediatr., 75:708, 1969.

South American Blastomycosis (Paracoccidioidomycosis)

Azevedo, P. C.: Algumas considerações sôbre a blastomicose Sul-Americana e seu agente etiológico. Tese, Faculdade de Odontologia do Pará, Belém-Pará-Brasil, 1954.

Batista, A. C., Shome, S. K., and Marques dos Santos, F.: Pathogenicity of Paracoccidioides brasiliensis isolated from soil. Publicação No. 373. Insto. de Micologia, Univ. do Recife, Brasil, 1962.

Fava Netto, C.: Estudos quantitativos sôbre a fixação do complemento no blastomicose Sul-Americana, com antígeno polissacarídico. Arq. Cir. Clin. Exp., 18:197, 1955.

Fava Netto, C.: Contribuição para o estudo imunológico da blastomicose de Lutz (blastomicose Sul-Americana). Rev. Inst. Adolfo Lutz, 21:99, 1961.

Fava Netto, C.: The immunology of South American blastomycosis. Mycopathologia, 26:349, 1965.

Lacaz, C. S.: South American blastomycosis. An. Fac. Med. Univ. São Paulo, 29:9, 1955.

Lythcott, G. I., and Edgcomb, J. H.: The occurrence of South American blastomycosis in Accra, Ghana. Lancet, 1:916, 1964.

Machado Filho, J., and Miranda, J. L.: Considerações relativas a 238 casos consecutivos de blastomicose Sul-Americana. O Hospital, 55:103, 1959.

Mackinnon, J. E., and others: Temperatura ambiental y blastomicosis Sudamericana. *An. Fac. Med. Montevideo*, 45:310, 1960.

Mackinnon, J.: On the importance of South American blastomycosis. *Mycopathologia*, 41:187, 1970.

Murray, H. W., Littman, M. I., et al.: Disseminated paracoccidioidomycosis (South American blastomycosis) in the United States. *Am. J. Med.*, 56:209, 1974.

Restrepo, A., Robledo, M., Gutierrez, F., Sanclemente, M., Castaneda, E., and Calle, G.: Paracoccidioidomycosis (South American blastomycosis). A study of 39 cases observed in Medellín, Colombia. *Am. J. Trop. Med. Hyg.*, 19:68, 1970.

Romero Rivas, O.: El granuloma apical dentario en la blastomicosis Sudamericana. *Arch. Peruanos Pat. Clin.*, 14:203, 1960.

Sampãio, S. de A. P.: Tratamento da blastomicose Sul-Americana com anfotericina B. Tese de concurso para a Cátedra de Dermatologia da Faculdade de Medicina da Universidade de São Paulo, Brasil, 1960.

Silva, M. E., and Kaplan, W.: Specific fluorescein-labeled antiglobulins for the yeast form of *Paracoccidioides brasiliensis*. *Am. J. Trop. Med. Hyg.*, 14:290, 1965.

Coccidioidomycosis

Ajello, L. (Ed.): *Coccidioidomycosis*. Tucson, University of Arizona Press, 1967.

Aronson, J. D., Saylor, R. M., and Carr, E. I.: Relationship of coccidioidomycosis to calcified pulmonary nodules. *Arch. Pathol.*, 34:31, 1942.

Aronstam, E. M., and Hopeman, A. R.: Surgical experiences with pulmonary coccidioidomycosis: a survey of 112 operative cases. *J. Thorac. Cardiovasc. Surg.*, 42:200, 1961.

Birsner, J. W.: Roentgen aspects of five hundred cases of pulmonary coccidioidomycosis. *Am. J. Roentgenol.*, 72:4, 1954.

Castleberry, M. W., Converse, J. L., and Del Favero, J. E.: Coccidioidomycosis transmission to infant monkey from its mother. *Arch. Pathol.*, 75:459, 1963.

Cohen, R., Bos, J., and Webb, P. A.: Co-existing coccidioidomycosis and tuberculosis in children. *Arch. Ped.*, 69:267, 1952.

Converse, J. L., and Reed, R. E.: Experimental epidemiology of coccidioidomycosis. *Bacteriol. Rev.*, 30:678, 1966.

Converse, J. L., Pakes, S. P., Snyder, E. M., and Castleberry, M. W.: Experimental primary cutaneous coccidioidomycosis in the monkey. *J. Bacteriol.*, 87:81, 1964.

Cotton, B. H., and Birsner, J. W.: Surgical treatment of pulmonary coccidioidomycosis. *J. Thorac. Cardiovasc. Surg.*, 38:435, 1959.

Dickson, E. C., and Gifford, M. A.: Coccidioides infection (coccidioidomycosis). *Arch. Intern. Med.*, 62:853, 1938.

Drips, W., Jr., and Smith, C. E.: Coccidioidomycosis. *J.A.M.A.*, 190:1010, 1964.

Eckmann, B. H., Schaefer, G. L., and Huppert, M.: Bedside interhuman transmission of coc-

cidioidomycosis via growth on fomites. An epidemic involving six persons. *Am. Rev. Resp. Dis.*, 89:175, 1964.

Egeberg, R. O.: Factors influencing the distribution of *Coccidioides immitis* in soil. *Recent Progress in Microbiology*, VIII:652, U. of Toronto Press (Canada), 1963.

Egeberg, R. O., and Ely, A. F.: *Coccidioides immitis* in the soil of the southern San Joaquin Valley. *Am. J. Med. Sci.*, 23:151, 1956.

Fiese, M. J.: *Coccidioidomycosis*. Springfield, Illinois, Charles C Thomas, 1958.

Kent, D. C., and Kendall, H. F.: Short term, low dosage amphotericin B therapy for residuals of coccidioidomycosis. *Dis. Chest*, 47:284, 1965.

Lipschultz, B. M., and Liston, H. E.: Steroid induced disseminated coccidioidomycosis. *Dis. Chest*, 46:355, 1964.

Medoff, G., and Kobayashi, G. S.: Amphotericin B. Old drug, new therapy. *J.A.M.A.*, 232:619, 1975.

Melick, D. W.: The surgical treatment of pulmonary coccidioidomycosis, with a comprehensive summary of the complications following this type of therapy. *Am. Rev. Tuberc.*, 77:17, 1958.

Puckett, T. F.: Hyphae of *Coccidioides immitis* in tissues of the human host. *Am. Rev. Tuberc.*, 70:320, 1954.

Sievers, M. L.: Coccidioidomycosis among Southwestern American Indians. *Am. Rev. Resp. Dis.*, 90:920, 1964.

Smith, C. E.: Diagnosis of pulmonary coccidioidal infections. *Calif. Med.*, 75:385, 1951.

Smith, C. E., Pappagianis, D., Levine, H. B., and Saito, M.: Human coccidioidomycosis. *Bacteriol. Rev.*, 25:310, 1961.

Smith, C. E., Saito, M. T., Beard, R. R., Rosenberger, H. G., and Whiting, E. G.: Histoplasmin sensitivity and coccidioidal infection. *Am. J. Public Health*, 39:722, 1949.

Smith, C. E., Saito, M. T., and Simons, S. A.: Pattern of 39,500 serologic tests in coccidioidomycosis. *J.A.M.A.*, 160:546, 1956.

Winn, W. A.: Recent advances in the therapy of coccidioidomycosis. In Dalldorf, G. (Ed.): *Fungi and Fungous Diseases*. Springfield, Illinois, Charles C Thomas, 1962, pp. 315–325.

Pulmonary Cryptococcosis

Abrahams, I., and Gilleran, T. G.: Studies on actively acquired resistance to experimental cryptococcosis in mice. *J. Immunol.*, 85:629, 1960.

Anderson, H. W.: Yeast-like fungi of the human intestinal tract. *J. Infect. Dis.*, 21:341, 1917.

Aschner, M., Mager, J., and Leibowitz, J.: Production of extracellular starch in cultures of capsulated yeasts. *Nature*, 156:295, 1945.

Baker, R. D., and Haugen, R. K.: Tissue changes and tissue diagnosis in cryptococcosis; a study of 26 cases. *Am. J. Clin. Pathol.*, 25:14, 1955.

Barron, C. N.: Cryptococcosis in animals. *J. Am. Vet. Med. Assoc.*, 127:125, 1955.

Benham, R. W.: Cryptococci—their identification by morphology and by serology. *J. Infect. Dis.*, 57:255, 1935.

Benham, R. W.: The genus Cryptococcus: the

present status and criteria for the identification of species. *Trans. N.Y. Acad. Sci.*, 17:418, 1955.

Benham, R. W., and Hopkins, A. M.: Yeastlike fungi found on the skin and in the intestines of normal subjects. *Arch. Derm. Syph.*, 28:532, 1933.

Bindschadler, D. D., and Bennett, J. E.: Serology of human cryptococcosis. *Ann. Intern. Med.*, 69:45, 1968.

Black, R. A., and Fisher, C. V.: Cryptococcic bronchopneumonia. *Am. J. Dis. Child.*, 54:81, 1937.

Carter, H. S., and Young, J. L.: Note on the isolation of *Cryptococcus neoformans* from a sample of milk. *J. Pathol. Bacteriol.*, 62:271, 1950.

Collins, V. P., Gelhorn, A., and Trimble, J. R.: The coincidence of cryptococcosis and disease of the reticulo-endothelial and lymphatic systems. *Cancer*, 4:883, 1951.

Cox, L. B., and Tolhurst, J. C.: *Human Torulosis; A Clinical, Pathological, and Microbiological Study with a Report of Thirteen Cases.* Melbourne, Australia, Melbourne University Press, 1946.

Debré, R., and others: Sur la torulose. Étude clinique et expérimentale (à propos d'un cas observé chez un enfant atteint de lymphogranulomatose maligne). *Ann. Paediatr.*, 168:1, 1947.

Drouhet, E., and Couteau, M.: Sur les variations sectorielles des colonies de *Torulopsis neoformans. Ann. Inst. Pasteur*, 80:456, 1951.

Durant, J. R., Epifano, L. B., and Eyer, S. W.: Pulmonary cryptococcosis: treatment with amphotericin B. *Ann. Intern. Med.*, 58:534, 1960.

Emmons, C. W.: The isolation from soil of fungi which cause disease in man. *Trans. N.Y. Acad. Sci.*, 14:51, 1951.

Emmons, C. W.: Isolation of *Cryptococcus neoformans* from soil. *J. Bacteriol.*, 62:685, 1951.

Emmons, C. W.: *Cryptococcus neoformans* strains from a severe outbreak of bovine mastitis. *Mycopathol. Mycol. Appl.*, 6:231, 1952.

Emmons, C. W.: Saprophytic sources of *Cryptococcus neoformans* associated with the pigeon (*Columbia livia*). *Am. J. Hyg.*, 62:227, 1955.

Evans, E. E.: The antigenic composition of *Cryptococcus neoformans*. I. A serologic classification by means of the capsular and agglutination reactions. *J. Immunol.*, 64:423, 1950.

Evans, E. E., Sorensen, L. J., and Walls, K. W.: The antigenic composition of *Cryptococcus neoformans*. V. A survey of cross-reactions among strains of Cryptococcus and other antigens. *J. Bacteriol.*, 66:287, 1953.

Gendel, B. R., Ende, M., and Norman, S. L.: Cryptococcosis; a review with special reference to apparent association with Hodgkin's disease. *Am. J. Med.*, 9:343, 1950.

Greening, R. R., and Menville, L. J.: Roentgen findings in torulosis; report of four cases. *Radiology*, 48:381, 1947.

Haugen, R. K., and Baker, R. D.: The pulmonary lesions in cryptococcosis, with special reference to subpleural nodules. *Am. J. Clin. Pathol.*, 24:1381, 1954.

Kapica, L., and Shaw, C. E.: Improvement in lab-oratory diagnosis of pulmonary cryptococcosis. *J. Can. Med. Assoc.*, 101:582, 1969.

Kaufman, L.: *Serology: Its Value in the Diagnosis of Coccidioidomycosis, Cryptococcosis and Histoplasmosis.* Proceedings of the International Symposium on Mycoses. Washington, D.C., P.A.H.O. Sci. Publ. No. 205, 1970, p. 96.

Linden, I. H., and Steffen, C. G.: Pulmonary cryptococcosis. *Am. Rev. Tuberc.*, 69:116, 1954.

Littman, M. L., and Schneierson, S. S.: *Cryptococcus neoformans* in pigeon excreta in New York City. *Am. J. Hyg.*, 69:49, 1959.

Littman, M. L., and Zimmerman, L. E.: *Cryptococcosis.* New York, Grune & Stratton, Inc., 1956.

Lodder, J., and Kreger-Van Rij, N. J. W.: *The Yeasts, a Taxonomic Study.* New York, Interscience Publishers, 1952.

Moody, A. M.: Asphyxial death due to pulmonary cryptococcosis; a case report. *Calif. Med.*, 67:105, 1947.

Neuhauser, E. B. D., and Tucker, A.: The roentgen changes produced by diffuse torulosis in the newborn. *Am. J. Roentgenol.*, 59:805, 1948.

Owen, M.: Generalized cryptococcosis simulating Hodgkin's disease. *Texas State J. Med.*, 35:767, 1940.

Pollock, A. Q., and Ward, L. M.: A hemagglutination test for cryptococcosis. *Am. J. Med.*, 32:6, 1962.

Procknow, J. J., Benfield, J. R., Rippon, J. W., Diener, C. F., and Archer, F. L.: Cryptococcal hepatitis presenting as a surgical emergency. *J.A.M.A.*, 191:269, 1965.

Reeves, D. L., Butt, E. M., and Hammack, R. W.: Torula infection of the lungs and central nervous system; report of six cases with three autopsies. *Arch. Intern. Med.*, 68:57, 1941.

Rinehart, J. F., and Abul-Haj, S. K.: An improved method for histologic demonstration of acid mucopolysaccharides in tissues. *Arch. Pathol.*, 52:189, 1951.

Seabury, J. H.: *The Treatment of Coccidioidomycosis, Cryptococcosis and Histoplasmosis.* International Symposium on Mycoses. Pan American Health Organization, 1970, p. 128.

Smith, C. D., Ritter, R., Larsh, H. W., and Furcolow, M. L.: Infection of white mice with air borne *Cryptococcus neoformans. J. Bacteriol.*, 87:1364, 1964.

Starr, K. W., and Geddes, B.: Pulmonary torulosis. *Aust. N. Z. J. Surg.*, 18:212, 1949.

Sunderland, W. A., Campbell, R. A., et al.: Pulmonary alveolar proteinosis and pulmonary cryptococcosis in an adolescent boy. *J. Pediatr.*, 80:450, 1972.

Susman, M. P.: Torula (Cryptococcus) infection of the lung. *Aust. N. Z. J. Surg.*, 23:296, 1954.

Takos, M. J.: Experimental cryptococcosis produced by the ingestion of virulent organisms. *N. Engl. J. Med.*, 254:598, 1956.

Takos, M. J., and Elton, N. W.: Spontaneous cryptococcosis of marmoset monkeys in Panama. *Arch. Pathol.*, 55:403, 1953.

Terplan, K.: Pathogenesis of cryptococcic

(Torula) meningitis. *Am. J. Pathol., 24*:712, 1948.

Tynes, B., Mason, K. N., Jennings, A. E., and Bennett, J. E.: Variant forms of pulmonary cryptococcosis. *Ann. Intern. Med., 69*:117, 1968.

Wickerham, L. J., and Burton, K. A.: Carbon assimilation tests for the classification of yeasts. *J. Bacteriol., 56*:363, 1948.

Zimmerman, L. E.: Fatal fungus infections complicating other diseases. *Am. J. Clin. Pathol., 25*:26, 1955.

Zimmerman, L. E., and Rappaport, H.: Occurrence of cryptococcosis in patients with malignant disease of reticuloendothelial system. *Am. J. Clin. Pathol., 24*:1050, 1954.

Opportunistic Fungus Infections

Abramowsky, C. R., Quinn, D., Bradford, W. D., and Conant, N. F.: Systemic infection by Fusarium in a burned child. *J. Pediatr., 84*:561, 1974.

Baker, R. D.: Leukopenia and therapy in leukemia as factors predisposing to fatal mycoses: mucormycosis, aspergillosis, and cryptococcosis. *Am. J. Clin. Pathol., 37*:358, 1962.

Baum, G. L.: Significance of *Candida albicans* in human sputum. *N. Engl. J. Med., 263*:70, 1960.

Berkel, I., Say, B., and Tinaztepe, B.: Pulmonary aspergillosis in a child with leukemia. Report of a case and a brief review of the pediatric literature. *N. Engl. J. Med., 269*:893, 1963.

Bodey, G. P., and Rosenbaum, B.: Effect of prophylactic measures on the microbial flora of patients in protected environment units. *Medicine, 53*:209, 1974.

Bonfanti-Garrido, R., Barroeta, S., and de Montilva, A.: The vaginal fungi in pregnant woman. *Mycopath. Mycol. Appl., 37*:39, 1969.

Borowski, J., Dziedzinszko, A., Mierzejewskki, W., Dubrzynska, T., and Iwanowski, K.: Epidemiology of *Candida albicans* infection in newborn infants. *Proc. Int. Symp. Med. Mycol.,* 1963, pp. 133–135.

Burrow, G. N., Salmon, R. B., and Nolan, J. P.: Successful treatment of cerebral mucormycosis with amphotericin B. *J.A.M.A., 183*:370, 1963.

Campbell, M. J., and Clayton, Y. M.: Bronchopulmonary aspergillosis. Correlation of the clinical and laboratory findings in 272 patients investigated for bronchopulmonary aspergillosis. *Am. Rev. Resp. Dis., 89*:186, 1964.

Cawley, E. P.: Aspergillosis and the aspergilli: report of a unique case of the disease. *Arch. Intern. Med., 80*:423, 1947.

Conen, P. E., Walker, G. R., Turner, J. A., and Field, P.: Invasive primary aspergillosis of the lung with cerebral metastasis and complete recovery. *Dis. Chest, 43*:88, 1962.

Crichlow, D. K., Traub, F. B., and Silver, W.: Aspergillosis due to *aspergillus fumigatus* in an infant. *Bacteriol. Proc., 60*:138, 1960.

Darja, M., and Davy, M. I.: Pulmonary mucormycosis with cultural identification. *Can. Med. Assoc. J., 89*:1235, 1963.

Ellis, C. A., and Spivak, M. L.: The significance of candidemia. *Ann. Intern. Med., 67*:511, 1967.

Finegold, S. M., Will, D., and Murray, J. F.: Aspergillosis. *Am. J. Med., 27*:463, 1959.

Gruhn, J. G., and Sanson, J.: Mycotic infections in leukemic patients at autopsy. *Cancer, 16*:61, 1963.

Harris, J. S.: Mucormycosis. *Pediatrics, 16*:857, 1955.

Hutter, R. V. P., and Collins, H. S.: The occurrence of opportunistic fungus infections in a cancer hospital. *Lab. Invest., 11*:1035, 1962.

Kaliski, S. R., Beene, M. L., and Mattman, L.: Geotrichum in the blood stream of an infant. *J.A.M.A., 148*:1207, 1952.

Kroetz, R. W., Leonard, J. J., and Everett, C. R.: Candida albicans endocarditis successfully treated with amphotericin B. *N. Engl. J. Med., 266*:592, 1962.

Louria, D. B., and Dineen, P.: Amphotericin B in treatment of disseminated moniliasis. *J.A.M.A., 174*:273, 1960.

Louria, D. B., Greenberg, S. M., and Molander, D. W.: Fungemia caused by certain nonpathogenic strains of the family cryptococcaceae. *N. Engl. J. Med., 263*:1281, 1960.

Lupin, A. M., Dascomb, H. E., Seabury, J. H., and McGinn, M.: Experience with Candida recovered from venous blood. *Antimicrob. Agents Chemother.,* 1961, pp. 10–19.

Mikkelsen, W. M., Brandt, R. L., and Harrell, E. R.: Sporotrichosis: report of 12 cases, including two with skeletal involvement. *Ann. Intern. Med., 47*:435, 1957.

Pepys, J., Riddle, R. W., Citron, K. M., Clayton, Y. M., and Short, E. I.: Clinical and immunologic significance of *Aspergillus fumigatus* in the sputum. *Am. Rev. Resp. Dis., 80*:167, 1959.

Ramirez-R., J.: Pulmonary aspergilloma: endobronchial treatment. *N. Engl. J. Med., 271*:1281, 1964.

Ridgeway, N. A., Whitcomb, F. C., Erickson, E. E., and Law, S. W.: Primary pulmonary sporotrichosis. *Am. J. Med., 32*:153, 1962.

Riley, H. D.: Systemic mycoses in children. I. *Curr. Probl. Pediatr., 2*:3, 1972.

Riley, H. D.: Systemic mycoses in children. II. *Curr. Probl. Pediatr., 3*:3, 1972.

Riopedre, R. N., Cesare, I. de Miatello, E., Caria, M. A., and Zapater, R. C.: Aislamiento de *Rhodotorula mucilagnosa* del l. c. r., heces, orina, exudado faringuo y piel de un lactante de tres meses. *Rev. Assoc. Med. Argent., 74*:1430, 1960.

Scott, S. M., Peasley, E. D., and Crymes, R. P.: Pulmonary sporotrichosis: report of two cases with cavitation. *N. Engl. J. Med., 265*:453, 1961.

Seabury, J. H., and Dascomb, H. E.: Results of the treatment of systemic mycoses. *J.A.M.A., 188*:509, 1964.

Seabury, J. H., and Samuels, M.: Pathogenetic spectrum of aspergillosis. *Am. J. Clin. Pathol., 40*:1, 1963.

Shelburne, P. F., and Carey, R. J.: *Rhodotorula fungemia* complicating staphylococcal endocarditis. *J.A.M.A., 180*:38, 1962.

Shurtleff, D. B., Peterson, W., and Sherris, J. C.: Systemic *Candida tropicalis* infection treated with amphotericin. *N. Engl. J. Med., 269*:1112, 1963.

Symmers, W. St. C.: Histopathologic aspects of the pathogenesis of some opportunistic fungal infections, as exemplified in the pathology of aspergillosis and the phycomycetoses. *Lab. Invest., 11*:1073, 1962.

Tashdjian, C. L., and Kozinn, P. J.: Laboratory and clinical studies on candidiasis in the newborn infant. *J. Pediatr., 50*:426, 1957.

Tassel, D., and Madoff, M. A.: Treatment of Candida sepsis and Cryptococcus meningitis with 5-fluorocytosine. *J.A.M.A., 206*:830, 1968.

Utz, J. P., German, J. L., Louria, D. B., Emmons, C. W., and Bartter, F. C.: Pulmonary aspergillosis with cavitation: iodide therapy associated with an unusual electrolyte disturbance. *N. Engl. J. Med., 260*:264, 1959.

Wickerham, L. J.: Apparent increase in frequency of infections involving *Torulopsis glabrata.* Procedure for its identification. *J.A.M.A., 165*:47, 1957.

Wickerham, L. J.: Taxonomy of yeasts. U.S. Dept. of Agr. Tech. Bull. 1029, 1961, pp. 1–61.

Young, R. C., Bennett, J. E., Geelhoed, G. W., and Levine, A. S.: Fungemia with compromised host resistance. A study of 70 cases. *Ann. Intern. Med., 80*:605, 1974.

Treatment of Systemic Mycoses

Bell, N. H., Andriole, V. T., Sabesin, S. M., and Utz, J. P.: On the nephrotoxicity of amphotericin B in man. *Am. J. Med., 33*:64, 1962.

Holt, R. J.: Laboratory tests of antifungal drugs. *J. Clin. Pathol., 28*:767, 1975.

Leikin, S., Parrott, R., and Randolph, J.: Clotrimazole treatment of chronic mucocutaneous candidiases. *J. Pediatr., 88*:864, 1976.

Lietman, P. S.: Commentary: clotrimazole. *J. Pediatr., 88*:908, 1976.

McCurdy, D. K., Frederic, M., and Elkinton, J. R.: Renal tubular acidosis due to amphotericin B. *N. Engl. J. Med., 278*:124, 1968.

Olivero, J. J., Lozano-Mendez, J., Ghafary, E. M., Ebnoyan, G., and Suki, W. N.: Mitigation of amphotericin B nephrotoxicity by mannitol. *Br. Med. J., 1*:550, 1975.

Patterson, R. M., and Ackerman, G. L.: Renal tubular acidosis due to amphotericin B nephrotoxicity. *Arch. Intern. Med., 127*:241, 1971.

Reynolds, E. S., Tomkeiwicz, Z. M., and Dammin, G. J.: The renal lesion related to amphotericin B treatment for coccidioidomycosis. *Med. Clin. North Am., 47*:1149, 1963.

Seabury, J. H.: Experience with amphotericin B. *Chemotherapia, 3*:2, 1961.

Seabury, J. H.: *The Treatment of Coccidioidomycosis, Cryptococcosis, and Histoplasmosis.* International Symposium on Mycoses. Pan American Health Organization, 1970, p. 128.

Seabury, J. H., and Dascomb, H. E.: Experience with amphotericin B for treatment of systemic mycoses. *Arch. Intern. Med., 102*:960, 1958.

Utz, J. P.: New drugs for the systemic mycoses: flucytosine and clotrimazole. *Bull. N.Y. Acad. Med., 51*:1103, 1975.

CHAPTER FIFTY-ONE

CYTOMEGALIC INCLUSION DISEASE

WILLIAM A. HOWARD, M.D.

Cytomegalic inclusion disease is a systemic infection characterized by the presence of intranuclear and intracytoplasmic inclusions in enlarged cells of many viscera; associated with these inclusions are varying degrees of inflammatory degeneration or necrosis. The disease in the newborn is apparently the result of an infection acquired in utero from an asymptomatically infected mother. Over 9 per cent of pregnant women excrete the virus from the cervix, with a progressive increase from trimester to trimester. While intrauterine cytomegalovirus infection may damage the fetus, there is no evidence that infection acquired at birth or in the immediate neonatal period is harmful. If the disease is not fatal, there is usually severe residual damage, especially of the central nervous system. Inapparent postnatally acquired infections are common in children and young adults. Because of the relatively recent development of adequate methods of diagnosis, much is yet to be learned about the frequency of cytomegalic inclusion disease and its clinical patterns in various age groups.

Incidence

Serologic studies, using neutralization and complement-fixation techniques, indicate that the virus responsible for the disease is widespread and occurs at all ages, although clinical cases are infrequent. Antibodies may be recognized in 70 per cent or more of newborn infants. This is roughly the same incidence as is found in young adults, indicating passage of the antibody through the placenta, and suggesting the occurrence of inapparent infections in adults. Neither a positive serologic reaction nor isolation of the virus necessarily warrants a diagnosis of cytomegalic inclusion disease, since the virus has been isolated from a number of fetuses and newborn infants dying from a variety of causes. An interesting finding is that virus isolation occurs approximately 20 times more frequently in institutionalized children and in contacts of children with viruria than in routine examination. Cytomegalic inclusion disease also has been found to occur with greater frequency in debilitated patients, those suffering from chronic illness and those with malignancy.

Etiology

Cytomegalic inclusion disease is caused by one of the group of cytomegaloviruses (CMV) formerly labeled human salivary gland viruses. The cytomegaloviruses are ether-sensitive DNA viruses measuring 120 to 130 microns in diameter, and are heat- and acid-labile. These physical properties, together with the pattern of cellular infection produced, indicate a close relation to the viruses of herpes simplex and varicella, and it is probable that the cytomegaloviruses will be classified with the herpesvirus group.

As a group, the human cytomegaloviruses are not antigenically homogeneous. At least three serologic types have been recognized, and it is possible that additional varieties may be isolated as more cases are studied. They may also infect humans, monkeys and other animals, including rodents.

Pathogenesis

Despite an apparently large reservoir of subclinical human infection, the mechanism by which the disease is spread from person to person is not readily apparent. The fetus in utero is infected by transplacental passage of the cytomegalovirus from a recently infected mother who herself has an inapparent infection. Transplacental infection usually results in clinical disease; infection occurring during passage through the birth canal at the time of delivery does not. The cytopathic and teratogenic effects of congenital cytomegalovirus infections may, in large part, be a function of the timing and duration of the infection in utero. Prospective studies suggest that infection in the first and second trimesters results in more severely infected infants; maternal infections in the third trimester may or may not involve the fetus.

The mother may continue to excrete virus in spite of the development of a good antibody titer. The presence of antibody apparently does not prevent virus multiplication, but it may prevent the disease from being transmitted in subsequent pregnancies. It is rare to have a succeeding infant afflicted, but this also is possible on the theoretical basis of infection with another serotype of cytomegalovirus.

There is a curious note in the contrasting behavior of the illness in the mother and in her severely affected infant. The latter may not only have a more severe infection, but may also develop a higher antibody titer, and excrete virus for a longer time (up to three to four years). This makes it appear that the adult host has a greater ability to terminate the infection. Medearis (1964) suggests that since en-dogenous interferon may be responsible for both the limitation and termination of viral infection, and since immature animals (including premature infants) have a deficient interferon-producing capacity, the presence of interferon produced by cytomegalovirus may play an important role in pathogenesis. This is a notable example of the modifying effect of host maturation on the response of individuals to infectious agents. Cell-mediated immunity may be depressed during pregnancy, allowing reactivation of the virus.

At autopsy, the widespread disturbance produced by cytomegalic inclusion disease becomes apparent. The virus has been found in salivary glands, lung, kidney, brain, liver, bone marrow and numerous other organs throughout the body. Generally the liver, kidney and lungs are the organs most heavily infected, but the brain is also heavily involved from the viewpoint of functional damage. In almost every instance, pulmonary involvement is recognized at autopsy, although clinical evidence may have been mild. The pulmonary changes are diffuse, but are principally those of an interstitial pneumonia, with numerous inclusions found in cells around the terminal air spaces. Occasional instances of placental involvement in cytomegalic inclusion disease have been reported; in Rosenstein and Navarette-Reyna's (1964) case, approximately 1 per cent of the villi showed focal necrosis, with neutrophils and nuclear debris. A few of the affected villi showed typical intranuclear inclusions.

It is now recognized that cytomegalovirus may produce infection in adults. It has occurred as a complication in patients with underlying immunologic deficiency, whether inherited, acquired or induced by immunosuppression, and in patients, both children and adults, with renal allografts (Fig. 1). Also, the heterophil-negative, mononucleosis-like illness, the postperfusion syndrome occurring after cardiac surgery, may be

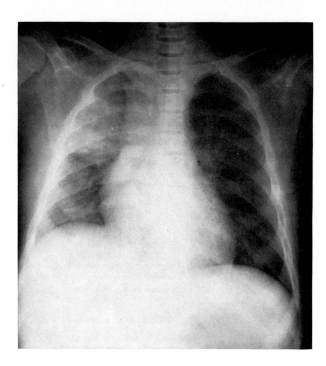

Figure 1. Cytomegalic inclusion disease following renal transplant. (Courtesy of David Hume, M. D., Medical College of Virginia, Richmond.)

due to cytomegalovirus. In each instance a hematologic origin is suggested, either from transfusions or from the transplanted kidney. Fine and his coworkers (1970) found histologic evidence of cytomegalovirus infection in 15 of 26 patients dying of pulmonary infections after organ transplantation.

Clinical Manifestations

Symptoms of the usually congenitally acquired form of cytomegalic inclusion disease appear within a matter of hours to a few days after birth in a prematurely born first child of an apparently healthy mother. Some of these mothers have reported the occurrence of a severe respiratory infection during pregnancy, leading to the supposition that this infection may be the original source of cytomegalovirus infection in the mother and her infant.

The most frequent and severe manifestations of cytomegalic inclusion disease are hepatosplenomegaly, jaundice and petechiae. Hepatosplenomegaly is nearly always present, is considerable,

and in survivors may persist into the second or third year of life. Jaundice may appear early, within the first 24 hours, and may be intense, persisting for several weeks. Direct bilirubin usually accounts for more than 50 per cent of the bilirubinemia, and the indirect fraction rarely rises above 20 mg. per 100 ml. Petechiae and purpuric areas relatable in part to thrombocytopenia are frequent findings. Petechiae present at the time of delivery should suggest the possibility of cytomegalic inclusion disease. A hemolytic anemia is often present. Symptoms of nervous system involvement appear early and include twitching, convulsions, motor abnormalities, chorioretinitis and cerebral calcifications in the subependymal region of the lateral ventricles (visible by roentgenogram). Microcephaly is present in most infants with the cogenital form of the disease, and may become apparent at any time up to one year of age. Spastic paralysis, seizures and blindness may result, and mental retardation is the rule in most survivors. Measured intelligence quotient levels in these retarded infants range from 30 to 50. Hanshaw (1964) has shown that 5 to 15 per cent of infants infected in utero sustain overt central nervous system damage. It is possible that long-term follow-up of infected but clinically normal infants may demonstrate covert, more subtle damage, with some sensorineural hearing loss, subnormal intelligence and a failure to reach their genetically determined potential.

Pulmonary manifestations are overshadowed by other striking symptoms, but in many of the severe, eventually fatal cases, pneumonia is diagnosed ante mortem, and is always found post mortem. X-ray examination may be helpful in severe involvement. In some infants in whom the disease appears later in the postnatal period, pneumonitis is the cause of persistent respiratory distress. In the early months of life, a pneumonic form with hepatosplenomegaly may be recognized, and cytomegalovirus has been found associated with *Pneumocystis carinii* pneumonia. The frequency of pulmonary involvement increases with age, and in adults it most commonly appears in patients with malignancy. The occurrence of viruria, hepatomegaly and abnormal liver function tests in children without any other underlying disease suggests that cytomegalic inclusion disease is clinically significant, that the process may localize in the liver, and that this may be a possible cause of sporadic cases of chronic hepatitis in childhood.

Diagnosis

Initially, the diagnosis could only be suspected during life and confirmed at autopsy by the finding of the typical enlarged inclusion-bearing cells in many tissues and organs of the body. Wyatt and coworkers (1950), observing that these large cells were almost invariably present in the renal tubules, and often seen lying free in the tubules, suggested that a search of the urinary sediment might aid in diagnosis during life. Fetterman in 1952 reported the first successful identification of these inclusion-bearing cells in urinary sediment, and in 1962, Blanc and Gaetz increased the accuracy of the technique by using millipore filter equipment to collect and concentrate cells in the urine before staining. The characteristically enlarged cells may be as large as 40 microns in diameter, while the intranuclear inclusions range in size from 10 to 15 microns. With hematoxylin-eosin stain, the intranuclear inclusion is amphophilic, and is separated from the nuclear membrane by a clear halo (owl's eye cell). Cytoplasmic inclusions are much smaller (4 microns) in size and less characteristic. It has been suggested that the cytologic diagnosis be based only on the finding of intranuclear inclusions, thereby avoiding a good deal of confusion. Cytologic diagnosis is more accurate in infancy, less so in older children and adults. Virus isolation is the most effective method of diagnosis, though viruria does not necessarily mean active disease; cytomegalovirus has been recovered in a high percentage of contacts of patients, and individuals institutionalized for other problems, all without clinical disease. Serologic diagnosis is hampered by lack of reference antisera in laboratory animals, the diverse strains of the virus, and the equivocal results obtained by complement-fixation.

Differential diagnosis runs the gamut of the hemorrhagic and hemolytic processes in the newborn, chiefly sepsis, erythroblastosis fetalis, neonatal thrombocytopenic purpura and congenital leukemia. The neurologic findings may be readily confused with the congenital form of *Toxoplasma gondii* infection. Less commonly, one may consider congenital syphilis and generalized herpes simplex infections.

Prognosis

Though cytomegalic inclusion disease is not necessarily fatal, the problem is a serious one, since a number of patients are left with crippling residual effects, as shown in the long-term follow-up studies of Berenberg and Nankervis (1970). The most significant of these are the neurologic sequelae, including microcephaly, mental retardation, paralysis, blindness and convulsions. It is probable that there are undiagnosed or inapparent infections that might raise the recovery rate, if all instances were recognized. In general, the prognosis for future pregnancies is good, since there is only one recorded instance of the infection occurring in a subsequent pregnancy in the same mother.

Treatment

No satisfactory treatment is available. Because of the high proportion of direct bilirubin present, exchange transfusions are seldom required in the management of severe jaundice in these infants. Corticosteroids have been used without apparent success, and it is unlikely that any drug administered postnatally would significantly influence the course of the disease in these infants damaged so severely in utero. Antibiotics may be used when sepsis cannot be ruled out, but have no effect on the underlying pathologic process. Gamma globulin administration has been without effect. More recently, floxuridine (5-fluorouracil-2-deoxyriboside, FUDR) has been demonstrated to have antiviral effects and has been reported to promote prompt resolution of cytomegalovirus infections in children with acute leukemia. Its use in one patient with congenital cytomegalic inclusion disease was unsuccessful. Idoxuridine and cytosine arabinoside as well as adenosine arabinoside have been used in treatment, the latter causing temporary suppression of viruria except in immunosuppressed patients. The interferon inducer Poly I – Poly C has been suggested as a possible therapeutic agent, but toxicity limits its use.

A vaccine has been suggested as a means of preventing cytomegalovirus infection, and neutralizing and complement-fixing antibodies have been observed following subcutaneous inoculation of a strain of cytomegalovirus passed through human diploid cell cultures. No virus was excreted, and no serious side-effects were noted. Certain obvious problems present themselves, such as the duration of antibody persistence, the effectiveness against other strains of the virus, and the possibility of association with human lymphoproliferative disease. Since most people eventually acquire the infection, it may be appropriate to say that the possible benefits of prevention of the disease and its neurologic sequelae may far outweigh the potential for neoplastic disease.

REFERENCES

Berenberg, W., and Nankervis, G.: Long term follow-up of cytomegalic inclusion disease in infancy. *Pediatrics, 46*:403, 1970.

Birnbaum, G., Lynch, J. L., Margileth, A. M., Lonergan, W. M., and Sever, J. L.: Cytomegalovirus in newborn infants. *J. Pediatr., 75*:789, 1969.

Blanc, W. A., and Gaetz, R.: Simplified millipore filter technic for cytologic diagnosis of cytomegalic inclusion disease in examination of the urine. *Pediatrics, 29*:61, 1962.

Cangir, A., Sullivan, M. P., Sutow, W. W., and Taylor, G.: Cytomegalovirus syndrome in children with acute leukemia. *J.A.M.A., 201*:612, 1967.

Editorial: *Lancet, 1*:845, 1974.

Emodi, G., and Just, M.: Impaired interferon response of children with cytomegalovirus disease. *Acta Paediatr. Scand., 63*:183, 1974.

Feigen, R. D., Schackelford, P. G., DeVivo, D. C., and Haymond, M. D.: Floxuridine treatment of congenital cytomegalic inclusion disease. *Pediatrics, 48*:318, 1971.

Fetterman, G. H.: A new laboratory aid in the clinical diagnosis of inclusion disease of infancy. *Am. J. Clin. Pathol., 22*:424, 1952.

Fine, R. N., Grushkin, C. M., Anand, S., Lieberman, E., and Wright, H. Y., Jr.: Cytomegalovirus in children — post renal transplantation *Am. J. Dis. Child., 120*:197, 1970.

Hanshaw, J. B.: Clinical significance of cytomegalovirus infection. *Postgrad. Med., 35*:472, 1964.

Hanshaw, J. B., and Simon, G.: Cytomegaloviruses in the urine of children with generalized neoplastic disease. *J. Pediatr., 58*:305, 1961.

Hayes, K., and Gibas, H.: Placental cytomegalovirus infection without fetal involvement following primary infection in pregnancy. *J. Pediatr., 79*:401, 1971.

Kantor, G. L., and Johnson, B. L., Jr.: Cytomegalic inclusion disease. *Ann. Intern. Med., 73*:333, 1970.

Kibrick, S.: Cytomegalic inclusion disease clinical rounds. *Clin. Pediatr., 3*:153, 1964.

Kluge, R. C., Wicksman, R. S., and Weller, T. H.: Cytomegalic inclusion disease of the newborn. Report of a case with persistent viruria. *Pediatrics, 25*:35, 1960.

Kramer, R. I., Cirone, V. C., and Moore, H.: Interstitial pneumonia due to Pneumocystis carinii, cytomegalic inclusion disease, and hypogammaglobulinemia occurring simultaneously in the same infant. *Pediatrics, 29*:816, 1962.

McAllister, R. M., Wright, H. T., Jr., and Tasem, W. M.: Cytomegalic inclusion disease in twins. *J. Pediatr., 64*:278, 1964.

Medearis, D. N., Jr.: Observations concerning human cytomegalovirus infection and disease. *Bull. Johns Hopkins Hosp., 114*:181, 1964.

Monif, G. R. G., Egan, E. A., II, Held, B., and Eitzman, D. V.: The correlation of maternal cytomegalovirus infection during varying stages in gestation with neonatal development. *J. Pediatr., 80*:17, 1972.

Naib, Z. M.: Cytologic diagnosis of cytomegalic inclusion body disease. *Am. J. Dis. Child., 105*:153, 1963.

Rosenstein, D. O., and Navarette-Reyna, A.: Cytomegalic inclusion disease. Observation of the characteristic inclusion bodies in the placenta. *Am. J. Obstet. Gynecol., 89*:220, 1964.

Rowe, W. P., Hartley, J. W., Cramblett, H. G., and Mastrotta, F.: Detection of human salivary gland virus in mouth and urine of children. *Am. J. Hyg., 67*:57, 1958.

Stagno, S., Reynolds, D., Tsiantos, A., Fucillo, D. A., Smith, R., Tiller, M., and Alford, C. A., Jr.: Cervical cytomegalovirus excretion in pregnant and non-pregnant women; suppression in early gestation. *J. Infect. Dis., 131*:522, 1975.

Weller, T. H., and Hanshaw, J. B.: Virologic and clinical observations on cytomegalic inclusion disease. *N. Engl. J. Med., 266*:1233, 1963.

Weller, T. H., Hanshaw, J. B., and Scott, D. E.: Serologic differentiation of viruses responsible for cytomegalic inclusion disease. *Virology, 12*:132, 1960.

Wyatt, J. P., Saxton, J., Lee, R. S., and Pinkerton, H.: Generalized cytomegalic inclusion disease. *J. Pediatr., 36*:271, 1958.

CHAPTER FIFTY-TWO

PSITTACOSIS (ORNITHOSIS)

ROBERT H. HIGH, M.D.

Psittacosis is an acute infectious disease occurring naturally in many species of birds and transmissible to humans. Early reports suggested that the disease was chiefly spread from birds of the psittacine group, such as parrots and parakeets; hence the term "psittacosis." More recent studies have shown that many species of birds, both wild and domesticated, can be infected. These include pigeons, chickens, turkeys, ducks, pheasants, finches and others, and some authors, therefore, prefer to designate the infection as ornithosis. Spread from human to human can also occur during the acute phase of a pulmonary infection. In this chapter, the traditional term "psittacosis" will be retained.

The infectious agent is generally regarded as one of the chlamydiae, antigenically related viruses that are included in the psittacosis—lymphogranuloma venereum and trachoma group of agents, a group that is intermediate between rickettsiae and viruses. Some doubt that the psittacosis agent is a true virus. Regardless of the eventual resolution of the classification of the organism, it is known that psittacosis can be grown in tissue cultures and on the yolk sac of embryonated eggs. Coccoid-shaped elementary bodies appear to be the causative agent. When grown in tissue culture, inclusion bodies develop in the cells.

In birds, the agent has been recovered from nasal secretions, blood, liver, spleen, feces and feathers presumably contaminated with nasal secretions or feces. Many apparently healthy birds harbor the agent, and birds that have recovered from the infection can continue to shed the agent for long periods. Isolation of the agent from human beings has been made chiefly from secretions from the respiratory tract. The carrier state may persist for long periods of time in human patients who have recovered from psittacosis. The same or a closely related agent has been recovered from other mammalian species.

Humans acquire the infection by handling sick or well birds, from inhalation of dust contaminated with fecal droppings or from handling feathers. The portal of entry is the respiratory tract. Since infected human patients shed the agent in their respiratory tract secretions, person-to-person spread is also possible. Indeed, small outbreaks have occurred in hospital personnel caring for patients with psittacosis. Laboratory workers processing live preparations of the agent have likewise become infected. Because of this fact, many laboratories do not attempt direct isolation of the psittacosis agents.

Psittacosis is most common in those caring for birds, such as workers in aviaries, or in those who keep birds as pets. In 1970, three cases were associated with aviaries in zoos; two were in employees, and one was in a visitor to the aviary. It may also occur in those working with feathers or in those processing domestic fowls for market. Most cases have been noted in adults, but children are not immune, and infections during childhood have been documented (Table 1).

The actual frequency of psittacosis in this country cannot be stated, since many of the mild cases are not accurately diagnosed and some cases are not

TABLE 1. THIRTY-SIX CASES OF HUMAN PSITTACOSIS BY AGE AND SEX DISTRIBUTION, UNITED STATES, 1970*

Age (Years)	Sex		Total	Per Cent of Total
	MALE	FEMALE		
0–9	0	1	1	2.8
10–19	2	0	2	5.6
20–29	0	2	2	5.6
30–39	7	3	10	28.0
40–49	6	5	11	30.6
50–59	3	1	4	11.1
60–69	1	1	2	5.6
70+	1	2	3	8.3
Unknown	0	1	1	2.8
Total	20	16	36	
Per Cent of Total	55.5	44.4	99.9	100.4

*Provisional Data.
Source: Case reports submitted to Center for Disease Control.

reported to the health departments. The United States Public Health Service includes psittacosis among "notifiable diseases of low frequency."

In 1970, a total of 36 cases of human psittacosis were reported, 23 less than were reported in 1969 (see Table 2). New York reported the largest number of cases (eight), and California reported seven cases; together they accounted for 42 per cent of the total. Parakeets were the most probable source of infection in 28 per cent of the total cases (Table 3). Parrots were the most probable source of infection in four cases (11.1 per cent) in 1970, compared with eight (14 per cent) in 1969. In 1970, four cases were attributed to pigeons and two to chickens.

As indicated by the data shown in Figure 1, there is no seasonal peak of incidence.

According to the U.S. Public Health Service as reported by the Center for Disease Control, the figures for 1972 were as follows (Morbidity and Mortality Weekly Reports, 1973):

Seventeen states reported 38 human cases of psittacosis with onsets in 1972 to CDC. In addition, 3 cases with onsets in late 1971 were reported in 1972, increasing the 1971 case total from 33 to 36. Epidemiologic data were received on 33 of the 38 human cases recorded in 1972 and on all of the late 1971 cases.

Reports were obtained from all 50 states and Puerto Rico. Of the states reporting cases in 1972, 8 reported an increase over 1971, 4 reported a decrease, and 5 reported no change in the number of cases over the previous year. Connecticut reported the largest number of cases (6), followed by Texas (5), California (4), and Kansas (4).

Of the 32 cases for which the date of onset was known, most (5 each) occurred in March and July. However, there was no apparent seasonal variation in the onset of the disease, as almost equal numbers of cases occurred in every quarter of the year.

Of the 33 cases for which age and sex were known, 29 were in adults, and the remaining 4 were in children ages 2, 8, 9, and 9½ years. Fifteen cases occurred in males, 18 in females.

Parakeets were the most probable source of infection in 10 cases (30 per cent), while pigeons accounted for 6 cases (18 per cent). A total of 16 cases occurred in persons who did not own birds, 10 of whom were exposed to birds either at work or in their neighborhoods; in 6 cases no known exposure was reported. Four other cases occurred in pet shop employees whose most probable exposure was at the shop. (Reported by the Office of Veterinary Public Health Services, Bureau of Epidemiology, CDC.)

According to the U.S. Public Health Service, 164 cases in humans were reported in 1974. Only very occasional deaths from psittacosis have been reported (Morbidity and Mortality Weekly Reports, 1974).

In human beings and monkeys, unlike birds, the disease does not cause widespread visceral involvement, but tends to be localized in the lungs, where a diffuse interstitial pneumonia is produced. Some pleural reaction may occur. The pathologic changes are not pathognomonic for psittacosis, since similar changes occur with other viral infections of the lungs. The liver may show focal necrosis, and the spleen may be enlarged.

The clinical manifestations of psitta-

TABLE 2.   HUMAN PSITTACOSIS—UNITED STATES, 1961–1970*

State	1961	1962	1963	1964	1965	1966	1967	1968	1969	1970*	Total	10-Year Rank
Alabama	0	0	0	0	0	0	0	0	1	0	1	23
Alaska	0	1	0	0	0	0	0	0	0	0	1	23
Arizona	0	1	1	0	1	0	0	1	0	0	4	20
Arkansas	0	0	0	1	0	0	0	0	0	1	2	22
California	10	10	14	14	12	6	2	9	15	7	99	1
Colorado	0	2	0	0	0	0	0	0	0	0	2	22
Connecticut	2	6	3	0	2	1	2	3	6	1	26	7
Delaware	1	0	0	0	0	0	0	0	0	0	1	23
Dist. of Col.	0	0	0	0	0	0	0	0	0	0	0	24
Florida	0	0	0	1	1	0	1	0	2	0	5	19
Georgia	2	0	3	4	0	0	0	1	1	1	12	13
Hawaii	0	0	0	0	0	0	0	0	0	0	0	24
Idaho	1	0	0	0	0	0	0	0	0	0	1	23
Illinois	7	4	11	6	5	1	0	1	0	0	35	5
Indiana	0	1	0	0	0	0	0	0	0	1	2	22
Iowa	0	0	0	1	0	0	1	0	0	0	2	22
Kansas	0	0	0	0	0	1	1	0	0	1	3	21
Kentucky	0	0	1	0	1	0	0	0	0	0	2	22
Louisiana	0	0	0	0	0	0	1	0	4	0	5	19
Maine	0	0	0	0	1	0	0	0	0	0	1	23
Maryland	0	1	0	0	2	0	0	0	5	2	10	15
Massachusetts	3	1	2	2	1	4	5	1	0	0	19	11
Michigan	2	3	4	3	1	0	1	6	1	3	24	8
Minnesota	2	4	1	1	5	3	2	0	4	1	23	9
Mississippi	0	0	0	0	0	0	0	0	0	0	0	24
Missouri	0	4	0	0	0	0	0	0	0	0	4	20
Montana	0	2	1	0	0	0	2	0	0	0	5	19
Nebraska	0	0	0	0	0	0	0	0	0	0	0	24
Nevada	0	0	0	0	0	0	0	0	0	0	0	24
New Hampshire	0	0	0	0	0	1	1	0	0	0	2	22
New Jersey	1	1	0	3	0	1	0	1	0	2	9	16
New Mexico	0	0	0	0	0	0	0	1	1	0	2	22
New York	6	6	5	2	4	1	3	6	4	8	45	4
North Carolina	1	3	1	1	1	1	0	1	1	1	11	14
North Dakota	0	0	0	0	0	0	0	0	0	0	0	24
Ohio	0	1	2	3	2	1	1	3	4	1	18	12
Oklahoma	0	0	0	0	0	0	1	0	0	0	1	23
Oregon	2	1	2	1	1	1	0	0	1	0	9	16
Pennsylvania	6	5	0	2	1	4	3	1	5	1	28	6
Rhode Island	0	0	0	0	0	0	0	0	0	0	0	24
South Carolina	0	0	0	0	0	0	0	0	0	0	0	24
South Dakota	1	0	0	0	0	0	0	0	0	0	1	23
Tennessee	6	1	1	2	4	3	3	2	0	0	22	10
Texas	23	0	17	1	8	12	9	6	0	3	79	2
Utah	3	1	2	0	2	0	0	0	0	0	8	17
Vermont	0	0	0	0	0	0	0	0	0	0	0	24
Virginia	1	0	0	1	1	2	0	0	0	0	5	19
Washington	2	0	0	0	2	1	1	0	1	0	7	18
West Virginia	1	0	1	0	0	0	0	1	0	0	3	21
Wisconsin	18	20	4	4	3	6	1	1	3	2	62	3
Wyoming	0	1	0	0	0	0	0	0	0	0	1	23
Total	101	80	76	53	61	50	41	45	59	36	602	

*Provisional Data
Source: Case reports submitted to Center for Disease Control, Morbidity and Mortality Weekly Report.

TABLE 3. THIRTY-SIX CASES OF HUMAN PSITTACOSIS BY MOST PROBABLE SOURCE OF INFECTION AND EXPOSURE CLASSIFICATION, UNITED STATES, 1970*

Exposure Classification	Most Probable Source of Infection											
	Parakeet	Pigeon	Canary	Parrot	Chicken	Turkey	Birds, Variety or Unspecified	Cockatiel	Lovebird	Unknown or No Known Exposure	Total	Per Cent of Total
Pet Bird Owner	9	1		2			3	1			16	44.4
Pet Bird Dealer							2				2	5.6
Pet Bird Breeder	1	1									2	5.6
Poultry Related		1			2						3	8.3
Other		1		2			5				8	22.2
Unknown										5	5	13.9
Total	10	4	0	4	2	0	10	1	0	5	36	100.1
Per Cent of Total	27.8	11.1	0	11.1	5.6	0	27.8	2.8	0	13.9		100.0

*Provisional Data
Source: Case reports submitted to Center for Disease Control.

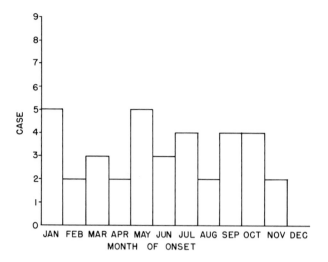

Figure 1. Cases of human psittacosis by month of onset, in the United States, 1970 (provisional data). Source: case reports submitted to Center for Disease Control.

cosis vary considerably in severity, ranging from a mild influenza-like or "grippelike" illness to severe pneumonia. The manifestations of psittacosis are not sufficiently distinctive to permit a diagnosis on clinical grounds. The diagnosis may be suspected when there is a history of exposure to birds, sick or well, but the diagnosis can be confirmed only by appropriate laboratory studies.

The incubation period varies from several days to two weeks. The onset is usually abrupt with fever, malaise, myalgia, photophobia and chills. Cough may develop as a manifestation of the diffuse pneumonia, but this symptom is often not a prominent one. Epistaxis occurs, and occasionally a rash appears which resembles that seen in typhoid fever. Children may have nonspecific neurologic manifestations such as delirium and convulsions. The fever, in the untreated case, tends to be high during the first week or so and then gradually falls to reach normal by the end of the second or third week of the disease.

Physical examination does not show any characteristic abnormalities. The pulse may be slow despite fever. Examination of the lungs may reveal the signs associated with diffuse pneumonia, but the extent of involvement is usually not in keeping with that noted by roentgenographic examination.

Chest roentgenograms reveal the presence of a diffuse bronchopneumonia or interstitial pneumonitis. The abnormalities are not pathognomonic and are seen in other viral pulmonary infections.

Laboratory studies, other than specific serologic tests, are not helpful in establishing the diagnosis of psittacosis. The diagnosis can be confirmed by specific complement-fixation or agglutination tests performed on acute and convalescent phase serum specimens. The first specimen should be obtained early in the clinical course, and the convalescent one should be obtained during the second or third week of the disease. A rise in titer of fourfold or more is considered diagnostic. As mentioned previously, many laboratories do not attempt direct isolation of the agent because of the hazard of infection in the personnel.

The most effective therapy at present is the administration of tetracycline in daily doses of about 50 mg. per kilogram. The duration of treatment should be about two weeks or for ten days after the temperature has become normal. It is recognized that the infrequent occurrence of this infection makes the appraisal of treatment difficult, and these recommendations are somewhat arbitrary. The remainder of treatment is the application of the usual supportive and symptomatic management of diffuse pneumonia, such as the administration of oxygen, analgesics, parenteral fluids, and the like.

REFERENCES

Brunell, P. A.: Psittacosis. In Gellis, S. S., and Kagan, B. M. (Eds.): *Current Pediatric Therapy* 7. Philadelphia, W.B. Saunders Company, 1976, p. 616.

Dean, D. J., and others: Psittacosis in man and birds. *Public Health Rep.*, 79:101, 1964.

Haig, D. A., and others: Occurrence of ornithosis in the wood pigeon. *Nature (London)*, 200:381, 1963.

Hodes, H. L.: Ornithosis (psittacosis). In Holt, L. E., Jr., McIntosh, R., and Barnett, H. L.: *Pediatrics*. 13th Ed. New York, Appleton-Century-Crofts, Inc., 1962, pp. 1155–1156.

Morbidity and Mortality Weekly Reports: 22:355, 1973.

Morbidity and Mortality Weekly Reports: 23:2, 1974.

Report of the Committee on Infectious Diseases. 17th Ed. American Academy of Pediatrics, Evanston, Illinois, 1974, p. 126.

CHAPTER FIFTY-THREE

Q FEVER

ROBERT H. HIGH, M.D.

Q fever is an acute infectious disease caused by infection with *Rickettsia burnetii*, also called *Coxiella burnetii*. The disease was originally described in Australia in 1935 but has subsequently been recognized as having a worldwide distribution. It is not common in this country except in California, where many domesticated animals are infected in certain endemic areas. However, it has been reported in many other states. In 1974, 57 cases were reported to the Center for Disease Control. All reported cases were in western states, with about one-half reported from California. This number does not represent the true frequency, since reporting of this disease is optional. Q fever differs from the other major rickettsial infections in several respects: a rash is not present, the primary clinical manifestations are those of pulmonary infection, and it usually is not spread by arthropod vectors.

Q fever occurs as a natural infection in cattle, sheep, goats and many wild animals. Ticks may become infected and can pass the organism to subsequent generations through the ova. Experimental infections have been produced by the bite of ticks, but this mode of spread is not usual for human infections. Ticks may play a significant role in the transmission of this disease to animals. The rickettsiae are excreted from animals in milk, urine, fetal membranes and discharges, and the rickettsiae are also present in meat from infected animals. The infected animals usually do not appear to be sick.

Humans usually acquire Q fever by the inhalation of dust, particles of straw and the like contaminated by animal discharges, by contamination with fetal membranes and discharges during the birth of calves or lambs, from contact with infected meat or by the ingestion of infected milk. Commercial pasteurization of milk does not necessarily kill all the rickettsiae. Person-to-person transmission is not likely but can occur.

Outbreaks of Q fever have occurred chiefly in slaughterhouse workers and in the employees of tanneries or processing plants for wool and other animal hair. During World War II, outbreaks occurred in the United States military personnel in Italy. Most of the epidemics were caused by the inhalation of infected dust. The organism is resistant to destruction by drying and can remain viable in dust for long periods.

The epidemiology of Q fever is such that children are not commonly exposed except in rural areas or by drinking infected milk.

The clinical manifestations develop after an incubation period of two to almost four weeks. Studies, chiefly in military personnel, suggest an average incubation period of 17 to 19 days. Mild cases may simulate mild influenza and are diagnosed only by serologic studies. The usual manifestations in the typical case include the fairly abrupt onset of fever, malaise and chilliness, and a prominent early complaint is that of severe headache, often frontal, which is worsened by movement of the eyes. A nonproductive cough may develop toward the end of the first week. Chest pain and the production of slightly blood-tinged sputum may occur. Rales and signs of consolidation may be heard when the lungs are examined. A rash does not appear.

The illness tends to have a febrile course for one to two weeks followed by gradual improvement. Convalescence may be moderately prolonged. Complications are rare, and recovery is expected.

Roentgenographic examinations of the chest often show diffuse parenchymal infiltrations, which are usually more extensive than is suggested by the findings of the physical examination. Serofibrinous pleurisy is sometimes present. Enlargement of the hilar and mediastinal lymph nodes is not expected. Resolution of the pneumonia is slow, sometimes requiring several weeks before a normal x-ray appearance is noted.

The diagnosis may be confirmed by isolation of *R. burnetii* from the blood, urine or sputum during the early stages of the disease, using animal inoculation of guinea pigs, monkeys or mice or by inoculation of embryonated eggs. These methods of isolation are not readily available and offer the possibility of infection of the laboratory personnel. Serologic tests, using acute and convalescent phase sera, are the most widely recommended studies. Complement-fixing antibody tests and agglutination tests using antigens from *R. burnetii* are available. It should be stressed that the Weil-Felix reaction is not positive in Q fever. Other laboratory findings are not useful in the diagnosis of this disease.

Treatment with tetracycline in daily oral doses of 50 to 100 mg. per kilogram is recommended until the patient has been free of fever for several days. Since tetracycline does not kill the rickettsiae, some recommend two courses of treatment of five days' duration separated by a period of five days

without treatment. Improvement is usually rapid, and relapse uncommon. Chloramphenicol is also effective in treating Q fever, but it offers no advantage over tetracycline. Chloramphenicol administration is more hazardous than the program described above. Symptomatic treatment of headache, chest pain and the like may be indicated.

The preventive aspects of Q fever, like those of other rickettsial diseases, are complex and without adequate solution at present. In theory, milk from infected cattle should not be used, but the difficulty in identifying these animals, which do not appear ill, makes such a procedure impractical. Pasteurization of milk from suspected infected herds should be at higher temperatures or for longer periods than usual. Endemic areas should be defined so that patients from them who present the symptoms and findings described above may be diagnosed promptly.

REFERENCES

Gold, E., and Robbins, F. C.: Q fever. In Nelson, W. E. (Ed.): *Textbook of Pediatrics.* 9th Ed. Philadelphia, W.B. Saunders Company, 1969, pp. 703–704.

Hughes, W. T.: Q fever. In Gellis, S. S., and Kagan, B. M. (Eds.): *Current Pediatric Therapy 4.* Philadelphia, W.B. Saunders Company, 1970, p. 888.

Luoto, L., and others: Q fever vaccination of human volunteers. I. The serologic and skin-test response following subcutaneous injection. *Am. J. Hyg.,* 78:1, 1963.

Morbidity and Mortality Weekly Reports: 23:32, 1974.

Peterson, J. C.: Q Fever. In Holt, L. E., Jr., Mc Intosh, R., and Barnett, H. L. (Eds.): *Pediatrics.* 13th Ed. New York, Appleton-Century-Crofts, Inc., 1962, pp. 1166–1167.

Wisniewski, H. J., and Krumbiegel, E. R.: Q fever in the Milwaukee area. *Arch. Environ. Health, 21*:58, 1970.

Wisseman, C. L.: Progress report on the development of Q fever vaccines. *Milit. Med., 129*:389, 1964.

CHAPTER FIFTY-FOUR

TULAREMIA

William A. Howard, M.D.

Tularemia is primarily a septicemic disease of rodents; it may be transmitted to humans by the handling of infected material or by the bite of certain insect vectors. The disease is generally considered to be fatal to the animal hosts, but of 39 rabbits trapped during the study of one epidemic, 15 were found to possess agglutinating antibodies to the causative organism. Tularemia was first described in ground squirrels in Tulare County, California, in 1912 by McCoy of the United States Public Health Service, and the first human case was described by Wherry in 1914.

Incidence

Tularemia probably has worldwide distribution and is found in all those parts of the United States and Canada where rodents and small game abound. The disease is also reported regularly in Europe and the USSR. Sporadic cases are the rule, although the disease may appear occasionally in epidemic form, such as the outbreak in Vermont in 1968, when 72 cases were identified and the group of 38 cases that occurred in Utah in 1971. From 1960 through 1968, a total of 2594 cases were reported in the United States, with 23 deaths, a marked drop from the peak incidence of 2291 cases reported in 1939. Most recent figures show 121 cases reported in 1975, with 62 reported for the first six months of 1976. The majority of cases are now reported from the central states, both north and south, with relatively few from the Mountain and Pacific states, representing a major shift in geographic distri-

bution from the west to the central and eastern parts of the country. A special susceptibility to tularemia is noted among laboratory workers handling the infecting agent.

Etiology

The disease is caused by *Francisella tularensis (Pasteurella tularensis)*, a small nonmotile, gram-negative, coccoid bacillus, 0.3 to 0.7 micron in length. The organism is readily destroyed by heating at 56°C. for ten minutes, and by most disinfectants, including one part per million of chlorine in drinking water. This probably accounts for the rarity of the gastrointestinal, oropharyngeal and glandular varieties of the disease in the United States, since potentially infected foods are nearly always cooked before being eaten, and chlorination of water is the rule.

Pathogenesis

Although tularemia is usually found in rodents, including the rabbit and the hare, the organism may infect the deer, fox, coyote, woodchuck, sheep, skunk, squirrel, opossum, water rat, cat, dog, and many other animals. Birds and quail may also harbor *F. tularensis.* The disease is transmitted from animal to animal by several species of ticks of the family Ixodidae, including the rabbit tick *(Haemaphysalis leporis-palustris)*, the brown dog tick *(Rhipicephalus sanguineus)*, as well as members of the species Ixodes and Amblyomma.

Transmission from animals to humans may also be mediated by members of the family Ixodidae, most commonly the American dog tick *(Dermacentor variabilis)*, the Rocky Mountain wood tick *(D. andersoni)*, the Pacific coast tick *(D. occidentalis)* and the southern lone star tick *(Amblyomma americanum)*. In the tick, the infection is perpetuated by transmission through the egg, and the organism is present in both the gut and hemocele. The deer fly *(Chrysops discalis)* transmits tularemia in the northwestern United States, and it is probable that other tabanid flies are responsible for the spread of the disease in the USSR. In Russia, the common mosquitoes *Aedes aegypti* and *Culex apicalis* have been implicated as vectors. To date, mosquito transmission has not been reported in this country, but with the recognized mosquito population of the United States, this remains a distinct possibility. *Francisella tularensis* has survived for 50 days in *Anopheles maculipennis*. Squirrel and rabbit fleas may also be vectors in occasional instances. In the Utah epidemic, there was some evidence that biting gnats of the genus *Culicoides* were implicated in the rodent to human transmission.

Naturally acquired infection is almost always obtained by the handling of infected small game, primarily rabbits. Rarely, it may be caused by the bite of an infected tick or by the crushing of a tick on the skin. The organism seems able to penetrate the unbroken skin, and a remarkably small number of bacteria (10 to 50) are regularly capable of causing the infection in the experimental subject. Person-to-person transmission has not been recorded, but laboratory infections are common.

Francisella tularensis is an intracellular parasite, and recent evidence indicates that host resistance to tularemia may be dependent primarily on a cellular immune response, with humoral factors (circulating antibody) appearing to be of secondary importance. Recovery usually results in lifelong immunity.

Clinical Manifestations

Tularemia has been more prevalent during the fall and winter months, coincident with the hunting season. However, with the increase in the number of cases apparently transmitted by arthropods, an increasing incidence is being observed during the summer months, when these vectors are most prevalent. The incubation period of the disease is nearly always less than two weeks and usually less than one week. Depending on the portal of entry and the mode of infection, six clinical types are described: (1) ulceroglandular (most common), (2) oculoglandular, (3) oropharyngeal, (4) pulmonic, (5) glandular, and (6) intestinal (typhoidal).

There obviously may be some overlapping, and some reports indicate that a high percentage of patients, regardless of the type of clinical picture, will have roentgenographic evidence of lung involvement.

In naturally occurring infections, mostly from handling infected animals, approximately 90 per cent are of the ulceroglandular type, while laboratory infections are almost always of the pneumonic variety. In natural infections, the onset is abrupt, with chills, temperature as high as 105 or 106°F., headache and vomiting. Evidence of the portal of entry may not be present for the first 24 hours, though regional lymphadenopathy may be evident. The initiating lesion begins as a localized inflammatory area, 2 to 3 cm. in diameter, with a central papule. The lesion progresses to central necrosis with abscess formation and ulceration. The regional lymph nodes become enlarged, firm, reddened and tender, and may undergo abscess formation, requiring surgical drainage. Other systemic symptoms include generalized muscular aches and pains, prostration, sweating and somnolence. Skin rashes may be present and vary from macules and papules to petechiae. Hepatosplenomegaly may be observed. Variations occur, depending upon the portal of entry, and ulcers may be found on the tonsils, pharynx or conjunctiva. Corneal ulcers have also been reported.

Many patients have evidence of pulmonary involvement both clinically and

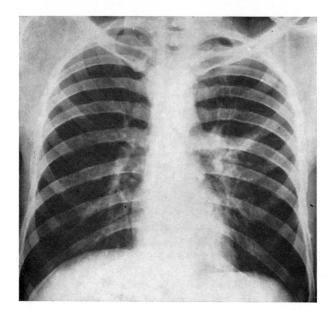

Figure 1. Tularemia. (Courtesy of Walter T. Hughes, M.D., Johns Hopkins Hospital, Baltimore, Maryland.)

on roentgenogram, often with an associated hilar adenopathy (Fig. 1). In obscure pulmonary lesions, one should consider tularemia, since the portal of entry may not be obvious, and primary lesions may not be found. Infection acquired by laboratory workers is nearly always of the pulmonic variety, and respiratory symptoms include dry cough, sore throat, substernal discomfort and pleuritic pain. Physical signs may include those of bronchopneumonia. Roentgenographic findings may be indicative of patchy bronchopneumonia, pleural effusion, peribronchial thickening and nodular infiltration. Residual changes include fibrosis and an apparent increase in calcification.

The oropharyngeal type usually results from the ingestion of contaminated food or water and may involve more than one member of the family since there is a common source of infection. This form produces the characteristic ulcerations in the mouth, throat or tonsils, with cervical adenitis and occasionally exudate or pseudomembrane on the tonsils.

Eye involvement causes lacrimation, photophobia, itching and swelling of the eyelids, and enlargement of the preauricular lymph nodes. Rarely, corneal ulcers may cause permanent impairment of vision.

Diagnosis

The presence of tularemia usually may be suspected when the patient gives a history of contact with some sort of small wild animal, usually a rabbit. This, combined with the classic appearance of the ulceroglandular form of the disease, may suggest the proper diagnosis. The leukocyte count may be as high as 14,000 to 16,000 per cubic milliliter at the onset, and the erythrocyte sedimentation rate and C-reactive protein level are usually slightly elevated. Laboratory confirmation may be obtained by the isolation of the causative agent from material from ulcers or buboes cultured on glucose-cystine blood agar. Animal inoculation is also an effective way of establishing the diagnosis. Unfortunately, both methods carry a high degree of risk to laboratory personnel, and are not normally recommended. Blood drawn early in the disease and three to four weeks after onset may be used for comparative complement-fixation, fluorescent antibody studies, hemagglutination inhibition and antibody neutralizing studies. Agglutination titers of 1:80 to 1:160 are considered diagnostic, but a definite rise in titer in the convalescent blood is more conclusive. Titers of 1:1280 may be reached four to eight weeks after onset of the disease.

The intradermal skin test for tularemia is a valuable diagnostic tool, since it becomes positive in the first seven to fourteen days of the disease and is often positive on the first day the patient presents to the physician. The test is evidence of the development of delayed hypersensitivity, suggesting that cell-mediated immunity plays a prominent part in development of host resistance. The test may be read in 48 to 72 hours, and induration measuring greater than 5 mm. indicates a positive response. It rarely causes a rise in the agglutination titer and may remain positive for many years.

The ulceroglandular form of the disease must be differentiated from lymphadenitis due to pyogenic organisms, from infectious mononucleosis, and from other infections that produce an initial skin lesion followed by regional lymph node involvement, such as sporotrichosis, plague and anthrax. The rarer oropharyngeal form must be distinguished from herpes simplex mucous membrane involvement, herpangina, and the oral manifestations of blood dyscrasias. Pneumonic involvement resembling tularemia may occur in Mycoplasma infections, tuberculosis, brucellosis, sepsis, rat-bite fever, psittacosis, relapsing fever, histoplasmosis and Salmonella infections.

Pathology

In addition to the local lesion, pathologic findings include enlarged regional lymph nodes that contain focal lesions with central suppurative necrosis, characteristically bordered by a granulomatous infiltrate consisting of epithelioid cells and multinucleated giant cells of the foreign body type. In addition, there are focal necrotic lesions in various organs throughout the body, especially the liver, spleen, kidney,

lungs and bone marrow. Polymorphonuclear leukocytes are plentiful in the center of these lesions, while in older lesions evidence of fibrosis is usually present.

Complications

Involvement of the respiratory tract occurs most commonly and includes bronchopneumonia, chronic bronchitis, and pleural effusion. Encephalitis and meningitis have been reported, and painful arthritis may occur. Other rare complications include thrombophlebitis, osteomyelitis, peritonitis and pericarditis.

Prevention

Tularemia is most effectively prevented by the avoidance of contact with infected wild game and with various insect vectors. One should reject for use and destroy by burying or burning any game with evidence of liver involvement, such as abscesses or spots. Vaccine prophylaxis has been used in laboratory workers, but is rarely indicated for children. The killed vaccine does not appear to prevent local infection, but may prevent the resulting systemic infection or may modify the severity of the disease. The viable attenuated vaccine recently in use appears to offer protection against respiratory challenge in experimental subjects, and appears to be the material of choice. The causative agent is not destroyed by digestive processes in the stomach, and recent successful trials of an oral attenuated vaccine in both monkeys and humans suggest that this might eventually become the vaccine of choice for the individual at high risk from infection. In spite of the routine use of vaccines in laboratory workers, there are now over 200 cases of tularemia recorded in this group.

Treatment

Streptomycin is the most effective drug in the treatment of tularemia. It is bactericidal at concentrations of 1.9 micrograms per milliliter; if the strain is resistant to the drug, it will remain resistant regardless of concentration. Dosage in children should be 20 to 40 mg. per kilogram per day in divided doses, the total dosage not to exceed 1 gm. daily. Treatment is continued for seven to ten days; relapses have not been observed with this plan of therapy. The later in the course of the disease that streptomycin is started, the slower will be the response.

The tetracyclines are also effective drugs in the treatment. Because they are bacteriostatic, relapses are common if they are begun too early in the course of the disease, before host immune response has been initiated. Relapses respond promptly, however, to a second course of the drug. Tetracyclines are used in a dosage of 20 to 40 mg. per kilogram per day in divided doses orally, or 12 to 20 mg. per kilogram per day intramuscularly or intravenously for at least ten days. Chloramphenicol in dosage of 50 to 100 mg. per kilogram per day orally or intramuscularly may be used when the other drugs are for any reason contraindicated.

For the individual case, general supportive measures are used for fever and pain, including the use of acetylsalicylic acid, analgesics and sedatives. Local treatment is largely symptomatic, with emphasis on the maintenance of cleanliness. Surgical intervention with the drainage of suppurative processes may be necessary, but may be accompanied by systemic reactions. Isolation is generally not considered necessary, although exudates and dressings should be handled with rubber gloves. Ocular lesions may be treated with saline soaks, and topical atropine may be used for corneal ulcers.

Untreated, the majority of patients will recover in six to eight weeks, but with a rather protracted convalescence. Suitable antibiotic therapy greatly shor-tens both the duration and severity of the infectious process.

REFERENCES

Anderson, R. A.: Oculoglandular tularemia. *J. Iowa Med. Soc.*, *60*:21, 1970.

Archer, V. W., Blackford, S. D., and Wissler, J. E.: Pulmonary manifestations in human tularemia. *J.A.M.A.*, *104*:895, 1935.

Brooks, G. P., and Buchanan, T. M.: Tularemia in the United States. *J. Infect. Dis.*, *121*:359, 1970.

Buchanan, T. M., Brooks, G. F., and Brachman, P. S.: The tularemia skin test. *Ann. Intern. Med.*, *74*:336, 1971.

Burroughs, A. L., Holdenried, R., Longanecker, D. B., and Meyer, K. F.: A field study of latent tularemia in rodents with a list of all known naturally infected vertebrates. *J. Infect. Dis.*, *76*:115, 1945.

Faust, E. C., and Russell, P. F.: Tularemia. In *Clinical Parasitology*, 7th Ed. Philadelphia, Lea & Febiger, 1964, p. 762.

Gould, S. E., Hinerman, D. L., Batsakis, J. G., and Beamer, P. R.: Diagnostic patterns in diseases of the reticulo-endothelial system. Tularemia. *Am. J. Clin. Pathol.*, *41*:419, 1964.

Hughes, W. T.: Tularemia in children. *J. Pediatr.*, *62*:495, 1963.

Klock, L. E., Olsen, P. F., and Fukushima, T.: Tularemia epidemic assocated with the deer fly. *J.A.M.A.*, *226*:149, 1973.

Ljung, O.: Intradermal and agglutination tests in tularemia. *Acta Med. Scand.*, *160*:149, 1958.

Ljung, O.: The intradermal test in tularemia. *Acta Med. Scand.*, *160*:135, 1958.

Miller, R. P., and Bates, J. H.: Pleuropulmnary tularemia—a review of 29 cases. *Am. Rev. Resp. Dis.*, *99*:31, 1969.

Morbidity and Mortality Weekly Reports: 25:209, 1976.

Overholt, E. L., Tigertt, W. D., Kadall, P. J., and Ward, M. K.: An analysis of forty-two cases of laboratory acquired tularemia. *Am. J. Med.*, *30*:785, 1961.

Pankey, G. A.: Tularemia. In Gellis, S. S., and Kagan, B. M.(eds.): *Current Pediatric Therapy 7.* Philadelphia, W. B. Saunders Company, 1976.

Parker, R. T., Lister, L. M. Bauer, R. E., Hall, H. E., and Woodward, T. E.: Use of chloramphenicol in experimental and human tularemia. *J.A.M.A.*, *143*:7, 1950.

Saslaw, S., Eigelsbach, H. T., Wilson, H. E., Prior, J. A., and Carhart, S.: Tularemia vaccine study. I. Intracutaneous challenge. *Arch. Intern. Med.*, *107*:689, 1961.

CHAPTER FIFTY-FIVE

VARICELLA PNEUMONIA

Rosa Lee Nemir, M.D.

Varicella, a highly contagious viral disease of childhood, has taken on new interest and importance in recent years. Since the early detailed reports of fatalities from pneumonia in congenital varicella and in adults following varicella infection, the literature has been filled with accounts of chickenpox pneumonia and descriptions of disseminated varicella occurring at all ages, with some fatalities.

The virus that causes varicella has been fully described, and is the same as that which causes herpes zoster. The virus of *variola*, on the other hand, can be distinguished from varicella by both its cytologic characteristics and its pathologic lesions. The clinical manifestations produced by each of these two viruses differ also—an interesting point, especially since the name "varicella" is the diminutive of variola.

Pathology

In the acute phase of the pneumonia, the pulmonary pathologic lesions may be found in the parenchyma, the interstitial tissues, the trachea (mucosal erosion) and the pleural surfaces. The lungs are congested, and the alveoli are filled with protein-rich edema fluid resembling that seen in hyaline membrane disease. Many small hemorrhagic areas are described. The outstanding microscopic findings in the lungs are the cellular exudate in which large mononuclear cells predominate, proliferation of septal cells to form a prominent alveolar lining, alveolar necrosis and vascular damage. Arteriolitis and occasional infiltration of the small vessel walls may be found. Evidence for

viral infection is supported by the frequency of type A inclusion bodies (Fig. 1) and the absence or rarity of bacteria on staining. The many patchy lobular lesions radiating out from the hilus into all lobes of the lung may show coalescence. In uncomplicated varicella there is no mediastinal or hilar adenopathy, a helpful point in differentiation from tuberculosis.

Disseminated nodular lesions of varying sizes are found in many organs of the body in addition to the skin, namely, in the liver, lung, spleen, adrenal glands, gastrointestinal tract, renal pelvis, bladder and pancreas. The central portion of these lesions shows necrosis. Vesicular and, in the healed state, papular or nodular lesions may be seen on the surface of the pleura. Effusion in both pleural and pericardial cavities has been observed at autopsy and in x-ray films.

Oppenheimer (1944), in her report on the pathologic features of congenital varicella, added to these observations the description of foci of necrosis containing intranuclear inclusion bodies in the thymus and lesions on the placenta.

In the *healed* or *late* stage of varicella pneumonia, the pathologic characteristics of the focus in the lung and on the pleural surface and its progression from the soft nodular lesion to calcification have been described in adults. Knyvett (1965) contributed to present-day knowledge by reporting the pathologic changes found in pulmonary resections for other diseases or those found at autopsy on patients dying of unrelated causes. Calcified foci visualized in the chest roentgenogram were also associated in the same lung with

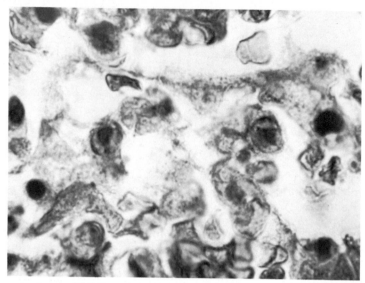

Figure 1.   Intranuclear inclusions in sloughed alveolar septal cells (× 1200) in an infant.

other small areas surrounded by an outer fibrous tissue capsule, enclosing granular eosinophilic material resembling the caseous material found in tuberculous tissue. Stains for *Histoplasma capsulatum* and acid-fast bacilli were negative. These foci were much more frequent in the bases of the lung. Caseous nodules were found with and without calcium.

Epidemiology

This highly contagious disease spreads by droplet infection from contact, with a usual incubation period of 14 to 16 days and varying from 10 to 21 days. Infection by way of the maternal blood stream to the fetus also occurs. Varicella infection in the pregnant woman may produce abortion, prematurity and, rarely (nine cases reported), congenital anomalies in the baby. Both the mother and the newborn may show the lesions of chickenpox varying in severity from a mild to a rapidly fulminating course ending in death and usually involving the lung. Fish (1960) described four such instances that were fatal for both mother and infant. There is no evidence at

present that pregnancy increases susceptibility to varicella, but when varicella occurs in the pregnant patient, the disease is very serious, especially in the presence of pneumonia, and the prognosis is guarded.

Varicella, a disease of childhood, may occur at any age. When adults contract the disease, pulmonary complications may develop, ranging from mild to serious; therefore, recognition of the susceptibility of adults is important. An infected child should be isolated promptly, and adults with no previous history of varicella infection—especially pregnant women and any patient under corticosteroid therapy—should be protected from exposure.

Occasionally, the history of the spreading of varicella to contacts is helpful in differentiating variola from acute fulminating hemorrhagic varicella. Fitz and Meiklejohn (1956) found it necessary to vaccinate 70 contacts of one such patient whose diagnosis was later clarified when variola antibodies failed to develop.

Although one attack of varicella is believed to confer lifelong immunity, Shee and Fehrsen (1953) have described the recurrence of varicella one month after the first attack in a nine-year-old boy. Reactivation of dormant varicella virus in the tissues was believed to be related to cortisone treatment that was given immediately after the first crop of chickenpox lesions to control giant urticaria thought to have been induced by penicillin.

Incidence

It is difficult to give a statistical analysis of the frequency of pneumonia in patients with varicella, a frequent and mild contagious disease of childhood usually not requiring hospitalization. Bastin and coworkers (1963) reported only three cases of pneumonia among 2225 children and 143 adults over the period from January 1960 to June 1962.

It is likely that varicella pneumonia is more prevalent than was previously realized. This appears to be even more probable, since we now know that this pneumonia in its mild form is unassociated with physical findings in the lungs and there may be no symptoms of pulmonary disease. These instances of mild pneumonia may be recognized only by roentgenograms. An unusual opportunity for a study of such cases in military patients with varicella was the basis of a report by Weber and Pellecchia (1965). All the men with pox lesions were hospitalized and received a chest roentgenogram. In the 110 patients, the majority mildly ill, 16.3 per cent had pneumonia demonstrable by roentgenogram. The incidence of pneumonia in adults is variously stated as between 16 and 33 per cent, with an estimated mortality of 20 per cent. This latter figure will obviously decrease as more mildly ill patients with pneumonia are recognized.

Congenital varicella is rare, and the extent of disease when it develops is related to the protection provided by transport of varicella zoster antibody across the placenta. Ehrlich and coworkers (1958) pointed out that congenital varicella developing between the fifth and tenth days after birth appears to be more severe than chickenpox, which develops earlier. Transplacental antibodies may ameliorate the infection in the latter instance. In their review of the literature, they found a mortality rate of almost 25 per cent (four deaths in the group of 17 infants).

Clinical Features

Pneumonia as a complication of varicella may be viral (varicella virus) or bacterial in origin. Typically, the viral pneumonia parallels the rash, whereas the bacterial pneumonia usually occurs later in the course of the disease with recrudescence of fever and the development of respiratory signs. The diagnosis of bacterial pneumonia may be established by obtaining pathogens from cultures of the nasopharynx or blood, by finding foci of bacterial infection, by laboratory aids such as the white blood cell count and sedimentation rate, and by x-ray examination of the lungs. There is no uniform roentgenographic picture in bacterial infection, in contrast to varicella viral pneumonia. The symptoms and signs of bacterial pneumonia vary with the organisms responsible; hemolytic *Staphylococcus aureus*, *Hemophilus influenzae*, beta hemolytic streptococcus and pneumococcus are the predominant bacteria involved.

The earliest large study, made by Bullowa and Wishik (1935) of 2534 patients, reported a very small incidence (5.2 per cent) of complications of any sort with varicella; only 0.5 per cent were diagnosed as pneumonia, and these were associated with secondary bacterial infection.

Varicella pneumonia is more frequent among adults than among children. Pulmonary and respiratory tract complications do occur in children, however, not only as congenital varicella in full-term infants and prematures, but also in older children, some of whom fail to survive. In some of these, autopsy reports have verified the clinical diagnosis. Moreover, autopsy specimens from adults dying of varicella infection have clearly shown mucosal damage in the tracheobronchial tree. This suggests that many of the young patients with tracheobronchitis or bronchiolitis may be ill from the effects of the varicella virus itself and not from some other agent, such as bacteria normally found in the respiratory passages.

The first signs of pulmonary involvement by the varicella virus appear between the second and fifth days. They include cough, increasing in severity, some dyspnea, and occasionally fever and cyanosis. These signs may progress rapidly to fatal termination within a few days after onset, but usually they disappear after five to seven days. Approximately one-fourth of the patients complain of chest pain. In adults, especially, blood-streaked sticky sputum and hemoptysis may be a disturbing feature. The physical findings in the lungs depend in part on the degree of coalescence of the patchy nodular areas. When the latter occurs, some dullness and diminished breath sounds may be heard. The most common findings are wheezes, rhonchi, and scattered, fine or moist rales. The paucity of physical findings in the lungs as compared with the extent of the pathologic changes noted in the x-ray film is well known (Fig. 2). In rare instances, a pleural friction rub may be present. Varicella lesions on the pleura and pleural effusion described pathological-ly may well account for the occasional physical findings of pleurisy. Pleural effusion of varying degrees has been described and usually clears rapidly without complications. The pleural fluid was bacteria free. The majority of patients have minimal lung involvement, and in general, the pulmonary infection is more frequently diagnosed by roentgenogram than by physical findings.

The severity of the pneumonia parallels the progression of the skin lesions, which in some instances may be confluent and hemorrhagic. Mermelstein and Freireich (1961) have noted that all patients requiring oxygen had widespread rash. It has been emphasized repeatedly that pulmonary complications of varicella are more frequent than the clinicians may suspect from physical examination of the lung alone; x-ray examination of the lungs may show extensive pathologic changes even though the physical examination gives negative results.

The range of severity is indicated in a study of 453 patients made by Weinstein and Meade (1956), 41 of whom developed respiratory tract disease. They classified pulmonary complications into three groups. In type I, viral respiratory involvement concerned patients whose respiratory disease was mild and subsided rapidly without treatment; most of these patients were children, and many had laryngotracheobronchitis. Type II included more severely ill patients who had an exten-

Figure 2. Typical varicella pneumonia. *A*, Roentgenogram of the lungs on the day of admission of a 20-year-old male showing diffuse mottling bilaterally. Note the normal mediastinum.

This patient was admitted for a sore throat, cough and pain in the chest for 24 hours. Difficulty in breathing and swallowing was present for 12 hours. Extensive vesicular rash characteristic of varicella developed during the previous five days. The body on admission was covered with macular, pustular and crusted lesions; there were vesicles on the hard palate and tonsils, the temperature was 102° F., respirations were slow (20 per minute) and comfortable, and the white blood cell count was normal. No pathogens were found in the nose and throat cultures. Tine test was positive. *B*, Five days later the mottlings in the lungs have cleared. The patient was afebrile and symptom-free within 36 hours with symptomatic treatment only. Although the tine test was positive, the rapid clearing eliminates the diagnosis of miliary tuberculosis. The first x-ray picture of the lung (*A*) appearing at the height of the rash and the prompt clearing are characteristic of varicella pneumonia.

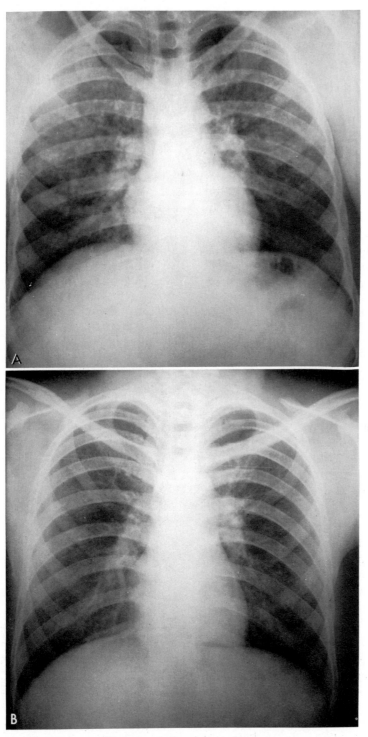

Figure 2. *See legend on opposite page.*

sive rash and distressing cough. Almost all of those in this group had fever ranging from 102° to 105° F. Auscultation of the lungs gave normal results, and the patients recovered without specific treatment. The roentgenographic findings in the lungs varied from extensive interstitial infiltration to minimal lung changes, e.g., peribronchial thickening with occasional hilar enlargement. Type III included patients whose main complaint was respiratory distress and who were severely ill with definite primary varicella pneumonia and extensive skin rash, often suggesting variola, and whose illness lasted for a period ranging from one day to two weeks. In all these, the authors reported typical roentgenographic findings of numerous, soft, rounded infiltrates scattered throughout the lungs, and hilar lymphadenopathy. Treatment of some patients with various antibiotics had no apparent effect on the course of the disease as compared with the untreated patients.

In similar manner, in a review of three clinical categories graded according to severity, Sargent and coworkers (1967) reported the outcome for 20 patients—16 adults and four children. There were six deaths; two were adults, and all four children died. Two of the latter group died with staphylococcal sepsis, substantiating the frequent observation that pneumonia in children with varicella is often associated with secondary bacterial infection. The other two children died from varicella viral pneumonia and evidence of disseminated viremia affecting the brain and other organs.

Diagnosis and Laboratory Aids

The clinical diagnosis of varicella with its typical location and progression of skin lesions is usually relatively simple. Variola, a rare disease today, must be considered in acute fulminating cases. Laboratory aids such as isolation of type A inclusion bodies from the sputum of patients with varicella pneumonia as described by Williams and Capers (1959) may be used when indicated. The cultural and basic differences of variola and varicella viruses may be pursued if ultimate confirmatory evidence is desired. The varicella virus may be cultured from the vesicles of chickenpox. Complement-fixing antibodies to varicella virus appear rapidly, beginning on the fourth day. A serologic test for measurement of antibody to varicella zoster virus by immune adherence hemagglutination described by Gershon and associates (1976) is specific, rapid and easily performed.

The differentiation of herpes zoster infection from varicella is much more difficult. The discovery of contact cases of varicella may be helpful, although contact of a patient with one of these two diseases may trigger the appearance of the other. Pek and Gikas (1965) have reported a fatal herpes zoster pneumonia occurring in a patient with Hodgkin's disease. The clinical and pathologic picture was indistinguishable from varicella pneumonia.

In uncomplicated chickenpox pneumonia, the white blood cell count is normal, although an occasional leukocyte count of 20,000 per cu. mm. with polymorphonuclear increase may be found. The erythrocyte sedimentation rate is rarely elevated and the cold agglutinin and streptococcus MG titers are negative, the bacterial cultures of the nose and throat are negative or show normal flora, blood cultures are negative, and blood clotting time, even in hemorrhagic cases, is normal.

The most helpful diagnostic aid is the roentgenogram of the lungs. The typical widespread, nodular soft densities of varying sizes in all five lobes of the lungs, usually more prominent in the bases and in the hilar regions, are characteristic, but not pathognomonic. A long list of diseases, notably among them tuberculosis, sarcoidosis and histoplasmosis, have been considered in the differential diagnosis. In varicella pneumonia there are increased bronchovascular markings and increased prominence of root shadows. We have never seen enlargement of the superior mediastinum in these patients as is often present in childhood tuberculosis with miliary or bronchogenic spread (see Chapter 46, Tuberculosis). The knowledge of a previously normal chest roentgenogram and the early and rapid, although partial, regression paralleling the course of the skin lesion is a diagnostic feature of varicella infection. The lobular infiltrate clears quickly; increased bronchovascular markings persist longer. The roentgenogram is usually normal within six weeks, although complete return to normal may require months.

In considering tuberculosis in the differential diagnosis, it must be remembered that there is an anergy or diminished tuberculin reaction during the acute varicella infection. Usually within one month to six weeks, the tuberculin reaction once more becomes a valuable aid in diagnosis.

Pulmonary function studies by Bocles, Ehrenkranz and Marks (1964) in ten adult patients with varicella pneumonia disclosed a significant diffusion defect, with abnormal alveolar capillary exchange persisting long after clinical recovery and roentgenogram clearing. Similar observations were not found in a control group of eight varicella patients without pneumonia.

Dahlström and coworkers (1969) also studied the pulmonary function of eight patients whose healed varicella infection had already produced calcification. The mean values of the static lung volume and the dynamic ventilatory capacity did not deviate significantly from the findings in normal subjects. As a group, the oxygen saturation was slightly lowered. In five patients, there was evidence of increased pulmonary shunting when breathing 100 per cent oxygen. The arterial carbon dioxide tension was low, indicating hyperventilation. The authors suggest that these findings indicate extensive lung disease, such as fibrosis, in addition to the apparent calcification.

Complications

As previously mentioned, pleurisy with effusion may be found in patients with varicella pneumonia. Claudy (1947) described at autopsy the typical varicella "pock" lesions on the surface of the pleura of an infant. A pathologic report of pericarditis in a child with rheumatic fever dying from varicella has been noted. More recently Tatter and coworkers (1964) reported a fatality in a three-year-old child with pancarditis six days after the onset of varicella and unassociated with any other disease. At autopsy, intranuclear inclusion bodies were found in the heart muscle; the lungs showed minimal pathologic changes. Clinically, pericarditis has been reported in adults. Mandelbaum and Terk (1959), in describing pericarditis in an adult who recovered in eight days, noted that it was proved only by electrocardiographic changes. This case indicates that pericarditis may occur without serious consequences and suggests that it may be diagnosed more often if electrocardiograms are made more frequently in these patients.

Other complications reported in patients with varicella pneumonia have been heart failure with shock, orchitis, nephritis, encephalitis, Waterhouse-Friderichsen syndrome, conjunctivitis and iritis, and laryngitis (one case reported as croup). All these and other reports testify to the diffuse spread of the varicella virus at the time of the lung infection.

Late Pulmonary Sequelae

From New Zealand, a country that has not reported histoplasmin infections, MacKay and Cairney (1960) described calcification of the lung following varicella in seven adult patients. Their theory that this calcification was etiologically related to varicella (tuberculosis was ruled out) was supported by the pathologic finding in one adult with carcinoma of the lung who required pneumonectomy shortly after varicella. Caseation was found in the central area of the calcified lesion.

From Australia, Abrahams and co-workers (1964), and later Knyvett (1965), published a series of articles on the nature and frequency of calcifications in the lung. These patients were adults in the healed stage of varicella pneumonia. Jones and Cameron (1969) described a fatal disseminated varicella infection in a 19-month-old child with nephrosis. Pulmonary calcifications were found to have developed during the active phase of this varicella infection, an exceptionally early appearance for varicella calcification.

The usual time for visualization of pulmonary calcifications by roentgenogram is three to five years following varicella, the earliest reported being two years. This calcification continues over the years, being present even 13 years later. Retrospective studies of some of the patients with calcific foci place the varicella infection in childhood. Characteristically, the calcific nodules are 1 to 3 mm. in diameter, irregular, multiple, usually basal and bilateral. Sequential pathologic studies from surgical material have also revealed the presence of other lesions in the lung consisting of small nodular irregular shadows with a fibrotic capsule and containing material with no calcification or in various stages of its development.

Differential diagnosis of these *late pulmonary* sequelae includes the gamut of diseases producing calcifications. Tuberculosis is more likely to produce calcification in the hilar or mediastinal lymph nodes; it may also cause calcification in the liver, spleen or superficial lymph nodes. Not all of these are seen in patients who have recovered from varicella. The presence of a positive tuberculin reaction need not necessarily relate etiologically to these foci, but a positive histoplasmin test (a much rarer occurrence) in patients from endemic areas requires careful evaluation. The calcific lesions of histoplasmosis are more variable in size and sometimes involve hilar nodes.

Treatment

There is no specific treatment for varicella pneumonia. Supportive therapy is directed primarily toward the use of properly humidified and administered oxygen as indicated to relieve cyanosis. In severely ill patients with respiratory distress, nasal oxygen or endotracheal oxygen with intermittent positive pressure breathing may be required. In a few patients, these measures will not maintain adequate arterial blood oxygenation, and tracheotomy, together with positive pressure breathing, may be necessary. Antibiotic therapy is indicated only for the treatment of secondary bacterial infections demonstrated by throat or blood cultures.

Severely ill patients with varicella pneumonia who were immunologically compromised have been treated with the experimental drug vidarabine (formerly adenine arabinoside), with some success. This purine nucleoside is effective in tissue culture against varicella zoster virus.

Corticosteroids are not indicated in the treatment of varicella pneumonia, but their necessary use in the therapy of concomitant disease may continue. In exceptionally severe cases of varicella, steroids have been used without untoward effect, e.g., in very ill patients with hemorrhagic lesions, in an adult with pericarditis, and in a seven-year-old girl with rheumatic carditis during varicella infection. However, the reactivation of the virus, as described earlier, is always a possibility.

Preventive Treatment

There is need for prevention or modification of varicella in susceptible, exposed immunocompromised persons. Varicella infection may spread rapidly and produce serious and fatal disease in such patients. These are patients with congenital or acquired defects in cell-mediated immunity, patients with malignancy, such as lymphomas or leukemia, patients with organ transplants, and those receiving immunosuppressive chemotherapeutic drugs or irradiation therapy. In addition, patients at high risk of contracting infection include those treated with large doses of corticosteroids, and newborn infants whose mothers contract varicella within four days of delivery. Fortunately for these patients, passive immunization may be achieved by one of two methods, immune serum globulin (ISG) or the more effective zoster immune globulin (ZIG).

A study by Ross in 1962 on household contacts showed that large amounts of immune serum globulin (ISG) given within the first three days of exposure modified the varicella infection in normal children.

Zoster immune globulin (ZIG) prepared from patients recovering from zoster infections was developed by Brunell and associates (1969). In a double-blind study in family groups of exposed normal children, they demonstrated complete protection for those who received ZIG, whereas those who received immune serum globulin (ISG) developed varicella. This difference is explained by the 10- to 20-fold greater amount of VZ antibody in ZIG as compared with ISG.

In a test of the value of ZIG, Gershon and associates (1974) treated a group of immunocompromised children. Modification of the disease (not prevention) was obtained if ZIG was given 72 hours after exposure in doses of approximately 0.25 ml. per kilogram. A valuable and limited therapeutic agent, zoster immune globulin (ZIG) may be obtained from the Center for Communicable Diseases, Atlanta, Georgia, for susceptible children of high risk who have had close contact to varicella or herpes zoster. Consultants from whom ZIG may be obtained are listed in the current *Report of the Committee on Infectious Diseases*, American Academy of Pediatrics.

REFERENCES

Abler, C.: Neonatal varicella. *Am. J. Dis. Child.*, 107:492, 1964.

Abrahams, E. W., Evans, C., Knyvett, A. F., and

Stringer, R. E.: Varicella pneumonia: a possible cause of subsequent pulmonary calcification. *Med. J. Aust.*, 2:781, 1964.

Alkiewicz, J. A., and Wójcińska, G.: Gangrenous varicellae with pulmonary changes in a four-year-old child. *Dermatol. Monatsschr.*, 156:259, 1970.

Almeida, J. D., Howatson, A. F., and Williams, M. G.: Morphology of varicella (chickenpox) virus. *Virology*, 16:353, 1962.

Andrews, C. H., and others: Virus infecting vertebrates: present knowledge and ignorance. *Virology*, 15:52, 1961.

Aronson, M. D., Phillips, C. F., Gump, D. W., Albertini, R. J., and Phillips, C. A.: Vidararine therapy for severe herpesvirus infections. An unusual syndrome of chronic varicella and transient immunologic deficiency. *J.A.M.A.*, 235:1339, 1976.

Asano, Y., Yazaki, T., and Ito, S.: Letter: Contact infection from live varicella vaccine recipients. *Lancet (London)*, 1:965, 1976.

Asano, Y., Nakayama, H., Yazaki, T., et al.: Protection against varicella in family contacts by immediate inoculation with live varicella vaccine. *Pediatrics*, 59:3, 1977.

Asano, Y., Nakayama, H., Yazaki, T., et al.; Protective efficacy of vaccination in four episodes of natural varicella and zoster in the ward. *Pediatrics*, 59:8, 1977.

Baroody, N. B., Jr., Baroody, W. G., Jr., and Cakell, B. B.: Varicella pneumonia in pregnancy; report of case treated with corticosteroids. *Am. Pract.*, 12:739, 1961.

Bassetti, D., Giacchino, R., and Dimic, E.: Varicella pneumonia in an agammaglobulinemic patient cured by cytosine-arabinoside. *Panminerva Med.*, 16:177, 1974.

Bastin, R., Binard, C., and Phav-Sany: Les manifestations pulmonaires au cours de la varicelle. *Presse Méd.*, 71:1873, 1963.

Belsey, M. A.: Tuberculosis and varicella infections in children. *Arch. Dis. Child.*, 113:444, 1967.

Bereston, E. S., and Robinson, R. C.: Herpes zoster and varicella in identical twins. *Arch. Dermatol.*, 83:503, 1961.

Bocles, J. S., Ehrenkranz, N. J., and Marks, A.: Abnormalities of respiratory function in varicella pneumonia. *Ann. Intern. Med.*, 60:183, 1964.

Brody, J. A., Overfield, T., and Hammes, L. M.: Depression of the tuberculin reaction by viral vaccines. *N. Engl. J. Med.*, 271:1294, 1964.

Brunell, P. A.: Placental transfer of varicella-zoster antibody. *Pediatrics*, 38:1034, 1966.

Brunell, P. A.: Varicella-zoster infections in pregnancy. *J.A.M.A.*, 199:315, 1967.

Brunell, P. A., Ross, A., Miller, L. H., and Kuo, B.: Prevention of varicella by zoster immune globulin. *N. Engl. J. Med.*, 280:1191, 1969.

Brunell, P. A.: Commentary. Protection against varicella. *Pediatrics*, 59:1, 1977.

Bullowa, J. G. M., and Wishik, S. M.: Complications of varicella. I. Their occurrence among 2,534 patients. *Am. J. Dis. Child.*, 49:923, 1935.

Cheatham, W. J., Weller, T. H., Dolan, T. F., Jr., and Dower, J. C.: Varicella; report of 2 fatal cases with necropsy, virus isolation, and serologic studies. *Am. J. Pathol., 32*:1015, 1956.

Cimons, I. M., Lacher, M. J., LaMonte, C. S., Lewitt, L., Cady, B., and Beattie, E. J., Jr.: Treatment of varicella pneumonia. *J.A.M.A., 206*:372, 1968.

Claudy, W. D.: Pneumonia associated with varicella; review of literature and report of fatal case with autopsy. *Arch. Intern. Med., 80*:185, 1947.

Dahlström, G., Hillerdal, O., Nordbring, F., and Uusitalo, A.: Pulmonary calcifications following varicella and their effect on respiratory function. *Scand. J. Resp. Dis., 48*:249, 1969.

Darke, C. S., and Middleton, R. S. W.: Calcification of the lungs after chickenpox. *Br. J. Dis. Chest, 61*:198, 1967.

DiMase, J. D., Groover, R., and Allen, J. E.: Artificial respiration in the therapy of primary varicella pneumonia. *N. Engl. J. Med., 261*:553, 1959.

Downie, A. W.: Chickenpox and zoster. *Br. Med. Bull., 15*:197, 1959.

Drips, R. C.: Varicella in a term pregnancy complicated by postpartum varicella pneumonia and varicella in the newborn infant. *Obstet. Gynecol., 22*:771, 1963.

Editorial: Chickenpox and pregnancy. *J.A.M.A., 173*:1030, 1960.

Ehrlich, R. M., Turner, J. A., and Clarke, M.: Neonatal varicella; a case report with isolation of the virus. *J. Pediatr., 53*:139, 1958.

Eisenbud, M.: Chickenpox with visceral involvement. *Am. J. Med., 12*:740, 1952.

Endress, Z. F., and Schnell, F. R.: Varicella pneumonitis. *Radiology, 66*:723, 1956.

Esswein, J. G., and DiDomenico, V. P.: Hemorrhagic varicella pneumonia. *Ann. Intern. Med., 53*:607, 1960.

Farrell, G. F., and Banshoff, A. M., Jr.: Primary varicella pneumonia, *W. Va. Med. J., 60*:204, 1964.

Fish, S. A.: Maternal death due to disseminated varicella. *J.A.M.A., 173*:978, 1960.

Fitz, R. H., and Meiklejohn, G.: Varicella pneumonia in adults. *Am. J. Med. Sci., 232*:489, 1956.

Frank, L.: Varicella pneumonitis; report of case with autopsy observations. *Arch. Pathol., 50*:450, 1950.

Frey, H. M., Bialkin, G., and Gershon, A.: Congenital varicella: case report of a serologically proved long-term survivor. *Pediatrics, 59*:120, 1977.

Gable, J. J., Jr.: Primary chickenpox (varicella) pneumonia; report of two cases seen in the private practice of internal medicine. *Ann. Intern. Med., 51*:583, 1959.

Geeves, R. B., Lindsay, D. A., and Robertson, T. I.: Varicella pneumonia in pregnancy with varicella neonatorum: report of a case followed by severe digital clubbing. *Aust. N.Z. J. Med., 1*:63, 1971.

Geiser, C. F., Bishop, Y., Myers, M., Jaffe, N., and Yankee, R.: Prophylaxis of varicella in children with neoplastic disease: comparative results with zoster immune plasma and gamma globulin. *Cancer, 35*:1027, 1975.

Gershon, A. A., Steinberg, S., and Brunell, P. A.: Zoster immune globulin. *N. Engl. J. Med., 290*:243, 1974.

Gershon, A. A., Kalter, Z. A., and Steinberg, S.: Detection of antibody to varicella-zoster virus by immune adherence hemagglutination. *Proc. Soc. Exp. Biol. Med., 151*:762, 1976.

Glick, N., Levin, S., and Nelson, K.: Recurrent pulmonary infarction in adult chickenpox pneumonia. *J.A.M.A., 222*:173, 1972.

Good, R. A., Vernier, R. L., and Smith, R. T.: Serious untoward reactions to therapy with cortisone and adrenocorticotropin in pediatric practice. *Pediatrics, 19*:272, 1957.

Grayson, C. E., and Bradley, E. J.: Disseminated chickenpox (pneumonia and nephritis). *J.A.M.A., 134*:1237, 1947.

Haggerty, R. J., and Eley, R. C.: Letters to the editors: Varicella and cortisone. *Pediatrics, 18*:160, 1956.

Harris, R. E., and Rhodes, E. R.: Varicella pneumonia complicating pregnancy. Report of a case and review of literature, *Obstet. Gynecol., 25*:734, 1965.

Helmly, R. B., Smith, J. O., Jr., and Eisen, B.: Chickenpox with pneumonia and pericarditis. *J.A.M.A., 186*:870, 1963.

Hughes, W. T.: Fatal infections in childhood leukemia. *Am. J. Dis. Child., 122*:283, 1971.

Johnson, H. N.: Visceral lesions associated with varicella. *Arch. Pathol., 30*:292, 1940.

Johnson, M. T., Buchanan, R. A., Luby, J. P., and Mikulec, D.: Treatment of varicella-zoster virus infections with adenine arartinode. *J. Infect. Dis., 131*:225, 1975.

Jones, E. L., and Cameron, A. H.: Pulmonary calcification in viral pneumonia. *J. Clin. Pathol., 22*:361, 1969.

Knyvett, A. F.: Pulmonary calcifications following varicella. *Am. Rev. Resp. Dis., 92*:210, 1965.

Knyvett, A. F.: The pulmonary lesions of chickenpox. *Q. J. Med., 35*:313, 1966.

Knyvett, A. F.: The relation between tobacco smoking and pulmonary chickenpox. *Med. J. Aust., 22*:1197, 1967.

Krugman, S., Goodrich, C. H., and Ward, R.: Primary varicella pneumonia. *N. Engl. J. Med., 257*:843, 1957.

Laforet, E. G., and Lynch, C. L., Jr.: Multiple congenital defects following maternal varicella. Report of a case. *N. Engl. J. Med., 236*:534, 1947.

Levine, A. S., Graw, R. G., Jr., and Young, R. C.: Management of infections in patients with leukemia and lymphoma: current concepts and experimental approaches. *Semin. Hematol., 9*:141, 1972.

Lobes, L. A., Jr., and Cherry, J. D.: Fatal measles pneumonia in a child with chickenpox pneumonia. *J.A.M.A., 223*:1143, 1973.

Loebl, W. Y., and Taylor, C. E. D.: Treatment of varicella. *Lancet, 1*:1037, 1966.

Lucchesi, P. F., LaBoccetta, A. C., and Peale, A.

R.: Varicella neonatorum. *Am. J. Dis. Child.*, *73*:44, 1947.

MacKay, J. B., and Cairney, P.: Pulmonary calcification following varicella. *N. Z. Med. J.*, *59*:453, 1960.

Mandelbaum, T., and Terk, B. H.: Pericarditis in association with chickenpox. *J.A.M.A.*, *170*:191, 1959.

Mendelow, D. A., and Lewis, G. C., Jr.: Varicella pneumonia during pregnancy. *Obstet. Gynecol.*, *33*:98, 1969.

Mermelstein, R. H., and Freireich, A. W.: Varicella pneumonia. *Ann. Intern. Med.*, *55*:456, 1961.

Montgomery, R. R., and Olafsson, M.: Waterhouse-Friderichsen syndrome in varicella. *Ann. Intern. Med.*, *53*:576, 1960.

Newman, C. G. H.: Perinatal varicella. *Lancet*, *2*:1159, 1965.

O'Neil, R. R.: Congenital varicella. *Am. J. Dis. Child.*, *104*:391, 1962.

Oppenheimer, E. H.: Congenital chickenpox with disseminated visceral lesions. *Bull. Johns Hopkins Hosp.*, *74*:240, 1944.

Pearson, H. E.: Parturition varicella-zoster. *Obstet. Gynecol.*, *23*:21, 1964.

Pek, S., and Gikas, P. W.: Pneumonia due to herpes zoster. Report of a case and review of the literature. *Ann. Intern. Med.*, *62*:350, 1965.

Pickard, R. E.: Varicella pneumonia in pregnancy. *Am. J. Obstet. Gynecol.*, *101*:504, 1968.

Raider, L.: Calcification in chickenpox pneumonia. *Chest*, *60*:504, 1971.

Ranney, E. K., Norman, M. G., and Silver, M. D.: Varicella pneumonitis. *Can. Med. Assoc. J.*, *96*:445, 1967.

Rosecan, M., Baumgarten, W., Jr., and Charles, B. H.: Varicella pneumonia with shock and heart failure. *Ann. Intern. Med.*, *38*:830, 1953.

Ross, A. H.: Modification of chickenpox in family contacts by administration of gamma globulin. *N. Engl. J. Med.*, *267*:369, 1962.

Sargent, E. N., Carson, M. J., and Reilly, E. D.: Varicella pneumonia. A report of 20 cases, with postmortem examination in six. *Calif. Med.*, *107*:141, 1967.

Saslaw, S., Prior, J. A., and Wiseman, B. K.: Varicella pneumonia. *Arch. Intern. Med.*, *91*:35, 1953.

Schleussing, H.: Nekrosen im Leber, Milz, und Nebennieren bei nicht vereiterten Varicellen. *Verh. Dtsch. Ges. Pathol.*, *22*:228, 1927.

Shee, J. C., and Fehrsen, P.: Reactivation of varicella virus by cortisone therapy. *Br. Med. J.*, *2*:82, 1953.

Southard, M. E.: Roentgen findings in chickenpox pneumonia; review of literature; report of 5 cases. *Am. J. Roentgenol.*, *76*:533, 1956.

Starr, S., and Berkovich, S.: The depression of tuberculin reactivity during chickenpox. *Pediatrics*, *33*:769, 1964.

Strachman, J.: Uveitis associated with chickenpox. *J. Pediatr.*, *46*:327, 1955.

Tan, D. Y. M., Kaufman, S. A., and Levene, G.: Primary chickenpox pneumonia. *Am. J. Roentgenol.*, *76*:527, 1956.

Tatter, D., Gerard, P. W., Silverman, A. H., Wang, C., and Pearson, H. E.: Fatal varicella pancarditis in a child. *Am. J. Dis. Child.*, *108*:88, 1964.

Taylor-Robinson, D.: Herpes zoster occurring in a patient with chickenpox. *Br. Med. J.*, *5187*:1713, 1960.

Tidstrom, B.: Varicella pneumonia. Treatment with tracheostomy and mechanical endotracheal positive-pressure ventilation. *Scand. J. Resp. Dis.*, *48*:40, 1967.

Tomlinson, A. H.: The incidence of complement-fixing antibody to varicella-zoster virus in hospital patients and blood donors. *J. Hyg. (Camb.)*, *68*:411, 1970.

Triebwasser, J. H., Harris, R. E., Bryant, R. E., and Rhoades, E. R.: Varicella pneumonia in adults. Report of seven cases and a review of literature. *Medicine (Balt.)*, *46*:409, 1967.

Trimble, G. X.: Attenuation of chickenpox with gamma globulin. *Can. Med. Assoc. J.*, *77*:698, 1957.

Valdés-Dapena, M. A.: Unusual pulmonary infections in immunodeficiency. *Ann. Clin. Lab. Sci.*, *3*:224, 1973.

Waddington, H. K.: Congenital chickenpox; report of a case in twins. *Obstet Gynecol.*, *7*:319, 1956.

Wallis, K., Gross, M., and Herczeg, E.: Varicella as the cause of death in an infant affected by lymphopenic thymic dysplasia with dysgammaglobulinemia. *Acta Paediatr. Scand.*, *61*:98, 1972.

Waring, J. J., Neubuerger, K. T., and Geever, E. F.: Severe forms of chickenpox in adults with autopsy observation in case with associated pneumonia and encephalitis. *Arch. Intern. Med.*, *69*:384, 1942.

Weber, D. M., and Pellecchia, J. A.: Varicella pneumonia. Study of prevalence in adult men. *J.A.M.A.*, *192*:572, 1965.

Weinstein, L., and Meade, R. H.: Respiratory manifestations of chickenpox. *Arch. Intern. Med.*, *98*:91, 1956.

Wesselhoeft, C., and Pearson, C. M.: Orchitis in the course of severe chickenpox with pneumonitis, followed by testicular atrophy. *N. Engl. J. Med.*, *242*:651, 1950.

Williams, B., and Capers, T. H.: The demonstration of intranuclear inclusion bodies in sputum from a patient with varicella pneumonia. *Am. J. Med.*, *27*:836, 1959.

CHAPTER FIFTY-SIX

MEASLES PNEUMONIA

Rosa Lee Nemir, M.D.

Measles, the most common contagious exanthematous disease of childhood, known since ancient times, continues to cause a serious problem in many parts of the world. With the use of protective measles vaccine, a dramatic decline in both morbidity and mortality has been achieved in countries such as the United States and Great Britain. These successes with vaccines, both live attenuated and killed, are made possible because of the isolation of measles virus in tissue culture by Enders and Peebles (1954) and shortly afterward by Cohen and coworkers (1955).

Measles pneumonia, caused by the measles virus alone, may occur early in the disease. More commonly, pneumonia may occur later, after the fading of the rash, when it is associated with secondary bacterial invaders. Bronchitis, laryngotracheitis and even bronchiolitis may be manifestations of a severe attack of measles. The acute inflammatory process throughout the bronchial tree may produce special symptoms of laryngeal obstruction, resulting in the clinical and alarming picture of croup. Tracheolaryngitis is a part of the measles infection; therefore, accurately speaking, clinical "croup" in measles represents tracheolaryngitis of increased severity. The ensuing discussion is confined to measles pneumonia, the leading cause of death from measles.

Pathology

All epithelial cells of the respiratory tract from the nasal mucosa to the bronchioles are inflamed (Fig. 1). Hyperplasia of the lymphoid tissue is found. There is an interstitial pneumonia with peribronchial infiltration by mononuclear cells (Fig. 2). Two types of giant cells are found: large multinucleated syncytial cells containing inclusion bodies, and the Warthin-Finkeldey cell, found in the lymph nodes and the reticuloendothelial system, probably formed by the clumping and fusion of lymphoid cells and rarely showing inclusion bodies. The first, the epithelial multinucleated cell, has been described in "giant cell" pneumonia (see Chapter 57, Giant Cell Pneumonia) the second giant cell is pathognomonic for measles. These Warthin-Finkeldey cells were first described in the tonsils and appendix; subsequently, they have been found in lymph nodes throughout the respiratory and gastrointestinal tracts, and in the spleen, thymus and bone marrow. Recognition of the multinucleated epithelial giant cells in pathologic sections is credited to the careful descriptions of Denton (1925). The first description in tissues of the tongue was made by Semsbroth (1939).

The alveoli may become filled with the syncytial giant cells, and these, together with desquamated, degenerative cells, may line the alveolar wall in a manner similar to a hyaline membrane (Fig. 3). In some instances, obstructions to bronchioles may occur, resulting in hyperaeration and bullae.

Pathogenesis

By both experimental and epidemiologic evidence, measles is a respiratory disease, beginning with infection in the upper respiratory tract and in the con-

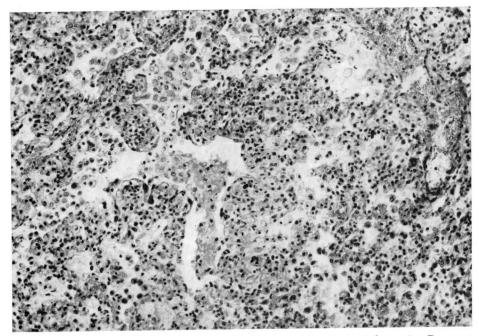

Figure 1. Measles pneumonia. Section of lung showing extensive interstitial inflammation. Desquamated bronchial epithelium, giant cells and mononuclear cells in alveoli and ducts. (H. and E., × 150.) (Courtesy of Dr. Renata Dische, Department of Pediatric Pathology, New York University School of Medicine.)

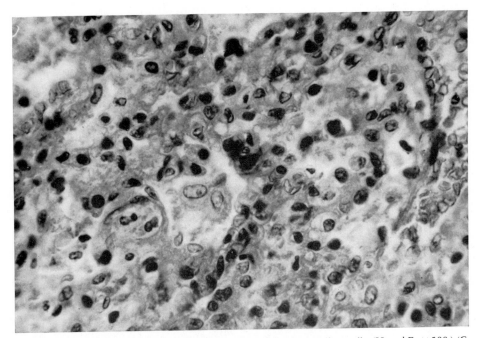

Figure 2. Measles pneumonia. Alveolar septa infiltrated by mononuclear cells. (H. and E., × 500.) (Courtesy of Dr. Renata Dische, Department of Pediatric Pathology, New York University School of Medicine.)

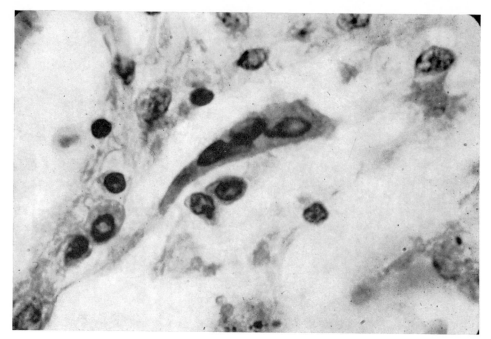

Figure 3.   Measles pneumonia. Giant cell lining alveolus. (H. and E., × 1500.) (Courtesy of Dr. Renata Dische, Department of Pediatric Pathology, New York University School of Medicine.)

junctivae. The infectious droplets from the nasopharyngeal secretions of an acute case lodge on the respiratory epithelium of the new host. The progress of infection thereafter has been ably described by Grist (1950). As Anderson and Goldberger (1911) showed experimentally, the virus invades the blood stream, producing a viremia. As the virus progresses to the reticuloendothelial system, generalized lymphadenopathy develops. This first viremia was demonstrated by Enders and coworkers (1959) by inoculating monkeys with measles virus from tissue culture. They recovered the virus from the blood within five to seven days after inoculation. Using blood from patients with measles to inoculate monkeys, Sergiev and coworkers (1960) recovered the virus as early as the third day. There is a short period of decrease in virus titer in the blood after inoculation, followed by a demonstrable viremia (the second viremia) starting six to 11 days before the appearance of the rash, and persisting for a day or two

after the appearance of the rash. The prodromal signs of measles – fever, coryza and conjunctivitis – usually occur 10 to 12 days after the initial infection and during this second viremia. Measles virus may be cultured from the respiratory tract during the early prodromal period of respiratory infection. Early infection of the epithelial cells of the respiratory tract and the lymphatic nodes, including those in the hilar and mediastinal areas, has been demonstrated by experimental measles in monkeys. Sherman and Ruckle (1959) isolated interstitial pneumonia virus from the lung, as well as from other tissues, of a patient dying during the prodromal stage of the disease.

By applying these observations clinically, tracheobronchitis is usually found at this time, and pneumonia is found occasionally. Roentgenograms taken during the first days of the rash show increased hilar markings that correlate with the peribronchial infiltration present in the first few days of the posteruptive stage of measles.

During the eruptive stage of measles, the inflamed epithelial lining of the respiratory tract with its disturbed physiology is ripe for secondary bacterial infection and the consequent development of bacterial complications. Accumulated bronchial secretions, desquamated giant cells and epithelial cells often fill the lumen of the bronchi and produce obstruction of the bronchial tree, thus promoting areas of atelectasis, areas of hyperaeration, and the growth of bacterial pathogens in pulmonary tissues, resulting in superimposed bacterial pneumonia.

Incidence

The frequency of *pulmonary complications* varies from epidemic to epidemic and from country to country, and currently is heavily influenced by the extensive use of measles virus vaccine licensed for use in 1963.

The dramatic decline in measles in the United States from 400,000 in 1963 to 39,585 in 1976 is a testimonial to the efficacy of the measles virus vaccine and its implementation. Many other countries have been equally successful. In a 1969 publication, 85 to 95 per cent protection was achieved in two epidemics in Great Britain, and in Poland in 1968, the lowest mortality rate from measles in the past 20 years (0.3 per 100,000) was reported and attributed to the widescale use of measles vaccination.

Epidemics in developed countries are still occurring despite the availability of measles vaccine for immunization. In Canada, such an epidemic in Winnipeg in 1973 affected 688 children, 73 of whom had previously been immunized, some before one year of age. In the United States, three reports may be cited. One epidemic reported from Aberdeen, S.D., between October 1970 and mid-January 1971 resulted in 292 cases (patients 1 to 14 years of age). Another epidemic reported from the Naval Hospital, Great Lakes, Illinois, in the winter of 1974 listed 32 naval recruits, 17 to 27 years of age, admitted for acute measles. Fifty per cent of the latter group had measles pneumonia. The third epidemic occurred in St. Louis during the winter and spring of 1970–1971 and resulted in an estimated 10,000 cases; 44 per cent of these were vaccine failures.

A serious epidemic in Auckland, New Zealand, 1971–1972, led to hospitalization of 114 patients with measles, one-half of whom had pneumonia. There were three deaths from pneumonia, one due to measles virus alone and showing typical giant cell pathologic changes at autopsy. The other two cases were complicated by additional infection and histologic evidence of adenoviral infection, identified from postmortem lung biopsy in one patient as adenovirus type 7.

In many underdeveloped countries, measles is still a common and serious disease. Morley (1962) reported on a large group of Nigerian children ill with measles (1283 over a three-year period) in which approximately one-half had bronchopneumonia and 28 per cent of these died; Morley attributed the high fatality rate in part to the severe malnutrition in these Nigerian children. Many observers in Africa have called attention to the frequency with which measles precipitates kwashiorkor. Bwibo (1970), during a five-year period (1963–1968) in Uganda, also related the high mortality rate from measles of 8.6 to 13.5 per cent to severe malnutrition. One-half of the 83 deaths in this series were complicated by bronchopneumonia.

Factors Affecting Susceptibility and Severity

A study of the effect of *malnutrition* on the antibody response to live attenuated measles vaccine was made in 20 malnourished children and 20 matched healthy controls (Chandra, 1975). Serum and IgA antibody levels were studied. In the malnourished group, the time of first appearance of secretory IgA antibody was delayed and the maximum level reached was lower.

These findings suggest that impaired antibody response may contribute to the severity and fatality from measles infection. The adverse effect of dehydration and malnutrition on patients with measles has been frequently emphasized by reports for the tropics and frequently described in patients terminating fatally.

Previously unexposed and isolated populations are highly susceptible to measles infection. Such infection is frequently severe, with an associated high mortality rate, chiefly due to pulmonary complications.

Christensen and others (1952–1953), reporting on the measles epidemic in southern Greenland in 1951, noted that half of the pulmonary complications developed early in the course of disease, in direct connection with the rash, and during the prodromal period; the other half developed late in the disease. Fatalities from measles pneumonia largely occur late in the course of the disease and are due to secondary bacterial infection. Antibiotic therapy is effective against these complications. The fall in mortality rate before measles immunization was in large measure due to control of these late bacterial infections. Deaths from measles (all causes) in the United States in 1974 were 20, compared with 552 in 1959.

Patients with immunologic deficits, whether genetic or related to disease, may have severe and often fatal measles. Illustrating the former is a report of a boy with dysgammaglobulinemia who developed disseminated measles following attenuated measles vaccine and died of giant cell pneumonia seven weeks later (Mawhinney and coworkers, 1971). Patients with leukemia and lymphoma have increased susceptibility to infection by the measles virus because of lowered resistance as a function of their disease and as a function of their therapy, whether antimetabolites, chemotherapy or irradiation. Several deaths from measles pneumonia in such children have been reported, one in a 70-year-old woman

receiving long-term chemotherapy for leukemia. In the latter patient, measles virus was identified by electron microscopy (Akhtar and Young, 1973).

Respiratory Symptoms and Signs

Inflammation of the conjunctivae and mucous membrane of the nasopharynx may occur even at the time of the initial invasion of the virus, with mild transient respiratory symptoms and the horizontal red lines in the conjunctivae described by Papp (1956). In general, however, the first signs of measles infection occur later, during the prodromal period, after an average incubation period of 10 to 12 days. These signs include profuse mucoserous nasal discharge, sneezing, excessive tearing and photophobia, a mild irritating cough, Koplik spots and some fever. As the rash develops, the fever mounts and the inflammation in the tracheobronchial tree progresses. Cough increases and often develops a "barking" quality. Transient musical and occasional moist rales and rhonchi may be heard in the lungs.

Most patients recover within a few days, although a mild cough may linger for a while. In some patients, a recrudescence of the disease or an increasing severity of the initial symptoms is noted with increase in the fever. These patients must be examined carefully for evidence of complications, encephalitis, otitis media, lymphadenitis, sinusitis and pulmonary disease—either bronchitis, tracheobronchitis, bronchiolitis or pneumonia. Excessive mucoid and mucopurulent secretions may be found in the posterior pharyngeal spaces. A hoarse voice or barking cough may call attention to increased infection in the larynx. Physical findings suggesting obstruction of bronchi, either partial or complete, may be obtained. Hyperresonance and decreased breath sounds suggest areas of hyperaeration and large bullae. These areas may clear quickly if they are due to endobronchial obstruction from mucoid secretions and desquamated epithelial material, or they may remain longer if they are also associated with bronchopneumonia and peribronchial inflammation. Similarly, complete obstruction with segmental collapse may clear readily or remain longer, depending on the underlying disease.

Bacterial pneumonia during the course of measles may be detected not only by means of laboratory aids described previously, but also by clinical observations of the patients. An increase in respiratory distress, and areas of consolidation, for example, found in examination of the lungs, suggest the presence of bacterial pneumonia in measles.

Diagnosis

When pneumonia occurs during the typical clinical picture of measles, there is usually no difficulty in making the diagnosis. In most instances, when the diagnosis of measles is not clear, laboratory and immunologic aids may be helpful.

Antibody formation in measles can be measured by the hemagglutination inhibition test, by the complement-fixing antibodies, which appear within two to three days, and by the neutralizing antibodies, which appear as the rash begins to subside, often as early as the fourth day after the appearance of the rash.

The measles epidemic in Greenland in 1951, a virgin area for measles infection, furnished a unique opportunity for the study of antibody titers. Bech (1962) showed that one-third of 71 patients had complement-fixing antibodies on the first day after the onset of the exanthem. Within a short time, the titers reached high levels; on the second postexanthematous day, the majority had titers of 1:32 to 1:512.

The usual antibody response, however, may be suppressed in patients who are debilitated or have long-standing disease, notably leukemia. Determination of antibody titer may differentiate the immune person from the nonimmune. Bech showed a more rapid rise in antibody level in immune persons after exposure to measles. The newborn infant receives transplacental antibodies from an immune mother; these antibodies usually persist for the first five months of life (Krugman and coworkers, 1965).

Fluorescent antibody technique may enable us to make an early presumptive diagnosis. It may be helpful when the disease is atypical, in experimental work, or when a retrospective or necropsy diagnosis of the origin is to be made, or in the clarification of the agent of giant cell pneumonia.

In the prodromal period of measles, typical multinucleated giant cells, sometimes containing inclusion bodies, may be demonstrated in smears from nasal secretions, and from nasal, conjunctival and buccal tissue, including areas over Koplik's spots (Tompkins and Macaulay, 1955). The appearance of these giant epithelial cells before the exanthem may be of diagnostic assistance. They rapidly decrease, disappearing on the fifth to seventh day, although they may be found in the urine some days later. The specificity of these cells in nasal secretions has been established for humans (Mottet and Szanton, 1961); similar cells have been found in dogs with distemper. The practicality and usefulness of this test were demonstrated in Africa, where the dark pigmented skin of patients made recognition of exanthem and diagnosis more difficult and where early diagnosis to prevent spread of infection was also important (Lightwood and Nolan, 1970).

Measles pneumonia of viral origin alone occurs early in the course of the disease. Later bacterial infection may produce symptoms of pulmonary disease. Certain tests are diagnostically helpful, such as white blood cell counts, bacterial cultures, erythrocyte sedimentation test, and radiograms. For example, the white blood cell count shifts from the usual leukopenia with slight lymphocytosis at the onset of disease to a leukocytosis with polymorphonuclear increase as secondary bacterial infections occur. The most common bacterial invaders of the respiratory tract are the staphylococcus, hemolytic streptococcus, pneumococcus and *Hemophilus influenzae.* These were reported as etiologic agents by Weinstein and Franklin (1949) in their study of 163 children with measles, 25 per cent of whom had pneumonia.

A roentgenogram of the chest is essential in the diagnosis of pulmonary complications in measles (Fig. 4). Since the tracheobronchial tree (Figs. 5 and 6) and bronchopulmonary lymph nodes

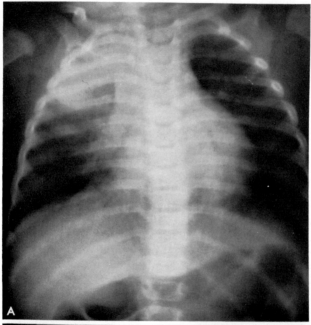

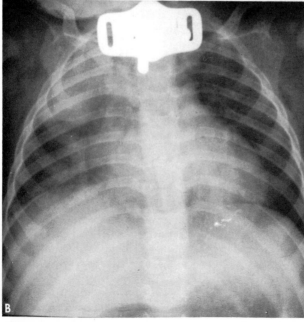

Figure 4. *A,* Roentgenogram of chest, taken on admission three days after onset of measles rash, showing homogeneous density in the right upper lobe and some prominence of the right root. *B,* Three days after admission and two days after tracheostomy. Respiratory distress was relieved, although the right upper lobe pulmonary shadow remains.

are always infected in measles, it is logical to assume that the chest roentgenogram will show some evidence of this involvement.

Our experience on the Pediatric Service at Bellevue Hospital is that the majority of chest roentgenograms show a picture commonly seen in viral pneumonia (Fig. 7). There are increased bronchovascular markings radiating out from the hilar areas, especially into the lower lobes, and enlargement of the bronchopulmonary nodes in the hilar areas. These radiographic findings may persist several weeks after recovery from measles. Rarely, pronounced enlargement in the superior mediastinum is seen, similar to that in childhood tuberculosis.

When bronchopneumonia becomes established, the areas of increased density may coalesce. Patchy areas of unequal aerations with blebs and atelectasis may appear and disappear; emphysematous blebs may also be a complication. These findings are not specific for measles and are found in common with other viral bronchopneumonias. Occasionally segmental collapse occurs, but usually clears as the infection subsides.

The radiologic lung changes of 897 cases from Manchester, England, seen from January 1948 to June 1955 were categorized by Fawcitt and Parry (1957). In addition to the above findings, they reported hilar gland enlargement in 63 per cent.

At present, with antibiotics readily available, the majority of pulmonary lesions are due to measles virus alone. Roentgenographic evidence of superimposed bacterial pulmonary infection will vary, depending on the type of invading organism.

A persisting pulmonary shadow in the roentgenogram that does not coincide with the criteria for a bacterial pneumonia (negative bacterial cultures and so on) may be due to a collapsed segment or lobe of the lung, secondary either to the measles infection or to

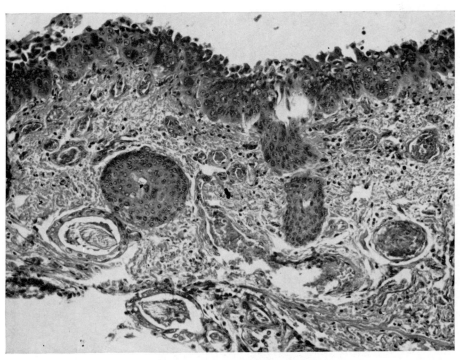

Figure 5. Measles tracheitis (×150).

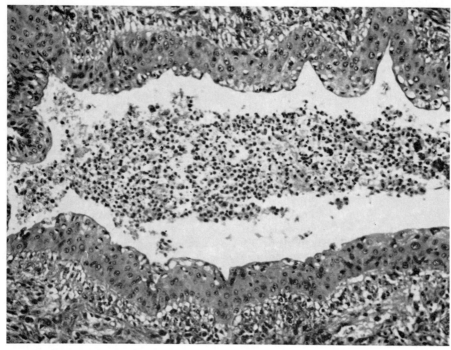

Figure 6. Extensive bronchitis and squamous cell metaplasia seen in autopsy material of a patient dying of measles pneumonia (× 150).

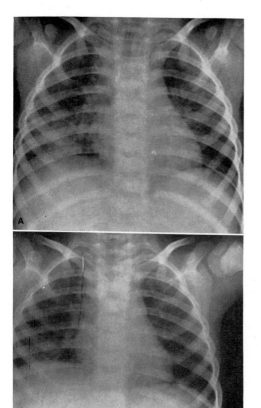

Figure 7. *A,* Four days after admission, pulmonary infiltration is seen in the right base above the diaphragm. There are also mottled soft lesions of irregular size in the right lung near the hilus and in the left upper lobe. *B,* There is complete clearing of the lungs six days later.

tuberculous bronchopulmonary nodes; or it may represent a tuberculous pulmonary infiltrate. Tuberculosis cannot be ruled out on the basis of a negative tuberculin skin test alone. The skin reaction to tuberculin is greatly decreased during the period of active measles infection (Fig. 8); therefore, a tuberculin test should be repeated three to six weeks later.

DIAGNOSIS OF MEASLES PNEUMONIA WITHOUT RASH. The verification of such an entity was made by Enders and his coworkers (1959b) when they cultured measles virus from three children dying of "giant cell" pneumonia. All of them were ill with other serious conditions, cystic fibrosis, leukemia and Letterer-Siwe disease. A 1959 report in a 12-month-old infant added another instance of pulmonary disease without rash, diagnosed as measles at autopsy. This baby had been exposed to measles shortly before the fatal illness. Similar reports continue to appear. Immuno-

logic studies and nasal secretion smears for giant epithelial cells described previously may be of diagnostic value in such instances.

The question of the relation of measles to distemper virus infections and especially to giant cell pneumonia (Hecht's disease) is provocative. Measles virus vaccine has been used successfully in protecting dogs from distemper and appears to be superior to the conventional distemper vaccine or to gamma globulin (Ablett, 1970). With regard to giant cell pneumonia and measles, the histopathologic similarity described by Pinkerton and coworkers (1945) initiated many subsequent articles and studies, and Janigan (1961) concluded that the measles virus is a specific etiologic agent in giant cell pneumonia. Measles virus was isolated from the lung of a child whose autopsy was described as showing giant cell pneumonia. Three weeks previously this patient had a measles rash (McLean and co-

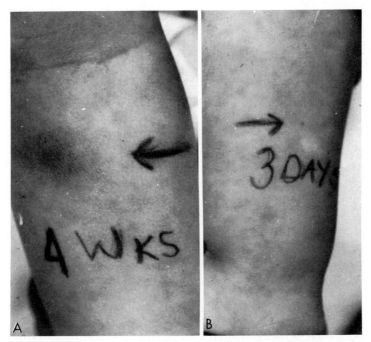

Figure 8.   Tuberculin test on a patient with tuberculosis admitted to the hospital for measles. *A,* The pigmented areas resulting from an intermediate PPD given four weeks before onset of measles. *B,* Negative result to similar tuberculin test three days after onset of measles. The positive tuberculin reaction returned 17 days after the measles rash.

workers, 1966). A full discussion of giant cell pneumonia is given in Chapter 57.

Complications

Obstructive lesions in the diseased lower respiratory tract may lead to *mediastinal emphysema*, although this is not a common complication. There were three in the 897 patients studied by Fawcitt and Parry (1957), and occasional other references are found in the literature.

The mechanism for the development of mediastinal emphysema has been described by Macklin and Macklin (1944). Rupture of diseased alveoli with blebs and the coalescence of adjacent blebs into large bullae form the framework for pulmonary interstitial emphysema. The trapped air follows the path of least resistance and proceeds along the sheaths of blood vessels and adjacent bronchi either toward the mediastinum and along the structures upward to the mediastinum and around the heart, the usual route, or peripherally to the pleura, producing a pneumothorax.

Atelectasis in single or multiple lobes of the lungs occurs in patients of all ages with measles, although less frequently than in patients with pertussis. Fawcitt and Parry obtained roentgenographic evidence of atelectasis in 28.4 per cent of the patients in their series, practically all of whom were over one year of age. If atelectasis persists for a time and secondary bacterial infection occurs, bronchiectasis may be the ultimate outcome (see Chapter 25). A patient with long-standing atelectasis should be considered a potential candidate for bronchiectasis. If clinical signs and impairment of health corroborate the suspicion of lung damage, bronchograms should be obtained.

With the possible exception of staphylococcal infections, *empyema* is a rare complication today when broad-spectrum antibiotic therapy is available. In contrast, in the 1937 pathologic study by Degen of 100 cases of measles, empyema was described in 13 per cent and pleurisy in 27 per cent. In this same study, four patients were described with exudative pericarditis.

The deleterious effect of measles on active tuberculosis has been common knowledge. On our Children's Tuberculosis Ward at Bellevue Hospital prior to 1960, there were many instances of tuberculous meningitis, bronchogenic spread of tuberculosis, and miliary tuberculosis following measles. Recognizing the possible flare-up of tuberculosis precipitated by measles, we have stressed the importance of isoniazid (INH) therapy "to cover" this period of greater susceptibility. We have arbitrarily suggested a three-week period of therapy for children known to be positive tuberculin reactors who are not receiving therapy. (For further details see Chapter 46.)

A most instructive documentation of the effect of measles on tuberculosis was made during the Greenland epidemic in 1951 by Bech (1962). Of 352 radiograms taken on patients one month prior to the epidemic and found negative, 19 showed pulmonary infiltration on reexamination three months later. Acid-fast bacilli were found in the sputum of 13 of these.

Re-evaluation of these and other long accepted data is the subject of an editorial (Flick, 1976) in which the author suggests that "if measles does have a deleterious influence on tuberculosis, it is probably at low frequency in most populations." In our experience, it is true that spread of tuberculous disease associated with measles as seen two or more decades ago before the widespread use of INH is very rare.

A second effect of measles and the administration of measles vaccine on tuberculosis is the suppression of tuberculin sensitivity as measured by the tuberculin reaction (Helms and Helms, 1958; Starr and Berkovich, 1964; Brody and coworkers, 1964). Clinically, we are quite familiar with this phenomenon. Considerable variation in time occurs in the return of tuberculin sensitivity, ranging from ten days to five weeks, with an average of 18 days after the onset of the rash.

Treatment

Symptomatic care of patients with measles should be carefully supervised; whenever complications arise, close observation and appropriate specific therapy must be provided. Bendz and Engström (1953), for example, reported the risk of asphyxiation in measles encephalitis. Cough may require medication, but we are cautious in the use of codeine mixtures. Humidified atmosphere is helpful for tracheitis. Patients with signs of obstructive laryngotracheitis should be observed closely, preferably in a hospital, where tracheostomy may be done if the symptoms of increased respiratory distress and restlessness suggest impending serious obstruction.

There is no specific treatment for measles interstitial pneumonia. Humidity and oxygen therapy are used as indicated for anoxia. Antibiotic therapy as a preventive measure is not desirable routinely; in fact, possible harm may result from its use by superimposed infection. Bacterial cultures in the severely ill patient should be taken early in the course of disease as a guide to therapy in the event of complications.

The treatment of bacterial pneumonia is described in Chapters 18 and 19. Careful and repeated cultures of the nasopharynx and blood help to determine the choice of therapeutic agents.

Prevention

Nonimmune persons known to have been exposed within a period of four days should be protected with gamma globulin.

Extensive use of measles virus vaccine in a worldwide program has shown that measles immunization is safe, effective and long-lasting. Krugman (1971), in a ten-year follow-up of children immunized with live measles vaccine, observed clinical protection against measles and a rise in protective antibody titer when these children were exposed in epidemics even eight and one-half years later. Many studies in this country and elsewhere have reflected the high level of immunity (95 to 98 per cent) obtained from a live measles vaccination. It is hoped that a concerted, well designed worldwide immunization program will continue in an effort to eradicate this disease.

ATYPICAL MEASLES PNEUMONIA
In Children Previously Immunized With Killed Measles Virus Vaccine

The dramatic results achieved in the control of measles can be attributed to the use of measles vaccine. Two vaccines were licensed for use in the United States in 1963: live attenuated measles virus vaccine (Edmonston B type), and formalin-inactivated alum-precipitated vaccine, now no longer used. This latter killed virus vaccine originally was given to patients in whom live virus was postulated to have a possible harmful effect. These were children receiving immunodepressant drugs, such as corticosteroids or antimetabolites, or those acutely ill or infected with disease that would be affected adversely by live measles virus, e.g., tuberculosis.

Withdrawal of killed vaccine followed the report of Rauh and Schmidt in 1965. They described the findings in 125 children immunized two and one half years previously with killed virus vaccine when they were intimately exposed in an epidemic of clinical measles. Fifty-four of these children developed some form of measles, predominantly a modified form. Most surprising was the *atypical measles* seen in eight (6.4 per cent) of those infected. The atypical features were an unusual rash (in appearance, location and progression), a severe pneumonia, and the absence of catarrhal symptoms and conjunctivitis, commonly seen in patients with measles. The rash progressed from extremities toward the body (caudocephalad) rather than the usual sequence of face to body and extremities (cephalocaudad).

Similar reports of small numbers of these atypical measles continued to appear in this country, in Canada, and in Sweden. In atypical measles reported from the three countries, more than half had pneumonia, a much higher incidence than in natural measles infection. Three patients who failed to develop a rash had atypical measles pneumonia as confirmed by increase in antibody titer to measles.

These atypical reactions to measles infection have been attributed to delayed hypersensitivity and to Arthus reaction. The administration of killed measles vaccine (KMV) results in delayed hypersensitivity to measles virus antigen and to specific serum antibodies. With the passage of time, the vaccinée may lose more of his protective antibody than of his virus hypersensitivity. When subsequently exposed to wild measles virus, he may then have an exaggerated Arthus type reaction on the pulmonary mucus membranes; this may explain the severe and frequent atypical pneumonia. Bellanti and colleagues (1969), in a comparative study of children receiving attenuated and inactivated measles vaccines, reported a difference in antibody responses. Recipients of inactivated measles virus showed a reduced amount of nasal secretory gamma A antibody while producing adequate serum antibodies. The differences in the antibody response of the respiratory tract may account for the altered or atypical response of the child receiving inactivated vaccine to measles virus infection. An Arthus-like phenomenon is observed locally in skin reactions of vaccinées to KMV when retested with live measles virus.

Clinical Features

The onset is abrupt following exposure to measles virus, usually during epidemics. High fever, cough, headache, myalgia, and abdominal pain usually precede the rash by two or three days. Unlike typical measles, the rash appears first on the palms and soles and in the creases of the body and spreads to the trunk, often sparing the face. The progression of the rash is caudocephalad instead of cephalocaudad, i.e., face, hairline to trunk, and extremities. The exanthem is maculopapular with petechial and purpuric lesions, sometimes also vesicular in character without progression to crusting; it is occasionally urticarial. Edema of the extremities is often observed. Soon pulmonary symptoms and signs develop that suggest pneumonia, which can be confirmed by roentgenographic findings. Although the pneumonia is usually severe, all patients recover, and the pleural effusion, which occurs frequently, clears within a short time. The acute illness usually subsides within four to seven days.

Laboratory Findings

The white blood cell counts are low, ranging from 2700 to 10,000 per cu. mm. The differential count varies, sometimes showing a mild eosinophilia of 4 to 13 per cent, returning to normal in four to six days. The platelet count is normal, but occasional elevation of the erythrocyte sedimentation rate is found. The nasopharyngeal cultures show normal flora. Pleural fluid from one patient (Young and coworkers, 1970) was straw-colored and sterile, and contained some eosinophils.

Roentgenographic Findings

Evidence of pneumonia is chiefly that of a lobular infiltration, but occasionally more diffuse and segmental lesions are seen. Hilar adenopathy is a frequent finding, and pleural effusion is also common (Fulginitti and coworkers, 1967; Young and coworkers, 1970). In general, these pulmonary lesions clear completely, but Young described a residual 1.5 to 4 cm. nodular lesion in some of his patients, the lesion remaining for many months—one for as long as 30 months.

Treatment

No specific treatment is required once the diagnosis is clarified. Antibiotics and antipyretics given early in the disease did not alter its course.

Prevention

Since killed measles is no longer recommended, this type of atypical measles pneumonia should gradually disappear. This atypical measles syndrome, however, was described by Cherry and colleagues (1972) in six children who had previously received attenuated measles virus vaccine. Awareness of the clinical picture as herein described may be helpful to the clinician.

REFERENCES

Ablett, R. E.: Prophylaxis and clinical evaluation concerning measles virus for distemper immunization. *J. Am. Vet. Assoc., 156*:1766, 1970.

Adams, J. M., and Imagawa, D. T.: The relationship of canine distemper to human respiratory disease. *Pediatr. Clin. North Amer., 4*:193, 1957.

Akhtar, M., and Young, I.: Measles giant cell pneumonia in an adult following long-term chemotherapy. *Arch. Pathol., 96*:145, 1973.

Anderson, J. F., and Goldberger, J.: The period of infectivity of the blood in measles. *J.A.M.A., 57*:113, 1911.

Archibold, W. R., Weller, R. O., and Meadow, S. R.: Measles pneumonia and the nature of the inclusion-bearing giant cells: a light and electron microscope study. *J. Pathol., 103*:27, 1971.

Baratta, R. O., Ginter, M. C., Price, M. A., Walker, J. W., Skinner, R. G., Prather, E. C., and David, J. K.: Measles (rubeola) in previously immunized children. *Pediatrics, 46*:397, 1970.

Barkin, R. M.: Measles mortality. Analysis of the primary cause of death. *Am. J. Dis. Child., 129*:307, 1975.

Barsky, P.: Measles: Winnipeg, 1973. *Can. Med. Assoc. J., 110*:931, 1974.

Beale, A. J.: A rapid cytological method for the diagnosis of measles. *J. Clin. Pathol., 12*:335, 1959.

Bech, V.: Studies on the development of complement fixing antibodies in measles patients. *J. Immunol., 83*:267, 1959.

Bech, V.: Measles epidemics in Greenland. *Am. J. Dis. Child., 103*:252, 1962.

Bellanti, J. A., Sanga, R. L., Klutinis, B., Brandt, B., and Artenstein, M. S.: Antibody responses in serum and nasal secretions of children immunized with inactivated and attenuated measles-virus vaccines. *N. Engl. J. Med., 280*: 628, 1969.

Bendz, P., and Engström, C. G.: Risk of death from asphyxiation in measles encephalitis. *Am. J. Dis. Child., 86*:772, 1953.

Black, F. L., Woodall, J., and Pinheiro, De P.: Measles vaccine reactions in a virgin population. *Am. J. Epidemiol., 89*:168, 1969.

Blake, F. G., and Trask, J. D., Jr.: Studies on measles. II. Symptomatology and pathology in monkeys experimentally infected. *J. Exp. Med., 33*:413, 1921.

Bolande, R. P.: Inclusion-bearing cells in the urine in certain viral infections. *Pediatrics, 24*:7, 1959.

Breitfeld, V., Hashida, Y., Sherman, F. E., Odagiri, K., and Yunis, E. J.: Fatal measles infection in children with leukemia. *Lab. Invest., 28*:279, 1973.

Brodsky, A. L.: Atypical measles. Severe illness in recipients of killed measles virus vaccine upon exposure to natural infection. *J.A.M.A., 222*:1415, 1972.

Brody, J. A., and McAlister, R.: Depression of tuberculin sensitivity following measles vaccination. *Am. Rev. Resp. Dis., 90*:607, 1964.

Brody, J. A., Overfield, T., and Hammes, L. M.: Depression of the tuberculin reaction by viral vaccines. *N. Engl. J. Med., 271*:1294, 1964.

Buser, F.: Side reaction to measles vaccination suggesting the Arthus phenomenon. *N. Engl. J. Med., 277*:250, 1967.

Bwibo, N. O.: Measles in Uganda. An analysis of children with measles admitted to Mulago Hospital. *Trop. Geogr. Med., 22*:167, 1970.

Carlstrom, G.: Neutralization of canine distemper virus by serum of patients convalescent from measles. *Lancet, 273*:344, 1957.

Chandra, R. K.: Reduced secretory antibody response to live attenuated measles and poliovirus vaccines in malnourished children. *Br. Med. J., 2*:583, 1975.

Cherry, J. D., Feigen, R. D., Lopes, L. A., Jr., and Shackelford, P. G.: Atypical measles in children previously immunized with attenuated measles virus vaccines. *Pediatrics, 50*:712, 1972.

Christensen, P. E., and others: An epidemic of measles in Southern Greenland, 1951. *Acta Med. Scand., 144*:430, 1952–1953.

Cohen, S. M., Gordon, I., Rapp, F., Macaulay, J. C., and Buckley, S. M.: Fluorescent antibody and complement fixation tests of agents isolated in tissue culture from measles patients. *Proc. Soc. Exp. Biol. Med., 90*:118, 1955.

Cooch, J. W.: Measles in U.S. Army recruits. *Am. J. Dis. Child., 103*:264, 1962.

Corkett, E. U.: The visceral lesions in measles. *Am. J. Pathol., 21*:905, 1945.

Crawford, K., Joseph, J. M., Mellin, H., Richardson, J. H., and Busch, L. A.: From the National Communicable Disease Center. Current status of measles in the United States. *J. Infect. Dis., 121*:234, 1970.

DeBuse, P. J., Lewis, M. G., and Mugerwa, J. W.: Pulmonary complications of measles in Uganda. *J. Trop. Pediatr., 16*:197, 1970.

DeCarlo, J., Jr., and Startzman, H. H., Jr.: The roentgen study of the chest in measles. *Radiology, 63*:849, 1954.

Degen, J. A.: Visceral pathology in measles; a clinicopathologic study of 100 fatal cases. *Am. J. Med. Sci., 194*:104, 1937.

Denton, J.: The pathology of fatal measles. *Am. J. Med. Sci., 169*:531, 1925.

Dover, A. S., Escobar, J. A., Dueñas, A. L., and Leal, E. C.: Pneumonia associated with measles. *J.A.M.A., 234*:612, 1975.

Dudgeon, J. A.: Measles vaccines. *Br. Med. Bull., 25*:153, 1969.

Editorial: Pneumonia in atypical measles. *Br. Med. J., 2*:235, 1971.

Enders, J. F.: Development of attenuated measles-virus vaccines. *Am. J. Dis. Child., 103*:335, 1962.

Enders, J. F., and Peebles, T. C.: Propagation in tissue cultures of cytopathogenic agents from patients with measles. *Proc. Soc. Exp. Biol. Med., 86*:277, 1954.

Enders, J. F., Katz, S. L., and Medearis, D. N.: Recent advances in knowledge of the measles virus. In *Perspective in Virology.* Vol. I. New York, John Wiley & Sons, Inc., 1959a, pp. 103–120.

Enders, J. F., McCarthy, K., Mitus, A., and Cheatham, W. J.: Isolation of measles virus at autopsy in cases of giant-cell pneumonia without rash. *N. Engl. J. Med., 261*:875, 1959b.

Escobar, J. A., Dover, A. S., Dueñas, A., Leal, T. M. E., Medina, P., Arguello, A., de Gaiter, M., Greer, D. L., Spillman, R., and Reyes, M. A.: Etiology of respiratory tract infections in children in Cali, Columbia. *Pediatrics, 57*:123, 1976.

Fawcitt, J., and Parry, H. E.: Lung changes in pertussis and measles in childhood. A review of 1894 cases with a follow-up study of the pulmonary complications. *Br. J. Radiol., 30*:76, 1957.

Feyrter, F.: Über die Histopathologie der Masern des Menschen. *Wien. Z. Inn. Med., 28*:Suppl. 1, 1947.

Finkeldey, W.: Über Riesenzellbefunde in den Gaumenmandeln, zugleich ein Beitrag zur Histopathologie der Mandelveranderungen im Maserninkubationsstadium. *Virchows Arch. Pathol. Anat., 281*:323, 1931.

Flick, J. A.: Editorial: Does measles really predispose to tuberculosis? *Am. Rev. Resp. Dis., 114*:257, 1976.

Fulginiti, V. A., and Arthur, J. H.: Altered reactivity to measles virus: skin test reactivity and antibody response to measles virus antigens in recipients of killed measles virus vaccine. *J. Pediatr., 75*:609, 1969.

Fulginiti, V. A., Eller, J. J., Downie, A. W., and Kempe, C. H.: Altered reactivity to measles virus. Atypical measles in children previously immunized with inactivated measles virus vaccines. *J.A.M.A., 202*:1075, 1967.

Garcia, A. G. P.: Fetal infection in chickenpox and alastrium with histopathological study of the placenta. *Pediatrics, 32*:895, 1963.

Gordon, J. E., Jansen, A. A. J., and Ascoli, W.: Measles in rural Guatemala. *J. Pediatr., 66*:779, 1965.

Grist, N. R.: The pathogenesis of measles: review of the literature and discussion of the problem. *Glasgow Med. J., 31*:431, 1950.

Helms, S., and Helms, P.: Tuberculin sensitivity during measles. *Acta Tuberc. Scand., 35*:166, 1958.

Hers, J. F.: Fluorescent antibody techniques in respiratory viral diseases. *Am. Rev. Resp. Dis., 88*:316, 1963.

Hong Kong Measles Vaccine Committee. Two-year follow-up study of measles vaccine antibodies. *Med. J. Aust., 1*:532, 1970.

Janigan, D. T.: Giant cell pneumonia and measles: an analytical review. *Can. Med. Assoc. J., 85*:741, 1961.

Jones, O. R.: Measles: a case of emphysema correspondence. *Am. Rev. Resp. Dis., 87*:597, 1963.

Josan, R., Suciu, O., Iepureau, A., and Marina, M.: On the gravity of the complications of measles after the epidemic that occurred in the winter of 1968–1969 in patients hospitalized in the infectious disease clinic of Cluj. *Pediatria (Bucur.), 19*:41, 1970.

Karelitz, S., and others: Inactivated measles virus vaccine. Subsequent challenge with attenuated live virus vaccine. *J.A.M.A., 184*:673, 1963.

Karzon, D. T., Rush, D., and Winkelstein, W., Jr.: Immunization with inactivated measles virus vaccine: effect of booster dose and response to natural challenge. *Pediatrics, 36*:40, 1965.

Koffler, D.: Giant cell pneumonia. *Arch. Pathol., 78*:267, 1964.

Kohn, J. L., and Koiransky, H.: Roentgenographic reexamination of the chests of children from six to ten months after measles. *Am. J. Dis. Child., 41*:500, 1931.

Kohn, J. L., and Koiransky, H.: Relation of measles and tuberculosis in young children. A clinical and roentgenographic study. *Am. J. Dis. Child., 44*:1187, 1932.

Krugman, S.: Present status of measles and rubella immunization in the United States: a medical progress report. *J. Pediatr., 78*:1, 1971.

Krugman, S., Giles, J. P., Friedman, H., and Stone, S.: Studies on immunity to measles. *J. Pediatr., 66*:471, 1965.

Lennon, R. G., Isacson, P., Rosales, T., Elsea, W. R., Karzon, D. T., and Winkelstein, W., Jr.: Skin tests with measles and poliomyelitis vaccines in recipients of inactivated measles virus vaccine. Delayed dermal hypersensitivity. *J.A.M.A., 200*:275, 1967.

Levine, A. S., Graw, R. G., Jr., and Young, R. C.: Management of infections in patients with leukemia and lymphoma: current concepts and experimental approaches. *Semin. Hematol., 9*:141, 1972.

Levitt, L. P., Case, G. E., Neill, J. S., Casey, H. L., Adler, P., Ferreri, S., and Witte, J. J.: Determination of measles immunity after a mass immunization campaign. *Public Health Rep., 85*:261, 1970.

Lightwood, R., and Nolan, R.: Epithelial giant cells in measles as an aid in diagnosis. *J. Pediatr., 77*:59, 1970.

McCarthy, K.: Measles. *Br. Med. Bull., 15*:201, 1959.

McLean, D. M., Best, J. M., Smith, P. A., Larke, R. P. B., and McNaughton, G. A.: Viral infections of Toronto children during 1965. II. Measles encephalitis and other complications. *Can. Med. Assoc. J., 94*:905, 1966.

McLean, D. M., Kettyls, G. D. M., Kingston, J., Moore, P. S., Paris, R. P., and Rigg, J. M.: Atypical measles following immunization with killed measles vaccine. *Can. Med. Assoc. J., 103*:743, 1970.

Macklin, M. T., and Macklin, C. C.: Malignant interstitial emphysema of the lungs and mediastinum as an important occult complication in many respiratory diseases and other conditions: an interpretation of the clinical literature in the light of laboratory experience. *Medicine, 23*:281, 1944.

Mawhinney, H., Allen, I. V., Beare, J. M., Bridges, J. M., Connolly, J. H., Haire, M., Nevin, N. O., Neill, D. W., and Hobbs, J. R.: Dysgammaglobulinemia complicated by disseminated measles. *Br. Med. J., 2*:380, 1971.

Miller, D. L.: Frequency of complications of measles, 1963. *Br. Med. J., 2*:75, 1964.

Mitus, A., Enders, J. F., Craig, J. M., and Holloway, A.: Persistence of measles virus and depression of antibody formation in patients with giant-cell pneumonia after measles. *N. Engl. J. Med., 261*:882, 1959.

Morley, D. C.: Measles in Nigeria. *Am. J. Dis. Child., 103*:230, 1962.

Morley, D. C.: Severe measles in tropics. I. *Br. Med. J., 1*:297, 1969.

Mottet, N. K., and Szanton, V.: Exfoliated measles giant cells in nasal secretions. *Arch. Pathol., 72*:434, 1961.

Nader, P. R., Horwitz, M. S., and Rousseau, J.: Atypical exanthem following exposure to natural measles. Eleven cases in children previously inoculated with killed vaccine. *J. Pediatr., 72*:22, 1968.

Naruszewicz-Lesiuk, D.: Measles in Poland in the years 1962–1968 as viewed against the background of the epidemiologic situation throughout the world. *Przegl. Epidemiol., 24*:1, 1970. (Pol.)

National Communicable Disease Center: *Morbidity and Mortality Weekly Report, 24*:2, 1976.

Neel, J. V., Centerwall, W. R., Chagnon, N. A., and Casey, H. L.: Notes on the effect of measles and measles vaccine in a virgin-soil population of South American Indians. *Am. J. Epidemiol., 91*:418, 1970.

Norrby, E.: Hemagglutination by measles virus: a simple procedure for production of high potency antigen for hemagglutination-inhibition (HI) tests. *Proc. Soc. Exp. Biol. Med., 111*:814, 1962.

Norrby, E., Lagercrantz, R., and Gard, S.: Measles vaccination. IV. Responses to two different types of preparations given as a fourth dose of vaccine. *Br. Med. J., 1*:813, 1965.

Norrby, E., Lagercrantz, R., and Gard, S.: Measles vaccination. V. The booster effect of purified hemagglutinin in children previously immunized with this product or formalin-killed vaccine. *Acta Paediatr. Scand., 55*:73, 1966.

Norrby, E., Lagercrantz, R., and Gard, S.: Measles vaccination. VI. Serological and clinical follow-up analysis 18 months after a booster injection. *Acta Paediatr. Scand., 55*:457, 1966.

Olson, R. W., and Hodges, G. R.: Measles pneumonia. Bacterial suprainfection as a complicating factor. *J.A.M.A., 232*:363, 1975.

Panum, P. L.: Observations during the epidemic of measles on the Faroe Islands in the year 1846. Translated by Mrs. A. S. Hatcher, United States Public Health Service. *Medical Classics, 3*:829, 1939.

Papp, K.: Experiences prouvant que la voie d'infection de la rougeole est la contamination de la muqueuse conjonctivale. *Rev. Immunol., 20*: 27, 1956.

Pinkerton, H., Smiley, W. L., and Anderson, W. A. D.: Giant cell pneumonia with inclusion; a lesion common to Hecht's disease, distemper and measles. *Am. J. Pathol., 21*:1, 1945.

Rauh, L. W., and Schmidt, R.: Measles immunization with killed virus vaccine. *Am. J. Dis. Child., 109*:232, 1965.

Ristori, C., Boccardo, H., Borgono, J. M., and Armijo, R.: Medical importance of measles in Chile. *Am. J. Dis. Child., 103*:236, 1962.

Rossipal, E., Falk, W., and Zanger, J.: Atypical measles with giant cell pneumonia under treatment with chlorambucil (author's translation). *Verh. Dtsch. Ges. Pathol., 56*:388, 1972.

Ruckle, G., and Rogers, K. D.: Studies with measles virus. II. Isolation of virus and immunologic studies in persons who have had the natural disease. *J. Immunol., 78*:341, 1957.

Schaffner, W., Schluederberg, A. E. S., and Byrne, E. B.: Clinical epidemiology of sporadic measles in a highly immunized population. *N. Engl. J. Med., 279*:783, 1968.

Scott, F. F. McN., and Bononno, D. E.: Reactions to live-measles-virus vaccine in children previously inoculated with killed-virus vaccine. *N. Engl. J. Med., 227*:248, 1967.

Semsbroth, K. H.: Multinucleate epithelial giant cells with inclusion bodies with prodromal measles: report of an autopsy. *Arch. Pathol., 28*:386, 1939.

Sergiev, P. G., Ryazantseva, N. E., and Shroit, I. G.: The dynamics of pathological processes in experimental measles in monkeys. *Acta Virol.,* 4:265, 1960.

Sherman, F. E., and Ruckle, G.: In vivo and in vitro cellular changes specific for measles. *Arch. Pathol.,* 65:587, 1959.

Siegal, M., Fuerst, H. T., and Peress, N. S.: Comparative fetal mortality in maternal virus diseases: a prospective study in rubella, measles, mumps, chickenpox and hepatitis. *N. Engl. J. Med.,* 274:768, 1966.

Starr, S., and Berkovich, S.: Effects of measles, gamma-globulin-modified measles, and vaccine measles on tuberculin test. *N. Engl. J. Med.,* 270:386, 1964.

Steele, B. T.: Measles in Auckland, 1971–72. *N.Z. J. Med.,* 77:293, 1973.

Stokes, J., Jr., Maris, E. P., and Gellis, S. S.: Chemical, clinical, and immunological studies in the products of human plasma fractionation. XI. The use of concentrated normal human serum gamma globulin (human immune serum globulin) in the prophylaxis and treatment of measles. *J. Clin. Invest.,* 23:531, 1944.

Tompkins, V., and Macaulay, J. C.: A characteristic cell in nasal secretions during prodromal measles. *J.A.M.A.,* 157:711, 1955.

Warthin, A. S.: Occurrence of numerous large giant cells in the tonsils and pharyngeal mucosa in the prodromal stage of measles. Report of four cases. *Arch. Pathol.,* 11:864, 1931.

Weinstein, L.: Failure of chemotherapy to prevent the bacterial complications of measles. *N. Engl. J. Med.,* 253:679, 1955.

Weinstein, L., and Franklin, W.: The pneumonia of measles. *Am. J. Med. Sci.,* 217:314, 1949.

Young, L. W., Smith, D. I., and Glasgow, L. A.: Pneumonia of atypical measles. Residual nodular lesions. *Am. J. Roentgenol.,* 110:439, 1970.

Zweiman, B., Pappagianis, D., Maibach, H., and Hildreth, E. A.: Effect of measles immunization on tuberculin hypersensitivity and *in vitro* lymphocyte reactivity. *Int. Arch. Allergy,* 40:834, 1971.

CHAPTER FIFTY-SEVEN

GIANT CELL PNEUMONIA

Samuel Stone, M.D.

Giant cell interstitial pneumonia was first described by Hecht, who in 1910 reported autopsy findings in 27 children. In 19 of these cases there was an antecedent history of measles. Clinically, the disease cannot be distinguished from other pneumonias. The diagnosis depends solely upon the histologic examination of lung tissue.

Pathologically, the lungs show an interstitial pneumonia characterized by the presence of epithelial giant cells with intranuclear and intracytoplasmic inclusions (Fig. 1). There is a preponderance of mononuclear cells in the infiltrate, squamous metaplasia of the bronchial and bronchiolar epithelium, and proliferation of alveolar lining cells. Occasionally giant cells may appear in organs other than the lungs.

The nature of the etiologic agent has remained obscure until recently. In many cases there has been a history of measles immediately preceding the pneumonia. In the absence of clinical evidence of measles, the disease has been referred to as Hecht's pneumonia. Some observers have found morphologic similarities between giant cell pneumonia and the pneumonia found in fatal measles. Other investigators have also been impressed with the morphologic and certain clinical similarities between giant cell pneumonia in human patients and distemper infections in animals. Up to 1958, it was the impression of workers that when clinical measles was present in association with giant cell pneumonia, the lesions were directly attributable to the measles virus. But since not all patients dying with giant cell pneumonia had clinical measles, the pneumonia was often re-ferred to as Hecht's pneumonia, and another virus was felt to be the cause.

The most valuable contribution in elucidating the causation of this disease was made by McCarthy, Enders, Mitus and their group (McCarthy and co-workers, 1958; Enders and coworkers, 1959). A virus indistinguishable from the measles virus was isolated at autopsy from each of three cases of giant cell pneumonia. There had been no clinical manifestations of measles in these patients. All had other serious illnesses such as mucoviscidosis, leukemia and Letterer-Siwe disease. This report suggests that in cases of giant cell pneumonia occurring in the course of other serious disease, but with no clinical measles, the host response to the measles infection is altered. Although giant cell pneumonia in patients who did not have clinical measles has been called "Hecht's pneumonia," there are no morphologic differences between such cases and the giant cell pneumonia of measles. It is likely that "Hecht's pneumonia" is caused by the measles virus in persons who do not exhibit the rash. The reason for this atypical host response is not clear, although it has been reported in patients already affected with chronic debilitating disease and with impaired immune response.

These observers also reported four children with leukemia who had typical measles followed by pneumonia; two of these children died, and autopsy showed typical features of giant cell pneumonia that had been provisionally diagnosed during life. Agents identified as measles virus were isolated during life and from tissues taken at autopsy. In these two cases, the measles

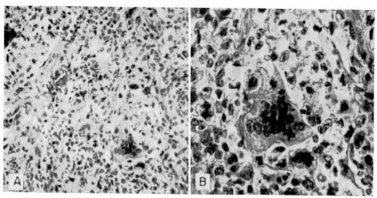

Figure 1. Photomicrographs from a lung section of a baby with primary pneumonitis, illustrating a low-power (*A*) and a high-power (*B*) magnification of the general pathologic state with characteristic multi-nucleated giant cells. (From Adams, J. M., and Imagawa, D. T.: *Pediatr. Clin. North Am.,* 4:193, 1957.)

virus persisted for an unusually long period in the upper respiratory tract, and the patients also failed to respond in the normal manner by formation of specific antibodies. The virus persisted in these two cases for several weeks after the onset of the measles rash. This is in sharp contrast to the rapid disappearance of the agent from the throats of normal children suffering from measles. As a rule, attempts to isolate the virus from normal children 48 hours or longer after the rash are unsuccessful. In the two survivors, measles virus persisted for an unusually long period in one, and the antibody response was depressed in both. Presumably, giant cell pneumonia was also present in these two children.

From the practical standpoint, laboratory diagnostic methods now available for the detection of measles virus may permit the clinical recognition of giant cell pneumonia. It is especially important to make this diagnosis regarding therapy and prevention of measles in contacts, since the virus may persist and be a source of contagion for considerable periods after the initial infection. The survival of two patients who received large doses of gamma globulin at the time of exposure suggests that this material may be of value in the modification of subsequent measles pneumonitis. Furthermore, it is possible that large quantities of anti-body administered intravenously in the form of measles convalescent plasma may mitigate this condition. Since, in children with acute leukemia, measles infection may present as a mild disease typical in course or as a fatal giant cell pneumonia, it is important to offer these children protection. Administration of attenuated live measles vaccine of Enders to children with acute leukemia appears to be contraindicated. The use of large doses of gamma globulin for passive immunization is preferable.

Giant cell pneumonia is now known to affect children with underlying disease of the reticuloendothelial or the hematopoietic system or those treated with antimetabolites as well as those with altered immune states.

REFERENCES

Adams, J. M., and Imagawa, D. T.: The relationship of canine distemper to human respiratory disease. *Pediatr. Clin. North Am.,* 4:193, 1957.

Akhtar, M., and Young, I.: Measles giant cell pneumonia in an adult following long-term chemotherapy. *Arch Pathol.,* 96:145, 1973.

Archibald, R. W. R., Weller, R. O., and Meadow, S. R.: Measles pneumonia and the nature of the inclusion-bearing giant cells: a light and electron microscopic study. *J. Pathol.,* 103:27, 1971.

Breitfeld, V., Hashida, Y., et al.: Fatal measles infection in children with leukemia. *Lab. Invest.,* 28:279, 1973.

Enders, J. F., McCarthy, K., Mitus, A., and

Cheatham, W. J.: Isolation of measles virus at autopsy in cases of giant-cell pneumonia. *N. Engl. J. Med., 261*:875, 1959.

Hecht, V.: Die Riesenzellenpneumonia im Kindesalter, eine historische-experimentelle Studie. *Beitr. Pathol. Anat. Allg. Pathol., 48*:263, 1910.

Janigan, D. T.: Giant-cell pneumonia and measles: an analytical review. *Can. Med. Assoc. J., 85*:741, 1961.

Koffler, D.: Giant cell pneumonia . Fluorescent antibody and histochemical studies on alveolar giant cells. *Arch. Pathol., 78*:267, 1964.

Lipsey, A. I.,Kahn, M. J., and Bolande, R. P.: Pathologic variants of congenital hypogammaglobulinemia: an analysis of three patients dying of measles. *Pediatrics, 39*:659, 1967.

Mawhinney, H., Allen, I. V., et al.: Dysgammaglobulinemia complicated by disseminated measles. *Br. Med. J., 2*:380, 1971.

McCarthy, K., Mitus, A., Cheatham, W., and Peebles, T. C.: Isolation of virus of measles from three fatal cases of giant cell pneumonia. *Am. J. Dis. Child., 96*:500, 1958.

McConnell, E. M.: Giant-cell pneumonia in an adult. *Br. Med. J., 2*:289, 1961.

Meadow, S. R., Weller, R. O., and Archibald, R. W. R.: Fatal systemic measles in a child receiving cyclophosphamide for nephrotic syndrome. *Lancet, 2*:876, 1969.

Mitus, A., Enders, J. F., Craig, J. M., and Holloway, A.: Persistence of measles virus and depression of antibody formation in patients with giant-cell pneumonia after measles. *N. Engl. J. Med., 261*:882, 1959.

Mitus, A., Holloway, A., Evans, A. E., and Enders, J. F.: Attenuated measles vaccine in children with acute leukemia. *Am. J. Dis. Child., 103*:413, 1962.

Pinkerton, H., Smiley, W. L., and Anderson, W. A. D.: Giant-cell pneumonia with inclusions. *Pediatrics, 10*:681, 1952.

CHAPTER FIFTY-EIGHT

PERTUSSIS PNEUMONIA

Rosa Lee Nemir, M.D.

Pneumonia due to *Bordetella pertussis*, formerly called *Hemophilus pertussis*, usually occurs during the paroxysmal stage of the disease. Pertussis may cause interstitial pneumonia, or in association with secondary bacterial invaders may produce bronchopneumonia.

Incidence

The frequency and severity of pertussis have diminished greatly in recent years. The mortality rate in the United States declined from two per 100,000 population in 1945 to 0.5 in 1960. Deaths from pertussis in this country fell from 55 persons in 1965 to 14 in 1974. The morbidity rate fell even more. Unfortunately, 10 per cent of these infections occur during the first year of life, a time when the mortality rate is highest and pneumonia is most likely to develop.

Most of the pathologic and clinical studies on this disease were made at a time when pertussis was more prevalent and more severe. Indeed, the National Health Survey in 1963–1964 no longer lists pertussis separately, but includes it in the category of "common childhood disease." This decline in prevalence and severity began before 1940, when pertussis vaccine immunization was introduced, but accelerated rapidly in the years that followed.

Pertussis is still a reportable disease in the United States. The statistical reports, although not a true index of prevalence of the disease because of failure to report mild cases, are nevertheless impressive. A continuing decline is seen in the morbidity rate (14,809 in 1960 to 1738 in 1975) and in the mortality rate (177 in 1960 to 14 in 1974). However, the curve downward has not always been a steady one, resulting in reinvestigation of the effectiveness of both the immunization program and the pertussis vaccine, its potency, composition and coverage for serotypes.

The incidence of *pneumonia* as a complication of pertussis is not usually indicated in large statistical or official records. In addition, there is a paucity of literature in recent years on pulmonary complications of pertussis even though pneumonia is the most frequent complication, excluding otitis media, and the most common cause of death.

In 1965, Jernelius reported 58 cases of bronchopneumonia or atelectasis among 602 pertussis patients observed between the years 1951 and 1953 in the Stockholm Hospital for Infectious Diseases. This 10 per cent incidence corresponds to the rate reported from England in 1947 by Oswald. In Glasgow, in 1946–1947, Lees (1950) reported a 20 per cent incidence of bronchopneumonia in 150 patients. Before the advent of antibiotics, pneumonia produced by secondary bacterial invaders was probably more frequent.

A report of 190 children with pertussis seen between 1959 and 1966 in Dallas, Texas, included severely ill patients with atelectasis (the most frequent pulmonary complication in this group) and pneumonia. Two of the three deaths were from bacterial pneumonia; one was due to Pseudomonas and the other to Staphylococcus. The third infant died from asphyxia during a paroxysm of coughing (Brooksaler and Nelson, 1967).

During a similar period, 1950 to 1970, in Hamburg, Germany, Ehrengut and Sturm (1975) reported pneumonia due to pertussis in 1674 patients among the 9240 inpatients under 15 years of age admitted for pertussis. The fatality rate from pneumonia in this group dropped from 2.2 per cent in the first period to 0.4 per cent in the second, 1961 to 1970. These observations suggest a less severe pertussis and are correlated with decreased frequency of hospital admissions and of the development of complications such as bronchiectasis in those who recovered.

Pathology

In pertussis, the entire mucosal lining of the respiratory tract is congested, edematous and infiltrated with cells. Characteristic lesions consist of necrosis of basilar midzonal portions of bronchial epithelium with clumps of organisms in the cilia of the bronchial and tracheal epithelium (Mallory and Horner, 1912–1913). The presence of pneumonia is indicated both by polymorphonuclear leukocytic infiltration of the bronchial walls and by the peribronchial collar of mononuclear cells (Fig. 1). The alveolar walls are thickened and are also infiltrated by mononuclear cells. Viscous mucus, so characteristic of pertussis, may fill the bronchi or bronchioles. Atelectasis is common, and distention of alveoli with bleb formation occurs often. Early in the disease, edema and hemorrhage may be found in the parenchyma. Terminal pneumonia may be produced by *B. pertussis* alone or in combination with secondary bacterial invaders, the latter accounting for pus, cellular debris and mucus within the alveolus. The interstitial pneumonia in pertussis is similar to that of influenza and other viral infections.

Enlargement of tracheal and bronchial lymph nodes, if present, is not

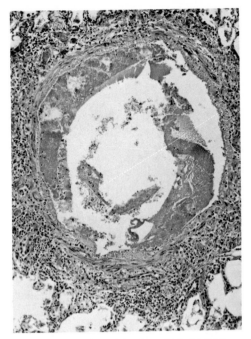

Figure 1.   Necrotizing bronchitis. (× 100.)

impressive clinically or in the roentgenograms and does not approach that seen in primary tuberculosis.

Pathogenesis

Inflammation of the mucosal lining of the trachea and bronchi is an essential part of the disease. The thick, tenacious mucus is not easily expelled, and its stagnation or presence in the bronchi produces obstruction of various degrees. The paroxysmal cough is associated with peribronchial mononuclear infiltration. Cyanosis often occurs after a long bout of coughing and is associated with obstruction to the airways by mucus, spasm and congestion. Any secondary bacterial or viral invaders will alter the clinical picture.

Clinical Features

Pneumonia develops during the paroxysmal stage. When there is a sudden reappearance of fever in pertussis, a pulmonary complication must always be considered. Rales are found early, followed by dullness and bronchial breathing. The cough often becomes less paroxysmal, the respiratory rate increases out of proportion to the temperature elevation, and dyspnea becomes apparent. If sufficient pulmonary tissue is involved, cyanosis alternating with pallor may be observed, and occasionally apnea is noted, especially post-tussic. The disease is more severe and the mortality rate is higher in infants under one year of age.

Scattered areas of airway obstruction, partial or total, are regularly a part of the pathologic picture of pertussis and may alter the physical findings associated with areas of collapse or consolidation. Blebs may coalesce and rupture, peripherally to produce pneumothorax or centrally to cause mediastinal emphysema (Fig. 2). The latter may be discovered by crepitus in the tissues of the neck and chest if the air escapes from the mediastinum along the great vessels. The physical findings of hyperresonance, the possible shift of mediastinal structures, the increased respira-

tory distress and finally the chest roentgenogram confirm the diagnosis.

Restlessness and irritability are associated with anoxia. Fatigue from bouts of coughing and loss of weight associated with vomiting are also observed.

Diagnosis

Aids to diagnosis consist of blood cell counts, immunologic tests and roentgen examination of the lungs. A clinical history of exposure to pertussis, or infection in a sibling, and the lack of or inadequacy of pertussis immunization all lend support to the diagnosis of pertussis as a cause of the presenting pulmonary disease. The white blood cell count is particularly high (as much as 100,000 per cubic millimeter), except in young infants, with a decided lymphocytosis (all normal cells). Immunization does not always prevent pertussis, but it does prevent a severe infection, and pneumonia is less likely to develop.

Accurate diagnosis can be made by bacterial culture on appropriate Bordet-Gengou medium using nasopharyngeal swabs. B. pertussis may be cultured in the early preparoxysmal stage in a high percentage of cases. Antibiotic therapy greatly reduces the likelihood of obtaining a positive culture; so also does previous immunization with pertussis vaccine. A positive culture is more likely to be obtained from patients who have been ill less than three weeks.

A valuable, specific and more rapid diagnostic test for B. pertussis utilizes the fluorescent antibody technique on material obtained by nasopharyngeal swabs. Such specimens may be sent from distant areas by airmail for fluorescent antibody study elsewhere. The test is a practical one for most laboratories, and a positive result can often be obtained more promptly than by means of culture. A combination of both bacterial culture and fluorescent antibody test is the best diagnostic approach, especially for early and untreated cases.

Antibodies produced by B. pertussis

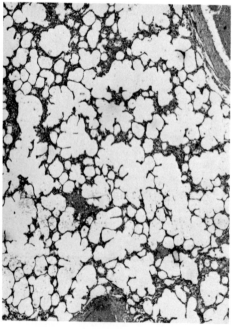

Figure 2. Emphysema. (× 30.)

infection include humoral antibodies, agglutinins and antihemagglutinins, complement-fixing and mouse protection antibodies, and opsonocytophagic antibodies; the last appear in the third week of disease. A positive intradermal reaction to the injection of agglutinogen in the convalescent stage of pertussis may be valuable in detecting sensitivity to the disease, thereby casting doubt on the diagnosis.

In a 1970 cooperative study of 223 children with respiratory infection in Dundee, Edinburgh, and Glasgow, Scotland, immunologic tests and cultures were used to diagnose patients. Approximately one-half were found to have pertussis by one of several tests used. Paired sera for tests by complement-fixation and agglutination technique and nasopharyngeal swabs for cultures were obtained. There was high correlation between the two immunologic tests used. Positive cultures for *B. pertussis* were obtained from 59 patients (28 per cent of the group) and were higher in the young patients. From those infants under six months of age, positive cultures were more frequently found than a positive serologic reaction, indicating a poor or delayed antibody response by the young infant. Conversely, in those over one year of age, a positive serologic reaction for pertussis occurred more frequently than did positive cultures.

Roentgen Diagnosis

The majority of patients show some changes in the chest roentgenogram during pertussis infection. The extent of pulmonary lesions seen on the chest roentgenogram is directly related to the severity of the disease.

Patients with mild illness may show only some decrease in radiotranslucency of the lung fields and increased bronchopulmonary markings. As pneumonia becomes clinically apparent, these infiltrations along the larger bronchi increase and produce a picture of interstitial pneumonia. These shadows radiate from the hilus overlying the heart and may obscure the cardiac borders, especially when the pneumonia is severe (Fig. 3). Occasional emphysematous areas and small scattered areas of increased density may be found in the lung parenchyma. Some of these clear quickly and may represent patchy areas of alveolar collapse; others may represent alveolar infiltration due to *B. pertussis* or intercurrent bacterial infection. An associated febrile illness is usually present in the latter instance. Lobar consolidation is rarely seen and is most often a combination of pertussis and other bacterial infection. Rarely, mediastinal emphysema with infiltration of air pockets into the subcutaneous tissue of the neck and chest as well as the mediastinum may be present. Pneumothorax is also rare.

Segmental collapse is more frequent in the older child than in the infant; it also occurs more often in severe cases. The segments affected are usually the lower lobes, frequently the right middle lobe, and rarely the upper lobes. Occasionally, bilateral segmental collapse is encountered. The left lower lobe is affected somewhat more frequently than the right, apparently because of the sharper angulation of the left main bronchus and its proximity to the arch of the aorta and the pulmonary artery. James and coworkers (1956) found collapse of the right middle lobe most common.

In general, the segment or segments re-expand as the patient improves, usually within a few weeks. The age of the patient is also a factor in the speed of expansion; infants reaerate rather quickly. Persistent collapse is uncommon in infants and in young children below the age of five years. Today, long-standing collapsed segments are much less frequent, but it is important to recognize such complications when they occur. Prolonged periods of collapse may be associated with the development of bronchiectasis.

In establishing the diagnosis of collapse by roentgenography, both posteroanterior and lateral films are needed. The collapsed segment or lobe

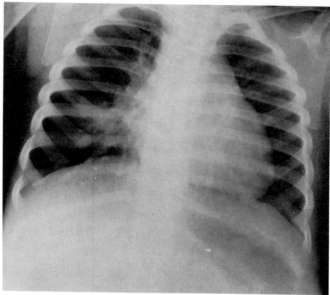

Figure 3. Roentgenogram of chest showing increased bronchovascular markings and pulmonary density obscuring the right heart border.

is visualized as a dense shadow, frequently smaller than the normal lobe; however, very early, after obstruction, the lobe may be swollen and larger than normal with distorted convex fissure lines.

Differential Diagnosis

Pertussis in its typical form is easily identified. Difficulty may arise when the disease is modified by the partial protection of an old immunization. In the very young infant, a whoop is usually not present in pertussis; a paroxysmal cough in such a patient should arouse suspicion. Pertussis is simulated almost exactly, but to a milder degree, by *B. parapertussis*. Although it is customary to think of parapertussis as a mild disease, fatal pneumonia due to *B. parapertussis* was described in two children by Zuelzer and Wheeler (1946).

The cough attributed to pertussis may be observed in patients infected with another member of the Bordetella group, *B. bronchiseptica*, and occasionally in cases of *Hemophilus influenzae*. Hoarseness is characteristic of *H. influenzae* infections, not of pertussis. Di Sant'Ag-

nese (1955) calls attention to the similarity of the pertussis cough to the paroxysms of patients with cystic fibrosis of the pancreas, a disease with frequent protean pulmonary complications.

Some patients with extensive bronchopneumonia and interstitial pneumonia unassociated with *B. pertussis* may also have paroxysmal, spasmodic cough without whoop or vomiting. These patients usually have extensive physical findings in the lungs consisting of many scattered rales and suffer from much respiratory difficulty. These patients continue to be quite ill between the bouts of coughing, with rapid and often shallow respirations. A pertussoid eosinophilic pneumonia with a pertussis-like cough (see p. 994) has been described in very young infants. A similar syndrome associated with adenovirus type 2 was reported in 1964 by Olson and coworkers. Two years later, adenovirus type 5 was isolated from the lungs of a child dying of a similar *pertussis syndrome*. The pathologic examination of the lung revealed a necrotizing bronchiolitis accompanied by cytopathic findings in the lung parenchyma typical of adenovirus infection, including giant cells containing intranuclear inclusion bodies (Collier and co-workers, 1966). Laboratory studies and a careful history of onset and progression of signs and symptoms should clarify the diagnosis.

Occasionally, patients with enlarged tuberculous bronchopulmonary glands have a paroxysmal spasmodic cough similar to that noted in pertussis; there may also be an associated collapse of a segment of the lung. In this instance pressure by enlarged lymph nodes causes the obstruction; in pertussis, obstruction results from the thick mucus within the bronchus. The presence of a whoop in pertussis and a barking metallic cough in tuberculosis may aid in diagnosis. Cyanosis, rather than suffusion of the face, is more commonly associated with the paroxysmal coughing of the tuberculous child, and vomiting is rare. Nasopharyngeal cultures for B. pertussis, the white blood cell count and lymphocytosis, tuberculin tests, pertussis antibody studies and the chest roentgenogram are helpful aids. Enlarged mediastinal nodes are rare in pertussis. Physical findings in the chest of a child with tuberculosis are often negative except for a localized wheeze at the site of obstruction.

Complications

Collapse occurs so frequently in pertussis, with or without pneumonia, that it is perhaps improper to consider it under the category of complication. Indeed, pertussis, until the past decade, was the most frequent cause of pulmonary collapse in children. It is more frequent when the disease is severe and may exceptionally persist for several months. Bronchoscopic examination may be required to assist in airway clearance.

Bronchiectasis is a late complication of pertussis pneumonia, and is apt to follow atelectasis. All observers agree that long-standing collapse produces irreversible damage to the bronchi and leads to bronchiectasis. The exact

length of time required to produce this change is not known.

Biering (1956) made follow-up observations on 62 children seen in the Blegdam Hospital nine years previously and found only one with bronchiectasis. The rarity of this complication is certainly in line with our experience in recent years. We have not observed symptoms suggesting bronchiectasis.

A long-term follow-up study of children who had pertussis in the Baltimore City Hospitals between 1949 and 1953 was made to determine the incidence of pulmonary impairment. There was no evidence of chronic lung disease by physical examination or on the roentgenogram (White and co-workers, 1964).

Pulmonary function studies of 49 children with pertussis complicated by bronchopneumonia or atelectasis were made by Jernelius (1965) seven to ten years later. Significantly lower static lung volumes than the predicted normal values were found. The maximum breathing capacity and the intrapulmonary gas mixing showed normal values.

Because of the constant coughing with increased intrapulmonary pressure and the intense venous congestion with each paroxysm, pertussis may conceivably reactivate or spread pulmonary tuberculous foci. In our experience, this is rare today.

Treatment

A number of antibiotics have been tried for their therapeutic value in clearing the respiratory tract of B. pertussis (thus preventing the spread of infection) and for their effect on the course of the disease. Erythromycin is the most effective for this purpose and is the first choice, followed by the alternate choice of ampicillin. Antibiotic therapy should be continued for not less than seven days, preferably for ten days.

When intercurrent bacterial infections are suspected, an antibiotic selected by the clinician in accordance with his best judgment may be used until bacterial cultures and other aids to diagnosis clarify the etiologic pathogen. Hyperimmune pertussis gamma globulin administered intramuscularly has been used for seriously ill patients, but the efficacy of such therapy is not established.

For some severely ill patients, oxygen with increased humidity is indicated. Selection of medication for cough must be made with care. Sedatives depressing the respiratory center are to be avoided. Good nursing care is of paramount importance because of the danger of asphyxia during bouts of coughing, when the bronchi are filled with tenacious mucus, and because of the possibility of aspiration following vomiting. Gentle suction, performed promptly, relieves the airways. Infants, especially, require the most careful watching because of vomiting in the prone position, with its danger of aspiration of vomitus, and because of discomfort, cyanosis from coughing, and emotional fatigue and distress. Small frequent feedings may be effective in maintaining nutrition, and attention must be given to providing adequate fluid intake.

Prognosis

Pneumonia is the common cause of death from pertussis and is an especially serious complication during infancy. Approximately one-half of the pertussis deaths in the United States within the past decade occurred in infants under six months. A leukemoid reaction, lymphocytosis of more than 50,000 per cu. mm., is another factor apparently associated with severe pneumonia and a poor prognosis. In one series of eight such patients, all save one had pneumonia and two of them died (Brooksaler and Nelson, 1967).

The present low incidence of severe pertussis, with great decline in fatality and, therefore, in pneumonia associated with pertussis, can be attributed, in large measure, to the widespread use of prophylactic vaccine and to im-

proved methods of treatment. Other possible factors are greater host resistance, possible decreased virulence of the infecting agent, and environmental factors that affect either host resistance or activity of the infecting agent.

Prevention

Pertussis vaccine, although highly effective, does not furnish absolute immunity. Early diagnosis and prompt therapy with an antibiotic (erythromycin) in those patients suspected of infection prevent the spread of disease. Fortunately, there is good evidence for the absence of a carrier state; persons exposed to pertussis do not become carriers of B. pertussis, although they may develop mild, unrecognized infection. With continuing vigilance in the preventive immunization program and with continuing research in the field of vaccine production and related problem areas, pertussis and the pneumonia it causes should continue to decline.

REFERENCES

Abbott, J. D., Preston, N. W., and Mackay, R. I.: Agglutinin response to pertussis vaccination in the child. Br. Med. J., 1:86, 1971.

Barnhard, H. J., and Kniker, W. T.: Roentgenologic findings in pertussis with particular emphasis on the "shaggy heart" sign. Am. J. Roentgenol., 84:445, 1960.

Bass, J. W., Klenk, E. L., Kotheimer, J. B., Linnemann, C. C., and Smith, M. H. D.: Antimicrobial treatment of pertussis. J. Pediatr., 75:768, 1969.

Biering, A.: Childhood pneumonia, including pertussis pneumonia and bronchiectasis. A follow-up study of 151 patients. Acta Pediatr., 45:348, 1956.

Botsztejn, A. von: Die pertussoide, eosinophile Pneumonie des Säuglings. Ann. Paed. (Basel), 157:28, 1941.

Bousfield, G.: Whooping-cough immunization. Br. Med. J., 1:238, 1970.

Brooksaler, F., and Nelson, J. D.: Pertussis. A reappraisal and report of 190 confirmed cases. Am. J. Dis. Child., 114:389, 1967.

Chalvardjian, N.: The laboratory diagnosis of whooping cough by fluorescent antibody and by culture methods. Can. Med. Assoc. J., 95:263, 1966.

Collier, A. M., Conner, J. D., and Irving, W. R.: Generalized type 5 adenovirus infection associated with the pertussis syndrome. *J. Pediatr.*, 69:1073, 1966.

Diagnosis of whooping cough: Comparison of serological tests with isolation of *Bordetella pertussis*. A combined Scottish study. *Br. Med. J.*, 4:637, 1970.

Donaldson, P., and Whitaker, J.: Diagnosis of pertussis by fluorescent antibody staining of nasopharyngeal smears. *Am. J. Dis. Child.*, 99:423, 1960.

Ehrengut, W., and Sturm, H.: Pertussis and its complications—analysis of hospitalized patients in Hamburg 1950–1970. *Immunol. Infekt.*, 3:269, 1975.

Fawcitt, J., and Parry, H. E.: Lung changes in pertussis and measles in childhood. A review of 1894 cases with a follow-up study of the pulmonary complications. *Br. J. Radiol.*, 39:76, 1957.

Felton, H. M., and Flosdorf, E. W.: The detection of susceptibility to whooping cough. I. Institutional experience with the pertussis agglutinogen as skin test reagent. *J. Pediatr.*, 29:677, 1946.

Gallavan, M., and Goodpasture, E. W.: Infection of chick embryos with *H. pertussis* reproducing pulmonary lesions of whooping cough. *Am. J. Pathol.*, 13:927, 1937.

Immunization against whooping cough. (Leading article). *Br. Med. J.*, 4:316, 1969.

James, U., Brimblecombe, F. S. W., and Wells, J. W.: The natural history of pulmonary collapse in childhood. *Q. J. Med.*, No. 97, p. 121, 1956.

Jernelius, H.: Pertussis with pulmonary complications—a follow-up study. *Acta Paediatr.*, 53:247, 1965.

Kohn, J. L., Schwartz, I., Greenbaum, J., and Daly, M. M. I.: Roentgenograms of the chest taken during pertussis. *Am. J. Dis. Child.*, 67:463, 1944.

Lees, A. W.: Atelectasis and bronchiectasis in pertussis. *Br. Med. J.*, 2:1138, 1950.

Linnemann, C. C., Bass, J. W., and Smith, M. H. D.: The carrier state in pertussis. *Am. J. Epidemiol.*, 88:422, 1968.

Mallory, F. B., and Horner, A. A.: The histological lesion in the respiratory tract. *J. Mod. Res.*, 27:115, 1912–1913.

Nelson, J. D., Tanaka, R., and Pauls, F. P.: Fluorescent antibody diagnosis of infections. *J.A.M.A.*, 188:1121, 1964.

Nelson, J. D., Matteck, B. M., and McNabb, J.: Susceptibility of *Bordetella pertussis* to ampicillin. *J. Pediatr.*, 68:222, 1966.

Nicholson, D. P.: Pulmonary collapse in pertussis. *Arch. Dis. Child.*, 24:29, 1949.

Ocklitz, H. W., Weppe, C. M., and Lemmer, U.: Serologische Untersuchungen bei kulturell und mit der Immunfluoreszenz bestätigter Pertussis. *Arch. Kinderheilk.*, 179:154, 1969.

Olson, L. C.: Comments. In Gellis, S.: Editorial note. *Yearbook Pediatrics*, 1967–1968, p. 97.

Olson, L. C., Miller, G., and Hanshaw, J. B.: Acute infectious lymphocytosis presenting as a pertussis-like illness: its association with adenovirus type 12. *Lancet*, 1:200, 1964.

Oswald, N. C.: Collapse of the lower lobes of the lungs in children. *Proc. R. Soc. Med.*, 40:736, 1949.

Polk, L. D.: Pertussis vaccination. New thoughts on an old vaccine. *Clin. Pediatr. (Phila.)*, 9:313, 1970.

Preston, N. W.: Protection by pertussis vaccine. Little cause for concern. *Lancet*, 1:1065, 1976.

Preuss, H. J., and Padelt, H.: Radiological aspects of pertussis and measles pneumonia from 1959 to 1969. *Radiol. Diagn. (Berl.)*, 11:655, 1970.

Public Health Laboratory Service Whooping Cough Committee and Working Party: Efficacy of whooping-cough vaccines used in the United Kingdom before 1968. *Br. Med. J.*, 4:329, 1969.

Rich, A. R.: The etiology and pathogenesis of whooping cough. *Bull. Johns Hopkins Hosp.*, 51:346, 1932.

Sant'Agnese, P. A. di: The pulmonary manifestations of fibrocystic disease of the pancreas. *Dis. Chest*, 27:654, 1955.

Standfast, A. F. B.: Pertussis, typhoid-paratyphoid and cholera vaccines. *Br. Med. Bull.*, 25:189, 1969.

United States Department of Health, Education, and Welfare: Center for Disease Control, Morbidity and Mortality. Annual Supplement. Summary 1975, 24:2–4 (August), 1976.

Whitaker, J. A., Donaldson, P., and Nelson, J. D.: Diagnosis of pertussis by the fluorescent-antibody method. *N. Engl. J. Med.*, 263:850, 1960.

White, R., Finberg, L., and Tramer, A.: The modern morbidity of pertussis in infants. *Pediatrics*, 33:705, 1964.

Zamora, A. F., Chiozza, A., and Alonso, A. T.: Complications de la coqueluche a traves de 500 casos observados en el servicio de clinica epidemiologica de la casa Cuna. *Rev. Assoc. Méd. Argent.*, 76:121, 1962.

Zuelzer, W. W., and Wheeler, W. E.: Parapertussis pneumonia. A report of 2 fatal cases. *J. Pediatr.*, 29:493, 1946.

CHAPTER FIFTY-NINE

PERTUSSOID EOSINOPHILIC PNEUMONIA

Rosa Lee Nemir, M.D.

Pertussoid eosinophilic pneumonia is a term that was first used by Botsztejn in 1941 to describe a subacute, benign illness characterized by a pertussis-like cough associated with lymphocytosis and eosinophilia; the syndrome occurred in very young infants. Since this first report there has been a publication by Biro (1960) from the same hospital in Zurich; Biro has also described two additional cases.

Etiology and Incidence

Reluctance to publish reports of similar patients seen in the United States is related to inability to offer an etiologic agent. Sporadic patients fitting this category have been seen on the Children's Service at Bellevue Hospital. In personal communication with Dr. James Bass, presently at Walter Reed Hospital, Washington, D.C., a report of many infants (over 15) with the clinical picture of pertussoid eosinophilic pneumonia was obtained. Bass observed these infants in Honolulu when he was Chief of Pediatrics at the Tripler Army Medical Center. Five of these patients were studied for a viral etiologic agent. From two of these, advenovirus type 2 was isolated from stools and nasopharyngeal material, and the acute and convalescent sera showed a fourfold rise in antibody titer.

Four infants under four months of age with the clinical picture of pertussoid eosinophilic pneumonia have been reported from Washington, D.C., and in these, an etiologic agent was not identified (Oetgen, 1977). Infectious agents, such as viral, bacterial and mycoplasmal, were not found in cultures of these patients; however, immunoglobulin studies showing significant elevations of IgM levels in all and of IgG levels in two patients suggest an infectious etiologic agent.

The pertussoid eosinophilic pneumonia syndrome recently was described in eight infants, all under three months of age, seen in a hospital in Chicago and studied by Beem and Saxon (1976). *Chlamydia trachomatis* was obtained from nasopharyngeal cultures in all eight infants, although only five had conjunctivitis by either history or examination. A control study of the presence and significance of *Chlamydia trachomatis* in other patients was made by the authors. It appears clear that Chlamydia is etiologically related to the pneumonia, being present in 100 per cent of the pneumonia patients and in 10 to 15 per cent of infants hospitalized for reasons other than pulmonary disease. Pertussoid eosinophilic pneumonia may represent, as the authors suggest, "a special case within the larger setting of chlamydial respiratory disease and chlamydial pneumonia." In this series, elevated levels of IgG and IgM were also found.

A further possibility must be considered, namely, that Chlamydia may produce disease singly or in combination with a second agent by altering the infectivity of the lung, making it possible for superinfection to occur.

Clinical Features

The patients so far described vary in age from three weeks to four months.

There is gradual development of the symptoms, which consist of bouts of coughing spells associated with tachypnea and very little, if any, temperature elevation. The patients are only moderately ill, and all reported patients have recovered. The physical findings in the lungs vary from negative findings and occasional rales to signs indicating bronchopneumonia.

The distinguishing feature of the syndrome is the absolute and relative lymphocytosis and eosinophilia. These blood changes parallel the pneumonia, which subsides slowly, often persisting several weeks and varying from three to eight weeks.

The roentgenograms uniformly show increased bronchovascular markings bilaterally radiating out from the hili and filling the inner half of the lung fields and obscuring the heart borders. In the original description, pleurisy was diagnosed from the visualization of the horizontal fissures in the roentgenogram of the lungs. Biro (1960) proposed a new title for this syndrome, *interstitial pertussoid eosinophilic pneumonia*, because the roentgenograms of the lungs were characteristic of an interstitial pneumonia, which is produced by many agents with or without eosinophilia.

Course

The disease runs a subacute course after the initial few days of severe dyspnea and cough. The symptoms disappear before the roentgenograms of the lungs become normal. It requires three to eight weeks before the radiograms show final resolution of the pneumonia. The absolute eosinophilia is highest early in the disease, within the first week to ten days, and is usually normal within a month. Leukocytosis is rarely above 18,000, although an occasional count of 22,000 to 28,000 white blood cells has been reported.

Treatment and Prognosis

All the patients so far reported have recovered despite their prematurity, small size, and the severity of the dyspnea at onset. Treatment is nonspecific, supportive and symptomatic, directed toward relief of the cough and the respiratory symptoms. Biro in 1960 varied his treatment from a purely symptomatic one to the use of penicillin, streptomycin, and broad-spectrum antibiotics, singly or in combination. There appeared to be no difference in the response to the various therapeutic regimens in this group of 12 patients. Subsequent experience is similar.

Comment

The question of the relation of pertussoid eosinophilic pneumonia to the pertussis syndrome merits discussion. There is no pathologic material for study, and etiologic agents for each are not entirely clarified. Eosinophilia is not uniformly described in the pertussis syndrome, but follow-up blood counts were frequently not done, thus failing to demonstrate the eosinophilia that may be seen late in this syndrome. Of course, many patients with the eosinophilia pertussis syndrome do not have demonstrable pneumonia.

PERTUSSIS SYNDROME

In 1964, Olson and coworkers reported an illness similar to the above-mentioned syndrome in a family of nine; they called it acute lymphocytosis with eosinophilia, presenting as a pertussis-like illness. In all these patients, *Bordetella pertussis* could not be cultured on Bordet-Gengou media. They did isolate *adenovirus type 2* from throat swabs of these children, and showed in all members of the family a marked and significant complement-fixing antibody rise persisting for months.

Two years later, Collier and coworkers (1966) described a similar disease, which they called the *pertussis syndrome*, in two siblings, one of whom died during a seizure. *Adenovirus type 5* was cultured from the autopsy material of the lungs, liver and kidney. The pathologic pulmonary condition, a necrotizing bronchiolitis, corresponded to that previously described in adenovirus pneumonitis. The surviving one-year-old sibling also had a typical whoop and leukocytosis of 30,000 per cu. milliliter; half of these were small lymphocytes and 30 per cent were eosinophils. Convalescent sera from this patient and his other siblings were negative for *B. pertussis* antibodies.

In both series, eosinophilia was found during convalescence, a time when blood cell counts are done less often. This fact may account for the failure of many clinicians to detect a feature of the syndrome. The age of the patient may also be a factor; all of the original cases of pertussoid eosinophilic pneumonia occurred in young infants.

The relationship between the pertussis syndrome and adenovirus infections has been the subject of several studies. One consisted of a 30-month study of patients with the clinical picture of whooping cough (Connor, 1970). From 11 of 13 patients, adenovirus types 1, 2, 3 or 5 were cultured; moreover, cultures and agglutination test for *B. pertussis* and *B. parapertussis* were negative. The comparable isolation rate in 200 children of a control group was 2 to 3 per cent. Leukemoid reaction with lymphocytosis was a feature of these illnesses, and eosinophilia was found during convalescence in several patients. Clinically, the majority of those under two years of age had bronchitis, and three had pneumonia (one interstitial, two middle lobe disease). Radiologic evidence of bronchiolitic disease was found in seven, and bilateral interstitial pneumonia was found in three.

Two subsequent reports, by contrast, suggest that the adenovirus in the per-tussis syndrome is not the sole or even the most significant etiologic agent producing the disease syndrome, and that *Bordetella pertussis* must be sought with great care. In one report from the United States, 19 such patients are described, only 7 of whom had evidence of adenovirus infection, while 14 had positive cultures for *B. pertussis* (13) or *B. parapertussis* (1) (Klenk and associates, 1972). The authors suggest concurrent bacterial and viral infection may be responsible for the disease in these patients.

The second study from Canada covers a four-year observation of 201 children with "the whooping cough syndrome" (Islur and associates, 1975). *Bordetella pertussis* was isolated from nasopharyngeal cultures in 139 patients, and viruses were also isolated from one-fifth of these. Those patients with negative cultures for *B. pertussis* also had viral isolations in one-fifth of the cases. Thus, once more, both viral and bacterial agents are implicated etiologically, with emphasis by the authors on the significance of *B. pertussis*.

It becomes clear that the differential diagnosis of bacterial pertussis due to *B. pertussis* and the pertussis syndrome associated with adenovirus is dependent not on clinical signs but on appropriate microbiologic studies.

The foregoing reports have reopened an old discussion of the relation of virus infections to whooping cough and have stimulated a series of editorials in this country and Great Britain. The earliest pathologic descriptions of a viral type disease in the pertussis syndrome was made by Rich (1932) and later Rich and associates (1932). Shortly afterward, McCordock and Smith (1934) described inclusion bodies in similar instances at autopsy. In recent years, these findings have been reported in fatalities of definite adenoviral pulmonary disease, clinically diagnosed as pneumonia.

The clinical similarity of the pertussis syndrome and pertussoid eosinophilic pneumonia is provocative. The crucial difference may well be the age of the patients in the latter category, all under four months of age. Etiologic agents do evoke different reactions in the very young infant. Future studies to identify causative agents should center around the syndromes within the first months of life.

REFERENCES

Bass, J. W.: Personal communications, 1976.

Beem, M. O., and Saxon, E.: Pneumonia in infants infected with *Chlamydia trachomatis. Pediatr. Res., 10*:395, 1976.

Beem, M. C., and Saxon, B. S.: Respiratory tract colonization and a distinctive pneumonia syndrome in infants infected with *Chlamydia trachomatis. N. Engl. J. Med., 296*:306, 1977.

Biro, Z.: Twelve more cases of interstitial pertussoid eosinophilic pneumonia in infants. *Helvet. Paediatr. Acta, 15*:135, 1960.

Biro, Z.: Personal communication, 1970.

Blattner, R. J.: The whooping cough syndrome. *J. Pediatr., 65*:150, 1964.

Botsztejn, A. von: Die pertussoïde, eosinophile Pneumonie des Säuglings. *Ann. Pediatr. (Basel), 157*:28, 1941.

Calder, M. A., et al.: What causes whooping cough? *Lancet, 2*:1079, 1970.

Cocchi, P.: Letters to the Editor, Pertussis syndrome. *N. Engl. J. Med., 283*:1175, 1970.

Collier, A. M., Connor, J. D., and Irving, W. R., Jr.: Generalized type 5 adenovirus. Infection associated with the pertussis syndrome. *J. Pediatr., 69*:1073, 1966.

Connor, J. D.: Evidence for an etiologic role of adenoviral infection in pertussis syndrome. *N. Engl. J. Med., 283*:390, 1970.

Connor, J. D.: Letters to the Editor. Pertussis syndrome. *N. Engl. J. Med., 283*:1174, 1970.

Editorial: What causes whooping cough? *Lancet, 2*:917, 1970.

Islur, J., Anglin, C. S., and Middleton, P. J.: The whooping cough syndrome: a continuing pediatrics problem. *Clin. Pediatr., 14*:171, 1975.

Klenk, E. L., Gaultney, J. V., and Bass, J. W.: Bacteriologically proved pertussis and adenovirus infection. *Am. J. Child., 124*:203, 1972.

Leading Article: Whooping cough due to adenovirus. *Br. Med. J., 4*:570, 1970.

Love, W. C., et al.: What causes whooping cough? *Lancet, 2*:1142, 1970.

McCordock, H. A.: Intranuclear inclusions in pertussis. *Proc. Soc. Exp. Biol., 29*:1288, 1932.

McCordock, H. A., and Smith, M. G.: Intranuclear inclusions: incidence and possible significance in whooping cough and in a variety of other conditions. *Am. J. Dis. Child., 47*:771, 1934.

Nelson, J. D.: Whooping cough—viral or bacterial disease? *N. Engl. J. Med., 283*:428, 1970.

Oetgen, W. J.: Pertussoid eosinophilic pneumonia; pulmonary infiltrates with eosinophilia in very young infants. *Chest, 71*:492, 1977.

Olson, L. C., Miller, G., and Hanshaw, J. B.: Acute infectious lymphocytosis presenting as a pertussis-like illness: its association with adenovirus type 12. *Lancet, 1*:200, 1964.

Olson, L. C.: Comments in Gellis, S. Editorial note *Yearbook Pediatrics*, 1967–1968, p. 97.

Rich, A. R.: On the etiology and pathogenesis of whooping cough. *Bull. Johns Hopkins Hosp., 51*:346, 1932.

Rich, A. R., Long, P. H., Brown, J. H., Bliss, E. A., and Holt, L. E., Jr.: Experiments upon the cause of whooping cough. *Science, 76*:330, 1932.

Wigger, H. J., and Blanc, W. A.: Fatal hepatic and bronchial necrosis in adenovirus infection with thymic alymphoplasia. *N. Engl. J. Med., 275*:870, 1966.

CHAPTER SIXTY

SALMONELLA PNEUMONIA

Rosa Lee Nemir, M.D.

Although typhoid bacilli were isolated from the sputum in 1884, the pulmonary manifestations of salmonella infections have received little attention. Salmon and Smith published the first reports of salmonella infections in 1886, and as early as 1895 Osler described pulmonary lesions in typhoid fever. Jehle again called attention to the presence of typhoid bacilli in the sputum of 15 patients in 1902. Shortly thereafter, reports of various types of lung disease due to infections with the typhoid bacillus appeared, and recognition of a similar pulmonary disease produced by the paratyphoid organism followed.

Etiology

Data have been collected, and classifications of the ever-increasing Salmonella groups have been drawn up in this country and elsewhere. In 1962 Huckstept reported the existence of approximately 700 types. Among the most frequently encountered types in this country are S. typhimurium, montevideo, newport, heidelberg, thompson, oranienburg, paratyphi B, and enteritidis. Of these, S. choleraesuis (paratyphoid group C_1), previously called S. suipestifer, is the type most often associated with pulmonary complications. S. typhimurium is the organism most commonly responsible for infection, but pulmonary complications with this organism are less common; however, it has been cultured from the pleural fluid in an appreciable number of cases.

The frequency of serotypes varies in different years within a country and from country to country. A more recent type, S. agona, has become widespread. It was responsible for one outbreak in France (minced horse meat), one in Scotland (poultry), and eight in the United States (pork, beef, chicken and mayonnaise), where, in 1975, 1333 isolates were reported, an increase of 300 over the previous year. A ten-year review (1959 to 1968) of the incidence in humans and animals in N.E. Scotland brings to light the high percentage of S. typhimurium (61 per cent of the total), "a rather higher percentage than that reported for the whole of the United States of America in 1967, which was 29.4 per cent"; it remains the same for 1975.

Some of the more recent sources of infection in humans include pets such as turtles (tortoises and terrapins), cage birds, dogs and cats. These become infected by eating contaminated foods. These animals have been found to excrete salmonella for a long period of time and, thus, intermittently may be infectious to humans, especially children.

Pathology and Pathogenesis

In an early textbook of pathology, MacCallum (1925) stated that "lobar and lobular pneumonia may accompany typhoid fever, the former rarely, the latter as a common terminal infection. Lobar pneumonia caused by B. typhosus has a peculiarly hemorrhagic character. . . . In the bronchopneumonia the typhoid bacillus may cause the lesions and appear in the sputum. . . . In the pharynx and larynx there is

998

sometimes an extensive diphtheritic and haemorrhagic inflammation in the late stage of disease." Today, the last-named lesion is exceedingly rare, and other pulmonary manifestations, such as pulmonary thrombi, lung abscess, pleurisy and empyema, have been added to the list.

The etiologic relation of Salmonella to pulmonary lesions has been demonstrated by culture of the bacilli from sputum, from bronchial secretions, from pus from abscess, and from pleural fluid. *S. choleraesuis* is most often identified with sepsis and lung disease.

The organisms usually enter the body through the mouth by the ingestion of contaminated food or water, rarely through the handling of contaminated toys or other objects. An unusual epidemic in a newborn nursery was traced to the contamination of resuscitators and suction machines. The trap water fluid was found to harbor *S. montevideo* and *S. bareilly* in each of two epidemics, and it was thought that the infection was disseminated in the nursery by the inhalation of contaminated air.

Bronchitis is the most common pulmonary manifestation, especially in *S. typhi* infections. Bronchopneumonia and pulmonary congestion are next in frequency. Lobar pneumonia due to the Salmonella agent alone may also occur, and Bullowa (1928) first reported lobar pneumonia due to *S. suipestifer* (now called *S. choleraesuis*) in an adult; the organism was isolated on culture of the blood and sputum, and by postmortem lung puncture.

The pathogenesis may be described as follows. Lesions may begin in the mucous membranes of the bronchopulmonary tree, producing tracheobronchitis, bronchitis or subsequently bronchopneumonia. The parenchyma may be infected by way of the blood stream, producing separate areas of inflammatory reaction, which, by necrosis and excavation, result in abscess formation. Pulmonary thrombi may be produced, resulting in pulmonary infarction. The

bones, particularly the ribs and the cartilages, are often the target of focal salmonella infections; pleurisy and empyema may result from the spread of infection from these foci into the pleura. One such case of empyema and bronchopleural fistula has been reported in an adult 11 years after a gunshot wound in the chest. Empyema and, rarely, bronchopleural fistula may result from the rupture of a pulmonary abscess into the pleura. Some of these pulmonary manifestations, such as abscess or empyema, are late complications of salmonella infection. In patients with empyema, subsequent pneumonitis may occur.

Pleural fluid varies from purulent to serofibrinous or hemorrhagic, the latter two being more frequent, and salmonellae are often cultured from these fluids.

Incidence

The chief pulmonary manifestations of salmonella infection, especially with *S. typhi*, are bronchitis and secondary bronchopneumonia. Pneumonia and the more serious manifestations of lung disease have always been uncommon, and since the advent of the antibiotics have decreased still further. In an analysis of 95 cases of bacteriologically proved salmonellosis (45 children), Eisenberg and associates (1955) did not find a single instance of abscess, pneumonia or other localizing bacterial infection among the children.

Reported fatalities from salmonella pulmonary disease in children are rare and usually are associated with underlying serious disease, such as neoplastic disease, sickle cell anemia or conditions requiring corticosteroid therapy on a long-term basis. The difficulty of determining the extent of the Salmonella infection is shown in a report by Szanton (1957) of an epidemic of *Salmonella oranienburg* in a newborn nursery. An infant 144 days old died on arrival at the hospital, and necropsy revealed bronchitis and bronchiolitis. In New

York City for the year 1965–1966, there were 28 newborn infants with salmonellosis, five of whom died. The pathologic findings of this epidemiologic report were not given (Cherubin and associates, 1969).

In other countries where salmonella infection is more frequent, the incidence of pulmonary infection and mortality is also low. Rowland, in 1961, reporting his experience in Iran with 191 children with typhoid fever treated with chloramphenicol, reported no instances of pneumonia. In 1948 Kao, reporting from China, described two deaths from typhoid fever and bronchopneumonia among 126 cases of sulfadiazine-treated children.

In a review of salmonellosis in the United States during 1963–1975, the average annual incidence among human beings was ten cases per 100,000 population. There was a small increase in the last five years, resulting in 11.1 cases per 100,000. Among persons under ten years of age, the incidence of salmonellosis unaccountably showed a rise, particularly for those under one year of age, and the fatality rate was highest in this age group and in those over 69 years of age. This study offered no description of fatalities or of the complications, such as pneumonia.

In an outbreak of typhoid fever (traced to a meat counter, and infected canned corned beef) in Aberdeen in 1964, 507 patients were infected; of these, 86 were children under 12 years of age. Four of these children had mild bronchitis, a surprisingly low incidence of pulmonary involvement according to one of the reporters, whose experience in India was associated with "more frequent and prominent respiratory symptoms."

Clinical Features

The clinical pattern of salmonella infection has been categorized as follows: (1) gastroenteritis, the most common; (2) typhoid-like or septic syndrome; (3)

focal manifestations; and (4) the carrier state involving apparently healthy persons who harbor the infection and may serve as a reservoir.

Bronchitis or tracheobronchitis may occur during any one of the first types of involvement. Nelson and Pijper (1951), in a series of 876 patients with salmonella infections in Pretoria, South Africa, and Goulder and coworkers (1942) in this country, list the presence of bronchitis in 30 per cent of the patients. Both series include children. Our own early experience on the Children's Medical Service, Bellevue Hospital, is similar; however, today there is a decreased incidence of S. typhi infections, and such pulmonary complications are rare.

Cough, usually resulting from a simple tracheitis or tracheobronchitis, is one of the most frequent symptoms. The accompanying signs and symptoms include fever (varying in degree), abdominal pain or tenderness, headache, drowsiness or irritability, and occasionally mild chest pain aggravated by coughing. When rales appear, the diagnosis of bronchitis is assured. Diarrhea may not be present; indeed, in S. typhi infections in children, constipation is more frequent. Hepatomegaly and splenomegaly are often present.

The pulmonary complications of bronchopneumonia, "lobar" pneumonia, abscess formation and pleural infections usually occur after the first week of infection. They may appear during the period of acute infection, especially with bronchopneumonia and disseminated pneumonia, and are often associated with septicemia and, not infrequently, osteomyelitis. Bronchopneumonia usually follows shortly after the appearance of the early symptoms of salmonella infection. There may be a new elevation in temperature following defervescence or absence of fever, increasing cough, and the occurrence of chest pain following cough; physical findings include scattered transient rales and some patchy areas of altered breath sounds. The physical findings are not characteristic and differ from other pulmonary infections in only one way; the sputum frequently is hemorrhagic or blood-streaked. There have been few descriptions of abscess formation or pleural complications in children. Focal manifestations of salmonella infection occur later in the course of the disease, sometimes years afterward, and may include lung abscess or pleurisy and empyema.

Diagnosis

In order to establish the diagnosis of salmonella infection, cultures should be made from the stools, urine and blood, and to clarify the origin of pulmonary complications, cultures from the sputum, pleural fluid and bronchial aspirations should be included. Occasionally, cultures of the cerebrospinal fluid are made. Diarrhea must not be the only indication for suspicion. A successful isolation of Salmonella is more likely during the first week of illness. Agglutination reactions to both O and H antigens, suitably grouped, furnish valuable evidence and were positive in more than 90 per cent of the 876 cases observed by Nelson and Pijper (1951). Serums for groups C and E Salmonella should be included in the diagnostic antigens, since group C, especially *S. choleraesuis*, is the most frequently involved agent in pulmonary complications.

Other laboratory aids, such as white blood cell counts, are of little aid in diagnosis. Leukopenia may be present, but the white blood cell count may vary, with elevations as high as 22,000 per cubic millimeter.

The findings noted in the roentgenogram of the chest in salmonella infections vary with the underlying pathologic condition. Increased bronchovascular markings may be seen in bronchopneumonia. When bacteremia is present and the parenchyma is infected by dissemination, mottled areas of infiltrate resembling miliary tuberculosis have been described. In patients with known salmonella septicemia, examination of the chest roentgenogram for focal involvement of the bony structures, especially ribs, may be rewarding. These lesions may be forerunners of pleural infection.

Certain diseases predispose the patient to infection by Salmonella. Bennett and Hook (1959) have given an excellent discussion of host factors and of the disease and nutritional status predisposing the patient to such infections. Among the more frequent are malaria, relapsing fever, bartonellosis, viral hepatitis, sickle cell anemia and postoperative complications. Such patients merit diagnostic tests for salmonellae when evidence of infection appears and when unexplained chest disease is found.

In a study of patients with sickle cell anemia hospitalized for bacterial infection over a ten-year period (1958–1968), salmonellosis was responsible for seven illnesses. Three of these were infants who had Salmonella pneumonia. Salmonella was second to the pneumococcus as a cause of bacteremia in the 166 patients studied in this series (Barrett-Connor, 1971).

Treatment

Treatment for pulmonary manifestations is the same as for other salmonella infections. Both chloramphenicol and ampicillin are effective drugs, both have been associated with the rapid development of resistant strains, and neither drug affects the emergence of the carrier rate. The necessity for obtaining antibiotic sensitivity studies on the isolated organism in choosing the therapeutic agent is obvious. Also, ampicillin should not be given to penicillin-allergic patients. A new experimental drug, trimethoprim-sulfamethoxazole (TMP-SMX), has been used with some success.

In the case of purulent complications, empyema or lung abscess, it is also important to test the sensitivity of the organism isolated by culture.

Usually there is a prompt clinical response within a few days following antibiotic therapy, an average of four days in children. When *Salmonella choleraesuis* is cultured, it is desirable to continue treatment longer than usual because of the high invasiveness and fatality rate, including those deaths resulting from pulmonary infections. Short periods of therapy may be responsible for the later appearance of pulmonary complications.

Corticosteroid therapy should be reserved for the very toxic patient; then it may be used in conjunction with antibiotics. A controlled study by Rowland (1961), in which one-half of the patients received prednisolone, indicated that the addition of a corticosteroid affected neither the incidence of complications nor the relapse rate.

The management of lung abscess, pleural effusion or empyema is much the same as when these complications are produced by other organisms. These serious complications require longer therapy, but in time usually respond to medical treatment. Adequate medical therapy should always precede any decision as to the necessity for surgical intervention.

The Carrier State

Thomson (1955), in a study of pathogenic bacilli in feces, has pointed out that infants and young children, as well as adults, can act as symptomless carriers, excreting large numbers of pathogens; however, the frequency is much lower in children.

Jones and Pantin (1956), studying an outbreak of *S. paratyphoid* B in a maternity home where adults and child contacts became infected, found that infants remained carriers longer than older children or adults. Three infants were still excreting *S. paratyphoid* B nine months after infection. Chloramphenicol was valuable in combating symptoms, but had no effect on the carrier state.

Bille and coworkers (1964) reported one case of an infant infected at birth from the maternal amniotic fluid. The newborn did not become ill, but at ten weeks of age, long after its mother had become negative, the infant was still excreting *S. newport.*

Similarly, an *S. newport* outbreak in a premature nursery began with an infant whose mother was apparently a symptomless carrier, following an illness a few months prior to delivery. Eleven other premature infants were infected in the nursery; one of these died, and two became asymptomatic carriers. In this epidemic, as in others, the antibiotic treatment of the asymptomatic carrier was evaluated by long-term observation of stool cultures after ampicillin treatment. Despite ampicillin therapy, eight months after the initial infection, the carrier state persisted in 40 per cent of the infants.

The extent of spread of salmonella infection in a newborn nursery became apparent in Finland. An outbreak in a nursery infecting 77 cases was traced to a nurse, an asymptomatic carrier, who prepared milk foods for newborn babies in the Helsinki maternity clinic. She had been infected while traveling in the Eastern Mediterranean area. The need for constant vigilance in screening food handlers and personnel in nurseries as possible carriers is apparent.

Prognosis

There are several factors that determine the prognosis in salmonella infections. These include the speed and accuracy of diagnosis, appropriate selection of therapeutic agents, the general health and age of the patient, the extent or massiveness of bacterial invasion, and the type of Salmonella organism. That age is a factor is shown by the figures computed by Saphra (1950) from 174 fatalities; in infants, the mortality rate was 5.8 per cent; the rate was 2 per cent in those from ages one to 50 years; and for patients past 50 years of age, the mortality rate was 15 per cent.

Saphra and Winter (1957) also

found that the fatality rate of *S. choleraesuis* infections was 21.3 per cent as compared with 5.3 per cent for the total group (174 cases). Twenty patients, who failed to survive, had pneumonia or pleurisy *(S. choleraesuis,* cultured from seven cases). In the report by MacCready and coworkers (1957), of 37 fatalities (1.4 per cent) among 2605, *S. choleraesuis* was responsible for five (16 per cent) deaths in 31 patients. The high invasiveness of *S. choleraesuis* was suggested by the observations of these authors that ten of the 31 bacterial isolations came from the blood stream.

In summary, it appears that pulmonary manifestations other than bronchitis are rare in salmonella infections, and that in general the prognosis is good. It must be pointed out that with the exception of *S. typhi* infections, salmonella diseases appear to be increasing in incidence. The reported incidence in the United States was 6929 in 1960 and 23,445 in 1975. This indicates a need for increased alertness, not only for the initial salmonella infections, but also for their possible complications.

REFERENCES

Abram, J. H.: Paratyphoid infections of the pleura. *Lancet, 2*:283, 1919.

Abrams, I. F., Cochran, W. D., Holmes, L. B., Marsh, E. B., and Moore, J. W.: A *Salmonella newport* outbreak in a premature nursery with a one-year follow-up. Effect of ampicillin following bacteriologic failure of response to kanamycin. *Pediatrics, 37*:616, 1966.

Adler, J. L., Anderson, R. L., Boring, J. R., III, and Nahmias, A. J.: A protracted hospital-associated outbreak of salmonellosis due to multiple-antibiotic-resistant strain of *Salmonella indiana. J. Pediatr., 77*:970, 1970.

Aserkoff, B., Schroeder, S. A., and Brachma, P. S.: Salmonellosis in the United States — a five-year review. *Am. J. Epidemiol., 92*:13, 1970.

Baker, E. F., Jr., Anderson, H. W., and Allard, J.: Epidemiological aspects of turtle-associated salmonellosis. *Arch. Environ. Health, 24*:1, 1972.

Balkin, S. S.: Bronchopneumonia empyema, pneumothorax and bacteremia due to Salmonella (var. kunzendorf) treated with chloramphenicol. *Am. J. Med., 21*:974, 1956.

Barrett-Connor, E: Bacterial infection and sickle cell anemia. An analysis of 250 infections of 166 patients and a review of the literature. *Medicine, 50*:97, 1971.

Basch, S.: Report of a case of typhoid fever complicated by a pure typhoid pneumonia and pulmonary abscess. *Med. Rec., 87*:539, 1915.

Bennett, I. L., Jr., and Hook, E. W. Infectious diseases (some aspects of salmonellosis). *Am. Rev. Med., 10*:1, 1959.

Bille, B., Melbin, T., and Nordbring, F.: An extensive outbreak of gastroenteritis caused by *Salmonella newport.* I. Some observations on 745 known cases. *Acta Med. Scand., 175*:557, 1964.

Bokra, S. T.: Chronic empyema due to *Salmonella oranienburg* complication of old chest wound. *Can. Med. Assoc. J., 78*:599, 1958.

Bornstein, S., and Schwarz, H.: Salmonella infection in infants and children. *Am. J. Med. Sci., 204*:546, 1942.

Brodie, J., and Porter, I. A.: Salmonellosis in man and animals in N.E. Scotland. A ten year review — 1959–1968. *Health Bull. (Edinb.), 28*:37, 1970.

Buchanan, N., Berger, H., and Van Hoogstraten, R. C. J.: Subdural empyema caused by *Salmonella typhimurium. S. Afr. Med. J., 47*:1345, 1973.

Bullowa, J. G. M.: *Bacillus suipestifer* (Hog cholera) infection of the lung. *Med. Clin. North Am., 12*:691, 1928.

Cherubin, C. E., Fodor, T., Denmark, L. L., Master, C. S., Fuerst, H. T., and Winter, J. W.: Symptoms, septicemia and death in salmonellosis. *Am. J. Epidemiol., 90*:285, 1969.

Cohen, L., Fink, H., and Gray, I.: *Salmonella suipestifer* bacteremia with pericarditis, pneumonitis and pleural effusion (report of a case). *J.A.M.A., 107*:331, 1936.

Delon, P. J.: Salmonella surveillance in 1973. *W.H.O. Chron., 30*:240, 1976.

DeMatteis, A., and Armani, G.: *Salmonella typhi* pneumonia without intestinal lesions. *J. Pathol., Bacteriol., 94*:464, 1967.

Dixon, J. M. S.: Effect of antibiotic treatment on duration of excretion of *Salmonella typhimurium* by children. *Br. Med. J., 2*:1343, 1965.

Eisenberg, G. M., Palazzolo, A. J., and Flippin, H. F.: Clinical and microbiologic aspects of salmonellosis. A study of ninety-five cases in adults and children. *N. Engl. J. Med., 253*:90, 1955.

Finley, F. G.: Typhoid pleurisy. *Can. Med. Assoc. J., 2*:764, 1912.

Fuchs, P. C.: Nonenteric salmonella infections. *Am. J. Clin. Pathol., 54*:428, 1970.

Galloway, H., Clark, N. S., and Blackhall, M.: Pediatric aspects of the Aberdeen typhoid outbreak. *Arch. Dis. Child., 41*:63, 1966.

Goulder, N. E., Kingsland, M. F., and Janeway, C. A.: Suipestifer infection in Boston. Report of 11 cases with autopsy findings in case of bacterial endocarditis due to this organism and study of agglutination reactions in this infection. *N. Engl. J. Med., 226*:127, 1942.

Hahne, O. H.: Lung Abscess due to *Salmonella typhi. Am. Rev. Resp. Dis., 89*:566, 1964.

Harvey, A. M.: *Salmonella suipestifer* infection in human beings. *Arch. Intern. Med.,* 59:118, 1937.

Harvill, T. H.: Typhoid pulmonary abscess. *J.A.M.A.,* 119:494, 1942.

Hirsch, W., Sapiro-Hirsch, R., Berger, A., Winter, St. T., Mayer, G., and Merzbach, D.: *Salmonella edinburgh* infection in children. A protracted hospital epidemic due to a multiple-drug-resistant strain. *Lancet,* 2:828, 1965.

Huckstept, R. L.: *Typhoid Fever and Other Salmonella Infections.* Edinburg, E. and S. Livingstone, Ltd., 1962, p. 282.

Ibrahim, A. A. E.: Bacteriophage typing of salmonella. I. Isolation and host range study of bacteriophages. *Appl. Microbiol.,* 18:444, 1969.

Ibrahim, A. A. E.: Bacteriophage typing of salmonellae. II. New bacteriophage typing scheme. *Appl. Microbiol.,* 18:748, 1969.

Jameson, H. P., and Signy, A.: A case of paratyphoid B infection with purpura and specific bronchopneumonia. *Arch. Dis. Child.,* 34:238, 1928–1929.

Jehle, L.: Ueber den Nachweis von Typhusbacillen in Sputum der Typhenkranker. *Wien. Klin. Wochenschr.,* 25:232, 1902.

Johnson, D. H., Rosenthal, A., and Nadas, A. S.: Bacterial endocarditis in children under two years of age. *Am. J. Dis. Child.,* 129:183, 1975.

Jones, D. M., and Pantin, C. G.: Neonatal diarrhea due to salmonella. *J. Clin. Pathol.,* 9:128, 1956.

Kao, Y.-E.: A study of typhoid fever in children in Kweichow. *Chinese Med. J.,* 66:391, 1948.

Kaufmann, A. F., Feeley, J. C., and DeWitt, W. E.: Salmonella excretion by turtles. *Pub. Health Rep.,* 82:840, 1967.

Kuncaitis, J., and Okutan, A.: Empyema due to *Salmonella typhimurium. Am. Rev. Resp. Dis.,* 83:741, 1961.

Kuttner, A. G., and Zepp, H. D.: *Salmonella suipestifer* infections in man. *J.A.M.A.,* 101:269, 1933.

Layles, A. M.: Human infection with *salmonella choleraesuis. Br. Med. J.,* 1:1284, 1957.

Licari, J. J., and Potter, N. N.: Salmonella survival during spray drying and subsequent handling of skim milk powder. I. Salmonella enumeration. *J. Dairy Sci.,* 53:865, 1970.

MacCallum, A. G.: *A Textbook of Pathology.* 3rd Ed. Philadelphia, W. B. Saunders Company, 1925, p. 613.

MacCready, R. A., Reardon, J. P., and Saphra, I.: Salmonellosis in Massachusetts. A sixteen year experience. *N. Engl. J. Med.,* 256:1121, 1957.

McCracken, G. H., and Eichenwald, H. F.: Antimicrobial therapy: therapeutic recommendations and a review of newer drugs. I. Therapy of infectious conditions. *J. Pediatr.,* 85:297, 1974.

McLean, I. W., Jr., Schwab, J. L., Hillegas, A. B., and Schlingman, A. S.: Susceptibility of microorganisms to chloramphenicol (chloromycetin). *J. Clin. Invest.,* 28:953, 1949.

Minet, J.: Congestions pulmonaires à bacilles paratyphiques. *Bull. Acad. Méd.,* 35:196, 1916.

Minor, G. R., and White, M. L., Jr.: Some unusual thoracic complications of typhoid and salmonella infections. *Ann. Intern. Med.,* 24:27, 1946.

Naidu, P. S. L., and Satyavathi, S.: Salmonella species at aberrant sites—a review. *Indian J. Med. Sci.,* 28:149, 1974.

Nelson, H., and Pijper, A.: Typhoid and paratyphoid fevers. *In* Banks, H. S., (Ed.): *Modern Practices in Infectious Fevers.* New York, Paul B. Hoeber, Inc., 1951, pp. 349–375.

Okubadejo, O. A., Montefiore, D. G., and Hamilton, G.: Multiple drug resistance in salmonella group G. Serotypes associated with a high incidence of human infections. *J. Trop. Med. Hyg.,* 74:167, 1971.

Oprée, W.: Infection with enteritis salmonella at nonintestinal sites. *Dtsch. Med. Wochenschr.,* 100:1425, 1975.

Osler, W.: Typhoid fever. II. Special features. Symptoms and complications. *Johns Hopkins Hosp. Rec.,* 5:283, 1895.

Perkins, J. C., Devetski, R. L., and Dowling, H. F.: Ampicillin in the treatment of *salmonella* carriers. *Arch. Intern. Med.,* 113:528, 1966.

Robinson, C. C.: The role of the typhoid bacillus in the pulmonary complications of typhoid fever. *J. Infect. Dis.,* 2:498, 1905.

Roque and Bandel: *Lyon Méd.,* 100:578, 1903.

Rosenstein, B. J.: Salmonellosis in infants and children: epidemiologic and therapeutic considerations. *J. Pediatr.,* 70:1, 1967.

Rowland, H. A.: The treatment of typhoid fever. *J. Trop. Med. Hyg.,* 64:101, 1961.

Rowland, H. A.: The complications of typhoid fever. *J. Trop. Med. Hyg.,* 64:142, 1961.

Rubenstein, A. D., and Fowler, R. N.: Salmonellosis of the newborn with transmission by delivery room resuscitators. *Am. J. Pub. Health,* 45:1109, 1955.

Sachs, J., and Antine, W.: Salmonella infection in man. A report of five cases with autopsies in two cases and a review of the clinical aspects. *Am. J. Med. Sci.,* 208:633, 1944.

Sahli: *Mitt Klin. Med. Inst. Schweiz.,* 1:749, 1894.

Salmon, D. E., and Smith, T.: Investigations in swine plague, annual report. Bureau Animal Ind., U.S. Department of Agriculture, 1886.

Saphra, I.: Fatalities in salmonella infections. *Am. J. Med. Sci.,* 220:74, 1950.

Saphra, I., and Wassermann, M.: *Salmonella choleraesuis:* clinical and epidemiological evaluation of 329 infections identified between 1940 and 1954 in New York Salmonella Center. *Am. J. Med. Sci.,* 228:525, 1954.

Saphra, I., and Winter, J. W.: Clinical manifestations of salmonellosis in man. An evaluation of 779 human new infections identified at the New York Salmonella Center. *N. Engl. J. Med.,* 256:1128, 1957.

Simon, H. J., and Miller, R. C.: Ampicillin in the treatment of chronic typhoid carriers. Report of 15 treated cases and a review of the literature. *N. Engl. J. Med.,* 247:807, 1966.

Solomon, S., Subramaniam, S., and Madanagopolan, N.: In vitro sensitivity of enteric bacteria to epicillin chloramphenicol, ampicillin and furazolidone. *Curr. Med. Res. Opin.*, 4:229, 1976.

Stuart, B. M., and Pullen, R. L.: Typhoid: clinical analysis of three hundred and sixty cases. *Arch. Intern. Med.*, 78:629, 1946.

Szanton, V. L.: Epidemic salmonellosis. A 30-month study of 80 cases of *Salmonella oranienburg* infection. *Pediatrics*, 20:794, 1957.

Thomson, S.: The number of pathogenic bacilli in faeces in intestinal diseases. *J. Hyg.*, 53:217, 1955.

United States Department of Health, Education and Welfare: Center for Disease Control. Morbidity and Mortality. Annual Suppl. Summary. Vol. 24: August 1976.

United States Department of Health, Education and Welfare: Center for Disease Control. Salmonella Surveillance, Report 126, Annual Summary 1975, issue September 1976.

Weiss, W., Eisenberg, G. M., and Flippin, H. F.: Salmonella pleuropulmonary disease. *Am. J. Med. Sci.*, 233:487, 1957.

Westerlund, N. C., and Bierman, A. H.: Salmonellosis. Report of an unusual case. *Am. J. Clin. Pathol.*, 53:92, 1970.

Whitby, J. M. F.: Ampicillin in treatment of *salmonella typhi* carriers. *Lancet* 2:71, 1964.

Wilfret, C. M., and Gutman, L. T.: Pharmacokinetics of trimethoprim-sulfamethoxazole in children. *Can. Med. Assoc. J.*, 112:738, 1975.

Williams, L. P., Jr., and Helsdon, H. L.: Pet turtles as cause of human salmonellosis. *J.A.M.A.*, 192:347, 1965.

Wolfe, M. S., Armstrong, D., Louria, D. B., and Blevins, A.: Salmonellosis in patients with neoplastic disease. *Arch. Intern. Med.*, 128:546, 1971.

Zollar, L. M., Krause, H. E., and Mufson, M. A.: Microbiologic studies on young infants with lower respiratory tract disease. *Am. J. Dis. Child.*, 126:56, 1973.

CHAPTER SIXTY-ONE

RHEUMATIC PNEUMONIA

Rosa Lee Nemir, M.D.

Rheumatic fever, the center of much attention and study some decades ago, has been steadily receding into the background as a frequent cause of childhood disease. The therapeutic use of the sulfones and antibiotics, particularly penicillin, against the group A streptococcus, which is generally accepted as the underlying etiologic agent in rheumatic fever, has been largely responsible for this change. Therefore, rheumatic pneumonia, the pulmonary manifestation of the infection, is also less frequently diagnosed. However, this does not mean that either rheumatic fever or rheumatic pneumonia has been entirely conquered. Unrecognized, subacute attacks of infection still occur, and there is evidence that rheumatic pneumonitis may precede recognized rheumatic carditis or arthritis. Such pulmonary infections are most likely to receive various nonrheumatic diagnoses without challenge. This is particularly true because there is no pathognomonic sign or test for rheumatic pneumonia, and more especially because the pneumonia, like the rheumatic fever itself, follows the streptococcal infection after a short latent period.

Incidence

The frequency of rheumatic pneumonia is difficult to determine; for a long time there has been much discussion as to its actual existence. Now sufficient carefully documented pathologic material has accumulated to substantiate the diagnosis of rheumatic pneumonia, thus implicating the lung as one of the organ systems affected in the total rheumatic disease pattern. In the opinion of Scott and coworkers (1959), the lung is commonly involved in varying degrees. Reporting an analysis of 87 children (three to 16 years of age) who died during the acute active rheumatic infection, between 1919 and 1954, these writers found 54 cases of rheumatic pneumonia, an overall incidence of 62 per cent. Over a third of these (39 per cent) had only slight pulmonary involvement; half (54 per cent) showed moderate rheumatic pulmonary disease. On the other hand, Griffith and coworkers in 1946 reported an 11.3 per cent incidence of rheumatic pneumonia based on the autopsy analysis of 119 fatal cases from the 1046 patients in the United States Naval Hospital. The experience of Neubuerger and colleagues (1944) with postmortem material is similar; they found an incidence of 12.7 per cent among 63 patients, some with quiescent and others with active rheumatic disease. Brown and associates (1958) accumulated from the literature references as to the frequency of pneumonia and pleurisy from 1844 to 1954. They reported a frequency range from 27.8 per cent to less than 1 per cent. These figures are based in part on clinical impressions, and serve best to indicate the difficulty in diagnosis and the long-standing attempts to clarify the relation of the pulmonary findings to the rheumatic infection.

The decreasing severity of rheumatic fever in recent years noted by clinicians in North America and Europe suggests that rheumatic pneumonia, a manifestation of severe rheumatic infection, will be seen even more rarely. A 40-

year review (1927–1967) from the Soviet Union of the frequency of pulmonary disease found in rheumatic fever provides evidence of the milder course of the disease in the past 15 to 20 years, when the pulmonary lesions were not impressive. In contrast, there was a 5 to 10 per cent involvement of the respiratory system in the lungs or serous surfaces "in the prewar years and the first years after the war" (Kovaleva and coworkers, 1970).

Similarly, a review of mortality rates between 1940 and 1965 in Nashville and Davidson County, Tennessee, showed a decline in death rate for ages under 29 years per 100,000 from 6.56 in 1940–1945 to 1.6 in 1946–1955 and again to 0.09 in 1956–1965. No mention was made of rheumatic complications, such as pneumonia (Quinn and coworkers, 1970).

In Czechoslovakia, the changing picture in rheumatic fever is indicated by a report of the incidence of first and recurrent attacks between 1961 and 1968. Recurrent attacks decreased to approximately one-seventh the frequency (from 37 per 100,000 in 1961 to 5.7 per 100,000 in 1968), and first attacks decreased to almost one-third the frequency (Sitaj and coworkers, 1970).

Rheumatic pneumonia continues to be rare. Single cases are reported from Argentina and Spain because of this rarity. The data from these patients who recovered were comprehensive and convincing. Similarly, single fatal cases with pathologic changes are reported. From New York, a case of pneumonitis with pleural effusion in a 12-year-old child dying shortly after an acute attack of rheumatic carditis was verified by autopsy findings. From Phoenix, Arizonia, a report of rheumatic pneumonia in a 13-year-old boy describes the failure to respond to antibiotic and steroid therapy, resulting in death within one month. The autopsy revealed lesions characteristic of rheumatic disease in the lungs and heart. From Washington, D.C., two of the three children described with the clinical picture of rheumatic pneumonia

terminated fatally. Classic pathologic findings of rheumatic pneumonia were demonstrated.

However, the difficulty of differentiating rheumatic pneumonia from congestive heart failure is well known and often impossible without pathologic evidence. It is therefore reasonable to speculate on the possible existence of such pneumonias in the cases of fatality from congestive heart disease. Pilapil and Watson (1971), describing the course of rheumatic fever in 104 children under 16 years of age seen between 1956 and 1965, mention the development of congestive heart failure in 31.7 per cent, but no reference was made to rheumatic pneumonia even though there was a 23 per cent mortality rate for the series and a 34 per cent mortality rate for those patients with carditis.

Pulmonary edema and rheumatic pneumonia may and do coexist, as is described by Mahajan and colleagues (1973) in one of seven Indian patients with "uncommon manifestations of rheumatic fever." The autopsy report of this child confirmed the diagnosis of rheumatic pneumonia together with bilateral pulmonary edema. In this series, two other children ill with recurrent rheumatic fever and pulmonary disease recovered. One had pneumonia complicated by pericardial and pleural effusion; the other had pleurisy with heart failure.

Pathologic Features

The first histologic description of rheumatic pneumonia was made in 1928 by Naish. In gross appearance, the lung is characteristically larger than normal, with dark red areas due to hemorrhage (unilateral and bilateral) scattered in various parts of the lung, usually hilar or peripheral. The lungs are elastic and resilient on palpation with a consistency comparable to India rubber (Hadfield, 1938). On microscopic examination, the following features are found: alveolar hemorrhage, necrosis of alveolar walls, and arteriolitis and vasculitis with occasional thrombosis in alveolar capillaries, hyaline membrane lining of alveoli and alveolar ducts and alveolar proliferation of mononuclear fibroblast cells, sometimes called Masson bodies (see Figs. 2 to 4). The pleura may show fibrinous exudate, usually without effusion. None of these lesions is pathognomonic.

Many pathologists have contributed to the present understanding of the pulmonary findings in rheumatic pneumonitis. Scott and coworkers (1959) thought that the most satisfactory criterion for diagnosis was the focal mononuclear, fibrinous intra-alveolar or intraductal exudate containing protein-rich fluid. Lustock and Kuzma (1956) have called attention to unusual bronchiolar changes in which the epithelial cells are desquamated, often stripped completely from the bronchi, and also to the presence of eosinophilic granular necrosis of the lamina. This destruction of the bronchial wall and mucosa was also described by Fraser (1930). Von Glahn and Pappenheimer (1926) reported the presence of arteriolitis in the smaller pulmonary arterial vessels. The cellular tissue mass filling the alveoli and alveolar ducts described by Masson (1937) was given the name "Masson bodies" by Neubuerger and his associates (1944), and though there is a difference of opinion in this regard, it is possible that "Masson bodies" are the equivalent of a modified form of Aschoff nodules.

The best explanation for the lung changes is that proposed by Rich and Gregory (1943); these workers attributed the lung changes to a sensitivity phenomenon secondary to arteriolar damage. They were able to reproduce in animals pathologic lesions of the heart identical with those seen in patients with rheumatic pneumonitis. Van Wijk (1948), Mossberger (1947) and Jensen (1946) have all attributed the pneumonia to an allergic basis. It appears likely, then, that there is capillary endothelial injury, and the hyaline membrane, a predominant feature of rheumatic pneumonia, can best be explained on the basis of capillary injury with the seepage of fibrinogen into the alveoli, where it is converted to fibrin.

With the acceptance of group A streptococcus as the etiologic agent of rheumatic fever, the development of pneumonia as an allergic reaction to this organism seems the most attractive explanation for the pathologic changes, especially for the alveolar exudative membrane, for the reputed severity of the lung manifestations, and for the transitory, rapidly changing radiographic findings in which the pulmonary lesions appear to move from one area of the lung to another, not unlike the clinical picture of Loeffler's pneumonia. Even the transient development of pleural fluid is compatible with this theory.

A review of the pulmonary disease found in 24 patients dying of acute rheumatic fever between the years 1949 and 1970 (Grunow and Esterly, 1972) conforms to the descriptions above, except for the lesser frequency of vascular changes. Arteriolitis, seen in only four cases, was complicated in three of these by acute pneumonia. One-third of the 24 patients, three to 25 years of age, did show thromboemboli in arteries and arterioles, and in many there were associated areas of pneumonia. Aschoff bodies were described in 21 of these patients, and pericarditis in 15. In only two was there evidence of nonrheumatic lung disease. Influenza virus was cultured from one, and intranuclear inclusion bodies were seen from another, suggesting infection with cytomegalic inclusion disease.

Clinical Features

With the foregoing descriptions of the pulmonary pathologic condition in mind, especially the asphyxiating hyaline membrane and the hemorrhagic alveolar exudate, the predominant symptoms of dyspnea, tachypnea, tachycardia (usually out of proportion to the general appearance of illness and to the amount of fever), persistent cough and blood-streaked sputum are readily understandable. Chest pain and restlessness are frequent, and cyanosis may develop. The presence, degree and duration of fever are variable. It is usually intermittent and irregular, ranging from 101° to 105°F., gradually tapering off to normal. The onset of pneumonia may be mild, simulating an upper respiratory tract infection, or it may appear as a sudden acute attack of dyspnea. The latter is particularly evident if there is a concurrent acute carditis. Other symptoms and signs referable to rheumatic infection elsewhere in the body may be present if carditis or arthritis is also manifest, e.g., arthralgia, swelling of joints, gallop rhythm, heart murmur, skin manifestations or, rarely, chorea.

At one time, on the Children's Rheumatic Fever Service at Bellevue Hospital, the diagnosis of rheumatic pneumonia was withheld unless there was also other evidence of active rheumatic infection, especially carditis. The rapidity with which carditis may develop was highlighted in two reports of rheumatic fever in very young children. One, from Boston, included ten children, 19 months to three years of age, all with severe rheumatic fever; nine of these had carditis, eight of whom developed congestive heart failure. In the chest roentgenogram, bronchopneumonia or atelectasis was described in three, and passive pulmonary vascular engorgement in seven. In the tropics, carditis appeared in 79.4 per cent of the 68 children with rheumatic fever under five years of age (two under one year at the onset of infection). Again, congestive heart failure was a frequent occurrence in the young patients. Today, there is evidence that rheumatic pneumonia may precede other forms of rheumatic infection. This argument has been presented by Rubin and Rubin (1961) and documented by Jensen (1946).

Griffith and coworkers (1946) have produced evidence that rheumatic pneumonia is more apt to develop in conjunction with acute rheumatic fever, and Seldin and colleagues (1947) found that pneumonia may occur at any time from four days to 12 months after the onset of rheumatic fever. On the basis of Griffith's observations, the following classification of rheumatic pneumonitis is offered: (1) primary acute pneumonitis, often the presenting manifestation of rheumatic fever; (2) secondary acute pneumonitis occurring during the course of rheumatic fever, often the polycyclic type; and (3) subclinical pneumonitis, when the pulmonary infection may be overlooked entirely. There are few symptoms or signs. The diagnosis is dependent on the study and interpretation of the pulmonary findings in the roentgenograms. Evidence of streptococcal group A infection helps to establish the diagnosis of rheumatic pneumonitis.

A summary of the dominant symptoms of rheumatic pneumonitis (dyspnea, tachypnea, cough with sputum that is occasionally blood-streaked and usually bacteria-free, and chest pain) clearly indicates the importance of a careful assembling of diagnostic data for rheumatic pneumonitis by physical examination, by laboratory tests and certainly by a study of the chest roentgenograms. Often, the x-ray films, supplemented by appropriate laboratory tests or history of previous streptococcal infection, give support to the diagnosis.

Physical examination of such a patient may reveal a sick child whose pulmonary symptoms are greater than the demonstrable lung findings. There is often a paucity of the latter. Debré and coworkers (1937) have pointed out that pulmonary lesions may exist in the absence of clinical signs. In the early stage, there may be dullness and diminished breath sounds, progressing to flatness and bronchial breathing, depending on the extent of the lung involvement and amount of pleural reaction. Occasionally fine or moist rales, usually transitory, are heard, and a friction rub, pleural or pericardial, is common. Pleurisy, although short-lived and transient, is common and may or may not be associated with pleural effusion. If the effusion is present, displacement of the heart and mediastinum may or may not occur. Associated findings of active carditis, such as gallop rhythm, newly developed murmurs, muffled heart sounds and pericardial friction rub, may be heard.

Laboratory Findings

The leukocyte count is high, the erythrocyte sedimentation rate is increased, the C-reactive protein is positive, and there is a moderate anemia just as in active rheumatic fever. Bacteriologic study of the blood, nose and throat usually gives negative results. Tests for the reaction to a recent streptococcal infection should always be made, especially the antistreptolysin O titer (ASO) and, when possible, other tests for streptococcal antibodies, such as antihyaluronidase (AH) and antistreptokinase (ASK). These tests are positive in a very high proportion of patients early in the rheumatic attack—the period when rheumatic pneumonia is most apt to occur. Other antibody tests, such as anti-nicotinamide-adenine-dinucleotidase (anti-NADase) and anti-desoxyribonuclease B (anti-DNAse B), may be helpful and are more easily performed. Comparative readings of serial tests are helpful diagnostically and also serve as a measure of successful response to therapy. Electrocardiographic studies made at frequent intervals are important in relating and finding evidence of an active carditis. Although pleural effusion may be suspected from the roentgenogram of the chest, a pleural tap may be unsuccessful. The fluid, when found, is sterile and often sanguineous.

The roentgenogram of the lung shows the rapid appearance and disappearance of hazy-edged densities in the periphery or the central portion of the lungs, usually in the left midlung and the right upper lobe, although there are often bilateral shadows. Pleurisy, when present, is commonly transitory. The radiographic shadows may vary from increased bronchovascular markings to a large homogeneous segmental density and may even include small, soft, mottled shadows resembling miliary tuberculosis. Lobar shadows are rare and are usually transitory. The apices and bases of the lungs are relatively clear. The size of the heart should be carefully observed on each roentgenogram. It frequently shows an enlarging cardiac silhouette and occasionally exhibits the presence of pericarditis.

Differential Diagnosis

Since there is no pathognomonic sign of rheumatic pneumonitis, and since rheumatic fever patients with quiescent or active infection are subject to intercurrent infections, it is easy to understand why a differential diagnosis is difficult. Nevertheless, antemortem diagnosis can be established if careful attention is given to the possibility. The list of disease processes simulating rheumatic pneumonitis is long; only the more important ones will be listed. Foremost among them are viral pneumonitis, congestive heart failure, bacterial pneumonia and Loeffler's pneumonia (reacting to antigens other than to the streptococcus).

The greatest difficulty in diagnosing rheumatic pneumonitis lies in distinguishing between viral pneumonitis on the one hand and pulmonary edema on the other, especially in patients severely ill with carditis. With improved diagnostic techniques, these forms of pneumonopathy, as well as bacterial and other infections, may be more readily differentiated now than they were two decades ago. There are new, refined methods not only for bacteriologic cultures of group A streptococci and other organisms, available even for office practice, but also for the identification of respiratory viral infections, whether by tissue culture techniques, by fluorescent antibody tests, or by immunologic methods such as complement-fixing antibody tests or viral neutralization tests.

Figure 1 is an example of rheumatic

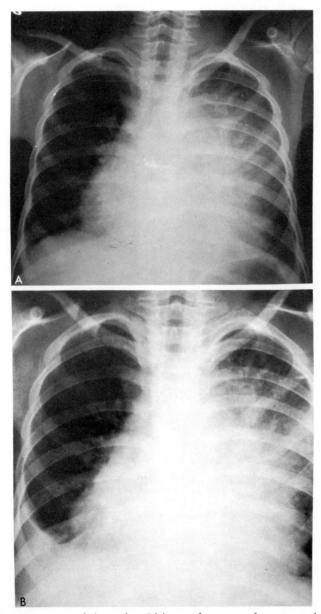

Figure 1. *A,* Roentgenogram of chest taken 24 hours after onset of symptoms shows a fuzzy-edged, homogeneous nonsegmental shadow in the middle third of the lung. The cardiac silhouette seems enlarged to right and left. Trachea is in the midline. In the original film a fine, pleural line may be seen extending bilaterally from the costophrenic angle upward two interspaces. *B,* The left pulmonary shadow is unchanged. The right costophrenic angle is obliterated by a small triangular shadow consistent with pleural fluid. The cardiac shadow is somewhat larger bilaterally; this may be due to pericardial fluid.

Illustration continued on the following page

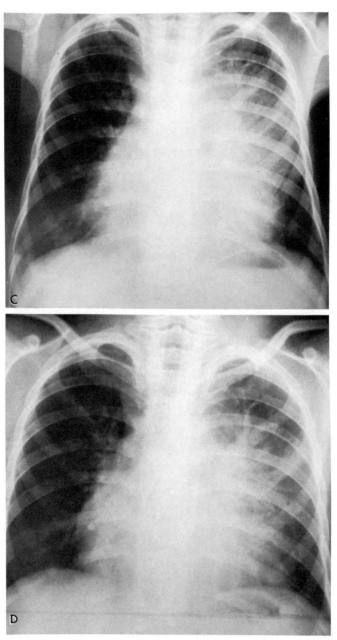

Figure 1 *Continued.* *C,* Almost complete clearing at the right base on the third day. No tap was done. Note obliteration of right costophrenic angle and a fine oblique fissure line above diaphragm extending to right heart border in the cardiohepatic angle. *D,* The right diaphragm and costophrenic angle are clear. The pulmonary shadow in left midlung shows some clearing at the periphery, 20 days after onset of symptoms. The cardiac silhouette seems smaller. The left border especially is obscured by fuzzy, mottled pulmonary infiltrate and increased bronchovascular shadows.

pneumonitis as the presenting symptom of rheumatic involvement in a patient. For such a person, prophylactic penicillin therapy is a wise choice, since the prevention of serious rheumatic cardiac damage can thereby be prevented. The opportunity to prevent recurrent rheumatic illness should not be overlooked.

Subacute and unrecognized streptococcal infections still occur. It is in these patients that the physician must be most alert to the possibility of rheumatic infection when the proper respiratory symptoms present themselves. Rabinowitz, as early as 1926, suggested that rheumatic pneumonia may occur in patients with subacute infection before carditis is clearly diagnosed.

Some of the salient features in the diseases most commonly requiring differentiation are given in Table 1. Addi-

tional aids from the laboratory include blood cultures, bacteriologic cultures from the nose and throat, cold agglutinin tests, antistreptolysin O titers, related tests and electrocardiograms. All of these may aid in clarifying the diagnosis.

Additional observations of diagnostic value from a clinical standpoint are the frequency of pleuritic pain, the unusual degree of dyspnea and the presence of blood-tinged sputum (when, indeed, sputum is available).

There may be other evidences of rheumatic fever, including skin manifestations such as erythema nodosum, erythema marginatum and an undifferentiated rash (also possibly erythema marginatum). Chorea is rarely reported with rheumatic pneumonitis.

Therapeutic trial and response are often revealing. Patients with pulmo-

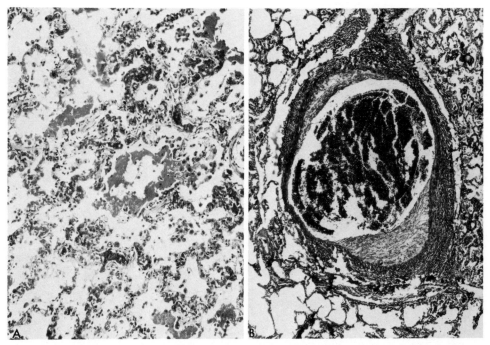

Figure 2. A four-year-old girl was admitted to the rheumatic fever ward in Bellevue Hospital with acute arthritis and active carditis. She was digitalized and treated with salicylates and improved thereafter. Three months later, fever, substernal pain and pericarditis developed. Rales were also heard in the chest. She was in acute respiratory distress and died four months after admission. The final diagnosis was rheumatic myocarditis, endocarditis of the tricuspid and mitral valves, and hypertrophy and dilatation of the heart with organizing fibrinous pericarditis. The lungs showed some pathologic features described in rheumatic pneumonia. *A,* Hyaline membranes and congestion (× 150). *B,* Arterial thrombus, organized (× 30).

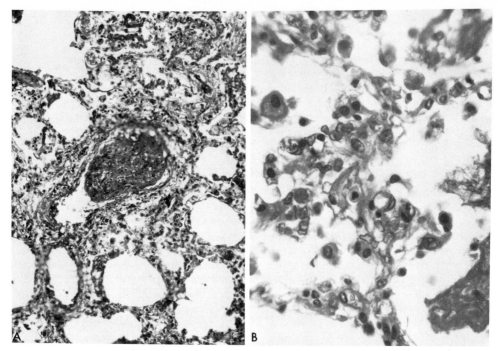

Figure 3. A 15-year-old Puerto Rican girl who died within 12 days after admission to Bellevue Hospital. Her clinical diagnosis was active rheumatic heart disease with enlarged heart, mitral stenosis and insufficiency and bronchopneumonia. At autopsy she was found to have rheumatic myocarditis; endocarditis of the mitral, aortic and tricuspid valves; rheumatic pericarditis and arteritis. In the lungs there was congestion, pulmonary embolism and rheumatic pneumonia with hyaline membranes. *A*, Pulmonary thromboembolus, acute (× 150). *B*, Exudate of mononuclear cells (× 500).

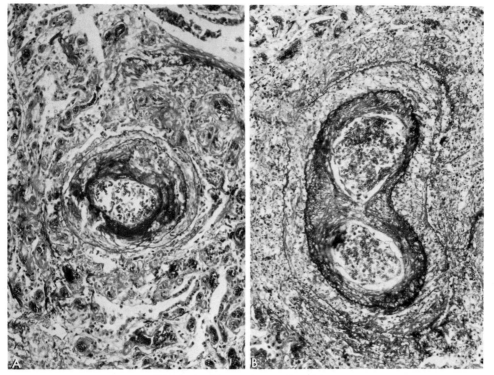

Figure 4. Rheumatic arteritis (× 100).

TABLE 1. DIFFERENTIAL DIAGNOSIS OF RHEUMATIC PNEUMONIA, ACUTE PULMONARY EDEMA,* BACTERIAL PNEUMONIA AND VIRAL OR PRIMARY ATYPICAL PNEUMONIA

		Bacterial Pneumonia	Viral or PAP Pneumonia	Rheumatic Pneumonia	Pulmonary Edema
PHYSICAL FINDINGS	Clinical history	Upper respiratory infection, immediately preceding infection	Insidious onset usually with respiratory symptoms	Preceding beta hemolytic streptococcus infection; often previous rheumatic fever	Usually previous rheumatic fever and often associated carditis
	Predominant presenting symptom	High fever, occasionally hacking cough	Frequent cough	Respiratory distress	Respiratory distress (with edema peripherally and liver enlargement)
	Lungs	Segmental, constant over the area, corresponding to roentgenogram lesions; rales follow signs of consolidation	Nonsegmental, variable, inconstant signs. Rales predominate and precede signs of consolidation when present	Nonsegmental, fleeting minimal findings, dull and diminished to bronchial breath sounds, few rales	Nonsegmental, bilateral findings at bases, rales, pleural fluid ± fluid elsewhere, edema, ascites
	Pleurisy ± fluid	Positive with fluid; tap often productive and culture positive	Rarely occurs; when present, cultures are sterile	Frequent, migratory and bilateral as fibrinous pleurisy ± fluid, transient and sterile	Common with fluid
	Heart	Normal (tachycardia)	Normal	Usually active carditis, occasionally pericarditis; often enlarged heart	Not necessarily active carditis; enlarged always
CHEST FILM	Location and type of lesions	Segmental, homogeneous, dense shadow, develops early	Nonsegmental, lesions scattered, often bilateral, different degrees of density and extent	Nonsegmental, migratory, fleeting, soft hazy shadows from hilus, often bilateral	Nonsegmental, dense, diffuse, extensive shadows usually bilateral from hilus
	Pleurisy	Fibrinous moderately frequent Effusion occasionally	Fibrinous and interlobar	Frequent, fleeting ± pericarditis	Pleural fluid frequent
	Heart	Normal	Rare otherwise Normal	Sometimes enlarged at beginning, may increase in size	Abnormal always, frequently large
	Duration of pulmonary shadow	Resolves shortly (few days) after effective antibiotic therapy	Slowly resolving, unrelated to therapy	Short time clearing unrelated to any therapy	Often responsive to diuretics and cardiac therapy Watch heart shadow
	Relation to physical examination	Corresponds	Scattered, transient, often not found over roengenogram shadow	Corresponds	Corresponds

*In patients with rheumatic heart disease.

nary edema may show prompt response to the use of digitalis, diuretics, oxygen and other supportive measures; this response is not seen in uncomplicated rheumatic pneumonitis.

Treatment

Supportive therapy should be given for the respiratory distress, for the chest pain and for the restlessness so frequently seen. Oxygen is usually required. Digitalis should be given as indicated.

Various therapeutic agents, such as salicylates, sulfonamides (which were actually harmful) and β-dimethylamino-ethylbenzhydryl ether (Benadryl), have been used without success.

There is evidence that corticosteroid therapy may be helpful, especially since it is indicated for the majority of patients with severe carditis, which so frequently accompanies the pneumonia.

Prognosis

There is fairly uniform opinion that rheumatic pneumonitis has a grave prognosis. One must be constantly alert to the possibility of widespread pulmonary involvement; it appears that this finding has prognostic significance, especially in the initial attack. For those who survive, pulmonary damage may occur later in the form of chronic interstitial fibrosis.

It has been shown that the prophylactic therapy of streptococcal infections and the continuous prophylactic penicillin therapy are associated with a decrease in the recurrence of rheumatic fever itself, and therefore of rheumatic pneumonitis. Prompt and early use of penicillin in the treatment of acute rheumatic fever will eliminate foci of streptococci and thereby lessen its antigenic elaboration. The use of corticosteroids during the acute phase is also helpful, to a greater degree than salicylates, in diminishing inflammation in acute rheumatic processes. Early diagnosis of rheumatic fever must be

made in time for the prophylaxis of complications to be effective. In some instances, however when the first rheumatic manifestation is the occurrence of pulmonary signs and symptoms instead of the classic joint and cardiac ones, arriving at the correct diagnosis may be virtually impossible in the absence of cardiac manifestations or other signs pointing to its rheumatic origin.

Prevention

The prevention of the first attack of rheumatic fever is largely dependent on control of beta hemolytic streptococcal infections in the community. Among school children, the carrier rate during epidemics is reported to be 20 to 25 per cent during the winter months. More frequent cultures for beta hemolytic streptococcus in patients with exudative pharyngitis and in contacts of such patients in schools are essential in the control program.

The success of the long-term prophylaxis of rheumatic fever is in large measure dependent on patient compliance. The reliability of patients cannot always be prejudged, but a study from Baltimore offers one criterion using the results of weekly urine tests for penicillin excretion. Three positive specimens suggest a 75 per cent compliance, and conversely, with three negative specimens, the noncompliance probability is 90 per cent (Gordis and coworkers, 1969c). Parent and patient education concerning the nature of rheumatic fever and the importance of prophylactic antibiotic therapy is an essential part of the preventive therapeutic program.

REFERENCES

Brown, G., Goldring, D., and Behrer, M. R.: Rheumatic pneumonia. *J. Pediatr.*, 52:598, 1958.

Burch, G. E.: Annotations: trends in the incidence of disease in the United States. *Am. Heart J.*, 88:807, 1974.

Czoniczer, G., Amezcua, F., Pelargonio, S., and Massell, B. F. L.: Therapy of severe rheumatic carditis. Comparison of adrenocortical steroids and aspirin. *Circulation, 29*:813, 1964.

Daugherty, S. C., and Schmidt, W. C.: Current considerations regarding the prevention of primary and recurrent rheumatic fever. *Med. Clin. North Am., 47*:1301, 1963.

Debré, R., Marie, J. Bernard, J., and Normand, E.: Pneumonie rhumatismale. *Presse Méd., 45*:273, 1937.

Findlay, I. I., and Fowler, R. S.: The changing pattern of rheumatic fever in childhood. *Can. Med. Assoc. J., 94*:1027, 1966.

Franken, R. A., Campana, J. O., Attab Filho, P., Okuyama, M. H., and Stecca, J.: Rheumatic pneumonia: anatomo-clinical study of 15 cases. *Rev. Paul. Med., 81*:231, 1973.

Fraser, A. D.: The Aschoff nodule in rheumatic pneumonia. *Lancet, 1*:70, 1930.

Gaspary, F. V., Nannini, L., Crespo, C. F., and Alonso, H. O.: Rheumatic pneumonitis apropos of a case. *Prensa Med. Argent., 53*:1597, 1968.

Geever, E. F., Neubuerger, K. T., and Rutledge, E. K.: Atypical pulmonary inflammatory reactions. *Dis. Chest, 19*:325, 1951.

Glahn, W. C. von, and Pappenheimer, A. M.: Specific lesions of peripheral blood vessels in rheumatism. *Am. J. Pathol., 2*:235, 1926.

Goldring, D., Behrer, M. R., Brown, G., and Elliott, G.: Rheumatic fever: report on the clinical and laboratory findings in twenty-three patients. *J. Pediatr., 53*:547, 1958.

Goldring, D., Behrer, M. R., Thomas, W., Elliott, G., and Brown, G.: Rheumatic pneumonia in children. *Postgrad. Med., 26*:739, 1959.

Gordis, L., Lilienfeld, A., and Rodriquez, R.: Studies in the epidemiology and preventability of rheumatic fever. I. Demographic factors and the incidence of acute attacks. *J. Chron. Dis., 21*:645, 1969a.

Gordis, L., Lilienfeld, A., and Rodriquez, R.: Studies in the epidemiology and preventability of rheumatic fever. II. Socio-economic factors and the incidence of acute attack. *J. Chron. Dis., 21*:655, 1969b.

Gordis, L., Markowitz, M., and Lilienfeld, A. M.: Studies in epidemiology and preventability of rheumatic fever. IV. Qualitative determination of compliance in children on oral penicillin prophylaxis. *Pediatrics, 43*:173, 1969c.

Griffith, G. C., Phillips, A. W., and Asher, C.: Pneumonitis occurring in rheumatic fever. *Am. J. Med. Sci., 212*:22, 1946.

Grunow, W. A., and Esterly, J. R.: Rheumatic pneumonitis. *Chest, 61*:298, 1972.

Hadfield, G.: The rheumatic lung. *Lancet, 2*:710, 1938.

Harris, T. N., Friedman, S., Needleman, H. L., and Saltzman, H. A.: Therapeutic effects of ACTH and cortisone in rheumatic fever: cardiologic observations in a controlled series of 100 cases. *Pediatrics, 17*:11, 1956a.

Harris, T. N., Needleman, H. L., Harris, S., and Friedman, S.: Antistreptolysin and streptococcal antihyaluronidase titers in sera of hormone-

treated and control patients with acute rheumatic fever. *Pediatrics, 17*:29, 1956b.

Herbut, P. A., and Manges, W. E.: The "Masson body" in rheumatic pneumonia. *Am. J. Pathol., 21*:741, 1945.

Honma, M.: A case of rheumatic pneumonitis. *J. Therapy (Tokyo), 45*:1169, 1963.

Jackson, H.: Rheumatic fever control measures; acceptance of routine pharyngeal cultures. *Am. J. Dis. Child., 115*:570, 1968.

Jensen, C. R.: Non-suppurative post-streptococcal (rheumatic) pneumonia. *Arch. Intern. Med., 77*:237, 1946.

Kovaleva, E. V., Belousova, M. A., and Dementieva, N. G.: Diseases of the organs of respiration in children with rheumatism at various periods of time from 1927 to 1967. *Vopr. Okhr. Materin. Det., 15*:8, 1970.

Krzanowska, E.: Pulmonary lesions in the course of rheumatic disease. *Gruzlica, 39*:559, 1971.

Lepskaya, E. S., Yaneva, T., and Ivanova, M.: Clinico-roentgenological diagnosis of pulmonary rheumocarditis of children. *Vopr. Revm., 8*:52, 1968.

Lustock, M. J., and Kuzma, J. F.: Rheumatic fever pneumonitis: a clinical and pathological study of 35 cases. *Ann. Intern. Med., 44*:337, 1956.

Mahajan, C. M., Bidwai, P. S., Walia, B. N. S., and Berry, J. N.: Some uncommon manifestations of rheumatic fever. *Indian J. Pediatr., 40*:102, 1973.

Markowitz, M.: Eradication of rheumatic fever: an unfulfilled hope. *Circulation, 41*:1077, 1970.

Marti Garcia, J. L., Candel Delgado, J. M., Guijarro Morales, A., Mateos Muller, J., and Martin Navajas, J. A.: Rheumatic pneumonitis. *Rev. Clin. Esp., 136*:551, 1975.

Massell, B. F., Fyler, D. C., and Roy, S. B.: Clinical picture of rheumatic fever: diagnosis, immediate prognosis, course and therapeutic implications. *Am. J. Cardiol., 1*:436, 1958.

Masson, P., Riopelle, J. L., and Martin, P.: Poumon rheumatismal. *Ann. Anat. Pathol. Med. Chir., 14*:359, 1937.

Massumi, R. A., and Legier, J. F.: Rheumatic pneumonitis. *Circulation, 33*:417, 1966.

Mossberger, J. I.: Rheumatic pneumonia: report of two cases. *J. Pediatr., 30*:113, 1947.

Naish, A. E.: The rheumatic lung. *Lancet, 2*:10, 1928.

Neubuerger, K. T., Geever, E. F., and Rutledge, E. K.: Rheumatic pneumonia. *Arch. Pathol., 37*:1, 1944.

Nittono, F., and Hoshiyama, J.: Necropsy findings in rheumatic pneumonia. *Jap. J. Med. Sci. Pathol., 5*:315, 1940.

Paul, J. R.: Pleural and pulmonary lesions in rheumatic fever. *Medicine, 7*:383, 1928.

Pilapil, V. R., and Watson, D. G.: Rheumatic fever in Mississippi. 104 cases seen over a decade. *J.A.M.A., 215*:1627, 1971.

Quinn, R. W., Sprague, H. A., and Quinn, J. L.: Mortality rates for rheumatic heart disease, 1940–65. *Public Health Rep., 85*:1091, 1970.

Rabinowitz, M. A.: Rheumatic pneumonia. *J.A.M.A., 87*:142, 1926.

Rich, A. R., and Gregory, J. E.: Experimental evidence that lesions with the basic characteristics of rheumatic carditis can result from anaphylactic hypersensitivity. *Bull. Johns Hopkins Hosp., 73*:239, 1943.

Rich, A. R., and Gregory, J. E.: Further experimental cardiac lesions of the rheumatic type produced by anaphylactic hypersensitivity. *Bull. Johns Hopkins Hosp., 75*:115, 1944.

Rosenthal, A., Czoniczer, G., and Massell, B. F.: Rheumatic fever under 3 years of age: report of 10 cases. *Pediatrics, 41*:612, 1968.

Rubin, E. H., and Rubin, M.: Rheumatic fever pneumonia. In *Thoracic Diseases.* Philadelphia, W. B. Saunders Company, 1961, pp. 770–771.

Scott, R. F., Thomas, W. A., and Kissane, J. M.: Rheumatic pneumonitis: pathologic features. *J. Pediatr., 54*:60, 1959.

Seldin, D. W., Kaplan, H. S., and Bunting, H.: Rheumatic pneumonia. *Ann. Intern. Med., 26*:496, 1947.

Serlin, S. P.: Rheumatic pneumonia: the need for a new approach. *Pediatrics, 56*:1075, 1975.

Shopfner, C. E., and Seife, M.: Rheumatic carditis and hemorrhagic pneumonitis treated with ACTH. *U.S. Armed Forces Med. J., 3*:819, 1952.

Sitaj, S., Urbanek, T., and Bosmansky, K.: Some aspects of epidemiology and surveillance of rheumatic fever. *Acta Rheumatol. Scand., 16*:30, 1970.

Taranta, A.: Factors influencing recurrent rheumatic fever. *Ann. Rev. Med., 18*:159, 1967.

Taranta, A., and Moody, M. D.: Diagnosis of streptococcal pharyngitis and rheumatic fever. *Pediatr. Clin. North Am., 18*:125, 1971.

United States Department of Health, Education, and Welfare: Center for Disease Control, Morbidity and Mortality. Annual Supplement. Summary 1975, *24*:2–5 (August), 1976.

Van Wijk, E.: Rheumatic pneumonia. *Acta Paediatr., 35*:108, 1948.

Von Glahn, W. C., and Pappenheimer, A. M.: Specific lesions of peripheral blood vessels in rheumatism. *Am. J. Pathol., 2*:235, 1926.

Wilson, M. G., Lim, W. N., and Birch, A. M.: Decline of rheumatic fever: recurrence rates of rheumatic fever among 782 children for twenty-one consecutive calendar years (1936–1956). *J. Chron. Dis., 7*:183, 1958.

CHAPTER SIXTY-TWO

VISCERAL LARVA MIGRANS

WILLIAM A. HOWARD, M. D.

Visceral larva migrans is the term applied to a clinical syndrome consisting of eosinophilia, hepatomegaly and pneumonitis, that results from the invasion of and prolonged migration through human viscera by nematode larvae normally parasitic to lower animals. Although aberrant human ascarid and hookworm larvae may occasionally produce the disease, the most common cause appears to be the dog ascarid, *Toxocara canis*, and possibly the cat ascarid, *T. cati*. The disease is widespread and apparently may occur anywhere that infected dogs are present, cases being reported from North and South America, England and Europe. One Canadian report indicates that 43 per cent of stools of stray dogs tested were found to contain ova of *Toxocara canis*.

Etiology

The etiologic agent, *Toxocara canis* (and possibly *T. cati*), is a common parasite of dogs, but is only accidentally infective to humans, who are unnatural hosts. *T. canis* in dogs produces lesions and symptoms similar to those of *Ascaris lumbricoides* infection in humans, to which it is related, since both are members of the superfamily Ascaridoidea. The adult male Toxocara is approximately 4 to 6 cm. long, while the female may be 10 cm. or more in length. The ova of this parasite measure 75 by 85 microns, and are passed unembryonated into the soil in the feces of the infected animal. Although the dog and the cat are the most likely sources of human infection, it is possible that the fox is a natural host. True intestinal infection with adult worms in humans has not been substantiated.

Pathogenesis

The unembryonated ova of *T. canis* are passed onto the soil, and under suitable conditions of temperature and humidity become embryonated and infective for the accidental intermediate human host, usually a small child with pica who is a dirt-eater. The ingested, embryonated eggs pass through the stomach, and their larvae hatch in the upper levels of the small intestine. The freed larvae penetrate the intestinal wall and migrate through blood and lymph channels to the liver, lungs, brain and other organs. In these areas the larvae are attacked by a host cell reaction of granulomatous nature, which effectively blocks their further migration. The larvae do not grow or molt, but become encapsulated and remain alive and infective for indefinite periods. The term "paratenic" has been suggested to describe the intermediate host role of humans, and also the many small mammals that serve as reservoirs of infection for the natural host. Since the larvae cannot complete their migration through the lungs to the tracheobronchial tree, there is no opportunity for *T. canis* to mature in the human intestine. The liver-lung-trachea migration of Ascaris and Necator in humans should not be included in the term "visceral larva migrans."

The immune response to such helminthic infections is caused primarily by, and operates against, larval migration stages in tissues. Lesions produced by various nematode larvae in tissues of immunologically responsive hosts are strikingly similar in different hosts and in different tissues, all resembling the eosinophilic granuloma. The tissue reaction, including the peripheral eosinophilia, is proportional in both intensity and promptness to the immune state and the degree of foreignness of the host. It has been suggested that the encapsulating granulomas may not be a host reaction but instead are under the control of the parasites and are induced by them to provide for their biologic needs during the long periods of survival (paratenesis).

Clinical Manifestations

Clinical symptoms are derived primarily from the number and location of the granulomatous lesions and from the allergic response of the human host to the presence of the nematode larvae. Visceral larva migrans occurs primarily in the young child under the age of four or five years who has a history of pica and dirt-eating and has ample opportunity for contact with dogs. The usual early signs and symptoms include mild anorexia, failure to gain weight, low-grade fever, anemia, eosinophilia and hepatomegaly of varying degree. There may be evidence of bronchitis, pneumonitis or asthma. More severe involvement may produce gross liver enlargement, abdominal pain, pains in muscles and joints, weight loss, high intermittent fever, severe pulmonary involvement, and various neurologic disturbances. The eye may be involved with iritis, choroiditis and ocular hemorrhage.

Relative eosinophilia is usually pronounced, ranging from 50 to 90 per cent, but unless above 30 per cent, the diagnosis may be questionable. Leukocytosis is common and may be extreme, above 100,000 cells per cubic millimeter.

Hepatomegaly is an almost constant finding, since the liver is the first organ invaded and is usually most heavily involved; this finding is absent in only the mildest infections. Fever, regardless of degree, may be associated with profuse sweating.

Pulmonic involvement is manifested clinically as bronchitis, pneumonitis or asthma in approximately 20 per cent of the cases, but pulmonary infiltrates are found in as many as 50 per cent of those patients who have chest roentgenograms. These lesions may represent actual migration of larvae, since studies in fatal cases have shown larval granulomatoses in the lungs as well as in other tissues. An occasional patient may show severe pulmonary involvement with widespread pneumonia, high fever and roentgenogram findings similar to those seen in miliary tuberculosis.

Neurologic disturbances are reported in severe cases. The author has observed a young black boy with epilepsy in whom a presumptive diagnosis of visceral larva migrans was made on the basis of a history of pica and dirt-eating, close association with dogs, and a 56 per cent blood eosinophilia. Encephalitis has also been reported as occurring in *T. canis* infection.

Other laboratory findings in visceral larva migrans include hypergammaglobulinemia, which may involve any or all of the IgG, IgA and IgM classes. Serum IgE levels above 900 I.U. per milliliter have been found in 60 per cent of the few patients tested. Anti-A and anti-B isohemagglutinins are usually elevated, sometimes to a striking degree. Levels of serum albumin are normal, but the sedimentation rate is elevated, and albuminuria is common. Most liver function tests have been reported as normal or equivocal, with the exception of the cephalin flocculation test, which may be elevated. Transaminase levels have not been recorded. The bone marrow shows a pronounced eosinophilia.

Complications

Eye involvement, occurring without the usual findings of eosinophilia and hepatomegaly, may prove serious. There may be iritis, choroiditis, retinal detachment, fibrous tumors and keratitis. In some instances, the appearance of the eye may be suspicious of retinoblastoma, and occasionally diagnosis can be made only after removal of the eye.

Pica is associated not only with visceral larva migrans but also with lead poisoning, and the finding of refractory anemia, eosinophilia and abdominal pain may be part of either picture. Cases are reported in which both conditions have existed simultaneously, with disastrous results.

Course and Prognosis

The clinical course of visceral larva migrans may be divided into three stages. During stage I, usually lasting several weeks, there is increasing eosinophilia, low-grade fever, and episodes of bronchitis, pneumonia and asthma. Stage II, lasting approximately one month, encompasses the cardinal signs of eosinophilia, hepatomegaly, pulmonary involvement, hyperglobulinemia and intermittent high fever. This is followed by stage III, the period of recovery, which may last as long as one to two years, although eventual returns to normal may be expected. A few patients die, either because of a massive involvement or because of a severe hypersensitivity reaction to the parasite.

Diagnosis

The diagnosis of visceral larva migrans is based upon the clinical history of pica, dirt-eating and adequate exposure to dogs, plus the clinical findings of chronic sustained eosinophilia, hepatomegaly and hypergammaglobulinemia. Additional findings may be referable to other organs involved, including the brain, the eye and the lung. Accurate diagnosis is still most readily made by biopsy of a lesion, usually of the liver, and the finding of the typical nematode larva in an eosinophilic granuloma. Toxocara ES (excretory-secretory) antigen has been used successfully in hemagglutination and soluble antigen fluorescent antibody tests for the serodiagnosis of Toxocara infection. A recently developed capillary tube precipitin test using crude Toxocara antigen has proved diagnostic in 76 of 80 patients, and may be useful where the more elaborate fluorescent antibody technique is not available. Occasional cross reactions with Ascaris may occur, but this can be eliminated by absorption with Ascaris antigen.

Differential diagnosis should include the visceral lesions that may be produced by a number of other nematode worms, including *Ascaris lumbricoides, Ancylostoma braziliense, Ancylostoma caninum, Strongyloides stercoralis,* as well as immature stages of certain spiroid nematodes and filarial worms. Invasion of the liver by *Fasciola hepatica,* a nematode worm, or *Capillaria hepatica,* a trematode, might also be included. It is apparent that *Toxocara canis* may be one cause of the picture of Loeffler's syndrome of transient pulmonary infiltrations and eosinophilia, but other causes may mimic the picture. Also to be considered in the diagnosis are trichinosis, hepatitis, leukemia, familial eosinophilia, tropical eosinophilia, tuberculosis, asthma, lead poisoning, and the leukemoid reaction occurring in certain severe bacterial pneumonias.

Treatment

No satisfactory treatment for visceral larva migrans is recognized at present. Diethylcarbamazine (Hetrazan) in doses of 10 to 30 mg. per kilogram per day for 14 days has been suggested, but has proved disappointing. Thiabendazole, successfully used in cutaneous larva migrans (creeping eruption), in a dosage of 25 to 100 mg. per kilogram per day has been used for the visceral form in a few cases with good results and apparent absence of any evidence of toxic effects. The usual dosage is 25 to 50 mg. per kilogram per day in two to three divided doses for seven to ten days, with the course of treatment being repeated in four weeks. The author has treated one patient in this manner, with rapid disappearance of symptoms and subsidence of the eosinophilia after four months. Adrenocorticosteroids in adequate dosage may be lifesaving for patients who are highly sensitive to the larval nematode, especially those with severe pneumonitis. Otherwise, treatment is primarily symptomatic and supportive, with stress on the correction of the anemia.

Preventive measures are of particular importance and include regular deworming of all household cat and dog pets. Puppies should not be allowed in living quarters until they are trained, and nursing bitches should be confined to a special and easily cleaned area.

REFERENCES

Aur, R. J. A., Pratt, C. B., and Johnson, W. W.: Thiabendazole in visceral larva migrans. *Am. J. Dis. Child., 121*:226, 1971.

Beaver, P. C.: The nature of visceral larva migrans. *J. Parasitol., 55*:3, 1969.

Beaver, P. C., Snyder, C. H., Carrera, G. M., Dent, J. H., and Lafferty, J. W.: Chronic eosinophilia due to visceral larva migrans. *Pediatrics, 9*:7, 1952.

Brain, L., and Allen, B.: Encephalitis due to infection with *Toxocara canis*. Reports of a suspected case. *Lancet, 1*:1355, 1964.

Chandra, R. K.: Visceral larva migrans. *Indian J. Pediatr., 30*:388, 1963.

Dafalla, A. A.: The serodiagnosis of human toxocariasis by the capillary-tube precipitin test. *Trans. R. Soc. Trop. Med. Hyg., 69*:146, 1975.

de Savigny, D. H.: In vitro maintenance of *Toxocara canis* larvae and a simple method for the production of Toxocara ES antigen for use in serodiagnostic tests for visceral larva migrans. *J. Parasitol. 61*:781, 1975.

Faust, E. C., and Russell, P. F.: *Clinical Parasitology.* Philadelphia, Lea & Febiger, 1964.

Friedman, S., and Hervade, A. R.: Severe myocarditis with recovery in a child with visceral larva migrans. *J. Pediatr., 56*:91, 1960.

Galvin, T. J.: Experimental *Toxocara canis* infections in chickens and pigeons. *J. Parasitol., 50*:124, 1964.

Jacklin, H. N., and Holt, L. B.: Ocular localization in larva migrans. *N. C. Med. J., 31*:55, 1970.

Karpinski, F. E., Jr., Everts-Saurez, E. Z., and Sawitz, W. G.: Larval granulomatosis (Visceral larva migrans).*Am. J. Dis. Child., 92*:34, 1956.

Patterson, R., Huntley, C. C., Roberts, M., and Irons, J. S.: Visceral larva migrans: immunoglobulins, precipitating antibodies and detection of IgG and IgM antibodies against *Ascaris* antigen. *Am. J. Trop. Med. Hyg., 24*:465, 1975.

Seah, S. K. K., Hucal, G., and Law, C.: Dogs and intestinal parasites: a public health problem. *Can. Med. Assoc. J., 112*:1191, 1975.

Smith, M. H. D., and Beaver, P. C.: Persistence and distribution of Toxocara larvae in the tissues of children and mice. *Pediatrics, 12*:491, 1953.

Snyder, C. H.: Visceral larva migrans. *Pediatrics, 28*:85, 1961.

Vinke, B.: Application of haemagglutination test for visceral larva migrans in adult. *Trop. Geogr. Med., 16*:43, 1964.

Woodruff, A. W., and Thacher, C. K. M.: Infections with animal helminths. *Br. Med. J., 1*:1001, 1964.

CHAPTER SIXTY-THREE

LOEFFLER'S SYNDROME

WILLIAM A. HOWARD, M. D.

In 1932, Loeffler described a group of patients whose chest roentgenograms showed shadows of variable structures and fleeting density, accompanied by a moderate eosinophilia (10 to 20 per cent) and mild systemic symptoms. This combination of symptoms was generally called Loeffler's syndrome and was presumed to be benign and of short duration, usually a matter of a few weeks. Although no etiologic agent was established, infection with *Ascaris lumbricoides* was known to be present in some of Loeffler's cases. A year later, Weingarten reported the same pulmonary and blood findings in cases of tropical eosinophilia from India. Since that time a number of other similar clinical pictures have been described and the many variants are now often grouped together under the terms "eosinophilic pneumonopathy" or "pulmonary infiltrates with eosinophilia," the PIE syndrome. The term "hypereosinophilic syndrome" has been proposed for the broad spectrum of disease states varying from Loeffler's original syndrome to disseminated eosinophilic collagen disease and eosinophilic leukemia. We have retained the older term of Loeffler's syndrome because of its familiarity to the pediatrician.

Classification

Crofton and his associates (1952) proposed the following classification of this heterogeneous group, though it obviously goes far beyond Loeffler's original concept:

GROUP I. SIMPLE PULMONARY INVOLVEMENT WITH EOSINOPHILIA, OR LOEFFLER'S SYNDROME. This group is limited to those cases in which pulmonary infiltration persists for no more than one month, with mild or absent systemic symptoms.

GROUP II. PROLONGED PULMONARY EOSINOPHILIA. Here the duration is two to six months with definite symptoms and occasional recurrences, but with ultimate recovery. It is not common in children.

GROUP III. TROPICAL EOSINOPHILIA (EOSINOPHILIC LUNG, WEINGARTEN'S SYNDROME). This term is now reserved for those cases of eosinophilic pneumonia due to the presence of degenerating microfilariae found in eosinophilic granulomas in the lung in the absence of circulating adult filarial worms. This has given rise to the designation of *occult filariasis* for this form of the syndrome. Pulmonary symptoms are mild to moderate, there is a characteristic marked eosinophilia, and, without treatment, the course is prolonged.

GROUP IV. PULMONARY EOSINOPHILIA WITH ASTHMA. This is an attempt to place asthmatics in the group of eosinophilic pneumonopathies whenever they have pulmonary infiltrates that may be shifting in nature.

GROUP V. POLYARTERITIS NODOSA. These patients usually are severely ill, with an asthmatic component and a poor prognosis.

Etiology and Pathogenesis

In many cases of Loeffler's syndrome, no specific etiologic agent can be demonstrated. The classic syndrome appears to occur more often in individuals with a personal and family history

1023

of allergy. When a specific cause has been found, it most often appears to be infection with parasitic nematodes, usually Ascaris or Toxocara, although amebiasis, trichinosis and filarial infections may give a similar picture. It may be difficult to determine the presence of a nematode worm in the patient, since in the case of Ascaris the pulmonary phase may occur some days or weeks before ova from adult worms will be found in the stool.

The larval forms of Toxocara become encysted in the tissue, including the lungs, and never reach the intestinal tract to develop into mature worms passing diagnostic ova, such as occurs in the dog. The filarial worms associated with eosinophilic lung have not been isolated or identified, but they are believed to be either *Wuchereria bancrofti* or a species of Brugia. While the presence of the degenerating microfilariae in the lung presupposes the presence of adult filarial worms, their absence is explained on the basis of their rapid elimination by host immune responses. Such a process would also help to explain the marked and constant eosinophilia.

A number of cases of Loeffler's syndrome caused by a variety of drugs and chemicals have now been reported. The list includes nitrofurantoin, para-aminosalicylic acid, hydralazine, mecamylamine, penicillin, imipramine, mephenesin and chlorpropamide, and the list will probably lengthen.

Clinical Manifestations

In general the symptoms are very mild or absent, even in the presence of fairly large pulmonary lesions. There may be a cough or wheeze, and occasionally scattered rales may be heard. On the roentgenogram, the pulmonary lesions are usually simple infiltrations, pneumonic or occasionally atelectatic, somewhat similar in appearance to those caused by tuberculosis (Figs. 1 to 3). In other instances, the roentgeno-

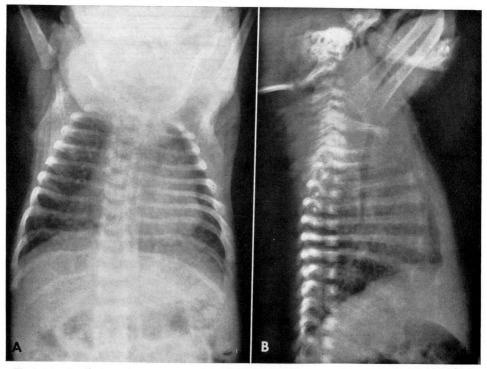

Figure 1. Loeffler's syndrome. Increased density at the right lung base. (Courtesy of John Kirkpatrick, M.D., Children's Hospital Medical Center, Boston.)

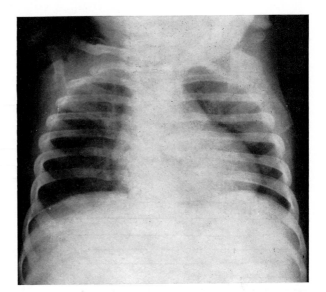

Figure 2. Loeffler's syndrome. X-ray film negative two weeks after admission film. (Courtesy of John Kirkpatrick, M.D., Children's Hospital Medical Center, Boston.)

graphic findings may resemble bronchopneumonia or a viral pneumonitis. Within a few days these lesions begin to clear, but new involvement appears in other areas. Pulmonary function studies in patients with tropical pulmonary eosinophilia often show a reduction in vital capacity as well as a significant lowering of the FEV_1. In most instances these values return to normal within weeks or months after recovery, whether spontaneous or after therapy.

There may be a moderate leukocytosis, and eosinophils range from 10 to 50 per cent. IgE levels ranging from 350 to 10,000 ng. per milliliter, with a mean of 2355 ng. per milliliter, have been observed in patients with tropical eosinophilia (occult filariasis), and there is evidence that similar elevations may be found in patients with overt filarial involvement. When Toxocara infection is the underlying cause, hepatomegaly is usually present.

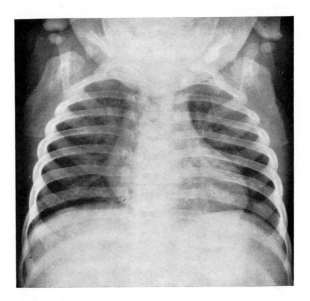

Figure 3. Loeffler's syndrome. Film one month after Figure 2, showing area of infiltration at the right lung base. (Courtesy of John Kirkpatrick, M.D., Children's Hospital Medical Center, Boston.)

Pathology

In the rare case observed at autopsy, the principal findings have been irregular bronchopneumonic foci and small areas of alveolar exudate with many eosinophils. Giant cells of the foreign body type, such as are seen in visceral larva migrans, may also be seen. The presence of degenerating microfilariae in pulmonary eosinophilic granulomas appears pathognomonic of tropical eosinophilia or eosinophilic lung. Vascular damage is rare except in those instances where polyarteritis is present.

Diagnosis

Diagnosis is dependent upon roentgenographic evidence of transient and migratory pulmonary infiltrations with eosinophilia and only mild systemic manifestations. A consideration of possible etiologic agents should include a careful history of recent drug ingestion and a careful search for parasites. Among those responsible besides Ascaris and Toxocara are included the hookworms, Strongyloides infection, filarial worms (Brugia malayi, B. palangi, Wuchereria bancrofti), and trichinosis. Pulmonary involvement with Aspergillus may give a similar radiographic picture at times, but the presence of asthma, a positive skin test to Aspergillus, and identification of mycelia in the sputum will serve to establish the diagnosis of allergic bronchopulmonary aspergillosis. A careful search should be made for tubercle bacilli in the sputum, and a tuberculin test result that remains negative will be helpful in differentiation. The possibility of polyarteritis should be kept in mind. Skin tests to Ascaris antigen may occasionally be helpful in diagnosis. Leukocyte alkaline phosphate determination may be helpful in differentiating the hypereosinophilic syndrome from acute eosinophilic leukemia.

Treatment

Typically, Loeffler's syndrome is self limited, and treatment may not be necessary. Where evidence of filarial infec-

tion exists, diethylcarbamazine (Hetrazan) may be used for seven to ten days in doses of 6 mg. per kilogram per day in three divided doses. The same drug may be used in Ascaris infection, giving 15 mg. per kilogram as a single dose on four successive mornings. Therapy of parasitic infestations of the intestinal tract will have no significant effect on the pulmonary phase of the disease.

If pulmonary lesions are bothersome or cough or wheeze is significant, rapid resolution of the pulmonary process can be produced by administration of a suitable corticosteroid preparation. These should be used only when the presence of tuberculosis has been excluded.

REFERENCES

Bell, R. J. M.: Pulmonary infiltrations with eosinophilia caused by chlorpropamide. *Lancet*, 1:1249, 1964.

Crofton, J. W., Livingston, J. L., Oswald, N. C. and Roberts, A. T. M.: Pulmonary eosinophilia. *Thorax*, 7:1, 1952.

Danaraj, T.J., Pacheco, G., Shanmugaratnam, K., and Beaver, P. C.: The etiology and pathology of eosinophilic lung (tropical eosinophilia). *Am. J. Trop. Med. Hyg.*, 15:183, 1966.

Incaprera, F. P.: Pulmonary eosinophilia. *Am. Rev. Resp. Dis.*, 84:730, 1961.

Loeffler, W.: Zur Differential-Diagnose der Lungeninfiltrierungen. II. Ueber fluchtige Succedan-Infiltrate (mit Eosinophilie). *Beitr. Klin. Tuberk.*, 79:368, 1932.

Mark, L.: Loeffler's syndrome. *Dis. Chest.*, 25:128, 1954.

Neva, F. A., Kaplan, A. P., Pacheco, G., Gray, L., and Danaraj, T. J.: Tropical eosinophilia. *J. Allergy Clin. Immunol.*, 55:422, 1976.

Poh, S. C.: The course of lung function in treated tropical pulmonary eosinophilia. *Thorax*, 29:710, 1974.

Quinlan, C. D., and Mitchell, D. M.: The hypereosinophilic syndrome. *J. Ir. Med. Assoc.*, 63:186, 1970.

Rutenberg, A. M., Rosales, C. L., and Bennett, J. M.: An improved histochemical method for the demonstration of leukocyte alkaline phosphatase. Clinical application. *J. Lab. Clin. Med.*, 65:698, 1965.

Scheer, E. H.: Loeffler's syndrome. *Arch. Pediatr.*, 68:407, 1951.

Weingarten, R. J.: Tropical eosinophilia. *Lancet*, 1:103, 1943.

Wilson, I. C., Gambill, J. M., and Sandifer, M. G.: Loeffler's syndrome occurring during imipramine therapy. *Am. J. Psychiatry*, 119:892, 1963.

CHAPTER SIXTY-FOUR

IDIOPATHIC HISTIOCYTOSIS (HISTIOCYTOSIS X)

ROBERT H. HIGH, M.D.

The terms "idiopathic histiocytosis" or "histiocytosis X," and many others such as systemic reticuloendotheliosis, histiocytic reticuloendotheliosis, nonlipoid reticuloendotheliosis, and nonlipoid histiocytosis, have been used to designate a group of several diseases with varying clinical patterns that have in common proliferation of the histiocytes in the tissues. These diseases, all of unknown origin, include the following in order of decreasing severity of morbidity and mortality: (1) the Letterer-Siwe syndrome, (2) the Hand-Schüller-Christian syndrome, (3) eosinophilic granuloma of bone and (4) histiocytic infiltrations of atypical distribution often involving one organ, such as the skin, the lungs, the lymph nodes and others, in varying degrees. Although some object to grouping these disturbances together, there seems to be a general consensus that they represent a spectrum of clinical patterns of related processes of unknown causation. These diseases are not malignant, not hereditary, not familial and not infectious in origin. They are not related to the lipoid reticuloendothelioses such as Gaucher's and Niemann-Pick diseases.

Consideration is given to these obscure diseases because all of them except eosinophilic granuloma of the bone can produce pulmonary infiltrations that may cause some of the symptoms and, at times, fatalities. Pulmonary infiltrations are most commonly associated with Letter-Siwe disease, less commonly associated with Hand-Schüller-Chris-

tian disease, and only occasionally noted in the group designated as "histiocytic infiltrations of atypical distribution." The great variability of the clinical manifestations and pathologic changes in these diseases precludes discussion here. Attention is directed only to the pulmonary component of these disturbances.

Because of the wide variations in the gross and histologic appearances of the lungs, the following descriptions are intended to include, in a general way, only the most important changes. Many details are not mentioned. Histiocytic infiltrations occur in the lungs, chiefly in the interlobular or interalveolar septa or in the perivascular, peribronchial or subpleural tissues. These collections can be of sufficient size to produce nodules in the lungs. Sometimes dilatation of the terminal bronchioles and alveoli develops secondary to the peribronchial infiltrates. This process leads to the development of microcysts, which are sometimes the origin of interstitial emphysema, pneumomediastinum or pneumothorax (Fig. 1).

In addition to the histiocytic infiltrations, there may also be infiltrations of eosinophils and fibroblasts. Lymphocytes and plasma cells may be present.

The development of pulmonary infiltrations in these diseases is usually a sign of ominous prognostic importance. Extensive pulmonary infiltrates are commonly found in the fatal cases even though the pulmonary involvement was not the cause of death.

The clinical manifestations of the

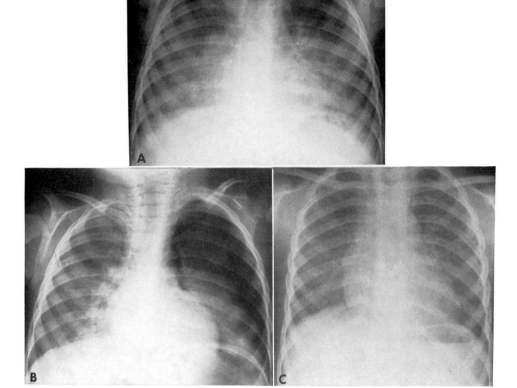

Figure 1. *A* (5/3/63), Diffuse bilateral pulmonary infiltrates. *B,* Left pneumothorax secondary to rupture of microcysts. *C* (3/12/65), Considerable resolution 22 months later after alternating weekly doses of vincristine and cyclophosphamide (Cytoxan).

pulmonary histiocytic infiltrations are added to those of the primary problem and may be minor or major, depending upon the extensiveness of the process. Cough and chest pain may be present, and these may be associated with tachypnea, dyspnea and cyanosis. Physical examination seldom reveals the presence of rales or abnormal percussion changes, although evidence of localized or generalized emphysema may be noted. Inspiratory retraction may be present. Rupture of the microcysts can lead to the development of interstitial emphysema, pneumomediastinum or pneumothorax, which produce the changes noted previously. In general, the abnormalities apparent by physical examination are far less than the extent

of the infiltrations demonstrable by roentgenographic examination.

Roentgenographic examination of the chest shows variable findings, depending upon the distribution and size of the histiocytic infiltrations. It may be within normal limits or may show evidence of overaeration. When the infiltrations are of sufficient size, generalized hazy densities much like those noted in fulminating miliary tuberculosis are produced. Sometimes discrete nodules are apparent. The roentgenographic abnormalities are not pathognomonic. Examination of other areas, especially the skull and long bones, is indicated when such diffuse densities are noted in the chest roentgenograms.

In this group of diseases, as in most

diseases of obscure origin, therapy is largely empiric and supportive and is directed toward the relief of symptoms. Irradiation of the chest may relieve some of the symptoms, and subsequent roentgenographic studies may show some resolution of the infiltrations. The administration of adrenocorticosteroids, the alkylating agents or the antimetabolic agents such as aminopterin may retard the progression of the disease, and sometimes recovery, or at least long-term survival, occurs (Fig 2).

The most hopeful therapeutic program at present is the administration of one of the several alkaloid derivatives of the periwinkle plant (*Vinca rosea* Linn). The intravenous administration of vincristine sulfate at weekly intervals for long periods of time seems to be especially beneficial in patients with Letterer-Siwe disease. Lahey (1975), reporting for a group of cooperative investigators who treated generalized histiocytosis, Letterer-Siwe disease and Hand-Schüller-Christian syndrome with vinblastine, vinblastine and prednisone, or prednisone and 6-mercaptopurine, noted very favorable results.

These investigators observed 83 patients and noted that 65, or 71 per cent, were alive with good or complete remissions ten months to six and one-half years from the onset of the disease. The average survival time was three and two-thirds years. Some had residual disabilities, such as short stature, diabetes insipidus, exophthalmos, vertebral compression, pulmonary fibrosis or combinations thereof. Others have noted good results employing a therapeutic program using an adrenocorticosteroid, usually prednisone, and an antimetabolic agent such as cyclophosphamide.

Therapy of the pulmonary aspects of the idiopathic histiocytoses is often a minor part of the treatment, especially when the process has a systemic distribution.

It is not possible to state a prognosis for a group of diseases as heterogeneous as those considered here. They are not uniformly fatal. Evaluation of the initial clinical manifestations and of the histologic appearance of tissues may give general indications of the possible outcome. Such appraisals are far

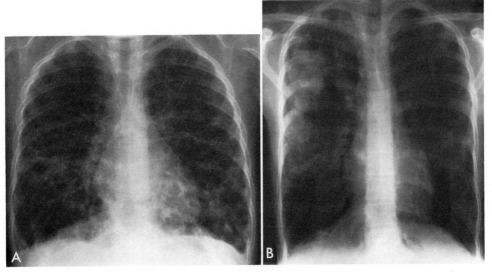

Figure 2. Histiocytosis X diagnosed by biopsy of osseous lesions in November 1962 at age of 2 years and 10 months. Treated with irradiation and prednisone. *A,* Essentially asymptomatic. Note extensive "honeycombing" of lungs secondary to cystic changes and fibrosis (one year after diagnosis). *B,* Multiple right upper lobe densities in cystic lesions. Note air-fluid levels. Presumed to be secondary to infection with Aspergillus species (ten years after diagnosis).

from reliable, since some patients with apparently fulminating disease have had the process become quiescent and have survived for long periods. In general terms, the severity of these disturbances in decreasing order of morbidity and mortality is as follows: (1) Letterer-Siwe syndrome, (2) Hand-Schüller-Christian syndrome, (3) eosinophilic granuloma of bone and (4) histiocytic infiltrations of atypical distribution. The prognosis appears to be best correlated with the extent of visceral involvement and the histologic appearance of the involved tissues. In the future, it may be possible to develop a system of staging of these diseases, such as is now available for Hodgkin's disease and others, which will be a better indicator of the prognosis.

REFERENCES

Crocker, A. C.: The histiocytosis syndrome. In Gellis, S. S., and Kagan, B. M. (Eds.): *Current Pediatric Therapy* 7. Philadelphia, W. B. Saunders Company, 1976, p. 719.

Holinger, P. H., Slaughter, D. P., and Novak, F. J.: Unusual tumors obstructing the lower respiratory tract of infants and children. *Trans. Am. Acad. Ophthalmol.*, 54:223, 1950.

Lahey, M. E.: Histiocytosis X—comparison of three treatment regimens. *J. Pediatr.*, 87, 179, 1975.

Lahey, M. E.: Histiocytosis X—an analysis of prognostic factors. *J. Pediatr.*, 87:185, 1975.

CHAPTER SIXTY-FIVE

PULMONARY INVOLVEMENT IN THE RHEUMATIC DISORDERS (SO-CALLED COLLAGEN DISEASES) OF CHILDHOOD

Bernhard H. Singsen, M.D., and Arnold C. G. Platzker, M.D.

Until the causes of all of the so-called collagen diseases are known, any classification of this group of syndromes will be no more than descriptive. A number of descriptive terms have been employed, including collagen diseases, connective tissue diseases and rheumatic diseases, but none of these is totally adequate. However, it is becoming increasingly evident that most rheumatic diseases are not primarily diseases of collagen or connective tissues.

Several observations about the rheumatic diseases are apparent. They may be characterized as chronic or chronic-recurrent diseases of tissue inflammation of unknown pathogenesis. With rare exception, meticulous investigation has not revealed an infectious cause for the rheumatic diseases. Whipple's disease, some cases of Reiter's syndrome, and specific viral diseases such as hepatitis, rubella and mononucleosis have an infectious cause but are mediated

Deep appreciation is expressed to the many physicians who contributed to the preparation of materials for this manuscript: Fred Lee (radiology), Benjamin Landing (pathology), Margaret O'Neal, Stuart Foster, M.S., and Daisy Bautista, B.S. (pulmonary physiology), and Virgil Hanson, Helen Kornreich, Bram Bernstein, and Karen Koster King (rheumatology).

through immunologic mechanisms. Many lines of evidence favor the chronic or recurrent presence of one or many antigens to stimulate the apparently immune-mediated inflammation common to the rheumatic diseases. Infectious agents, particularly undetected viral genomes, or long-departed viruses that have contributed genetic material to alter the host immunologic response remain favorite candidates for these unknown antigens.

A simplified schematic may help to explain the chronicity of inflammation characteristic of the rheumatic diseases. Figure 1 shows three major activities: the process from injury to healing, the phagocytosis by neutrophils of various foreign materials, and the stimulation of the immune system by antigens. Central to an understanding of inflammation is the potential within the inflammatory system for amplification and re-amplification. It is widely presumed that the persistence of as yet unrecognized antigens leads to the chronic inflammation that characterizes most of the rheumatic diseases. One can readily see from the schematic that this persistence leads to continuous Ag-Ab-C' formation, stimulates continuous phagocytosis and cellular toxicity, and thus constantly re-amplifies the processes causing injury.

The majority of the rheumatic diseases in both children and adults exhibit serologic abnormalities. Clearly, these serologic abnormalities result from antigenic stimulation of the humoral immune system, displayed on the right side of Figure 1. These serologic changes suggest that the patients have an altered immunologic status, but it is important to stress that the observed abnormalities need not have either specific diagnostic or etiologic significance. As an example, it is known that much of the nephritis of systemic lupus erythematosus (SLE) is due to the deposition of soluble DNA—anti-DNA antibody–complement complexes in the kidney. However, it is not clear what causes the presence of soluble DNA, or why it persists in the circulation. The injection of soluble DNA into normal ex-

perimental animals does not lead to the development of antinuclear antibodies (including anti-DNA antibodies), and does not cause nephritis. Further, although the presence of high titers of antinuclear antibodies (ANA) may be highly suggestive of SLE, their presence is by no means diagnostic of, or restricted to, this condition.

Table 1 shows the relative prevalence of ANA and rheumatoid factor (RF) in a recent survey of children from the rheumatic disease clinics of Children's Hospital of Los Angeles. Evidence of altered immunologic status is present in all of the diseases tested, and the results highlight the lack of diagnostic specificity of RF or ANA.

The clinical features of the various rheumatic diseases are in many respects similar, and in the past have superficially been described as "overlapping," much in the fashion that serologic fea-

TISSUE INJURY, INFLAMMATION, AND IMMUNE MECHANISMS

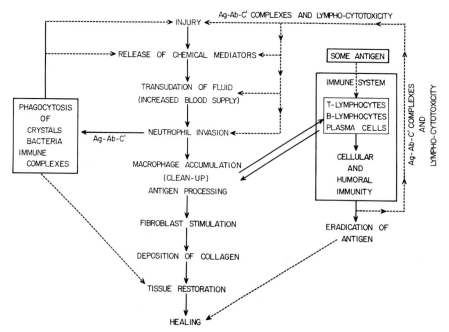

Figure 1.   Simplified schematic showing three simultaneously occurring aspects of inflammation and healing, including the roles of cellular and humoral immunity, the process of phagocytosis and the direct sequence of tissue healing. A major consequence of this system is the capability for chronic inflammation if antigens, immune complexes or crystals are persistently or intermittently present. (This schematic was designed by and supplied through the courtesy of Virgil Hanson, M.D.)

TABLE 1.   RHEUMATOID FACTOR (RF) AND ANTINUCLEAR ANTIBODIES (ANA) IN CHILDHOOD

Diagnosis	Number of Patients	% Positive	
		RF	ANA
Systemic lupus erythematosus	108	5	95
Juvenile rheumatoid arthritis	110	25	28
Dermatomyositis	20	0	55
Scleroderma	19	25	47
Ulcerative colitis	34	11	23
Mixed connective tissue disease	14	64	100
Controls	49	0	6

tures appear to overlap. It is true that many of the rheumatic diseases share gross, common denominators, but it is equally true that careful study, particularly of the clinical characteristics, allows delineation of the differences. As an example, the majority of the rheumatic diseases exhibit arthritis, without demonstrable infectious cause, at some time during the disease course. But careful examination and follow-up reveals marked differences—e.g., the chronic, slowly progressive, erosive changes of juvenile rheumatoid arthritis (JRA), contrasted with the recurrent synovitis without destructive potential of SLE, versus the early synovitis of childhood scleroderma and dermatomyositis. Similarly, recent investigation of JRA, in conjunction with lymphocyte tissue typing (HLA), has further defined the subtypes present in the pauciarticular group of childhood arthritides (Schaller and coworkers, 1976). As another example, mixed connective tissue disease (MCTD) is coming to be recognized as a distinct entity with typical, but slowly evolving, characteristics (Singsen and coworkers, 1977). But here again, anti-ribonucleoprotein antibodies are not a serologic property exclusive to MCTD (Notman and associates, 1975), and further investigation may define subclasses of MCTD, or additional distinct "overlap" syndromes with special, but not exclusive, serologic characteristics.

More than 100 distinct syndromes are known to be associated with arthri-

tis in childhood, including metabolic disorders and numerous miscellaneous conditions. Among these are the rheumatic diseases of childhood presented in Table 2. These latter diseases were the subject of a recent extensive conference, the proceedings of which are available to the reader who desires an understanding of the pediatric rheumatic diseases beyond the scope of this chapter (Schaller and Hanson, 1977).

In the following sections, the diseases are presented roughly in the order of the likelihood and the severity of pulmonary involvement due to the primary disease process. Beyond the initial

TABLE 2.   THE RHEUMATIC DISEASES OF CHILDHOOD

Systemic lupus erythematosus (SLE)
Scleroderma
Dermatomyositis
Juvenile rheumatoid arthritis (JRA)
Mixed connective tissue disease (MCTD)
Wegener's granulomatosis
Periarteritis nodosa
Systemic vasculitis
Henoch-Schönlein purpura
Stevens-Johnson syndrome
Mucocutaneous lymph node syndrome (MCLS)
Ulcerative colitis
Regional enteritis
Ankylosing spondylitis
Reiter's syndrome
Psoriatic arthritis
Behçet's syndrome
Sjögren's syndrome
Familial Mediterranean fever (FMF)
Acute rheumatic fever (see Chapter 61)
Sarcoidosis (see Chapter 48)

six diseases, which are dealt with in detail, is a large group of distinctly identifiable pediatric rheumatic disease syndromes. We have not recognized pulmonary involvement, nor is it described in the pediatric literature, in diseases such as Stevens-Johnson syndrome, Henoch-Schönlein purpura, mucocutaneous lymph node syndrome, or allergic (systemic) vasculitis. And yet, the character of the recognized pathologic processes of these entities suggests that pulmonary involvement might occur. Where appropriate, pulmonary involvement in the adult presentation of these and other rheumatic diseases will be noted.

Finally, it is important to distinguish between the pediatric and adult forms of the rheumatic diseases. In some situations, such as ankylosing spondylitis, the disease appears to extend as a direct continuum from childhood to adult life, with earlier detection increasingly extending the diagnosis to younger age groups. But in numerous other instances, the pediatric rheumatic diseases are not just "little people's" versions of the adult form. Examples of differences present between childhood and adult versions include the prevalence of linear and focal forms of scleroderma to the relative exclusion of the systemic form in childhood, the greater morbidity and mortality of childhood SLE, the prominence of pauciarticular JRA (often with iridocyclitis), the unique histologic characteristics of vasculitis associated with childhood dermatomyositis, and so forth. Therefore, it is not unreasonable to speculate that the type and severity of pulmonary involvement in the pediatric rheumatic diseases may differ also.

The investigation of pathologic pulmonary processes in the rheumatic diseases of childhood remains nascent at present. To our knowledge, there are no extensive studies of the pulmonary histopathologic changes in any of the childhood rheumatic diseases, nor, perhaps more important, are there published serial studies of pulmonary function over the course of most of the pediatric rheumatic diseases. It is hoped that this chapter will be a small step toward further knowledge in this area.

SYSTEMIC LUPUS ERYTHEMATOSUS

Systemic lupus erythematosus (SLE) in childhood, as in the adult, is characterized by highly variable clinical and serologic manifestations. It is a diffuse and chronic inflammatory process that may affect any organ system. Establishing a diagnosis of SLE may be aided by the preliminary criteria for the classification of SLE of the American Rheumatism Association (Cohen and coworkers, 1971). SLE in childhood has been the subject of many excellent reports; those of Meislin and Rothfield (1968) and Kornreich and coworkers (1977) are particularly suggested for further review.

Awareness of pleuropulmonary involvement in SLE has existed since the nineteenth century, but little attention was paid to specific pulmonary manifestations until 1952 (Bagenstoss, 1952; Harvey and coworkers, 1954; Purnell and coworkers, 1955). Since that time, investigation has expanded rapidly in three directions: pulmonary function studies, histopathology, and chest roentgenographic patterns.

In 1965, Huang and coworkers studied the pulmonary function of 28 adults with SLE. Four groups were studied, including eight patients with a past or present history of pleural involvement; nine patients with a past or present history of parenchymal disease; three patients with a past or present history of both pleural and parenchymal involvement; and eight patients with no past or present evidence of pulmonary disease. The high incidence of abnormal lung function was unexpected and included abnormal diffusing capacity for carbon monoxide

(D_LCO) in 89 per cent of patients tested. Forced vital capacity was abnormal in 79 per cent, inspiratory capacity was decreased in 87 per cent and total lung capacity was decreased in 61 per cent. Most significant was the observation that pulmonary function abnormalities were present in almost two-thirds of patients without current clinical or roentgenographic evidence of pulmonary disease.

Similar findings were observed by Gold and Jennings (1966) and by Laitinen and coworkers (1973), who suggested that the single-breath carbon monoxide test (D_LCO) was the most sensitive indicator of pulmonary dysfunction in SLE. More recent studies have debated, with inconclusive results, the contribution of cigarette smoking to observed dysfunction (Hunt and coworkers, 1975; Chick and colleagues, 1976). Unfortunately, serial pulmonary function studies from the onset of SLE have not been performed.

The present authors have performed pulmonary function studies in 20 children with SLE (mean age at testing: 15.5 years). All patients with clinical or roentgenographic evidence of pulmonary disease at the time of study were excluded. The findings included abnormal D_LCO in 25 per cent, pulmonary restrictive defects in 35 per cent, abnormal P_{O_2} in 10 per cent, and an obstructive defect in 5 per cent. These preliminary results may suggest that pulmonary abnormalities are less common in children with SLE, or may merely reflect a shorter disease duration and less exposure to environmental hazards.

Numerous histopathologic descriptions of SLE pulmonary disease are available, but the changes are disappointing in their lack of specificity. According to Purnell and associates (1955), interstitial pneumonitis, pleuritis with effusions and atelectasis are the most common pathologic changes. Gross and coworkers (1971) observed bronchopneumonia, interstitial pneumonia, alveolar hemorrhage and chronic pleural thickening all to occur in more than 50 per cent of cases in an autopsy series. Another major finding included the lack of significant interstitial fibrosis, despite the almost constant presence of interstitial thickening and inflammatory infiltrates. However, 100 per cent of their 44 patients had evidence of distal airway alterations, including bronchiolar dilatation, alveolar simplification and focal panacinar emphysema. It was speculated that these changes might contribute to decreased diffusing capacity and to ventilation-perfusion inequalities. Only 19 per cent of these patients had pulmonary vascular lesions, in comparison with 40 per cent in another report (Fayemi, 1975). In this latter investigation, Fayemi stressed that correlation between clinical and pathologic findings is poor because primary histologic changes are commonly obscured by congestive heart failure, infection and uremia.

Between 1961 and 1976 there were 21 deaths due to SLE among a clinic population of 130 patients followed at the Children's Hospital of Los Angeles. A preliminary review of the pulmonary histopathologic findings in association with Benjamin Landing, M.D., revealed many of the pathologic changes to be similar to those observed in adults. One striking observation was that during the most recent five-year period, eight of ten deaths occurred as a direct result of pulmonary compromise. Among the 21 children, vascular lesions were uncommon, but unexpected pulmonary hemosiderosis and alveolitis obliterans (mucoid or hyaline-like round collections within the alveolus) each occurred in one-third of cases. Acute bronchopneumonia was present in 57 per cent of the lungs reviewed.

Cultures were taken from the lungs at postmortem examination in 15 cases, and all 21 were reviewed histologically for specific, nonbacterial pathogens; the results are shown in Table 3. They indicate that infection is a common denominator in childhood SLE pulmo-

TABLE 3.   PATHOGENS IN THE LUNGS OF 21 CHILDREN DYING FROM SLE

Klebsiella aerobacter	5	Candida albicans	3
Escherichia coli	4	Aspergillus species	3
Alpha streptococcus	3	Cytomegalic inclusion virus	3
Alpha enterococcus	2	Pneumocystis carinii	3
Staphylococcus epidermidis	2	Cryptococcus neoformans	1
Pseudomonas aeruginosa	1	Allescheria boydii	1
Proteus mirabilis	1		
Staphylococcus aureus	1		

nary involvement, and confirm the findings of several adult series. Staples and coworkers (1974) showed that infection rate and the number of disseminated infections increase in lupus patients with increasing steroid doses and with decreasing renal function. However, those patients with normal renal function and no, or small dose, steroid therapy also had a significantly higher infection rate than controls did. The authors suggested that a defect in neutrophil function was at least partially responsible for their findings. Other reports have described deep fungal infections (Sieving and coworkers, 1975), and related their occurrence to immunosuppressive therapy or SLE-related deficits in cell-mediated immunity (Paty and coworkers, 1975).

The chest roentgenographic patterns encountered in patients with SLE are widely varied, and their proper evaluation presents a formidable challenge to the radiologist and clinician. The implication of early roentgenographic studies was that patients with SLE commonly develop a primary lung disease, which may be called "lupus pneumonitis" (Alarcon-Segovia and Alarcon, 1961). Conversely, Dubois and Tuffanelli (1964) noted only a 0.9 per cent incidence of pulmonary involvement due to SLE, but 31 per cent of their patients were found to develop bacterial pneumonias as a secondary complication. Levin (1971) attempted to resolve this conflict with an evaluation of the clinical histories and chest roentgenograms of 111 patients with SLE. He noted that 38 patients had pleural involvement, and many of these had patchy atelec-

tasis on the involved side. Sixteen developed superimposed pulmonary infection, and four developed uremic pulmonary edema. True "lupus pneumonitis" by roentgenographic criteria developed in only three individuals (2.7 per cent). These patients were symptomatic, with dyspnea, cough or chest pain, and showed patchy infiltration of small nodules (without evidence of congestive heart failure or pleuritis) on chest roentgenograms.

The following case reports illustrate three types and degrees of SLE pulmonary involvement. An approach to diagnosis and therapy, which can, with some modification, be extended to pulmonary involvement in each of the childhood rheumatic diseases, is then presented.

Case 1

This four-year-old female was first seen in May 1972 with a three-month history of progressive malaise, fever, arthralgias and rash over the trunk and extremities. Examination revealed an anxious, febrile girl with an erythematous maculopapular eruption over the trunk and thighs. Moderate lymphadenopathy and hepatosplenomegaly were present. The lungs were clear, but tachypnea was present. The heart showed cardiomegaly and a grade II/VI systolic ejection murmur. Arthritis of the elbows, wrists and knees was present.

Laboratory findings included a white blood cell count (WBC) of 11,800/mm.^{3}, hemoglobin (Hgb) 8.8 gm./100 ml., erythrocyte sedimentation rate (ESR) of 130 mm./hr., positive direct and indirect Coombs tests, serum albumin 2.9 gm./100 ml., and serum globulin 5.2 gm./100 ml.; serum antinuclear antibodies were strongly positive, and rheumatoid factor was present in a titer of 1:160. Serum IgG was 3525 mg./100 ml. (normal: 550–1100 mg./100 ml.), and the serum C3 was less than 10 mg./100 ml. (normal: 60–140 mg./100 ml.). Creatinine clearance was 47 ml./min./1.73 m^2. A urinalysis revealed 2+ proteinuria, 25 to 30 WBC/hpf, 75 to 100 RBC/hpf, and granular and hyaline casts. A chest roentgenogram showed moderate cardiomegaly with slightly increased pulmonary vascularity. An electrocardiogram and echocardiogram were both normal.

A diagnosis of SLE with renal disease and mild myocarditis was made, and she was begun on prednisolone, 35 mg. per day, and hydroxychloroquine, 100 mg. per day. A renal biopsy revealed histologic evidence of severe proliferative glomerulonephritis with diffuse, chronic interstitial nephritis. Diuretics were begun because of progressive edema and hypertension.

By August 1972, the patient's serum C3 had returned to 133 mg./100 ml., the ANA was only mildly positive. One episode of mild pneumonitis resolved following treatment with oral ampicillin. The next 18 months were marked by active nephritis and varying degrees of rash and arthritis. Despite continuous prednisolone therapy (15 to 40 mg. every other day), her serum C3 progressively fell to 30 mg./100 ml.

In February 1974, the patient, now 6½ years old, was readmitted with fever and headaches. The cerebrospinal fluid protein was 30 mg./100 ml., but an electroencephalogram revealed mild, diffuse dysfunction. A repeat renal biopsy showed diffuse, proliferative lupus nephritis with positive immunofluorescence for IgG, M, A, E, C3 and fibrin. A urine protein was 4.1 gr./24 hr. Cyclophosphamide, 50 mg. per day, was begun, and the prednisolone was increased to 30 mg. per day; serum C3 and ANA slowly reverted to normal.

In June and August of 1974, the patient was admitted because of fever and pneumonia. Cyclophosphamide was discontinued. Clinical and roentgenographic resolution of both episodes followed administration of intravenous cephalothin. Serum C3 and C4 were normal during both episodes, and the ANA was negative. The ANA again became positive in December 1974, and remained so for the remainder of her illness. Active renal disease continued, with fluctuating serum C3 and C4 levels, proteinuria and an active urine sediment.

In October 1975, the patient developed fever and a left lower lobe pneumonia, which responded to intravenous cephalothin. In December, she developed *H. influenzae* cellulitis of the left arm, pericarditis and central nervous system involvement with chorea. Intravenous ampicillin and dexamethasone, 1.5 mg. every 6 hours, were successfully employed. A chest roentgenogram showed clear lung fields. Hypertension was present, and her serum BUN rose to 66 mg./100 ml., and her creatinine to 1.5 mg./100 ml.

On January 9, 1976, the patient developed fever, cough, and chest pain. Mild cardiomegaly was present on chest roentgenogram. On January 12, 1976, myocarditis was detected, and she received diuretics and antibiotics; dexamethasone was increased to 2.0 mg. every 6 hours. On the following day, tachypnea, nasal flaring, grunting respirations, and bilateral rales were present. A chest roentgenogram revealed bilateral infiltrates suggestive of congestive heart failure (CHF), pneumonia or pulmonary hemorrhage (Fig. 2). Arterial blood gases (ABG) included pH 7.40, P$_{O_2}$ 56, P$_{CO_2}$ 30, and base excess −6. Increasing amounts of blood-tinged sputum were produced. Therapy for CHF was begun, and methylprednisolone, 500 mg., was given. Progressive respiratory distress occurred, and the patient was placed on a respirator with F$_{IO_2}$ 85

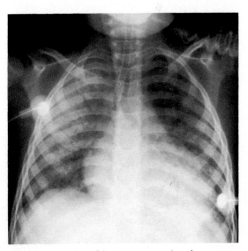

Figure 2. Portable anteroposterior chest roentgenogram showing bilateral parenchymal infiltrates consistent with diffuse, intra-alveolar hemorrhage or edema. The heart is large in its transverse diameter. The small pneumomediastinum and interstitial emphysema in the neck present in the original film are not well reproduced.

per cent, rate 20, PEEP 4; ABG were: pH 7.45, P_{O_2} 57, P_{CO_2} 37, base excess +2. On January 15, 1976, rapid clinical deterioration occurred, and the patient expired following a cardiac arrest.

Postmortem examination of the heart showed histologic changes due to hypertension, focal vasculitis of the right side of the heart, mild epicarditis and myocardial edema. The lungs revealed massive alveolar hemorrhage with few residual aerated sacs. Focal necrotizing pneumonitis and increased interstitial inflammatory cell infiltrates were present. Panacinar edema, alveolar septal decrease, and fibrinoid swelling of arteriolar walls were all occasionally observed.

This case represents the apparent rapid onset of primary lupus pneumonitis leading to diffuse alveolar hemorrhage and death. Congestive heart failure and superimposed pulmonary infection were major diagnostic and therapeutic complications.

Case 2

This nine-year-old female first became ill in April 1970, when she developed skin rash, nephritis and myocarditis, with congestive heart failure that necessitated digitalis and diuretic therapy. In September 1970, she was first seen at Children's Hospital of Los Angeles, where she was found to have spiking fever, characteristic malar rash of SLE, malaise and arthralgias. Laboratory findings included profuse proteinuria and an active urine sediment. The ANA was positive, and anti-DNA antibodies were present; serum C3 was below normal.

There was no clinical or roentgenographic evidence of pulmonary disease.

Up to the present time, her course has been marked by persistent hypocomplementemia (C3 and C4) and long periods of very active skin rash. Her nephritis remitted five months after she was first seen, and has never recurred. Since the onset of her SLE, this teenager has been troubled by relapsing but slowly progressive neurologic manifestations, including peripheral neuritis, mood swings, deterioration of fine motor coordination, brief episodes of psychosis, and persistent headaches. A recent cerebrospinal fluid protein was 76 mg./100 ml. (normal: less than 45 mg./100 ml.).

The neurologic manifestations and several episodes of severe oropharyngeal rash have necessitated the intermittent use of cyclophosphamide or azathioprine and the continued use of prednisolone in doses ranging from 7.5 to 90 mg. per day. The patient is moderately cushingoid, and has marked striae. Hypertension has not been a management problem, perhaps because of the long-standing absence of clinically evident renal disease.

Numerous chest roentgenograms have been obtained throughout her disease course. Slight thickening and prominence of lung markings were first observed in September 1971, and have not appreciably changed to the present (October 1976) (Fig. 3).

Pulmonary function studies were performed in August 1976, and the results are displayed below:

Vital capacity (VC) and its subdivisions are mildly to moderately reduced (Table 4). The functional residual capacity (FRC), re-

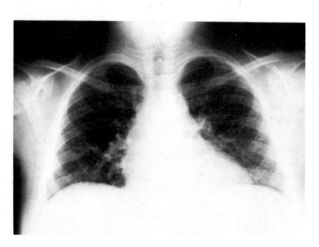

Figure 3. Chest roentgenogram showing a poor inspiratory effort with resultant prominent cardiac silhouette. The lungs show diffuse reticular changes suggestive of chronic pulmonary fibrosis. There are no pleural effusions or acute infiltrates.

TABLE 4. CASE 2

	Normal Range	Predicted Mean	August 1976 Measured (% mean)
VC (L)	1.9–3.3	2.6	1.6 (64%)
FRC (L)	1.0–2.1	1.5	0.9 (58%)
RV (L)	0.4–1.1	0.7	0.5 (69%)
TLC (L)	2.5–4.1	3.3	2.2 (65%)
FEV$_1$ (L)	2.0–2.9	2.5	1.5 (61%)
FEV$_1$/FVC (%)	72–100	86.0	87.0
MMEF (L/min)	122–258	190.0	109.0 (57%)
CV (L)		0.2	0.3
CV/VC (%)		7.0	19.0
N$_2$ (40) (%)		1.5	0.5
D$_L$CO (ml/min/mm Hg)	12.1–25.3	18.7	12.0
P$_{O_2}$ (mm Hg)		97.0	82.0
P$_{CO_2}$ (mm Hg)		37–43	30.0
pH		7.37–7.43	7.40

sidual volume (RV) and total lung capacity (TLC) show similar reductions in volume. The one-second forced vital capacity (FEV$_1$), although reduced, reflects the reduction in VC. Thus, the one-second forced vital capacity expressed as a percentage of the forced vital capacity (FEV$_1$/FVC) is well within the normal range. The maximal expiratory flow-volume curve (MMEF) has a normal configuration with normal expired flow rates at all lung volumes. The closing volume (CV) and closing capacity are increased. The distribution of ventilation as measured by the single-breath oxygen and the 40-breath nitrogen washout curve (N$_2$(40)) fall well within the normal limits. The single-breath diffusion capacity for carbon monoxide (D$_L$CO) is reduced from the predicted mean but is just within one standard deviation. The arterial oxygen tension (P$_{O_2}$) is within the normal range, and the

P$_{CO_2}$ and pH reflect a compensated respiratory alkalosis.

EXERCISE

Oxygen consumption at rest falls within the normal range (Table 5); however, the CO$_2$ production expressed as a fraction of the oxygen consumption is elevated. Minute respiratory volume is increased as a function of respiratory rate. Wasted ventilation and the wasted ventilation–tidal volume ratio are within the normal range. After six minutes of exercise at 150 kilogram-meters per minute, there is moderate hypoxia and approximately a threefold increase in the oxygen consumption. The respiratory quotient falls. Minute respiratory volume increases approximately threefold, and the respiratory rate doubles. Wasted ventilation increases, while the wasted ventilation–tidal volume ratio remains unchanged. Twelve minutes after the beginning of exercise and

TABLE 5. CASE 2

		Exercise Load: 150 kgM./min.	Exercise Load: 250 kgM./min.	Recovery
Arterial blood	rest	6 minutes	6 minutes	4 minutes
O$_2$ tension (mm. Hg)	86	72	64	88
CO$_2$ tension (mm. Hg)	32	29		29
pH	7.43	7.42	7.41	7.41
O$_2$ consumption (L/min.)	0.129	0.415	0.550	
R (CO$_2$/O$_2$)	1.03	0.87	0.98	
Minute vol. resp. (L/min.)	11.9	32.9	45.3	
Resp. rate (breaths/min.)	28.3	48.0	58.0	
Heart rate (beats/min.)	100.0	148.0	178.0	
Wasted vent. (L)	0.17	0.28	0.29	
VD/VT	0.41	0.41	0.38	

six minutes after increasing the rate to 250 kilogram-meters per minute, the patient experiences complete exhaustion. The arterial P_{O_2} has fallen further. The oxygen consumption has increased to $4\frac{1}{2}$ times above the baseline level, and there is balance of carbon dioxide production and oxygen consumption. Minute respiratory volume is now 4 times baseline levels. The respiratory rate is increased by 20 per cent from the first exercise load, and the heart rate is 178 per minute. Wasted ventilation remains relatively unchanged, and wasted ventilation–tidal volume ratio is also unchanged. Four minutes after cessation of exercise, the P_{O_2} has risen to the normal range, whereas the carbon dioxide tension remains markedly depressed.

This patient has moderately severe restrictive lung disease with intact airway function. The elevated closing volume and closing capacity may reflect basilar vascular congestion causing expiratory closure of the airway at relatively large lung volumes. The diffusing capacity is slightly decreased, reflecting some reduction in the pulmonary capillary blood volume consistent with either moderate restrictive lung disease or complicating pulmonary vascular or interstitial lung disease. The magnitude of the patient's lung disorder is brought into clear perspective with relatively low loads of exercise. At this point, the patient cannot reduce the wasted ventilation by recruitment of further pulmonary vascular bed for gas exchange. This supports the speculation of pulmonary vascular or interstitial lung disease and/or abnormal matching of pulmonary ventilation and perfusion.

This patient represents slowly progressive chronic respiratory insufficiency with parenchymal fibrosis due to SLE, without known antecedent pulmonary infection or episodes of primary lupus pneumonitis.

Case 3

This 15-year-old girl was admitted to Children's Hospital of Los Angeles on October 28, 1971, with a diagnosis of SLE and a history of progressive weight loss, anorexia, fatigue, anemia, frequent epistaxis, and urinary frequency during the previous month. Physical examination revealed a thin female with arthritis but no rash; the lungs were clear. The blood pressure was 100/70. Laboratory data included Hgb 8.1 gm./100 ml., WBC 7200/mm.[3], ESR 152 mm./hr., and weakly reactive VDRL; ANA was 4+, including anti-DNA antibodies. Serum C3 was less than 10 mg./100 ml., BUN 67 mg./100 ml., and creatinine 1.9 mg./100 ml.; urinalysis showed 1 to 3 WBC and 15 to 20 RBC/hpf. A 24-hour urine contained 2.5 gr. of protein.

On the day following admission, pericarditis, with tachycardia and fever, was detected, and prednisolone, 15 mg. every 6 hours, was begun. A chest roentgenogram revealed slight cardiomegaly but clear lung fields. Following several transfusions of packed red blood cells for severe anemia, a renal biopsy was performed and revealed diffuse lupus glomerulonephritis. Prednisolone was increased to 25 mg. every 6 hours.

On November 14, the patient was discovered to have severe chest pain, dyspnea and orthopnea; there was no fever. Examination showed a heart rate of 160/min., and respiratory rate was 60/min.; breath sounds were diminished on the right, and bilateral rales were present. The cardiac examination was normal, but the liver was descended 5 cm. A chest roentgenogram demonstrated cardiomegaly and a diffuse alveolar process with prominence on the right and posteriorly (Fig. 4 *A*). Blood and sputum cultures were obtained, and intravenous antibiotics and hydrocortisone, 100 mg. every 6 hours, were begun. A cardiology consultation was obtained, and digitalis and intravenous diuretics were added because of apparent right-sided heart failure secondary to severe pneumonitis. Hydrocortisone was increased to 150 mg. every 6 hours. Oxygen by mask was delivered at 10 liters/min.

By November 16, improvement had occurred, with a decrease in the cardiac and respiratory rates, and dyspnea was less pronounced. A sputum smear for *Pneumocystis carinii* was negative. The next four days were marked by great improvement in the patient's respiratory status, although roentgenographic evidence of clearing of infiltrates was delayed (Fig. 4 *B*). Prednisolone was substituted at 25 mg. every 6 hours, given orally, and oxygen was discontinued. All cultures were negative, and the intravenous antibiotics were discontinued. The impression was that the patient had experienced severe, primary lupus pneumonitis with rapid improvement in response to large corticosteroid doses.

Shortly after the pulmonary episode, the patient was begun on oral cyclophospha-

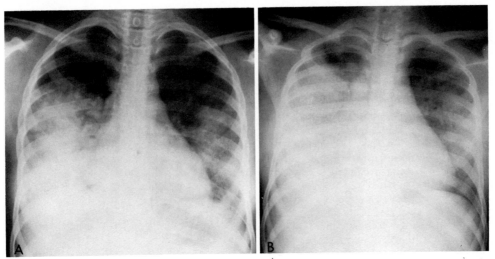

Figure 4. *A*, The heart is slightly enlarged in the transverse diameter. There is a diffuse, bilateral alveolar process, which is more pronounced on the right. This pattern is not etiologically specific and may reflect hemorrhage, edema or infection. *B*, There is no appreciable change in heart size. The bilateral alveolar infiltrates have progressed and the right diaphragm is obscured, despite the clinical evidence of improvement.

mide because of a severe peripheral neuropathy and very active, diffuse lupus nephritis. Her subsequent course included occasional arthralgias, mild intermittent rash and moderate fatigue, but was marked by a complete remission of active renal disease. Histologic confirmation was obtained in January 1973. She has subsequently developed severe, recurrent hemorrhagic cystitis believed to be due to cyclophosphamide therapy. She also continues to have a slightly positive ANA, anti-DNA antibodies, and hypocomplementemia, despite the absence of clinically signifi-

cant disease. No further episodes of pulmonary involvement have occurred.

Pulmonary function studies were performed in August 1976 to assess whether significant functional sequelae existed (Table 6). The patient stated she had smoked two to three cigarettes per day for four years, and seven per day during the previous year.

The vital capacity had its subdivisions fall within the normal range, as do the functional residual capacity, residual volume, and total lung capacity. The one-second forced vital capacity, expressed as a per-

TABLE 6.   CASE 3

	Normal Range	Predicted Mean	August 1976 Measured (% pred.)
VC (L)	1.9–3.3	2.6	2.2 (84%)
FRC (L)	1.0–2.1	1.5	1.3 (83%)
RV (L)	0.4–1.1	0.7	0.7 (90%)
TLC (L)	2.5–4.1	3.3	2.8 (86%)
FEV_1 (L)	2.0–2.9	2.5	1.9 (77%)
FEV_1/FVC (%)	72–100	86.0	91.0
MMEF (L/min)	122–258	190.0	155.0 (82%)
CV (L)		0.2	0.2
CV/VC (%)		7.0	10.0
N_2 (40) (%)		1.5	1.0
D_LCO (ml/min/mm Hg)	12.1–25.3	18.7	12.7
P_{O_2} (mm Hg)		95.0	114.0
P_{CO_2} (mm Hg)		37–43	28.0
pH		7.37–7.43	7.42

centage of the forced vital capacity, and the maximal expiratory flow, measured at all lung volumes, are normal. The closing volume and closing capacity fall within the predicted range, and the indices of uniformity of alveolar ventilation — the single-breath oxygen test and the 40-breath nitrogen washout test — suggest a normal distribution of ventilation. The diffusing capacity for carbon monoxide. measured by the single-breath method, is reduced from the mean and falls just within one standard deviation below the predicted mean. Arterial blood has normal oxygen tension, a mild uncompensated metabolic acidosis, and an acute respiratory alkalosis.

While the lung volumes, mechanics of ventilation, and distribution of ventilation fall well within the normal range predicted for the patient, she does have a reduced diffusing capacity. There is a four-year smoking history, but the study does not reveal any evidence of small airways disease, although the contour of the maximal expiratory flow-volume curve does suggest reduction in expired flow at low lung volumes. The arterial blood gas, although reflecting marked hyperventilation, has an acceptable oxygen tension and a normal alveolar-arterial oxygen difference. The measurement of arterial blood gases and wasted ventilation both at rest and during graded exercise will be performed to define whether there is evidence of underlying interstitial disease.

DIAGNOSTIC AND THERAPEUTIC CONSIDERATIONS

Three broad classifications of SLE pulmonary disease in childhood can be delineated: (1) mild to moderate progressive impairment in pulmonary function without clinical symptoms or significant roentgenographic findings (Case 2); (2) slow progression of pulmonary symptoms with roentgenographic findings; (3) rapid onset of severe pulmonary distress. The first category should be watched closely, with an awareness that worsening function may predispose to later infection. The latter two categories will be treated as different in degree only.

Pulmonary disease management should always start with a comprehensive assessment of general SLE disease activity. Falling serum complement levels and increasing titers of ANA or anti-DNA antibody suggest increased disease activity, as do increased rash, arthralgia, myalgia or evidence of internal organ derangement. In this setting, persistent low-grade fever, or spiking fever, is common. However, fever may be absent with moderate to large doses of corticosteroids.

The rapid onset of fever, cough and tachypnea is almost invariably due to infection, and following appropriate bacterial, fungal and viral cultures, broad-spectrum antibiotics should be started. Three rapidly occurring exceptions to this rule should be noted. Spontaneous hemothorax is a rare complication of primary SLE pulmonary involvement (Mulkey and Hudson, 1974). The presence of frothy, blood-tinged sputum usually suggests alveolar hemorrhage due to SLE (Case 1) (Gould and Soriano, 1975), and may respond to intravenous methylprednisolone, 100 to 500 mg. once per day for one to three days, or immunosuppressive drugs. If dyspnea and chest pain are prominent findings, primary SLE pneumonitis (Case 3) should be considered. In this rare situation, a combination of antibiotics and increased doses of corticosteroids are appropriate. In these latter circumstances, the potential for secondary infection is great, and the patient should be watched carefully.

Exceptional diagnostic difficulty may be encountered in those children with a rapid onset of symptoms who do not respond to antibiotics within 72 hours, and in those who have the slow progression (days to weeks) of pulmonary symptoms and roentgenographic findings. In our experience, cultures from these patients are commonly negative or contradictory, and accurate interpretation of chest roentgenograms is extremely difficult. Frequently, when a child becomes rapidly ill with major pulmonary manifestations, the concomitants of pneumonia, uremia, cardiomegaly due to myocarditis, pericarditis or fluid retention, pulmonary edema, or mild to moderate pleuritis may combine to make roentgenographic distinctions difficult. At this point, a multi-disciplinary team approach, including cardiology, radiology, nephrology, infectious diseases, pulmonary diseases and rheumatology, should be mandatory.

The temptation to change or continue antibiotics, to markedly increase corticosteroid doses, or to add immunosuppressive agents should be tempered by the knowledge that either course may lead to pulmonary or systemic superinfection. At this point, lung biopsy may be strongly considered. Techniques such as percutaneous or open lung biopsy (Bandt and coworkers, 1962; Gaensler and coworkers, 1964), endobronchial brush biopsy (Fry and Manalo-Estrella, 1970) and transbronchoscopic lung biopsy (Anderson and coworkers, 1970) all have their proponents, but none of these procedures is without significant risk (Bandt and coworkers, 1962; Gaensler and coworkers, 1964).

Finally, it is critically important to recognize that there are several possible causes of abnormal bleeding in SLE. Abnormalities of prothrombin time or partial thromboplastin time and thrombocytopenia are common. In addition, abnormal template bleeding times are frequent, even when the former three coagulation parameters are normal. All four tests should be performed prior to biopsy.

SCLERODERMA

Scleroderma (systemic sclerosis) is the rheumatic disease most frequently associated with severe pulmonary involvement. However, the prevalence of pulmonary disease in children may be lower than in adults because a different spectrum of scleroderma is encountered. Scleroderma is usually divided into two major categories: progressive systemic sclerosis (PSS), and "localized" scleroderma. Morphea and linear scleroderma are the major subdivisions of "localized" scleroderma. Several excellent discussions of PSS in adults leave the impression that PSS is more prevalent than are localized forms of scleroderma in adults (Tuffanelli and Winkelmann, 1961, Rodnan 1972); the opposite appears true in children (Dabich and coworkers, 1974). Our experience at the Children's Hospital of Los Angeles during the past 15 years includes 48 children with scleroderma. Thirteen (27 per cent) had PSS, 19 had predominantly linear scleroderma (40 per cent) and 16 (33 per cent) developed morphea (Kornreich and coworkers, 1977). The clinical course of PSS in children appears indistinguishable from that in adults, and includes the slow but relentless progression of major internal organ involvement, most predominantly in the heart, intestines, kidneys and lungs. Raynaud's phenomenon, severe skin changes and articular disability are also predominant but not life-threatening complications (D'Angelo and coworkers, 1969).

The most common histologic finding in scleroderma is extensive fibrosis with hyperplasia of connective tissue, which may be the result of overproduction of collagen, but impressive vascular and inflammatory lesions are also frequently evident. Serologic abnormalities, including the presence of rheumatoid factor, ANA, antibodies to DNA and elevated immunoglobulin levels, occur in between one-quarter and one-half of adults and children with scleroderma (Kornreich and coworkers, 1977); these findings may improve our understanding of the pathogenesis of the disease.

Pulmonary involvement in childhood PSS has received little attention because the findings are generally considered identical with those found in adults. In autopsy series, the lungs are affected in almost 90 per cent of adults with PSS (D'Angelo and coworkers, 1969); the predominant histologic changes consist of interstitial and peribronchial fibrosis, subpleural cystic changes and pleural thickening (Weaver and coworkers, 1968a; D'Angelo and coworkers, 1969). Vascular lesions are also prominent and frequent, and may include intimal proliferation and medial hypertrophy of small pulmonary arteries and arterioles that do not correlate with the severity of interstitial fibrosis. In early lesions, material rich in acid mucopolysaccharides is increased in the intima of small muscular arteries. However, extensive sclerosis may be a late finding, particularly in those patients with pulmonary hypertension and cor pulmonale (Trell and Lindstrom, 1971).

Impairment in the diffusing capacity of carbon monoxide is usually the earliest physiologic abnormality and frequently can be found prior to clinical or roentgenographic evidence of pulmonary disease (Huang and Lyons, 1966; Laitinen and coworkers, 1973). In many cases, evidence of decreased lung compliance and reduced vital capacity develops as the scleroderma progresses, and these restrictive changes may be related to interstitial and peribronchial fibrosis. Obstructive lung disease, including reduced maximal breathing capacity and increased residual volume, may become prominent late in the disease course. Almost invariably, these patients develop significant exercise intolerance; however, these changes rarely appear to be the dominant cause of death unless pulmonary hypertension leads to cor pulmonale and cardiac failure. Therefore, it may be convenient, as suggested by Trell and Lindstrom (1971), to discern three types of pulmonary involvement in PSS: (1) predominant lung fibrosis with a slow obliteration of the vascular bed and slowly progressive cor pulmonale; (2) combined pulmonary parenchymal and vascular lesions; and (3) predominant pulmonary vascular involvement associated with rapidly lethal right ventricular failure.

Chest roentgenograms may reveal linear or nodular densities with accentuation in the lower lung fields (Weaver and coworkers, 1968a), or may exhibit a more diffuse pattern of fibrosis. Cardiomegaly, vascular congestion and pleural thickening are also frequently observed abnormalities. The following is an illustrative case.

Case 4

This 18-year-old girl was first seen in September 1974 with a past history of "arthritis" at four years of age, and the onset of progressive systemic sclerosis at six years of age. The initial symptoms of skin involvement, Raynaud's phenomenon and dysphagia were treated with prednisone, 2.5 mg. three times per day for two months, without improvement. Growth failure was noted prior to steroid therapy and persisted after steroids were discontinued. At age 10 years, the patient was evaluated at another medical center, where a skin biopsy revealed increased fibrosis with reduced cellularity of the dermis; atrophic sweat glands surrounded by "constricting" collagen fibers were present. A chest roentgenogram demonstrated very little subcutaneous tissue, marked emphysema and severe interstitial fibrosis. Cysts were present in both lower lung fields.

When first seen at Children's Hospital of Los Angeles in 1974, the patient was suffering from shortness of breath, dyspnea on exertion, alternating constipation and diarrhea and severe Raynaud's phenomenon. Examination revealed a very thin female with generalized atrophic skin with variable hypo- and hyperpigmentation. She had poor chest expansion, inter- and supracostal retractions, mild nasal flaring, and fine rales at both bases on auscultation. The cardiac and abdominal examinations were not remarkable. Generalized muscle wasting and numerous severe flexion contractures were evident.

Laboratory studies included negative ANA and RF, normal CBC, BUN and creatinine, and severely abnormal barium enema; the chest roentgenogram revealed advanced parenchymal fibrosis. Serial pulmonary function studies were performed during the final two years of her disease course, and one study is presented below.

Various therapies, including D-penicillamine under experimental protocol and corticosteroids, were employed without success. Her course was marked by progressive cough, shortness of breath and dyspnea on exertion, and the continuous administration of oxygen was required by October 1975. Because of long-standing hypercapnia, oxygen was maintained at only 30 per cent to prevent loss of O_2 drive to ventilation; arterial blood gases at this time included: pH 7.37, P_{CO_2} 55, P_{O_2} 75, base excess -9. In late October the patient developed pneumonia, cor pulmonale and congestive heart failure, which responded well to intravenous gentamicin and methicillin, diuretics and oral Lanoxin. The chest roentgenogram revealed progressive fibrosis (Fig. 5); severe hypoxia and hypercapnia were also present.

In March 1976, she was readmitted to the hospital following a spontaneous right pneumothorax. Thoracotomy and insertion of a chest tube were performed. Partial lung expansion occurred, but during the next two months, all attempts to remove the chest tube were followed by reaccumulations of air in the right thorax. A right-sided empyema developed, in addition to progressive weakness and severe decubitus ulcers due to immobility. She exhibited advancing psychiatric disability with disassociation from events around her. Strength, endurance and respiratory status continued to deteriorate, but a chest roentgenogram showed no cardiomegaly and only a 10 per cent right pneumothorax. The patient experienced a sudden cardiorespiratory arrest and died in August 1976.

PULMONARY FUNCTION STUDIES (Table 7) The VC and its subdivisions are severely

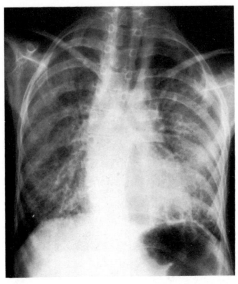

Figure 5. Advanced scleroderma lung with chronic pulmonary fibrosis in a reticulated, honeycomb pattern more prominent in the lower lobes. The heart is minimally enlarged, gaseous distention of the proximal and distal thirds of the esophagus is present, and there is a moderate right convex scoliosis.

attenuated. The RV, FRC and TLC are markedly reduced as a reflection of the reduction in vital capacity. While the one-second forced vital capacity is moderately reduced, it falls well within the normal range when expressed as a percentage of the forced vital capacity. Maximal expiratory flow, measured at all lung volumes, falls well within the normal range when corrected for the reduction in vital capacity.

TABLE 7.   CASE 4

	Normal Range	Predicted Mean	March 1975 Measured (% pred.)
VC (L)	2.6–4.2	2.6	0.6 (21%)
FRC (L)	1.2–2.7	1.6	0.7 (46%)
RV (L)	0.5–1.3	0.7	0.5 (64%)
TLC (L)	3.3–5.2	3.4	1.0 (30%)
FEV₁ (L)	2.5–3.8	2.4	1.5 (20%)
FEV₁/FVC (%)	72–100	89.0	91.0
MMEF (L/min)	166–302	177.0	63.0 (35%)
CV (L)			
CV/VC (%)			
N₂ (40) (%)			
D$_L$CO (ml/min/mm Hg)	15.0–31.3	14.7	2.2
P$_{O_2}$ (mm Hg)		93.0	57.9
P$_{CO_2}$ (mm Hg)		37–43	30.5
pH		7.37–7.43	7.39

The diffusing capacity for carbon monoxide, measured by the steady state method, reveals a major reduction in the ability to transport carbon monoxide into the pulmonary capillary blood volume.

This patient has such marked restrictions of the lung volume and pulmonary capillary blood volume that her ability to diffuse carbon monoxide into the alveolar capillary blood is drastically reduced.

DERMATOMYOSITIS

Childhood dermatomyositis is a chronic inflammatory disease primarily of skin and muscle, but it is increasingly being recognized also to have significant internal organ involvement. Dermatomyositis in childhood is a syndrome distinct from the adult form of the disease, and has been described as a systemic angiopathy in the classic histopathologic studies of Banker and Victor (1966). Proximal muscle weakness and a characteristic erythematous or violaceous rash around the eyes and over the malar eminences, over the extensor surfaces of the elbows and knees, and over the metacarpophalangeal and proximal interphalangeal joints are the most common presenting features. Laboratory confirmation of the diagnosis includes elevated serum muscle enzymes, characteristic electromyographic changes, and histologic findings on muscle biopsy, which may include muscle fiber degeneration, sarcolemmal nuclear proliferation, mononuclear cell infiltrates around muscle fibers, and vascular changes including prominent perivascular infiltrates and the occlusion of small vessels by intimal proliferation and fibrin thrombi.

The recent description of several large series of childhood dermatomyositis suggests that prognosis has significantly improved in the past ten years (Sullivan and coworkers, 1972; Hanson, 1976). In all probability, this improvement is due to the sustained use of corticosteroids for as long as clinical

or serologic evidence of muscle disease persists, and to an increased awareness of the potential for life-threatening internal organ involvement, particularly in the gastrointestinal tract (Banker and Victor, 1966) heart (Singsen and coworkers, 1976), and lungs (Tedford and coworkers, 1977). It is becoming clear that childhood dermatomyositis is a diffuse or systemic angiopathy, and that the vascular changes noted may be found in many major organs at some time during the disease course (Banker and Victor, 1966).

Diffuse interstitial pulmonary fibrosis is a well documented complication of adult polymyositis and dermatomyositis. Twenty histologically confirmed cases of pulmonary fibrosis (fibrosing alveolitis) have been observed, with the incidence estimated to vary from 1.5 to 5 per cent (Duncan and coworkers, 1974; Frazier and Miller, 1974). The clinical presentation may be one of acute onset of fever, dyspnea and cough, or may be insidious with only mild, slowly progressive respiratory symptoms. The roentgenographic pattern is usually that of a diffuse interstitial process. This pattern is occasionally noted by accident in an adult with dermatomyositis and no pulmonary symptoms.

Restrictive pulmonary defects and diminished $D_L CO$ are typical pulmonary function abnormalities in most cases tested, but these frequently do not progress. Various authors differ as to the efficacy of corticosteroid therapy (Camp and coworkers, 1972; Frazier and Miller, 1974), but particularly in the patient with an acute onset or early chronic fibrosis, a trial of corticosteroids appears warranted (Weaver and coworkers, 1968b). Histologic examination of the lungs most commonly reveals alveolar septal thickening and fibrosis, with the infiltration of chronic inflammatory cells. Vasculitis is usually not a feature, but cyst formation, perhaps due to dissolution of alveolar septal walls, has been observed (Hyun and coworkers, 1962).

In childhood dermatomyositis, roentgenographic evidence of pulmonary fibrosis has been reported in four children (Dubowitz and Dubowitz, 1964; Gwinn and Lee, 1975; Tedford and coworkers, 1977); two of these had histologic confirmation (Gwinn and Lee, 1975; Tedford and coworkers, 1977). Spontaneous pneumothorax has occurred in three cases, including one as a terminal event (Park and Nyhan, 1975; Tedford and coworkers, 1977). It has been suggested that pneumothorax may be a complication of the basic disease process (Tedford and coworkers, 1977).

The second, perhaps more common, type of pulmonary involvement relates to thoracic muscle weakness, impaired swallowing, and poor airway toilet in children with active early dermatomyositis, or rarely in those with end-stage disease. In both situations, aspiration pneumonia is a possible complication (Bitnum and coworkers, 1964). In this latter situation, antibiotic therapy should be started after appropriate cultures are taken. In the acute onset situation, with active muscle disease, vigorous therapy with corticosteroids should be pursued to improve strength, but it should be recognized that such patients are at an increased risk for developing secondary bacterial or fungal infections.

Case 5.

This 21-year-old female was well until 1967 (age 12 years), when she developed rash, anorexia and weight loss. The rash was red and scaly over the metacarpophalangeal and proximal interphalangeal joints; a violaceous discoloration of the upper eyelids was also present. The following six months were marked by progressive proximal muscle weakness of the quadriceps, neck and abdominal flexors. A muscle biopsy in January 1968 revealed muscle fiber degeneration, sarcolemmal nuclear proliferation, and vascular intimal thickening with perivascular infiltration of chronic inflammatory cells. Serum muscle enzymes were elevated.

The institution of prednisolone therapy was associated with almost complete resolution of the patient's rash and muscle weakness over the following four months. Prednisolone doses, varying from 5 to 15 mg. per day, were required during the next four years to maintain control of the dermatomyositis. Numerous complications occurred during the course of her disease, including vasculitis of the fingertips and progressive Raynaud's phenomenon, which began in 1969 and resulted in the autoamputation of several fingertips. Mild, but progressive and generalized, calcinosis was first detected in 1970, and in 1973 perforation of the nasal septum occurred. A biopsy of the adjacent mucosa revealed vasculitis, fibrosis and chronic inflammatory infiltrates.

In 1973 (age 18 years) this girl developed a nonproductive cough and was found upon examination of the chest to have fine, bi-basilar rales. Serial chest roentgenograms from 1969 to 1973 were reviewed and showed "progressive interstitial markings" suggestive of slowly increasing pulmonary fibrosis.

A spontaneous left pneumothorax occurred in November 1974 in association with an exacerbation of the Raynaud's phenomenon and worsening vasculitis of several fingertips. The patient was not receiving corticosteroids at this time. Thoracotomy, for chest tube placement and open lung biopsy, was performed. The lung revealed histologic evidence of pleural and interstitial fibrosis with focal, subpleural chronic pneumonitis. Irregular patterns of aeration, centrilobular emphysema and perivascular fibrosis of the parenchyma were present, but no obliterative vascular lesions were observed.

Prednisolone, 5 mg. four times per day, was begun, and over the next six weeks resolution of the pneumothorax and decrease in the vasculitis of the fingertips were observed. The subsequent two years of her disease course were marked by numerous complications, including severe muscle atrophy and flexion contractures, limited exercise tolerance, repeated hospitalizations for recurrent pneumonias and pneumothoraces, and an unexplained episode of abdominal pain without evidence of gastrointestinal involvement. Worsening depression and withdrawal from reality occurred, and several episodes of psychosis with catatonia responded poorly to medication and psy-

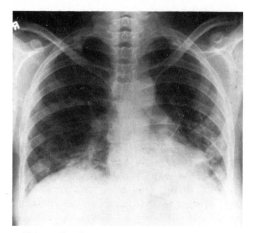

Figure 6. Dermatomyositis with chronic pulmonary fibrosis of two years' duration. The heart is normal in size, and soft tissue calcifications are present in both axillae. Interstitial thickening and cystic changes are bilateral and most pronounced at the bases.

severely reduced. Her FRC, RV and TLC are within one standard deviation of the mean, with the residual volume equal to the mean predicted value. The one-second forced vital capacity, expressed as a percentage of the forced vital capacity, is well within the normal range, as is the maximal expiratory flow measured at all lung volumes. Distribution of ventilation falls within the normal range. The $D_L CO$, measured by the steady state method, is reduced to less than 50 per cent of the predicted value. The arterial blood reveals moderate hypoxia, an enlarged alveolar-arterial oxygen difference, and a marked acute and chronic alveolar hyperventilation in face of a mild metabolic acidosis.

This patient has a very severe, restrictive lung disorder, compromised alveolar volume and alveolar surface area, and reduction in the alveolar capillary blood volume resulting in hypoxia.

chotherapy. An elevated cerebrospinal fluid protein and an electroencephalogram showing diffuse slowing were suggestive of cerebral dysfunction, perhaps due to dermatomyositis. However, the patient became increasingly resistant to further hospitalization or corticosteroid therapy. The pulmonary fibrosis slowly continued to advance, as seen on a chest roentgenogram of July 1, 1976 (Fig. 6). In August 1976, the patient died at home from cardiorespiratory failure. No postmortem examination was performed. The data from serial pulmonary function studies are shown in Table 8 and presented below:

This patient's VC and its subdivisions are

JUVENILE RHEUMATOID ARTHRITIS

As noted in the introduction to this chapter, there are in excess of 100 medical conditions known to be associated with arthritis. Among these, juvenile rheumatoid arthritis (JRA) is the most widespread and well known, afflicting perhaps 175,000 children in the United States alone (Calabro, 1972). The terms "JRA," "juvenile chronic

TABLE 8.   CASE 5

	Normal Range	Predicted Mean	June 1976 Measured (% pred.)
VC (L)	2.6–4.2	3.3	1.3 (38%)
FRC (L)	1.2–2.7	2.0	1.4 (71%)
RV (L)	0.5–1.3	0.9	1.1 (116%)
TLC (L)	3.3–5.2	4.2	2.3 (55%)
FEV_1 (L)	2.5–3.8	3.1	1.2 (38%)
FEV_1/FVC (%)	72–100	86.0	87.0
MMEF (L/min)	166–302	234.0	78.0 (33%)
CV (L)		0.3	
CV/VC (%)		8.0	
N_2 (40) (%)		1.5	1.3
$D_L CO$ (ml/min/mm Hg)	15.0–31.3	23.1	8.1
P_{O_2} (mm Hg)		93.0	62.0
P_{CO_2} (mm Hg)	37–43	25.0	
pH	7.37–7.43	7.45	

polyarthritis (JCP)" and "Still's disease" are frequently used interchangeably by physicians, but even among pediatric specialists in the field of rheumatology, the distinctions are blurred and controversy about correct nomenclature continues. What is clear is that the term "Still's disease" should be reserved for the acute systemic onset type associated with spiking fever, typical rash and a variety of internal organ derangements. The remaining two major groups within JRA or JCP are the polyarticular and pauciarticular types, both defined after a minimum three-month observation period. Until causes and subtle differential diagnostic points are better understood, some children with arthritis associated with inflammatory bowel disease, ankylosing spondylitis, psoriatic arthritis and Reiter's syndrome will undoubtedly continue to be included in surveys of children with JRA or JCP. The interested reader is referred to several recent excellent monographs regarding progress and controversy in this fascinating field (Calabro, 1972; Ansell, 1976; Jayson, 1976; Schaller and Hanson, 1977).

Rheumatoid lung involvement in the child is exceptionally rare, and appears almost exclusively limited to those with a systemic onset (Calabro, 1972). Pneumonitis and pleuritis may accompany early systemic manifestations, and are most frequently associated with myocardial or pericardial involvement (Jayson, 1976). Occasionally, asymptomatic pleural involvement will be observed as an incidental finding on chest roentgenogram (Jayson, 1976). One child with JRA, pulmonary arteritis and pulmonary hypertension has been reported (Jordan and Snyder, 1964).

Lung involvement in adults with rheumatoid arthritis is more common than in children; the various major types are briefly mentioned so the reader will be aware of possible alternative forms in childhood. The three major types commonly recognized include pleural effusions, pleural and pulmonary rheumatoid nodules and diffuse interstitial pneumonitis and fibrosis (Martel and coworkers, 1968; Steinberg, 1975). Frequently, the pleural effusions are transient and asymptomatic, but they may also be associated with pleural granulomas (Martel and coworkers, 1968). Similarly, interstitial nodules may be transient, but are frequently associated with high serum titers of rheumatoid factor. Historical and clinical findings are frequently of little value in diagnosing interstitial lung disease, but a combination of chest roentgenogram and testing of diffusing capacity for carbon monoxide in one preliminary study found one-third of 30 adults to be abnormal (Popper and coworkers, 1972).

One additional form of progressive, severe pulmonary impairment should also be recognized. In adults, as well as in children, marked thoracolumbar spine and sternoclavicular joint disease may lead to severe thoracic cage deformities and restrictive pulmonary defects.

Case 6

This six-year-old girl was first hospitalized at Children's Hospital of Los Angeles in October 1974 with a three-year history of polyarticular JRA following a systemic onset. Despite previous therapy with aspirin, gold and corticosteroids, she had become nonambulatory owing to severe lower extremity joint disease. Exceptionally poor weight gain was observed, and cricoarytenoid joint involvement was associated with partial vocal cord paralysis. In addition, moderate scoliosis (convex to the right), dorsal kyphosis and a bell-shaped rib cage were present (Fig. 7).

Because of very active synovial inflammation, marked muscle wasting, severe flexion contractures and respiratory insufficiency, this child received intensive in-patient physical and occupational therapy in the rehabilitation center for eight months. Indomethacin and ibuprofen were added to her therapeutic regimen. Efforts to achieve ambulatory status were successful, but progressive weight-bearing was associated with

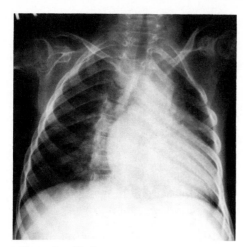

Figure 7. The bones are severely demineralized. Moderate right convex scoliosis is present, and the heart is moderately enlarged and projected to the left. The rib cage is noticeably bell-shaped in contour. A severe pectus carinatum cannot be appreciated in this view.   The lung fields are clear.

rapid advancement of the scoliosis from 10 degrees to 85 degrees, and marked decrease in the patient's respiratory reserve. Pulmonary function studies were obtained and are displayed below. Placement of a Harrington rod was considered, but the patient appeared an unacceptable operative risk; in addition, the osteoporotic spine appeared too frail to retain the rod.

D-penicillamine was substituted for weekly intramuscular Myochrysine therapy, but was without success. However, a Milwaukee brace appeared to arrest the progression of the kyphoscoliosis. Recently, the addition of oral chlorambucil has been associated with a marked reduction in joint disease activity, increased exercise tolerance and improved pulmonary function.

This girl's VC and its subdivisions are reduced to greater than two standard deviations below the predicted mean (Table 9). The one-second forced vital capacity expressed as a percentage of the forced vital capacity is normal, as is the maximal expiratory flow volume curve, after correction for the reduction in VC. A resting arterial blood sample reveals mild reduction in the P_{O_2}, increased alveolar-arterial oxygen difference, and a compensated alveolar hyperventilation.

This patient has evidence of severe restrictive lung disease, but has normal airway function. While her maximal expiratory flow rates at all lung volumes are reduced, they fall within the normal range when corrected for the degree of restrictive lung disease. The restrictive lung disease is so severe that alveolar volume and probably pulmonary perfusion have been compromised. Thus, the patient has mild hypoxia despite sustained alveolar hyperventilation. All of these findings are attributed to the severe chest wall deformity and scoliosis resulting from her arthritic condition.

MIXED CONNECTIVE TISSUE DISEASE

Most rheumatologists have long recognized a variety of unusual syndromes

TABLE 9. CASE 6

	Normal Range	Predicted Mean	January 1975 Measured (% pred.)
VC (L)	0.7–1.1	0.9	0.35 (38%)
FRC (L)	0.3–0.7	0.5	
RV (L)	0.2–0.4	0.3	
TLC (L)	0.9–1.4	1.2	
FEV$_1$ (L)	0.7–1.0	0.8	0.3 (42%)
FEV$_1$/FVC (%)	72–100	86.0	100.0
MMEF (L/min)	22–114	46.0	47.0 (104%)
CV (L)			
CV/VC (%)			
N$_2$ (40) (%)			
D$_L$CO (ml/min/mm Hg)			
P$_{O_2}$ (mm Hg)		100.0	69.0
P$_{CO_2}$ (mm Hg)	37–43	34.0
pH	7.37–7.43		7.39

characterized by overlapping features of several rheumatic diseases. However, in 1972, Sharp and coworkers first described mixed connective tissue disease (MCTD) as a distinct entity that exhibited overlapping clinical features of SLE, dermatomyositis and scleroderma, and distinctive serologic findings including high titers of speckled ANA and antibody against a ribonucleoprotein antigen (RNP). A subsequent survey of 100 adults with MCTD showed that among its particular characteristics were a high frequency of Raynaud's phenomenon, arthralgias and arthritis, sausage-shaped fingers, and rashes suggestive of SLE, dermatomyositis and scleroderma. The 5 per cent incidence of significant renal disease was unusually low, and MCTD appeared markedly responsive to small doses of corticosteroid therapy (Sharp, 1974–1975).

In the initial report, the youngest patient was 13 years of age, and in 1973 a brief report described an 11-year-old girl with MCTD (Sanders and coworkers, 1973). Recently, 14 additional children with MCTD have been investigated, and their serologic findings were compared with those from 127 children with other rheumatic diseases (Singsen and coworkers, 1977). In most respects, the children with MCTD (median age, 10.5 years) were similar to their adult counterpart, but differed in exhibiting more frequent arthritis, significant cardiac (64 per cent) and renal (43 per cent) involvement, and severe thrombocytopenia (43 per cent). The larger and more prolonged doses of corticosteroids required in these children and the death of four from hemorrhage or septicemia may suggest a more severe prognosis in childhood MCTD.

The first survey of MCTD in adults noted "abnormal diffusing capacity" in 67 per cent of 43 patients tested (Sharp, 1974–1975). More recently, Harmon and associates (1976) fully evaluated 24 patients through histories of unexplained dyspnea, physi-cal examination, chest roentgenograms and pulmonary function tests (PFT). Thirteen of the 24 patients had no symptoms, but only four were negative for all parameters. Five of the 13 had abnormal PFTs, one had only an abnormal chest roentgenogram, and three had both abnormal PFTs and chest roentgenograms. Thus, nine of 13 asymptomatic patients (69 per cent) had pulmonary disease. The remaining 11 symptomatic patients all had abnormal PFTs and chest roentgenograms. The PFTs in both groups always included decreased diffusion capacity by the single-breath carbon monoxide method (30 to 70 per cent of normal), and frequently reduced lung volumes. The chest roentgenograms revealed diffuse infiltrates and occasional volume loss or pleural disease; these findings are similar to the roentgenographic findings of Silver and coworkers (1976). Of the 24 fully evaluated patients, 20 (84 per cent) had pulmonary disease. Serial studies in 14 of these patients showed 12 to have significant improvement following corticosteroid treatment.

Case 7

This 15-year-old girl was first seen in May 1976 with a seven-month history of arthralgias and swelling of the hands, substernal chest pain and shortness of breath, malar rash, malaise and a 20-pound weight loss. She was diagnosed elsewhere as having SLE and begun on prednisolone, 5 mg. three times per day.

History upon admission to Children's Hospital of Los Angeles also revealed evidence of Raynaud's phenomenon, chronic constipation and dysphagia. Physical examination revealed the skin to be clear; arthritis was present at the wrists, knees and ankles. "Sausage fingers" were present, along with mild Raynaud's phenomenon. The lungs were clear and the cardiac examination was normal.

Laboratory data included a white blood cell count of 4200/mm³. Creatinine phosphokinase was 464 IU (normal: 0–100); a speckled ANA, titer 1:256, was detected. Antibody against RNP was present in a titer

TABLE 10.   CASE 7

	Normal Range	Predicted Mean	May 1976 Measured (% pred.)
VC (L)	2.4–4.1	3.3	2.5 (78%)
FRC (L)	1.2–2.7	1.9	1.6 (81%)
RV (L)	0.5–1.3	0.9	0.6 (70%)
TLC (L)	3.2–5.1	4.2	3.2 (76%)
FEV$_1$ (L)	2.5–3.7	3.1	2.2 (72%)
FEV$_1$/FVC (%)	72–100	86.0	93.0
MMEF (L/min)	163–299	231.0	226.0 (98%)
CV (L)		0.2	0.2
CV/VC (%)		7.9	7.0
N$_2$ (40) (%)		1.5	0.5
D$_L$CO (ml/min/mm Hg)	14.8–30.8	22.8	14.3
P$_{O_2}$ (mm Hg)		97.0	106.0
P$_{CO_2}$ (mm Hg)		37–43	32.0
pH		7.37–7.43	7.45

of $1:2.0 \times 10^7$. A barium esophagram showed diminished peristalsis and dilation of the distal third, and a barium enema showed pseudodiverticula at the hepatic and splenic flexures. A chest roentgenogram and ventilation-perfusion lung scan were both interpreted as normal, but pulmonary function testing revealed significant abnormalities, which are discussed below. A diagnosis of MCTD was considered confirmed because of overlapping clinical and laboratory features of SLE, dermatomyositis and scleroderma.

Hydroxychloroquine, 400 mg. per day, and prednisone, 40 mg. per day, were effective in controlling the patient's disease activity. Seven months later she was receiving prednisone, 15 mg. per day, and had no respiratory or articular complaints. She continues to have Raynaud's phenomenon, intermittent myalgias and dysphagia.

This patient's VC and its subdivisions, while reduced from predicted values, fall within one standard deviation of the mean (Table 10). The FRC and RV approximate the mean predicted value; the TLC is reduced, but within one standard deviation of the mean. The one-second forced vital capacity expressed as a percentage of the forced vital capacity is normal, as is the maximal expiratory flow rate when measured at all lung volumes. The distribution of ventilation, measured by the single-breath oxygen test, and 40-second nitrogen washout test are normal. The CV also falls within the normal range. The D$_L$CO is reduced. A resting arterial blood sample has a normal oxygen tension and alveolar-arterial oxygen difference and reveals a partially compensated alveolar hyperventilation.

This patient has mild restrictive lung disease and evidence of interstitial disease. The shortness of breath that she has experienced might be due in greater part to the interstitial rather than the restrictive component, since the latter is only mild. Thus, measurement of ventilation and blood gases during exercise should be a very valuable method for assessment of the pulmonary response to therapy.

WEGENER'S GRANULOMATOSIS

Wegener's granulomatosis (WG) is a necrotizing, granulomatous vasculitis that may occur in a localized form involving the upper and lower respiratory tract, or in a more common form that additionally includes renal involvement (Wolff and coworkers, 1974). Controversy continues as to whether midline granulomas, limited WG and generalized WG are separate clinicopathologic entities or represent an interrelated disease spectrum. The former is supported by the apparently differing responses to therapy (Schechter and coworkers, 1976). However, the similarity of many of the clinical and histologic features of WG to other vasculitic, granulomatous or infectious disorders may cause difficulty in establishing the correct diagnosis (Fauci and Wolff, 1973).

Rhinorrhea, sinus pain, fever, arthralgias or arthritis, cough, hemoptysis and skin rashes or ulcerations are the most common presenting signs and symptoms of WG. Renal involvement is usually late in the disease course, rather than a presenting finding, but once begun may progress rapidly to death. The histologic findings are widely varied, but characteristically include necrotizing granulomas with or without vasculitis. Almost all organ systems can be involved, but the nasopharynx, sinuses, kidneys, skin, joints and lungs predominate (Wolff and coworkers, 1974).

Wegener's granulomatosis is particularly rare in children. Only four patients under the age of 15 years have been described (Roback and coworkers, 1969); however, knowledge of WG is now widespread, and therefore many isolated cases may remain unreported.

Pulmonary involvement in WG may begin with fever, persistent cough, chest pain or hemoptysis, or may first be detected upon observing infiltrates on the chest roentgenogram of the asymptomatic patient. The roentgenographic manifestations have no characteristic localization of lesions and may take the form of multiple or solitary nodular densities or infiltrates. Lesions may vary in size from less than 1 to more than 10 cm., and may have vague or sharply demarcated borders. The lesions may be unilateral or bilateral, may cavitate, and frequently are transient and fleeting. However, associated atelectasis, pleural effusions, mediastinal lymph node enlargement and calcification of lesions are rare (Landman and Burgener).

The prognosis for Wegener's granulomatosis is usually guarded, with renal failure remaining the most frequent cause of death. Previously, corticosteroids were the primary form of therapy, but appeared responsible only for doubling the mean duration of survival to approximately 12 months (Hollander and Manning, 1967). Recently, numerous investigators have described the advantages of cytotoxic chemotherapy for WG (Hollander and Manning, 1967; Kaplan and coworkers, 1968; Isreal and Patchefsky, 1975; Reza and coworkers, 1975). Cyclophosphamide has been the most impressive agent used, and induced remission in all 10 patients from one study (Reza and coworkers, 1975). The mean duration of remission was 38 months; two patients were disease-free for seven years, and the one patient who relapsed responded to a second course of therapy. However, cyclophosphamide is very toxic and should be used only by those experienced in its administration. Chlorambucil has also been used with success and may be indicated as a first cytotoxic drug because of its fewer side-effects (Isreal and Patchefsky, 1975). The following case illustrates the protean nature of WG, an excellent response to cyclophosphamide, and late findings of pulmonary function studies.

Case 8

This 12-year-old female was first hospitalized in December 1973 with a five-month history of fatigue, weight loss, progressive cough, gingival inflammation and a slowly enlarging submandibular mass. There was no history of dyspnea or hemoptysis. Physical examination revealed generalized granulomatous inflammation of the mouth, obstruction of the left nose with a mass, and a 7 by 7 cm. mass in the right submandibular area. The skin showed occasional small nodules on the legs; the lungs were clear to percussion and auscultation.

Laboratory determinations included a normal chest roentgenogram, absent serum ANA and RF, normal serum creatinine, BUN and quantitative immunoglobulins, and a normal 24-hour urine for protein and creatinine clearance.

A skin biopsy from the left leg revealed a necrotizing dermal granuloma consistent with Wegener's granulomatosis; there was no evidence of vasculitis. One month later the onset of hematuria and a diminished creatinine clearance prompted a per-

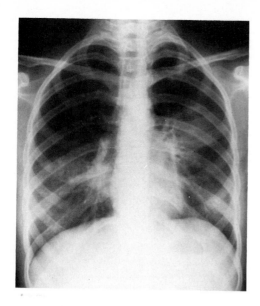

Figure 8. The heart is small and the left border is obscured by a lingular, segmental infiltrate. Patchy infiltrates are also present in the left upper and right middle lung zones, where cystic pneumatoceles or cavities are seen.

cutaneous renal biopsy, which revealed extracapillary proliferative and necrotizing glomerulonephritis without evidence of granulomas or vasculitis. All biopsy specimens were cultured, and were negative for tuberculosis and other pathogens.

Prednisolone and cyclophosphamide were started two weeks after admission, when progressive respiratory distress occurred owing to upper airway insufficiency. Serial chest roentgenograms also revealed progressive hilar prominences, perihilar infiltrates, and diffuse, enlarging nodules. Several weeks later pneumonia developed, intravenous antibiotics were begun, and the cyclophosphamide and prednisolone were

discontinued. Following resolution of the pneumonia, cyclophosphamide and prednisolone were restarted and given without further complications. One year later, the patient was in total remission except for residual bronchial stenosis, which required repeated dilatations.

The patient has now been disease-free and off medications for two years. In December 1976, a chest roentgenogram demonstrated multiple cavitations with accompanying infiltrates of the left perihilar and midlung regions; lingular and right middle lobe infiltrates were also present (Fig. 8). Pulmonary function studies were performed at this time.

TABLE 11. CASE 8

	Normal Range	Predicted Mean	December 1976 Measured (% pred.)
VC (L)	2.6–4.4	3.5	2.3 (66%)
FRC (L)	1.3–2.9	2.1	1.4 (69%)
RV (L)	0.5–1.4	1.0	0.8 (83%)
TLC (L)	3.4–5.5	4.6	3.1 (69%)
FEV_1 (L)	2.7–4.0	3.3	1.7 (51%)
FEV_1/FVC (%)	72–100	86.0	68.0
MMEF (L/min)	75–311	243.0	92.0 (38%)
CV (L)		0.2	
CV/VC (%)		7.0	
N_2 (40) (%)		1.5	4.0
P_{O_2} (mm Hg)		97.0	97.0
P_{CO_2} (mm Hg)		37–43	30.0
pH		7.37–7.43	7.43

This patient's VC and its subdivisions are moderately reduced, and there is a similar reduction in the FRC, RV and TLC (Table 11). However, the helium gas dilution method utilized to measure these parameters may significantly underestimate the size of these compartments in patients with obstructive airways disease. The one-second forced vital capacity is reduced to a larger degree than is the VC. Thus, the FEV_1 expressed as a percentage of the forced vital capacity is reduced. There is a marked reduction in the midmaximal expiratory flow rate and the expiratory flow rate measured at all lung volumes. The peak inspiratory flow rate is also markedly reduced. The phase IV closing volume measurement is indeterminate due to a marked slope in the phase III component and absence of an alveolar plateau. Uniformity of ventilation, as measured by the single-breath oxygen test and the N_2 (40), is abnormal. The single-breath D_LCO falls within the normal range when corrected for the reduction in VC. A specimen of arterial blood reveals moderately acute hyperventilation and a normal arterial oxygen tension. The alveolar-arterial oxygen difference is within the normal range. After inhalation of an aerosol of isoproterenol, there is moderate improvement in the VC and the one-second forced vital capacity expressed as a percentage of the FVC. Midmaximal end-expiratory flow rates and the maximal expiratory flow rates measured at all lung volumes also improve. This girl has mild to moderate restrictive lung disease and reversible obstructive airways disease. While the restrictive component is consistent with a diagnosis of Wegener's granulomatosis, the reversible airway obstructive disease is atypical and might not be related to this disorder.

There is no evidence from this study of pulmonary vasculitis. This might be demonstrable only with measurement of ventilation, ventilatory dead space, and arterial blood gases during exercise.

VASCULITIS SYNDROMES

Numerous classifications of the primary, nonspecific vasculitides have been described. The disease patterns most probably represent a continuum of pathologic changes ranging from necrosis and granuloma formation to various forms of angiitis, with the clinical presentation relating to the size and location of affected vessels. Table 12 is an extensive but by no means inclusive list of the vasculitides (with references). Several of these are described elsewhere in this text.

PERIARTERITIS NODOSA

Periarteritis nodosa (PAN) is a disease of inflammation and necrosis of medium and small-sized muscular arte-

TABLE 12. VASCULITIDES, WITH REFERENCES

Periarteritis nodosa (Fager and coworkers, 1951; Rose and Spencer, 1957; Roberts and Fetterman, 1963; Alarcon-Segovia and Brown, 1964; Winkelmann and Ditto, 1964; Frohnert and Sheps, 1967; Wedgwood and Schaller, 1969; Levin, 1970; Melam and Patterson, 1971; Arms and coworkers, 1972; Shulman and Harvey, 1972; Reimold and coworkers, 1976)

Henoch-Schönlein purpura (Allen and coworkers, 1960; Wedgwood and Schaller, 1969)

Wegener's granulomatosis (Hollander and Manning, 1967; Kaplan and coworkers, 1968; Roback and coworkers, 1969; Fauci and Wolff, 1973; Wolff and coworkers, 1974; Isreal and coworkers, 1975; Reza and coworkers, 1975; Schechter and coworkers, 1976; Landman and Burgener)

Stevens-Johnson syndrome (Rallison and coworkers, 1961; Wedgwood and Schaller, 1969)

Erythema nodosum (Wedgwood and Schaller, 1969; Shulman and Harvey, 1972)

Takayasu's arteritis (Warshaw and Spach, 1965; Bonventre, 1974)

Churg-Strauss vasculitis (Arms and coworkers, 1972)

Loeffler's syndrome (see Chapter 63)

Goodpasture's syndrome

Idiopathic pulmonary hemosiderosis (see Chapter 36)

Temporal arteritis (Shulman and Harvey, 1972)

Serum sickness (Shulman and Harvey, 1972)

Hypersensitivity angiitis, "systemic vasculitis" (Zeek, 1953; McCoombs, 1965)

Mucocutaneous lymph node syndrome (Kawasaki and coworkers, 1974)

ries, which may also be known as poly-arteritis because of the relative rarity of nodular lesions (Shulman and Harvey, 1972). Almost any organ in the body can be affected, but the kidneys, heart and lungs are most common, with liver, spleen, gastrointestinal tract, adrenals, testes, brain and peripheral nerves somewhat less commonly involved. The cause is not known, but PAN has been reported following drug exposure and is felt to have a hypersensitivity etiology. Clinical manifestations are varied, but frequently include fever, weight loss, arthritis, abdominal pain, renal disease and hypertension. Cutaneous disease is also frequent.

PAN in childhood is rare but well described both in forms resembling the adult disease course and in infantile polyarteritis (Roberts and Fetterman, 1963; Wedgwood and Schaller, 1969; Dabich and coworkers, 1974; Reimold and coworkers, 1976). In older children, differentiation from other rheumatic disorders may be difficult, and if muscle or testicular biopsies are not helpful, the diagnosis is usually made at autopsy. The prognosis is poor, with death commonly associated with heart or renal failure, or marked central nervous system or gastrointestinal disease. One recent report suggests that a combination of corticosteroids and immunosuppressives may improve prognosis (Reimold and coworkers, 1976), but correctly stresses that the rarity of childhood PAN makes the efficacy of any treatment regimen difficult to evaluate.

Polyarteritis in infants is an uncommon but characteristic illness that usually presents with signs suggestive of a viral illness. However, the disease persists, and cardiac involvement then predominates (Roberts and Fetterman, 1963; Wedgwood and Schaller, 1969). Unfortunately, the diagnosis is most frequently confirmed at autopsy, where pericarditis, aneurysms and thromboses of coronary arteries, and myocardial infarcts are commonly found. Pulmonary involvement is rare in infantile polyarteritis.

Pulmonary involvement in the vasculitides, and particularly in PAN, has been classified histopathologically (Alarcon-Segovia and Brown, 1964) and clinically (Arms and coworkers, 1972), and discussed in terms of therapeutic response (Levin, 1970). In adult PAN, respiratory disease was noted in 24 per cent of one series (Winkelmann and Ditto, 1964), and in 38 per cent of another (Frohnert and Sheps, 1967). In both reports, findings on chest roentgenograms were not consistent or diagnostic, in contrast to the report of Levin (1970), and neither group of investigators could clearly link prognosis to the presence or absence of pulmonary involvement, as previously suggested (Rose and Spencer, 1957). No studies of pulmonary function in any of the vasculitides are available to our knowledge. Many investigators concur that the incidence of secondary pulmonary infection is low in these patients, except in the terminal stages of illness, but superimposed pulmonary edema of cardiac or renal origin appears frequently.

Pulmonary involvement in children with PAN has been documented in isolated case reports but is probably quite rare (Fager and coworkers, 1959; Levin, 1970; Melam and Patterson, 1971; Reimold and coworkers, 1976). Both prednisone and azathioprine have been reported to lead to improvement of respiratory symptoms in some cases.

Most investigators concur that hypersensitivity to usually unrecognized antigens plays a dominant role in the vasculitides. Only rarely, such as in the well known examples of serum sickness and Stevens-Johnson syndrome, can a specific etiologic agent be identified. Beyond polyarteritis, Wegener's granulomatosis, Loeffler's and Goodpasture s syndromes and idiopathic pulmonary hemosiderosis, the primary vasculitides are only rarely associated with pulmonary disease. The character of the recognized histopathologic changes in the primary vasculitides suggests that pulmonary disease might occur, but in our clinical experience it has been rare.

SUMMARY

It has become evident that a majority of the rheumatic diseases can and do have pulmonary involvement at some time during their course. The most common initial events appear to be pleural inflammation and vasculitis or granulomatous parenchymal involvement, frequently resulting in slowly progressive interstitial fibrosis. However, pulmonary function studies in adults with various rheumatic diseases frequently suggest that pulmonary impairment occurs without obvious antecedent respiratory tract events. Our preliminary investigations, and data from others, suggest that the same is true in the childhood rheumatic diseases.

In conclusion, it is important to recall that most of the childhood rheumatic diseases are known to be associated with, or are suspected to have, defects in humoral or cell-mediated immunity, or both. In addition, many of these children are receiving corticosteroids or immunosuppressive agents. For these reasons, it is imperative that infection be the first consideration when any sudden change in respiratory status occurs. Complete cultures should always be taken and appropriate antimicrobial therapy begun, unless exceptionally clear-cut evidence points to a noninfectious cause. The addition of, or change in the doses of, corticosteroids or immunosuppressives should almost invariably occur only after appropriate cultures are known to be negative.

It is not clear what role chronic pulmonary impairment plays in the apparently increased incidence of lung infections in the childhood rheumatic diseases. For this reason, detailed serial pulmonary function studies and correlation with immune status, medications in use and the incidence of pulmonary infections in the childhood rheumatic diseases appear important areas for further study.

REFERENCES

Alarcon-Segovia, D., and Alarcon, D. G.: Pleuropulmonary manifestations of systemic lupus erythematosus. *Dis. Chest,* 39:7, 1961.

Alarcon-Segovia, D., and Brown, A. L.: Classification and etiologic aspects of necrotizing angiitides: An analytic approach to a confused subject with a critical review of the evidence for hypersensitivity in polyarteritis nodosa. *Mayo Clin. Proc.,* 39:205, 1964.

Allen, D. M., Diamond, L. K., and Howell, D. A.: Anaphylactoid purpura in children (Schönlein-Henoch syndrome): review with a follow-up of the renal complications. *Am. J Dis. Child.,* 99:833, 1960.

Anderson, H. A., Fontana, R. S., Sanderson, D. R., and Harrison, E. G.: Transbronchoscopic lung biopsy in diffuse pulmonary disease: results in 300 cases. *Med. Clin. North Am.,* 54:951, 1970.

Ansell, B. M. (Ed.): Rheumatic disorders in childhood. In *Clinics in Rheumatic Diseases.* Philadelphia, W. B. Saunders Company, 1976, pp. 303–494.

Arms, R. A., Dines, D. E., and DeRemee, R. A.: Pulmonary vasculitides: importance of the clinical and pathologic differentiation. *Minn. Med.,* 55:871, 1972.

Bagenstoss, A. H.: Visceral lesions in disseminated lupus erythematosus. *Proc. Mayo Clin.,* 27:412, 1952.

Bandt, P. D., Blank, N., and Castellino, R. A.: Needle diagnosis of pneumonitis. *J.A.M.A.,* 220:1578, 1972.

Banker, B. O., and Victor, M.: Dermatomyositis (systemic angiopathy) of childhood. *Medicine* 45:261, 1966.

Bitnum, S., Daeschner, E. W., Travis, L. B., et al.: Dermatomyositis. *J. Pediatr.,* 64:101, 1964.

Bonventre, M. V.: Takayasu's disease, revisited. *N.Y. State J. Med.,* 74:1960, 1974.

Calabro, J. J.: Juvenile rheumatoid arthritis. In Hollander, J. L., and McCarty, D. J. (Eds.): *Arthritis and Allied Conditions.* 8th Ed. Philadelphia, Lea and Febiger, 1972, p. 387.

Camp, A. V., Lane, D. J., and Mowat, A. G.: Dermatomyositis with parenchymal lung involvement. *Br. Med. J.,* 1:155, 1972.

Chick, T. W., DeHoratins, R. J., Skipper, B. E., and Messner, R. P.: Pulmonary dysfunction in systemic lupus erythematosus without pulmonary symptoms. *J. Rheumatol.,* 3:262, 1976.

Cohen, A. S., Reynolds, W. E., Franklin, E. C., et

al.: Preliminary criteria for the classification of systemic lupus erythematosus. *Bull. Rheum. Dis.,* *21*:643, 1971.

Dabich, L., Sullivan, D. B., and Cassidy, J. T.: Scleroderma in the child. *J. Pediatr., 85*:770, 1974.

D'Angelo, W. A., Fries, J. F., Masi, A. T., and Shulman, L. E.: Pathologic observations in systemic sclerosis (scleroderma): a study of fifty-eight autopsy cases and fifty-eight matched controls. *Am. J. Med. 46*:428, 1969.

Dubois, E. L., and Tuffanelli, D. L.: Clinical manifestations of systemic lupus erythematosus. *J.A.M.A., 190*:104, 1964.

Dubowitz, L. M., and Dubowitz, V.: Acute dermatomyositis presenting with pulmonary manifestations. *Arch. Dis. Child., 39*:293, 1964.

Duncan, P. E., Griffin, J. P., Gareia, A., et al.: Fibrosing alveolitis in polymyositis. *Am. J. Med., 57*:621, 1974.

Fager, D. B., Bigler, J. A., and Simonds, J. P.: Polyarteritis nodosa in infancy and childhood. *J. Pediatr., 39*:65, 1951.

Fauci, A. S., and Wolff, S. M.: Wegener's granulomatosis: studies in eighteen patients and a review of the literature. *Medicine, 52*:535, 1973.

Fayemi, A. O.: The lung in systemic lupus erythematosus: a clinicopathologic study of 20 cases. *Mt. Sinai. J. Med., 42*:110, 1975.

Frazier, A. R., and Miller, R. D.: Interstitial pneumonitis in association with polymyositis and dermatomyositis. *Chest, 65*:403, 1974.

Frohnert, P. P., and Sheps, S. G.: Long-term follow-up study of periarteritis nodosa. *Am. J. Med., 43*:8, 1967.

Fry, W. A., and Manalo-Estrella, P.: Bronchial brushing. *Surg. Gynecol. Obstet., 130*:67, 1970.

Gaensler, E. A., Moister, V. B., and Hamm, J.: Open lung biopsy in diffuse pulmonary disease. *N. Engl. J. Med., 270*:1319, 1964.

Gold, W. M., and Jennings, D. B.: Pulmonary function in patients with systemic lupus erythematosus. *Am. Rev. Resp. Dis., 93*:556, 1966.

Gould, D. B., and Soriano, R. Z.: Acute alveolar hemorrhage in lupus erythematosus. *Ann. Intern. Med., 83*:836, 1975.

Gross, M., Esterly, J. R., and Earle, R. H.: Pulmonary alterations in systemic lupus erythematosus. *Am. Rev. Resp. Dis., 105*:572, 1971.

Gwinn, J. L., and Lee, F. A.: Radiological case of the month: dermatomyositis with interstitial lung disease and soft tissue calcification. *Am. J. Dis. Child., 129*:703, 1975.

Hanson, V.: Dermatomyositis, scleroderma and polyarteritis nodosa. In Ansell, B. M. (Ed.): *Clinics in Rheumatic Disease.* Philadelphia, W. B. Saunders Company, 1976, p. 445.

Harmon, C., Wolfe, F., Lillard, S., Held, C., Cordon, R., and Sharp, G. C.: Pulmonary involvement in mixed connective tissue disease (MCTD). *Arthritis Rheum., 19*:801, 1976.

Harvey, A. M., Shulman, L. E., Tumulty, P. A., et al.: Systemic lupus erythematosus: review of the literature and clinical analysis of 138 cases. *Medicine, 33*:291, 1954.

Hollander, D., and Manning, R. T.: The use of alkylating agents in the treatment of Wegener's granulomatosis. *Ann. Intern. Med., 67*:393, 1967.

Huang, C. T., and Lyons, H. A.: Comparison of pulmonary function in patients with systemic lupus erythematosus, scleroderma and rheumatoid arthritis. *Am. Rev. Resp. Dis., 93*:865, 1966.

Huang, C. T., Hennigar, G. R., and Lyons, H. A.: Pulmonary dysfunction in systemic lupus erythematosus. *N. Engl. J. Med., 272*:288, 1965.

Hunt, R., Turner, R., Collins, R., and McLean, R.: Cardiopulmonary manifestatons of systemic lupus erythematosus. *Arthritis Rheum., 18*:524, 1975.

Hyun, B. H., Diggs, C. L., and Toone, E. C.: Dermatomyositis with cystic fibrosis (honeycombing) of the lung. *Dis. Chest, 42*:451, 1962.

Isreal, H. L., and Patchefsky, A. S.: Treatment of Wegener's granulomatosis of lung. *Am. J. Med., 58*:671, 1975.

Jayson, M., IV (Ed.): *Still's Disease: Juvenile Chronic Polyarthritis.* New York, Academic Press, 1976, pp. 1–289.

Jordan, J. D., and Synder, C. H.: Rheumatoid disease of the lung and cor pulmonale. *Am. J. Dis. Child., 108*:174, 1964.

Kaplan, S. R., Hayslett, J. R., and Calabresi, P.: Treatment of advanced Wegener's granulomatosis with azathioprine and duazomycin A. *N. Engl. J. Med., 178*:239, 1968.

Kawasaki, T., Kosaki, R., Okawa, S., et al.: A new infantile acute febrile mucocutaneous lymph node syndrome (MLNS) prevailing in Japan. *Pediatrics, 54*:271, 1974.

Kornreich, H.: Systemic lupus erythematosus in childhood. In Ansell, B. M. (Ed.): *Clinics in Rheumatic Diseases:* Philadelphia, W. B. Saunders Company, 1976, p. 429.

Kornreich, H. K., King, K. K., Bernstein, B. H., Singsen, B. H., and Hanson, V.: Scleroderma in childhood. *Arthritis Rheum.* (Suppl.), *20*:343, 1977.

Laitinen, O., Salorinne, Y., and Poppius, H.: Respiratory function in systemic lupus erythematosus, scleroderma, and rheumatoid arthritis. *Ann. Rheum. Dis., 32*:531, 1973.

Landman, S., and Burgener, F.: Pulmonary manifestations in Wegener's granulomatosis.

Levin, D. C.: Pulmonary abnormalities in the necrotizing vasculitides and their rapid response to steroids. *Radiology, 97*:521, 1970.

Levin, D. C.: Proper interpretation of pulmonary roentgen changes in systemic lupus erythematosus. *Am. J. Roentgenol., 111*:510, 1971.

Martel, W., Abell, M. R., Mikkelson, W. M., and Whitehouse, W. M.: Pulmonary and pleural lesions in rheumatoid disease. *Radiology, 90*:641, 1968.

McCombs, R. P.: Systemic "allergic" vasculitis: clinical and pathological relationships. *J.A.M.A., 194*:1059, 1965.

Meislin, A. G., and Rothfield, N. F.: Systemic lupus erythematosus in childhood. *Pediatr., 42*:37, 1968.

Melam, H., and Patterson, R.: Periarteritis nodosa: a remission achieved with combined prednisone and azathioprine therapy. *Am. J. Dis. Child.*, 121:424, 1971.

Mulkey, D., and Hudson, L.: Massive spontaneous unilateral hemothorax in systemic lupus erythematosus. *Am. J. Med.*, 56:570, 1974.

Notman, D. D., Kurata, N., and Tan, E. M.: Profiles of antinuclear antibodies in systemic rheumatic diseases. *Ann. Intern. Med.*, 83:464, 1975.

Park, S., and Nyhan, W. L.: Fatal pulmonary involvement in dermatomyositis. *Am. J. Dis. Child.*, 129:723, 1975.

Paty, J. G., Sienknecht, C. W., Townes, A. S., Hanissian, A. S., Miller, J. B., and Masi, A. T.: Impaired cell-mediated immunity in systemic lupus erythematosus (SLE): a controlled study of 23 untreated patients. *Am. J. Med.*, 59:769, 1975.

Popper, M. S., Bogdonoff, M. L., and Hughes, R. L.: Interstitial rheumatoid lung disease: a reassessment and review of the literature. *Chest*, 62:243, 1972.

Purnell, D. C., Bagenstoss, A. H., and Olsen, A. M.: Pulmonary lesions in disseminated lupus erythematosus. *Ann. Intern. Med.*, 42:619, 1955.

Rallison, M. L., Carlisle, R. E., Lee, R. E., Vernier, R. L., and Good, R. A.: Lupus erythematosus and Stevens-Johnson syndrome. *Am. J. Dis. Child.*, 101:725, 1961.

Reimold, E. W., Weinberg, A. G., Fink, C. W., and Battles, N. D.: Polyarteritis in children. *Am. J. Dis. Child.*, 130:534, 1976.

Reza, M. J., Dornfeld, L., Goldberg, L. S., Bluestone, R., and Pearson, C. M.: Wegener's granulomatosis: long-term follow-up of patients treated with cyclophosphamide. *Arthritis Rheum.*, 18:501, 1975.

Roback, S. A., Herdman, R. C., Hoyer, J., and Good, R. A.: Wegener's granulomatosis in a child: observations on pathogenesis and treatment. *Am. J. Dis. Child.*, 118:608, 1969.

Roberts, F. B., and Fetterman, G. H.: Polyarteritis nodosa in infancy. *J. Pediatr.*, 63:519, 1963.

Rodnan, G. P.: Progressive systemic sclerosis (scleroderma). In Hollander, J. L., and McCarty, D. J. (Eds.): *Arthritis and Allied Conditions.* 8th Ed. Philadelphia, Lea and Febiger, 1972, p. 962.

Rose, G. A., and Spencer, H.: Polyarteritis nodosa. *Q. J. Med.*, 26:43, 1957.

Sanders, D. Y., Huntley, C. C., and Sharp, G. C.: Mixed connective tissue disease in a child. *J. Pediatr.*, 83:642, 1973.

Schaller, J. G., and Hanson, V. (Eds.): Proceedings of the first ARA conference on the rheumatic diseases of childhood. *Arthritis Rheum.*, 1977, pp. 145–636 (Suppl.).

Schaller, J. G., Ochs, H. D., Thomas, E. D., et al.: Histocompatibility antigens in childhood-onset arthritis. *J. Pediatr.* 88:929, 1976.

Schechter, S. L., Bole, G. G., and Walker, S. E.: Midline granuloma and Wegener's granulomatosis: Clinical and therapeutic considerations. *J. Rheumatol.*, 3:241, 1976.

Sharp, G. C.: Mixed connective tissue disease. *Bull. Rheum. Dis.*, 25:828, 1974–1975.

Sharp, G. C., Irvin, W. S., Tan, E. M., Gould, R. G., and Holman, H. R.: Mixed connective tissue disease—an apparently distinct rheumatic disease syndrome associated with a specific antibody to an extractable nuclear antigen (ENA). *Am. J. Med.*, 52:148, 1972.

Shulman, L. E., and Harvey, A. M.: Polyarteritis and other arteritic syndromes. In Hollander, J. L., and McCarty, D. J. (Eds.): *Arthritis and Allied Conditions.* Philadelphia, Lea and Febiger, 1972, p. 918.

Sieving, R. R., Kaufman, C. A., and Watanakunakorn, C.: Deep fungal infection in systemic lupus erythematosus—three cases reported, literature reviewed. *J. Rheumatol.*, 2:61, 1975.

Silver, T. M., Farber, S. J., Bole, G. G., and Martel, W.: Radiological features of mixed connective tissue disease and scleroderma–systemic lupus erythematosus overlap. *Radiology*, 120:269, 1976.

Singsen, B. H., Goldreyer, B., Stanton, R., and Hanson, V.: Childhood polymyositis with cardiac conduction defects. *Am. J. Dis. Child.*, 130:72, 1976.

Singsen, B. H., Bernstein, B. H., Kornreich, H. K., King, K. K., Hanson, V., and Tan, E. M.: Mixed connective tissue disease (MCTD) in childhood: a clinical and serological survey. *J. Pediatr.*, 1977 (in press).

Staples, P. J., Gerding, D. N., Decker, J. L., and Gordon, R. S.: Incidence of infection in systemic lupus erythematosus. *Arthritis Rheum.*, 17:1, 1974.

Steinberg, C. L.: Rheumatoid lung disease: granulomas, fibrosis, pulmonary effusion. *N.Y. State J. Med.*, 75:854, 1975.

Sullivan, D. B., Cassidy, J. T., Petty, R. E., and Burt, A.: Prognosis in childhood dermatomyositis. *J. Pediatr.*, 80:555, 1972.

Tedford, J. C., Singsen, B. H., and Hanson, V.: Spontaneous pneumothorax: an early and late complication of juvenile dermatomyositis. (in press.)

Trell, E., and Lindstrom, C.: Pulmonary hypertension in systemic sclerosis. *Ann. Rheum. Dis.* 30:390, 1971.

Tuffanelli, D. L., and Winkelmann, R. K.: Systemic scleroderma: a clinical study of 727 cases. *Arch. Dermatol.*, 84:359, 1961.

Warshaw, J. B., and Spach, M. S.: Takayasu's disease (primary aortitis) in childhood: case report with review of literature. *Pediatrics*, 35:620, 1965.

Weaver, A. L., Divertie, M. B., and Titus, J. L.: Pulmonary scleroderma. *Dis. Chest*, 54:490, 1968a.

Weaver, A. L., Brundage, B. H., Nelson, R. A., and Bischoff, M. B.: Pulmonary involvement in polymyositis: report of a case with response to corticosteroid therapy. *Arthritis Rheum., 11*:765, 1968b.

Wedgwood, R. J., and Schaller, J.: Diseases of connective tissue. In Nelson, W. E., Vaughan, V. C., and McKay, R. J. (eds.): *Textbook of Pediatrics.* Philadelphia, W. B. Saunders Company, 1969, p. 511.

Winkelmann, R. K., and Ditto, W. B.: Cutaneous and visceral syndromes of necrotizing or "allergic angiitis": a study of 38 cases. *Medicine, 43*:59, 1964.

Wolff, S. M., Fauci, A. S., Horn, R. G., and Dale, D. C.: Wegener's granulomatosis. *Ann. Intern. Med., 81*:513, 1974.

Zeek, D. M.: Periarteritis nodosa and other forms of necrotizing angiitis. *N. Engl. J. Med., 248*:764, 1953.

CHAPTER SIXTY-SIX

FAMILIAL DYSAUTONOMIA

Felicia B. Axelrod, M.D., and Joseph Dancis, M.D.

In 1949, five children were reported with "central autonomic dysfunction with defective lacrimation." Since then, over 200 patients with familial dysautonomia, or Riley-Day syndrome, have been reported in the United States and Canada. In order to provide a background for discussion of the pulmonary manifestations, a brief general description of the disease will be presented.

Genetics

Familial dysautonomia is an inherited disorder resulting from the expression of an autosomal recessive gene. In studies of the inheritance pattern of 200 patients in America and 30 in Israel, it was found that the disease was limited to Jews of Ashkenazi origin. This suggests that the mutation took place after the migration of the Jews from Spain to central and eastern Europe at the end of the fifteenth century. In this population, the disease incidence is approximately one per 10,000 to 20,000, indicating a gene frequency of one per 100 to 140.

Pathology

The primary pathologic defect is neurologic. The sympathetic and sensory ganglia are small, with a diminished number of neurons. The submucosal neurons and axons in the tongue are poorly organized and reduced in number, and the fungiform and circumvallate papillae, in which the taste buds are normally found, are rudimentary. Sural nerve biopsies have revealed a thin nerve with very few nonmyelinated fibers, and a considerable reduction in small-diameter myelinated fibers. These fibers subserve pain detection.

Pulmonary disease and scoliosis are frequent complications (see section on Respiratory Problems). Corneal abrasions, ulcers and scarring are common.

Clinical Manifestations

The symptoms are protean and there is considerable variation among individuals. A relatively typical history is that of an infant who shortly after birth is recognized to have problems with sucking or swallowing. Other presenting complaints may be frequent unexplained fevers and slow motor and physical development. Respiratory infections are common. Feeding problems usually become less frequent by one to two years of age and are replaced in prominence by the "dysautonomic crisis": attacks of vomiting, fever, hypertension, excessive sweating and a blotchy erythema, lasting hours or days. A relative insensitivity to pain predisposes to burns, fractures, corneal abrasions and other types of trauma. The older dysautonomic may often be recognized by a peculiar pinched face with a transverse mouth, an awkward gait, short stature, nasal speech and exotropia.

Diagnosis

The most distinctive clinical sign is the *absence or marked diminution of overflow tearing*. When this is supported by other evidence of autonomic and sensory disturbance, such as postural hypotension, absence of patellar jerks and poor taste discrimination, the diagnosis is virtually assured. There are, in addition, three simple objective tests that aid in confirming the diagnosis.

HISTAMINE TEST. In the normal child, the intradermal injection of histamine, 1:1000 (1:10,000 may be more distinctive in infants), produces intense pain and erythema followed within minutes by the development of a central wheal surrounded by the axon flare, a zone of erythema 1 to 3 cm. in radius, which is maintained for more than ten minutes. In the dysautonomic, the pain is greatly reduced and there is no axon flare. No false-negative responses have been observed (dysautonomics with a normal flare), and the only false-positive reaction requiring serious consideration occurs in congenital sensory neuropathy. That entity is easily excluded by the following two signs.

METHACHOLINE (MECHOLYL) TEST. The instillation of methacholine 2.5 per cent into the conjunctival sac produces a miosis in almost all cases of familial dysautonomia and has no observable effect on the normal pupil. This is a sign of parasympathetic denervation and will be reproduced by any condition with such denervation.

ABSENCE OF FUNGIFORM PAPILLAE ON THE TONGUE. This unusual sign is associated with markedly impaired taste discrimination. To date, there have been only three reported cases of familial dysautonomia in which fungiform papillae have been clinically visible.

Respiratory Problems

FUNCTIONAL DEFECTS. There is a decreased sensitivity to breathing increased concentrations of carbon dioxide in the air (4 per cent CO_2). With hypercapnia, the minute ventilation does not increase as much as in the normal child, and respiratory acidosis results. When exposed to moderate hypoxia (12 per cent O_2 inhalations), the normal subject responds with a slight increase in minute ventilation and only a moderate fall in O_2 saturation, without visible disturbance to the patient. In the dysautonomic, the O_2 saturation rapidly falls to a very low level, despite an appropriate increase in minute ventilation. This results in cyanosis and, in some instances, syncope and convulsions (see Fig. 1). The systemic hypotension that complicates hypoxia in the dysautonomic probably contributes to the dramatic symptoms.

The abnormal response to hypoxia and the insensitivity to hypercapnia may help explain the following alarming clinical situations. During a flight on a commercial airplane with a pressurized cabin, a 12-year-old dysautonomic became comatose and convulsed. At a later date, this same boy was admitted to the hospital, comatose, with pneumonia; his Pa_{CO2} was 75 mm. Hg and his Pa_{O2} was 78 mm. Hg. Several youngsters have drowned during underwater swimming. In one such instance, a child was demonstrating his breathholding ability!

Abnormal breathing patterns become evident during sleep. The occasional deep respirations seen in the normal individual are infrequent, and periods of apnea of 15 seconds and longer have been noted.

PULMONARY DISEASE. Recurrent pneumonias are frequent. Repeated aspiration is probably the major factor in producing pulmonary disease. The disturbance in swallowing has been clearly demonstrated by cine-esophagrams. The dysautonomic child has difficulty in forming a bolus of food and then in directing the food properly. It can be misdirected into the trachea, eustachian tubes or nasopharynx (see Fig. 2). There is also dysfunction at the cardiac-esophageal junction resembling chalasia; this may result in regurgitation and sometimes in postprandial aspiration. Chronic pulmonary disease, i.e., atelectasis, bronchiectasis and abscess, is common. Diffuse fibrosis may occur in the absence of clinical history of recurrent pneumonia. Vital capacity is reduced.

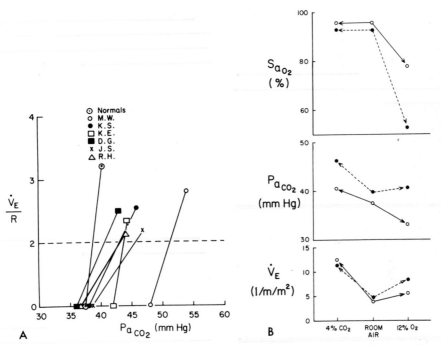

Figure 1. *A*, The relation between arterial P_{CO_2} (Pa_{CO_2}) and the increase in minute ventilation. The average of the results in five control subjects is presented as one line; the dysautonomic responses are presented individually. The greater slope in dysautonomia indicates that a greater change in Pa_{CO_2} is necessary to produce a corresponding increase in minute ventilation. *B*, Average values for arterial oxygen saturation (Sa_{O_2}), partial pressure of arterial CO_2 (Pa_{CO_2}) and minute ventilation (Ve) in five control subjects (solid line) and in six dysautonomic patients (broken line) while breathing, respectively, room air, 4 per cent CO_2 in air, and 12 per cent O_2. (*A* and *B* reprinted with approval of publishers from Filler, J., Smith, A. A., Stone, S., and Dancis, J.: *J. Pediatr.*, 66:509, 1965.)

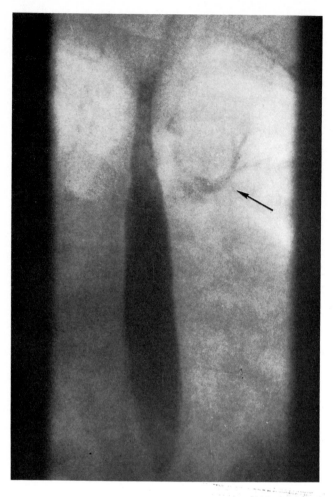

Figure 2. Posteroanterior view of barium swallow in dysautonomic. Note the barium that has been aspirated into the upper (left) stem bronchus. (Roentgenogram obtained through courtesy of Dr. Melvin Becker.)

Scoliosis of variable degree occurs in 95 per cent of dysautonomics over the age of ten years. On occasion, it is so severe as to further limit an already compromised pulmonary function (see Fig. 3). Cor pulmonale may complicate the final stages of decompensation.

Prognosis

Few of these patients reach adulthood, and none has yet lived beyond the age of 35. Pulmonary disease is the most frequent cause of death. Life expectancy is gradually improving with better care. A 26-year-old woman with dysautonomia has given birth to a clinically normal infant.

Treatment

Treatment of the pulmonary complications of familial dysautonomia is generally the same as that of any disorder complicated by acute and chronic pulmonary disease. This is adequately described elsewhere in this book. There are a few distinctive features, however, that deserve emphasis. The frequency of subtle clinical signs warrants a high index of suspicion for atelectasis, pneumonia and lung abscess. Fever, cyanosis or listlessness may be the only warning signs. Radiographic examination and early antibiotic therapy are commonly indicated. Cultures should be taken but may be confusing because the offending organisms may not be the usual

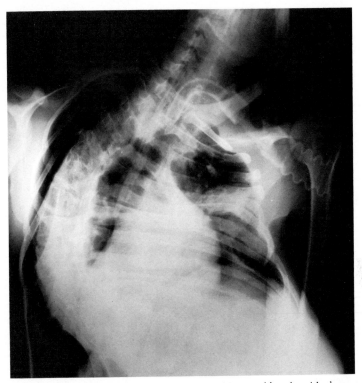

Figure 3.   Posteroanterior view of severe scoliosis in a 21-year-old male with dysautonomia. Chronic atelectasis and fibrosis are apparent in left lung. Tracheostomy was required for adequate ventilation of patient.

pathogens. In the severely ill child, blood gases must be monitored to detect CO_2 accumulation, which may require assisted ventilation. Suctioning and the elimination of milk from the diet may help the child who accumulates a lot of secretions in the nasopharynx. Very infrequently, a gastrostomy has been performed when aspiration regularly followed feeding. When the child is old enough to cooperate, a positive pressure respirator is used to improve lung expansion. Two patients who suffer from frequent apneic episodes have been tracheostomized to permit mechanical ventilation during sleep.

The pulmonary pathologic condition is generally diffuse, and surgery is rarely indicated. However, good results have been achieved in lobectomy performed in a three-year-old child with localized bronchiectasis, and nine patients have now had corrective surgery for scoliosis. During general anesthesia, careful attention must be given to avoid hypoxia and hypercapnia. The serious complication of hypotension, followed by cardiac arrest, may be prevented by infusions of volume expanders and epinephrine or norepinephrine as necessary.

Activity at high altitudes and underwater swimming should be prohibited. During flying, precautions should be taken to have oxygen available. It may be advisable to instruct parents in mouth-to-mouth resuscitation as a simple way to assist ventilation mechanically.

REFERENCES

Axelrod, F. B., Nachtigal, R., and Dancis, J.: Familial dysautonomia: diagnosis, pathogenesis and management. *Adv. Pediatr.*, *21*:75, 1974.

Brunt, P. W., and McKusick, V. A.: Familial dysautonomia—a report of genetic and clinical studies, with a review of the literature. *Medicine, 49*:343, 1970.

Dancis, J., and Smith, A. A.: Current concepts: familial dysautonomia. *N. Engl. J. Med., 274*:207, 1966.

Edelman, N. H., Cherniack, N. S., Lahini, S., Richards, E., and Fishman, A. P.: Effects of abnormal sympathetic nervous function upon the ventilatory response to hypoxia. *J. Clin. Invest., 49*:1153, 1970.

Filler, J., Smith, A. A., Stone, S., and Dancis, J.: Respiratory control in familial dysautonomia. *J. Pediatr., 66*:509, 1965.

Gyepes, M. T., and Linde, L. M.: Familial dysautonomia: the mechanism of aspiration. *Radiology, 91*:471, 1968.

Moses, S. W., Rotem, Y., Jagoda, N., Talmor, N., Eichhorn, F., and Levin, S.: A clinical, genetic and biochemical study of familial dysautonomia in Israel. *Isr. J. Med. Sci., 3*:358, 1967.

Riley, C. M., Day, R. L., Greely, D. McL., and Langford, W. S.: Central autonomic dysfunction with defective lacrimation. *Pediatrics, 3*:468, 1949.

Smith, A. A., and Dancis, J.: Response to intradermal histamine in familial dysautonomia—a diagnostic test. *J. Pediatr., 63*:889, 1963.

Smith, A. A., Dancis, J., and Breinin, G.: Ocular responses to autonomic drugs in familial dysautonomia. *Invest. Ophthalmol., 4*:358, 1965.

CHAPTER SIXTY-SEVEN

CHRONIC GRANULOMATOUS DISEASE OF CHILDHOOD

BYUNG HAK PARK, M.D.,
BEULAH HOLMES GRAY, PH.D.,
and ROBERT A. GOOD, M.D., PH.D.

Fatal (chronic) granulomatous disease of childhood (Good and coworkers, 1968) was first described by Berendes and colleagues (1957) and Bridges and coworkers (1959) as a distinct clinical entity of unknown causation. This disease is characterized by recurrent infections with low-grade pathogens, formation of suppurative granulomas, and normal humoral and cellular immunity. The usual onset of symptoms is early in life (one patient died at six days of age), the disease is generally chronic (the oldest known survivor at present is 27 years old) and the outcome was thought to be fatal—the result of overwhelming infection.

Since the original report, similar cases have been presented and various names have been used, i.e., progressive septic granulomatous disease (Carson and coworkers, 1965), chronic granulomatous disease (Baehner and Nathan, 1967) and congenital dysphagocytosis (Macfarlane and coworkers, 1968). We use the term "chronic granulomatous disease" (CGD) clinically for purposes of relieving parental apprehension.

Eighty-three years after Mechnikoff's theory of phagocytosis (1883), Holmes and coworkers (1966a) clearly demonstrated in CGD patients that a defect in phagocytic function is a major cause of the inadequacy in host defense against invading organisms. Thus, major advances in the theory of phagocytosis, as well as in the understanding of the pathogenesis of CGD, were made, and this disease became a unique "experiment of Nature" for the study of phagocytosis.

The respiratory tract is almost always involved in these patients and presents complex clinical manifestations.

Clinical Features

The hallmark of this disease is the occurrence, in the same lesions, of septic purulent inflammation due to catalase-positive, low-grade pyogenic bacteria (Table 1) and the formation of granulomas in response to these infections.

The clinical problems experienced early in life by these patients include infection of the skin, persistent purulent

---

TABLE 1. A CLASSIFICATION OF BACTERIA ACCORDING TO THE BACTERICIDAL CAPACITY OF LEUKOCYTES FROM PATIENTS WITH FATAL GRANULOMATOUS DISEASE

Bacteria that are not killed (catalase-positive)
Coagulase-positive staphylococci
Escherichia coli
Aerobacter aerogenes
Paracolon hafnia (Klebsiella)
Serratia marcescens

Bacteria that are killed (catalase-negative)
Lactobacillus acidophilus
Streptococcus viridans
Diplococcus pneumoniae
Streptococcus faecalis

rhinitis and lymphadenopathy in a well nourished infant of otherwise normal appearance (Table 2).

Johnston and Baehner (1971) reviewed data on 92 patients with CGD, including four new ones. Marked lymphadenopathy was noted in 87 patients, and in 79 of these the lymph nodes suppurated and drained pus. Pneumonitis or pneumonia occurred in 80 patients. Hepatomegaly was found in 77 patients, and splenomegaly in 68; these findings were noted in all but three patients who reached the age of six years. Of the 85 patients whose age at onset of disease was known, 84 had shown their first symptoms by age two years. There were 45 reported deaths, 34 before the age of seven years. Overwhelming pulmonary disease was the primary cause of death in 21 of 38 patients in whom the cause of death was stated. Septicemia led to death in 11 patients.

The skin lesion is characterized by granulomatous eruption surrounding impetigo; it progresses slowly to suppuration. The healing process is also extremely slow, resulting in a granulomatous nodular appearance, and the granulomatous nodules may persist for months. These lesions may be found in any part of the body, the face and neck being the more frequent sites. Purulent rhinitis and otitis are characteristic clinical features of this disease. They occur very frequently and represent recurrent clinical problems. With adequate local and systemic anti-biotic therapy, the lesion of the external nostrils clears up slowly only to recur within a few days after the treatment is discontinued.

Lymphadenitis is another common clinical feature and occurs in the majority of patients during the course of the disease. This is characteristically chronic, suppurative and granulomatous, and very often requires surgical drainage. Swelling and induration of cervical, axillary and inguinal lymph nodes are most frequently seen, but involvement of hilar and mesenteric lymph nodes also occurs with great frequency.

In the common form of this disease, the family history usually reveals strong evidence of x-linked recessive inheritance (see below) (Bridges and coworkers, 1959; Carson and coworkers, 1965; Windhorst and associates, 1967, 1968; Baehner and Nathan, 1968).

On physical examination, hepatosplenomegaly is observed in the majority of patients. An increased anteroposterior diameter of the chest can be found in those patients with chronic fibrotic lungs.

The most prominent pulmonary lesions include an extensive infiltration of the lung parenchyma and prominent hilar adenopathy demonstrable on roentgenogram (Fig. 1). In addition, bronchopneumonia, often combined with lobar pneumonia, pleural effusion, pleural thickening, pulmonary abscess and atelectasis of the right middle lobe, may be seen. An extensive reticulonodular infiltration often leads to pulmonary insufficiency and death.

The pneumonia characteristically begins as a hilar infiltration; it is bronchial and may be unilateral or bilateral or may be basilar. In spite of extensive antibiotic treatment, these lesions may regress very slowly over a period of weeks to months or may frequently progress to involve an entire lobe (Figs. 2 and 3). An unusual manifestation of pulmonary involvement that is frequently observed in these patients is the so-called encapsulated pneumonia (Wolfson and coworkers, 1968). This

TABLE 2.   CLINICAL FEATURES OF FATAL GRANULOMATOUS DISEASE

Recurrent infections with low-grade pathogens starting early in life.

Chronic suppurative granulomatous lesions of the skin and lymph nodes.

Hepatosplenomegaly—parenchymatous granuloma and liver abscess.

Progressive pulmonary disease—granulomatous infiltration, abscess, empyema.

Granulomatous septic osteomyelitis.

Pericarditis.

Normal cellular and humoral immune response.

Familial occurrence.

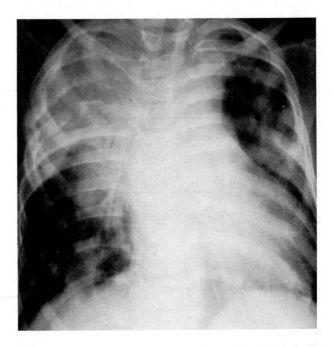

Figure 1. Roentgenogram of chest from a patient with chronic granulomatous disease showing extensive involvement of right lung. This patient died of overwhelming infection.

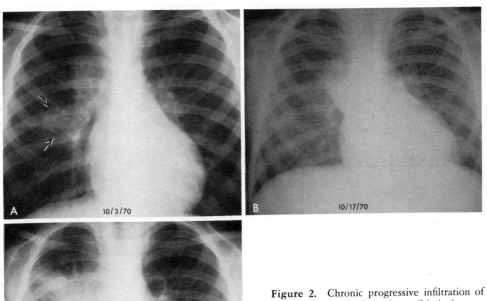

Figure 2. Chronic progressive infiltration of the right lung despite intensive antibiotic therapy. Right upper lobe was resected in order to control the infection. *A,* An early stage of infiltration with typical "encapsulated pneumonia" (shown by arrow). *B* and *C,* Progression of the lesion.

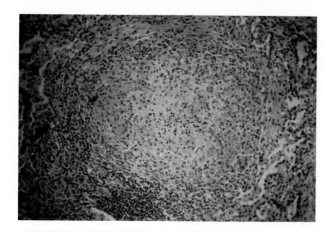

Figure 3. A typical granuloma of lung tissue removed from the patient shown in Figure 2 (approximately 400 × magnification).

pneumonia is characteristically seen on roentgenogram as a homogeneous, discrete and relatively round lesion; it may occur singly or in groups of two to three infiltrates (Fig. 2A). The size and contour of the lesions may change within a few days or remain unchanged for a period of weeks or months. Discoid atelectasis, thickening of the bronchi, air bronchogram, "honeycombing" and loss of lobar volume are occasionally observed. When underlying reticulation of the lungs persists, the pulmonary function may be correspondingly impaired.

Hepatic abscess, mesenteric lymphadenitis, osteomyelitis and oophoritis are also frequent manifestations. Anemia is often seen and may be an early sign of parenchymal infection.

Laboratory Findings

The intensive search for the organisms that are usually associated with the production of parenchymal granulomatous infiltration (mycobacteria, fungus and others) is to no avail. Although organisms usually considered to be true high-grade bacterial, viral or fungal pathogens rarely cause the lesions, the organisms frequently associated with the lesions generally are low-grade pyogenic pathogens (Table 1). It is striking that those organisms infecting the patients and causing clinical illness can be grouped together as catalase-producing organisms.

Immunologic study has revealed normal or slightly elevated circulating immunoglobulins, vigorous antibody responses to active immunization and normal cellular immunity.

The clinical dilemma involved in pathogenesis, i.e., the apparent deficiency of host defense against infection despite normal immunity, has provoked an extensive search for the mechanism underlying deficiency of bodily defense. The first major breakthrough in this clinical dilemma was made by Holmes and colleagues (1966a), who reported that the leukocytes of CGD patients failed to kill ingested bacteria (Fig. 4). In the course of these studies, these investigators showed that bacteria ingested by the phagocytic cells of these patients are actually protected from antibiotics present in high concentrations outside of phagocytes (Holmes and coworkers, 1966b). The exhaustive studies of Quie and associates (1967) and Kaplan and colleagues (1968) established that CGD leukocytes were unable to kill a number of organisms that are usually associated with the lesions, but that catalase-negative organisms, which cause little clinical difficulty in these patients, are killed in a normal manner by their leukocytes (Table 1).

The demonstration of the bacterici-

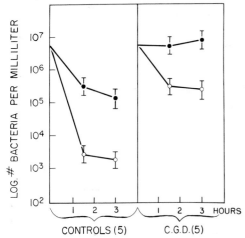

Figure 4. Bactericidal test of leukocytes. *Staphylococcus aureus* 502A was incubated with leukocytes, and the number of surviving bacteria was determined by colony count at intervals. Closed circles: no antibiotics were added. Open circles: penicillin and streptomycin were added at 15 minutes of incubation. CGD = Chronic granulomatous disease. The number of patients or controls is shown in parentheses.

dal defect in the leukocytes of CGD patients led Holmes and coworkers (1967) to study the metabolic response of leukoctyes during phagocytosis. It was clearly shown that the leukocytes of patients with CGD have deficiencies of the metabolic stimulation associated with phagocytosis (Table 3). Associated with the diminished bactericidal capacity is a decreased iodide binding of organisms ingested by CGD leukocytes (Klebanoff and White, 1969; Pincus and Klebanoff, 1971). Iodination of bacteria appears to require the myeloperoxidase present in lysosomal granules plus hydrogen peroxide, and this combination is bactericidal in a cell-free system. Recently, a defect in superoxide dismutase activity has been reported (Curnutte and coworkers, 1975) in the leukocytes of CGD patients.

Baehner and Nathan (1967, 1968) and Baehner and Karnovsky (1969) reported that the leukocytes of CGD patients have a deficiency of NADH oxidase and fail to reduce nitroblue tetrazolium (NBT) dye during phagocytosis. Holmes and coworkers (1970), however, did not find the NADH oxidase deficiency. Hohn and Lehrer (1975) described a defect of NADPH oxidase deficiency, which, to our view, also may be secondary to the abnormality of the metabolic changes by a more fundamental abnormality. Glutathione peroxidase of the leukocytes was, however, found to be deficient in female patients (Holmes and coworkers, 1970). The glucose-6-phosphate dehydrogenase (G-6-PD) of leukocytes from the male patients has been reported to be less stable at 4 and 38°C. than the G-6-PD of normal leukocytes (Bellanti and coworkers, 1970), but this abnormality is probably secondary rather than primary.

Some patients with CGD may have red cells with a very rare Kell system phenotype (Giblett and coworkers, 1971). Transfusion of such patients

TABLE 3.   RELATIONSHIP BETWEEN KX ANTIGEN,
MCLEOD KELL PHENOTYPE, AND CHRONIC
GRANULOMATOUS DISEASE

		KX Antigen	
	Kell Phenotype	Red Cell	Neutrophils
Non-CGD	Normal	+	+
Non-CGD	McLeod	−	+
CGD male (x-linked)	Normal	+	−
CGD male (x-linked)	McLeod	−	−
CGD (autosomal recessive)	Normal	+	+

Adapted from Marsh, W. L., Uretsky, C., and Douglas, S. D.: *J. Pediatr.,* 87:1117, 1975.

may stimulate the formation of antibodies against all of the common antigens of the Kell system, which makes it extremely difficult to find a subsequent blood donor. The majority of patients with CGD, however, do not have red cells with this peculiar Kell phenotype. The patient originally described to have this rare blood type (McLeod Kell phenotypes) (Allen and coworkers, 1961) did not have manifestations of CGD. Further studies of this relationship by March and colleagues (1975a, 1975b) yielded an important observation that may help understand the cellular defect in the x-linked form of CGD. In Table 3 we summarize Marsh's study. Marsh has defined a surface membrane component of definitive antigenicity that he calls Kx. This antigen is present on the surface of neutrophils, monocytes and red blood cells, but not on the lymphocytes, of normal persons. Persons with McLeod Kell phenotype lack the Kx antigen on their red cells. Such persons, however, have Kx in normal amounts on their neutrophils and monocytes. The majority of x-linked forms of male CGD patients lack the Kx membrane antigen on their neutrophils and monocytes but have normal Kell system phenotypes on their red cells. CGD patients with the rare McLeod Kell phenotype mentioned previously lack Kx on their red cells, neutrophils and monocytes. Patients with the autosomal recessive form of CGD did not have a defect of the Kx antigen. It seems entirely possible that the reported enzymatic abnormalities in this disease may be secondary to a membrane abnormality associated with the absence of Kx. This may render the membrane ineffective in triggering the metabolic response necessary for effective killing of ingested organisms.

Quie and coworkers (1967) presented electron microscopic evidence that phagocytosis of bacteria by CGD leukocytes was not accompanied by the vigorous degranulation that occurs in normal leukocytes. However, evidence that granule lysis is normal in the patients' leukocytes has been presented by others (Kauder and coworkers, 1968; Baehner and Karnovsky, 1969; Elsbach and coworkers, 1969; Ulevitch and coworkers, 1974). Recent reports (Gold and associates, 1974) indicate that the kinetics of degranulation may be abnormal.

Even though no satisfactory explanation, at the enzymatic level, for the metabolic abnormalities observed in CGD has been forthcoming, the diminished hydrogen peroxide production by CGD cells appears to be of major importance in the bactericidal defect. The enzyme responsible for the transfer of ions from reduced pyridine nucleotide to NBT dye seems to be localized in the granules of the cytoplasm (Park, 1971). This enzyme is present and normal in the granules of the leukocytes from CGD patients. The failure of NBT dye reduction by the leukocytes of CGD patients may, in fact, be due to an anomaly in the rupture of the particular granule containing this enzyme. Delayed granule rupture and release of myeloperoxidase may also be a crucial factor in the bactericidal defect. A strikingly reduced activity of an enzyme in the plasma membrane of the neutrophils has been described in male patients with CGD by Segal and Peters (1976). This enzyme, located in the plasma membrane of normal neutrophils, reduces NBT dye when NADH is present at lower, more physiological levels than is customarily used for the NADH-dependent oxidase assay. The relation of this enzyme and its activation to the Kx antigen would be a study of great interest.

Inheritance

At present, at least four separate groups of patients with the leukocyte bactericidal defect have been identified. The first is the group described by Berendes and colleagues (1957) and subsequently by others; this group represents the classic form of this disease.

Males are selectively involved, and the mothers as well as approximately half of the sisters and the maternal grandmothers of affected patients are detectable as carriers. In both the bactericidal tests and the NBT test, the leukocytes of carriers (of the defect) were shown to be intermediate between CGD patients and normal controls (Windhorst and coworkers, 1967, 1968). However, recent reports (Biggar and coworkers, 1976) indicate that the carriers may have varying degrees of abnormality ranging from near normal to the level of CGD. This is what would be predicted if random inactivation of one or the other x chromosome of somatic cells (Lyon's hypothesis) occurs in the neutrophils of CGD.

(2) In the second group, the defect appears to be inherited as an autosomal recessive trait, and both male and female patients with this defect have now been defined (Quie and coworkers, 1968; Baehner and Nathan, 1968; Azimi and coworkers, 1968; Chandra and coworkers, 1969; Malawista and Gifford, 1975). These patients present a clinical picture similar to that of the first group but often somewhat less severe in its clinical expression. Holmes and colleagues (1970) reported that leukocyte glutathione peroxidase was deficient in two of these patients, while the parents of one of these families had glutathione peroxidase values approximately one-half that of normal activity. Matsuda and coworkers (1976) reported glutathione peroxidase deficiency in a male patient with chronic granulomatous disease.

(3) The third group is represented by the cases originally described by Ford and colleagues (1962) and studied by Rodey and associates (1970). The latter authors reported that a bactericidal activity of leukocytes was defective in females with lipochrome histiocytosis. Levels of glutathione peroxidase in the leukocytes of these patients were normal (Holmes, unpublished data). The finding that the patients were female and that the mother did not show leukocyte functional deficiencies established that this disease is not of x-linked inheritance. Although these findings are compatible with an autosomal recessive inheritance, they did not establish the Mendelian nature of this cellular defect.

(4) The fourth form is represented by the patients reported by Cooper and coworkers (1970) and by Gray and coworkers (1973), in which a complete absence of glucose-6-phosphate dehydrogenase was associated with defective bactericidal activity of the patients' leukocytes. The mode of inheritance of this defect is not clear, but it probably represents an inborn error transmitted as an autosomal recessive trait.

Diagnosis

History and physical examination will reveal the characteristic clinical features of this disease. By the use of a simple screening test (Park and Good, 1970), it is now possible to make a prompt presumptive diagnosis. In this test, the total absence of reduced NBT dye in the leukocytes of patients is observed in each of the four groups of patients thus far defined. This initial screening test should be followed by a more elaborate functional and metabolic study of the leukocytes. The demonstration of a defect in bactericidal function of leukocytes establishes the diagnosis (Windhorst and coworkers, 1968).

Treatment

The new knowledge of granulomatous disease is useful in making the diagnosis at an early stage of the disease. The recognition of the bacteria in the lesions as potential pathogens permits an appreciation of the significance of low-grade pyogenic pathogens in each infection. This knowledge of the potential causative organisms facilitates the prompt use of appropriate antibiotics and chemotherapy at an earlier time than was previously the case. Because of this progress in diagnosis and treatment, the disease is much better managed and not nearly as lethal as it once was. Nonetheless, chronic granulomatous disease continues to have a high mortality owing to occurrence of overwhelming infection.

Treatment with gamma globulin, leukocyte transfusion, vitamin A to facilitate degranulation, and methylene blue to initiate pentose pathway activity in leukocytes of patients with this disease has been tried without clinical benefit. Continuous administration of nafcillin has been advocated, and some clinical benefit has been ascribed to this prophylactic antibiotic regimen (Philippart and coworkers, 1972). However, we have chosen not to give continuous antibiotic therapy to our patients with CGD, primarily because gram-negative bacteria and fungi have usually been responsible for infections leading to hospitalization and requiring specific antibiotic therapy or surgical excision, or both. Two of the three deaths in CGD patients of the Minnesota series since 1966 were due to pulmonary infections with Aspergillus, and the third was due to disseminated Pseudomonas infection. Early surgical drainage, excision of extending lesions and, at times, even radical surgery can be helpful and may be necessary for the clinical management of the infections. Close supervision of patients, early recognition of the characteristic symptoms and signs of each infection, and the prompt initiation of specific antibiotic therapy constitute the most effective present-day treatment of this group of diseases. It was reported that sulfisoxazole could partially correct the functional abnormality of the leukocytes of patients with CGD (Johnston and coworkers, 1975). Prolonged treatment using trimethoprim-sulfamethoxazole, although it does not correct the cellular defect as was originally thought, has been useful clinically (Pyesmany and Cameron, 1973).

Ideally, correction of the inborn error of metabolism by cellular engineering, for example by using bone marrow transplantation, should cure this disease. Although not clearly documented, this approach has been claimed to work for CGD by Hobbs (unpublished data) and, with perfection of bone marrow transplantation, could become the treatment of choice. At present, however, the risks of marrow transplantation seem too great for treatment of this disease, which is usually well managed these days if the responsible physician understands the disease and the organism likely to cause trouble, and is available to provide vigorous antibiotic therapy or chemotherapy when these are needed.

REFERENCES

Allen, F. H., Jr., Krabbe, S. M. R., and Corcoran, P. A.: A new phenotype (McLeod) in the Kell blood group system. *Vox Sang.*, 6:555, 1961.

Azimi, P. H., Bodenbender, J. G., Hintz, R. L., and Kontras, S. B.: Chronic granulomatous disease in three female siblings. *J.A.M.A.*, 206:2865, 1968.

Baehner, R. L., and Karnovsky, M. L.: Deficiency of reduced nicotinamide-adenine dinucleotide oxidase in chronic granulomatous disease of childhood. *Science*, 162:1277, 1968.

Baehner, R. L., and Karnovsky, M. L.: Degranulation of leukocytes in chronic granulomatous disease. *J. Clin. Invest.*, 48:187, 1969.

Baehner, R. L., and Nathan, D. G.: Leukocyte oxidase. *Science*, 155:835, 1967.

Baehner, R. L., and Nathan, D. G.: Quantitative nitroblue tetrazolium test in chronic granulomatous disease. *N. Engl. J. Med.*, 278:971, 1968.

Bellanti, J. A., Cantz, B. E., and Schlegel, R. J.: Accelerated decay of glucose-6-phosphate dehydrogenase activity in chronic granulomatous disease. *Pediatr. Res.*, 4:405, 1970.

Berendes, H., Bridges, R. A., and Good, R. A.: A fatal granulomatosis of childhood. *Minn. Med.*, 40:309, 1957.

Biggar, W. D., Buron, S., Holmes, B.: Chronic granulomatous disease in an adult male: a proposed x-linked defect. *J. Pediatr.*, 88:63, 1976.

Bridges, R. A., Berendes, H., and Good, R. A.: A fatal granulomatous disease of childhood. *Am. J. Dis. Child.*, 97:387, 1959.

Carson, J. M., Chadwick, D. L., Brubacker, C. A., Cleland, R. S., and Landing, B. H.: Thirteen boys with progressive septic granulomatosis. *Pediatrics*, 35:405, 1965.

Chandra, R. K., Cope, W. A., and Soothill, J. R.: Chronic granulomatous disease. *Lancet*, 2:71, 1969.

Cooper, M. R., DeChatelet, L. R., McCall, C. E., LaVia, M. F., Spurr, C. L., and Baehner, R. L.: Leucocyte G-6-PD deficiency. *Lancet*, 2:110, 1970.

Curnutte, J. H., Kipnes, R. S., and Babior, B. M.: Defect in pyridine nucleotide dependent superoxide production by a particulate fraction from the granulocytes of patients with chronic granulomatous disease. *N. Engl. J. Med.*, 293:628, 1975.

Elsbach, P., Zucker-Franklin, D., and Sansaricq, C.: Increased lecithin synthesis during phagocytosis by normal leukocytes and by leukocytes of a patient with chronic granulomatous disease. *N. Engl. J. Med.*, 280:1319, 1969.

Ford, D. K., Price, G. E., Charles, F. A. C., and Vassar, P. S.: Familial lipochrome pigmentation of histiocytes with hyperglobulinemia, pulmonary infiltration, splenomegaly, arthritis and susceptibility to infection. *Am. J. Med.*, 33:478, 1962.

Giblett, E. R., Klebanoff, S. J., Pincus, S. H., Swanson, J., Park, B. H., and McCullough, J.: Kell phenotypes in chronic granulomatous disease: a potential transfusion hazard. *Lancet*, 1:1235, 1971.

Gold, S. B., Hanes, D. M., Stites, D. P., and Fudenberg, H. H.: Abnormal kinetics of degranulation in chronic granulomatous disease. *N. Engl. J. Med.*, 291:332, 1974.

Good, R. A.: Progress toward a cellular engineering. *J.A.M.A.*, 214:1289, 1970.

Good, R. A., Quie, P. G., Windhorst, D. B., Page, A. R., Rodey, G. E., White, J., Wolfson, J. J., and Holmes, B.: Fatal (chronic) granulomatous disease of childhood. *Semin. Hematol.*, 5:215, 1968.

Gray, G. R., Stamatoyannopoulos, G., Naiman, S. C., Kliman, M. R., Klebanoff, S. J., Austin, T., Yoshida, A., and Robinson, G. C. F.: Neutrophil dysfunction, chronic granulomatous disease and nonspherocytic haemolytic anemia caused by complete deficiency of glucose-6-phosphate dehydrogenase. *Lancet*, 2:530, 1973.

Hohn, D. C., and Lehrer, R. I.: NADPH oxidase deficiency in x-linked chronic granulomatous disease. *J. Clin. Invest.*, 55:707, 1975.

Holmes, B., Page, A. R., and Good, R. A.: Studies of the metabolic activity of leukocytes from patients with a genetic abnormality of phagocytic function. *J. Clin. Invest.*, 46:1422, 1967.

Holmes, B., Park, B. H., Malawista, S. E., Nelson, D. L., Quie, P. G., and Good, R. A.: Chronic granulomatosis disease in females. *N. Engl. J. Med.*, 283:217, 1970.

Holmes, B., Quie, P. G., Windhorst, D. B., and Good, R. A.: Fatal granulomatous disease of childhood. *Lancet*, 1:1225, 1966a.

Holmes, B., Quie, P. G., Windhorst, D. B., Pollara, B., and Good, R. A.: Protection of phagocytized bacteria from the killing action of antibiotics. *Nature (London)*, 210:1131, 1966b.

Johnston, R. B., and Baehner, R. L.: Chronic granulomatous disease: correlation between pathogenesis and clinical findings. *Pediatrics*, 48:730, 1971.

Johnston, R. B., and McMurray, J. S.: Chronic familial granulomatosis. *Am. J. Dis. Child.*, 114:370, 1970.

Johnston, R. B., Wilfert, C. M., Buckley, R. H., Webb, L. S., DeChatelet, L. R., and McCall, C. E.: Enhanced bactericidal activity of phagocytes from patients with chronic granulomatous disease in the presence of sulphisoxazole. *Lancet*, 1:824, 1975.

Kaplan, E. L., Laxdal, T., and Quie, P. G.: Studies of polymorphonuclear leukocytes from patients with chronic granulomatous disease of childhood. *Pediatrics*, 41:591, 1968.

Karnovsky, M. L.: The metabolism of leukocytes. *Semin. Hematol.*, 5:156, 1968.

Kauder, E., Kahle, L. L., Moreno, H., and Parten, p. C.: Leukocyte degranulation and vacuole formation in patients with chronic granulomatous disease of childhood. *J. Clin. Invest.*, 47:1753, 1968.

Klebanoff, S. J., and White, L. R.: Iodination defect in the leukocytes of a patient with chronic granulomatous disease of childhood. *N. Engl. J. Med.*, 280:460, 1969.

Macfarlane, P. S., Speirs, A. L., and Sommerville, R. G.: Fatal granulomatous disease of childhood and benign lymphocytic infiltration of the skin (congenital dysphagocytosis). *Lancet*, 1:844, 1968.

Malawista, S. E., and Gifford, R. H.: Chronic granulomatous disease of childhood (CGD) with leukocyte glutathione peroxidase (LGP) deficiency in a brother and sister: a likely autosomal recessive inheritance. *Clin. Res.*, 23:416a, 1975.

Marsh, W. L., Oyen, R., Nichols, M. E., and Allen, F. H., Jr.: Chronic granulomatous disease and the Kell blood groups. *Br. J. Haematol.*, 29:247, 1975a.

Marsh, W. L., Uretsky, C., and Douglas, S. D.: Antigens of the Kell blood group system on neutrophils and monocytes: their relation to chronic granulomatous disease (CGD). *J. Pediatr.*, 87:1117, 1975b.

Matsuda, I., Oka, Y., Taniguchi, N., Furuyama, M., Kodama, S., Arashima, S., and Mitsuyama, T.: Leukocyte glutathione peroxidase deficiency in a male patient with chronic granulomatous disease. *J. Pediatr.*, 88:581, 1976.

Mechnikoff, E.: Untersuchungen uber die mesodermalen Phagocyten einiger Wirbeltiere. *Biol. Central Bl.*, 3:560, 1883.

Park, B. H.: The use and limitation of NBT reduction test as a diagnostic aid. *J. Pediatr.*, 78:376, 1971.

Park, B. H., and Good, R. A.: NBT test stimulated. *Lancet*, 2:616, 1970.

Philippart, A. I., Colodny, A. H., and Baehner, R. L.: Continuous antibiotic therapy in chronic granulomatous disease: preliminary communications. *Pediatrics*, 50:923, 1972.

Pincus, S. H., and Klebanoff, S. J.: Quantitative leukocyte iodination. *N. Engl. J. Med.*, 284:744, 1971.

Pyesmany, A. F., and Cameron, D. L.: Septrin-induced stimulation of granulocyte metabolism in chronic granulomatous disease (CGD). Abstract. *Pediatr. Res.,* 7:143, 1975.

Quie, P. G., Kaplan, E. L., Page, A. R., Gruskay, F. L., and Malawista, S. E.: Defective polymorphonuclear leukocyte function and chronic granulomatous disease in two female children. *N. Engl. J. Med.,* 279:967, 1968.

Quie, P. G., White, J. G., Holmes, B., and Good, R. A.: In vitro bactericidal capacity of human polymorphonuclear leukocytes. *J. Clin. Invest.,* 46:668, 1967.

Rodey, G. E., Holmes, B., Park, B. H., Ford, D., and Good, R. A.: Leukocyte function in lipochrome histiocytosis. *Am. J. Med.,* 49:322, 1970.

Segal, A. W., and Peters, T. J.: Characterization of the enzyme defect in chronic granulomatous disease. *Lancet,* 1:1363, 1976.

Ulevitch, R. J., Henson, P., Holmes, B., and Good, R. A.: An in vitro study of exocytosis of neutrophil granule enzymes in chronic granulomatous disease neutrophils. *J. Immunol.,* 112:1383, 1974.

Windhorst, D. B., Holmes, B., and Good, R. A.: A newly defined x-linked trait in man with demonstration of the Lyon effect in carrier females. *Lancet,* 1:737, 1967.

Windhorst, D. B., Page, A. R., Holmes, B., Quie, P. G., and Good, R. A.: The pattern of genetic transmission of the leukocyte defect in fatal granulomatous disease of childhood. *J. Clin. Invest.,* 47:1026, 1968.

Wolfson, J., Quie, P. G., Laxdal, S. D., and Good, R. A.: Roentgenologic manifestations in children with a genetic defect of polymorphonuclear leukocyte function. *Radiology,* 91:37, 1968.

CHAPTER SIXTY-EIGHT

DISORDERS OF THE RESPIRATORY TRACT DUE TO TRAUMA

ARNOLD M. SALZBERG, M.D., and JAMES W. BROOKS, M.D.

The incidence of thoracic trauma in the infant and the child is exceedingly low and is usually confined to automobile accidents, the battered child syndrome and falls from a considerable height. Stab and bullet wounds are rare. Nevertheless, the complete spectrum of chest trauma has been recorded and includes pneumothorax, hemothorax, destruction of the integrity of the chest wall and diaphragm, thoracic visceral damage and combined thoracoabdominal injuries (Fig. 1).

As in the adult, the significance of thoracic trauma parallels the pulmonary, cardiac and systemic dysfunction that follows, and in the pediatric age group, because of chest wall resiliency, physiologic aberrations can occur with trauma that does not fracture or penetrate. The interruption of satisfactory respiration and circulation secondary to chest injury is frequently complicated by blood loss and hypotension, and all three factors must be quickly reversed for survival. Shock from hemorrhage can usually be managed by intelligent, arithmetic specific replacement, which is monitored by serial blood pressures, hematocrit, central venous pressure, blood gas analysis and, if necessary, blood volume determinations, and pulmonary artery catheterization with a Swan-Ganz catheter for more precise information relating to pulmonary capillary wedge pressures and cardiac output. Restoration of the normal cardio-pulmonary function fundamentally depends on a clear airway, intact chest and diaphragm and unrestricted heart-lung dynamics. This, in most instances, can be accomplished by maneuvers other than thoracotomy.

STERNAL FRACTURES

Fractures of the sternum in infancy and childhood follow high compression crush injuries, and are usually associated with other thoracic and orthopedic problems elsewhere.

On physical examination there is local tenderness, ecchymosis and sometimes a peculiar concavity or paradoxical respiratory movement, but usually the sternal segments are well aligned without much displacement. Dyspnea, cyanosis, tachycardia and hypotension may be evidence of an underlying contused heart.

Cardiac tamponade and acute traumatic myocardial damage must be ruled out by various studies, including serial electrocardiograms, echocardiograms, sonography and careful monitoring of venous blood pressure. If the bony deformity is minimal, appropriate posture will suffice. Markedly displaced fragments are reduced under general anesthesia by the closed or open technique in order to prevent a traumatic pectus excavatum. Violent paradoxical

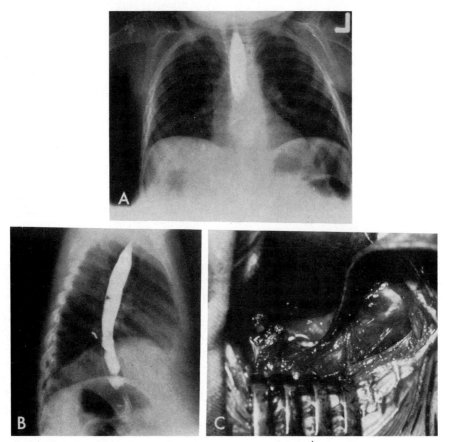

Figure 1. The posterior chest wall of this eight-year-old boy was penetrated by an object that was apparently accelerated by a power mower operating eight feet away. *A* and *B*, Posteroanterior and lateral chest films with barium in the esophagus demonstrate an opaque foreign body in the posterior mediastinum. *C*, Through an extrapleural approach a curved nail, seen just below the stump of the resected rib, and lying on the aorta, was removed from the posterior mediastinum.

respirations can be controlled by operative fixation or preferably by assisted mechanical respiration through an artificial airway.

FRACTURED RIBS

Rib fractures are unusual in pediatrics because of the extreme flexibility of the osseous and cartilaginous framework of the thorax. Crush and direct blow injuries are the usual etiologic factors. In addition, manual compression of the lateral chest wall, rickets, tumors and osteogenesis imperfecta have been incriminated. Multiple fractures of the middle ribs can be seen in the battered child syndrome (Fig. 2). The upper ribs are protected by the scapula and related muscles, and the lower ones are quite resilient.

Violence to the chest wall may produce pulmonary and cardiac lacerations and contusions, and a variety of pneumothoraces or hemothorax. Critical respiratory distress may also follow multiple anterior rib fractures, in which the integrity of the thoracic cage is destroyed and the involved chest becomes flail (Fig. 3). This unsupported area of the chest wall moves inward with inspiration and outward with expiration, and these paradoxical respiratory excursions inexorably lead to dyspnea (Fig.

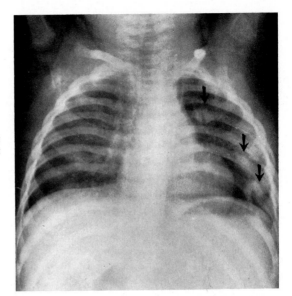

Figure 2. Multiple fractures of the left fourth and fifth ribs and fracture of the left clavicle in a battered child.

4). The explosive expiration of coughing is dissipated and made ineffectual by the paradoxical movement and intercostal pain. In effect, the ideal preparation for the respiratory distress syndrome, airway obstruction, atelec-

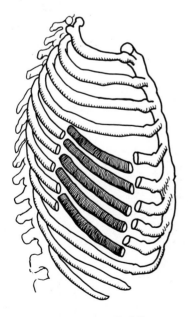

FRACTURED RIBS

Figure 3. Illustration of five ribs broken in two places with loss of chest wall stability and resultant paradoxical or "flail chest" wall.

tasis and pneumonia has been established.

The clinical picture includes local pain that is aggravated by motion. Tenderness is elicited by pressure applied directly over the fracture or elsewhere on the same rib. The fracture site may be edematous and ecchymotic. These minimal findings with simple, restricted fractures can be expanded to the severest form of ventilatory distress with a flail chest and lung injury.

Chest roentgenograms demonstrate the extent and displacement of the fractures and underlying visceral damage.

Treatment of the uncomplicated fracture involves control of pain in order to permit unrestricted respiration. Displacement requires no therapy. With severe fractures, the alleviation of pain and restoration of cough are important and can be provided by analgesics, physiotherapy and intermittent positive pressure breathing mechanisms. Thoracentesis and insertion of intercostal tubes should be done promptly for pneumothorax and hemothorax, and shock should be managed by appropriate replacement therapy and oxygen (Figs. 5 and 6).

Paradoxical respiratory excursions with flail chest must be brought under

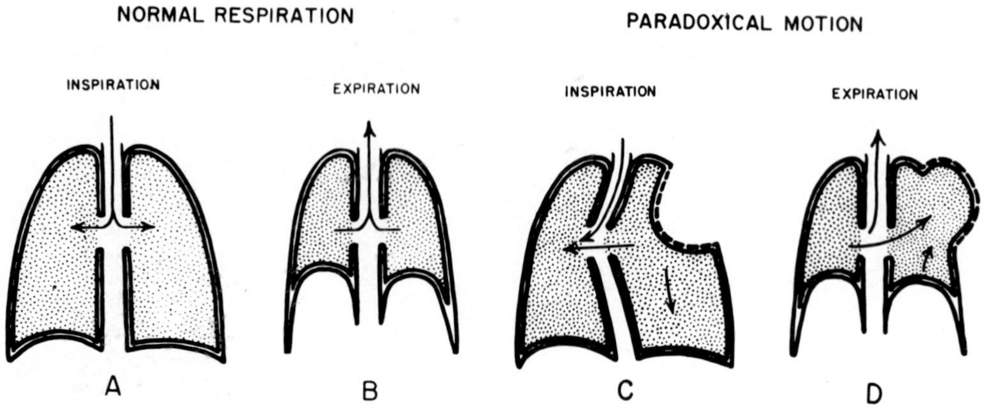

NORMAL RESPIRATION   PARADOXICAL MOTION

INSPIRATION   EXPIRATION   INSPIRATION   EXPIRATION

A   B   C   D

Figure 4.   Diagram of action of normal chest compared with "flail chest" during phases of respiratory cycle.

prompt control to help prevent the respiratory distress syndrome, which may be the morbid pulmonary complication (Fig. 7).

Controlled, mechanical respiration through an endotracheal tube has been used for paradox and respiratory insufficiency. In spite of vigorous therapy, secretions cannot be avoided and are attacked by tracheal catheterization and bronchoscopy. Tracheostomy, then, becomes useful in providing an avenue for the control of profuse secretions, diminishing the dead space and bypassing an obstructed airway (Fig. 8). Me-

chanical respiration can be applied and maintained through the tracheostomy for several weeks.

During the first year of life, tracheostomy is a morbid operation and should be avoided, if possible. Secretions may be difficult to aspirate, and the small tracheostomy tube becomes easily plugged; distal infection, often with staphylococci, is poorly handled, and withdrawal of the tracheostomy tube, at times, is a precarious and unpredictable adventure. Nevertheless, even in this age group, and certainly later, tracheostomy can be mandatory and life-

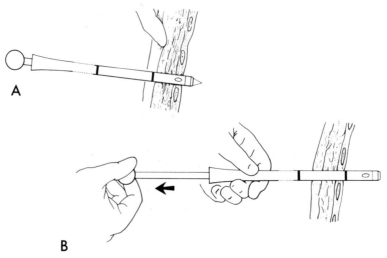

A

B

Figure 5.   Trocar technique of chest tube insertion.

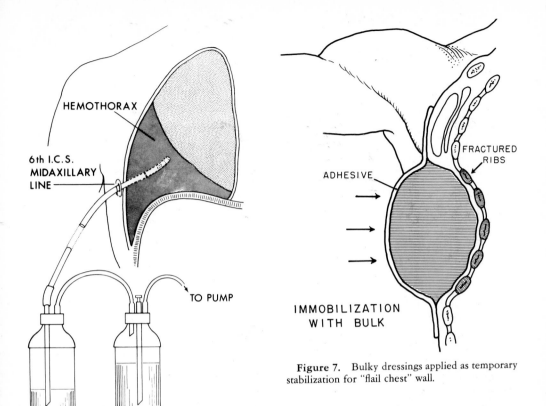

Figure 6. Classic set-up for closed drainage of pleural space.

Figure 7. Bulky dressings applied as temporary stabilization for "flail chest" wall.

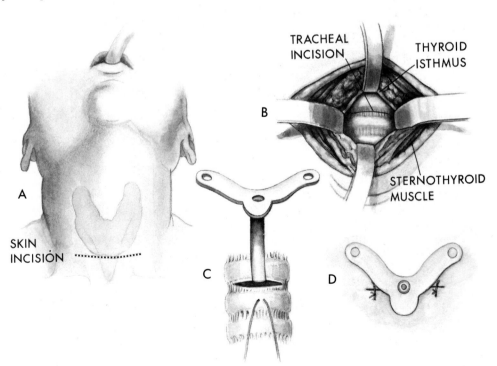

Figure 8. Techniques of tracheostomy performed over oral endotracheal tube. Note transverse skin incision in *A* and suture on lower tracheal flaps to facilitate subsequent tube changes (*C*).

saving in specific instances of chest trauma.

The decision for tracheostomy in cases of chest injury can often be made on the basis of (1) a mechanically obstructed airway that cannot be managed more conservatively and (2) flail chest. The unstable, paradoxing chest wall can be controlled for long periods of time by assisted positive pressure respirations through a short uncuffed silastic tracheostomy tube.

Often, however, the decision for tracheostomy is first broached in the presence of minimal dyspnea. In this situation, use of blood gas studies can augment the clinical impression and intercept clinical respiratory failure. Serial measurements of pH and arterial carbon dioxide tension are a satisfactory chemical guide to imminent ventilatory distress and the need for and efficiency of assisted or controlled mechanical respiration, since normal values rule out the presence of anoxia.

TRAUMATIC PNEUMOTHORAX

Traumatic tension and open pneumothorax are rare in infants and children, in whom a very mobile mediastinum would compound the usual cardiorespiratory distress. Both types of injuries are formidable and require specific maneuvers to reverse a malignant chain of events.

The creation of a tension pneumothorax in which intrapleural pressures approach or exceed atmospheric pressures requires a valvular mechanism through which air entering the pleura exceeds the amount escaping. The positive intrapleural pressure is dissipated by a mediastinal shift, which compresses the opposite lung in the presence of ipsilateral pulmonary collapse, and angulates the great vessels entering and leaving the heart. Intrapleural tension can be increased by traumatic hemothorax, and respiratory exchange

and cardiac output are critically diminished by this form of mediastinal tamponade.

The etiologic possibilities, in addition to chest wall and lung trauma, include rupture of the esophagus, a pulmonary cyst, an emphysematous lobe and postoperative bronchial fistula. These latter sources of tension pneumothorax almost always require thoracotomy for control.

The clinical finding may include external evidence of a wound, tachypnea, dyspnea, cyanosis with hyperresonance, absent or transmitted breath sounds and dislocation of the trachea and apical cardiac impulse. The hemithoraces may be asymmetrical, with the involved side larger.

A confirmatory x-ray film is comforting, but often cannot be afforded in this thoracic emergency. Fiberoptic transillumination may be helpful. Plastic needle aspiration or chest tube insertion is indicated for tension or a pneumothorax exceeding 25 per cent. Prompt relief and pulmonary expansion can be anticipated if the source of the intrapleural air has been controlled. Obviously, a traumatic valvular defect in the chest wall can be occluded. If the pulmonary air leak persists or recurs, the possibility of further tension pneumothorax is circumvented by the insertion of one or more intercostal tubes connected to waterseal drainage with mild suction. Most instances of traumatic tension pneumothorax will require tube drainage for permanent decompression, although the needle is indispensable for its emergency management. Stubborn bronchopleural fistulas that continue to remain widely patent in spite of adequate intercostal tube deflation may close with a therapeutic pneumoperitoneum. If this fails, thoracotomy may be required.

An open, sucking pneumothorax in which atmospheric air has direct, unimpeded entrance into and exit from a relatively free pleural space is a second, equally urgent thoracic emergency (Fig. 9). This is almost invariably accom-

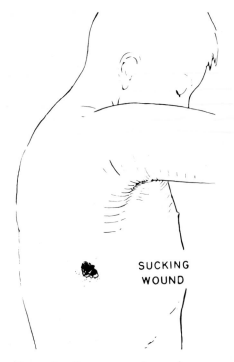

Figure 9. Open pneumothorax due to traumatic chest wall defect allowing ingress and egress of air into and from pleural cavity.

plished through a good-sized traumatic hole in the chest wall. Ingress of air during inspiration and egress during expiration produce an extreme degree of paradoxical respiration and mediastinal flutter, which is partially regulated by the size of the chest wall defect in comparison with the circumference of the trachea. If a considerable segment of chest wall is absent, more air is exchanged at this site than through the trachea, since pressures are similar. Inspiration collapses the ipsilateral lung and drives its alveolar air into the opposite side. During expiration, the air returns across the carina. In addition, the mediastinum becomes a widely swinging pendulum compressing uninjured lung on inspiration and lung on the injured side during expiration (Fig. 10). Obviously, under these circumstances, little effective ventilation is taking place because of the tremendous increase in the pulmonary dead space and decreased tidal exchange. A totally ineffective cough completes the clinical picture.

The diagnosis is readily made by inspection of the thoracic wound and the peculiar sound of air going in and coming out of the chest.

The emergency management of this critical situation demands prompt occlusion of the chest wall defect by bulky sterile dressings (Fig. 11) and measures to prevent conversion of this open pneumothorax into an equally aggravating tension pneumothorax, which can occur if the underlying lung has been traumatized. In this regard, Haynes (1952) has emphasized the importance of simultaneous pleural decompression by closed intercostal tube drainage. After systemic stablization, more formal surgical debridement,

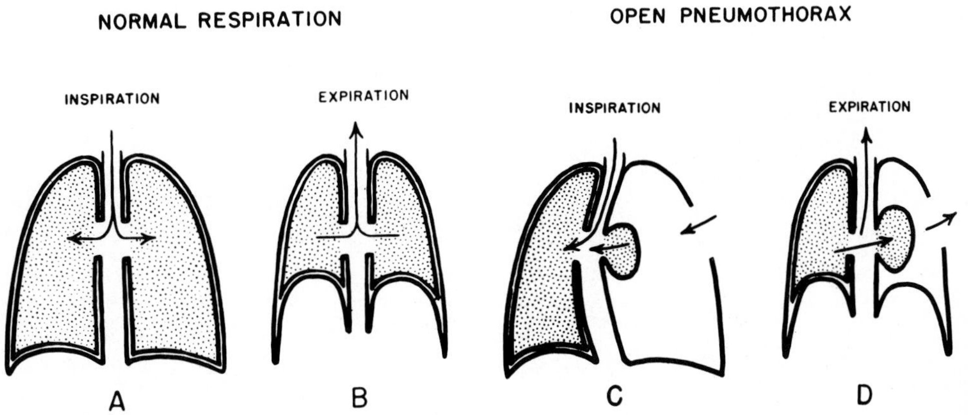

SUCKING WOUND

NORMAL RESPIRATION   OPEN PNEUMOTHORAX

INSPIRATION   EXPIRATION   INSPIRATION   EXPIRATION

A   B   C   D

Figure 10. Changes in normal respiratory pattern brought about by open, sucking thoracic wall injury.

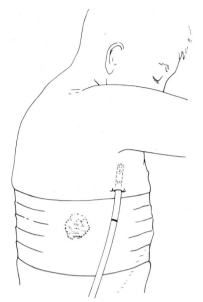

Figure 11. Temporary occlusive chest wall dressing applied to sucking wound with underwater intercostal chest tube drainage. Once period of emergency is over, operative debridement and closure of chest wound is necessary.

reconstruction and closure can be done in the operating room.

Subcutaneous emphysema usually results from injury to the pulmonary ven-

tilatory system (Fig. 12). The possibility of gastrointestinal tract injury or gas-forming bacilli must not be overlooked.

HEMOTHORAX

Blood in the pleural cavity is perhaps the commonest sequela of thoracic trauma, regardless of type. The source of the bleeding is either systemic (high pressure) from the chest wall, or pulmonary (low pressure). Hemorrhage from pulmonary vessels is usually self-limiting unless major tributaries have been transected.

Intrapleural blood eventually clots and becomes organized fibrous tissue (Fig. 13). Prior to this, pulmonary compression and mediastinal displacement, with reduced vital capacity and atrial filling, can occur. With the development of a fibrothorax, the changes in cardiorespiratory dynamics become chronic as the lung becomes incarcerated and the chest wall immobilized. Finally, empyema from secondary contamination is always a threat in the presence of a pleural space filled with blood.

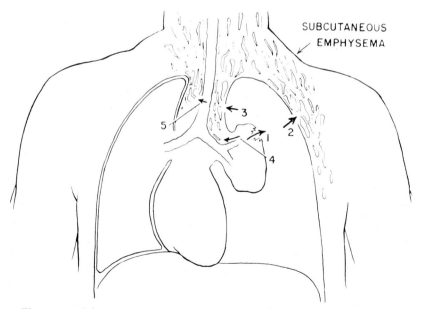

Figure 12. Subcutaneous emphysema resulting from injury to pulmonary system.

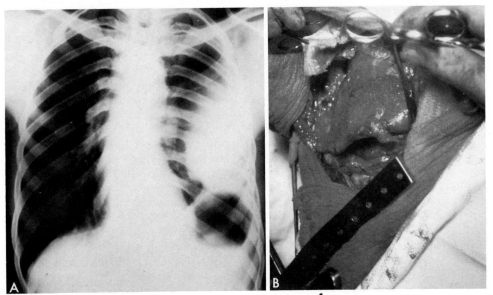

Figure 13. *A,* Clotted hemothorax. *B,* Operative decortication of pleural peel of improperly treated hemothorax.

The acute findings are those of blood loss compounded by respiratory distress and perhaps hemoptysis. The trachea and apical impulse are dislocated, the percussion note is flat, and the breath sounds are indistinct. The actual diagnosis is confirmed by thoracentesis after adequate x-ray studies, if time allows.

It has been established that aspiration of a hemothorax and expansion of the underlying lung do not instigate additional bleeding. Accordingly, the local management of hemothorax is prompt, continuous and total evacuation without air replacement. The dead space is abolished, and without it empyema cannot occur. Such evacuation is best accomplished by chest tube insertion (Fig. 6). Clotting is circumvented, and pulmonary function is restored by pulmonary expansion. Further extensive bleeding must be controlled by operation. Obviously, systemic resuscitation has not been overlooked.

In spite of vigorous initial therapy, clotting, loculation and infection may supervene. A rare patient eventually comes to decortication.

TRACHEOBRONCHIAL TRAUMA

Rupture of the trachea or bronchus in the infant and the child is usually preceded by a severe compression injury of the chest or sharp blow to the anterior part of the neck. This discontinuity of a major airway is characterized by intrathoracic tension phenomena; later, stricture at the site of rupture leading to loss of lung function by sepsis and atelectasis.

Violently progressive interstitial emphysema, pneumomediastinum, tension pneumothorax and hemoptysis are fairly specific. Upper rib fractures usually occur on the involved side, but certainly are not constant in children with partial tracheal or bronchial transection.

Conventional chest roentgenograms and the air tracheobronchogram can suggest the diagnosis in the presence of a compatible clinical picture, but bronchoscopic demonstration of the rupture is usually necessary. The diagnosis may not be suspected during the acute phase of smaller transections of major or minor bronchi, but becomes obvious when late stricture with distal atelectasis and chronic pneumonitis is related retrospectively to a history of fairly severe chest trauma.

The initial management of bronchial rupture is concerned with the maintenance of a patent airway and decompression of the pleura and mediastinum by one or more intercostal tubes connected to closed drainage. Confirmatory endoscopy and elective bronchoplasty within several months are followed by little or no loss of pulmonary function distal to the narrowed segment (Weisel and Jake 1953; Mahaffey and coworkers, 1956). Emergency bronchoscopy and immediate repair of the defect are preferred to a course of delayed recognition and repair, since morbidity can thus be circumvented.

Severe lacerations of the trachea can be immeasurably helped by bypassing the glottis with an artificial airway during the acute phase while preparing the patient for emergency tracheal repair. Smaller tears may heal spontaneously with tracheostomy alone; others will result in stricture and require later tracheorrhaphy.

PULMONARY COMPRESSION INJURY (TRAUMATIC ASPHYXIA)

Explosive blasts compress flexible ribs, the sternum and cartilages against the lungs with sudden, violent increase in intra-alveolar pressure. Alveolar disruption, interstitial emphysema and pneumothorax may follow if the glottis is closed when the compression occurs. Distribution of this force to the great, valveless veins of the mediastinum leads to venous distention, extravasation of blood and purplish edema of the head, neck and upper extremities ("traumatic asphyxia"). The pulmonary contusion is represented patholog-

ically by edema, hemorrhage and atelectasis.

Clinically, there may be dyspnea, cough, chest pain and hemoptysis. The face and the neck can be grotesquely swollen with crepitus and submucous and subconjunctival hemorrhage (Fig. 14). There need not be evidence of external trauma or fractured ribs in a child, and, accordingly, the indication for chest roentgenogram is merely the possible history of a blast, acceleration (fall) or deceleration (automobile) injury. Unilateral or bilateral pulmonary hematoma, hemothorax, pneumothorax and pneumomediastinum can be seen.

With mild injuries, the subcutaneous emphysema and purplish hue gradually and spontaneously disappear over several days. Patients with more serious blast injuries are treated initially for anoxia and hypotension, and attention is then directed toward the wet lung, atelectasis and pleural complications.

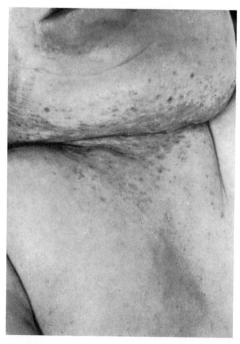

Figure 14. Subcutaneous hemorrhage and emphysema of the face and chest in an infant involved in an automobile accident. There were bilateral pulmonary contusions, but no fractured ribs.

Rapid progression of the mediastinal and subcutaneous emphysema would implicate a serious disruption of the trachea, bronchi or lungs and perhaps require intercostal tube drainage or even thoracotomy.

POST-TRAUMATIC ATELECTASIS (WET LUNG)

With pulmonary contusion from any source, production of tracheobronchial secretions is stimulated, but elimination is impeded by airway obstruction, pain and depression of cough. The addition of hemorrhage to these accumulated secretions produces atelectasis in the damaged lung and inevitable infection — a syndrome aptly called wet lung.

The clinical findings are dyspnea and cyanosis, an incessant, unproductive little cough with wheezing and audible rattling, and gross rhonchi and rales. Chest roentgenograms show varying degrees of unilateral and bilateral atelectasis.

The syndrome demands vigorous treatment to avoid morbidity and mortality. This should be started, in a preventive sense, in all instances of chest trauma, by frequent changes of position, insistence on coughing, small amounts of depressant drugs, oxygen, humidification, antibiotics, and the use of mechanical ventilation, diuretics, intravenous colloid and minimal hydration. If a child with chest trauma will not cough, tracheal catheterization, popularized by Haight (1938), should be instituted prior to the appearance of early signs of the wet lung syndrome. Failure of this step should be followed in quick succession by bronchoscopy and an endotracheal tube or tracheostomy if endoscopic aspiration is required too frequently. Spencer (1964) has emphasized the advantages of endoscopy through the tracheal stoma.

The adult respiratory distress syndrome following critical illness, surgery or trauma with congestion, edema, hemorrhage, pneumonia and pulmonary fibrosis is rarely, if ever, seen in pediatric practice.

CARDIAC TRAUMA

Cardiac wounds should be suspected after penetration of any part of the chest, lower part of the neck or upper part of the abdomen. The possibility of heart injury also exists in the presence of blunt trauma to the anterior or left hemithorax with laceration by fractured sternum or ribs or severe compression between the sternum and the vertebral column. Blood loss with perforation varies between exsanguination internally or externally and minimal bleeding with or without acute cardiac tamponade. Tamponade usually follows trauma to the myocardium with intact pleura bilaterally. The hemopericardium cannot decompress into the pleura or externally, since the pericardial wound is dislocated from the soft tissue wound of entrance by the pericardial blood. This increased intrapericardial pressure constricts the heart and great veins, and the venous return and cardiac output are critically impaired.

The physical findings with acute tamponade are often classic. The veins of the neck and upper extremity may be distended. The heart sounds are distant and perhaps inaudible. The systolic pressure is depressed, the pulse pressure is narrow, and the pulse rate is relatively slow in spite of the lowered blood pressure.

The venous pressure is a valuable laboratory determination and will be elevated. Fluoroscopy demonstrates an inactive cardiac silhouette whose margins may not be widened. Sonography may be helpful.

With this picture, in addition to systemic resuscitation, emergency aspiration of the pericardial sac through a left costoxiphoid approach should be performed while the operating suite is being prepared. Aspiration of small amounts of blood can restore cardiopulmonary dynamics. If bleeding and tamponade recur promptly, thoracotomy is indicated (Fig. 15).

Nonpenetrating trauma can produce varying degrees of myocardial contusions ranging from a small area of edema to a ruptured chamber. The chest pain and tachycardia may be dif-ficult to evaluate without evidence of cardiac failure. Immediate and serial electrocardiograms and enzyme determinations are essential for the emergency and late diagnosis of myocardial damage secondary to trauma (Fig. 16).

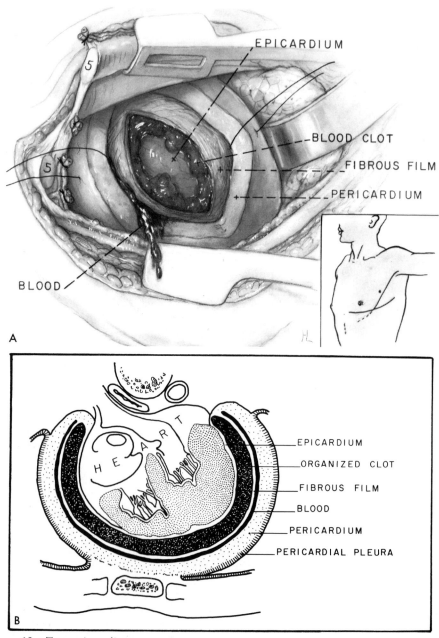

Figure 15. Traumatic cardiac tamponade relieved by open thoracotomy five days following trauma and after two partially relieving pericardiocenteses.

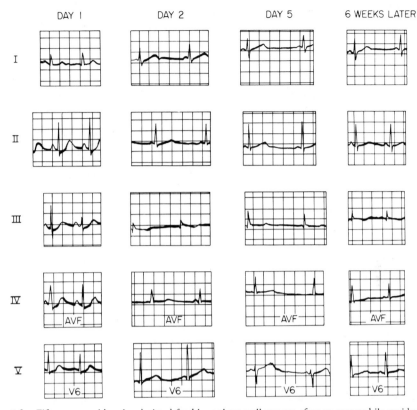

Figure 16.   Fifteen year old male admitted for blunt chest wall trauma after an automobile accident. Note progressive ST and T changes with marked depression immediately after the accident. There was improvement in the ST segment and flattening of the T waves on Day 2 and reversal to normal in later tracings. (Dr. C. McCue.)

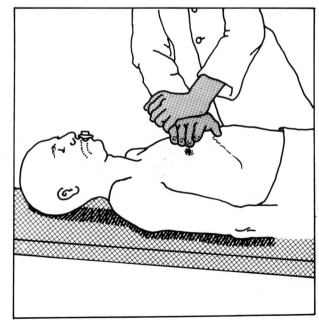

Figure 17.   External cardiac massage.

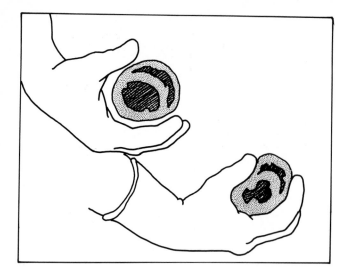

Figure 18. Internal cardiac massage.

Figure 19. Internal cardiac massage.

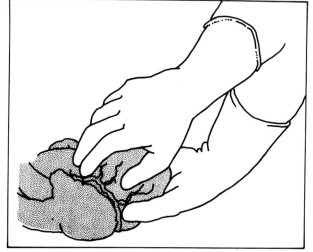

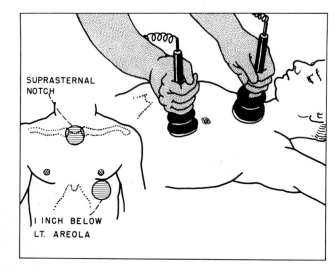

Figure 20. Electrode application for external cardiac defibrillation.

The treatment can follow the standard regimen for coronary occlusion with the exclusion of anticoagulants, and complete rehabilitation can be anticipated. Late complications include chronic constrictive pericarditis, congestive heart failure and ventricular aneurysm.

In this regard, physicians attending the acutely injured in the emergency ward must be prepared to institute prompt external cardiac massage (Fig. 17), internal cardiac massage (Figs. 18 and 19) or cardiac defibrillation (Fig. 20).

INJURIES TO THE ESOPHAGUS

Perforation of the esophagus in the pediatric age group can begin in the delivery room from extreme positive pressure resuscitation or aspiration with a stiff catheter. Later in infancy and childhood, rupture can follow ingestion of lye or a solid foreign body, esophagoscopy, and dilatation, usually without a guiding string. Spontaneous rupture proximal to an esophageal web has been described. Stab and gunshot wounds, as in the adult, can perforate the esophagus.

Clinically, hyperthermia, hypotension and chest and neck pain mirror the mediastinitis. Pneumomediastinum, tension pneumothorax, subcutaneous emphysema and hematemesis may be seen.

Plain chest roentgenograms followed by a contrast esophagogram and thoracentesis may demonstrate the tension sequelae, esophageal defect and perhaps high acid fluid.

The tension pneumothorax must be quickly decompressed and followed promptly by closure of the esophageal defect, mediastinal drainage and massive antibiotics.

THORACOABDOMINAL INJURIES

In the infant and the child, combined injury to the thorax and abdomen, in-

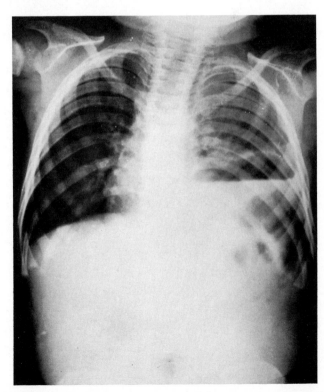

Figure 21. Blunt traumatic rupture of left hemidiaphragm—unrecognized. Death one hour later from acute gastric dilatation of intrathoracic stomach (same physiologic effects as tension pneumothorax).

cluding ruptured diaphragm, is usually preceded by a violent traffic accident or other forms of sudden, jolting impact. Splenic and hepatic lacerations commonly occur with minimal external evidence of injury and need not be associated with fractured ribs or soft tissue mutilation.

Clinically, upper abdominal tenderness, rigidity and rebound tenderness almost uniformly accompany lower chest trauma and are explained by the abdominal distribution of the intercostal nerves. Therefore, peritoneal irritation, of itself, is not conclusive evidence of a combined or abdominal in-

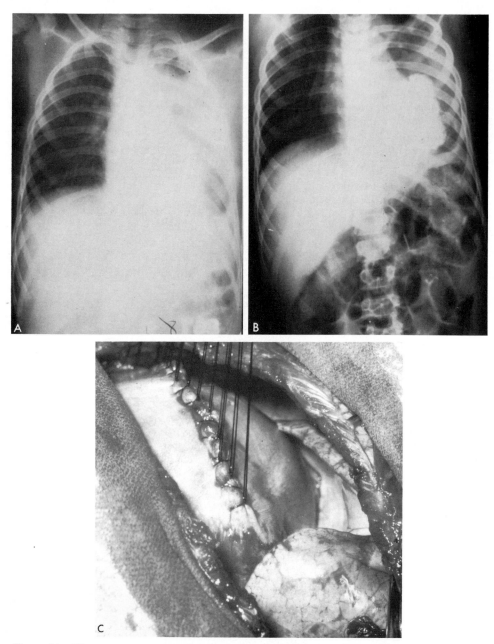

Figure 22. Blunt traumatic rupture of left hemidiaphragm (*A*) with barium swallow confirmation (*B*), and final closure at operation (*C*).

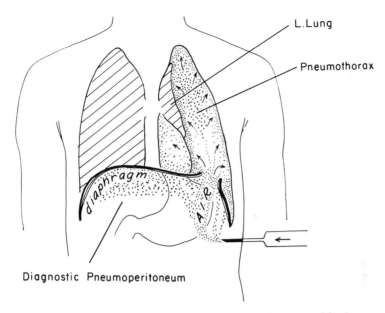

Figure 23. Diagnostic pneumoperitoneum in suspected rupture of diaphragm.

jury. Careful repeated examinations correlated with laboratory data are necessary for the diagnosis of intra-abdominal perforation or hemorrhage in the presence of chest trauma. Aspiration of the peritoneum may have a place and perhaps should be used more often.

A ruptured diaphragm can occur with minimal soft tissue injury, and there may be chest pain, dyspnea and hypotension. On inspection, the involved chest wall lags during inspiration, and percussion can be dull or hyperresonant (Fig. 21). Chest roentgenograms may not show fractured ribs. There is usually mediastinal shift to the right, since in 90 per cent of the cases the posterolateral left leaf of the diaphragm is torn in a radial manner (Fig. 22). At times, a pneumoperitoneum is seen or a diagnostic pneumoperitoneum may disprove a suspected rupture of the diaphragm (Fig. 23).

The preliminary management of combined chest-abdominal injuries must provide an adequate airway and circulation, gastric decompression and evaluation and control of other injuries. Intra-abdominal hemorrhage and perforation with thoracic and abdominal soiling is an obvious indication for immediate exploration. Ideally, a ruptured diaphragm should be repaired as soon as systemic stabilization has occurred.

REFERENCES

Avery, E. E., Morch, E. T., and Benson, D. W.: Critically crushed chests. *J. Thorac. Surg., 32*:291, 1856.

Berry, F. B.: Chest injuries. *Surg. Gynecol. Obstet., 70*:413, 1940.

Betts, R. H.: Thoraco-abdominal injuries: report of twenty-nine operated cases. *Ann. Surg., 122*:793, 1945.

Blades, B., and Salzberg, A. M.: The importance of tracheostomy in acute ventilatory distress. *Milit. Surg., 114*:184, 1954.

Burke, J., and Jacobs, T. T.: Penetrating wounds of the chest. *Ann. Surg., 123*:363, 1946.

Burke, J. F.: Early diagnosis of traumatic rupture of bronchus. *J.A.M.A., 181*:682, 1962.

Carter, B. N., and Guiseffi, J.: Tracheostomy—a useful procedure in thoracic surgery, with particular reference to its employment in crushing injuries of the thorax. *J. Thorac. Surg., 21*:495, 1951.

Carter, R., Wareham, E. E., and Brewer, L. A., III: Rupture of the bronchus following closed chest trauma. *Am. J. Surg., 104*:177, 1962.

Childress, M. E., and Grimes, O. F.: Immediate and remote sequelae in traumatic diaphragmatic hernia. *Surg. Gynecol. Obstet. 113*:573, 1961.

DeBakey, M. E. (Ed.): *The Year Book of General Surgery (1963–1964 Year Book Series).* Chicago, Year Book Medical Publishers, Inc., p. 186.

Edwards, H. C.: *Surgical Emergencies in Children.* Baltimore, William Wood and Company, 1963, p. 213.

Ellerton, D. G., McGough, E. C., Rasmussen, B., Sutton, R. B., and Hughes, R. K.: Pulmonary artery monitoring in critically ill surgical patients. *Am. J. Surg., 128*:791, 1974.

Flavell, G.: *An Introduction to Chest Surgery.* London, Oxford University Press, 1957, pp. 67, 68, 70, 71.

Fraser, J.: *Surgery of Childhood.* Vol. II. New York, William Wood and Company, 1926, p. 675.

Fryfogle, J. D.: Discussion of paper by R. L. Anderson: Rupture of the esophagus. *J. Thorac. Surg., 24*:369, 1952.

Graivier, L., and Freeark, R. J.: Traumatic diaphragmatic hernia. *Arch. Surg., 86*:33, 1963.

Haight, C.: Intratracheal suction in the management of postoperative pulmonary complications. *Ann. Surg., 107*:218, 1938.

Hayes, B. W., Jr.: Dangers of emergency occlusive dressing in sucking wounds of the chest. *J.A.M.A., 150*:1404, 1952.

Howell, J. F., Crawford, E. S., and Jordan, G. L.: Flail chest: analysis of 100 patients. *Am. J. Surg., 106*:628, 1963.

Johnson, J.: Battle wounds of the thoracic cavity. *Ann. Surg., 123*:321, 1946.

Keshishian, J. M., and Cox, P. A.: Diagnosis and management of strangulated diaphragmatic hernias. *Surg. Gynecol. Obstet., 115*:626, 1962.

Lindskog, G. E.: Some historical aspects of thoracic trauma. *J. Thorac. Cardiovasc. Surg., 42*:1, 1961.

Lucido, J. L., and Wall, C. A.: Rupture of diaphragm due to blunt trauma. *Arch. Surg., 86*:989, 1963.

Mahaffey, D. S., and others: Traumatic rupture of the left main bronchus successfully repaired eleven years after injury. *J. Thorac. Surg., 32*:312, 1956.

Maloney, J. V., Jr., and McDonald, L.: Treatment of trauma to thorax. *Am. J. Surg., 105*:484, 1963.

Melzig, E. P., Swank, M., and Salzberg, A. M.: Acute blunt traumatic rupture of the diaphragm in children. *Arch. Surg., 111*:1009, 1976.

Nealon, T. F., and Ching, N. P. H.: Trauma to the chest. In Sabiston, D. C., and Spencer, F. C. (Eds.): *Gibbon's Surgery of the Chest.* Philadelphia, W. B. Saunders Company, 1976, p. 306.

Paulson, D. L.: Traumatic Bronchial rupture with plastic repair. *J. Thorac. Surg., 22*:636, 1951.

Perry, J. F., and Galway, C. F.: Chest injury due to blunt trauma. *J. Thorac. Cardiovasc. Surg., 49*:684, 1965.

Pilcher, R. S.: Trachea, bronchi, lungs and pleura. In Brown, J. J. M. (Ed.): *Surgery of Childhood.* Baltimore, Williams & Wilkins Company, 1963, pp. 659, 660, 661, 664.

Ransdell, H. T., and others: Treatment of flail chest injuries with a piston respirator. *Am. J. Surg., 104*:22, 1962.

Richardson, W. R.: Thoracic emergencies in the newborn infant. *Am. J. Surg., 105*:524, 1963.

Said, S.: Personal communication.

Schwartz, A., and Borman, J. B.: Contusion of the lung in childhood. *Arch. Dis. Child., 36*:557, 1961.

Segal, S.: Endobronchial pressure as an aid to tracheobronchial aspiration. *Pediatrics, 35*:305, 1965.

Shaw, R. R., Paulson, D. L., and Kee, J. L., Jr.: Traumatic tracheal rupture.. *J. Thorac. Cardiovasc. Surg., 42*:281, 1961.

Spencer, F. C.: Treatment of chest injuries. *Curr. Probl. Surg.,* January 1964.

Strug, L. H., and others: Severe crushing injuries of the chest. *J. Thorac. Cardiovasc. Surg., 39*:166, 1960.

Swenson, O.: *Pediatric Surgery.* 2nd Ed. New York, Appleton-Century-Crofts, Inc., 1962, p. 150.

Taylor, S. F.: *Recent Advances in Surgery.* Boston, Little, Brown & Company, 1946, p. 143.

Warden, J. D., and Mucha, S. J.: Esophageal perforation due to trauma in the newborn. *Arch. Surg., 83*:813, 1961.

Webb, W. R.: Chest injuries. *J. La. Med. Soc., 116*:1, 1964.

Weisel, W., and Jake, R. J. L.: Anastomosis of right bronchus to trachea 46 days following complete bronchial rupture from external injury. *Ann. Surg., 137*:220, 1953.

White, M., and Dennison, W. M.: *Surgery in Infancy and Childhood, A Handbook for Medical Students and General Practitioners.* Edinburgh, E. & S. Livingstone, Ltd., 1958, p. 292.

White, P. D., and Glenby, B. S. In Brahdy L., and Kahn, S.: *Trauma and Disease.* Philadelphia, Lea & Febiger, 1937.

Zollinger, R. W., Creedon, P. J., and Sanguily, J.: Trauma in children in a general hospital. *Am. J. Surg., 104*:855, 1962.

INDEX

Note: Page numbers in *italics* indicate illustrations; references to tables include the designation (t).

Abdominal respiration, 94
Abscess
 peritonsillar, adenotonsillectomy for, 351
 pulmonary, 470–474, *471–473*
  aerobic (nonputrid), 472
  anaerobic (putrid), 472
 retropharyngeal, tuberculosis and, 830
Acid-base balance, 40
 carbon dioxide transport and, 37–41
 disturbances of, blood measurements in, 40(t)
 in cerebrospinal fluid and arterial blood, 55(t)
 interpretation of, 109(t)
Acidosis, acute respiratory, blood measurements in, 40, 40(t)
 metabolic, blood measurements in, 40, 40(t)
Actinomyces, 883
 media for isolation of, 882(t)
Actinomycosis, 883–889
 clinical manifestations of, 884, *885*
 epidemiology of, 886
 laboratory diagnosis of, 885, *886*
 pathogenesis of, 887
 pathology of, 887, *888*
 prevention of, 889
 treatment of, 887–889
Adenine arabinoside, in cytomegalic inclusion disease, 940
 in varicella pneumonia, 962
Adenitis, cervical, tonsillectomy for, 351
Adenoiditis, and tonsillitis, 347–352. See also *Tonsillitis, and adenoiditis.*
Adenoma, bronchial, 698, *699*
 parathyroid, 734
Adenotonsillectomy, complications of, 352
 indications for, 350
 results of, 352
Adenoviruses
 clinical aspects of, 417
 general properties of, 416
 in lungs of newborn, 296
 laboratory aspects of, 417
 pertussis syndrome and, 995–997
 pneumonia due to, 428
  pathology and pathogenesis of, 429

Adrenocorticosteroids, in sarcoidosis, 860
 in tuberculosis, 811
 in visceral larva migrans, 1021
Aerosol therapy, 123–127
 equipment for, 123, *124, 125*
 indications for, 126, 126(t)
Age, as factor in respiratory disease, 177–187
Air block, bronchopulmonary dysplasia and, 316
 in newborn, 280–283
Air bronchogram, 150, *151*
Air control systems, contamination of, pulmonary disease related to, 678, 678(t)
Air passages, foreign bodies in, 513–517
 diagnosis of, 513–515, *514, 515*
  results of, 517
  treatment of, 516, *516, 517*
Airway(s)
 conductance in, as function of age, 177–183, *178–182*
  in disease, 183–187, *184, 186*
 patency of, maintenance of, 200–202, 200(t)
  restoration of, 195
 resistance of. See *Resistance, airway.*
 upper, obstruction of, cor pulmonale and, 750
Alae nasi, flaring of, 87
Alkalosis, acute respiratory, blood measurements in, 40, 40(t)
 metabolic, blood measurements in, 40, 40(t)
Alpha₁-antitrypsin
 biology of, 594
 deficiency of, emphysema due to, 593–601. See also *Emphysema, due to alpha₁-antitrypsin deficiency.*
 genetics and incidence of, 594
 vs. asthma, 643
 measurement of, 594
 molecular abnormality of, 595
Altitude, high, pulmonary hypertension and, 753
Alveolar (air space) disease, radiographic appearance of, 155, *155*
Alveolar cell, flat, 62, *63*
 large, 62, *63*
Alveolar gases, 29

Alveolar surfactant, biosynthesis and secretion of surface-active lipoprotein for, 69
Alveolar ventilation, 25–30
Alveolitis
  cryptogenic (idiopathic) fibrosing, 518–522
    clinical manifestations of, 520, *521*
    complications of, 522
    course of, 522
    definition of, 518
    diagnosis of, 521
    etiology of, 520
    pathology, 518, *519*
    treatment of, 522
  extrinsic allergic, 73, 670–684. See also *Hypersensitivity pneumonitis.*
Amantadine, in treatment of influenza, 444
Amikacin, 338
  dosage schedule for, beyond newborn period, 342(t)
    in newborn, 340(t)
  in aerobic gram-negative bacillary pneumonia, 401
Aminoglycosides, 338
  dosage schedule for, beyond newborn period, 342(t)
    in newborn, 340(t)
Aminophylline, in treatment of asthma, 656(t), 658
Ammonium chloride, in treatment of asthma, 656(t)
Amoxicillin, 333
  dosage schedule for, beyond newborn period, 342(t)
Amphotericin B, 925
  dose of, 926
  duration of therapy with, 926
  in aspergillosis, 921
  in candidiasis, 923
  in coccidioidomycosis, 908
  in histoplasmosis, 876
  in North American blastomycosis, 898
  in phycomycosis, 924
  in pulmonary cryptococcosis, 917
  in South American blastomycosis, 902
  side effects of, 927
  toxicity of, 927
Ampicillin, 333, 338(t)
  dosage schedule for, beyond newborn period, 342(t)
    in newborn, 340(t)
  in *Hemophilus influenzae* pneumonia, 400
  in nocardiosis, 893
  in pertussis pneumonia, 991
  in pneumococcal pneumonia, 385
  in salmonella pneumonia, 1001
Amyotonia congenita, as cause of neonatal respiratory distress, 308
Angiography, in pulmonary disease, 136
  in pulmonary tumors, 705
Angioma, of trachea, 700
Antibiotics. See also names of specific drugs.
  direct instillation of, 344
  failure of therapy with, factors in, 344–346, 345(t)
  in bacterial pneumonias, 379

Antibiotics (*Continued*)
  in bacterial pneumonias, dosage schedules for, beyond newborn period, 342(t)–343(t)
    in infants and children, 341, 342(t)–343(t)
    in newborn, 339, 340(t)
  in cystic fibrosis, 779
  in renal insufficiency, dosage schedules for, 341
  oral, absorption of, food interference with, 341, 343(t)
  parenteral, administration of, 341
Antimicrobial therapy. See *Antibiotics,* and names of specific drugs.
Aortic arch, double or right, tracheal obstruction and, 228
Aplitest, for tuberculosis, 796
Apneic spells, 57, 88
APUD cell, *68,* 69
Arterial puncture, 108, *109*
Arteriovenous fistula, pulmonary, 252–254, *253*
Artery(ies)
  bronchial, radiographic appearance of, 153
  carotid, anomalous innominate or left, tracheal obstruction and, 228
  pulmonary, radiographic appearance of, 153
  radial, diagnostic puncture of, 108, *109*
  subclavian, aberrant right, esophageal obstruction and, 228
Arthritis, juvenile rheumatoid, pulmonary involvement in, 1048–1050, *1050*
Artificial respiration, 21–25
  apparatus for, 24
  principles of, 23
Artificial ventilation, 196
Aspergilloma, intracavitary, 919
Aspergillosis, 918–921, *920*
  allergic bronchopulmonary. See *Bronchopulmonary disease, allergic.*
  clinical picture of, 919
  laboratory diagnosis of, 920
  treatment of, 921
Aspergillus, media for isolation of, 882(t)
Asphyxia, in newborn, 276–278
  traumatic, 1086–1087, *1086*
Aspiration, transtracheal, in diagnosis of bronchiectasis, 455
  percutaneous, in diagnosis of bacterial pneumonia, 379
Aspiration syndrome, massive, 278–280, *279*
Asthma, 620–669
  allergic (atopic), 620, 633
  allergic rhinitis and, 635
  aspirin-induced, 637, 692
  blood values in, 638
  bronchial, 72
  bronchiectasis and, 455
  bronchiolitis and, 374
  clinical course of, 644
  clinical features of, 631–633, *632*
  clinical types of, 633–638, 633(t)
  complications of, 644, 645, *646, 647*
  continuous, 620
  differential diagnosis of, 642–644, 642(t)
  exercise-induced, 636
  extrinsic, 620
  gastric secretion in, 639

Asthma (*Continued*)
  incidence of, 620–622, 621(t), *621, 622*
  infectious, 635
  intractable, 620
  intrinsic, 620
  laboratory findings in, 638
  lung-damage type, 635
  meat-wrapper's, 689(t), 690
  morbidity of, 622, *622*, 623(t)
  mortality of, 623, 623(t)
  nasal secretion in, 638
  nonallergic (nonatopic), 620, 635
  pathogenesis of, 624–626
  pathology of, 626–629, *626–628*
  pathophysiology of, 629–631
  physical signs of, 632, *632*
  prognosis of, 648–650, 649(t)
  pulmonary edema in, 586
  respiratory dynamics in, 639–642, 640(t),
      641(t)
  spasmodic, 620
  sputum in, 638
  sweat levels in, 639
  symptoms of, 631
  treatment of, 650–664
    acute, 655–661
    long-range, 650–655
  with pulmonary eosinophilia, 1023
Atelectasis, 553–572
  as complication, of asthma, 646, *646*
    of measles pneumonia, 976
    of pneumococcal pneumonia, 385
  causes of, 553
  complications of, 564
  diagnosis of, 561–563
  due to bronchial obstruction, 556–560,
      556–559, 561
    signs and symptoms of, 560
  in tuberculosis, 819, *820, 821*
  incidence of, 555
  massive, 566–569
  nonobstructive, 565–566
  pathophysiology of, 553–555
  post-traumatic, 1087
  prognosis of, 564
  radiographic appearance of, *156*, 160, *162*
  total, *703, 704, 707*
  treatment of, 563
  vs. dysgenesis of lung, 161
Atresia, choanal, 303–304
  esophageal, 232–237, *233, 235, 237*, 301–303
Atropine, by aerosol, in reduction of exercise-
      induced bronchospasm, 637
Auscultation, segmental, 99–101
    differential, 102, 103(t)
Azathioprine, in treatment of isolated primary
      pulmonary hemosiderosis, 545
Azygos fissure, radiologic appearance of, 144, *144*

Bacillus(i)
  aerobic gram-negative, pneumonia due to,
      400–402
  gram-negative, drugs effective against, 331,
      338–339, 338(t)

Bacillus(i) (*Continued*)
  tubercle, 788, *788*
    recovery of, 805
Bacterial pneumonia
  antibiotic dosage schedule for, beyond new-
      born period, 342(t)–343(t)
    in infants and children, 341, 342(t)–343(t)
    in newborn infants, 339, 340(t)
  differential diagnosis of, 1015(t)
  gram-negative, 398–402
    aerobic bacillary, 400–402
    due to *Hemophilus influenzae*, 398–400, *399*
  gram-positive, 378–397
    diagnostic procedures for, 378
    meningococcal, 386
    metabolic disturbances and, 379
    pathogenesis of, role of viruses in, 378
    pneumococcal, 380–386. See also
        Pneumococcal pneumonia.
    staphylococcal, 388–396. See also
        Staphylococcal pneumonia.
    streptococcal, 386–388, *387*
    therapy of, 379
  in newborn, 292, *293, 294*
Bagassosis, 682
BCG vaccination, in prevention of tuberculosis,
      838, *839, 840*
  of infants of tuberculous mothers, 823, 823(t)
Beclomethasone, in treatment of asthma, 658(t),
      659, 660(t)
Beta adrenergic receptors, in asthma, 630
Biopsy
  lung, 107
    thoracotomy and, *709*, 710
  lymph node, 706, *708*
    peripheral, in sarcoidosis, 860
  of pleura and lymph nodes, in tuberculosis,
      805
  pleural, in empyema, 482
Biot's breathing, 88
Blastomyces, media for isolation of, 882(t)
Blastomyces brasiliensis, 899
Blastomyces dermatitidis, 893, *894, 896*
Blastomycosis
  North American, 893–898
    clinical disease in, 894, *895*
    epidemiology of, 897
    laboratory diagnosis of, 896, *896*
    pathogenesis of, 897
    pathology of, 897
    treatment of, 898
  South American, 899–902
    clinical disease in, 900, *900*
    epidemiology of, 901
    laboratory diagnosis of, 901
    pathogenesis of, 901
    pathology of, 901
    treatment of, 902
Blood, arterial, acid-base relationships in, 55(t)
Blood flow, pulmonary. See *Pulmonary
      circulation.*
Blood tests, in pulmonary tumors, 705
Blood transfusions, pulmonary hypersensitivity
      reactions to, 692
Bochdalek hernia, 219–222, *221, 222*
Bohr integration procedure, 31

Bone(s)
  eosinophilic granuloma of, 1027
  involvement of, in sarcoidosis, 858
  tuberculosis of, 836
    treatment of, 836(t)
Bone marrow, examination of, in pulmonary
  tumors, 705
Boyle's law, 4
Bradypnea, 83
Breath sounds, 101
Breathing
  Biot's, 88
  Cheyne-Stokes, 88
  labored, 80
  noisy, 80
  periodic, 56, 88
Breathing exercises, 119–121
  in cystic fibrosis, 781
Bronchial asthma, 72
Bronchial breath sounds, 101
Bronchial (postural) drainage, 109–119
  in cystic fibrosis, 781
  physical therapy and, 112–119
  positions for, 115–121
  table for, 122
Bronchial lavage, 127
Bronchial obstruction, atelectasis due to,
    556–560, 556–559, 561
  signs and symptoms of, 560
  relief of, in cystic fibrosis, 780
Bronchiectasis, 446–469, 704
  acquired, 447
  age distribution of, 185, 186
  as complication of pertussis pneumonia, 991
  asthma and, 455
  clinical features of, 451
  complications of, 458
  congenital, 446
  development of, factors associated with,
    446–449
  diagnosis of, 453
  diseases associated with, 455
  incidence of, 446
  irreversible, 448
  pathogenesis of, 449
  pathology of, 450
  prevention of, 459
  prognosis of, 458
  radiographic appearance of, 151, 151
  reversible, 448
  site of, 451
  treatment of, medical, 456
    surgical, 457
Bronchiolitis, 367–377
  age distribution of, 185, 186
  airway resistance in, 184, 185
  asthma and, 374
  clinical presentation of, 367, 368
  complications of, 373
  course of, 373
  diagnosis of, 371
  etiology of, 367
  pathology of, 369, 370
  pathophysiology of, 370
  pulmonary edema in, 587
  sequelae of, long-term, 375
  treatment of, 372

Bronchiolitis obliterans, 375–376, 528–529
Bronchitis, 361–366
  age distribution of, 185, 186
  allergic factors in, 364
  chemical factors in, 363
  infection as cause of, 362
    bacterial, 363
    fungal, 363
    viral, 362
  tuberculous, 818–823
    treatment of, 821–823
Bronchodilators, in treatment of asthma, 655,
  656(t), 657
Bronchofiberscope, 105
Bronchogenic carcinoma, 701
Bronchogenic cyst, 237–240, 238–240, 713–716,
  713–717
  congenital, 707
Bronchogram, air, 150, 151
  of pulmonary tumors, 706, 707
Bronchography, in diagnosis of bronchiectasis,
  454
  in pulmonary disease, 135
Bronchopleural fistula, radiologic assessment of,
  480, 481
Bronchopulmonary disease, allergic, 684–688
  clinical features of, 684
  diagnosis of, 688
  histologic studies of, 687, 688
  immunologic studies of, 685
  inhalation challenge studies of, 687
  laboratory features of, 685
  pulmonary function studies of, 685
  radiographic features of, 685, 686
  therapy of, 688
  vs. hypersensitivity pneumonitis, 684(t)
Bronchopulmonary dysplasia, 314–323
  mechanical ventilation and, 314–317
  patient management in, 321–323
  stages of, 314
    clinical-radiographic-histologic correlation
    in, 317–323, 317–320
Bronchoscopy, 105–107
  fiberoptic, in bronchiectasis, 454, 456
  in pulmonary abscess, 474
  in tuberculosis, 805
  of pulmonary tumors, 706
Bronchospasm, exercise-induced, 636
Bronchotomy, 129
Bronchovesicular breath sounds, 101
Bronchus(i)
  congenital stenosis of, 237
  diagnostic radiology of, 150–152, 151
  fibrosarcoma of, 701
  foreign body in, atelectasis and, 560, 561
    radiographic appearance of, 162
  lobar and segmental, distribution of, 110–114
  obstructive lesions of, in tuberculosis, 818–
    823, 819–822
    treatment of, 821–823
  papilloma of, 699
  rupture of, 1085

Candida, media for isolation of, 882(t)
Candidiasis, 921–923, 922
Capreomycin, in tuberculosis, 811

Carbenicillin, 334, 338(t)
  dosage schedule for, beyond newborn period,
    342(t)
  in newborn, 340(t)
  in aerobic gram-negative bacillary pneumonia,
    401
Carbon dioxide
  buffering and transport of, 37
  dissociation curve of, 38
    in vitro vs. in vivo, 41
  partial pressure of, in airway and blood, 26
    measurement of, clinical application of, 60
  transport of, acid-base balance and, 37–41
Carbon monoxide, in testing diffusing capacity,
    31
  poisoning with, as complication of smoke
    inhalation, 494
Carcinoma, bronchogenic, 701
Cardiac defibrillation, electrode application for,
    1090
Cardiac disease, congenital, 305–309
Cardiac failure, in newborn, 305
Cardiac massage, external, 194, 1089
  internal, 1090
Cardiac trauma, 1087–1091
Cardiac tumors, primary, 734
Carotid artery(ies), anomalous innominate or
    left, tracheal obstruction and, 228
Catheterization, transtracheal, 128
Cedar worker's disease, 689(t), 690
Ceelen-Gellerstedt's disease, 538
Cell(s)
  giant, in giant cell pneumonia, 984
    in measles pneumonia, 966, 967, 968
  pulmonary, 62–69
    alveolar macrophage, 62, 64
    APUD, 68, 69
    ciliated epithelial, 67, 67
    contractile interstitial, 64
    endothelial, 64, 65
    flat alveolar, 62, 63
    Kulchitsky, 67
    large alveolar, 62, 63
    mast, 64, 66
    mucus-secreting, 64
    neuroendocrine, 67
    smooth muscle, 64
  Warthin-Finkeldey, in measles pneumonia, 966
Central nervous system, hemorrhage into, as
    cause of respiratory symptoms in newborn,
    304–305
Cephalexin, 335, 335(t)
  dosage schedule for, beyond newborn period,
    342(t)
Cephaloglycine, 335(t)
Cephaloridine, 335, 335(t)
Cephalosporin(s), 335, 335(t)
  dosage schedule for, beyond newborn period,
    342(t)
  in cystic fibrosis, 779
Cephalothin, 335, 335(t), 338(t)
  dosage schedule for, beyond newborn period,
    342(t)
  in aerobic gram-negative bacillary pneumonia,
    401
Cephapirin, 335, 335(t)

Cephazolin, 335, 335(t)
  dosage schedule for, beyond newborn period,
    342(t)
Cephradine, 335, 335(t)
Cerebrospinal fluid, acid-base relationships in,
    55(t)
Charles's law, 4
Cheese worker's lung, 682
Chemodectoma, mediastinal, 731
Chemoreceptors, central, 54
  peripheral, 55
Chest
  configuration of, 92–94, 93, 94(t), 95(t), 96
  deformities of, cor pulmonale and, 751–753
  flail, due to fractured ribs, 1078, 1079, 1080
    stabilization of, 1081
  funnel, 214–217, 215, 216
  pain in, evaluation of, 81
  tumors of, 697–743
    cardiac, primary, 734
    diaphragmatic, 734
    mediastinal, 710–734, 711. See also
      Tumor(s), mediastinal.
    pericardial, 734
    pulmonary, 697–710. See also Tumor(s),
      pulmonary.
Chest tube, trocar technique of insertion, 1080
Chest wall, diagnostic radiology of, 142, 142
  tumors of, primary, 734–736, 735, 736
Cheyne-Stokes breathing, 88
Chloral hydrate, in treatment of asthma, 656(t)
Chlorambucil, in Wegener's granulomatosis, 1053
Chloramphenicol, 338(t), 339
  dosage schedule for, beyond newborn period,
    343(t)
    in newborn, 340(t)
  in actinomycosis, 888
  in aerobic gram-negative bacillary pneumonia,
    401
  in cystic fibrosis, 780
  in Hemophilus influenzae pneumonia, 400
  in Q fever, 949
  in salmonella pneumonia, 1001
  in tularemia, 954
Chlortetracycline, in cystic fibrosis, 779
Choanal atresia, 303–304
Chondroma, of chest wall, 735
Chondrosarcoma, of chest wall, 735
Chorioepithelioma, of lung, 702
Chyle, physical and chemical characteristics of,
    606(t)
Chylothorax, 225–226, 606
  management of, 609
Cleft(s), sternal, 213–214
Clindamycin, 336
  dosage schedule for, beyond newborn period,
    342(t)
  in treatment of staphylococcal pneumonia,
    394
Closing capacity, of lung, 20
Closing volume, of lung, 20
Clotrimazole, 929
  in aspergillosis, 921
  in candidiasis, 923
  in coccidioidomycosis, 909
  in phycomycosis, 924

Cloxacillin, 332, 333(t)
  dosage schedule for, beyond newborn period,
    342(t)
Clubbing, in respiratory disease, 82, 90, *90, 91*
  diseases associated with, 91(t)
Coccidioides, media for isolation of, 882(t)
Coccidioides immitis, 902, *903*
Coccidioidin skin test, in sarcoidosis, 860
Coccidioidomycosis, 902–910
  clinical disease in, 904, *905*
  epidemiology of, 907
  laboratory diagnosis of, 905
  pathogenesis of, 907
  pathology of, 907
  prevention of, 909
  treatment of, 908
Coffee worker's disease, 689(t), 690
Colistin, 339
  aerosol, in cystic fibrosis, 780
  dosage schedule for, beyond newborn period,
    343(t)
Collagen-vascular disease, pulmonary
    hemosiderosis as manifestation of, 549–550
Compliance, lung, 15, 16(t)
  airway resistance and, 20
Connective tissue, 67
Connective tissue disease, mixed, pulmonary
    involvement in, 1050–1052
Cor pulmonale, 747–759
  classification of, 747(t)
  hypoventilation in, extrinsic factors resulting
    in, 750–751
  parenchymal lung disease and, 747–750
  pulmonary vascular disease and, 753–756
Coronaviruses, clinical aspects of, 420
  laboratory diagnosis of, 421
Corticosteroids, in asthma, 659, 660(t)
  in salmonella pneumonia, 1002
Corticotropin, in sarcoidosis, 860
Cortisone, in asthma, 660(t), 661
Costal angle, lower, 95
Cough, evaluation of, 80
Countercurrent immunoelectrophoresis, in
    diagnosis of bacterial pneumonias, 379
  in diagnosis of *Hemophilus influenzae* pneu-
    monia, 400
  in examination of pleural liquid, 481
Cow milk, sensitivity to, with primary pulmonary
    hemosiderosis, 547–549
Crackles, classification of, 102(t)
Cromolyn, in reduction of exercise-induced
    bronchospasm, 637
  in treatment of asthma, 654, 658(t)
  pulmonary hypersensitivity reactions to, 692
Croup, 353–360
  clinical manifestations of, 357
  diagnosis of, 358
  etiology of, 353, 353(t), 354(t)
  incidence of, 353
  pathogenesis of, 355, *356*
  predisposition to, 355
  prognosis of, 358
  radiology of neck in, 140, *141*
  treatment of, 359
Cryptococcosis, pulmonary, 910–917
  clinical disease in, 911–913, *911, 912*
  epidemiology of, 915

Cryptococcosis (*Continued*)
  pulmonary, laboratory diagnosis of, 913, *914*
    pathogenesis of, 915
    pathology of, 915, *916*
    prevention of, 917
    treatment of, 917
Cryptococcus, media for isolation of, 882(t)
Cryptococcus neoformans, 910, *914*
Cyanosis, 35, 81
Cyclophosphamide, in Wegener's granuloma-
    tosis, 1053
Cycloserine, in tuberculosis, 811
Cyst(s)
  bronchogenic, 237–240, *238–240*, 713–716,
    713–717
    congenital, *707*
  congenital pulmonary, 242–244, *243, 244*
  esophageal, 716, *718, 719*
  gastroenteric, 717
  lung, in newborn, 299
  mediastinal, primary, 713–722
  pericardial celomic, 720, *721*
  thymic, *725, 726*
Cystic fibrosis, 74, 760–786
  bronchiectasis and, 448, 452, 456
  clinical evaluation of, 772, 774(t)
  complications of, 783, 784(t)
  diagnosis of, 767–771
    differential, 769(t)
    tests for, 772, *775–777*, 775(t)
    in adults, 778
  etiology of, 761
  genetics of, 762, *762, 763*
  incidence of, 760
  intestinal involvement in, 764, 765(t)
  liver in, 765
  pancreatic function in, testing of, 777
  pathogenesis of, 761
  pathology of, 763–767, *764, 766, 767*
  prognosis of, 783
  pulmonary function studies in, 773(t)
  pulmonary manifestations of, 770, *771*, 772(t)
  pulmonary resection in, results of, 782(t)
  respiratory tract in, 766, *766, 767*
  treatment of, 779–783
    with digestive system involvement, 782
    with pulmonary system involvement, 779
Cytomegalic inclusion disease, 936–941
  clinical manifestations of, 938
  diagnosis of, 939
  etiology of, 936
  incidence of, 936
  pathogenesis of, 937, *938*
  prognosis of, 939
  treatment of, 940
Cytosine arabinoside, in cytomegalic inclusion
    disease, 940

Dalton's law, 4
Dead space, alveolar, 25
  anatomic, 25
    measurement of, 28
  physiologic, 25
Deferoxamine, in treatment of isolated primary
    pulmonary hemosiderosis, 545

Defibrillation, cardiac, electrode application for, *1090*

Dermal-respiratory syndrome, 633

Dermatomyositis, pulmonary involvement in, 1046–1048, *1048*

Desquamative interstitial pneumonia, 523–527. See also *Pneumonia, desquamative interstitial.*

Diaphragm
  congenital eventration of, 222–224, *223*
  diagnostic radiology of, 143, *143*
  in respiration, 8–9
  paralysis of, cor pulmonale and, 752
  rupture of, diagnostic pneumoperitoneum for, *1093*
  tumors of, 734

Dicloxacillin, 332, 333(t)
  dosage schedule for, beyond newborn period, 342(t)

Diffusion, of gases, 30–32
  Fick's law of, 31
  measurement of, 31
  principles of, 30

Diphtheria, laryngeal, 358

Disodium cromoglycate, in treatment of asthma, 654

Doxycycline, in nocardiosis, 893

Drainage
  bronchial (postural), 109–119
    physical therapy and, 112–119
    positions for, 115–121
    table for, *122*
  intracavitary (Monaldi), 128
  of pleural space, 128
    closed, set-up for, *1081*
  of secretions, to maintain airway patency, 200

Drowning, 51, 498–510. See also *Near-drowning.*

Ductus arteriosus, patent, 75
  bronchopulmonary dysplasia and, 316

Dysautonomia, 57
  familial, 1061–1066. See also *Familial dysautonomia.*

Dysplasia, bronchopulmonary, 314–323. See also *Bronchopulmonary dysplasia.*

Dyspnea, 86

Eczema-prurigo-asthma syndrome, 633

Edema, pulmonary, 573–592. See also *Pulmonary edema.*

Emphysema, 74
  age distribution of, 185, *186*
  compensatory, radiographic appearance of, 163
  congenital lobar, 297–299, *298*
    radiographic appearance of, 162, *163*
  due to alpha₁-antitrypsin deficiency, 593–601
    clinical course of, 595–598, 596(t)
    diagnosis of, 598, *598, 599*
      differential, 599
    pathogenesis of, 595
    prognosis of, 600
    treatment of, 600
  in newborn, 280–283
    congenital lobar, 297–299, *298*
  lobar, 245–247, *246*

Emphysema (*Continued*)
  obstructive, *702, 703*
    in tuberculosis, 821, *822*
  pulmonary interstitial, 611, *611*
    management of, 617
  subcutaneous, *613*, 1084, *1084*

Empyema, 475–487
  as complication, of measles pneumonia, 976
    of pneumococcal pneumonia, 385
  chest roentgenogram in, 479, *479–481*
  diagnosis of, 478–483
  etiology of, 475–478, 476(t)
  examination of pleural liquid in, 480
  functional pathology of, 478
  management of, 483–486
    antimicrobial, 484(t), 485
    surgical, 485, 485(t)
  nontuberculous, bacteriology of, 477, 477(t)
  pathogenesis of, 475–478
  physical and chemical characteristics of, 481, 482(t)
  pleural biopsy in, 482
  prognosis of, 486

Endocrine glands, sarcoidosis and, 859

Endothelial cell, 64, *65*

Endotoxin (septic) shock, 74

Endotracheal intubation, bronchopulmonary dysplasia and, 316
  oral, tracheostomy over, technique of, *1081*

Enteroviruses, clinical aspects of, 414
  laboratory diagnosis of, 415

Enzyme worker's lung, 682

Eosinophilia, in sarcoidosis, 859
  pulmonary, prolonged, 1023
    with asthma, 1023
  tropical, 1023

Ephedrine, in treatment of asthma, 655, 656(t), 657(t)

Epiglottitis, acute, 357
  radiology of neck in, 141, *141*

Epinephrine, in treatment of asthma, 655, 656(t), 657(t)
  by aerosol, 652

Epithelium, ciliated, 67, *67*

Erythromycin, 336
  dosage schedule for, beyond newborn period, 342(t)
  in actinomycosis, 888
  in cystic fibrosis, 779
  in *Mycoplasma pneumoniae* infection, 437
  in pertussis pneumonia, 991
  in pneumococcal pneumonia, 385
  in staphylococcal pneumonia, 394

Esophagram, in pulmonary disease, 135

Esophagus, atresia of, 232–237, *233, 235, 237*, 301–303
  cysts of, 716, *718, 719*
  injuries to, 1091

Ethambutol, in atypical mycobacterial infection, 849
  in tuberculosis, 810

Ethionamide, in atypical mycobacterial infection, 849
  in tuberculosis, 810

Eupnea, 86

Ewing's tumor, 736

Expectorants, in treatment of asthma, 656(t)
Expiratory volume, measurement of, 12
Eye(s), lesions of, in sarcoidosis, 856

Failure to thrive, respiratory disease and, 82
Familial dysautonomia, 1061–1066
  clinical manifestations of, 1061
  diagnosis of, 1061
  genetics of, 1061
  pathology of, 1061
  prognosis of, 1064
  respiratory problems in, 1062, *1063–1065*
  treatment of, 1064
Farmer's lung, 682
Fibrocystic disease, age distribution of, 185, *186*
  airway resistance in, 185, *186*
Fibroma, of trachea, 700
Fibrosarcoma, of bronchus, 701
Fick's law, of gas diffusion, 31
Fissura sterni congenita, 213–214
Fistula
  bronchopleural, radiologic assessment of, 480,
    481
  pulmonary arteriovenous, 252–254, *253*
  tracheoesophageal, 301–303, *302, 303*
    as complication of tuberculosis, 830, *831,
      832*
    without esophageal atresia, 231–232, *232*
Flail chest, due to fractured ribs, 1078, *1079,
  1080*
  stabilization of, *1081*
Floxuridine, in cytomegalic inclusion disease,
  940
Flucytosine, 929
  in aspergillosis, 921
  in candidiasis, 923
  in pulmonary cryptococcosis, 917
  in pulmonary disease, 134
Foreign body(ies)
  bronchial, atelectasis and, 560, *561*
    radiographic appearance of, 162
  in air passages, 513–517
    diagnosis of, 513–515, *514, 515*
    results of, 517
    treatment of, 516, *516, 517*
Functional residual capacity, interpretation of,
  13, 13(t)
  measurement of, 12
Fungus(i), microbiologic diagnosis of, 880–883,
  882(t)
  opportunistic infections with, 917–925
Funnel chest, 214–217, *215, 216*

Ganglioneuroblastoma, mediastinal, 729
Ganglioneuroma, mediastinal, 729, *730*
Gantrisin, in cystic fibrosis, 780
Gas(es)
  alveolar, 29
  blood, interpretation of, 109(t)
  diffusion of, 30–32
    Fick's law of, 31
    measurement of, 31
    principles of, 30

Gas(es) (*Continued*)
  inefficient transfer of, 191(t)
    causes of, 193(t)
  properties of, 4–5
  variable values for, 3–4
Gentamicin, 338, 338(t)
  dosage schedule for, beyond newborn
    period, 342(t)
  in newborn, 340(t)
  in aerobic gram-negative bacillary pneumonia,
    401
Geotrichosis, 925
Ghon complex, 814, *815*
Giant cells, in giant cell pneumonia, *984*
  in measles pneumonia, 966, *967, 968*
Giant cell pneumonia, 528, 983–985, *984*
Glomerulonephritis, with primary pulmonary
  hemosiderosis, 546–547
Gomori methenamine–silver nitrate, for diagnosis of fungi, 881
Goodpasture's syndrome, 73, 546–547
Graham's law, 5
Gram's stain, for diagnosis of fungi, 881
Granuloma, eosinophilic, of bone, 1027
  swimming pool, 847
Granulomatosis, Wegener's, pulmonary involve-
  ment in, 1052–1055, *1054*
Granulomatous disease, chronic, of childhood,
  1067–1076
  clinical features of, 1067–1070, 1068(t),
    1069, 1070
  diagnosis of, 1073
  inheritance of, 1072
  laboratory findings in, 1070–1072, 1071(t)
  treatment of, 1073
Grunting, 81
  in respiratory disease, 88
Guaiphenesin, in treatment of asthma, 656(t)

Hamartoma, of lung, 697, *697*
Hamman-Rich syndrome, respiratory rate in, *85*
Hand-Schüller-Christian syndrome, 1027
Head-bobbing, in respiratory disease, 88
Head's paradoxical reflex, 54
Heaf test, for tuberculosis, 794, *796*
  apparatus for, *797*
Heart
  congenital disease of, 305–309
  defibrillation of, electrode application for,
    1090
  failure of, in newborn, 305
  massage of, external, 194, *1089*
    internal, *1090*
  sarcoid lesions of, 858
  trauma to, 1087–1091
  tumors of, primary, 734
Hecht's pneumonia, 983
Hemangioma, cavernous, of chest wall, 735
  of pericardium, 734
Hemoglobin dissociation curve, fetal, 34
Hemolytic disease, of newborn, pulmonary
  symptoms associated with, 307
Hemophilus influenzae, pneumonia due to, 398–
  400, *399*

Hemosiderosis, pulmonary, 538–552. See also
  Pulmonary hemosiderosis.
Hemothorax, 606, 1084–1085, *1085*
  management of, 609
Henderson-Hasselbalch equation, 38
Henry's law of diffusion, 5
Hering-Breuer reflex, 53
Hernia, congenital diaphragmatic, 300–301, *301*
    anterior (Morgagni), 218–219, *218*
    hiatal, 224–225, *225*
    of Bochdalek, 219–222, *221, 222*
    pulmonary, 242
Heroin addiction, bronchiectasis and, 456
  nonobstructive atelectasis in, 566
Hiatal hernia, congenital diaphragmatic, 224–
  225, *225*
Hila, pulmonary, assessment of size of, 152, *152*
Histamine test, for familial dysautonomia, 1062
Histiocytosis, idiopathic, 1027–1030, *1028, 1029*
Histoplasma, media for isolation of, 882(t)
Histoplasma capsulatum, 865, *866*
Histoplasmin, sensitivity to, 877, *878*
Histoplasmin skin test, in sarcoidosis, 860
Histoplasmosis, 865–878
  clinical manifestations of, 871–874, 871(t),
    872–875
  differential diagnosis of, 874
  geographic distribution of, 867, *867*
  history of, 865
  miliary, *868*
  pathology of, 867–871, *869–871*
  prognosis of, 875
  sensitivity to histoplasmin in, 877, *878*
  serologic tests for, 878
  treatment of, 876
History, medical, 77–83
    general aims of, 77–80
    of present and past illnesses, 80–82
    patient's environment and, 82
Hyaline membrane disease, 72, 283–290, *284,
  285, 289*
  atelectasis in, 161, *162*
  lung rupture in, 612
Hydrocarbon aspiration, lung injury from, 491–
  493
  clinical findings in, 492
  management of, 493
  pathology of, 491
  pathophysiology of, 491
Hydrocortisone, in asthma, 660(t), 661
Hydroxystilbamidine, in North American blastomycosis, 898
Hygroma, cystic, of mediastinum, 732, *732*
Hypercalcemia, in sarcoidosis, 859
Hypercapnia, infant response to, 56
  signs of, 89, 89(t)
Hyperglobulinemia, in sarcoidosis, 859
Hyperpnea, 85
Hypersensitivity, cell-mediated, diseases related
  to, 73
  pulmonary, due to chemical agents and drugs,
    688–693
    clinical features of, 689, 689(t)
    laboratory features of, 690
Hypersensitivity pneumonitis, 670–684
  acute form, 671
  classification of, 671(t)

Hypersensitivity pneumonitis (*Continued*)
  clinical features of, 671, *672*, 672(t)
  diagnosis of, 677
  dietary, 671(t), 677
  due to hobbies, 671(t), 679
  environmental, 671(t), 678
  experimental studies of, 676
  histologic studies of, 676, *676*
  immunologic responses to, 674, *674*
  inhalation challenge studies of, 675
  insidious form, 672
  laboratory features of, 672, 672(t)
  occupational, 671(t), 682
  pulmonary function tests in, 673
  radiographic studies of, 673, *673*
  related to medication, 671(t), 683
  therapy of, 677
  vs. allergic bronchopulmonary disease, 684(t)
Hypertension, pulmonary, high altitude and,
  753
    primary, cor pulmonale and, 753
Hypervolemia, in newborn, pulmonary symptoms associated with, 307
Hypokalemia, as complication of amphotericin B
  therapy, 927
Hypopnea, 85
Hypostatic pneumonia, 511–512
Hypoventilation, causes of, 30(t)
  extrinsic factors resulting in, 750–751
  primary alveolar, 57
    cor pulmonale and, 752
Hypovolemia, in newborn, pulmonary symptoms associated with, 307
Hypoxia, causes of, 35(t)
  infant response to, 56
  signs of, 89, 89(t)

Idoxuridine, in cytomegalic inclusion disease,
  940
Ileus, meconium, cystic fibrosis and, 764, 765(t),
  769
Immune serum globulin, in prevention of varicella pneumonia, 963
Indomethacin, for closure of patent ductus arteriosus, 75
Infant(s)
  antibiotic administration in, dosage schedules
    for, 341, 342(t)–343(t)
  bronchial drainage positions for, *120, 121*
  newborn. See *Newborn.*
  premature, chronic respiratory distress in,
    324–327
      clinical manifestations of, 324
      pathologic findings in, 326
      radiologic findings in, 325, *325, 326*
  tracheal palpation in, 91, *92*
Influenza, 442–445
  clinical features of, 444
  epidemiology of, 442
  immunity to, 442
  laboratory diagnosis of, 443
  pathogenesis of, 443
  treatment of, 444
Inhalation therapy, 122–127
Inspiratory volume, measurement of, 12

Intensive care, of respiratory disorders, 191–210. See also *Respiratory disorders, intensive care of.*
Intercostal spaces, retraction and bulging of, 86, *87*
Interstitial disease, diagnostic radiology of, 157, *159, 160*
Intestine, in cystic fibrosis, 764, 765(t)
Intracavitary (Monaldi) drainage, 128
Intubation, endotracheal, bronchopulmonary dysplasia and, 316
  nasotracheal, 203
Iodides, in aspergillosis, 921
  in asthma, 656(t)
Ipecac syrup, in asthma, 656(t)
Isoetharine, in asthma, 655, 658(t)
  by aerosol, 652
Isoniazid, in atypical mycobacterial infection, 849
  in tuberculosis, 808
Isoproterenol, in asthma, 655, 656(t), 657(t)
  by aerosol, 652
  toxic effect of, 624
  in cystic fibrosis, 780
  in status asthmaticus, 663
Isotope scanning, in pulmonary disease, 136, *136*

Joint(s), tuberculosis of, 836
  treatment of, 836(t)
Juvenile rheumatoid arthritis, pulmonary involvement in, 1048–1050, *1050*

Kanamycin, 338, 338(t)
  dosage schedule for, beyond newborn period, 342(t)
    in newborn, 340(t)
  in atypical mycobacterial infection, 850
  in tuberculosis, 811
Kartagener syndrome, 447
Kerley lines, in pulmonary edema, 153, *154*, 588, *589*
Kidney, in sarcoidosis, 858
  tuberculosis of, 836
    treatment of, 837(t)
Kulchitsky cell, of lung, 67
Kveim test, for sarcoidosis, 859
Kyphoscoliosis, cor pulmonale and, 751

Laryngeal diphtheria, 358
Laryngeal stridor, congenital, radiology of neck in, 141
Laryngitis, acute, 357
Laryngotracheitis, acute, 357
Laryngotracheobronchitis, acute, 357
Larynx, anatomy of, 354, *354, 355*
Leiomyoma, of lung, 700
Leiomyosarcoma, of lung, 701, *701*
Letterer-Siwe syndrome, 1027
Leukopenia, in sarcoidosis, 859

Lincomycin, 336
  dosage schedule for, beyond newborn period, 342(t)
  in cystic fibrosis, 779
Lipoma, mediastinal, 733
  of chest wall, 734
  of lung, 700
Liposarcoma, mediastinal, 733
Litten's phenomenon, 94
Liver, in cystic fibrosis, 765
  in sarcoidosis, 858
Lobar emphysema, 245–247, *246*
  congenital, 297–299, *298*
Locked lung syndrome, 652
Loeffler's syndrome, 1023–1026
  classification of, 1023
  clinical manifestations of, 1024, *1024, 1025*
  diagnosis of, 1026
  etiology of, 1023
  pathogenesis of, 1023
  pathology of, 1026
  treatment of, 1026
Lung(s). See also entries beginning *Pulmonary.*
  adenomatoid malformation of, congenital cystic, 250–251, *251*
  agenesis of, 299–300, *300*
  auscultation of, 99–101
  biopsy of, 107
    thoracotomy and, *709, 710*
  biosynthesis and secretion of surface-active lipoprotein by, 69
  boundaries of, 96, *97*
  chorioepithelioma of, 702
  collapse of, massive, 566–569
    as complication of asthma, 647, *647*
  compliance of, 15, 16(t)
    airway resistance and, 20
  conductance in, as function of age, 177–183, *178–182*
    in disease, 183–187, *184, 186*
  cysts of, in newborn, 299
  defense of, against infectious agents and foreign particles, 70
  disease of. See *Pulmonary disease* and names of specific diseases.
  disorders of, neonatal, assisted ventilation in, 309–312
  divisions of, 96, *98, 98*
  dysgenesis of, vs. atelectasis, 161
  elasticity of, 14
  embryology of, 5, *6*
  eosinophilic, 1023
  fetal, at term, 6
  fluid accumulation in, forces responsible for, 576–580, *576*. See also *Pulmonary edema.*
  gas exchange in, adequacy of, 89
  ground-glass appearance of, 157, *159*
  growth of, 5–11
  hamartoma of, 697, *697*
  hereditary diseases of, 78, 79(t)
  histology of, 5, *7*
  honeycomb, 157, *159*
    in bronchiectasis, 454
  hypoplasia of, 299–300
  idiopathic hyperlucent, radiographic appearance of, 163

Lung(s) (*Continued*)
  in sarcoidosis, 854, *855–857*
  infections of, in newborn, 292–296, *293–295*
  injury to, from hydrocarbon aspiration, 491–493
    from smoke inhalation, 493–497
  leiomyoma of, 700
  leiomyosarcoma of, 701, *701*
  lipoma of, 700
  lobes of, *98*
    weight of, 8
  localization of disease in, 90–103
  metabolic and endocrine functions of, 62–76
    cells in, 62–69. See also *Cell(s), pulmonary.*
  metabolism, synthesis, and release of vaso-active hormones by, 70, 70(t)
  morphology of, 5–11
  movement of liquid in, 50, *50*
  postnatal, 8, *9, 10*
  puncture of, diagnostic, 107
    in bacterial pneumonia, 379
  resection of tissue of, 131
  resistance of, 16
  segments of, *99*
  surface tension of, 14, *15*
  systemic neoplasms affecting, 702
  wet, 1087
  zones of, 50
Lung volumes, 11–14
  decreased, diagnostic radiology of, 160–162, *162*
  increased, diagnostic radiology of, 162–163, *163*
  interpretation of, 12, 13(t)
  measurement of, 12
Lupus erythematosus, systemic, pulmonary involvement in, 1034–1043, *1037, 1038, 1041*
    diagnostic and therapeutic considerations for, 1042
Lymph nodes
  biopsy of, 706, *708*
  mediastinal, abnormalities of, 731
  peripheral, in sarcoidosis, 856
    biopsy of, 860
  superficial, tuberculosis of, 831–833
    treatment of, 833, 833(t)
Lymphadenitis, chronic suppurative, due to atypical mycobacteria, 846, *846*
Lymphadenopathy, peripheral, in sarcoidosis, 856, *857*
Lymphangiectasis, congenital pulmonary, 251
Lymphoid interstitial pneumonia, 527–528
  clinical features of, 527
  prognosis of, 528
  radiologic changes in, 528
  treatment of, 528

Macrophage, alveolar, 62, *64*
Malt worker's disease, 682
Mantoux test, for tuberculosis, 793, *793, 795*
Maple bark disease, 682
Mast cell, 64, *66*

Measles pneumonia, 966–982
  atypical, 977–979
    clinical features of, 978
    laboratory findings in, 978
    prevention of, 979
    roentgenographic findings in, 978
    treatment of, 979
  complications of, 976
  diagnosis of, 971–976, *972–974*
    without rash, 975
  incidence of, 969
  pathogenesis of, 966
  pathology of, 966, *967, 968*
  prevention of, 977
  respiratory symptoms and signs of, 970
  severity of, factors affecting, 969
  susceptibility to, factors affecting, 969
  treatment of, 977
Meat-wrapper's asthma, 689(t), 690
Mechanical ventilation, 200(t), 203–207. See also *Ventilation, mechanical.*
Meconium, aspiration pneumonia of, 278–280, *279*
Meconium ileus, cystic fibrosis and, 764, 765(t), 769
Mediastinum, compartments of, 710, *710*
  diagnostic radiology of, 147–150, *147–149*
  tumors of, 710–734, *711*. See also *Tumor(s), mediastinal.*
Meningitis, as complication of pneumococcal pneumonia, 385
  tuberculous, 834–836
    treatment of, 836, 837(t)
Meningocele, intrathoracic, 721
Meningococcal pneumonia, 386
Metabolism, aerobic, 41
  anaerobic, 42
  temperature effects on, 43, *44*
Metal fume fever, 689(t), 690
Metaproterenol, in treatment of asthma, 655, 658(t)
  by aerosol, 652
Methacholine (mecholyl) test, for familial dysautonomia, 1062
Methicillin, 332, 333(t)
  dosage schedule for, beyond newborn period, 342(t)
  in newborn, 340(t)
  in staphylococcal pneumonia, 394
Methylxanthines, in reduction of exercise-induced bronchospasm, 637
Miconazole, 929
  in aspergillosis, 921
  in coccidioidomycosis, 909
Micrognathia, with glossoptosis, 303
Microlithiasis, idiopathic pulmonary alveolar, 535–537, *536*
Milk, hypersensitivity to, pulmonary disease and, 677
Mill worker's disease, 683
Minocycline, in nocardiosis, 893
Mist tent, for continuous aerosol therapy, *124*
  in cystic fibrosis, 781
Mixed connective tissue disease, pulmonary involvement in, 1050–1052
Monaldi drainage, 128

Monitoring, in respiratory disorders, 208–210
  electrical hazards and safety measures of,
    209
  of equipment function, 209
  of patient status, 208
Mono-Vacc test, for tuberculosis, 797, *798, 799*
Morgagni hernia, 218–219, *218*
Mucor, media for isolation of, 882(t)
Mucormycosis, 923–924
Mushroom worker's disease, 683
Mycobacteria, atypical
  characteristics of, 844
  classification of, 844, 845(t)
  infection with, 844–851
    clinical disease of, 846, *846*
    epidemiology of, 846
    incidence of, 846
    pathology of, 846
    sensitivity to tuberculin, 847
    treatment of, 849
  nonphotochromogens, 845
  photochromogens, 844
  rapid-growers, 845
  scotochromogens, 845
Mycoplasma pneumoniae infection, 433–441
  clinical manifestations of, 436
  diagnosis of, 437
  epidemiology of, 434
  immunology of, 435
  incidence of, 433
  laboratory findings in, 437
  management of, 437
  pathogenesis of, 436
  pathology of, 434
  prevention of, 441
  prognosis of, 441
  roentgenographic appearance of, 437, *438–440*
Mycosis(es), 879–935. See also names of specific
    infections.
  microbiologic diagnosis of, 880–883, 882(t)
  treatment of, 925–929
Mycostatin, in aspergillosis, 921
Myeloma, multiple, 701
Myxoma, cardiac, 734

Nafcillin, 332, 333(t)
  dosage schedule for, beyond newborn period,
    342(t)
  in newborn, 340(t)
Nasotracheal intubation, 203
Near-drowning, 498–510
  blood gas, acid-base, and pulmonary status
    changes in, 499–501
  blood volume and serum electrolytes in, 501
  cardiovascular system in, 503
  hemoglobin and hematocrit values in, 502
  neurologic function in, 503
  pathophysiology of, 499–504
  renal function in, 503
  therapy of, 504–510
Neck, radiology of, 139–142, *139–141*
Neomycin, aerosol, in cystic fibrosis, 780

Neoplasm, of thymus, 724
  systemic, affecting lung, 702
Nervous system, involvement of, in sarcoidosis,
    858
Neurilemoma, mediastinal, 728
Neuroblastoma, mediastinal, *728, 730*
Neuroendocrine cells, 67
Neurofibroma, mediastinal, 728, *729*
Neurogenic tumors, mediastinal, 728–731
Neuromuscular disease, cor pulmonale and, 751
Neuromuscular weakness, as cause of respiratory
    distress in newborn, 308
Newborn
  air block in, 280–283
  antibiotic administration in, dosage
    schedules for, 339, 340(t)
  asphyxia in, 276–278
  bacterial pneumonia in, 292, *293, 294*
  cardiac disease in, congenital, 305–309
  cardiac failure in, 305
  emphysema of, 280–283
    congenital lobar, 297–299, *298*
  hemolytic disease of, pulmonary symptoms
    associated with, 307
  hyaline membrane disease of, 283–290, *284,
    285, 289*
  lung cysts in, 299
  lung disorders of, assisted ventilation in, 309–
    312
  lung infections in, 292–296, *293–295*
  pneumatoceles in, 242, 299
  pneumomediastinum in, 280–283, *282*
  pneumothorax of, 280–283, *281*
  pulmonary edema in, 305, *305*
  pulmonary hemorrhage in, 296–297
  respiratory depression in, 276–278
  respiratory disorders in, 271–313. See also
    names of specific conditions.
  respiratory distress in, effects of transitional
    circulation on, 274–276
    evaluation of, 271–274
    neuromuscular weakness as cause of, 308
    nonpulmonary cases of, 304–305
  resuscitation of, 199, 276–278
  staphylococcal infection in, *295*, 296
  tachycardia in, paroxysmal atrial, 306
  tuberculosis of, 823–825
    effect of BCG vaccination of, 823(t)
    prophylactic regimen for, 824(t)
Nitrofurantoin, lung disease due to, 692
Nitrogen, partial pressure of, in airway and
    blood, *26*
Nocardia, 889, *889*
  media for isolation of, 882(t)
Nocardiosis, 889–893
  clinical disease in, 890, *891*
  epidemiology of, 891
  laboratory diagnosis of, 891
  pathogenesis of, 891
  pathology of, 891, *892*
  prevention of, 893
  treatment of, 892
North American blastomycosis, 893–898. See
  also *Blastomycosis, North American.*
Nystatin, in candidiasis, 923

Old tuberculin (OT), 792
Ondine's curse, 752
Ornithosis, 942–947
Orotracheal tube, specifications for, in pediatric age group, 196(t)
Orthomyxoviruses, 418
Orthopnea, 86
Otitis media, as complication, of pneumococcal pneumonia, 385
 of viral pneumonia, 430
 recurrent, adenoidectomy for, 351
Oxacillin, 332, 333(t)
 dosage schedule for, beyond newborn period, 342(t)
 in newborn, 340(t)
 in cystic fibrosis, 779
Oxygen
 arterial, management of saturation of, clinical application of, 60
 dissolved, oxyhemoglobin and, 32
 hyperbaric, therapy with, 37
 methods of administration of, 200(t), 202
 partial pressure of, in airway and blood, 27
 therapy with, 35–37, 122
  bronchopulmonary dysplasia and, 315
  hazards of high mixtures in, 36
  increased inspired mixtures for, 35
 transport of, 32–35
Oxygenation, artificial, 196
 methods of, 200(t), 202
Oxyhemoglobin dissociation curve, 33
 factors affecting, 34
Oxytetracycline, in cystic fibrosis, 779

Pain, chest, evaluation of, 81
Pancreas, functional evaluation of, in cystic fibrosis, 777
Pancreatic enzyme lung, 683
Papillae, fungiform, absence of, in familial dysautonomia, 1062
Papilloma, of trachea and bronchi, 699
Para-aminosalicylic acid, in atypical mycobacterial infection, 849
 in tuberculosis, 809
Paracoccidioides brasiliensis, 899, 899
Paracoccidioidomycosis, 899–902. See also Blastomycosis, South American.
Parainfluenza viruses, pneumonia due to, 426, 427, 427
 pathology and pathogenesis of, 429
Paramyxoviruses, 419
Paraneoplastic syndromes, 74, 75(t)
Patent ductus arteriosus, 75
 bronchopulmonary dysplasia and, 316
Pectus carinatum, 213
Pectus excavatum, 214–217, 215, 216
Penicillin(s), 331–335
 alternative antimicrobial agents for, 331, 335–338
 penicillinase-resistant, 332, 333(t)
  dosage schedules for, beyond newborn period, 342(t)
  in newborn, 340(t)
 sensitization to, 334

Penicillin(s) (Continued)
 toxicity of, 334
 use of probenecid with, 344
Penicillin G, 331
 aqueous, 331
 benzathine, 332
 dosage schedules for, beyond newborn period, 342(t)
  in newborn, 340(t)
 in pneumococcal pneumonia, 384
 in pulmonary abscess, 473
 in staphylococcal pneumonia, 394
 in streptococcal pneumonia, 388
 procaine, 332
Pentamidine isethionate, in Pneumocystis carinii pneumonitis, 410
Perfusion, relation to ventilation, 44–48
 intrinsic regulation of, 48
Periarteritis nodosa, pulmonary involvement in, 1055–1057
Pericardium, cavernous hemangioma of, 734
 cyst of, celomic, 720, 721
Periodic acid–Schiff stain, for diagnosis of fungi, 881
Pertussis pneumonia, 986–993
 clinical features of, 987, 988
 complications of, 991
 diagnosis of, 988
  differential, 990
  roentgen, 989, 990
 incidence of, 986
 pathogenesis of, 987
 pathology of, 987, 987
 prevention of, 992
 prognosis of, 992
 treatment of, 991
Pertussis syndrome, 995–997
Pertussoid eosinophilic pneumonia, 994–998
 clinical features of, 995
 course of, 995
 etiology of, 994
 incidence of, 994
 prognosis of, 995
 treatment of, 995
Pharmacologic agents, for respiratory resuscitation, 197(t), 198, 199(t)
Pharyngitis, streptococcal, 348
 viral, 348
Pharyngoconjunctival fever, due to adenoviruses, 417
Phenobarbital, in treatment of asthma, 656(t)
Pheochromocytoma, mediastinal, 731
Phosphatase, serum alkaline, in sarcoidosis, 859
Phrenic nerve, paralysis of, as cause of neonatal respiratory distress, 308
Phycomycosis, 923–924
Pickwickian syndrome, 57, 752
Picornaviruses, 414–416
Pigeon breast, 213
Pigeon breeder's disease, 679
 clinical course of, 672
 clinical features of, 680(t)
 histologic study of, 676
 roentgenogram of, 681
Pilocarpine iontophoresis, in cystic fibrosis, 773, 775–777

Pituitary snuff taker's lung, 683
Plasmacytoma, of chest wall, 736
Pleura, biopsy of, in empyema, 482
    in tuberculosis, 805
    diagnostic radiology of, 144–147, *144, 146*
Pleural effusion
    chyliform, 606
    chylous, 606, 606(t)
    exudate, 605, 605(t), 606(t)
    management of, 609
    radiographic appearance of, 145, *146*
    transudate, 605, 605(t), 606(t)
Pleural fissures, diagnostic radiology of, 144–
    147, *144, 146*
Pleural liquid, examination of, in pleurisy and
    empyema, 480
Pleural space
    air in, 610–619
        diagnosis of, 614–616, 614(t)
        etiology and pathogenesis of, 610–613,
            611–613
        functional pathology of, 613
        management of, 616–618
        prognosis of, 618
        secondary to lung rupture, 612, 612(t)
    drainage of, 128
        closed, set-up for, *1081*
    liquid in, 602–610
        anatomic features of, 602
        diagnosis of, 607–609, *607, 608*
        etiology and pathogenesis of, 604–606,
            605(t)
        functional pathology of, 606
        management of, 609
        physiology of, 602–604, 603(t)
Pleurisy, 475–487
    chest roentgenogram in, 479, *479–481*
    diagnosis of, 478–483
    dry (plastic), 475
    etiology of, 475–478, 476(t)
    examination of pleural liquid in, 480
    functional pathology of, 478
    management of, 483–486
        antimicrobial, 484(t), 485
        surgical, 485, 485(t)
    pathogenesis of, 475–478
    pleural biopsy in, 482
    prognosis of, 486
    tuberculous, with effusion, 826–829, *827*
        treatment of, 827, 827(t)
    with effusion, 475
        physical and chemical characteristics of,
            481, 482(t)
Pneumatocele, congenital, 242, 299
Pneumococcal pneumonia, 380–386
    bacteriology of, 380
    clinical features of, 382
    complications of, 385
    diagnosis of, 383
    epidemiology of, 381
    immunity to, 380
    management of, 384
    pathogenesis of, 381
    pathology of, 381
    prognosis of, 386
    roentgenographic appearance of, 383, *384*

Pneumocystis carinii pneumonitis, 403–411
    atypical, 411
    clinical features of, 403–405, *404, 405*
    diagnosis of, 407
    pathology of, 405, *406, 408, 409*
    predisposing factors to, 403
    treatment of, 410
Pneumomediastinum, 611, *613*
    in newborn, 280–283, *282*
    management of, 617
    radiographic appearance of, *146*, 150
Pneumonia
    aerobic gram-negative bacillary, 400–
        402
    bacterial. See *Bacterial pneumonia.*
    candidal, *922*
    desquamative interstitial, 523–527
        clinical features of, 526
        course of, 527
        etiology of, 526
        histologic features of, 523, *525*
        laboratory data in, 526
        radiologic findings in, *524,* 526
        treatment of, 527
    due to *Hemophilus influenzae,* 398–400, *399*
    due to *Mycoplasma pneumoniae,* 433–441. See
        also *Mycoplasma pneumoniae infection.*
    due to parainfluenza viruses, *426, 427, 427*
        pathology and pathogenesis of, 429
    due to Pseudomonas, 401
    due to *Serratia marcescens,* 401
    eosinophilic, 73
    giant cell, 528, 983–985, *984*
    Hecht's, 983
    hypostatic, 511–512
    intrauterine aspiration, 278–280, *279*
    intrauterine bacterial, 292, *293, 294*
    lymphoid interstitial, 527–528
        clinical features of, 527
        prognosis of, 528
        radiologic changes in, 528
        treatment of, 528
    measles, 966–982. See also *Measles pneumonia.*
    meconium aspiration, 278–280, *279*
    meningococcal, 386
    pertussis. 986–993. See also *Pertussis pneu-
        monia.*
    pertussoid eosinophilic, 994–998. See also
        Pertussoid eosinophilic pneumonia.
    pneumococcal, 380–386. See also *Pneumococcal
        pneumonia.*
    primary atypical, differential diagnosis of,
        1015(t)
    rheumatic, 1006–1018. See also *Rheumatic
        pneumonia.*
    salmonella, 998–1105. See also *Salmonella
        pneumonia.*
    staphylococcal, 388–396. See also *Staphylococ-
        cal pneumonia.*
    streptococcal, 386–388, *387*
    tuberculous, 818, *819*
    usual interstitial. See *Alveolitis, cryptogenic
        (idiopathic) fibrosing.*
    varicella, 955–965. See also *Varicella
        pneumonia.*
    viral, 423–432. See also *Viral pneumonia.*

Pneumonitis, desquamative interstitial, 749
  due to *Pneumocystis carinii*, 403–411. See also
    Pneumocystis carinii pneumonitis.
  hypersensitivity, 670–684. See also *Hypersensitivity pneumonitis.*
  interstitial, due to histoplasmosis, *870*
Pneumopericardium, 612
  management of, 617
Pneumoperitoneum, *613*
  diagnostic, 108
    in pulmonary tumors, 705, *706*
    in rupture of diaphragm, *1093*
  management of, 618
Pneumothorax, 610, *612*
  of newborn, 280–283, *281*
  radiographic appearance of, 145, *146*
  sucking, 1082, *1083*
    treatment of, 1083, *1084*
  tension, 1082
  traumatic, 1082–1084, *1083*
Poiseuille's law, 16
Poliomyelitis, as cause of neonatal respiratory
    distress, 308
Polyarteritis nodosa, 1023
Polyarthritis, juvenile chronic, 1049
Polymer fume fever, 689(t), 691
Polymyxin(s), 338(t), 339
  dosage schedule for, beyond newborn period,
    343(t)
Polypnea, 83
Polyposis, nasal, in cystic fibrosis, 768, *768*
Postural drainage, 109–119. See also *Bronchial
    (postural) drainage.*
Poultry worker's disease, 683
Prednisolone, in asthma, 660(t)
  in sarcoidosis, 861
Prednisone, in asthma, 660(t), 661
  in isolated primary pulmonary hemosiderosis,
    544, 545
  in sarcoidosis, 861
Probenecid, use of, with penicillins, 344
Prostaglandins, in asthma, 629
Proteinosis, pulmonary alveolar, 530–534
  clinical manifestations of, 532, *533*
  pathogenesis of, 531
  pathology of, 530, *531*
  prognosis of, 533
  treatment of, 533
Pseudobronchiectasis, 448
Pseudomonas, pneumonia due to, 401
Psittacosis, 942–947
  age and sex distribution of, 943(t)
Pulmonary abscess, 470–474, *471–473*
  aerobic (nonputrid), 472
  anaerobic (putrid), 472
Pulmonary agenesis, 240–242
Pulmonary aplasia, 240–242
Pulmonary cells, 62–69. See also *Cell(s), pulmonary.*
Pulmonary circulation, 48–52
  anatomy of, 48
  distribution of, measurement of, 47
  evaluation of, methods of, 51
  hemodynamics of, 49
  nonuniform, causes of, 47
  regulation of, 51

Pulmonary collapse, massive, 566–569
  as complication of asthma, 647, *647*
Pulmonary compression injury, 1086–1087, *1086*
Pulmonary consolidation, diagnostic radiology
    of, 154–157, *155, 156*
Pulmonary cysts, congenital, 242–244, *243, 244*
Pulmonary disease. See also *Respiratory disease.*
  associated with serum milk precipitins, 677
  diagnostic radiology of, 133–165. See also
    Radiology, diagnostic pulmonary.
  due to contamination of humidifying tents in
    home, 679
  interstitial, due to contamination of forced
    air systems, 678, 678(t)
  nonasthmatic allergic, 670–696
  obstructive, 78, 191(t)
    causes of, 192(t)
    chronic, thoracic index in, *96*
    cor pulmonale and, 747–749
  parenchymal, cor pulmonale and, 747–750
  restrictive, 78, 191(t)
    causes of, 193(t)
    cor pulmonale and, 749
  vascular, cor pulmonale and, 753–756
  veno-occlusive, 754–756, *755, 756*
Pulmonary edema, 573–592
  anatomic considerations of, 573–576, *574–576*
  causes of, 50, 50(t)
  diagnosis of, 588
    differential, 1015(t)
  diagnostic radiology of, 153, *154*
  etiology of, 581–586
  fluid movement in, forces responsible for,
    576–580, *576*
    interstitial, 577
    lymphatic clearance, 579
    microvascular filtration, 578
    surface tension, 579, *580*
    vascular, 577
  in asthma, 586
  in bronchiolitis, 587
  in neonatal respiratory distress syndrome, 587
  in newborn, 305, *305*
  pathophysiologic consequences of, 580
  radiographic findings in, 588, *589*
  safety factors against, 580
  therapy of, 589–591
Pulmonary function testing, 166–176
  clinical application of, 60–61
  equipment for, 167–169, 168(t)
  in cystic fibrosis, 773(t)
  in hypersensitivity pneumonitis, 673
  in tuberculosis, 805
  interpretation of, 171–176
  normal data for, 173(t)
  sensitivity of, 174(t)
  special considerations for, 166–169
  technique of, 169–171
  uses of, 166(t)
Pulmonary hemorrhage, in newborn, 296–297
Pulmonary hemosiderosis, 538–552
  as manifestation of diffuse collagen-vascular or
    purpuric disease, 549–550
  isolated primary, 538–546
    complications of, 543
    laboratory findings in, 539–542, *540, 541*

Pulmonary hemosiderosis (*Continued*)
  isolated primary, roentgenologic findings in,
      542–543, *543*
    symptoms and physical findings in, 538
    treatment of, 544
  primary, with cardiac or pancreatic involve-
      ment, 546
    with glomerulonephritis, 546–547
    with sensitivity to cow's milk, 547–549
  secondary to heart disease, 549
Pulmonary hernia, 242
Pulmonary hypersensitivity, due to chemical
      agents and drugs, 688–693
  clinical features of, 689, 689(t)
  laboratory features of, 690
Pulmonary hypertension, high altitude and, 753
  primary, cor pulmonale and, 753
Pulmonary hypoplasia, 240–242
Pulmonary lavage, 127
Pulmonary lymphangiectasis, congenital, 251
Pulmonary sequestration, 247–250, *248*, *249*
Pulmonary tumors, 697–710. See also *Tumor(s)*,
  pulmonary.
Pulmonary vessels, diagnostic radiology of, 152–
      154, *154*
Puncture, arterial, 108, *109*
  of lung, diagnostic, 107
    in bacterial pneumonia, 379
Purified protein derivative (PPD), 792
Purpuric disease, pulmonary hemosiderosis as
  manifestation of, 549–550
Pyopneumothorax, radiologic assessment of, 480
Pyrazinamide, in tuberculosis, 810
Pyrimethamine, in *Pneumocystis carinii* pneu-
  monitis, 410

Q fever, 948–949

Radial artery, diagnostic puncture of, 108, *109*
Radiation, hazards of, 134
Radiography, in pulmonary disease, 134
Radiology, diagnostic pulmonary, 133–165
  basic approach to, 133(t)
  hazards of, 134
  imaging methods of, 134–137
  interpretation of, technical factors affecting,
      137–138
  of bronchi, 150–152, *151*
  of chest wall, 142, *142*
  of diaphragm, 143, *143*
  of hila, 152, *152*
  of interstitial disease, 157, *159*, *160*
  of lung volume, decreased, 160–162, *162*
    increased, 162–163, *163*
  of mediastinum, 147–150, *147–149*
  of neck and thoracic inlet, 139–142
  of pleura and fissures, 144–147, *144*, *146*
  of pulmonary consolidation, 154–157, *155*,
      156
  of pulmonary vessels, 152–154, *154*
  of spine, 143, *143*

Rales, classification of, 101, 101(t)
Renal insufficiency, antibiotic dosage schedules
  in, 341
Residual volume, interpretation of, 13, 13(t)
  measurement of, 12
Resistance, airway, 16
  clinical evaluation of, 21, *22*
  compliance and, 20
  factors affecting, 19
  measurement of, 17
  sites of, 19
Respiration
  abdominal, 94
  artificial, 21–25
    apparatus for, 24
    principles of, 23
  depressants of, 58(t)
  depth of, 85
  derangements of, 56
  ease of, 86
  mechanics of, 14–25
    dynamic forces of, 16–21
    static-elastic forces of, 14–16
  muscles of, 8–11
    weakness of, as cause of neonatal respira-
        tory distress, 308
  pattern of, physical examination of, 83–88
  rate of, 83–85, *83*, 84(t), *85*
  regulation of, 52–59
    by chemical system, 54
    by neural system, 53
  rhythm of, 88
  stimuli of, 58(t)
  thoracic, 94
  tissue, 41–44
Respirator, requirements for, 24
Respiratory center, 53, *53*
  dysfunction of, cor pulmonale and, 752
Respiratory depression, in newborn, 276–
  278
Respiratory disease. See also *Pulmonary disease.*
  age as factor in, 177–187
  diagnostic procedures for, 105–109
  nonspecific signs of, 82
  physical examination in, 83–103
    for adequacy of gas exchange, 89
    for localization of disease, 90–103
    for pattern of respiration, 83–88
  therapeutic procedures for, 109–131
Respiratory disorders
  functional classification of, 191–192, 191(t)
  in newborn, 271–313. See also names of
    specific conditions.
  intensive care of, 191–210
    by monitoring, 208–210
    by resuscitation, 194–199
    continuing, 200–208
      principles of, 200(t)
    medical, 207
    surgical, 208
  monitoring in, 208–210
    electrical hazards and safety measures of,
        209
    of equipment function, 209
    of patient status, 208

Respiratory distress
  chronic, in premature infant, 324–327
    clinical manifestations of, 324
    pathologic findings in, 326
    radiologic findings in, 325, *325, 326*
  in newborn, effect of transitional circulation
    on, 274–276
  evaluation of, 271–274
  neuromuscular weakness as cause of, 308
  nonpulmonary causes of, 304–305
Respiratory distress syndrome, neonatal, 72,
    283–290, *284, 285, 289*
  atelectasis in, 161, *162*
  lung rupture in, 612
  pulmonary edema in, 587
  type II, 290–292
Respiratory failure, criteria of, 194(t)
  recognition of, 192–194
Respiratory illness, viral etiology of, 412–422
  laboratory diagnosis of, 413
Respiratory syncytial virus, 419–420
  pneumonia due to, 424, *425*
  pathology and pathogenesis of, 428
Respiratory tract
  disorders of, due to trauma, 1077–1094
  in cystic fibrosis, 766, *766, 767*
  infection of, due to *Mycoplasma pneumoniae*,
    433–441. See also *Mycoplasma pneumoniae*
    infection.
  lower, congenital malformations of, 213–270.
    See also names of specific conditions.
  non-gas exchange function of, 57
  viruses affecting, 412(t)
    laboratory diagnosis of, 413
    relative importance in illness, 413(t)
Resuscitation, 194–199
  airway patency for, 195
  by artificial ventilation and oxygenation, 196
  by external cardiac massage, 194
  equipment for, 195(t)
  pharmacologic agents for, 197(t), 198, 199(t)
  principles of, 195(t)
  pulmonary, in newborn, 276–278
Retrolental fibroplasia, as manifestation of
  oxygen toxicity, 36
Rhabdomyoma, cardiac, 734
Rheumatic disorders, of childhood, 1033(t)
  inflammation in, chronicity of, 1031, *1032*
  pulmonary involvement in, 1031–1060
  rheumatoid factor and antinuclear anti-
    bodies in, 1033(t)
Rheumatic pneumonia, 1006–1018
  clinical features of, 1008–1010
  differential diagnosis of, 1010–1016, 1015(t)
  incidence of, 1006
  laboratory findings in, 1010
  pathologic features of, 1007, *1013, 1014*
  prevention of, 1016
  prognosis of, 1016
  treatment of, 1016
Rhinoviruses, clinical aspects of, 413
  laboratory aspects of, 416
Rhizopus, media for isolation of, 882(t)
Rhodotorula mucilagnosa infection, 925
Rhonchi, classification of, 101, 101(t)

Rib(s)
  congenital absence of, 217–218, *217*
  fractures of, 1078–1082, *1079*
    flail chest and, 1078, *1079, 1080*
    stabilization of, *1081*
    treatment of, 1079, *1080, 1081*
Rifampin, in atypical mycobacterial infection,
    850
  in tuberculosis, 810
Riley-Day syndrome, 57, 1061

Sail sign, thymic, 148, *148*
Salbutamol, in treatment of asthma, 658(t)
Salmonella pneumonia, 998–1105
  carrier state of, 1002
  clinical features of, 1000
  diagnosis of, 1001
  etiology of, 998
  incidence of, 999
  pathogenesis of, 998
  pathology of, 998
  prognosis of, 1002
  treatment of, 1001
Sarcoidosis, 852–864
  age incidence of, 853
  clinical manifestations of, 854–859, 854(t),
    855–857
  clinical picture of, 859
  diagnostic procedures for, 859
  etiology of, 854
  geographic distribution of, 853
  heredity of, 853
  history of, 852
  immunology of, 854
  laboratory studies for, 859
  pathogenesis of, 854
  prognosis of, 860
  racial incidence of, 853
  sex distribution of, 853
  treatment of, 860
Sarcoma, primary, of heart, 734
  reticulum cell, of chest wall, *735*
Schwannoma, mediastinal, 728
Scleroderma, pulmonary involvement in,
    1043–1046, *1045*
Secretions, drainage of, to maintain airway
    patency, 200
Sedatives, for treatment of asthma, 656(t)
Segmental auscultation, 99–101
  differential, 102, 103(t)
Septic (endotoxin) shock, 74
Septicemia, fulminant pneumococcal, as com-
    plication of pneumonia, 385
Sequoiosis, 683
Serratia marcescens, pneumonia due to, 401
Shock, endotoxin (septic), 74
Sickle cell anemia, risk of pneumonia and, 385
Silhouette sign, 156, *156*
Sinusitis, as complication of pneumococcal
    pneumonia, 385
  bronchiectasis and, 455
Skin, lesions of, in sarcoidosis, 856
Skin tests, in pulmonary tumors, 705

Smoke inhalation, respiratory complications of,
        493–497
    clinical findings in, 495
    pathogenesis of, 493
    pathology of, 494
    pathophysiology of, 495
    treatment of, 496
    vs. pulmonary complications of surface
        burns, 497
South American blastomycosis, 899–902. See
    also *Blastomycosis, South American.*
Spine, diagnostic radiology of, 143, *143*
Spirometer, for pulmonary function testing,
        electronic, 168
    wedge, 168
Spleen, in sarcoidosis, 858
Sporothrix, media for isolation of, 882(t)
Sporotrichosis, 924
Sputum, examination of, in pulmonary tumors,
        704, *705*
    in asthma, 638
    in lung disease, 82
SRS-A (slow-reacting substance of anaphylaxis),
        629
Staphylococcal infection, in newborn, *295, 296*
Staphylococcal pneumonia, 388–396
    bacteriology of, 388
    clinical features of, 390
    diagnosis of, 391
    epidemiology of, 389
    immunity to, 388
    management of, 394
    pathogenesis of, 389
    prognosis of, 395
    roentgenographic appearance of, 391, *392,
        393*
Status asthmaticus, 620, 637
    respiratory dynamics in, 641
    treatment of, 661–664, 663(t), 665(t)
Sternum, cleft of, 213–214
    fractures of, 1077–1078
Stethoscope, bell-diaphragm, for segmental
        auscultation, 100
    double, *102,* 103
Still's disease, 1049
Streptococcal pneumonia, 386–388, *387*
Streptomycin, 338, 338(t)
    dosage schedule for, beyond newborn period,
        342(t)
    in atypical mycobacterial infection, 849
    in tuberculosis, 809
    in tularemia, 953
Subclavian artery, aberrant right, esophageal
        obstruction and, 228
Suberosis, 683
Subpulmonic effusion, radiographic appearance
        of, 145, *146*
Sulfadiazine, in nocardiosis, 892
Sulfisoxazole, in chronic granulomatous disease
        of childhood, 1074
Sulfonamide(s), 337
    in histoplasmosis, 877, *877*
    in nocardiosis, 892
    in *Pneumocystis carinii* pneumonitis, 410

Surface tension, of lung, 14, *15*
Surfactant, alveolar, biosynthesis and secretion
    of surface-active lipoprotein for, 69
Sweat chloride levels, in asthma, 639
    in cystic fibrosis, 705, 777
Sweat test, in cystic fibrosis, 772, *775–777*, 775(t)
Swyer-James-Macleod syndrome, radiographic
    appearance of, 163
Systemic disease, bronchiectasis and, 456
Systemic lupus erythematosus, pulmonary in-
        volvement in, 1034–1043, *1037, 1038,
        1041*
    diagnostic and therapeutic considerations
        for, 1042

Tachycardia, paroxysmal atrial, in newborn, 306
Tachypnea, 83
Tents, humidifying, contamination of, lung dis-
        ease due to, 679
    mist, for continuous aerosol therapy, *124*
        in cystic fibrosis, 781
Teratoid tumors, of mediastinum, 726–727, *727,
        728*
Teratoma, benign cystic, of mediastinum, 726
    of thymus, 726
Terbutaline, in treatment of asthma, 657, 658(t)
Tetanus, neonatal, as cause of respiratory
        distress, 308
Tetracycline(s), 337, 338(t)
    dosage schedule for, beyond newborn period,
        343(t)
    in actinomycosis, 888
    in *Mycoplasma pneumoniae* infection, 437
    in psittacosis, 946
    in Q fever, 949
    in tularemia, 954
THAM, in treatment of status asthmaticus, 662
Theophylline, in treatment of asthma, 657(t),
        658(t)
Thiabendazole, in visceral larva migrans, 1021
Thoracic index, in chronic obstructive lung
        disease, *96*
Thoracic inlet, radiology of, 139–142
Thoracoabdominal infection, pleurisy and, 476
Thoracoabdominal injuries, 1091–1093, *1091,
        1092*
Thoracotomy, for traumatic cardiac tamponade,
        1088
    lung biopsy and, *709,* 710
Thorax, configuration of, 92–94, *93,* 94(t), 95(t),
        96
    elastic properties of, 16
    relation of lungs to, 97
Thromboembolism, cor pulmonale and, 753
Thymoma, benign, *724,* 726
Thymus
    absence of, 148
    hyperplasia of, 722, *723*
    neoplasm of, 724
    radiographic appearance of, 148, *148, 149*
    teratoma of, 726
    tuberculosis of, 726

Thyroid, substernal, 733
Tidal volume, measurement of, 12
Tine test, tuberculin, 794, *797, 798*
Tissue, connective, 67
Tissue respiration, 41–44
Tobramycin, 338, 338(t)
    dosage schedule for, beyond newborn
        period, 342(t)
    in newborn, 340(t)
Toluene diisocyanate, pulmonary hypersen-
    sitivity to, 691
Tomography, in pulmonary disease, 135
Tonsillitis, and adenoiditis, 347–352
        acute, 347
        chronic, 350
        clinical manifestations of, 347–350
        pathogenesis of, 347
    recurrent, adenotonsillectomy for, 351
Tonsils, and adenoids, hypertrophied, pulmo-
        nary edema and, 583, *584*
    hypertrophied, adenotonsillectomy for, 351
Torulopsis glabrata infection, 925
Trachea
    agenesis of, 226
    angioma of, 700
    congenital stenosis of, 226, 227
    fibroma of, 700
    palpation of, 91, *92*
    papilloma of, 699
    rupture of, 1085
Tracheal breath sounds, 101
Tracheitis, measles, *973*
Tracheobronchial tree, anatomy of, *110–114*
    normal adult bronchogram of, *178*
    trauma to, 1085–1086
Tracheobronchomegaly, bronchiectasis and,
    447
Tracheoesophageal fistula, 301–303, *302, 303*
    as complication of tuberculosis, 830, *831, 832*
    without esophageal atresia, 231–232, *232*
Tracheomalacia, 227–228
Tracheostomy, 129, 203
    over oral endotracheal tube, technique of,
        1081
Transfusions, blood, pulmonary hypersensitivity
    reactions to, 692
Transtracheal aspiration, in diagnosis of
        bronchiectasis, 455
    percutaneous, in diagnosis of bacterial
        pneumonia, 379
Transtracheal catheterization, 128
Trauma, respiratory tract disorders due to,
    1077–1094
Trepopnea, 91
Triamcinolone, in sarcoidosis, 861
    in asthma, 660(t)
Trimethoprim-sulfamethoxazole, 338
    in chronic granulomatous disease of child-
        hood, 1074
    in nocardiosis, 893
    in *Pneumocystis carinii* pneumonitis, 410
    in salmonella pneumonia, 1001
    in South American blastomycosis, 902
Tuberculin, positive reaction to, treatment of,
    812, 813(t)

Tuberculin test, 792–801
    Aplitest, 796
    false-negative reactions to, 799
    false-positive reactions to, 798, *800*
    Heaf, 794, *796*
        apparatus for, *797*
    in measles pneumonia, 975
    in sarcoidosis, 860
    Mantoux, 793, *793, 795*
    Mono-Vacc, 797, *798, 799*
    positive reaction to, 812–813
    routine use of, 800, 801(t)
    tine, 794, *797, 798*
Tuberculosis, 787–843
    active, effect of measles on, 976
    age incidence of, 789
    allergy in, 790
    bronchiectasis and, 455, 456
    chronic pulmonary, *828, 829,* 829–830
        treatment of, 830, 830(t)
    classification of, 811–812
    diagnosis of, 792–805
        by biopsy of pleura and lymph nodes, 805
        by bronchoscopy, 805
        by history and physical examination, 801
        by pulmonary function tests, 805
        by recovery of tubercle bacilli, 805
        by tuberculin test, 792–801
        roentgenographic, 802–805, *803, 804*
    etiology of, 787
    epidemiology of, 788, 789(t)
    extrapulmonary, 831–838
    heredity of, 789
    in newborn, 823–825
        effect of BCG vaccination of, 823(t)
        prophylactic regimen for, 824(t)
    immunity to, 790
    incubation period of, 805
    intra-abdominal, 837
    lymph node–bronchial, 818–823
        treatment of, 821–823
    miliary, acute, 825–826, *825*
        treatment of, 826, 826(t)
    of bones and joints, 836
        treatment of, 836(t)
    of superficial lymph nodes, 831–833
        treatment of, 833, 833(t)
    of thymus gland, 726
    pathogenesis of, 790–792
    pathology of, 790–792, *791*
    pleurisy and, 476
    predisposing factors to, 789
    prevention of, 838–840
    primary pulmonary, 813–816, *814–817*
        treatment of, 816, 816(t)
    progressive primary pulmonary, 816–818
        treatment of, 818, 818(t)
    racial incidence of, 789
    renal, 836
        treatment of, 837(t)
    sex incidence of, 789
    treatment of, 806–811
        antimicrobial, 808–811
        general, 807
        preventive, 806

Tularemia, 950–954
  clinical manifestations of, 951, *952*
  complications of, 953
  diagnosis of, 952
  etiology of, 950
  incidence of, 950
  pathogenesis of, 950
  pathology of, 953
  prevention of, 953
  treatment of, 953
Tumor(s)
  cardiac, primary, 734
  desmoid, of chest wall, *736*
  diaphragmatic, 734
  mediastinal, 710–734, *711*
    cystic, 713–722
    diagnostic procedures for, 712
    gastrointestinal symptoms of, 711
    lymphatic, 732
    neurogenic, 728–731
    neurologic symptoms of, 711
    of lymph nodes, 731
    parathyroid, 733
    physical findings in, 712
    respiratory symptoms of, 711, *711*
    teratoid, 726–727
    thymic, 722–726
    thyroid, 733
    vascular, 732
    vascular symptoms of, 712
  mesodermal, benign parenchymal, 698
    polypoid intrabronchial, 698
  neurogenic intrapulmonic, 700
  pericardial, 734
  pulmonary, 697–710
    benign, 697–700
    malignant, 701–702
    metastatic, 702–703

Uveoparotid fever, in sarcoidosis, 858

Vancomycin, 338
  dosage schedule for, beyond newborn period,
    343(t)
Varicella pneumonia, 955–965
  clinical features of, 957–960, *959*
  complications of, 961
  diagnosis of, laboratory aids and, 960
  epidemiology of, 956
  incidence of, 957
  pathology of, 955, *956*
  pulmonary sequelae of, late, 961
  treatment of, 962
Vascular ring, 228–231, *229–231*, 301
  radiology of, 141, *142*
Vasculitis syndromes, pulmonary involvement
  in, 1055–1057, 1055(t)
Vasoactive hormones, nature and actions of,
  71(t)
  pulmonary metabolism, synthesis and release
    of, 70, 70(t)

Vein(s), pulmonary, radiographic appearance of,
  153
Veno-occlusive disease, pulmonary, 754–756,
  755, 756
Ventilation
  alveolar, 25–30
  artificial, 196
  assisted, in neonatal lung disorders, 309–312
  distribution of, measurement of, 45
  mechanical, 200(t), 203–207
    bronchopulmonary dysplasia and, 314–317
    complications of, 206, 206(t)
    selection of patients for, 203, 204(t)
  nonuniform, mechanism of, 46
  relation to perfusion, 44–48
    intrinsic regulation of, 48
Ventilator(s)
  mechanical, for neonatal lung disorders, 309–
    312
    types of, 204, 205(t)
  pressure-cycled, 204, 205(t)
  time-cycled, 204, 205(t)
  volume-cycled, 204, 205(t)
Vesicular breath sounds, 101
Vidarabine, in varicella pneumonia, 962
Viomycin, in tuberculosis, 811
Viral pneumonia, 423–432
  clinical manifestations of, 429
  complications of, 430
  diagnosis of, 430
    differential, 1015(t)
  epidemiology of, 424–428
  etiology of, 424, 424(t)
  incidence of, 423
  laboratory findings in, 430
  management of, 431
  pathogenesis of, 428
  pathology of, 428
  prevention of, 431
  prognosis of, 431
  roentgenographic appearance of, 430
Virus(es). See also names of specific viruses.
  affecting respiratory tract, 412(t)
    laboratory diagnosis of, 413
    relative importance in illness, 413(t)
  causing pneumonia, 424(t)
  influenza, 442
  role of, in pathogenesis of gram-positive
    bacterial pneumonia, 378
Visceral larva migrans, 1019–1022
  clinical manifestations of, 1020
  complications of, 1020
  course of, 1021
  diagnosis of, 1021
  etiology of, 1019
  pathogenesis of, 1019
  prognosis of, 1021
  treatment of, 1021
Vital capacity
  interpretation of, 12, 13(t)
  measurement of, 12
    clinical application of, 60
    maximal, 166, 167

Vocal cords, paralysis of, as cause of neonatal respiratory distress, 308

Warthin-Finkeldey cell, in measles pneumonia, 966
Wave sign, thymic, 148
Wegener's granulomatosis, pulmonary involvement in, 1052–1055, *1054*
Weingarten's syndrome, 1023
Wheezes, classification of, 102(t)
Wheezing, 81
  in respiratory disease, 88
Wilson-Mikity syndrome, 324–327

Wilson-Mikity syndrome (*Continued*)
  clinical manifestations of, 324
  pathologic findings in, 326
  radiologic findings in, 325, *325, 326*
Wright's stain, for diagnosis of fungi, 881

Xanthines, in treatment of asthma, 657, 657(t), 658(t)

Ziehl-Neelsen stain, for diagnosis of fungi, 881
Zoster immune globulin, in prevention of varicella pneumonia, 963